D1279653

HEALTH

MAN IN A CHANGING ENVIRONMENT

SECOND EDITION

ABOUT THE AUTHOR

Benjamin A. Kogan received his M.D. from Wayne State University College of Medicine and his M.S.P.H. and Dr.P.H. from the University of Michigan. An experienced classroom teacher, he is Professor of Health Science at California State University, Northridge, and Associate Clinical Professor of Community Medicine and Public Health, University of Southern California School of Medicine. Dr. Kogan is former Director of the Bureau of Medical Services of the County of Los Angeles Department of Health Services. He is the author of *Human Sexual Expression, Readings in Health Science,* and numerous articles on public health.

BENJAMIN A. KOGAN, M.D., Dr.P.H.

HEALTH

MAN IN A CHANGING ENVIRONMENT / SECOND EDITION

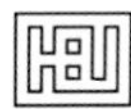

HARCOURT BRACE JOVANOVICH, INC.
New York Chicago San Francisco Atlanta

The following anatomical drawings are by Zena Bernstein:
Chapter 4 (Figure 9, left), Chapter 9 (Figures 2, 4, 7, 10, 11, 17),
Chapter 10 (Figures 4, 7, 8, 9, 14, 18, 20),
Chapter 13 (Figure 9), Chapter 16 (Figures 1, 3, 4, 6, 7, 8),
Chapter 22 (Figures 7, 12).

ISBN: 0-15-535583-X

Library of Congress Catalog Card Number: 73-15374

Printed in the United States of America

ACKNOWLEDGMENTS AND COPYRIGHTS

The author wishes to thank the companies and persons listed below for permission to use material in this book.

Textual Material and Tables

American Cancer Society, Inc., for Table 8-1, "Cancer: Estimated Casualty Figures for 1974, Warning Signals, and Safeguards," from the American Cancer Society, *'74 Cancer Facts & Figures.* Reprinted by permission of the American Cancer Society.

Bruno Bettelheim, for excerpts from Bruno Bettelheim, "Joey: A 'Mechanical Boy,'" *Scientific American*, Vol. 200, No. 3 (March 1959), pp. 117-27. Copyright © 1959 by Scientific American, Inc. All rights reserved.

Acknowledgments and copyrights for further textual material and tables and for illustrations continue at the back of the book on page xiii.

The second edition of this book is dedicated to
Ruby Pearson, Helen Nakagawa, Judith Greissman, and Gerald A. Heidbreder;
but it was written for the generation of
Brian C. Barbick.

preface

In February 1974, a startling experiment was announced that symbolizes a basic purpose of this book. Against the visual cortex of the brain of a totally blind Vietnam veteran, investigators placed an array of electrodes, coupling them with a television camera. Computer-controlled stimulation of the electrodes produced patterns of light (phosphenes) that the subject recognized and repeatedly reproduced (see page 767). The time will surely come when an electronic prosthesis will provide many blind persons with some artificial vision.

What broad meaning does this remarkable research lend to the Second Edition of *Health: Man in a Changing Environment?* The Preface of the First Edition began as follows:

> Man is in trouble. He is trapped in the web of his own technological triumphs. Never before has he known so much of both his inner mechanisms and his outer world. Yet never before has he been so oppressed by the imbalances between them. Since ecological balance is essential to human health, people need to know what is causing ecological imbalance. They must seek and find ways of achieving harmony between their slowly changing inner environment and their rapidly changing outer environment. This is the central and recurring theme of this book.

That theme remains unchanged. So does the author's attempt to meet the responsibility of presenting concrete evidence that human beings can solve the problems inherent in that theme. Whether these problems relate to pollution or psychosurgery, genetic engineering or population overgrowth, their solutions lie within the capacities of humankind. Testifying to this are the hundreds of new references in this Second Edition. Besides being a rich source for the student who wants to know more, these citations are meant to show that just as the human mind can conceive of a way to enable the blind to see, so can it seek and find ways to meet other challenges of healthful modern living. The human mind, then, is more than an evolutionary new growth, and in this there is a realistic reason for optimism.

In preparing the Second Edition, the author sought the advice of more than thirty health instructors across the nation. The diversity of their responses was heartening; the teaching of health science would have a gloomy future indeed were it conducted in the same way by all. There was, however, much agreement on certain suggestions for revision. Consequently, in addition to incorporating the results of recent research, this Second Edition includes a glossary, introductory outlines and concluding summaries for each chapter, new chapters on physical fitness and on the economics of health care, and expansion of many discussions, such as drug abuse, the cell and cancer research, sexuality, pregnancy, birth control, nutrition, and the sexually transmitted diseases. The material has been divided into eight parts containing a total of twenty-five shorter chapters; from these, the instructor can select those which meet the greatest needs of the students. To promote the decision-making abilities of the student, scrupulous attention has been paid to objectivity.

Thanks are due to John Leedom, M.D., Associate Professor of Medicine at the University of Southern California School of Medicine, who read the entire manuscript. Thanks are also due the staff of Harcourt Brace Jovanovich, Inc., especially Everett M. Sims, Cele Gardner, Paula F. Lewis, Alice Sanchez, Jeremiah Lighter, Helen Faye, Carla Hirst Wiltenburg, and John Holland. The author particularly wishes to acknowledge the contributions of all those who suggested ways in which the text might be revised and improved, including: Ross O. Armstrong, Department of Health, Physical Education, and Recreation, Chadron State College; Alice Bercseny, Department of Health Education, Los Angeles Trade-Technical College; Patricia Binding, Department of Health Education, Los Angeles Harbor College; Alan Briggs, Department of Health Science, Edmonds Community College; Lynne Bynum, Life Sciences Division, Monterey Peninsula College; Donald Carlucci, Department of Health Education, Los Angeles Harbor College; J. Alfred Chiscon, Department of Biological Sciences, Purdue University; Jack Criqui, Department of Health Science, Chabot College; Alan B. Davidson, Coordinator of Health Education, Kent Public Schools, Kent, Wash.; Robert Diller, Health Science Chairman, Cabrillo College; Donald A. Fusco, Coordinator of Health Education, Queensborough Community College; V. W. Greene, School of Public Health, University of Minnesota; Donovan Horn, Department of Physical Education and Recreation, Mississippi State University; Michael Hosokawa, Department of Health Education, University of Oregon; Jack Madigan, Department of Health Education, City College of San Francisco; Victor Petreshene, Health Education Coordinator, College of Marin; Nicholas J. Pisacano, University of Kentucky; James M. Pryde, Department of Health Sciences, American River College; Charles R. Schroeder, Department of Health, Physical Education, and Recreation, Memphis State University; Henny Shepherd, Department of Health Education, Los Angeles Pierce College; Morry Storseth, Department of Health Science, Seattle Central Community College; Muriel Svec, Department of Life Science, Santa Monica College; Kenneth Swearingen, Department of Health Education, El Camino College; Jack V. Toohey, Chairman, Health Education, Arizona State University; Robert E. Vanni, Department of Health Sciences, Western Illinois University; C. Harold Veenker, Health Education Section, Department of Physical Education for Men, Purdue University; Kenneth E. Veselak, Department of Health and Physical Education, Nassau Community College; Murray Vincent, Department of Health and Physical Education, University of South Carolina; William E. R. Whitely, Department of Health Sciences, California State University at Los Angeles; and Verne E. Zellmer, Department of Health Sciences, American River College. Finally, special thanks to Edith Heinemann, Director of the Alcoholism Nursing Program and Associate Professor in the Psychosocial Nursing Department, University of Washington, for her reading of the section on alcoholism.

However, it is the author who must accept total responsibility for errors; corrections would be most gratefully appreciated.

BENJAMIN A. KOGAN

contents

HEALTH

MAN IN A CHANGING ENVIRONMENT

SECOND EDITION

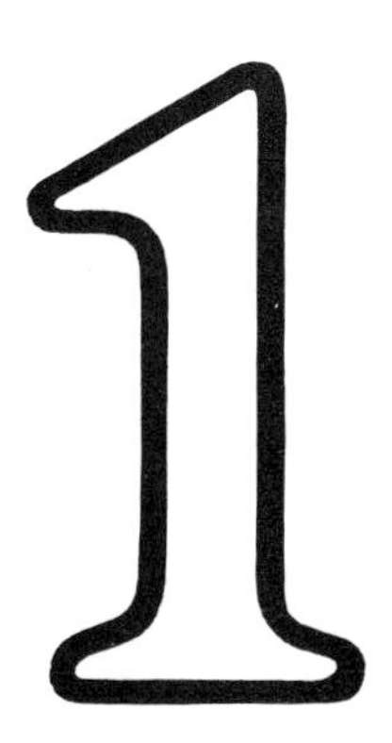

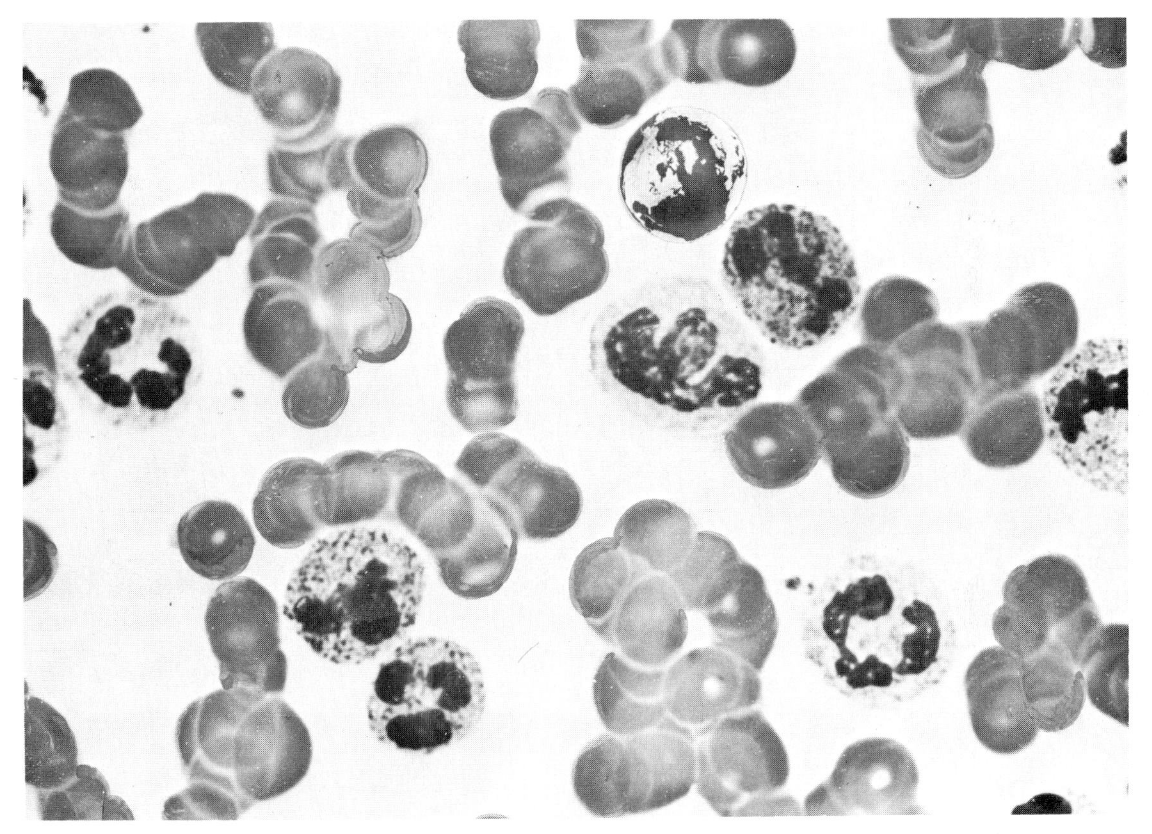

So complex is the earth, with so many parts invisibly connected, it is very like a cell.

man's health in a changing environment

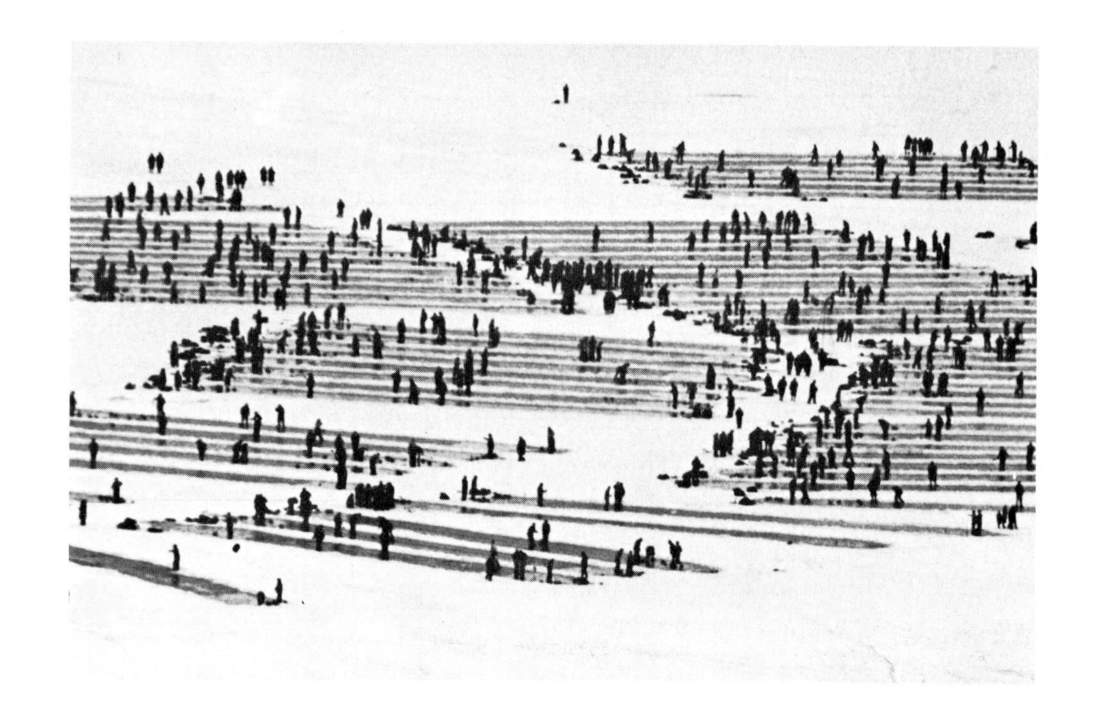

health: a fabric richly woven

1

the scale of health

What is health? Is it visible? Is it seen as a gleaming smile, for example? Not to those Asians who chew betel nuts to blacken their teeth for beauty. Or is health felt? Many people feel well yet harbor infectious illness. Perhaps a formula, something short and magical, like $E = mc^2$, could define health. But formulae such as Einstein's equation apply best not to men but to things. Since there is no human equation, there is no health equation. Health is as complex as man, as variable as life. An attempt to define health within strict limits is as idle as to seek the mind in the dissecting laboratory. This is its encompassing problem, its endless fascination.

Among the many existing definitions of health, there is this famous one devised by the World Health Organization: health is "a state of complete physical, mental and social well-being and not merely the absence of disease or infirmity." In its positive approach this definition has virtue: it is uncompromising. The mere absence of disease or infirmity is indeed not enough for health. The statement is also inclusive: man is not healthy unto himself; man and health are both of culture and society and are reciprocally influenced by the mind.

But has the World Health Organization provided a realistic definition or an idealistic policy? Even though they labor for a Utopia of health, WHO's most devoted workers (and they are legion) hardly expect to attain "complete physical, mental and social well-being" for everyone. They have given much, but they have not given a usable definition of health.

Any concept of health must be viewed as much with imagination as with words. Imagine, then, a scale or a ruler, of as yet unmeasured length. At one end of the scale is zero health (death); at the other end is perfect health, which as yet remains an unknown optimum. In developing this concept, Marston Bates points out that health is a "polar word" and "its meaning is relative only to some standard or scale."[1] Between the poles of death and perfect health are the many gradations of health—the scale is a continuum along which living things constantly move and shift directions.

Stand back and watch someone living on the scale of health. His life is a series of constantly changing happenings. So long as he breathes, so long as his heart beats, so long as his cells divide—so long does he constantly move on the health scale. His health, then, is a dynamic attribute of his life. From one moment to the next, it is never the same. Sometimes illness strikes. He moves toward the death end of the scale. Should he recover, he moves away from death—toward, but probably never reaching, perfect health.

An example? At about 6 A.M. one Sunday morning, a man who has been feeling below par develops a sudden shaking chill. At 10 A.M. the physician is called. Within the hour he arrives. By that time the man has had severe chills half a dozen times. A sharp pain knifes his right chest. His slight cough produces a rust-colored sputum. His breathing is labored. His oral temperature: 104° F. After examining the patient, the physician promptly hospitalizes him. X-ray and

[1] Marston Bates, "The Ecology of Health," in Iago Galdston, ed., *Medicine and Anthropology* (New York, 1959), p. 59.

other studies confirm the diagnosis: pneumonia. The man is perilously ill. He has been rapidly moving toward the death pole of the health scale. Apprehension fills his eyes.

Treatment is prompt. The patient is placed in an oxygen tent. Fluids are dripped into his veins. Antibiotics are administered. His doctor visits him several times every day. Nurses hover at his bedside. Efficiently they carry out the physician's directives. Slowly, the patient improves. He moves away from death toward a safer, healthier level on the scale. He regains his strength. Hopefully, brushing elbows with death has given him wisdom about living. He develops a good health regimen. He moves along the scale of health, approaching perfect health.

Things are never dull on the health scale. Something is always happening to every individual. It is affecting him and he is reacting to it individually. That is because each person is unique. Does this statement seem obvious? Actually it is neither understood nor accepted by everyone.

health and the individual

all men are not created equal —in health

"We hold these truths to be self-evident, that all men are created equal." Written in a passion for liberty, these words still give the nation purpose in time of trial. There is only one thing wrong with them: they are not true. All men are not created equal. On the scale of health each human being is born to a particular place and pace. No two people occupy the same place. All have individual speeds. When one considers the infinite genetic variations that exist in the more than 3 billion inhabitants of the earth, the concept of equal birth becomes ludicrous. Nobody has ever happened before. Nobody will ever happen again. One infant, born a symphony of nerve and muscle, is destined to run the hundred-yard dash in nine seconds. Another, palsied, will find walking five feet an agony. One human being may be born a congenital idiot, another a congenital genius. Differences may be much more subtle than this, and the variations may be hardly noticeable. It is good that men are not created equal, for only duplicates are equal. Men want freedom for themselves, not duplicates of themselves. (What the Founding Fathers meant was that all men are equal in the eyes of a divine personality. So it followed that opportunity should be made equal for all. With equal opportunity, men could attain the high responsibilities of freedom.) Of course, it has never been proved that there is either an innate difference or an innate equality in the intellectual ability of all people.

Nevertheless, creative individuality is a fact of life, and nowhere is this more evident than in the difficulty encountered in surgical transplants of tissue from one person to another. To achieve success, profound changes in both the transplanted tissue and the recipient are necessary.[2]

Lower on the biological scale, tissue transplants are less difficult. Skin from

[2]With few exceptions, such as the cornea of the eye, successful tissue transplants between people were, until recently, extremely rare. Foreign skin or organs that were not from twins or close relatives were usually rejected

one frog may be successfully grafted to any member of the same species. On a still lower level, different parts of two earthworms may be grafted together as long as all the segments point in the same direction.[3]

Viruses, which contain only materials for self-propagation, are at the bottom of the scale of "living things." Indeed, many experts place them in an intermediate position—between living creatures and nonliving things. Recently, scientists at the California Institute of Technology performed a remarkable experiment. They placed various parts of a number of viruses of the same type into a test tube. All of these viruses were genetically defective in some way. Some lacked genes to make heads, others had no genes for tails, still others had no "collar" genes, and so on. Mixing these incomplete viruses together in a test tube, the researchers were able to assemble a complete virus.[4] Compare this singular lack of individuality to the infinitely complex human being whose mother's skin may not ordinarily stay grafted to him.

On the basis of individuality human beings occupy the top position on the biological scale. Variety is possible not only in such obvious external features as height, eye color, and bone structure but in internal organs as well. Studies[5] of the human stomach, for example, show its numerous normal variations in size and shape. But what about the heart? Surely any deviation from a single heart structure would be fatal. Nonsense. Hearts vary so much in normal people that careful training and experience are needed to tell sick hearts from normal variations. No organ of any person is exactly like that of another person. It follows that the chemical functions of these organs differ from person to person. Human patterns of excretion, of glandular activity, of enzyme activity, and the very composition of the hair, skin, bone, stomach juices, saliva, and blood—all these vary from individual to individual.[6]

In sexual appetite enormous differences also exist. These are at least partly due to variations in such organs as the pituitary, sex, and adrenal glands. As one writer sees it, "When two men brought up in the same society differ in their sex activities by ten, one hundred, one thousand, or ten thousand fold, there is bound to be something back of the variation besides what their mammas, or some naughty boy, told them."[7]

Realizing the normally wide variations of people should make one cautious

by the recipient's immunological system (see pages 138–54). Thus a heart transplant, for example, still necessitates medical treatment to suppress the recipient's immunological system. This diminished immunity paved the way for the recipient's greater tendency to infection and, some believe, cancer. Simple skin transplants needed for severely burned patients were also often rejected unless they came from the patient himself, a twin, or a close relative. Now there is hope for change. It has been found that if skin or other tissues are grown in a laboratory medium especially prepared for culturing tissues before being grafted or transplanted, they are not treated as foreigners. They are not rejected by the recipient. Thus, a black mouse has accepted a white fur graft (see Figure 1-1), a rabbit has accepted a cultured human cornea, and burned human beings have accepted cultured foreign skin. Why is cultured foreign skin so acceptable? One theory: it is similar to the skin of an embryo. By degenerating into a more primitive, embryonic state, it loses some genetic information. Therefore, unlike fresh cells, cultured cells cannot make those uniquely individual compounds that a recipient's immunological system would consider foreign. ("A Major Advance in Preventing Rejection of Transplanted Tissue," *Science News*, Vol. 104, No. 1 [July 7, 1973], p. 4.)

[3] Roger J. Williams, *Free and Unequal* (Austin, Tex., 1953), p. 15.

[4] *Science News*, Vol. 91, No. 15 (April 1967), p. 356.

[5] Roger J. Williams, *Biochemical Individuality* (New York, 1956), pp. 21–30.

[6] *Ibid.*, Chapter IV.

[7] Roger J. Williams, *Free and Unequal*, p. 22.

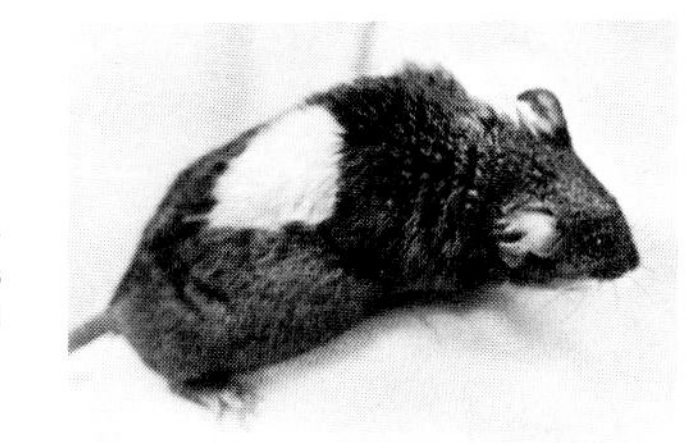

1-1 *White on black: skin graft on a mouse.*

about making hasty comparisons. Most people want to be a trifle different, but never beyond what is acceptable. To put it another way, they want to be acceptably extraordinary. In great measure, the desire to belong to a common group accounts for this. But on the health scale there is no common man. Thus one should not attempt to enforce one's personal health ideas on anyone else. Many ideas of health are personal: writers of health rules usually write about themselves. Eight hours sleep may be what some people need. Many people get along beautifully on six. Some need ten. "Drink milk" is good advice for most people, but there are those who are sickened by milk; they may even be allergic to it. "I can't start the day without a good breakfast," one person insists. Another finds the thought of a heavy breakfast nauseating. A singularly predictable trait of man is his unpredictability.

Health rules should be taken with a grain of salt, and only if salt suits the taste. For effective living, health rules must allow for individuality. A hundred years ago Thoreau wrote in *Walden,* "If a man does not keep pace with his companions, perhaps it is because he hears a different drummer. Let him step to the music which he hears, however measured or far away."

A poignant example both of human individuality and of the rich range within which a life can be lived under adverse health conditions is provided by the life of Mary Lamb, who grew to realize not only her limitations but also her potential. She was the gifted sister of the brilliant English essayist Charles Lamb. All their adult lives they lived together. Mary Lamb conducted a gracious home for her celebrated brother, skillfully entertaining his literary friends. She wrote with grace, too, collaborating with her brother on the classic *Tales Founded on the Plays of Shakespeare* (1807). She also suffered tragically from insanity.

A careful study[8] has been made of her case. Briefly, it is as follows. Her first mental attack occurred when she was thirty. It lasted a month. Two years later she had her second attack, and during it, killed her beloved mother. Only the intervention of a close friend of the family, an attorney, saved her from prosecution. For the rest of her life, she was placed in the care of her brother.

She lived to be eighty-two, a respected figure in English literature. Never, in the forty years that he cared for her, did her brother forsake her. (He died at sixty-nine.) A slight irritability would warn them both of an attack of insanity. She would then be placed into the straitjacket they always carried with them or would be immediately taken to a hospital. During the fifty-two years of her illness, she was hospitalized at least thirty-eight times. Between the eighth and ninth hospitalizations (and between her forty-second and forty-fourth birthdays), she collaborated with her brother in writing the *Shakespeare Tales.*

health and rhythm

Few facts about man are more enigmatic and individual than his rhythms. In a study of biological rhythms,[9] one researcher wrote of a Cambridge team that adjusted its schedule to the accumulation of water in the knee joints of its star player, whose illness occurred regularly every nine days and lasted for two or three days. This is a rather gross example; yet it illustrates that it is by means

[8] E. C. Ross, *The Ordeal of Bridget Elia: A Chronicle of the Lambs* (Norman, Okla., 1940).
[9] Curt Paul Richter, *Biological Clocks in Medicine and Psychiatry* (Springfield, Ill., 1965), p. 92.

of his biological rhythms that man adapts to much of his changing environment and becomes synchronized and in harmony with it. Genetic messages may direct these rhythms. Recent research indicates that the basic timing mechanism may lie in the chemical structure of some of the cell's nuclear DNA. This timing mechanism is what is meant by an ''inner biological clock.'' Its rhythm, integrated into every living cell, is part of the biological organization of the organism. Other research indicates the additional presence of a natural time rhythm, an ''outer cosmic clock,'' which is correlated with the relative position of earth, sun, and moon, as well as with other physical factors of the cosmos, such as cosmic radiation and magnetic fields.

Rhythm characterizes all life patterns. Whether rhythm is governed by the inner biological clock or the outer cosmic clock has become a question for avid research. That there is a relationship between the two seems indisputable. Raise a bean plant in darkness. Its leaves will develop no natural daily sleep movement. Expose it to but a flash of light and natural sleep movement will be induced. Returned to darkness, the leaves then persist in elevating each day at the same time as the single exposure to light. At sunrise the fiddler crab begins to blacken. In this way it is protected from both the sun's glare and its predators. At sunset its dark coat rapidly blanches to a cool silvery gray. Captured and kept in a dark room, it maintains this gray color. These examples illustrate how closely all creature life is related to the day and night changes on earth, which in turn depend on cosmic changes in the universe. Man's rhythms are no less marked. There are the obvious rhythms of a beating heart, of walking, sleeping, breathing, loving. And there are the more subtly secret rhythms of body functions. Within a twenty-four-hour cycle, for example, a person's temperature may vary from 1 to 1.5 degrees Fahrenheit. In the late afternoon or early evening, the ''normal'' temperature (98.6° F. orally) is normally maximal at 100.1° F. At four or five in the morning, it is normally minimal (97.6° F.). Rhythmical biological cycles that recur at approximately twenty-four-hour intervals are called *circadian.* Most people who travel by jet over several time zones in one day will testify to the fatigue (and even illness) resulting from interference with their timed cycles. A man leaves Chicago at 6 P.M. The flight takes eight hours, but he arrives in London when the English are having breakfast. For the Chicagoan it is bedtime. He may feel ill. How can he avoid this affront to his body rhythms? He can begin the trip rested. He should allow a day to adjust. He should avoid overeating.

Even attacks of illness seem to occur in a rhythmic cycle. Asthmatic and heart attacks are most common at 4 A.M.[10] Studies[11] of thousands of epileptics in England show that many patients tend to have an epileptic seizure at about the same time every day.

Were Mary Lamb's attacks rhythmic? Richter wrote: ''The attacks occurred with regularity over some periods, and with little regularity in others—possibly owing in part to failure of the records to show all the attacks.''[12]

[10] ''Biologic Rhythms,'' *Therapeutic Notes,* Vol. 74 (March–April 1947), p. 35.
[11] G. M. Griffiths and J. T. Fox, ''Rhythm in Epilepsy,'' cited in Curt Paul Richter, *Biological Clocks in Medicine and Psychiatry,* p. 60.
[12] Curt Paul Richter, *Biological Clocks in Medicine and Psychiatry,* pp. 60–61.

Periodicity has been observed among some patients with nervous diseases. For years a physician recorded a twenty-four-hour cycle in a hospitalized young woman with a nervous ailment of a particularly crippling nature.[13] During the day, although her mind was clear, she suffered the symptoms of the illness. She was unable to walk, speak clearly, or write legibly. She endured severe rigidity and tremors of her legs and arms. Every evening, at 9 P.M., she suddenly became quite well. She could walk, eat, drink, write, and talk. For two or three hours she was thus remarkably improved. Then she would relapse, remaining helpless until 9 P.M. the following evening.

Some emotionally ill patients have been noted to be very abnormal for twenty-four hours, then, within a few minutes, to become normal for twenty-four hours, and then, again within a few moments, to revert to abnormality. Such abnormal–normal transitions have occurred in certain patients in cycles ranging from a few days to as long as ten years.[14]

Every man maintains his own loom of life. Every man has his own patterned fabric of good health and disease. Yet these billions of different looms manufacture infinitely varying fabrics that must fit together into a functional harmony called mankind. And the same unified system of life exists not only between men but between mankind and all other life. Everything that lives has a rhythm that is synchronized with the individual rhythms of all that relates to it.

health is not human duplication: the limitations of averages

The complex rhythmic individuality of human beings should caution against total reliance on average health measurements. In proper perspective, averages are indispensable. Health workers use average measurements—such as height and weight, blood sugar content, and white cell counts—in a host of ways. However, many people do not fit into averages, nor can they be forced into them. For the average population, smog tolerance levels are valuable indices of whether the smog level is safe or not. But for those with severe chronic bronchitis, the same level may be dangerous. They may become ill and even die before the average tolerance to smog is reached. Those who set legal tolerances for smog levels must, then, set them low enough to protect the sick.

Man is individual, but neither man nor any other living creature moves along the scale of health alone. Life, health, sickness, recovery, and death are dynamically related episodes, shared by all that lives. But this sharing goes on in an all-inclusive environment. The environment molds, and, in turn, is molded, by all within it. To understand health one must be concerned with how man relates to his environment.

ecology: a system of environmental checks and balances

Consider a community of giant redwoods in northern California. The trees are cathedral. Away from the choking freeways, a man can observe a hurrying ant and not feel like one himself. The quiet is so pervasive that he does not think that much is happening there.

[13] *Ibid.*, p. 61.
[14] *Ibid.*

Yet, amidst the seeming serenity of the forest, as much is happening as on the freeways. From its roots each tree must slake its thirst and feed its outermost bud. At the tree's top each leaf must find light or die. With silent ferocity, each tree competes with every other for life. In living together, however, trees better resist wind and water erosion. A dense grove of trees prevents fallen leaves from being blown away, thus helping to maintain soil moisture and nutrients. About each tree, on it, and in it are numberless forms of life similarly striving for existence, competing with and yet adapting to one another. As Clarke wrote: "The community, as well as the individual organism, is 'something happening.'"[15]

So it is with man within his community. He is not rooted to one place, of course, but, like the tree, he competes with the rest of life for his place in the sun. Swarming inside of him and outside of him are countless other organisms, all competing, all adapting.

In discussing the environment, one is automatically involved in a major field of science—*ecology.* This word is derived from the Greek *oikos,* meaning "home" or "household," and *logos,* meaning "discourse." It is the mutual interaction between living things and their environmental household that is of interest to the ecologist. A key word in his vocabulary is *ecosystem,* a term so new that it did not even appear in *Webster's Unabridged Dictionary,* published just two decades ago. *Ecosystem* refers to the systematic, orderly combination or arrangement of living organisms mutually interacting with a shared environment. One may sharply define the area of an ecosystem even to the simplest unit of ecology. A single-celled bacterium thriving in the human gut has its own ecosystem. But the concept of an ecosystem may be wider. There are complex interrelationships between the bacterium and millions of other bacterial ecosystems within the gut. Nor could anyone deny a relationship between the bacterial ecosystems and those of their human hosts. So, innumerable ecosystems interrelated with one another can be distinguished. One may speak of the ecosystem of the Atlantic Ocean or of a man swimming in it, or of a bacterium swimming in him. Ecosystems cannot be separated from one another. They are interdependent, and all within them is interdependent too. Indeed, the basic chemicals comprising the genetic material within the nucleus of every human cell are similar to those in each living cell of all plant and animal life, and some of these chemicals are found in other parts of the universe. "We are brothers of the boulders," wrote the astronomer Harlow Shapley, "cousins of the clouds." This concept of a unified interdependence within the universe was movingly described more than half a century ago by the English poet Francis Thompson:

> All things by immortal power,
> Near or far,
> Hiddenly
> To each other linked are,
> That thou canst not stir a flower,
> Without troubling of a star.[16]

[15] George L. Clarke, *Elements of Ecology* (New York, 1966), p. 16.
[16] Francis Thompson, "The Mistress of Vision," from *Complete Poetical Works of Francis Thompson,* Vol. XXII (New York, 1900), p. 184.

nonhuman ecology: balance, imbalance, and counterbalance

There are many ways to regard a garden. One may admire the delicate turn of a petal or an armored ladybug resting on it. One patient Englishman looked even closer. While studying his own modest garden, he counted hundreds of different living species. In their harmonious garden environment they lived in ecological balance with one another. This does not mean they all survived their entire life span. Many, perhaps most, did not. However, in that orderly English garden community, no single species completely overran another. But were that garden to be permanently deprived of most of its sun, a profound ecological imbalance would result. Much life of the garden would die or leave. Yet, some plants and animals would prevail. Eventually, species needing less sun would begin to develop. Counterbalancing changes would be set in motion. In a now dimmer garden, a new ecological balance would be achieved. A new and shady ecosystem would have replaced the former sunny garden. But the principle of interrelatedness would remain unchanged.[17]

A question arises here. Does counterbalance always succeed in rectifying ecological imbalance? Is there no possible cataclysm as a result of overwhelming ecological change? In terms of life, ecological changes can indeed be cataclysmic. Ecosystems would still exist, but the changes within them could exclude life. As will be seen, this is the core of man's environmental health problem. He must maintain his garden in an ecological balance that averts the threat of cataclysm and assures him the opportunities of the good life.

the biotic drama within the ecosystem

All life, then, is imprisoned within a shared, weblike ecosystem. This creates for its inhabitants a life of paradox—of competition and dependency. Recall the pneumonia patient referred to previously. For the man's life to be saved, bacteria had to be killed. For life, life was sacrificed. Thus life and health for one species may spell disease and death for another. All living organisms are susceptible to parasitic invasion, and sometimes this invasion kills the host. This is all a part of the natural order. For the parasite (the bacterium that caused the pneumonia), the restoration of human health was not only unnatural, it was fatal. Another bacterial victim is shown in Figure 1-2.

1-2 *Debris of a bacterial cell victimized by the T2 virus. The viruses (the large round white objects) multiplied inside the host cell. The walls of the cell were destroyed and then the virus spilled out.* (×*23,850*)

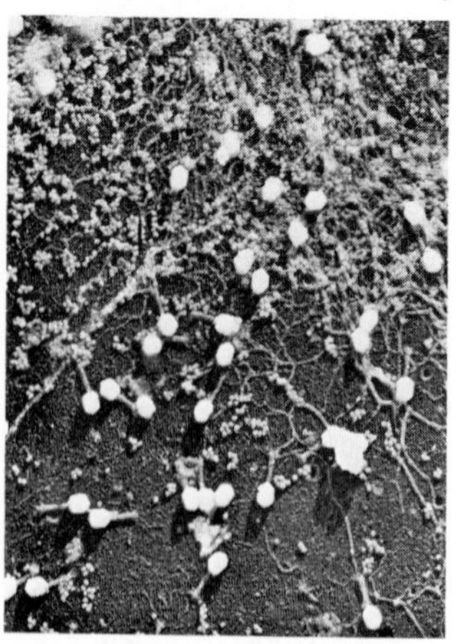

Clarke's reference to a distinguished study by Petrunkevitch unforgettably illustrates such a life and death relationship:

> When the female of the giant wasp *Pepsis marginata* is ready for egg laying, she somehow locates a tarantula *Cryptopholis portoricia,* and explores it with her antennae to make sure that it is the correct species. The larvae of each species of wasp can be nourished by only one species of tarantula. Although the tarantula could easily kill the wasp, it does not do so, and makes little attempt to escape. After the wasp has dug a grave for her intended victim, she stings it, drags it into the grave, and lays a single egg, which she attaches to the abdomen of the paralyzed monster. At hatching the wasp larva is only a tiny fraction of the bulk of the tarantula, but, by the time it is ready for metamorphosis and independent life, it has consumed all the soft tissue of the giant spider.[18]

[17] In the case of the individual cell, the nature of this interrelationship is different. For the cell to survive, there must be a physical and chemical *imbalance* between the inner cell and its outer environment, causing nutrients to enter the cell and wastes to leave it. Nevertheless, this very imbalance makes possible ecological balance within and between cells.

[18] George L. Clarke, *Elements of Ecology,* p. 387.

There is still more to this biotic drama. The permanent paralysis induced by the wasp sting does not promptly kill the tarantula. Initially, it is a living but helpless recipient of the wasp's egg. Only later does it become a source of food for the larva. Instinct serves the wasp well but the tarantula poorly.

But is ecological existence pure exploitation? By no means. The foraging Pederson shrimp (*Periclimenes pedersoni*) of the Bahamas, in taking food from a host fish, provides its host with a health-giving cleaning. Limbaugh described the process:

> The shrimp . . . climbs aboard and walks rapidly over the fish, checking irregularities, tugging at parasites with its claws and cleaning injured areas. The fish remains almost motionless during this inspection and allows the shrimp to make minor incisions in order to get at subcutaneous parasites. As the shrimp approaches the gill covers, the fish opens each one in turn and allows the shrimp to enter and forage among the gills. The shrimp is even permitted to enter and leave the fish's mouth cavity. Local fishes quickly learn the location of these shrimp. They line up or crowd around for their turn and often wait to be cleaned when the shrimp has retired into the hole.[19]

Symbiosis is the general term given to such close association of two dissimilar organisms. The results of this phenomenon range from mutual benefit to mutual destruction. There are occasions when symbiosis is essential for health. A mouse raised in a germ-free environment develops profound structural abnormalities of the digestive tract (Figure 1-3). If the mouse is brought into contact with proper bacteria, its anatomic abnormalities are quickly corrected.[20]

[19] Conrad Limbaugh, "Cleaning Symbiosis," *Scientific American*, Vol. 205, No. 2 (August 1961), p. 42.

[20] Recently, attention has been drawn to the "germ-free baby." Such babies have a rare genetic condition known as *combined immune deficiency disease*. The disease is believed to be carried by a sex-linked gene (page 521); like hemophilia (page 546), it affects only males. Such a child produces neither the antibodies (page

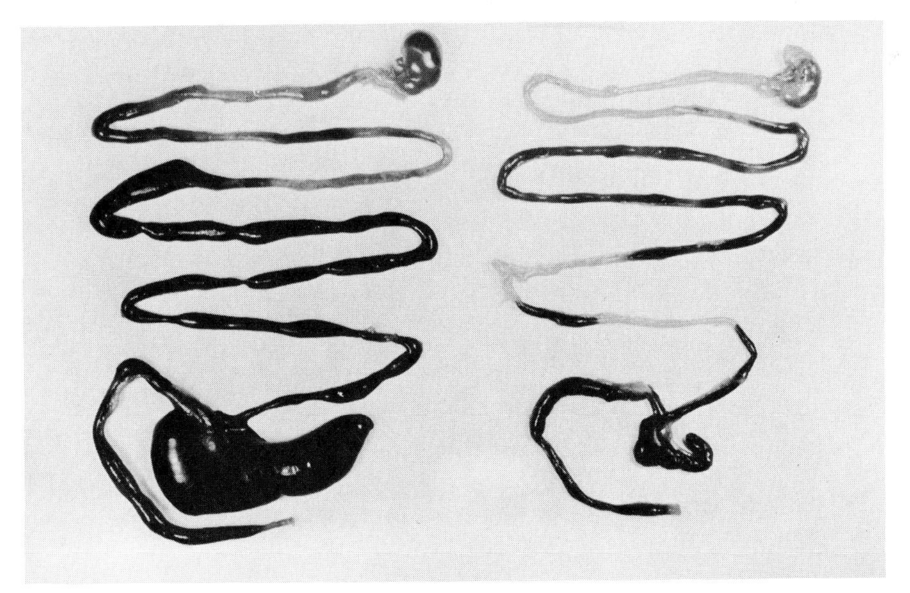

1-3 *Symbiosis: microbe and mouse may need each other—normal* (left) *and germ-free* (right) *digestive tracts of mice.*

As the giant wasp lives at the expense of the tarantula, as the Pederson shrimp relieves a fish of its parasites, as the mouse needs some germs to maintain health, so does man grow healthy and live in cooperation with or at the expense of a wide variety of living creatures. He consumes endless quantities of meat. Within his digestive tract are countless bacteria helping to maintain his health. Other bacteria he destroys with drugs. Both mammals and microbes may pay with their lives for man's will to live. Or they may cooperate with man in a joint struggle for survival. With this in mind, still another aspect can be added to the bipolar health scale. All life on the scale is interrelated; the life of one species may depend on either the life or the death of another. Frequently, the relationship is parasitic and exploitive; frequently, it is not. In this world man is not isolated. Yet in one major respect man's ecosystem is unique. For all other life the ecosystem is comprised of two interrelated dimensions—physical and biological. Man's ecosystem is complicated and enriched by a third dimension—*culture.*

to human ecology a third dimension is added: culture

Unique to man, culture is the sum of what he has learned. It is the substance of that sum that differentiates him from all other life, giving him singular adaptive powers. Like all other living things, man is subject to physical and biological stimuli. But his culture permits their planned alteration and, therefore, changes their effects. Man's cultural processes may also operate independently of the physical or biological stimuli that instigated them.

Within the pneumonia patient discussed earlier, there occurred a biological imbalance between his lung cells and a pneumonia-causing microbe. But it was to the patient that this imbalance was the greatest threat. For the invading microbes the man's sickness was a temporary boon, an opportunity to propagate its species. However, man's culture had provided that patient with penicillin. It turned the ecological tables. With the antibiotic, man created a disastrous ecological imbalance for the microbe. Combining with the patient's natural biological resistance, the antibiotic secured for the afflicted lung cells first counterbalance and finally ecological balance.

Consider this second example. Uranium miners have at least three times the incidence of lung cancer as other men in their age group. Exposed to undue amounts of radioactive uranium, a miner experiences biological changes in his lung cells. He develops lung cancer. Helplessly, he moves toward the death end of the health scale. But are not all people subjected to the physical stimulus of

---

141) nor the white blood cells (page 138) that fight disease-causing microorganisms. Without special attention, he will probably die of infection within six months after birth. The day before delivery, the mother is isolated and scrubbed with germicidal soap; she sleeps on sterile sheets, wears a sterile mask and gown, and prepares her own "germ-free" meals. She is delivered under special conditions, and the newborn is immediately placed in an isolator. He is fed germ-free food and cuddled by hands in sterile gloves that protrude into his germ-free domain. What is the future of the germ-free baby if he survives? Whether he will develop any anatomic problems is, as yet, unknown. Should this occur, however, one treatment might be to contaminate the child with microorganisms that have a known function. Drug therapy is also possible. It is believed that the immunological system of such babies is not completely absent, but slow in developing. In order to fight infection, a bone marrow transplant to provide immunity (see page 141) may be considered. How do physicians suspect that such a child might be born? A previous similar birth to that mother. ("Germ-Free Birth Offsets Immune Deficiency," *Journal of the American Medical Association,* Vol. 218, No. 11 [December 13, 1971], pp. 1631–33, 1637.)

some natural radiation? Yes. Some cells are damaged. Some cells die. With most people, however, the total radiation dose at any one time is small. There is time for cellular recovery and replacement, for restoration of the ecological balance.

The uranium miner is less fortunate. For a long time he has suffered an excessive dose of radiation. Adequate counterbalance is impossible. He is overwhelmed. He sickens critically. The biological events within him stimulate cultural changes that are reflected by his own responses and those of his loved ones. He must, for example, "be brave," and his family must attempt to conceal their anguish. Moreover, his society, which embraces him culturally, becomes deeply involved. Crusading newspaper articles anger the public. The miner dies. Coming into play now are cultural processes utterly unrelated to the original stimuli causing the tragedy. The miner is mourned in a certain way. His funeral is in strict accordance with cultural dicta. He is buried according to a rigid set of cultural rules. Bitterly, the miner's union pressures the officials in Washington. Public clamor is now vast, insistent. A cultural imbalance has occurred and must be set aright. To restore the cultural balance laws are passed. The original physical stimulus and biological effect happened deep in a mine. But the actual operation of the legislative process, a cultural event, occurred independently of them.

To what extent is man affected by imbalance in his ecosystems? Are his environmental competitors able to nullify his cultural powers? René Dubos has written:

> All living things, from men to the smallest microbe, live in association with other living things . . . an equilibrium is established which permits the different components of biological systems to live at peace together, indeed often to help one another. Whenever the equilibrium is disturbed by any means whatever, either internal or external, one of the components of the system is favored at the expense of the other . . . and then comes about the process of disease.[21]

[21] René Dubos, "The Germ Theory Revisited," quoted in *Harold G. Wolff's Stress and Disease,* rev. and ed. by Stewart Wolf and Helen Goodell, 2nd ed. (Springfield, Ill., 1968), p. 190.

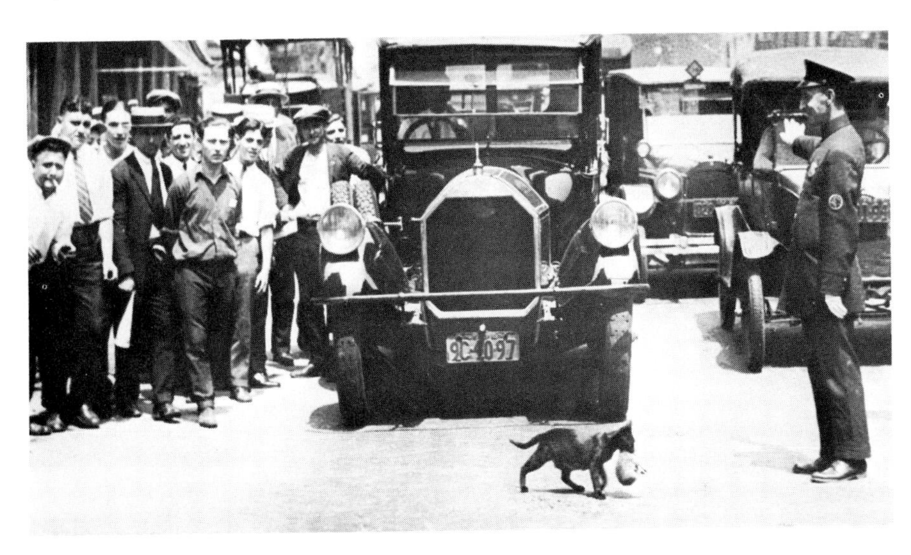

1-4 *"All living things . . . live in association with other living things."*

Study now some of mankind's challengers for environmental control. Their actions spell ecological imbalance for man. Their weapon is disease.

the staphylococcus versus man's penicillin: a world war

Staphylococcus aureus is a microorganism carried in the nose and throat by numberless people throughout the world—including those who work in hospitals. Most people who carry the germ, however, are unaffected by it. They are in a state of ecological balance with it.

Occasionally, however, the germ overcomes the resistance of its host. It then causes conditions such as pimples, boils, or eye infections. At one time, most staphylococci were exquisitely sensitive to penicillin. Small doses of the antibiotic destroyed vast numbers of these staphylococci. Doctors, therefore, saturated the environment of these microorganisms with this antibiotic. Most staphylococci could not live in the penicillin environment but a few could. They were resistant. The original penicillin-resistant staphylococci were not the result of change brought about by the antibiotic. The resistant bacteria were present in the original bacterial population. These resistant germs lived through the penicillin deluge. They multiplied enormously. Today, they are a spectre of infection in every hospital in the world. And staphylococci have developed resistance to antibiotics other than penicillin.[22]

Organisms of higher species also exhibit this resistance to man's connivance. Consider the louse.

of lice and men

Man struggles to control his environment. His ability to behave according to what he has learned molds his culture. Insects do not learn. Their environmental control is entirely by instinct. They have a society, not a culture. About three-fourths of the insect's brain is eye. It sees much, but learns nothing. Instinct governs it. Its sexual instincts, for example, generally depend on its exquisite sensitivity to odor. The scientist can isolate the insect sex chemical and spray it over an area. One can imagine the confusion of the male insect. He is completely surrounded by glamorous females who are not there. One would think the frustration enough to kill him. It is. Man, in this instance at least, has outwitted the insect.

But in his constant war with insects for environmental control, man is hardly the instant winner. Temporarily, at least, the humble body louse can thwart man. On the warm body of a human the louse can find comfort for some time. Left to its own devices, the louse gets free board, room, and transportation. It finds a transient ecological peace. The compliment goes unreturned. The satis-

[22] More than a decade ago, at Keio University in Tokyo, Dr. Tsutomu Watanabe identified a *resistance* (or *"R"*) *factor* in certain bacteria. It is made up of genes—DNA (Chapter 18). Many bacteria, such as those causing typhoid fever and infant diarrhea, can contain these resistant genes. By simple contact, antibiotic-resistant germs may transmit their resistance factor to germs of a different species. And one strain of bacteria can develop resistance to a variety of drugs. Such multiple drug resistance was a serious problem when U.S. travelers to Mexico developed typhoid fever during the summer of 1972. (Ruth M. Lawrence, Elliot Goldstein, and Paul D. Hoeprich, "Typhoid Fever Caused by Chloramphenicol-Resistant Organisms," *Journal of the American Medical Association,* Vol. 224, No. 6 [May 7, 1973], pp. 861–63.) Drug immunity can thus be spread to a whole population of different bacteria. How to meet this potential threat to antibiotic effectivity is a major problem of modern science. Although the connection between animal and human R factors is unclear, in 1972 the U.S. Food and Drug Administration curtailed the indiscriminate use of antibiotics in the feeds of those animals consumed by human beings. (Nicholas Wade, "US Restricts Antibiotics in Feeds," *New Scientist,* Vol. 53, No. 784 [February 24, 1972], p. 413.)

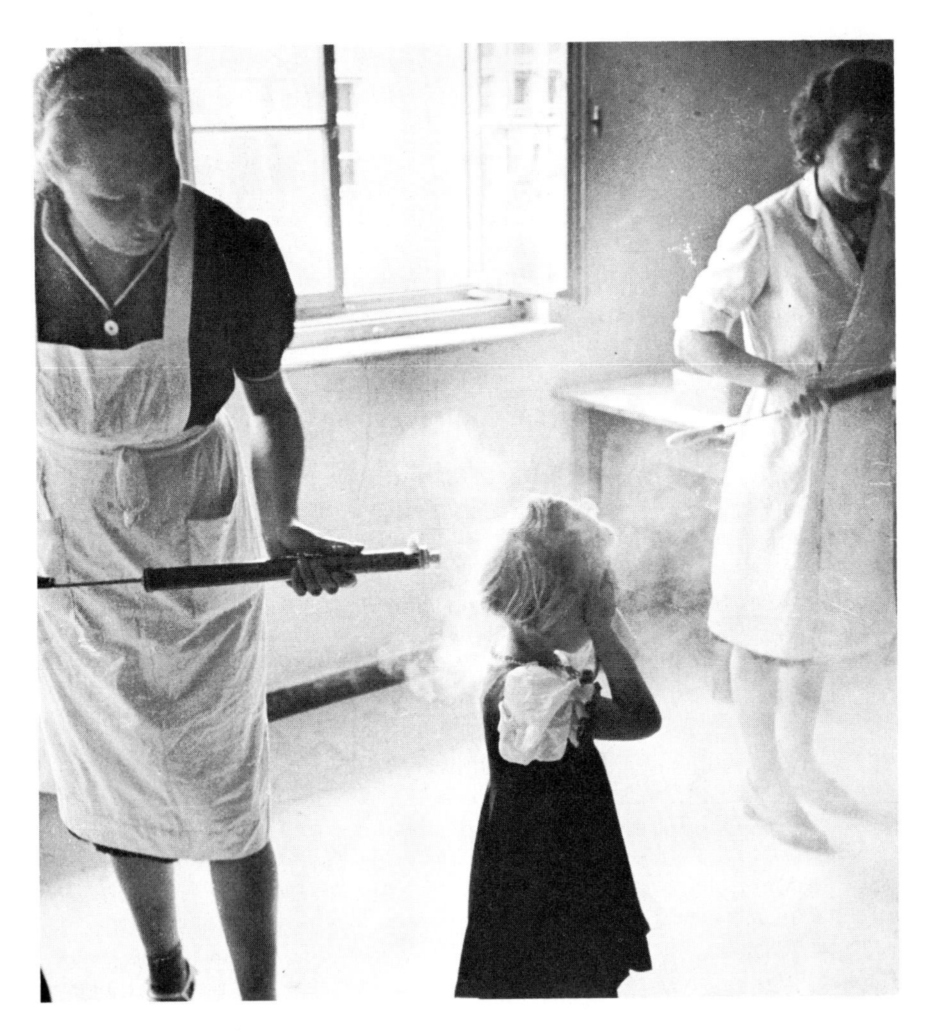

1-5 *A European child being deloused with DDT. Such spraying was commonplace during and just after the Second World War.*

faction is not mutual. In the first place, infestation by lice will make a person itch. Second, some lice can carry serious, even fatal, epidemic disease (typhus fever). Lice are notorious for their partiality to soldiers and their clothing. However, anybody will do. It was with some relief, therefore, that during the Second World War, DDT was found to be fatal to the body louse. For some time during and immediately after the war, soldiers and affected populations alike were effectively deloused with this agent (see Figure 1-5).

Imagine the consternation that occurred when, during the Korean War, it was found that DDT was useless in killing the body louse. The foot soldier had lost a valuable chemical ally. What had happened? During the Second World War, DDT had been introduced into the louse environment. That environment became more tolerable for humans, but intolerable for many lice. Most of the exposed lice died. Most—not all. Some lice lived. To understand why, one must remember that great numbers and varieties of lice exist. Enormous numbers of lice, with various genetic combinations, produced astronomic numbers of offspring. These offspring contained even greater numbers of genetic combinations. A few of these genetic combinations resulted in lice that were resistant to DDT. These DDT-resistant lice produced offspring with genetic combinations as resistant to DDT as their predecessors (some were even more resistant). In this way DDT acted as a selector of DDT-resistant lice. Since all the DDT-susceptible lice were killed, in the end only DDT-resistant lice were left. Adaptation to DDT meant survival of the louse.

This is a classic example of a biological (genetic) adaptation by an organism to a man-made change in physical environment. The adaptation by the louse profoundly affects man's culture. To completely defeat the body louse, to protect health, the ecology of lice and men will need to be changed even more.

of rain, potatoes, and tuberculosis

It is more than a hundred years since the Irish potato famine, but the scars of its deep societal wounds are still apparent. The famine was the result of an ecological imbalance. Climate, a physical factor in the Irish ecosystem, had not previously disturbed the biological balance between the potato (their "root of delight") and one of its parasites. Suddenly, climate did upset that subtle relationship. Like a house of cards, the whole ecosystem collapsed.

In 1845, a black cloud hung over Ireland. This is what had happened. The parasitic fungus *Phytophthora infestans* had long infested the Irish potato. This potato, originally an inedible tuber growing wild in the Andes, had been brought to Ireland as a new food. The fungus had come along. With careful farming and reasonably good weather, the fungus had been kept at bay. Ireland prospered and her population multiplied.

Then the crop failed. Why? For two basic reasons. First, by growing the best varieties, the Irish had refined the potato for edibility and yield. The tastier potato was now delicate. It could no longer resist a fungus as well as its hardy Andean ancestor could. Second, in 1845 the weather in Ireland was pitiless. Rain and fog upset the by-then delicate ecological-biological balance between

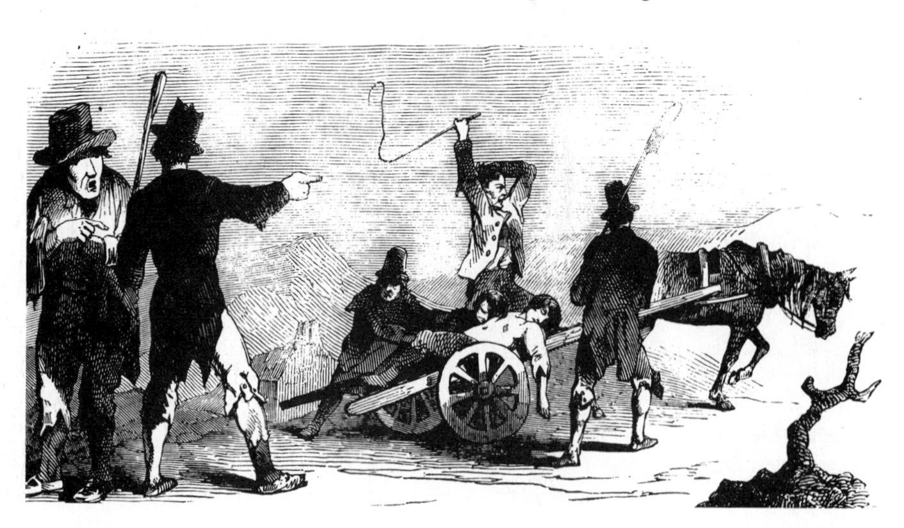

1-6 *A funeral during the Irish potato famine.*

potato and fungus. The potato was overwhelmed. It lay soaked, rotting. The crop was ruined, and so was Ireland.

The enormity of the calamity has been recorded in a masterpiece by Salaman.[23] More than a million people died of sheer hunger. Others were plagued by scurvy (from vitamin C deficiency), dysentery, and typhus. Insanity and blindness were rampant. The former was doubtless due to prolonged stress and lack of vitamins. The latter was probably caused by lack of decent nourishment.

Fearful people of Europe, then as now, looked to the New World. In desperate droves, the rural Irish, starved, disease-ridden, left Ireland for New York, Philadelphia, and Boston. There they met with other miseries. Accustomed to the pace and space of the Irish farm, they were forced into the congestion and speed of the cities. Their situation could not have been more conducive to the spread of tuberculosis. As Dubos points out, "The sudden and dramatic increase of tuberculosis mortality in the Philadelphia, New York and Boston areas around 1850 can be traced in large part to the Irish immigrants who settled in these cities at that time."[24]

So, because it rained in Ireland in 1845, tuberculosis increased in Boston and New York and Philadelphia in 1850. The arm of ecology is long. The physical change in the climate, resulting in a change in the biological balance between the potato and its fungal parasite, brought about vast physical, biological, and cultural imbalances affecting the health of human beings thousands of miles away.

But note this: in the succession of imbalances, there were counterbalances. The ecological scales were but temporarily tipped against man. In the end, he survived. And with his help, so did the Irish potato. Why? Because man is able to think, and to transmit his thoughts to the generations that follow him.

of unwelcome guests, their unprepared hosts, and imbalanced ecosystems

Much has been written of the friendly Indian reception given early European invaders of the New World. Perhaps there were isolated instances of such behavior. On the whole, however, the Europeans were met with bitter hostility. Had it not been for the Europeans' powerful ally, the Indians might have successfully, albeit temporarily, driven the invaders from the New World. That ally was disease. To the Indians, the Europeans brought grievous ecological imbalance.

So it was with the North American Indians when the English arrived in the seventeenth century. The Indians resisted, trying to rid their lands of the ruthless invaders. They failed. Their greatest enemy was the smallpox brought them from Europe. Modern celebrants of Thanksgiving Day portray the Puritan relationship with the Indian as pious and benevolent. Dubos tells a different story:

> Europeans soon became aware of the fact that smallpox was one of their most effective weapons against Indians, and they did not hesitate to spread the infection intentionally by means of contaminated blankets, always on the pretext that it helped destroy the enemies of the faith.[25]

[23] N. Redcliffe Salaman, *The History and Social Influence of the Potato* (Cambridge, Eng., 1949).
[24] René Dubos, *Mirage of Health* (Garden City, N.Y., 1961), p. 90.
[25] *Ibid.*, p. 189.

It has been estimated that of the 12 million seventeenth-century American Indians, 6 million died of smallpox.

Similar incidents have been recorded involving the effects of tuberculosis, venereal disease, scarlet fever, and polio on populations newly exposed to them. At various times both Polynesians and Africans have been cruelly decimated by these afflictions. But one need not seek out exotic countries to provide excellent examples of biological imbalance caused by the occurrence of a new infectious agent in a community.

In February and March 1966, type A2 influenza sent half a million Los Angeles school children to bed. They complained of headaches, sore throats, and coughing. Some had muscle pains. Oral temperatures rose as high as 104° F. Not many vomited or had diarrhea. Gastrointestinal symptoms are not usually part of the true influenza picture. Their parents, who had been adequately exposed to the virus some five years before, were immune and were hardly affected by the disease. The virus, absent in epidemic amounts from the Los Angeles area for five years, found a receptive host in the child. Why? In his preschool years, the Los Angeles child had had no opportunity to develop immunity. Almost two years later (in December 1968), a new A2 influenza virus variant, originating in Hong Kong, made millions of people sick. In this Los Angeles epidemic, both adults and children were affected. In this case neither had been previously exposed to the Hong Kong type of influenza A2 virus. The Hong Kong influenza virus had changed genetically from the previous influenza A2 virus. The population had not developed a resistance to this changed virus.

These examples demonstrate biological imbalance resulting from the introduction of a new microbe into a community. It is well to remember that a microorganism can exist in the human body quite harmlessly. However, man's activities, resulting in a changed ecosystem, can transform a harmless relationship into a destructive battle. An example is the yeastlike fungus *Candida albicans,* which usually inhabits the human intestine without harm. It can cause a disease of infants (rarely of adults) called *thrush.* This condition is characterized by whitish spots in the mouth. Oral antibiotics, such as penicillin, have been known to kill certain microorganisms in the intestine that keep the *Candida* in check. *Candidiasis,* an infection that occurs when there is an overgrowth of these fungi, can result in serious abscesses of organs such as the kidney or liver.

Sometimes, biological imbalances are purposely instigated by man to his own advantage. The rabbit of Australia is a case in point. Once these animals were a major agricultural pest. In an attempt to control them, ferrets and weasels, the natural enemies of the rabbit, were introduced into Australia. This attempt had little success. A virus was then tried, which caused a rabbit disease called *myxomatosis.* The introduction of the virus into Australia seemed to solve the problem. However, one is reminded of the genetic success achieved by the louse against DDT and by the staphylococci against penicillin. Already strains of rabbits resistant to the virus have appeared. Another method of rabbit control will be needed soon.[26]

[26] Marston Bates, *Animal Worlds* (New York, 1963), p. 296.

for balance, ecologic challenge alters man

Every creature characteristic, varying from the opening of a flower to the opening of a hand, is determined by both genes and environment (see Chapter 18). Formed and stored many millennia ago, the structured chemical pattern of man's uniquely arranged set of genes changes with the deliberate speed of evolution. The patterned detail of his genetic make-up changes as environmental conditions favor the selective activity of some genes over others. Genes and environment interplay in subtle concert to produce a creature with the best chance of meeting the particular environmental challenge. Thus man, by means of his genetic structure, remains in balance with his environment.

Can environmental stimulus alone produce rapid change? Yes. Normally, the human genetic pool changes little, if at all, from a single generation to the next. Yet, in the years since the Second World War, one environmental change, diet, has helped produce a whole generation of larger Japanese and Israeli children. Another recent environmental change accounts for the earlier sexual maturity of today's Western teen-ager. From his parents the modern teen-ager has inherited an unchanged reproductive system. But the culture within that modern ecosystem, independent of his genes, stimulates early marriage.

That environmental or ecological changes such as diet may have marked effects on future generations is shown by research indicating a close relationship between maternal stature and the death rates of newborns. "The deleterious effects of malnutrition in childhood will not be confined to the skeleton but must affect the development of the whole body, and thus the quality of the response to pregnancy."[27] The mother's reproductive capacity (profoundly influenced by her diet) plus the standards of her care are two basic factors in determining the viability of her newborn.

Another example: the environment of the Aymara Indians of the Peruvian Andes negatively influences their stature and reproductive maturity. Oxygen deficiency and cold are characteristic of the high Peruvian plateaus. Such stresses are associated with the lessened birth weight, slower growth rate, and diminished adolescent spurt of the children in that area. There, the earliest age at which any woman gives birth to a child is eighteen.[28]

The needs of man's ecosystem exert even more profound changes in his physical characteristics. The fair skin of Northwest Europeans affords them the maximum benefit of the little ultraviolet radiation that passes through the cloudy skies of their environment. Conversely, the dark skin of black people, evolved in the distant past, was doubtless protective. It guarded them against overexposure to the ultraviolet rays of the sun while allowing them to get enough of those rays so that synthesis of vitamin D could occur. Without adequate ultraviolet radiation from the sun, rickets results. It is of interest to note that black children who live in cities are somewhat more liable to rickets than white children in the same area. This is thought to be due to the filtering action of the skin pigment.[29] (Thus, rickets is not fundamentally a dietary deficiency disease resulting from the lack of vitamin D. "In actual fact rickets was the first

[27] Dugald Baird, "Perinatal Mortality," *The Lancet,* Vol. 1, No. 7593 (March 8, 1969), p. 511.
[28] Paul T. Baker, "Human Adaptation to High Altitudes," *Science,* Vol. 163, No. 3872 (March 14, 1969), p. 1156.
[29] Jacques M. May, *The Ecology of Human Disease* (New York, 1958), p. 5.

air-pollution disease."[30] Air pollution is discussed in Chapter 3, pages 52–53. Rickets is discussed further in Chapter 22, page 654.)

Eskimos (Figure 1-7) have short noses. Were their noses as long as those of the average desert dweller, there would surely be an epidemic of frozen noses in the Arctic. The Tongus and Mongoloids of eastern Siberia live in probably the coldest places in the world. They have short noses, narrow nasal passages, and flat faces. Their squat bodies are fat-padded to help keep them warm. In the African heat, a body frame so covered with fat would be a discomfort. To the Eskimo and the Siberian, it is essential for survival.

to meet their needs, creatures modify their ecosystems

Other living organisms may change their environment to suit themselves. The romantic little firefly has a characteristically unique code of flashing light. Seeing the signal of the flying male, the female firefly signals her response, thereby attracting him. In the deep darkness of the sea, some shrimp resist attack by producing a discharge of light that distracts or frightens the attacker. But, of all the creatures of this planet, none can modify his ecosystem so much as man. How his very ingenuity has produced ecosystems that threaten his health is explored in Chapters 3 and 4.

This first chapter, however, has reviewed some ways to regard health. An ever changing, rhythmic biotic adventure of varying individuals, health is a part of the weave of life, coloring it brightly here, subtly shading it there, obvious

[30] W. F. Loomis, "Rickets," *Scientific American,* Vol. 223, No. 6 (December 1970), p. 77.

1-7 *That man is molded by his environment is demonstrated by the Masai of East Africa* (left), *whose tall, lean bodies are admirably suited to the hot climate of that region, and by the Eskimos* (right), *whose squat, padded bodies, short, broad noses, and tough skin help them to survive their rigorous climate.*

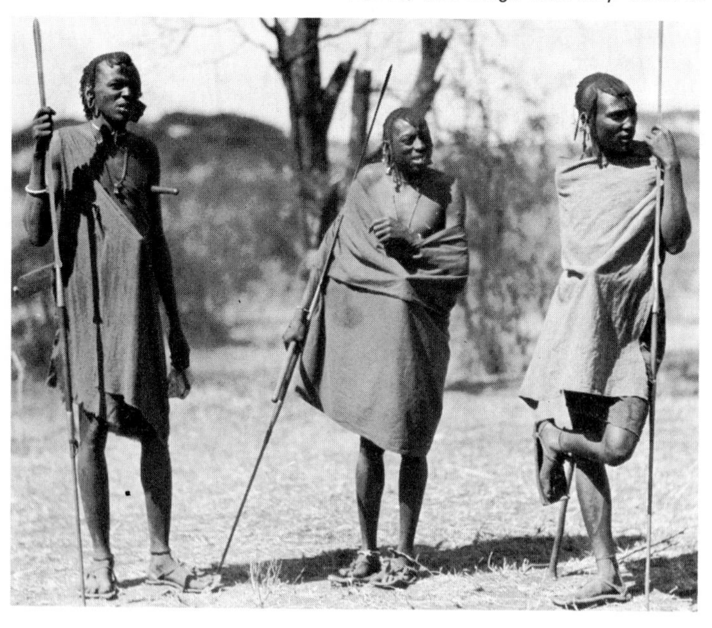

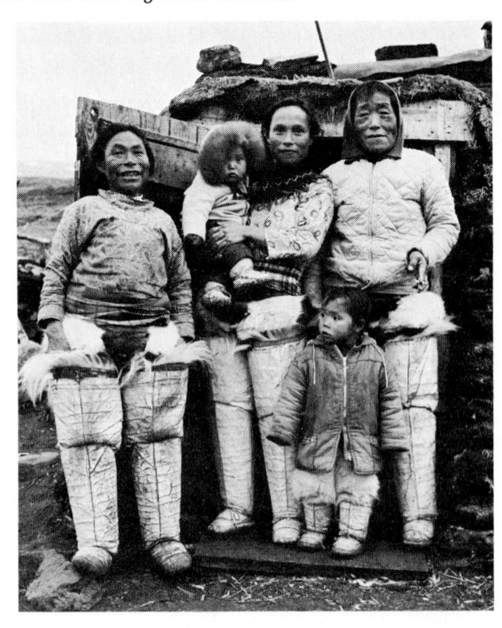

in one place, obscure—almost lost—in another. In holding the fabric to the light, one sees the infinite variety of health. So singular and so varied a pattern does mankind's all-pervasive culture give his ecosystems that it is the subject of the entire following chapter.

summary

The scale of health is a continuum, with death at one end and perfect health, an unknown optimum, at the other. Living things constantly move along, and shift directions on, the scale of health. Because each individual is unique, health rules must allow for variations in physical features and functions, biological cycles such as the *circadian rhythm* (page 7), and psychological condition. Each individual affects and is affected by his environment. *Ecology* (page 9) is the study of the orderly arrangement of living organisms mutually interacting with their shared environment—an arrangement called an *ecosystem* (page 9). One type of ecosystem involves *symbiosis*—the close association of two dissimilar organisms (page 11). All ecosystems have two interrelated dimensions—physical and biological. Only mankind adds a third dimension—culture (page 12), the sum of what mankind has learned, which enables him to alter physical and biological stimuli and thus to change their effects. One of mankind's greatest challenges is to maintain the balance of his ecosystem—neither to disrupt his environment nor to be overwhelmed by his competitors in that environment.

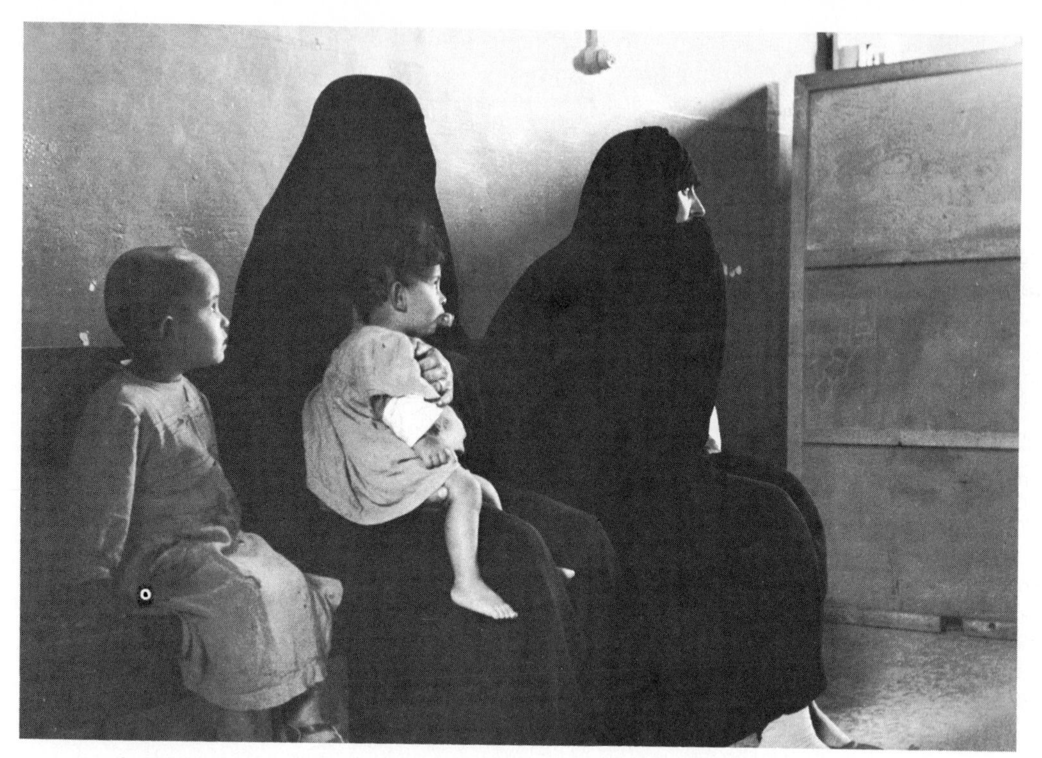

At a Syrian dispensary, children wait to be examined for favus, a scalp infection.

health and the community

2

culture and health

Up to this point a variety of rhythmic, balanced interrelationships between living things has been considered. The redwood tree struggling silently to survive, the selfless tarantula, the obliging Pederson shrimp, the greedy potato fungus, the stubborn staphylococcus resisting its antibiotic enemy, the devious louse changing genetically to foil man's clever chemicals, and man himself changing physically to meet his needs—all these speak of dynamic operations in the environment. They both remind man of the basic environmental threats challenging him and suggest possible ways of coping with these challenges. For example, in Chapter 1 it was noted that a certain species of wasp was able to propagate itself only by sacrificing a tarantula. Mankind's knowledge of such events as this, combined with his cultural achievements, enables him to manipulate ecosystems to his own benefit. In what way? Large milk supplies in California were recently found to be polluted by a pesticide. How did this happen? Cows eat alfalfa. Competing for their food were voracious alfalfa weevil larvae. Wanting milk, man brought his culture to bear on the side of the cow. To save the cow-food crop, alfalfa growers first used a pesticide. The weevil was eliminated. But the milk was polluted by the pesticide. Another method of destroying the weevil had to be found. Within the balance of the ecosystem lay the answer. It had been observed that certain wasps deposited their eggs inside the alfalfa weevil (Figure 2-1). Within the host, the eggs hatched and the weevil died. And so, into the weevil's ecosystem great numbers of wasps were deliberately let loose. By this manipulation of the environment, the threat of the alfalfa weevil was removed. No longer was there a need for dangerous pesticides. The milk pollution was eliminated.

Thus man's complex, learned culture enters into the simpler ecological picture of a biological relationship. Scientific skill is wholly learned and taught. But

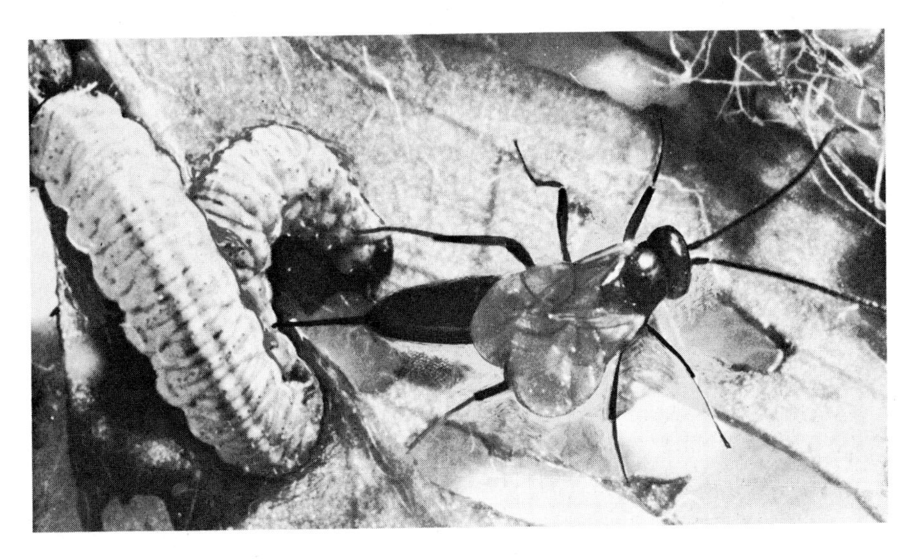

2-1 *The wasp and the weevil. A natural enemy of the alfalfa weevil and a friend of the alfalfa grower, the wasp deposits its eggs within the alfalfa weevil larva, as shown here. The eggs hatch within the host. The host dies.*

science, as much as any other aspect of culture, can harm as well as help man. His culture has brought him both health and disease. In distinguishing man from all else that lives, it has lent him power over all other life. Yet within his own ecosystem man has become his own worst enemy. To comprehend this ecological threat, man must examine mankind and the consequences of group living. Other creatures live successfully in groups. Why is man so different? To what extent does man's culture, patterned into the web of his ecosystem, control him? How does it create his health problems and yet at the same time offer him solutions? This chapter will seek answers to these questions. But first it might be well to examine the behavior of a species existing in a singularly successful society. "Go to the ant, thou sluggard; consider her ways, and be wise" (Proverbs 6:6). Man need not emulate the ant. It is inefficient, a slaveholder, and a thief. But ant society has so much in common with human society, as well as having so many instructive differences, that it merits a careful examination.

an insect sophisticate

A morsel to tempt the most finicky Mexican bride at her wedding breakfast might well be an insect honeyball. This delicacy is a collection of ants, swollen like tiny barrels, purposely stuffed by worker ants with honeydew. In times of short supply these cask ants provide food for worker ants. Being a living mason jar is but one of the countless ingenuities of the ant. For millions of years, several thousand recorded species of ants, the members of the family *Formicidae,* have scurried about on the face of the earth.

As the example of the cask ant shows, these insects have a caste structure. Ants maintain slaves and babysitters, keep cattle, engage in agriculture, construct cities, skyscrapers, and freeways, and have an elaborate and regular system of patrols. Soldiers (undeveloped females) defend the nest from outside invasion. Let a stray ant wander into a strange nest and he is attacked, but a prodigal, gone for weeks, is welcomed back. There is even a "doorkeeper" ant, whose head is fashioned into a plug to close nest entrances.[1]

Such coordinated devotion by the individual to the common societal good would be hard to surpass. But, as Dobzhansky stated, "Among the marvels of ant and termite societies, one thing is conspicuously absent. Nowhere is there a school for the young workers or soldiers!"[2] The ant's behavioral patterns are not learned.

man and learned culture

This is the crux of the difference between *Hominidae* and *Formicidae,* between human and ant society. For the insect, behavior is instinctual. The ant need not learn. Without training, it becomes expert at particular tasks when it reaches a given stage of development. The human must be trained, and only after prolonged growth and development does he achieve a certain ability. Moreover, what the ant does is suitable for its limited environment. In a new environment its inherited instinctual effort is useless or fatal. The human, however, can adapt to new environments. Paul has written:

[1] Theodosius Dobzhansky, *Evolution, Genetics, and Man* (New York, 1955), p. 343.
[2] *Ibid.*

> Should all the members of an ant community perish, for example, except one fertilized female, the lone survivor would be capable of rebuilding the entire social edifice in all its original complexity within the span of a few short generations. A society of humans could not similarly recover from catastrophe if all humans suddenly disappeared except one adult couple organically intact but innocent of knowledge and all other social learning . . . it would take tedious thousands of generations to rediscover the ways and wisdom needed to run any human society now in existence. This is because humans, unlike insects, order their lives and interpersonal relations largely by means of socially acquired signals.[3]

So human beings rely primarily on learned behavior, or culture, for survival. It is this acquired guidance, this cultural instruction, that enables man to constantly adapt to change. Insect societies do not change; human societies change constantly, and change makes progress possible.

Still another difference between human beings and life that is lower on the biological scale is the length of time required for the development of independence. No other creature must remain dependent so long as the human. Usually the insect has a brief period of immaturity followed by a relatively long period of productivity. While the young monkey busily forages in the supermarkets of nature, the human of the same age idly contemplates his fingers. For a man to mature requires almost one-third of his life span. He needs this time to learn the rules of adaptation to his culture. Also, man has an unusually long postreproductive life span. In the length of her life after menopause, the woman is unique among mammals. Nature grants humankind extra years in which to learn the demands of human culture and even more years in which to make use of this wisdom. But, in his developmental years, man picks up problems as well as wisdom. And, in his productive years, he creates even more problems for himself. In growing, he often flaws his health and thus his productive energy.

In *Childhood and Society,* Erikson has pointed to the price of "becoming": "It is human to have a long childhood; it is civilized to have an ever longer childhood. Long childhood makes a technical and mental virtuoso out of man, but it also leaves a lifelong residue of emotional immaturity in him."[4]

So, although man is unique in his learned behavior (culture), the process of his learning has a price. Too often the cost of some aspect of this culture is his health. The price will depend on his ability to create a balance between himself and his surroundings. The relationships between culture and environment and health are aptly stated by Mead: "In many cultures throughout the world, man is continuous with his environment. Therefore, he is not healthy unless his environment is 'healthy' or conversely, the well-being of his environment depends upon his acts."[5]

Health, then, helps to create culture and culture creates health, for man is not alone. But culture can be tyranny.

[3] Benjamin D. Paul, ed., *Health, Culture, and Community* (New York, 1955), p. 461.
[4] Erik H. Erikson, *Childhood and Society* (New York, 1950), from the Foreword.
[5] Margaret Mead, ed., *Cultural Patterns and Technical Change* (New York, 1955), pp. 217–18.

the power of culture

All men and their communities share a variety of problems. However, various cultures have various solutions to these similar problems.

In the face of sickness, every culture defines what must be done, by whom, with what, when, and so forth.[6] Herb medicines and antibiotic therapy are highly dissimilar treatments, but they are both specific. Even how to behave in the presence of illness is strictly prescribed by culture. In his autobiographical novel *Of Human Bondage* W. Somerset Maugham expressed this through the thoughts of the hero, Philip Carey, a medical student in an English hospital dispensary.

> Sometimes you saw an untaught stoicism which was profoundly moving. Once Philip saw a man, rough and illiterate, told his case was hopeless; and, self-controlled himself, he wondered at the splendid instinct which forced the fellow to keep a stiff upper-lip before strangers. But was it possible for him to be brave when he was by himself, face to face with his soul, or would he then surrender to despair?[7]

Clearly, this man's "stiff upper-lip before strangers" is ordered by his culture. He may tremble within, but to the outside world, his cultural world, he must show a brave face. So does culture at times force man into a cruel paradox. It gives him company and sustenance and yet it enforces loneliness, too. As the man becomes sicker, and even as he approaches death, his culture will still make demands based on set rules, which, so long as he is able, he will obey. Indeed, so it was with the previously mentioned uranium miner who died of lung cancer.

Death is the ultimate unknown. That men have been known to accept death and even to embrace it because their culture so dictates is remarkable. A community that believes in magic can literally condemn a man to death by pointing a bone at him. Malinowski described bone-pointing in Melanesia:

> For the sorcerer has, as an essential part of the ritual performance, not merely to point the bone dart at his victim, but with an intense expression of fury and hatred he has to thrust it in the air, turn and twist it as if to bore it in the wound, then pull it back with a sudden jerk. Thus not only is the act of violence, or stabbing, reproduced, but the passion of violence has to be enacted.[8]

Simmons and Wolff tell of the overwhelming impact of this condemnation on the damned individual.[9] To be read out of the living, to be considered already dead by one's own, means death. Terrified by belief in magic, utterly alone through loss of support from kin, excommunicated in an organized manner by the culture and society that sheltered him, the tragic figure undergoes profound physical changes. Sinking from trembling fear to choking terror to tormented collapse to mute agony and, finally, to utter resignation, the "boned" man awaits death. The members of the community who have forsaken him return,

[6] Ralph Linton, *The Study of Man,* cited in Leo J. Simmons and Harold G. Wolff, *Social Science in Medicine* (New York, 1954), pp. 74–75.
[7] W. Somerset Maugham, *Of Human Bondage* (Garden City, N.Y., 1915), pp. 497–98.
[8] Bronislaw Malinowski, *Magic, Science and Religion* (Garden City, N.Y., 1955), p. 71.
[9] Leo J. Simmons and Harold G. Wolff, *Social Science in Medicine,* pp. 92–94.

but only to organize his doom. The rules must yet and ever be obeyed. He is prepared for "death and ritual mourning." The condemned man utters no sound, partakes neither of food nor water.

He dies quietly. So overwhelming are the cultural powers of man.

To find "boning" in his own culture, the reader need merely be reminded of the torment of the "witches" of the sixteenth and seventeenth centuries and the activities of Nazi Germany some three decades ago.[10] Today, more subtle examples of "boning" are commonplace. And so are its consequences. In the first half of this century, as Wolff has pointed out, stomach ulcers became principally a male disorder.[11] Among the reasons for this phenomenon is increased male stress due to the changed relationship between the sexes. Millions of married women seek careers. Many a married woman who fails in an occupational venture need not endure societal condemnation; she may honorably return to being a full-time housewife. In the event of the husband's failure, no such escape is possible. Indeed the reverse is true. Cultural sanctions often endorse the public humiliation (or "boning") of a man who fails to provide for his family. "Thus while society's requirements of the male are essentially as stringent as before, the emotional support accorded him in return has become less."[12] Furthermore, those women who remain in the competitive world previously occupied largely by men suffer an increasing rate of "stress diseases," of which the stomach ulcer is but one.

The effect of "boning" on the modern adolescent is no less disturbing. Menninger wrote,

> It is logical to suggest that our adolescents' provocative behavior may be their way of saying to us, "I object." They may be telling us how they feel about our systematically segregating them from adult society . . . Nowhere are the starkness and the meagerness of this social isolation more apparent than in the lot of the 15-year-old. Except for going to school, virtually nothing that he can do is legal. He can't quit school, he can't work, he can't drink, he can't smoke, he can't drive in most states, he can't marry, he can't vote, he can't enlist, he can't gamble. He cannot, in fact, participate in any of the adult virtues, vices, or activities . . . this infantilizing of the adolescent provokes adventure-seeking, thrill-seeking, serious risk-taking behavior, such as taking drugs.[13]

This "enforced sidelining of the adolescent" ill prepares him for adulthood. Explaining his restrictions to him would be helpful.

Still another consequence of "boning" is to be found in ghetto rioting; this is how two investigators summarized the results of their 1967 survey done in Detroit and Newark:

[10] There are those who separate these actions from the people and attribute them rather to their leaders. But the British historian Trevor-Roper put this idea to rest in this way: "No ruler has ever carried out a policy of wholesale expulsion or destruction without the cooperation of society . . . Without general social support, the organs of isolation and expulsion cannot even be created." (H. R. Trevor-Roper, "Witches and Witchcraft," *Encounter,* Vol. 28, No. 5 [May 1967], p. 14.)

[11] *Harold G. Wolff's Stress and Disease,* rev. and ed. by Stewart Wolf and Helen Goodell, 2nd ed. (Springfield, Ill., 1968), pp. 216–17.

[12] *Ibid.,* p. 217.

[13] Roy Menninger, "What Troubles Our Troubled Youth?" *Mental Hygiene,* Vol. 52, No. 3 (July 1968), pp. 324–27.

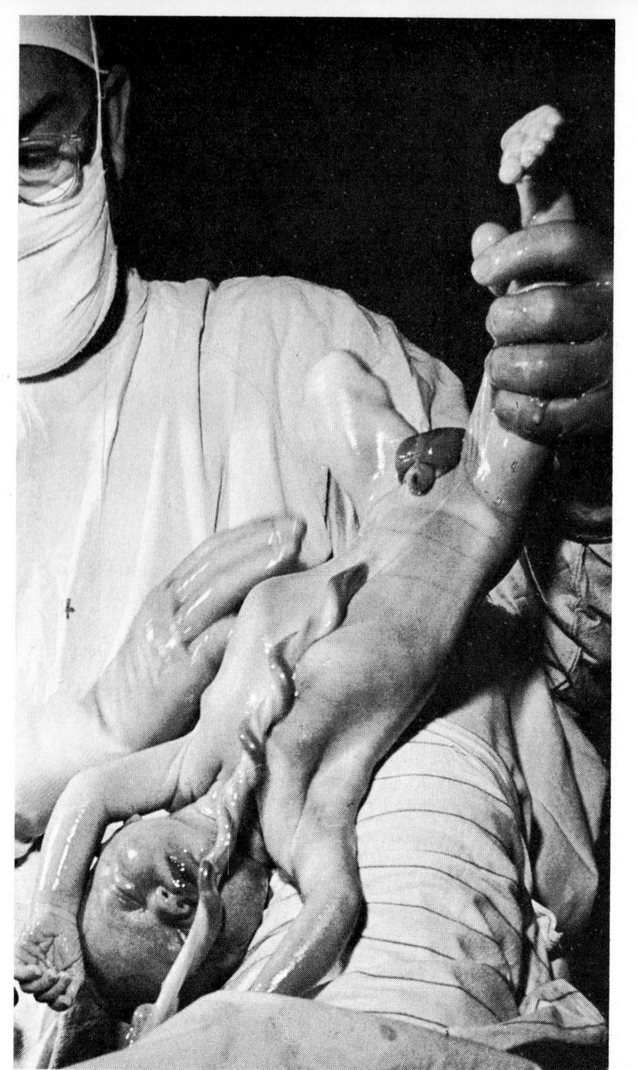

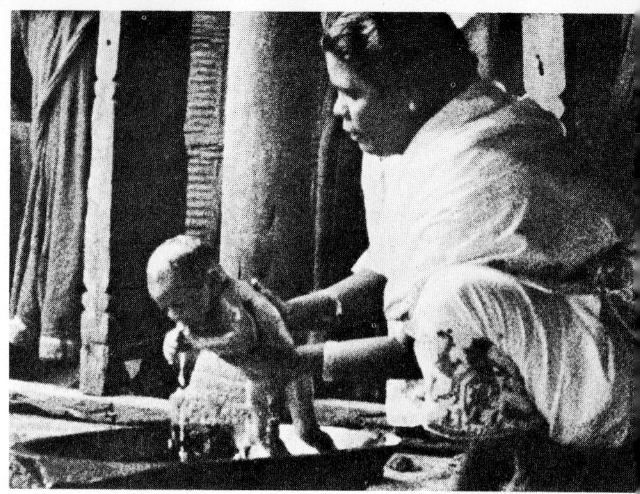

2-2 Culture and Health

Economics and health: a baby is born. The child pictured at top left is the beneficiary of all that modern science can offer the newborn; the infant at top right, born in an underdeveloped society, is washed off by a midwife.
Technology and health: the premature baby. This 19th-century incubator (bottom left) *was kept warm by hot water poured into a container behind the head of the bed. The hot water flowed into a canal under the mattress and was let out through a spigot at the foot of the bed. Today's incubator* (bottom right) *is designed to give the infant his best chance for life.*

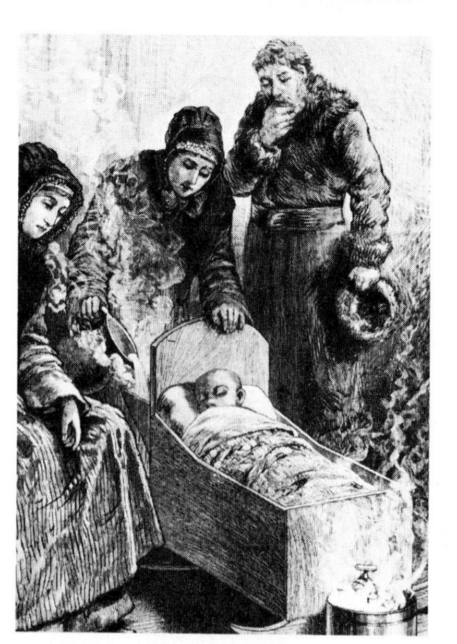

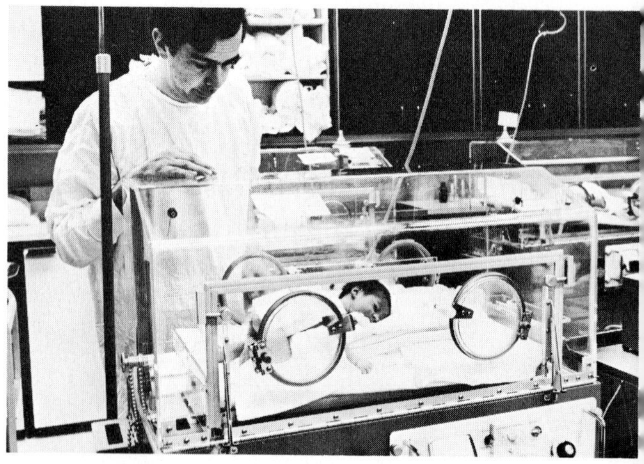

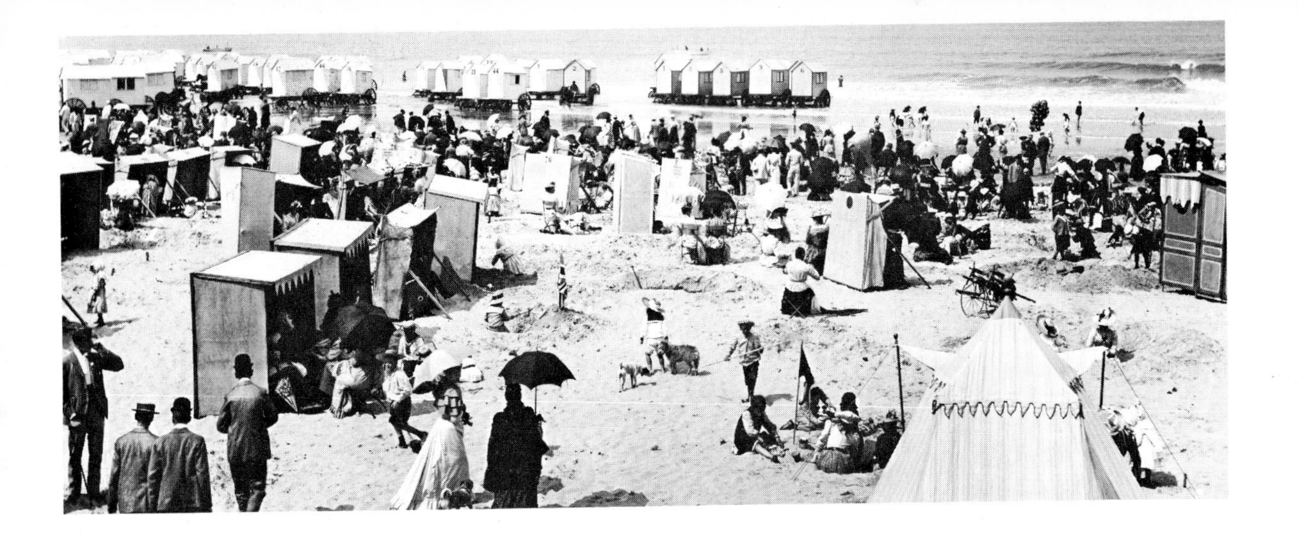

Fashion and health: the ecosystem of human skin. In Ostende, Belgium (top), *ladies were not to be seen in bathing costumes. They kept from public view by remaining in little changing cabins or "bathing boxes," which were drawn to the water by ponies. After a dip, the ladies resumed their ruffles while being wheeled back to the dry beach. The contemporary beach, by contrast* (bottom), *is a study in skin exposure. Modern bathing customs are a peril to some; prolonged overexposure, particularly of blonds, to the sun's ultraviolet light radiation may cause skin cancer.*

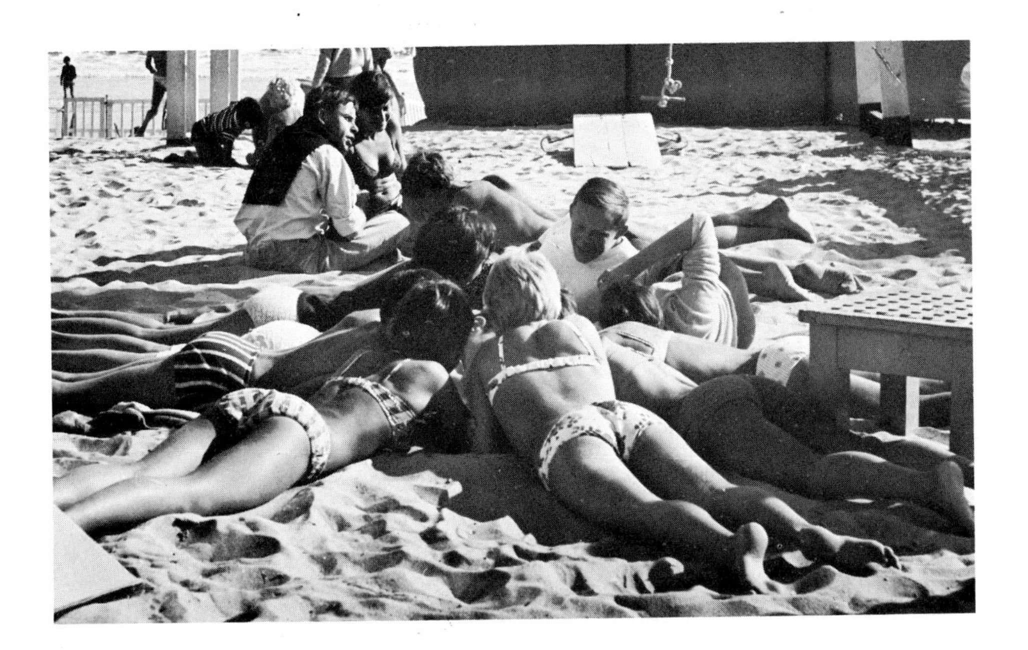

> One is led to conclude that the continued exclusion of Negroes from American economic and social life is the fundamental cause of riots. This exclusion is the result of arbitrary racial barriers rather than a lack of ability, motivation or aspiration on the part of the Negroes who perceive it as arbitrary and unjust.[14]

emotions and ecosystems

For the primitive, belief often means fear. Death from "boning," for example, could not occur without complete belief in magic. But in primitive cultures belief in the community is as strong as belief in magic. Only by community support can one be saved from evil happenings. When someone finds himself utterly forsaken by the community, he is lost.[15] The primitive community, in turn, fearful of inadequate control of its ecosystem, sticks together. Ecological threats can be best met by the group. In the primitive community, anxiety is a cohesive force.

Unlike the primitive, however, civilized man has brought the techniques of ecological control to a high state. Never in human history has man ordered his ecosystem about so successfully. This control is a triumph of Western civilization. And yet, both within and without, man is ridden with problems. His very creativity has boomeranged. Too often it has also meant the creation of disease.

Western man is threatened. Not only is he endangered by the results of his own ecological mismanagement (Chapters 3 and 4), but he is also tormented by confusions and doubts. He has created and developed emotional disorders that profoundly affect his adjustment to the physical, biological, and cultural aspects of his ecosystem. For example, a diabetic may, as a result of emotional distress, impair his ability to metabolize sugar. He may develop symptoms that can kill him if they remain uncontrolled. Even with the proper dosage of insulin, the diabetic may, in such circumstances, become listless, weak, and thirsty. He may vomit, experience extreme dizziness, and finally lapse into a coma. This critical situation is called diabetic crisis.

Although several factors, such as acute injuries, may be involved, the profound influence of emotional disturbance in precipitating diabetic crisis is undeniable. Conflicts with parents or relatives, a bitter quarrel with a friend, indeed any severe emotional upset, can precipitate a diabetic crisis. Why? Human beings normally respond to any stressful situation with an increased sugar metabolism. This response fulfills the body's sudden need for energy, a result of the psychic stress. With normal people, this increase is protective. To the diabetic, it is a hazard. His precarious, delicately attuned metabolism, exquisitely balanced by highly refined medication, cannot handle the rapidly elevated sugar supply. A disturbance in his interpersonal relationships may, therefore, cause him to go into the shock of a diabetic crisis. It may even cost him his life. The balance of his personal ecosystem—the balance between his drug

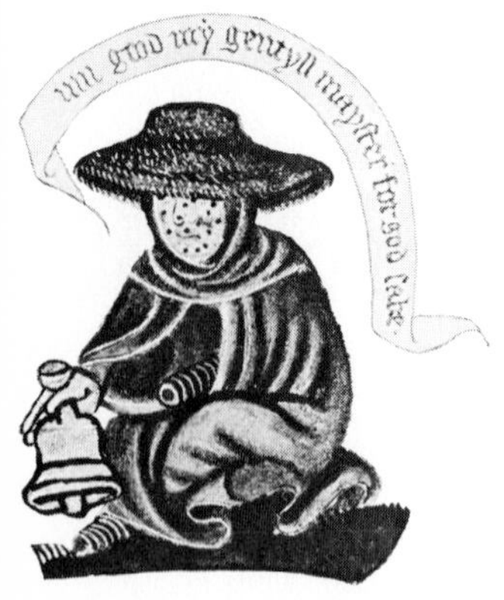

2-3 *Woman leper with a warning bell (late 14th or early 15th century).*

[14] Nathan S. Caplan and Jeffrey M. Paige, "A Study of Ghetto Rioters," *Scientific American,* Vol. 219, No. 2 (August 1968), p. 21.

[15] No better example of "boning" can be found than in the treatment of the leper in medieval Europe. Clad in a white shroud and with a grave cloth covering his garments, the leper was led to the church, where he kneeled in the place customarily used for putting the bodies of the dead. Then the clergy intoned over him the rites for the dead. The leper was then led to the lepers' cemetery, and there he knelt as earth was thrown over him three times. He was then excluded from ordinary communal life and often wore a bell to warn those who approached him. This cruel quarantine was partly responsible for the reduction of the disease in Europe.

and his sugar metabolism, between his emotions and his motions, between himself and those about him—so carefully engineered by decades of elegant medical research and centuries of cultural training, is sacrificed to the costly luxury of human disagreement.

cultural interpretation of symptoms

Symptom interpretation is closely related to culture. What would be considered illness in some communities might be considered the natural state in others. Among some people living in the southern United States and among Africans, diarrhea is not considered unusual. Many African mothers become concerned unless their children have six or seven bowel movements daily. Most observers would consider pinta an unsightly skin disease. Seen in some parts of South America, it is characterized by colored spots on the skin. But among the North Amazonian Indians pinta is so common that the disfigured are regarded as normal and the normal are considered sick. In that area, Indians without pinta are excluded from marriage.[16] Among the Thonga in Africa, the ever present intestinal worms are appreciated—the natives consider them essential for digestion. And, in the nineteenth century, malaria was so prevalent in the Mississippi Valley that the residents did not consider it a disease.

religion and health

For most of the world's religious people, faith has profound emotional connotations. But there is more to religion than emotion. Into its dogma have often been built pragmatic society-saving precepts—precepts that are often involved with health. For example, consider the question of the sacred cow in India. Newspapers are filled with stories of the starvation in that overpopulated country. In their history, Indians have endured dozens of famines. One has read of "starving fields" where people go to die. Yet the Hindu religion prohibits Indians from killing and eating cows. In that hungry country, cows consume 10 million tons of human food yearly. To practical Westerners, such a situation would be intolerable. Resistance to Indian aid is widespread.

But why do so many Indians reject beef? Is the religious concept of the sacred cow a product of stupidity? Foolishness? Ignorance? No. Without the bullock the Indian farm could not exist. In India cows produce the bullocks that pull the plows. Cows, even if old and ailing, produce lavish amounts of manure. For millions of Indians, manure is the only source of fertilizer and fuel. It also provides a usable building material.

What the Indian farmer has developed, ecologically speaking, is a cultural balance. To kill and eat the cows would feed several million Indians for a short while. But the resulting ecological imbalance would cause an agricultural catastrophe of incalculable dimensions. True, technological change will eventually alter the situation. But at this point the destruction of the cow—a major source of agricultural traction, fuel, manure, and building material—would be antilife, irreligious. And just as Moses forbade pork to the ancient Jews (to protect them, it is thought, from a serious disease, now known as trichinosis), so the Hindu

[16] Erwin W. Ackerknecht, "The Role of Medical History in Medical Education," cited in Irving Kenneth Zola, "Culture and Symptoms—An Analysis of Patients Presenting Complaints," *American Sociological Review*, Vol. 31, No. 5 (October 1969), p. 618.

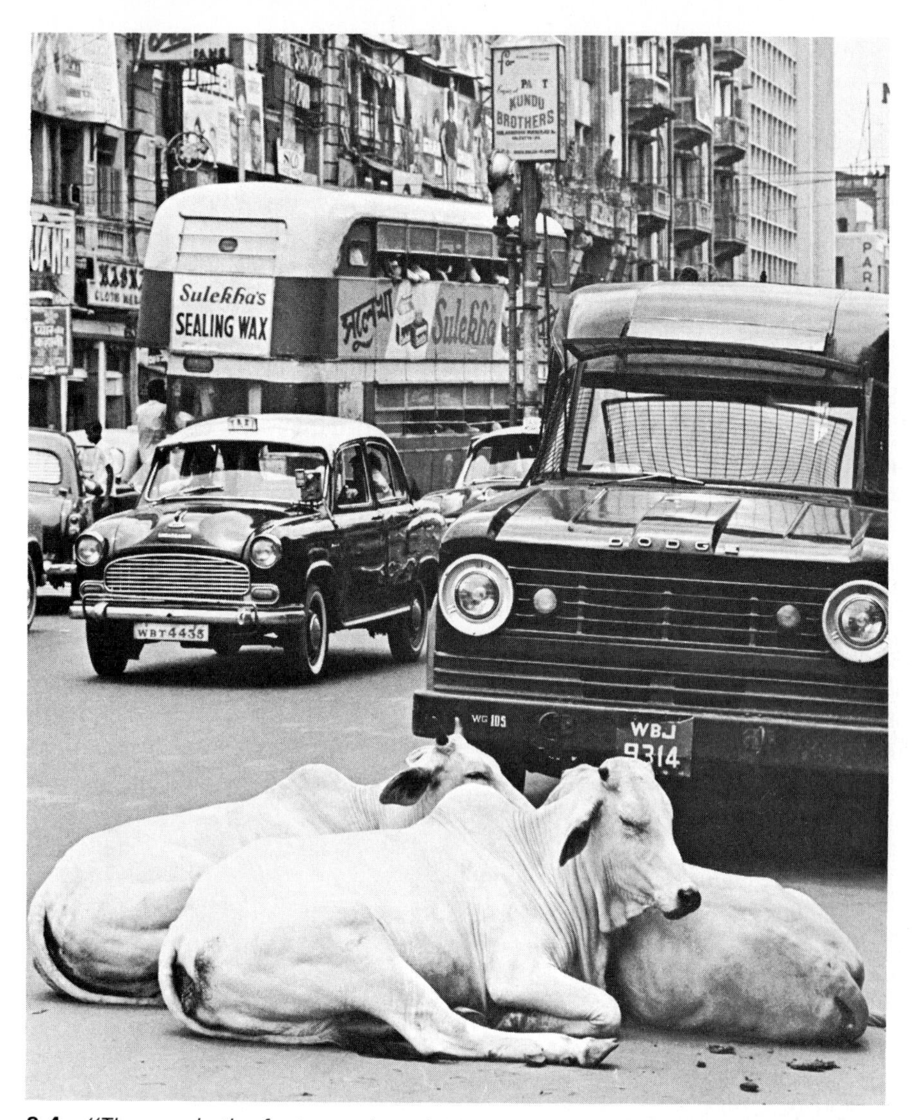

2-4 *"The cow is the foster mother of the human race," wrote Governor William Dempster Hoard (1836–1918), who did much to make Wisconsin a dairy state. "How many men . . . realize that they make merchandise out of the maternity of the dairy cow? . . . A man who would abuse a cow ought to be denied entrance into heaven." Hoard's reverence for the cow was based on economics. For basically the same reason, members of the Hindu faith have long revered cows as sacred. Here some sacred cows in New Delhi, India, block traffic until they have had their nap.*

religion forbids the destruction of the cow. To some extent, the Indian's refusal to eat a sacred cow could be compared to the Westerner's reaction to dogmeat. In some societies puppy-hams are a popular food. Some observers have suggested that Western man's reaction to this usually amiable animal borders on worship.

indifference and resistance to health programs

in its proper place, health is important

In the United States today, health workers are often confronted by a powerful obstacle to their efforts: indifference, even active resistance. What place does health have in life? And why do some people resist health measures?

"Although health is a common need and the effort to attain it represents a common drive it is actually of secondary rather than of primary importance."[17] If health is not a primary need, then what is? The basic human needs are generally considered to be food, shelter, and sexual expression. Only insofar as health furthers or thwarts the satisfaction of these needs do normal people pay much attention to it. It is to the hypochondriac that health is a continually central thought—an obsession. Indisputably, however, health is a superb adornment to life.

How does man consider death—the end of health—in his scheme of things? Freud called death the goal of all life. The Elizabethan poet John Donne bade "Death, be not proud." After they died, the ancient Roman emperors were customarily deified. It was recorded by the Roman historian Suetonius that Emperor Vespasian's last words were: "Woe's me. Methinks I'm turning into a god." During the First World War, British soldiers used to sing a song that asked, "O death, where is thy sting-a-ling-a-ling?" A modern wit spoke of death as "nature's way of telling you to slow down." Although such wry references to death are numerous, they merely emphasize man's sense of inadequacy in dealing with it. Death is a central event of life, before which all ordinary men stand in awe.

But does death stimulate universally similar reactions? The death of a child is instructive in this regard. In an old English churchyard, on the small gravestone of a three-week-old child, is this inscription:

> It is so soon that I am done for,
> I wonder what I was begun for.

These poignant lines reflect the deep and sharp pain caused by the death of a child. All scriptures—whether Hindu, Buddhist, Zoroastrian, Moslem, Confucianist, Taoist, or Judeo-Christian—cherish the child, and modern civilized societies are geared to nourish and protect the child. However, there have been tragic lapses when this was not so. Winslow wrote:

> Tyler in *Primitive Culture* relates the Thuringian tale that to make the castle of Liebenstein fast and impregnable, a child was bought for hard money of its mother and walled in. It was eating a cake while the masons were at work and it cried out, "Mother, I see thee still"; then later, "Mother, I see thee a little still"; and as they put in the last stone, "Mother, now I see thee no more."[18]

But one need not go back in history to find people who accept a child's death

[17] John J. Hanlon, *Principles of Public Health Administration* (St. Louis, 1969), p. 55.
[18] C.-E. A. Winslow, *The Conquest of Epidemic Disease* (Princeton, N.J., 1943), p. 4.

with equanimity. Hanlon, in discussing the customs of some developing societies, described the characteristics of the funeral of an infant or young child:

> Often there appears to be surprisingly little mourning; the physical appearance of the funeral procession, if anything, tends to be much brighter and, among some people, even rather cheerful. Songs may be sung, bands may play, and, when the small body is finally removed, there may be a somewhat enthusiastic social event with dining, drinking, dancing and indulgence in all other pleasures of the flesh.[19]

It is, to them, immutable economic logic. The loss of a child cannot be compared to that of a hunter. The unproven child is destined to a prolonged dependence unsuited to the emergencies of tribal life. The child is a consumer, not a contributor. The hunter, however, sustains the group by solving the immediate problem of hunger. And so the death of a great hunter is a signal for the women to wail and for the men to offer sacrifices.

poverty: the mother of diseases

Health, then, is an aspect of life that helps satisfy man's primary needs. As such, it merits serious (though not obsessive) concern. Yet in this culture, those who attempt to improve the public's health are often stymied by an indifference that does not necessarily stem from attitudes to health and death. This indifference is a mark of social disadvantage. It is an indifference born of poverty and bred by a hopeless sense of helplessness.

Every health worker is witness to this societal tragedy; no complete health survey fails to demonstrate it. A survey recently conducted by a large West Coast health department is illustrative. It had been part of the preplanning activity necessary for a campaign to promote immunization against "regular" measles (rubeola). A safe and effective vaccine was available. The year before, a similar effort had seemed to abort an epidemic. For protection against the disease, thousands of parents had brought their children either to their family doctors or to the health department. The new survey revealed that there were still large pockets in the community containing thousands of unvaccinated children. It was statistically certain that a high proportion of them had not had the disease. Lacking immunity by vaccination or by an attack of the illness, they were susceptible not only to the illness but to its serious complications.

The health workers studied a pin-studded map indicating areas of inadequate vaccination levels. They drew circles around a few pockets in the middle-class areas. The survey showed that relatively few children in these sections of the county were still susceptible to measles. The circles surrounding the areas of poverty enclosed the majority of the pins. Although health department workers had provided the vaccinations free of charge, the children of the poor were the least immunized. Here was the old story of the *behavioral* or *performance gap*—the gap between the preventive health services offered and those accepted. That gap between the available benefits of modern preventive care and the indifference to them by a large segment of the poor is hard to bridge.

[19] John J. Hanlon, *Principles of Public Health Administration,* p. 56.

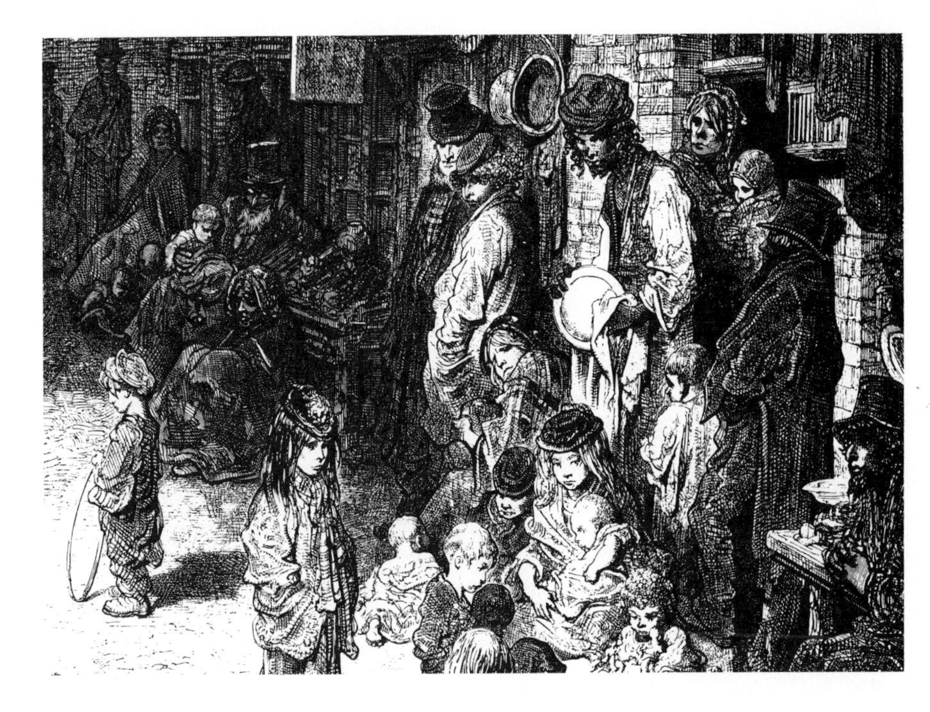

2-5 *Poverty: the mother of diseases. Gustave Doré's "Wentworth Street, Whitechapel."*

The great majority of poor people do take advantage of health facilities. Nor do they fail to understand the importance of health. Chancellor Lee of the University of California has pointed out that

> A recent Harris poll makes it very clear that poor people understand the relationship between their ill health and poverty. Health is one of their major concerns. Mr. Harris found that 59 percent of the poor blacks and 72 percent of poor whites give health a higher priority than having a good job, compared to 51 percent of Americans as a whole, and he wrote, "Good health to the poor is the lifeline to all else."[20]

But a large segment of the poor do not take advantage of available preventive health programs. Most of these people are part of what anthropologist Oscar Lewis has called "the culture of poverty."[21] The people in this culture feel deeply alienated from the major institutions of the surrounding society, generally have little or no effective community organization beyond the family, have a sharply curtailed period of childhood dependency, and often feel helpless and inferior. Lewis distinguishes between poverty and the culture of poverty. Despite their desperate circumstances, many of the poor of Africa, Asia, and South America, for example, have a sense of belonging to and participating with the larger group. Of the estimated 20 to 50 million poor people in the United States, only 20 percent (4 to 10 million) live in the culture of poverty.

In the United States, those in the culture of poverty are mostly blacks,

[20] Philip R. Lee, "The Problems of the Minorities Rest Not with Them, but with the White Majority," *California's Health,* Vol. 26, No. 11 (May 1969), p. 4.

[21] Oscar Lewis, "The Culture of Poverty," *Scientific American,* Vol. 215, No. 4 (October 1966), pp. 20–25.

Chicanos (Mexican-Americans), Puerto Ricans, American Indians, and Southern poor whites. And since the culture of poverty perpetuates itself, the children within it are most likely condemned to the behavioral gap too. In this country the largest number of people in the behavioral gap are black. They encounter a double lock on the door to societal opportunities—poverty and prejudice. While the fires of Watts were still burning, a resident of the area summed up the problem of alienation this way: "We have absentee leadership, absentee ministers, absentee landlords and absentee merchants. They provide what services they can during the day, and when the sun goes down in Watts, it's just us and the cops."[22] James Baldwin has been no less direct: "To be a Negro in this country," he has said, "and to be relatively conscious, is to be in a rage almost all of the time."[23] What does the black man want? He wants what the white man wants. Despite the deep sense of alienation within black and other minority communities, the vast majority still seek to avail themselves of societal opportunities. In this there is hope. Nevertheless, the alienation, born of white prejudice, felt by many members of this nation's racial minorities accounts for some of their resistance to government-sponsored health services.

The active participation of minority groups in all phases of health planning provides warmth and meaning to health services. Money alone will solve neither alienation nor the behavioral gap, for the problems are not merely economic. But money is essential to relieving them. High death rates among children and pregnant women, shorter adult life expectancies, malnutrition—these are among the bitter realities of the poor.[24]

Poverty is not the only cause of resistance to health programs. Sometimes it is due to an irrational refusal to accept scientifically proven information. Consider the following example.

"them dogs don't vote"

In a large western city, not long ago, it was unsafe for a child to play in the street, much less walk home from school. Rabid dogs roamed the streets, biting and possibly infecting any human being who happened across their path. A safe and effective vaccine to prevent rabies in dogs had long been available. All responsible scientific organizations supported compulsory vaccination of dogs. Yet for many years, a small, militant, seemingly well-financed minority successfully led the fight against rabies vaccinations of dogs. The advice of public health officials, distinguished deans of medical and veterinary schools, and other leading scientific figures in the community went unheeded.

It was usually children who paid. A child does not easily understand that a sick dog can carry death and must be left alone. And when he does understand this, his compassion usually gains the upper hand over his judgment. In that city, children had to be taught to fear dogs—sick dogs in particular. Frequently, both children and adults had to endure the fourteen to twenty-eight injections that constitute the antirabies preventive procedure. To survive rabies is medically rare; the preventive vaccine was the best procedure. However, it

[22] Gladwin Hill, *The New York Times* (August 28, 1965), p. 54.
[23] Quoted in Charles Silberman, *Crisis in Black and White* (New York, 1964), p. 36.
[24] For a discussion of malnutrition and retardation, see Chapter 22, pages 670–71.

caused paralysis about once every two thousand times it was used.[25] The following true story illustrates the dilemma.

Tommy, a nine-year-old newsboy, was brought to a physician by his mother because he had been bitten by a dog that "was acting funny—he was limping around and had a funny bark." The boy had tried to help the animal, and it had bitten him savagely on the hand. Before coming to the doctor, the mother had reported the dog bite to the health department. The doctor immediately telephoned the health department and asked their veterinarian about the animal. The dog had been caught. It was rabid. The bite in the child's thumb was a deep tear. The doctor washed the wound with soap and water for a long time, and then started the preventive injections against rabies.

After nine injections into the soft tissue around the umbilicus, the child developed a fever (103° F. orally), a headache, and a "'lectric like" feeling over the right ribs and arm. "See, doctor," he said, more curious than concerned, "I can't hold a pencil." The doctor saw only too well. The boy's symptoms heralded a treatment paralysis. He turned to the mother. "We will have to stop his treatments," he said slowly.

"But won't he get rabies?" Her voice rose. She fought to control it.

"He could. But right now, with this reaction from the vaccine, the chances of his getting rabies are not as great as the chances of a permanent treatment paralysis. It's a matter of measuring the risks. And there is a good chance, the best chance, that nothing at all will happen and he will be all right."

"When will we know?"

The doctor paused. He had seen two cases of human rabies. Now, as he regarded the boy, he remembered them. "In about a week or two we should know pretty well. But we can't be absolutely positive, not for some months."

After the distraught woman left with her child, the doctor telephoned a city councilman. He explained the case in detail. "Why don't you vote for rabies vaccination?" he asked. "It's even good for the dogs."

"Listen doc," the politician said bluntly, "when we took up this rabies vaccination thing, the council chambers were swarming with dog lovers. They raised a row. These days two things bring people to a council meeting—taxes and dogs. You know how many people came to talk for vaccination? One was this rundown botany professor whose sleeves are too long for him. The other was the president of the medical society, and nobody likes him because he drives a Cadillac. Where were you? There were twenty dog lovers for every kid lover. Everybody gets what he deserves. As for them sick dogs, well, them dogs don't vote."

The doctor telephoned the mother. "I just wanted to ask you," he said, "do you remember the council meeting on compulsory rabies vaccination last month? Were you there?"

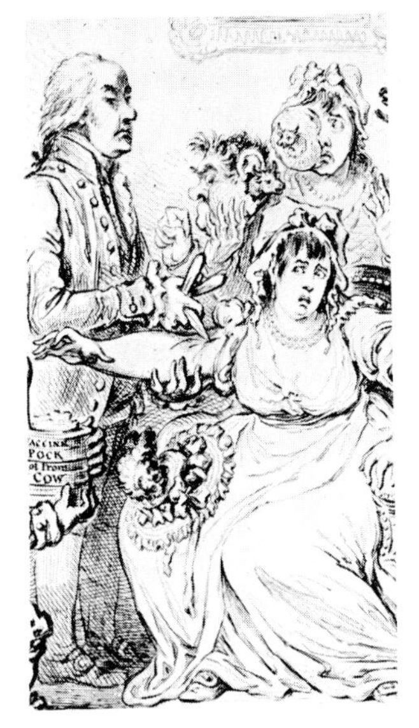

2-6 *A contemporary cartoon bitterly lampooning Edward Jenner, the developer of the vaccine to prevent smallpox. Too often have public health advances been met with such resistance.*

[25] A much safer and equally effective rabies virus vaccine made of rabies virus grown in duck embryos is now available. Moreover, an antirabies vaccine made from growing the virus in human tissue cells (see pages 155–56) is being tested. Preliminary results indicate that it is safer, less painful, and more effective than any previous rabies vaccine. (Tadeusz J. Witkor, Stanley A. Plotkin, and Doris W. Grella, "Human Cell Culture Rabies Vaccine," *Journal of the American Medical Association,* Vol. 224, No. 8 [May 21, 1973], pp. 1170–71.)

There was a long pause. ''I wasn't there,'' she said. ''I'm getting what I deserve.''

The child recovered, but his mother did not rest until, in the next year, compulsory rabies vaccination for dogs was the law in her town.

So it has been since this country began. Public health is sometimes accepted only after years of effort by an informed and a finally aroused citizenry. In colonial America, Cotton Mather was widely hated for his advocacy of protection against smallpox. Indeed, in 1791, a hand grenade was thrown into his house. Attached to it was this message: ''Cotton Mather, you Dog, Damn you, I'll inoculate you with this, and a Pox to you.''

Smallpox vaccination, rabies vaccination, water fluoridation and chlorination, milk pasteurization—these and a host of other health advances have been met with the bitter resistance of the misinformed. Though experience may teach the misinformed, too often the paths of experience are littered with the dead and disabled.

The first chapter of this book placed man on a health scale within a dynamic ecosystem. This second chapter has considered him within his culture. Alone among living creatures, man has added thought to instinct, culture to inherited impulse. Human health is inextricably tied to culture. It is profoundly affected not only by such basic cultural concerns as ethics, religion, money, and freedom but also by the environmental changes that man has continually wrought. Many of these changes he has used productively. As a primitive, the harnessing of fire brought him warmth and cooked food. As a sophisticate, the harnessing of the laser beam enabled him to perform delicate eye surgery. But the environmental changes of mankind are rarely unmixed blessings. Pesticides have multiplied man's crops, but now may threaten his well-being. The automobile has extended his world, but, too often, it has ended his life. Has man remained in healthful balance with his environment? Or has he, for temporary advantage, been too careless with his ecological future? These questions will be discussed in the next two chapters.

summary

The dimension of culture, which only mankind adds to the physical and biological dimensions of his ecosystem, can both create health problems and offer solutions to them. Because humans can learn, they can adapt to change, and change makes progress possible (page 24). Compared with life that is lower on the biological scale, humans take much longer to mature (because of the time required to learn the rules of adaptation to their culture), and humans have an unusually long post-reproductive life span in which they may use—or abuse—the knowledge they have acquired (page 25). Human culture, environment, and health are interrelated. Various cultures have different attitudes toward and ways of dealing with death, illness, and deviation from cultural rules (as in ''boning,'' page 26). Culture is also reflected in the influence of emotional distress on physical illness (page 30) and in the interpretation of symptoms (page 31). Religion is another cultural influence on health (page 31). Poverty, ignorance, and fear are rooted in cultural factors that often breed indifference or even resistance to programs of health care (pages 33–36).

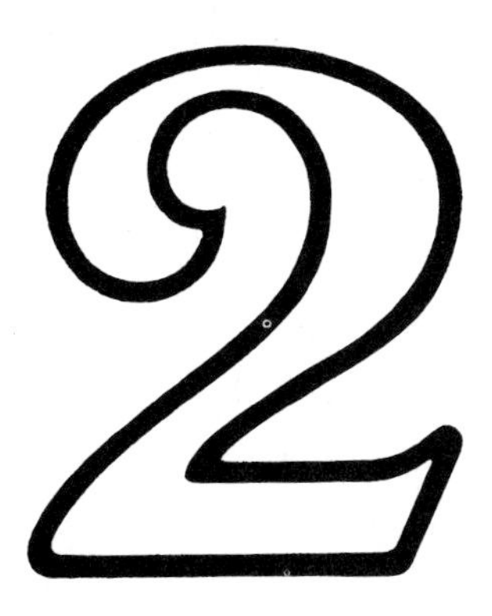

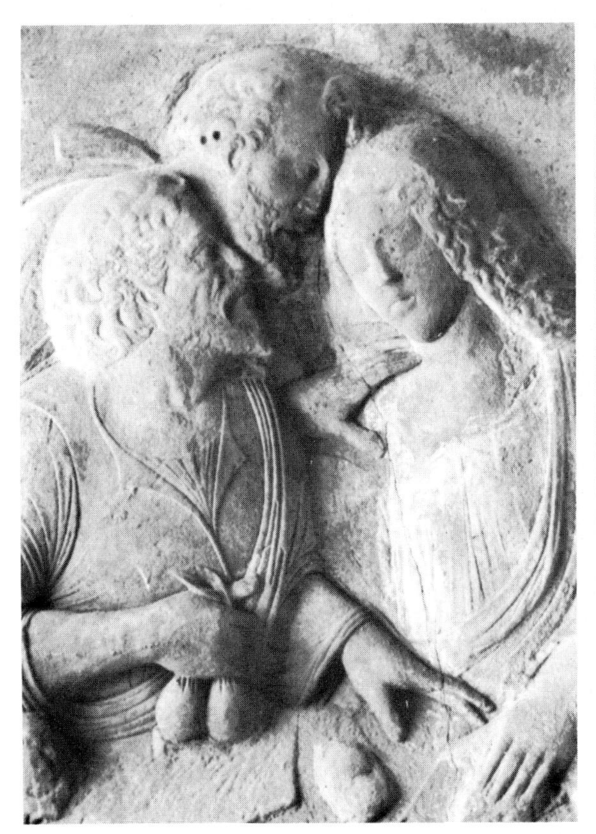

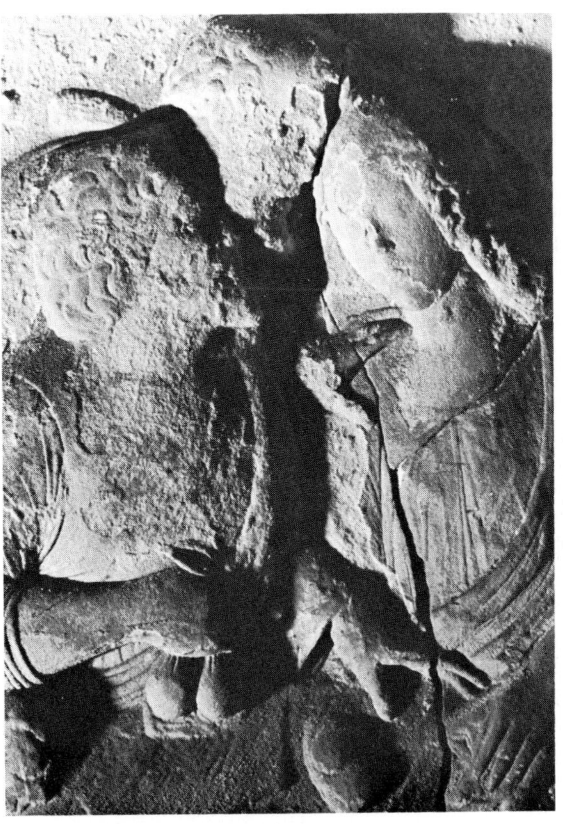

"If air pollution eats away stone, how does polluted air affect soft, friable lung tissue?" (*page 53*). *These pictures were taken in the increasingly industrial Italian city of Venice in 1900* (left) *and 1973* (right).

man versus man

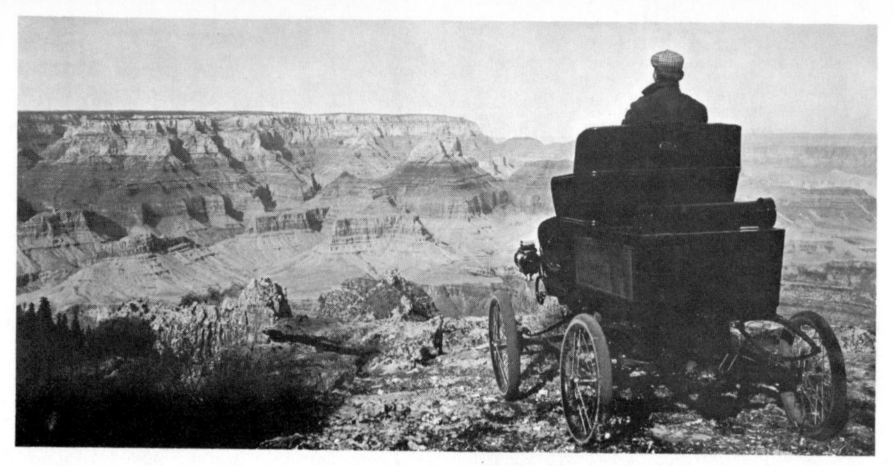

A clear view of the future?

waters of affliction, solid wastes, ill winds, and accidents

3

For the Lord thy God bringeth thee into a good land, a land of brooks of water, of fountains and depths that spring out of valleys and hills.[1]

samples from the polluted past

To live is to pollute. This condition of existence man shares with all creatures. Even, however, as evolution granted man greater gifts to control environment, so did it enable him to dirty it most. Beginning with the Neanderthal and Cro-Magnon peoples of the Paleolithic period (who have occupied 98 percent of the total human time on earth so far), man has constantly befouled the planet. In adapting and evolving, primitive man acquired thumbs, a complex brain, an erect posture, an accommodating digestive tract. Slowly, he learned how best to use them. His wants stimulated him. He was dissatisfied with vegetable roots. He wanted meat. Using his thumb, therefore, he grasped a lit torch and thought enough to set woods afire. The flames drove wild game out for the kill, but smoke filled the air. Much of earth was once forest. The trees failed to outlast man. Around the charred stumps, farmers planted their crops. People gathered. Little cities rose. Sharing one another's company, people also had to share one another's residues, and because they came to believe that sickness rose from filth, they sought ways of cleanliness.

"And the Lord God took the man, and put him into the garden of Eden to dress it and to keep it" (Genesis 2:15). Expelled from the storied garden, man presumably took his custodial function with him. But in this stewardship of nature, his performance left much to be desired. Still lacking humility, he considered the world to be his. "We make our greatest mistake when we believe that the world belongs to us. It does not—we belong to it."[2] Not comprehending this, man has polluted his environment ceaselessly, carelessly, and with abandon. Should he persist, he may ultimately find as little room for himself in the world as he found in Eden. Nor has his garbage been limited to earth. Today, the junk from man's spaceships orbits the globe. Human litter has even invaded the moon.

medieval smog and the reign of cholera

As a polluter man has an ancient record. More than twenty centuries before Christ, the lush Tigris-Euphrates Valley of southwestern Asia was beginning to be transformed into desert by the unwise irrigation procedures of that time.[3] Centuries passed. New lands were settled. Wars were fought. Early in European history English influence arose and spread. But the English homeland was cold country. The early English burned wood for warmth. Then wood became scarce. Englishmen were forced to seek elsewhere for heat's comfort. Perhaps they had heard that the Chinese had been using coal as a fuel for a thousand

[1] Deuteronomy 8:7.
[2] Phillip Kellerin, quoted in Robert and Leona Train Rienow, *Moment in the Sun* (New York, 1967), p. 33.
[3] "The Closing Circle," review by Paul R. Ehrlich and John P. Holdren, *Environment*, Vol. 14, No. 3 (April 1972), p. 24.

years. Tardily, Henry III permitted his shivering subjects to burn coal. This resulted in a formidable thirteenth-century English smog. To pacify the coughing, complaining barons, Henry's son Edward decreed death as punishment for coal burning while Parliament was in session, "lest the health of the Knights of the Shire should suffer during their residence in London."[4] One early Englishman certainly found coal unhealthful. In 1307, he was hanged for burning it.

London smog persisted as a dangerous nuisance, as is shown by these lines complaining about the fumes of "seacoale smoake" from a seventeenth-century book of collected verse:

> He[5] shewes that 'tis the seacoale smoake
> That allways London doth Inviron,
> Which doth our Lungs and Spiritts choake,
> Our hangings spoyle, and rust our Iron.
> Lett none att Fumifuge be scoffing
> Who heare att Church our Sunday's Coughing.[6]

Air pollution was hardly the only environmental problem of early England. The October 17, 1710, edition of *The Tatler* carried an especially pungent description of the turgid waters of the Thames River. It reads in part:

> Sweepings from butcher's stalls, dung, guts, and blood,
> Drown'd puppies, shaking sprats, all drenched in mud,
> Dead cats, and turnip tops, come tumbling down the flood.[7]

The whole area around the Thames became known as "the capital of cholera." It well deserved this name. In those days, this bacterial, waterborne disease was rampant in London.

Meanwhile, what had been going on in the New World?

on a basic use of waste

Some historians are fond of referring to pre-Columbian America as a virgin land. But it had been raped long before the Italian and his crew reached its shores. In ravaging the land, the early Central American Mayan Indians destroyed their civilization. First they burned the trees. Then they planted crops for quick harvest. They did not think to replenish the land with their excreta. This failure to use their own organic wastes cost them their survival as a great people. As soon as the unfed soil of their farms became too exhausted to provide more food, they moved. From place to place they went, from despoiled to unspoiled soil, always taking, never giving. Under ordinary conditions, nature needs three hundred to a thousand years to build one inch of topsoil. The Mayan method of agriculture gave nature neither time nor help to rebuild. Eventually exhausted, the soil could yield no more food. Kept on the move, constantly forced to reconstruct anew at each new site, in a thousand years the Mayans were also

[4] Eugene Ayres, "The Age of Fossil Fuels," in William L. Thomas, Jr., ed., *Man's Role in Changing the Face of the Earth* (Chicago, 1956), p. 368.
[5] This verse, among others, was dedicated to John Evelyn (1620–1706), whose work on London smog, *Fumifugium,* had attracted wide attention.
[6] Quoted in Marjorie Hope Nicolson, *Pepys' Diary and the New Science* (Charlottesville, Va., 1965), p. 149.
[7] N. J. Barton, *The Lost Rivers of London* (London, 1962), p. 106.

exhausted. Today, they are a people of monuments and memories. By contrast, the Chinese did not take food from their soil without feeding the soil their wastes. They survived.

The Mayans are an example of what not to do. The Oriental exemplifies what must be done.[8] "The function of all waste organic matter, animal and vegetable, is to maintain the fertility of the soil, and while man's ingenuity may produce wonderful as well as monstrous things, he is incapable of getting round this fundamental fact."[9] In considering waste control, it is well to remember this.

life in a new republic

"Why should cities be erected," Noah Webster asked mournfully, "if they are to be only the tombs of men?" The wise old man had not been unduly concerned. According to the May 3, 1799, issue of the *Aurora,* Philadelphians of the day were often "saluted with a great variety of fetid and disgusting smells . . . exhaled from the dead carcasses of animals, from stagnant waters, and from every species of filth that can be collected from the city, thrown in heaps as if . . . to promote the purposes of death."[10]

The decade following 1790 saw repeated yellow fever epidemics sweeping through North American cities. In 1793, more than 10 percent of the population of Philadelphia perished. A few years later New York was similarly afflicted. A few correctly guessed a relationship between the "clouds of musketoes" and the disease. Sheer fear stimulated the survivors to improve water supply and sewage disposal facilities. Large storm drainage systems had already been built. But these conduits had not been used for the disposal of human feces and urine. It was not until the nineteenth century that the idea of a water-carriage system for human excreta was accepted. This was "the major sanitary advance over the centuries."[11] By this means mankind could be separated from his disease-carrying waste.[12]

on the Spartan nature of early campus life

In the early nineteenth century it was common for underfed undergraduates at Harvard and Princeton to use a fork for more than eating. With it they would pin on the under surface of the dining table a few scraps of today's meat for tomorrow's dinner. Such property rights were rigidly respected by all but stray dogs. College cows often ate better than college men. They were pastured on most campuses, and, at Harvard, pigs were an animal garbage disposal system for commons. If college students turned up their noses in those days, there was, at least, good reason. Refuse was generally thrown out dormitory windows. The

[8] The modern Japanese, too, provide a lesson in frugality. During the Second World War, they carefully collected human and animal wastes and, like a priceless brew, carefully applied them to their private gardens. Because of the use of so dangerously infected a fertilizer, there was much typhoid. But starvation was rare.

[9] J. C. Wylie, *The Wastes of Civilization* (London, 1959), p. 124.

[10] Quoted in Nelson Manfred Blake, *Water for the Cities* (Syracuse, N.Y., 1956), p. 4.

[11] Abel Wolman, "Disposal of Man's Wastes," in William L. Thomas, Jr., ed., *Man's Role in Changing the Face of the Earth,* p. 808.

[12] Yet, at the same time as man learned to be rid of one waste, he created still another. On August 4, 1727, a German reporter in Paris wrote an article for his countrymen about "A certain mathematicus . . . [who] has invented a carriage for four persons, with which he will drive without horses through its own internal motion fourteen French miles in two hours." (Hermann Schreiber, *The History of Roads,* tr. by Stewart Thomson [London, 1961], p. 213.)

The Los Angeles-type smog was born.

lower floors stank and, it is presumed, were reserved for freshmen and other wanderers.[13]

the effluence of affluence

Now, almost two centuries later, the problems have changed but man's relationship to his environment has not improved; rather, it has deteriorated in proportion to the increase of his numbers and needs. For each pollution problem that has been solved, another crucial one has been created. More than half a century ago a distinguished university lecturer eloquently expressed a prophetic paradox. "I do suspect," he told his class, "that many of you young gentlemen may live to see a time for which neither by tradition nor experience are we particularly well prepared, because the struggle of the future is going to be who will survive prosperity, not adversity. We have had a long racial experience on surviving adversity, but what do we know about surviving prosperity?"[14]

Radiation. Accidents. Noise. Pesticides. Water pollution. Air pollution. An increasing list of major environmental hazards besets man. For a long time his clutter and waste have been gathering. Can he live in harmony while his excess pollution remains uncontrolled? No. Mankind must be in balance with all else in his ecosystem. Only at his peril does man violate its fragile web. And the time for his reconsideration is dangerously short. It is here pertinent to call to mind a portion of an inscription long ago placed on the road to Vesuvius, some three miles from Naples. It is dated 1631, a year in which that temperamental volcano blew its top once again, creating an air pollution that killed four thousand people.

> Posterity, posterity, this is your concern,
> one day enlightens the next, the next
> improves the third.
> Be attentive.[15]

water

> I am the Poem of Earth, said the voice of the rain,
> Eternal I rise impalpable out of the land and the bottomless sea,
> Upward to heaven, whence, vaguely form'd, altogether changed, and yet the same,
> I descend to lave the drouths, atomies, dust-layers of the globe,
> And all that in them without me were seeds only, latent, unborn;
> And forever, by day and night, I give back life to my own origin, and make pure and beautify it.[16]

3-1 *A fresh draught.*

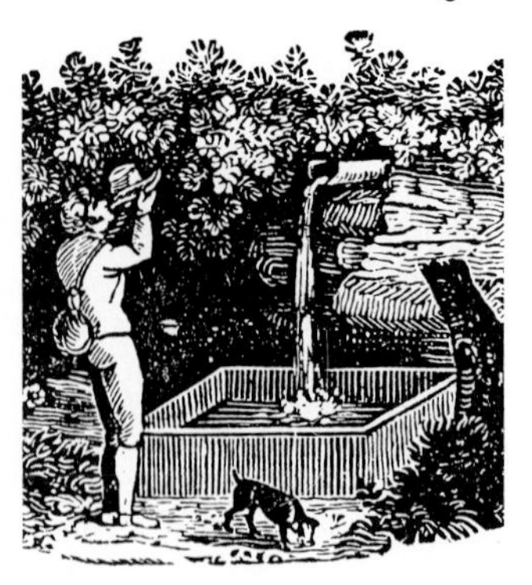

The poet Walt Whitman thus described the eternal water cycle. The rainfall

[13] Christian Gauss, "How Good Were the Good Old Days?" in A. C. Spectorsky, ed., *The College Years* (New York, 1958), pp. 81–88.
[14] Dr. Alan Gregg speaking of a lecture by Thomas Nixon Carver, quoted in William L. Thomas, Jr., ed., *Man's Role in Changing the Face of the Earth,* pp. 956–57.
[15] John Boyle, Earl of Orrery, *The Letters of Pliny the Younger with Observations on Each Letter,* 2nd ed., Vol. II (London, 1751), p. 59.
[16] Walt Whitman, "The Voice of the Rain," as quoted in *Scientist and Citizen,* Vol. 7, No. 2 (December 1964), p. 1.

moistening the earth is gathered up as vapor by the sun's warmth. Air cools. Vapors condense. Clouds form. Then the rain falls again. During its life-giving stay on earth, some rainfall seeps into the ground. In sinking, it is slowly filtered through sand and cleansed. The American Indian understood this purifying action of filtration. He did not drink from a polluted stream. Instead he scooped a hole near its bank and drank the water that filtered into it.

water purification

Water that does not seep underground flows from the mountains into rivulets and rivers, seeking—and eventually finding—the sea. In its course man draws from it. But first it must be made safe. In a water-treatment plant, this may be accomplished primarily by filtration and chlorination. Safe drinking water is one of the triumphs of modern public health. Even before chlorine was introduced into the United States as a water disinfectant (in 1908), filtration alone could provide considerable, though hardly enough, protection against waterborne disease. Among the most common of such diseases is typhoid fever. This infection is caused by a microbe that may be transmitted by human feces and urine. Pollution of drinking water or food by these human discharges can result in frequent typhoid fever epidemics. At the turn of this century, the annual national typhoid fever death rate was about 35 per 100,000. Pittsburgh and Cincinnati still used unfiltered water. Their typhoid fever death rates were three times the national average. Chlorination brought bacteriological safety to a degree previously unknown. It does not cost much more to purify highly polluted water than relatively safe water.

Today, some two-thirds of the population of this country is served by a completely safe public water supply. For countless other millions of the world's city dwellers, however, safe water is a dream, waterborne disease the bitter reality. For example, more than 8 million people are packed into four hundred square miles of Calcutta. (By contrast, the four hundred square miles of Los Angeles contain 3 million people.) Millions of Calcutta residents use unfiltered hydrant water for cleaning and drinking. As in Western countries two centuries ago, open sewers run through some streets. Cholera is common.

the uses of water

The people of the United States use water lavishly. Swimming pools and lawn sprinklers help make Beverly Hills residents this nation's greatest per capita water consumers. But the average citizen is hardly parsimonious with it. He will use no less than five gallons a day to shave, wash, and brush his teeth. Flushing the toilet once requires five to seven gallons. A minute under a running shower spends five gallons. Almost thirty gallons are used in a home load of laundry.

Agriculture is a huge water consumer. To grow one pound of flour requires 375 gallons of water. It takes about 5,000 gallons to can 100 cases of peas or corn. A one-acre orange grove requires 800,000 gallons of water. But the thirstiest of all is industry, and it often demands water of high purity. Making the paper for the Sunday newspaper consumes 150 gallons. Brewing one barrel of beer uses 1,000 gallons of water. For the aluminum in a bomber, 29 million gallons are needed. Water does not only sustain life; it is also needed to maintain a way of life.

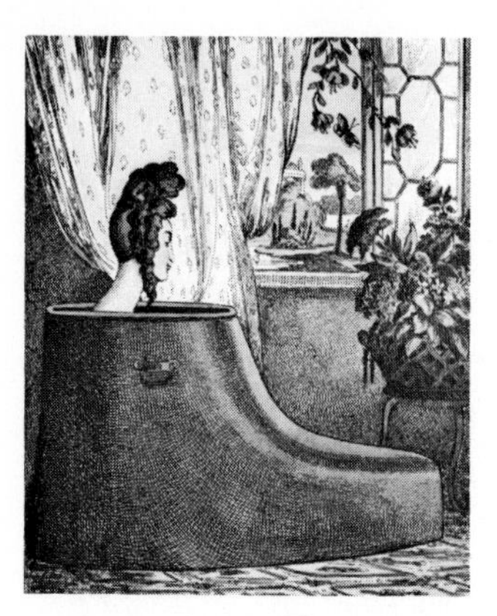

3-2 *An early 19th-century English bathtub.*

The total amount of the earth's water is not diminished by man's use of it. Nature's water cycle provides a constant supply. But water is unevenly distributed. In one part of the world, the people suffer drought; in another they fight flood. The western part of the United States is drier than the eastern. Los Angeles pipes water to its homes from hundreds of miles away. To obtain the water that daily drips from a leaky faucet in this country, a parched Asian, African, or Indian may need to walk a dozen miles. Man must keep water pollution to a minimum and learn to reuse purified water. In these ways he can protect himself against the whims of nature.

More than a generation has elapsed since the late humorist Robert Benchley attended Harvard. One day, during an examination on American diplomatic history, he was asked a question on the rights to the Newfoundland fisheries. Benchley worked around his ignorance this way: "This question has long been discussed from the American and British points of view, but has anyone ever considered the viewpoint of the fish?"[17] He gave that viewpoint and passed his exam.

Pollution of the waterways should be considered from the viewpoint of the fish. It is perhaps mankind's safest point of view, for the danger to fish is also one measure of man's danger.

waste reveals the era (and some tales of a tub)

Once used, urban water is a waste carrier. The character of that waste reflects the times. What can waste tell about the past? Are people of this civilization cleaner than their predecessors? Their remnant plumbing helps to tell. "There were more than one thousand baths in ancient Rome and that is more than were in London at the beginning of the last century."[18] Early urbanites of this nation found the opportunities for "all over" bathing extremely limited. The sixth president of the United States was no exception. In order to get a decent bath, John Quincy Adams had to sneak away from the White House before dawn and use the Potomac River. In his later years, Benjamin Franklin had lived more luxuriously. His tub was shaped like a lady's slipper (see Figure 3-2). Under the heel was a place for a charcoal heater and on the instep the great Colonial philosopher could prop a book. The soaps of Franklin's day were of a different composition than those used today. Clearly the bath wastes of the Colonial era were different from those of the modern bather. This was also true of laundry wastes. Detergents long ago replaced the strong lye soaps of another generation. Every new era has brought new wastes. Tissues have almost wholly replaced handkerchiefs. Leftovers from dinner, carefully preserved by the thrifty housewife of yesteryear, are now fed to the "electric pig." All this, and more, finds its way into sewage pipes. All reveal a changing era. All bring new problems to waste disposal engineers.

what happens to urban waste?

In some areas waste is just collected by sewer pipes that lead it unpurified to the nearest river. At least this removes the problem from immediate sight. A better answer is the modern sewage treatment plant. From toilet bowl, laundro-

[17] Richard M. Dorson, "Campus Folklore," in A. C. Spectorsky, ed., *The College Years,* p. 281.
[18] J. C. Wylie, *The Wastes of Civilization,* p. 11.

mat, bathtub, shower, and sink, waste leaves the home by pipes leading to main sewer lines. By these routes it reaches sewage treatment plants. Here, body waste and other pollutions are removed. How? In the plant, sewage is first passed through a screen. Large objects, such as sticks and rags, are caught. Then the sewage may be passed through a tank. Within the tank, solids settle, and in the absence of oxygen, organic solids are broken down. The sewage may then be filtered. Then, by means of oxidation, sewage is further broken down to even simpler constituents. Finally, a disinfectant such as chlorine is added. Using these methods, only reasonably safe sewage need be discharged into a natural waterway. But even modern cities frequently do not employ the best methods, or their methods are incomplete. A major modern problem has developed—the vast pollution of rivers, lakes, streams, and deep wells.

nonhuman waste pollution

But human wastes are not the only problem. In former times, animals providing man's food were widely distributed. When their waste was used for fertilizer it, too, was spread over a large area. Today hog and poultry production are concentrated, factory-like operations. Often cows are close to cities. "A cow generates as much manure as sixteen human beings; one hog produces nearly as much waste as two human beings; seven chickens create as much of a disposal problem as one person does. In total, farm animals produce ten times as much organic waste as the human population."[19] Disposal of animal waste has become a problem not often handled satisfactorily (see page 49). It is a topic of much federal Public Health Service concern.

To all these pollutions one must add over 500,000 different chemicals that find their way into U.S. streams. The dimensions of this nation's water pollution

[19] "Restoring the Quality of Our Environment," report of the Environmental Pollution Panel, quoted in Philip H. Abelson, "Man-Made Environmental Hazards: How Man Shapes His Environment," *American Journal of Public Health,* Vol. 58, No. 11 (November 1968), p. 2046.

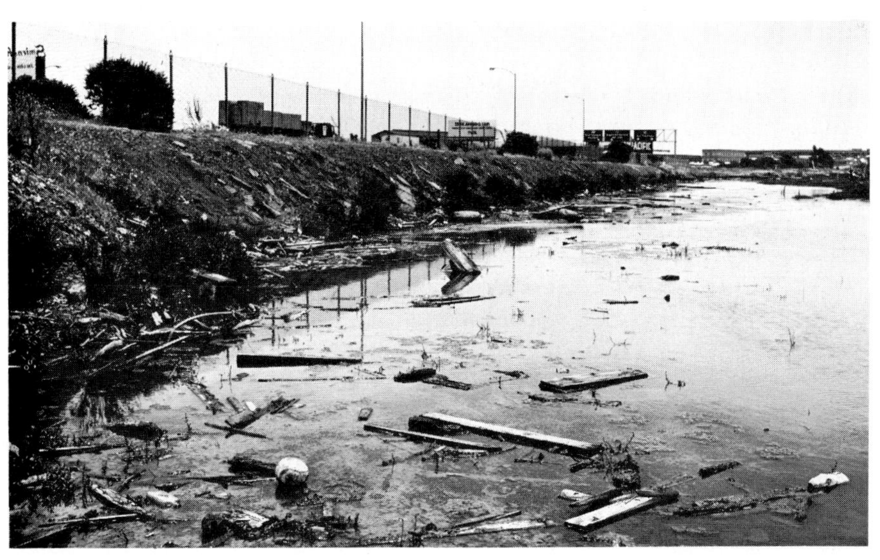

3-3 *Water pollution on the West Coast.*

are indeed enormous. And the threat to water life is more than biological and chemical. Modern industry is now creating a dangerous physical change in aquatic ecosystems.

thermal pollution

Rivers, lakes, streams, and other waters are now being used in certain cooling and condensing procedures in such industrial activities as the generation of electrical power. In these processes water temperature is raised, and in this way everything alive in the water is imperiled. Nuclear power plants require up to 40 percent more cooling water than traditional power plants. The Atomic Energy Commission estimates that by the turn of this century, the operational capacity of nuclear power plants will have increased two-hundred-and-fifty fold. This may become a threat to aquatic life; it will require the combined efforts of federal, state, and local governments to keep that threat from becoming a major hazard.

pollution of deep wells

In 1965 Congress passed the Water Quality Act and in 1966 it passed the Water Pollution Control Act. These are good pieces of legislation as far as they go, but they do not go far enough. They are largely concerned with the protection of surface water—rivers, lakes, and streams. Disposal of wastes in deep wells also needs controls. "Many [of these] wastes are highly toxic,"[20] containing a variety of substances from cyanides to radioactive wastes. Nor are the wastes always safely contained within their wells. Brine waste injected deep into Canadian earth has ended up in Michigan. And brine injection wells in Texas have spouted like geysers. Such wells may bring other dangers. Some experts believe that "disposal of waste fluids by injection into a deep well has triggered earthquakes near Denver, Colorado."[21] Yet even this experience may provide more than a warning of destruction. By injecting limited amounts of fluid deep into the earth in earthquake-prone areas, a gradual dislocation may be induced. This relieves pressure along a stressed fault line. It is hoped that such controlled, little earthquakes may prevent big ones.

pollution of surface waters: Lake Erie

The United States and Canada share the largest fresh-water reservoir on earth—the Great Lakes. Along their shores live some 14 percent of this country's population and almost a third of Canada's. By the end of the century the number of inhabitants is expected to double. This vast waterway extends for two thousand miles, from Duluth to the western end of the St. Lawrence River. It provides transportation, hydroelectric power, and food. It is an unparalleled water playground. Its worst enemy has been its greatest beneficiary—man.

In the recent past, municipal and industrial wastes threatened to turn vast areas of the Great Lakes into murky sewage pits. Among the most endangered of its waters was the once sparkling Lake Erie. If the lake was not dying some

[20] David M. Evans and Albert Bradford, "Under the Rug," *Environment,* Vol. 11, No. 8 (October 1969); p. 8. For an interesting discussion and bibliography about modern threats to human drinking water, see Janice Crossland and Virginia Brodine, "Drinking Water: Try Not to Think About What Comes from the Tap," *Environment,* Vol. 15, No. 3 (April 1973), pp. 11–19.

[21] J. H. Healy, W. W. Rubey, D. T. Griggs, and C. B. Raleigh, "The Denver Earthquakes," *Science,* Vol. 161, No. 3848 (September 27, 1968), pp. 1301–10.

years ago, it was certainly very sick. Its average depth is only 58 feet (compared to the 487 feet of Lake Superior); in so shallow a lake, pollutants, such as nitrates and phosphates, do not stay at the bottom; they tend to surface.[22] Huge amounts of agricultural fertilizers, containing phosphates, were blown off or run off or leached out of the soil into the lake. Nitrates and phosphates are food for algae. (Algae are a group of plants, such as seaweed, widely distributed in both fresh and salt water. In ordinary circumstances they are valuable in maintaining the balance of the ecosystem.) Great masses of algae overgrew in the lake, and when they died and began to decompose, the lake had to give up some oxygen to the process. Had the phosphate from agricultural fertilizers been the only pollution, the lake might have withstood their harmful presence for a long while. As time went by, however, pollutants in the lake became more complex. Phosphate-rich detergents were added to the fertilizer phosphates already in the lake. Acids and alkalis from industrial plants further depleted the lake's oxygen. How? They killed oxygen-producing organisms, and oxygen was used as these organisms decomposed. Also robbing the already damaged lake of its oxygen were the biological wastes of man and animal. Close to the shores of Lake Erie, for example, are cattle feedlots. They are a prime source of organic wastes. "The sewage produced by the concentration of cattle in a single feedlot can be equivalent to that from a city of 200,000 people"[23] (see page 47). Man's biological wastes compounded the danger to the lake, and they also endangered him. Not long ago, one-third of the beaches on Lake Erie's southern shore were closed to swimmers for the entire season. In former times, moreover, Lake Erie had abounded in delicious fish such as trout, whitefish, and lake herring. These were replaced by coarser and less valuable fish—carp, smelt, yellow perch, and sheepshead. The cost to the fishing industry was enormous. It was as if a part of ancient Egypt's doom might become true in these waters: "The fishers also shall mourn, and all they that cast angle into the brooks shall lament, and they that spread nets upon the waters shall languish" (Isaiah 19:8).

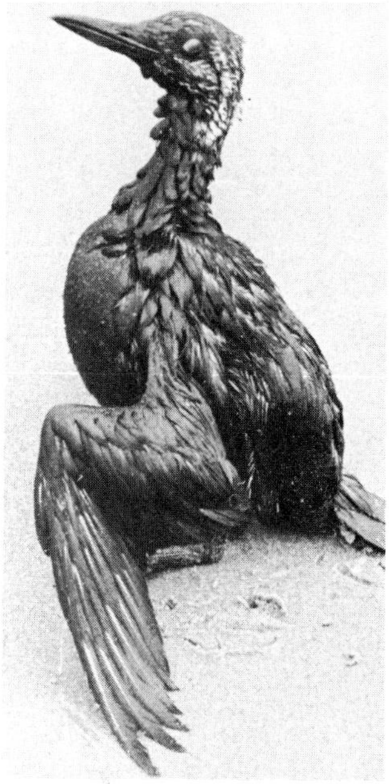

3-4 *An oil-soaked bird rescued from the Santa Barbara Channel in California after a disastrous oil spill in 1969.*

what is being done to save water resources?

On April 15, 1972, the Prime Minister of Canada and the President of the United States signed the detailed Great Lakes Water Quality Agreement. "The pact holds that the Lakes have a right to five freedoms: from toxic substances, nutrient overloading, oil, sludge, and noxious colors and odors."[24] This historic agreement "was the first pact between two nations designed to protect and resuscitate a shared environmental resource."[25]

Within the United States, efforts to control water pollution have taken on a new urgency. Not long ago Oregon's Willamette River was called "a giant septic tank" by the Public Health Service. Polluted from countless sources, it was a vast toilet flushed by water released from federal dams. Today, it is a magnificent model of what can be done by a crusading governor backed by an

[22] Edward J. Kormondy, "Lake Erie Is Aging but Effort Can Save It from Death," *Smithsonian,* Vol. 1, No. 9 (December 1970), p. 30.
[23] Alec Nisbett, "The Myths of Lake Erie," *New Scientist,* Vol. 53, No. 788 (March 23, 1972), p. 651.
[24] "Great Lakes Water Treaty Signed," *Science,* Vol. 176, No. 4033 (April 28, 1972), p. 390.
[25] *Ibid.*

interested people. Old laws were tightened; new laws passed. Now the Willamette serves the recreational, industrial, and agricultural needs of more than one and a half million Oregonians.[26]

Also receiving long overdue attention is the great Hudson River. "It was a happy thought," wrote Walt Whitman almost a hundred years ago, "to build the Hudson River railroad right along the shore."[27] Were he alive today he would surely regret these words. In 1965 and 1966, New York City experienced a gross water shortage. As restaurant waiters doled out precious glasses of water, 30,000 gallons of the Hudson flowed by the city every second. Why could not this water be used? Eight children provided a pitiful answer. They ate a watermelon they found floating in the river. Within a short time, they had typhoid fever. Into the river from which that watermelon came, flowed not only industrial wastes of all kinds, but also the feces and urine of more than 10 million people. Today, that situation is slowly changing. Enforcement of the old Refuse Act of 1899 has resulted in the successful prosecution of a score of polluters. Among the stipulations of the act is that private citizens who report violators be paid part of the fine.[28] Bounties for people who report polluters might help other cities with similar problems.

Industry is restudying its waste disposal processes. And it is making money doing it. Formerly dumped into rivers, animal- and fish-packing wastes are now used in pet-food preparations. Other industries use purified city sewage water. For almost thirty years the Bethlehem Steel Company plant at Sparrows Point, Maryland, near Baltimore, has used the processed and treated effluents of the sewage of almost a million people.[29] It is a magnificent example of waste water recycling that is beneficial to all—citizens and industry alike.

One of the most promising examples of water reuse, however, is provided by a small California community. Just thirteen thousand people live in Santee, California, and an annual average of only ten inches of rain falls upon them. A few years ago Santee was known (if at all) as a small town thirty miles from the big city—San Diego. Today, it is studied and praised by water experts across the nation. By passing their sewage through a modern treatment plant and then filtering the effluent, the people of Santee have reduced their water costs and created a lake for swimming, boating, and fishing. They are living the lines of Longfellow's *Evangeline:*

> its waters, returning
> Back to the springs, like the rain, shall fill them full of refreshment;
> That which the fountain sends forth returns again to the fountain.

[26] Ethel A. Starbird, "A River Restored: Oregon's Willamette," *National Geographic,* Vol. 141, No. 6 (June 1972), pp. 818–19.

[27] Walt Whitman, "Hudson River Sights," *Walt Whitman,* Selected and with Notes by Mark Van Doren (New York, 1945), p. 653.

[28] John G. Mitchell, "The Restoration of a River," *Saturday Review,* Vol. 55, No. 15 (April 8, 1972), p. 35.

[29] Abel Wolman, "Disposal of Man's Wastes," in William L. Thomas, Jr., ed., *Man's Role in Changing the Face of the Earth,* p. 814.

solid-waste disposal

The story is told of the indifferent housekeeper who, when asked what she did with her garbage, replied, "Oh, I just kick it around till it gets lost." Every year in the United States, 48 billion cans and 26 billion bottles are made; 86 billion pounds of paper products reach the market; 8 billion pounds of new plastics are produced; 6 million cars are scrapped and join the 25 to 40 million already stored in dumps.[30] Too often, much of this refuse just gets kicked around. The trouble is, it will not get lost. Getting rid of solid waste, moreover, is expensive. "It costs more to dispose of the *New York Sunday Times* than it does a subscriber to buy it."[31]

Most solid waste consists of food wastes (garbage) and rubbish from households, institutions, and commercial establishments. Abandoned automobiles, garden sweepings, pus-laden hospital bandages, and refrigerators—all these and more clog the ecosystem. In this country solid wastes do not usually transmit disease. True, their improper disposal breeds rats, insects, and vermin associated with illnesses such as plague and gastrointestinal infections. But today's danger of inadequate solid-waste disposal lies in its pollution possibilities.

There are a variety of ways of disposing of solid wastes. *Open-dump burning* promotes aerial garbage. *Dumping trash into water* merely aggravates an already serious mess. Trash has been called "our only growing resource."[32] Accordingly, many modern garbage disposal methods attempt to reuse solid wastes. *Burned in a modern incinerator,* some solid waste may be reduced to an ash that can be used in surfacing roads or in making building blocks. Even the heat of the incineration is increasingly being used to provide warmth for office buildings and swimming pools. Garbage is also used to *fill land.* The only hill in one U.S. city is a heap of garbage covered with layers of clay, dirt, and sod. In the winter it provides fine toboggan runs.

But land to fill is usually distant and limited. The farther away it is, the greater are transportation costs. Three better ways of dealing with refuse are *pulverization, compaction,* and *composting.* In *pulverization,* the waste—even stoves and sofas—is passed through shredders or pounded by a hammermill and broken down into smaller pieces that are easier to handle. *Compaction* goes a step further than pulverization. The refuse is squashed beyond the "yield point," so that it stays compressed. In Japan, where compaction is used extensively, bigger bales of compacted rubbish are sunk in the sea; smaller cubes are used for building river banks and sea walls. *Composting* is usually preceded by some pulverization. Bulky and heavy items are removed. The rest of the waste is permitted to rot in damp conditions. The process depends on the action of aerobic, or "oxygen-breathing," bacteria. The resultant material can be used

[30] Melvin W. First, "Urban Solid-Waste Management," *New England Journal of Medicine,* Vol. 275, No. 26 (December 29, 1966), pp. 1480–84.
[31] *Ibid.,* p. 1484.
[32] Robert R. Grinstead, "The New Resource," *Environment,* Vol. 12, No. 10 (December 1970), p. 3. For an excellent discussion of waste pollution, see Hinrich L. Bohn and Robert C. Cauthorn, "Pollution: The Problem of Misplaced Waste," *American Scientist,* Vol. 60, No. 5 (October 1972), pp. 561–65.

as a topsoil to cover garbage fills.[33] Other uses are now being sought for it.

Still another method of disposing of garbage is by decomposing it with heat. This is called *pyrolysis.* Waste is heated to high temperatures with little or no air present. The residue is composed of charcoal and mineral materials. The charcoal can be used as fuel. Combinations of various methods of disposal are proving feasible and profitable. In St. Louis, for example, the Union Electric Power Company, aided by the federal Environmental Protection Agency, feeds shredded refuse into a coal-burning power-generating system.[34] Thus, a home's refuse may be transformed into its bright lights. But the price of electric power may be more than can be seen on a monthly bill. Coal burning is a major source of air pollution (see page 56).

The inventor and designer R. Buckminster Fuller once remarked that "pollution is a resource that we are not exploiting."[35] As can be seen from the above innovations, that situation is being slowly rectified. The number of programs for the recycling of waste is increasing. Millions of bottles are collected and used in the production of more bottles.[36] In Omaha, recycled glass is used in a road-surfacing material called "glasphalt."[37] In the Norwich, Connecticut, area, old telephone directories are being recycled.[38] Scrap rubber may be reused in rubber products and as a fuel.[39] Animal wastes may be converted into methane gas, thus providing a supply of clean fuel that might one day almost double the nation's supply of natural gas.[40]

Across the country, scientists are studying the nation's solid wastes as a source not only of pollution but also of untapped wealth. Even automobiles and light steel products, such as refrigerators, may be recycled by being scrapped and then incorporated into steel production. In England, "Few of the 900,000 cars scrapped each year now fail to be recycled . . . one large company recently reclaimed an entire gas-works!"[41]

the dirty, dangerous skies

> O dark, dark, dark, amid the blaze of noon,
> Irrecoverably dark, total Eclipse
> Without all hope of day![42]

[33] Jon Tinker, "Must We Waste Rubbish?" *New Scientist,* Vol. 54, No. 796 (May 18, 1972), p. 389.

[34] Robert R. Grinstead, "Machinery for Trash Mining," *Environment,* Vol. 14, No. 4 (May 1972), p. 34.

[35] Quoted in Michael D. Pillburn, "New Beaches from Old Bottles," *Natural History,* Vol. 81, No. 4 (April 1972), p. 49.

[36] Recycling of glass is not a new idea. Today, antique collectors pay high prices for eighteenth-century American bottles. They are rare because they used to be collected to be melted and reused.

[37] Robert R. Grinstead, "Bottlenecks," *Environment,* Vol. 14, No. 3 (April 1972), p. 8.

[38] "Environmental Briefs," *Rodale's Environment Action Bulletin,* Vol. 3, No. 21 (May 20, 1972), p. 1.

[39] Robert R. Grinstead, "Bottlenecks," p. 13.

[40] Hinrich L. Bohn, "A Clean New Gas," *Environment,* Vol. 13, No. 10 (December 1971), p. 5. Because of the tremendous increase in U.S. fossil fuel consumption, considerable research has been directed toward the possibilities of changing organic solid wastes into synthetic fuels. Even if this is feasible, organic wastes will remain but a minor source of energy for many years. Among the reasons: problems of waste collection and the fact that more than half these wastes is actually water. (Thomas H. Maugh II, "Fuel from Wastes, a Minor Source of Energy," *Science,* Vol. 178, No. 4061 [November 10, 1972], pp. 599–602.)

[41] David Clutterbuck, "Wealth in Waste," *New Scientist,* Vol. 49, No. 734 (January 14, 1971), p. 58.

[42] John Milton, *Samson Agonistes,* lines 80–82.

"Cleopatra's Needle" refers to one of two Egyptian obelisks. Neither stone monument is in Egypt any more. One rests on the Thames embankment in London. The other, in New York's Central Park, is of present interest. Made in 1460 B.C., it was given to the city in 1881 by Ismail Pasha, the former khedive of Egypt. In less than a century, New York smog did what thirty-three centuries of Egyptian climate did not do—obscure the hieroglyphics on the obelisk.

Cleopatra's Needle is not the nation's only obelisk to be marred by polluted air. The discolored Washington Monument is dulled testimony to the aerial garbage that comes from the smoking District of Columbia garbage dump. There are other smog sources. There always are, whether the damage is to the Acropolis of Greece or to the Hilton of New York.

Some time ago a nagging question arose. If air pollution eats away stone, how does the seven to ten thousand quarts of polluted air each person inhales daily affect soft, friable lung tissue? In seeking an answer to this question, first consider the source and nature of this aerial rubbish.

London-type smog

The nineteenth-century English poet Percy Bysshe Shelley hated London. He suffered from a pulmonary ailment; perhaps his affliction caused him to write that "Hell is a city much like London—a populous and smoky city." What so troubled the ailing Shelley, and countless Londoners before and after him, is called *London-type smog.* The word "smog" probably originated from a 1901 scientific report attributing some 1,063 deaths in Glasgow and Edinburgh to "Smoke and Fog." London-type smog is not limited to the British Isles. It dims such industrialized communities as New York, Philadelphia, and Chicago. It is, as will be seen, quite different from Los Angeles-type smog, to be described below. However, it shares a basic feature with Los Angeles-type smog.

In both types of air pollution normal cleansing of air is prevented by a phenomenon called *temperature inversion.* Ordinarily, temperature decreases with altitude. For each thousand-foot rise in elevation, the air temperature drops about five degrees Fahrenheit. So, under usual conditions, the air at ground level is warmer than the air above. It is this difference in temperature that helps make possible the vertical air motion so necessary for cleansing man's ground-level air. But temperature inversion reverses (inverts) this ground-air cleansing situation. For a variety of meteorological reasons, a layer of warm air above traps a layer of cold air below. Over the affected area there is a blanket of warm air. In London-type smog this inversion layer of warmer air usually occurs at about three hundred or four hundred feet. In Los Angeles-type smog the warm-air blanket is higher—usually at a thousand feet and even more. The lower the inversion layer, the more severe the smog. Not until the cold layer of ground air is warmed enough by the sun to break the inversion, can the ground air escape and, with it, its accumulated pollutants. Thus it is temperature inversion that impedes dispersion of air pollutants. Temperature inversion phenomena cannot be controlled. Air pollution must be.

London-type smog came with coal. Smoking stacks meant employment. But coal burning released a product of its incomplete combustion, sulfur dioxide (SO_2) gas. Sunlight oxidized the SO_2 to sulfur trioxide (SO_3). When the sulfur

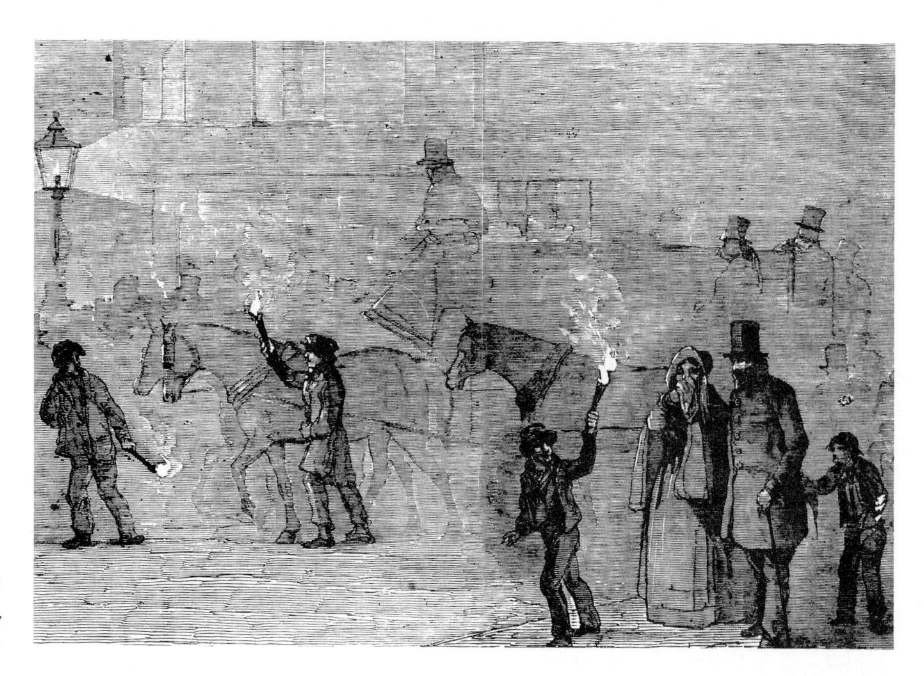

3-5 *Dickens' London: smoke and fog (smog), 1847.*

trioxide combined with air moisture (or fog), corrosive sulfuric acid (H_2SO_4) was formed. ($H_2O + SO_3 \rightarrow H_2SO_4$). There is an old laboratory ditty that has taken on a new relevance:

> We often think of Willie.
> Alas he is no more.
> For what he thought was H_2O
> Was H_2SO_4.

"Sulfuric acid is more irritating to the lungs than is sulfur dioxide, particularly if the acid is suspended in a fine mist of the sort encountered in London, according to the U.S. Public Health Service Air Quality Criteria for Sulfur Oxides."[43] So it is not the sulfuric acid in particles as large as raindrops that is presently causing concern; it is the misty day that could become hazardous. And as if this acid rain were not enough, the recipe for London-type smog also includes other poisonous gases such as benzopyrene and irritating particles of soot.

In the United States, the major source of London-type smog is from the burning of coal, oil, and natural gas to produce electric power. About one-fifth of the particulates (soot), one-fifth of the nitrogen oxides, and one-half of the sulfur oxides polluting the air are from this source. "In New York City, for instance, two-thirds of Consolidated Edison's oil-burning capacity has no emission controls at all and adds up to two tons of soot per hour in the urban air."[44]

[43] Gene E. Likens, F. Herbert Bormann, and Noye M. Johnson, "Acid Rain," *Environment,* Vol. 14, No. 2 (March 1972), p. 34.

[44] Anthony Wolff, "The Price of Power," *Harper's Magazine,* Vol. 244, No. 1464 (May 1972), p. 37.

Los Angeles-type smog

Los Angeles-type smog (''oxidizing'' or ''photochemical'' smog), unlike the London type, is a warm-weather irritant rarely associated with fog. It occurs in various regions of this country, as does the London type. Weather conditions and pollution (automobile and industrial) combine to produce it. Particularly during warm months, warm air enters the atmosphere at high levels. Caught beneath this warm blanket of air (the inversion layer) is the colder ground air. Every day 4 million cars in Los Angeles County consume 8 million gallons of gasoline. And a car does not have to be running to emit smog-contributing chemicals. Fuel tank and carburetor evaporations add to the smog misery. Morning traffic begins. Into the trapped, cold ground air each car belches or evaporates its pollutants. The pollutants cannot penetrate beyond the thermal inversion. They are trapped beneath the warm air inversion blanket. The sun rises. It is indispensable for the smog that is brewing. Its ultraviolet light reacts with the pollutant pall.

Many chemicals comprise this pollution. In the formation of photochemical smog the two most important chemical groups necessary are the *hydrocarbons* and the *oxides of nitrogen.* In sunlight, nitrogen dioxide (NO_2) is dissociated into a simpler compound, nitric oxide, and oxygen. This oxygen readily combines with hydrocarbons to produce a series of reactions that in turn lead to the production of compounds of which poisonous *ozone* is one. Ozone is one of the four Los Angeles air contaminants that can cause a smog alert.[45] The other three are nitrogen oxides, sulfur oxides, and carbon monoxides. Sulfur oxides are primary to London-type smog. *Carbon monoxide,* although not related to the formation of photochemical smog, is nevertheless an important part of Los Angeles' air pollution. It is also largely a product of the gasoline-burning automobile. Every gallon of gasoline consumed results in three pounds of this deadly gas. It causes harm by inactivating the blood's hemoglobin—the oxygen-transporting pigment of the red blood cells. Exposure to high levels of carbon monoxide can result in death. Depending on the length of time of exposure, a little more than one-tenth the lethal amount of carbon monoxide can risk the health of sensitive people. The headache, dizziness, and extreme fatigue noticed by traffic policemen in congested areas is not limited to them. Moreover, carbon monoxide is an added threat to both the cigarette-smoking driver and those about him. Cigarette smoke contains carbon monoxide. Heavy smoking and polluted air can combine to inactivate so much blood hemoglobin that driving functions are impaired. Still other chemicals are part of the Los Angeles-type smog. Some of these injure vegetation. (Los Angeles-type smog is causing an estimated $500 million damage to agriculture conducted near U.S. cities.) Other smog chemicals disintegrate rubber and women's nylon stockings. Still others occur in such low concentrations that they defy identification.

3-6 *A Los Angeles traffic policeman responds to the eye irritation caused by smog.*

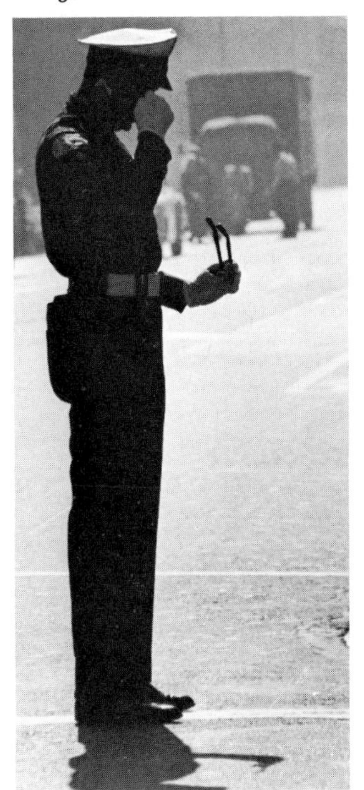

[45] There are several stages to a Los Angeles smog alert, ranked according to danger. In 1955, Los Angeles County experienced fifteen first-stage smog alerts. Today, these are about one-third as frequent. Ozone is the only chemical compound in the Los Angeles atmosphere to have caused a first-stage smog alert level. At this level, the concentration of ozone is safe, but corrective action may be indicated.

some air pollution disasters

Charles Dickens opened his novel *Bleak House* (1852–53) with this description of nineteenth-century London: "Smoke lowering down from chimney-pots, making a soft black drizzle, with flakes of soot in it as big as full-grown snow flakes—gone into mourning . . . for the sun . . . Fog everywhere . . . Fog in the eyes and throats of ancient Greenwich pensioners wheezing by the firesides." There had always been a lot of fussing about "the black skullcap" that covered London. An occasional committee coughed through an occasional meeting. Nobody did much.

Then came December 5, 1952. On that day a strangling black fog lay on London. People fought to breathe. In less than a day many were dead. On December 9, the last day of the chill killer-fog, the London *Times* published a warm-hearted article about "the fogs of ancient Britons." It was a cheery piece: "The countryside dissolves under the spell into a parody of fairyland . . . The farmer hears news of the great city with a comradely smile. The fog has not forgotten to pay him a visit."[46] In his dying thoughts, many a city Englishman might have included a vain hope that the fog had been less attentive. Four thousand people perished in that fog. Most were sufferers from chronic respiratory disease who were over forty-five years old. In those several days, more Londoners died from the smog than from the nineteenth-century cholera epidemic.

Evilly, fog had been curling, lurking about the dank streets of Donora, Pennsylvania, for some days, a pale yellow poison, before it snuffed out the life of its first victim. It was during October 1948. One-third of this coal town's 13,839 population became ill. Seventeen died. Close by, the people of Pittsburgh looked on, horrified, apprehensive.

What chemicals in the smog caused the London and Donora disasters? The findings give reason for somber concern. Dubos noted that "no single smog component was present in unusually high concentrations."[47] He wondered if it could be that the smog, ordinarily breathed by everyone a day or two at a time without being harmful, could become injurious, even lethal, to many people when inhaled for a few days longer. Since these events took place, more disquieting data have been gathered. For those in Donora affected by the 1948 smog attack, illness and death rates are higher than would otherwise have been expected.

the breath of death

Since they were disasters, the tragedies in London and Donora are widely known. The average person is not so aware that there are other evidences of smog's lethal possibilities. In November 1953, an air pollution blanketed New York City. Not until nine years later did a review of vital statistics reveal a startling fact. During that 1953 episode 200 more New Yorkers died than would have been expected to die in that period.[48] Other ominous data are being accu-

[46] Arie J. Haagen-Smit, "Atmospheric Ecology," *Archives of Environmental Health,* Vol. 11, No. 1 (July 1965), p. 87.

[47] René Dubos, *Man Adapting* (New Haven, Conn., 1965), p. 218.

[48] L. Greenburg, M. B. Jacobs, B. M. Drolette, F. Field, and M. M. Braverman, "Report of an Air Pollution Incident in New York City, November, 1953," *Public Health Reports,* Vol. 77, No. 1 (January 1962), pp. 7–16.

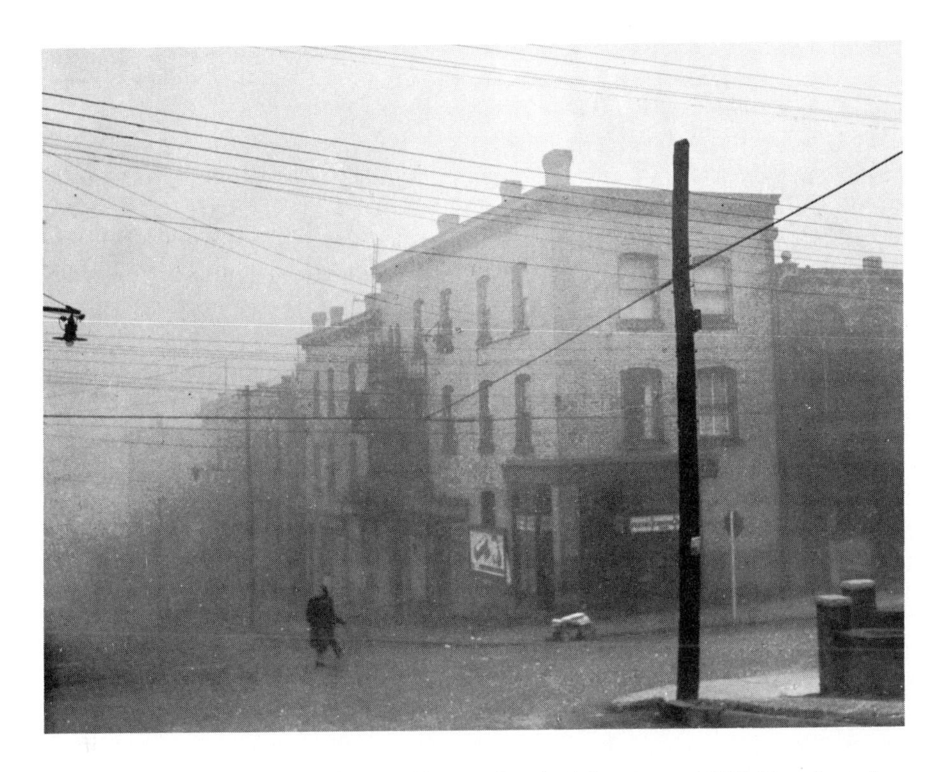

3-7 *Donora, Pennsylvania, during the 1948 air pollution disaster.*

mulated and analyzed. During and immediately following a 1966 Thanksgiving weekend attack of air pollution, there were 168 "excess" deaths in New York City.[49] Still another study points out that: "Examination of total deaths in New York City by day of occurrence shows periodic peaks in mortality which are associated with periods of high air pollution . . . fog is not a necessary part of this picture, and therefore the presence of these episodes is often not apparent at the time to most inhabitants."[50]

Confirmatory evidence that the Los Angeles-type smog is directly responsible for an increase in mortality is lacking. But there is much cause for concern. Recent years have seen a marked increase in the deaths, both in California and elsewhere in the nation, from emphysema, a crippling lung disease (pages 389–92). Some of this increase is doubtlessly due to improved diagnosis, but certainly not all. Physicians recall that those who died in Donora in 1948, and in London in 1952, were older people suffering from chronic ailments of the bronchi and lungs. These were startling episodes. Is prolonged exposure to lower levels of smog producing less dramatic but no less damaging results? In the past twenty years, U.S. death rates from bronchitis and asthma have also risen sharply. The specific relationship between these rises and smog is unknown. But one fact is known: smog can kill.

[49] M. Glasser, L. Greenburg, and F. Field, "Mortality and Morbidity During a Period of High Levels of Air Pollution, New York, Nov. 23 to 25, 1966," *Archives of Environmental Health,* Vol. 15, No. 6 (December 1967), p. 694.

[50] James McCarroll and William Bradley, "Excess Mortality as an Indicator of Health Effects of Air Pollution," *American Journal of Public Health,* Vol. 56, No. 11 (November 1966), p. 1942.

smog and sickness Smog is an insidious presence, aggravating the illness of countless people who are already chronically ill. And to those not already so disadvantaged, smog may silently bring the beginnings of a serious sickness. Many people, particularly those with chronic respiratory diseases such as asthma, suffer painfully during a smog attack. One study emphasizes that "there can be no doubt that a considerable effect is exerted by pollutions on hospital admissions for certain disease groupings."[51] Another study suggests "that susceptibility to, or duration of, common viral respiratory infections is increased . . . by exposure to . . . air pollutants."[52] Yet another researcher writes that "a review of factors relating atmospheric pollution to lung cancer warrants its incrimination as one of the dominant agents . . . associated with the disease."[53] Various investigations point to an "association between urban residence and lung cancer" and implicate "the atmosphere as one dominant factor in . . . lung cancer."[54] British research and studies in Japan[55] are no more encouraging. They point to "a possible influence on respiratory disease of children."[56] Nor should it be thought that air pollution merely worsens the already sick. There is "clear evidence that oxidant air pollution has an adverse effect on athletic performance in healthy adolescent males."[57]

Yet another hazard has been suggested. It is possible that one reason for the dangerously high level of poisonous lead in the blood of many urban children is their small height; they are nose-high to automobile exhaust fumes.[58]

These are grim reports. However, another factor must again be emphasized. Time. Citizens complain about immediate discomforts. A burning sensation of the eyes, a night of coughing—these will prompt an angry letter to an editor or mayor. But what of prolonged, subtle exposure to low levels of pollution? Perhaps this is the far deadlier enemy: "The most important among the . . . deleterious effects of air pollution are slow in developing . . . continued exposure to low levels of toxic agents will eventually result in . . . misery . . . increasing the medical load."[59]

Can air pollution be linked to lung cancer? That it may be is strongly suggested by a recent committee report of the National Research Council of the National Academy of Sciences. People living in urban areas have twice the incidence of lung cancer as do those living in nonurban areas. In those city areas where fossil-fuel products from industrial use pollute the air, the incidence of

[51] T. D. Sterling, J. J. Phair, S. V. Pollack, D. A. Schumsky, and I. De Grott, "Urban Morbidity and Air Pollution," *Archives of Environmental Health,* Vol. 13, No. 1 (August 1966), p. 169.

[52] F. Curtis Dohan, "Air Pollutants and Incidence of Respiratory Disease," *Archives of Environmental Health,* Vol. 3, No. 4 (October 1961), p. 394.

[53] Paul Kotin, "The Role of Atmospheric Pollution in the Pathogenesis of Pulmonary Cancer: A Review," *Cancer Research,* Vol. 16, No. 5 (June 1956), pp. 375–93.

[54] Paul Kotin and Hans L. Falk, "Polluted Urban Air and Related Environmental Factors in the Pathogenesis of Pulmonary Cancer," *Diseases of the Chest,* Vol. 45, No. 3 (March 1964), p. 244.

[55] T. Toyama, "Air Pollution and Health Effects in Japan," a paper read before the Sixth Air Pollution Medical Research Conference, California State Department of Public Health, January 28–29, 1963.

[56] "Air Pollution and Respiratory Infection in Children," an editorial in *The Lancet,* No. 7452 (June 25, 1966), p. 1409.

[57] W. S. Wayne, P. F. Wehrle, and R. E. Carroll, "Oxidant Air Pollution and Athletic Performance," *Journal of the American Medical Association,* Vol. 199, No. 12 (March 20, 1967), pp. 901–04.

[58] "Lead Poisoning in the Middle Class?" *Medical World News,* Vol. 12, No. 7 (February 19, 1971), p. 17.

[59] René Dubos, "Adapting to Pollution," *Scientist and Citizen,* Vol. 10, No. 1 (January–February 1968), pp. 2–3.

lung cancer is greatest. The older people are when they migrate to the United States, the closer are their lung cancer rates to those in their home countries; this suggests an environmental effect occurring early in life that promotes lung cancer development in later years. Of particular concern are a group of air pollutants called *polycyclic organic matter* (POM). Ninety percent of POM emissions are from coal- and wood-burning residential furnaces, coal refuse fires, and coke production from the iron and steel industries. POM is also implicated in skin cancer and other skin conditions, such as acne, among people who must work with fossil fuels.[60]

the secret enemy: carbon monoxide

"Secret path marks secret foe," wrote the English novelist and poet Sir Walter Scott in *The Lady of the Lake.* So it is with carbon monoxide. Invisible, odorless, tasteless, this poisonous gas does no harm in natural amounts. Concentrated in city streets and freeways, however, carbon monoxide often reaches high levels that last for hours and that affect the nervous system. At some busy city intersections, tanks of pure oxygen are available to provide traffic policemen with oxygen-breaks every half-hour. Otherwise, they endure symptoms such as severe headache, nausea, and giddiness.

Why? Ordinarily, oxygen from air is transferred via the lungs to the hemoglobin of the blood (see page 221). It is then transported to the cells of the body. When carbon monoxide is inhaled, it combines with the blood hemoglobin. Not only does it do so more readily than oxygen, but the resultant mixture is two hundred times more stable than the oxygen-hemoglobin combination. Thus, oxygen cannot easily displace the carbon monoxide. The result: tissues suffer oxygen hunger. The brain and other nervous tissues are the most sensitive in the body to oxygen deprivation. Once destroyed, adult brain cells do not regenerate. For this reason, those who do recover from severe carbon monoxide poisoning are frequently left with permanent brain damage. When death occurs from carbon monoxide poisoning, it is due to suffocation. One study suggests that, in this country, over five hundred people "die each year from carbon monoxide poisoning because their vehicles are defective due to deterioration, damage, or poor automotive design."[61] Cigarette smoking while driving is particularly hazardous. Combustion in the lighted tip of a cigarette occurs in a limited supply of oxygen. Every time he takes a puff, a smoker inhales a concentration of carbon monoxide that is as much as four hundred times the concentration that exists naturally in the air. From 5 to 15 percent of the hemoglobin of a heavy smoker may be bound by carbon monoxide.[62] Man-made pollution accounts for about 100 million tons of carbon monoxide in the air yearly. The major source of pollution is the automobile. In one year an automobile emits about 3,200 pounds of the gas. Converters have been made that

[60] "Nailing Lung Cancer to Air Pollution," *Science News,* Vol. 102, No. 12 (September 16, 1972), p. 183.
[61] Susan P. Baker, Russel H. Fisher, William C. Masemore, and Irving M. Sopher, "Fatal Unintentional Carbon Monoxide Poisoning in Motor Vehicles," *American Journal of Public Health,* Vol. 62, No. 11 (November 1972), p. 1463.
[62] Robert W. Medeiros, "Carbon Monoxide: The Invisible Enemy," *Chemistry,* Vol. 46, No. 1 (January 1973), p. 19.

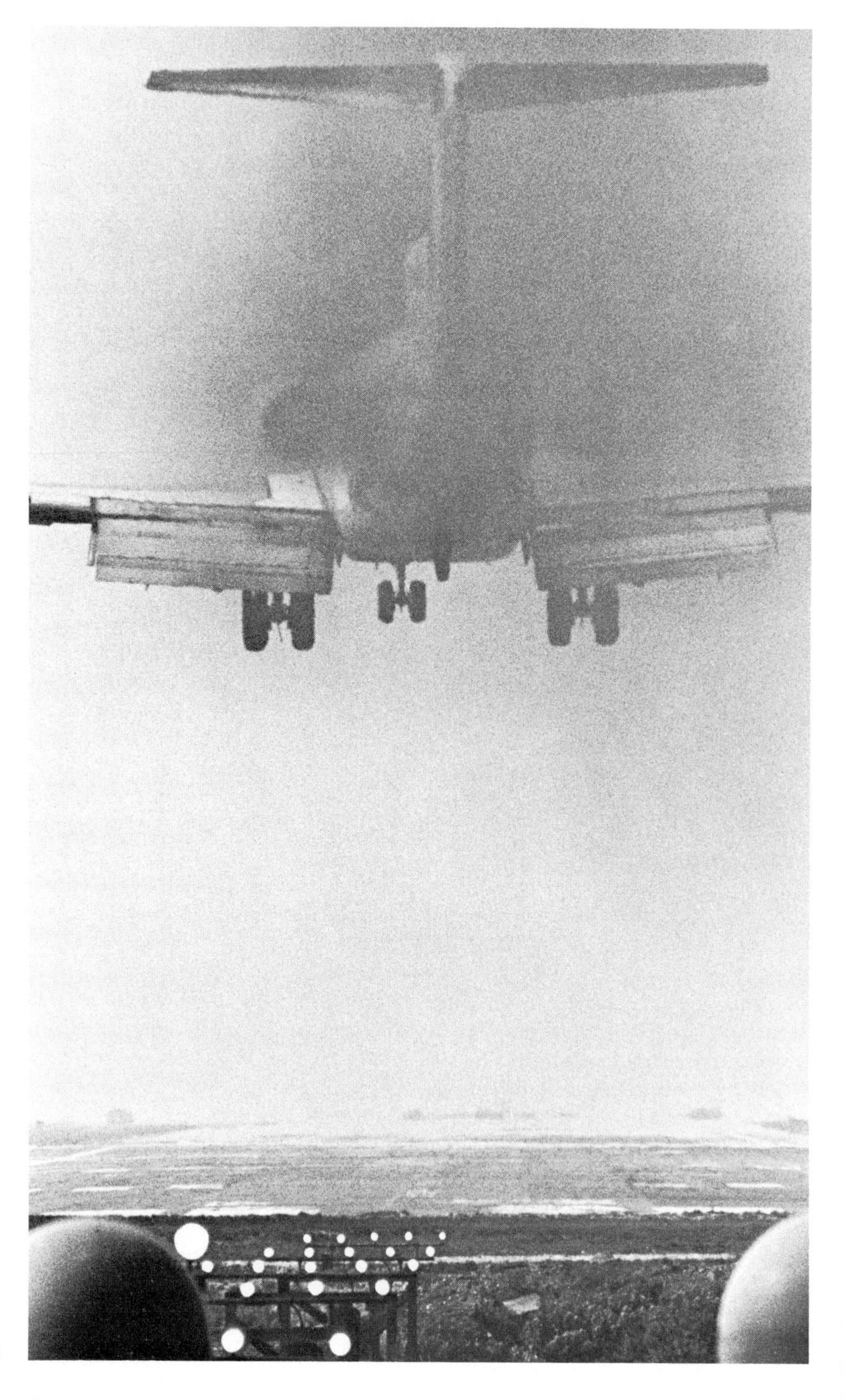

3-8

meet U.S. government emission standards, but usually they are impaired after about 5,000 miles of driving.

what must be done?

"We may have to find a new mode of transportation."[63] This statement was made on March 27, 1972, by the distinguished president of the National Academy of Sciences before a group of U.S. Senators. There is increasing opinion that automobile traffic will need to be restricted in many urban areas. On January 15, 1973, the director of the Environmental Protection Agency announced that, beginning in 1975, it would be necessary to ration gasoline in the South Coast Air Basin during the May-through-October smog season. In some areas even that would be insufficient because of pollutants, such as nitrous oxides, which come, not from the automobile, but from fuel-burning power plants (page 54). Ways of purifying fuel and of controlling emissions from stationary sources of pollution must also be found. In areas troubled by London-type smog, for example, the oxides of sulfur can be partly controlled with the cooperation of industry. Improvements in factory construction enable industrialists to dispose of sulfur pollutions without danger to surrounding populations. Moreover, various chemical processes may not only relieve the pollution problem but also benefit industry. From sulfur oxide gases, sulfuric acid and sulfur may be obtained and sold to a ready market.[64]

The major cause of air pollution, however, is the automobile. To the pollution caused by using gasoline as automobile fuel, man may yet be forced to seek a solution, "for by 2025—within the lives of many young people now entering college—world petroleum resources will be largely depleted."[65] Alternatives to the presently used internal combustion engine of the automobile are being actively sought. Steam or gas turbine engines are being built for experimental purposes. They present many mechanical problems, as does the automobile run on an electric battery. Recently, researchers have suggested adding a second flywheel behind the automobile engine to help propel the vehicle. The flywheel is a disc or a bar-shaped device that, when spun at high speed, will store energy. Should this device be perfected, it could help reduce auto emissions.[66]

A nonpolluting new means of transportation is the recently developed automated Personal Rapid Transport (PRT) system.[67] One type is a computer-controlled, driverless, rubber-tired minibus (for from four to forty passengers) on elevated guiderails. It has been described as a cross between an automatic elevator and a monorail. During rush hours, the minibus stops only at certain stations. At other times (as with an elevator), the passenger presses a call button at a station. Once aboard, he presses a destination button. In 1973, a 3.2-mile, relatively pollution-free PRT system opened connecting the three campuses of

[63] Quoted in Richard H. Gilluly, "Nitrogen Oxides, Autos, and Power Plants," *Science News,* Vol. 101, No. 16 (April 15, 1972), p. 252.

[64] "Diminishing the Role of Sulfur Oxides in Air Pollution," an editorial in *Science,* Vol. 157, No. 3794 (September 15, 1967), p. 1265.

[65] James I. Mattill, "The Growing Challenge," *Technology Review,* Vol. 75, No. 1 (October–November 1972), p. 4, citing Earl Cook, Dean of the College of Geosciences at Texas A & M University.

[66] Julian McCaull, "A Lift for the Auto," *Environment,* Vol. 13, No. 10 (December 1971), pp. 35–41.

[67] Joseph Hanlon, "Personal Rapid Transit Comes to the U.S.," *New Scientist,* Vol. 54, No. 797 (May 25, 1972), pp. 429–30.

West Virginia University. A somewhat similar PRT system is being built at the Dallas-Fort Worth Regional Airport. On a larger scale, San Francisco's computer-controlled subway system is attracting national attention.

auto pollution and the law

Eighty percent of Los Angeles' smog comes from motor vehicles. More than 4 million vehicles crowd its streets. Every year that number is increased by some 10 percent. Other cities, notably Chicago (which has more automobiles per square mile than Los Angeles), New York, and Detroit, have a similar problem. Two federal laws spell out this nation's program for control of air pollution: the Air Quality Act of 1967 and the Clean Air Amendments of 1970. It is apparent that the federal Environmental Protection Agency intends to enforce the Clean Air Amendments. These amendments establish strict standards for automobile emissions as well as for ambient (circulating) air. In June 1972, the Environmental Protection Agency ruled that the automobile industry must meet specified emission standards by 1975 and others by 1976.

air pollution and economics

Early in 1972, the White House Office of Science and Technology reported on the economics of auto emission control. "Air pollution," the report said in part, "—like so many other related problems of modern society—may be controllable only by drastic changes in our national patterns of private, commercial, and industrial activity."[68]

It is claimed that the cost of equipment to control pollution can only be reflected in higher prices and taxes for the average consumer. But is it not ultimately less expensive for the consumer to be rid of the pollution than to keep it? Air pollution alone costs the people of this nation an estimated $16 billion a year. It is difficult to compute the price the individual pays for air pollution. However, some limited information is available. For example, in 1971 some one hundred Texas dock-workers were made seriously ill by four chemical-plant pollution incidents. In cases like this, aside from their pain and inconvenience, the economic cost to the individual worker can be computed. In 1960 air pollution costs per capita were compared between heavily polluted Steubenville, Ohio, and less industrialized Uniontown, Pennsylvania; air pollution costs in Steubenville were $84 per capita higher.[69]

Will pollution abatement result in widespread unemployment? Marginal plants with old equipment are in danger of closing. Some unemployment (50,000 to 100,000 workers) will occur. "Hardest hit would be an estimated 50 to 150 one-industry small towns. [But since] jobs would also be created in pollution-abatement equipment industries, the net loss of jobs might be only 0.1 percent of current unemployment."[70] Federal programs are needed to deal specifically with unemployment resulting from environmental improvements.

[68] Quoted in Richard H. Gilluly, "Nitrogen Oxides, Autos, and Power Plants," p. 252.

[69] "Pollution and Economics: Measuring the Real Costs," *Science News*, Vol. 100, No. 5 (July 31, 1971), p. 76.

[70] "Pollution Abatement: Costs and Benefits," *Science News*, Vol. 101, No. 12 (March 18, 1972), p. 183.

a worldwide effort against pollution

The first global meeting on pollution was the United Nations Conference on the Human Environment, held in Stockholm in June 1972. One hundred and twelve nations sent 1,200 delegates. Two main results came of the conference: first, a declaration of recommendations and principles for action to prevent environmental abuse and, second, a proposal for the establishment of UN machinery to carry out an antipollution program. Among the 109 recommendations adopted by the conference (and later approved by the UN General Assembly) was one making nations responsible for pollution of areas outside their national jurisdictions. Another urged the development of international laws to provide compensation for those people in any country who are the victims of pollution from another country.[71]

the mobile epidemic

It doubtless never crossed his mind that his name would be inscribed in the record books. Yet, on September 13, 1899, when Mr. A. W. Bliss stepped off a New York trolley and was hit by a horseless carriage, he became the world's first auto fatality.[72] By 1974, in this country alone, more than 2 million people had died in automobile accidents. This is more than the total number of people that have died in all the wars of this nation's history.[73]

the mathematics of death

According to the National Safety Council, 117,000 people in this country died because of accidents in 1972. Almost half —56,600—died in motor-vehicle accidents.[74] In other words, on an average day, about 155 people died in motor-vehicle accidents. Traffic accidents also account for millions of injuries a year; over 14,600 people a day suffer injuries needing medical attention.[75]

Such large numbers often seem meaningless unless they are related to a personal experience. In Los Angeles, a twenty-six-year-old woman goes for a Sunday afternoon drive in the country with her husband and their two small

[71] John Walsh, "U.N. Environmental Program: Despite Hitch, Coming on Strong," *Science,* Vol. 178, No. 4066 (December 15, 1972), p. 1185. To the citizens of underdeveloped countries, the priority problems are malnutrition, poverty, and disease. Environmental pollution is secondary. (Terri Aaronson, "UN Environmental Agency Sent to Kenya," *New Scientist,* Vol. 57, No. 828 [January 11, 1973], pp. 72–73.) Moreover, leaders of these countries consider pollution to be the responsibility of those industrialized nations that cause it. Nevertheless, that Third World countries played an important and effective role at the Stockholm conference was demonstrated by the selection of Nairobi, Kenya, as the site of the administrative machinery of the UN environmental agency.

[72] "First Auto Crash Victim Died 72 Years Ago Today," *Journal of the American Medical Association,* Vol. 217, No. 11 (September 13, 1971), p. 1461.

[73] J. Robert Moskin, "Life and Death in Your Automobile," *World,* Vol. 2, No. 6 (March 13, 1973), p. 14. It was estimated that the two millionth U.S. automobile fatality occurred sometime on July 10, 1973. In addition to the killed, almost 16½ million people have been maimed or seriously injured in the past half-century.

[74] National Safety Council, *Accident Facts and Figures, 1973 Edition,* p. 3. Accidents in the home ranked second with 27,000 fatalities. In 1972, there were 23,500 deaths in public places (excluding motor-vehicle and work accidents, and 14,000 people in this country died in accidents that took place at work. (National Safety Council, *Accident Facts and Figures, 1973 Edition.*) These figures add up to more than the 117,000 total because of some overlapping: some work deaths involving motor vehicles are in both the work and motor-vehicle categories; also, some motor-vehicle deaths occurred on home premises and are in both the home and motor-vehicle categories.

[75] "Drinking Driver Target of New Safety Efforts," *American Medical News,* Vol. 15, No. 50 (December 18, 1972), p. 9.

3-9 *The official symbol for the United Nations Conference on the Human Environment, 1972.*

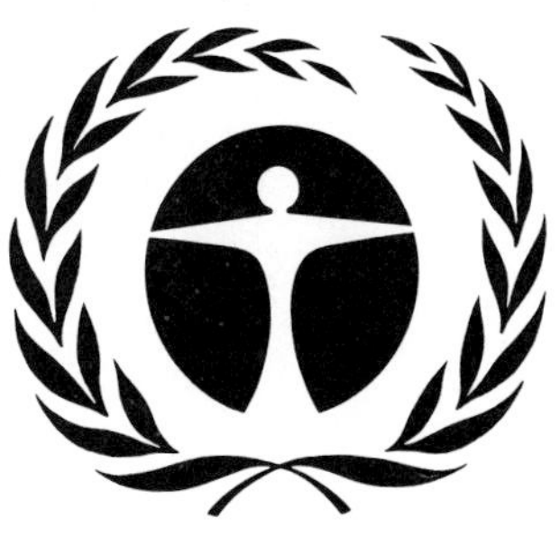

daughters, aged three and five. There are two more children on the way, for next month this woman is due to deliver twins. Throughout his wife's pregnancy her physician husband has been amused at the idea of twins. The couple has bantered a lot and has had fun shopping for baby clothes. Now the woman is tired and a trifle impatient. "I can't be comfortable with these seat belts anymore," she tells her husband good-naturedly, and lets them fall unfastened. Then, as if reminded, she turns to be certain of the children's seat belts.

Soon they are in the country. It is a fine day. Suddenly somebody is coming over the hill on the wrong side of the road. They are hit head-on. In the hospital, the man is repaired: seven stitches are needed for the scalp, five for his right cheek; some broken ribs are taped. Then he is told. The children are badly shaken up, that is all. But his wife has a crushing head injury. There is extensive brain damage. The twins are born and dead. That night the woman dies. She is, then, one of the 56,600 who died that year in an auto accident. So is the other driver. He was dead on admission to the hospital. The husband is counted with the millions who are disabled. That is part of the meaning of the numbers. Not the least interesting thing about them is how uninteresting they are to so many people.

How did it happen that this young woman was killed? One answer to this question is simply mathematical. There were two crashes, not one. The car was traveling 55 miles an hour. The first crash brought the car to a sudden halt. But for a fraction of a second the woman, unrestrained by a seat belt, continued traveling. She thus became a projectile heading for a second crash. Her knees crumpled against the heater. Her chest hit the dashboard. Her head struck the windshield, causing it to yield two inches. Her head collapsed two inches. Thus her head traveled four inches, or one-third of a foot, after hitting the windshield. What was the force of the impact? For this there is an equation:[76]

$$G = \frac{\text{miles per hour}^2}{30 \times \text{stopping distance in feet}} \text{ or } \frac{(55)^2}{30 \times \frac{1}{3}} = \frac{3{,}025}{10} = 302.5$$

The weight of that part of her upper body directly involved in the windshield blow is estimated at 20 percent of the weight of herself and her unborn babies (130 pounds), or 26 pounds. Multiplying 26 pounds by 302.5 G's equals 7,865 pounds—almost four tons. This was the average force with which her head impacted against the windshield.[77]

the emotionally distressed driver

In this particular accident there was a lone driver in the opposite car. That he had been a heavy drinker for two years is the basic reason for the disaster. "It is known that well over half of all fatally injured drivers had been drinking; among drivers found to be responsible for the fatal crash, two-thirds had

[76] "Fighting Death on Wheels," *Roche Medical Image,* Vol. 8, No. 6 (June 1966), p. 8. G is the force developed in slowing an object, measured in terms of the force of gravity. In the formula, 30 represents a constant developed from the acceleration due to gravity (32.2 feet per second per second) and the measurement units used (in this case, miles per hour and feet).

[77] In Sweden, many car occupants now wear helmets. There is nothing in this equation that would make this practice anything but eminently sensible.

been drinking, and in the one-car fatal crashes, seven out of ten had been drinking.''[78]

Further investigation of the accident involving the young woman revealed more about the lone drinking driver who was responsible for her death. As a teen-ager he had been somewhat impulsive but oddly conservative about driving. ''He liked to go on these long rides,'' his father later grieved quietly. ''Alone. All by himself. He'd say it relaxed him. Then he took to drinking. Then he wasn't good for driving or anything else.''

This history is not unusual. The ''graduation of the inexperienced, impulsive, but cautious beginner to a self-confident, financially independent, heavier drinking, and more dangerous young adult''[79] is an event that contributes to many an accident. Moreover, accidental death strikes young drivers harder than any other age group. In 1971, well over half the motor-vehicle fatalities (30,800 of the 54,700 total) were between the ages of fifteen and forty-four; 16,500 were killed who were between eighteen and forty-four. One study revealed a particularly high incidence of crashes for young males between eighteen and twenty years of age.[80]

The close relationship between emotional illness and fatal accidents has long intrigued investigators. In one study, depressions, suicidal tendencies, and delusions of persecution were all found to be much more common among drivers responsible for fatal accidents than in a control group.[81] ''It is clear,'' stated one health spokesman, ''that an individual whose mind is filled with rage over a personal problem is not, at the moment, the best choice to drive a car.''[82]

The increasing awareness of the relationship between accidents and emotional instability has led to much conjecture about the so-called accident-prone individual. There is not enough scientific data to support this general term.[83] An individual may be likely to have an accident in one circumstance but not in another.

prevention of accidents: cars and roads

Automobile accidents, like all other epidemics, must be considered in three interrelated aspects. The *host* or driver has already been discussed. Consider now the *agent* or automobile and the *environment* or roads.

seat belts

The experiments of Colonel Stapp in the New Mexico desert have demonstrated that a person who is adequately restrained is able to survive a 50-mile-per-hour

[78] H. Emerson Campbell, ''Traffic Deaths Go Up Again,'' *Journal of the American Medical Association,* Vol. 201, No. 11 (September 11, 1967), p. 861.
[79] Stanley H. Schuman *et al.,* ''Young Male Drivers: Impulse Expression, Accidents, and Violations,'' *Journal of the American Medical Association,* Vol. 200, No. 12 (June 19, 1967), p. 102.
[80] Stanley H. Schuman, Roberta McConochie, and Donald C. Pelz, ''Reduction of Driver Crashes in a Controlled Pilot Study,'' *Journal of the American Medical Association,* Vol. 218, No. 2 (October 11, 1971), p. 234.
[81] Melvin L. Selzer, Joseph E. Rogers, and Sue Kern, ''Fatal Accidents: The Role of Psychopathology, Social Stress, and Acute Disturbance,'' *American Journal of Psychiatry,* Vol. 124, No. 8 (January 1968), p. 53.
[82] George James, former Commissioner of Health of New York City, quoted in ''Chronic Disease, a Major Cause of Accidents.'' *Geriatric Focus,* Vol. 4, No. 4 (March 15, 1965), p. 1.
[83] ''Accident Proneness,'' an editorial in *Canadian Medical Association Journal,* Vol. 90, No. 10 (March 7, 1964), pp. 646–47.

head-on crash into a stone wall without sustaining any serious injuries.[84]

Like all accidents, the accident that killed the young woman and the drunk driver can teach. It is understandable that the young woman failed to fasten her seat belt. Yet, had she used seat belts, she and her unborn children might have been among the estimated 3,000 people in this country whose lives are saved each year by their use. (It is further estimated that a total of 8,000 to 10,000 lives would be saved each year if all passenger car occupants used seat belts at all times.) Lap and sash seat belts are more effective than lap belts alone.

A recent study[85] of 139 fatal automobile accidents, in which 177 people were killed, shows how the use of seat belts might have saved the lives of 63 of the 101 drivers who were killed. Of 28 drivers whose death resulted from ejection, 26 would probably have been saved by the use of the belts. Many facial injuries resulting from impact with the front door, steering assembly, and other parts of the car could also have been avoided. Nor, of course, were drivers the only victims who would have survived if they had used belts.

Unfortunately, at least two out of three people fail to use their safety belts and nine out of ten ignore the shoulder belts. Since January 1, 1972, all cars built for sale in this country must have a buzzer which sounds whenever the driver fails to fasten his seat belt. A flasher light emphasizes the warning.

air bags

The National Highway Safety Administration of the federal Department of Transportation has ruled that all automobiles built in the United States after August 15, 1975, must have a "passive restraint system" for all passengers. Passive restraints are automatic and are not so dependent on passenger participation as "active restraints." Thus, safety belts are active restraints; among the passive restraints now being tested are energy-absorbing steering wheels and air bags. Inflation of an air bag would be triggered by sensors on detecting an impact. The air bag would inflate to about three times the size of an ordinary bed pillow in about forty-thousandths of a second. It would then immediately begin to deflate.[86] In 1973, the air bag presented numerous problems. It was costly. It had to be engineered to be triggered only by serious impacts and not by curb bumps or bumps from other parking cars. It was noisy. Moreover, it was useful only in frontal impacts.[87] Despite these and other problems, two companies already consider their engineering problems to have been solved well enough to allow them to install air bags in some 1974 and 1975 models.

[84] Ross A. McFarland, "Injury—A Major Environmental Problem," *Archives of Environmental Health,* Vol. 19, No. 2 (August 1969), p. 253.

[85] Donald F. Huelke and Paul W. Gikas, "Causes of Deaths in Automobile Accidents," *Journal of the American Medical Association,* Vol. 203, No. 13 (March 25, 1968), p. 1106. That a pregnant woman should always wear a seat belt unless her physician says otherwise was confirmed by a study of 208 pregnant victims of severe auto accidents. This study revealed that "among unbelted . . . women . . . the death rate was 33 percent of those ejected from the car and 5 percent of those not ejected. The fetal death rate was 47 percent when the mother was ejected and 11 percent when she was not . . . Thus lap belts, which usually prevent ejection, may be recommended for pregnant travelers." (Warren M. Crosby and J. Paul Costiloe, "Safety of Lap-Belt Restraint for Pregnant Victims of Automobile Collisions," *New England Journal of Medicine,* Vol. 284 [March 25, 1971], p. 632.)

[86] "Researchers 'Rev Up' for Safer Driving," *Journal of the American Medical Association,* Vol. 219, No. 8 (February 21, 1972), p. 984.

[87] Murray Mackay, "Safer Cars by 1977," *New Scientist,* Vol. 53, No. 780 (January 27, 1972), pp. 211–12.

tires

In this country nineteen manufacturers make some twenty dozen brands of tires in such a variety of fabrics, plies, and treads as to confuse any buyer. Tires should be bought not according to price but according to intended use. A cross-country salesman will need tires different from a truck driver's, and the suburban shopper's needs are different yet.

Fabrics are built into the tire in plies (layers of fabric cords). It is not the number but rather the thickness of the plies or layers that determines fabric strength. And some kinds of fabric are safer than others. Rayon, an excellent cord material, is cheaper than nylon, but not as strong. Polyester is almost as strong as nylon and, when combined with the fiberglass belt, is considered a superior safety tire. Also important for safety is the tire tread, the outer grooved surface of the tire. On wet roads effective tread patterns may be invaluable. Modern patterns wipe dry that wet portion of the road upon which the tire rests at any moment, thus reducing the chances of skidding.

For a car restricted to suburban errands, an 80-level[88] rayon or nylon tire is adequate. Freeway and family vacation travel requires at least a 100-level rayon or polyester tire. Fast drivers or those traveling long distances with heavy loads will do well to invest in nylon, fiberglass belt, or radial tires. High-speed tires have special nylon cord, thin-tread construction. They should not be confused with the extremely durable, 200-level, thick-tread tire, which is usually the best tire a company makes. Because these retain heat, they are unsuitable for high speeds. Among the safest of all tires is the ''tire within a tire.'' Mandatory on a racetrack, it enables the driver with a puncture to get to a service station without further tire damage.

Correct air pressure is essential to tire care and safety. For the average car, 28–30 pounds are considered best. Lower pressures give softer but not safer rides. A slightly overloaded, underinflated tire traveling at 75 miles per hour will heat to 300 degrees! At 325 degrees rubber is a semiliquid. Overinflation in a tire will carry one just as close to disaster. The blow of a road object cannot be properly absorbed. As a result the fabric tears and the tire may blow out immediately, or, if the damage is slight, fail days later. Wheel alignment checks prevent tire wear and provide greater safety, as do tire rotations. When is a tire beyond repair? Molded into the patterns of most recently manufactured tires are tread-wear indicators. These are solid crossbars between the grooves. If these show, the tire should no longer be in use. For tires without built-in indicators, a penny can serve as an indicator. When the penny is inserted into the center groove, the date should not be visible.[89]

other car safety factors

Growing public clamor is stimulating safer automobile design. Nothing does more to persuade a businessman than the opinion of the consumer. ''The days

[88] Tires are still spoken of as quality level. A 100-level tire is one of a quality regarded as adequately safe for average driving.

[89] This section is based on an article by Don Macdonald, ''All About Tires,'' *Westways*, Vol. 61, No. 3 (March 1969), pp. 26, 31, 47.

of the flamboyant stylist are over, and increasingly cars will be engineered primarily to provide good crash protection.''[90] The recontoured and padded instrument panel, collapsible steering column, energy-absorbent materials in roof areas, securely fastened seats, rear windshield wipers and defrosters, improved seat locks, door locks with recessed handles, a stronger wall between the trunk area and the rear seat, removal of bumper projections, dual braking systems—these are some of the improvements being considered in reformed auto design. Of considerable help in decreasing facial cuts is a new windshield (Figure 3-10). Now required on all U.S.-built cars, it has a plastic interlayer between the two panes of glass. On being struck, ''the outer pane breaks first, reducing the immediate resistance to head impact forces. The . . . inner pane continues to flex, absorbing head impact energy before it break[s] into thousands of small, non-lacerating granules. The plastic interlayer is then free to 'balloon,' cushioning the head forces of the passenger.''[91] After an accident, the granules of glass from the inner pane are found in a small pile on the instrument panel. Recent research has suggested that big windows on two-door cars are a special hazard and should receive similar attention.[92] Of course, the danger is greater when the occupants do not use seat belts.

The 75,000-candlepower, sealed-beam headlight used in U.S. cars has not been improved much in thirty years; it has been described as obsolete for high-speed night driving. Two recommendations about lighting have been suggested (which must be checked against state laws): having special driving lights installed and, in heavy fog, switching on the flashers or driving with a turn signal on ''because being seen, particularly from the rear, is as important as being able to see.''[93]

It should be noted that the size of a car has an effect on the seriousness of an accident. Usually the occupant of a large car will sustain less injury in a crash than the occupant of a small car. When a large car strikes a small car, it is the small car that decelerates and deforms more rapidly. Thus the occupant of the small car also decelerates more rapidly and, in addition, is subjected to the greater deformity of the car.[94]

roads

Safer automobiles must be matched by better road engineering. Small highway improvements are often investments producing big dividends. By a program of such ''spot improvements,'' the County of Los Angeles has made driving safer for its millions of drivers. For example, in wet weather a section of the Hollywood Freeway was noted to be a skidding area. To combat this the pave-

[90] Murray Mackay, ''Safer Cars by 1977,'' p. 214.
[91] A press release from the Corning Glass Works Public Relations Department, November 26, 1968.
[92] ''Big Windows in New Autos Constitute a Safety Hazard,'' *Journal of the American Medical Association,* Vol. 217, No. 11 (September 13, 1971), p. 1460.
[93] John F. McDermott, ''Lights,'' *Hospital Tribune,* Vol. 6, No. 25 (December 18, 1972), p. 19.
[94] John M. Douglass, ''Protection of Automobile Occupants,'' *American Family Physician,* Vol. 4, No. 6 (December 1971), p. 121.

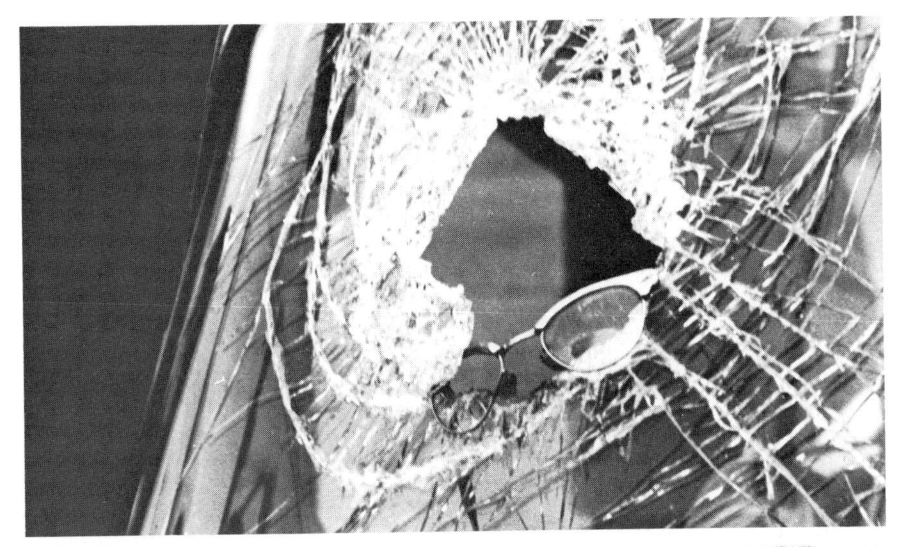

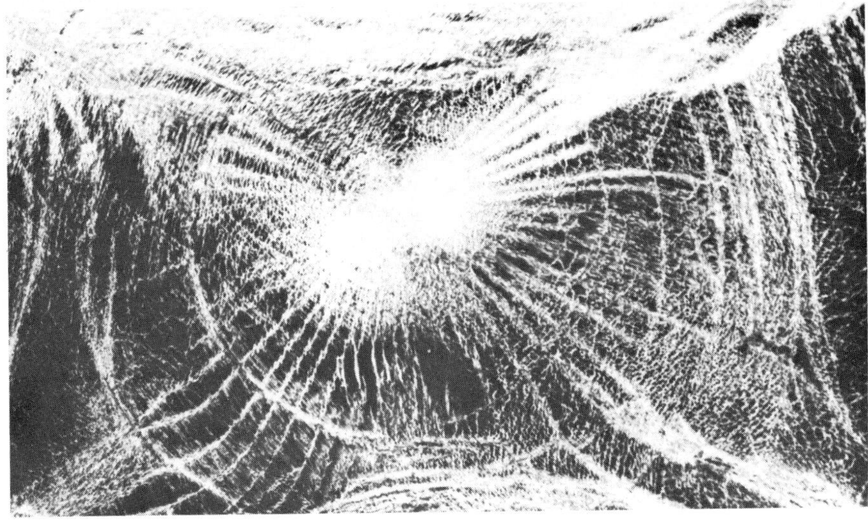

3-10 *After a crash, the eyeglasses of an Indianapolis woman dangle from the smashed windshield* (top). *Damage to her head was severe. A safety windshield* (bottom) *breaks into blunt-edged, nonlacerating granules.*

ment was regrooved. The result was almost a 90 percent reduction in accidents. A program in which locations of consistent accidents are studied and improved has spread throughout the state. Redesigned and relocated signs and land markings, adequate roadway widening, the construction of channeling islands—these are but a few of the spot improvements that in "before and after" studies have been shown to reduce accident fatalities by 53 percent and injuries by almost 25 percent.

who should not drive?

Ninety-five million automobiles swarm over the highways of this country. Every year that number increases by 9 million. One hundred and thirty-five million people are licensed to drive them. There is no dearth of advice on how to increase safety on the roads. One expert states that the fast driving of some women may be attributed to their high heels. ''They increase the leverage on the accelerator,'' he claims, ''when they 'sit up' very close to the wheel in order to avoid scuffing the backs of their high heeled shoes.''[95] Regardless of specific causes, it is undeniably true that the driving of some people is an accident on its way to happening. They should not drive.

''In Pennsylvania, a motorist was killed when he crashed into a tree. He was totally blind. An eight-year-old boy directed his driving.''[96] This is an extreme. But it is also extreme to renew licenses by mail, as do thirty states. Some states require an eye examination only with the first issuance of the driver's license, not for license renewal. Surely this practice reflects an unwarranted optimism about the efficiency of aging vision.

What about drivers who are ill? ''Half of the drivers who have heart attacks behind the wheel are unaware of their heart disease until the accident occurs.''[97] A group of serious accident risks can and should be medically identified, if only to protect them against themselves. As for alcoholic drivers, a strictly punitive approach has been tried and has failed. What is needed is early identification of such drivers, who should then be given therapy and be denied driving privileges until they are cured.

help for the injured

Once an accident has occurred, how quickly does help come? The accident in which the young woman and her unborn twins were killed happened in the open country, seventeen miles from a hospital. Emergency care was not quickly available. Rural areas are poor in emergency services. In an investigation of eight hundred California accidents, it was found that 90 percent of the fatally injured in rural areas died at the crash scene within an hour of the accident.[98] Only 37 percent of those fatally injured in urban areas were dead before they were moved by ambulance. Since rural accident victims often have to be transported twice as far as people injured in cities, more time elapses before they reach the hospital and receive treatment. And the length of time between injury and treatment may be a crucial factor in deciding the victim's fate.

pity the poor pedestrian

About 20 percent of traffic fatalities are pedestrians. ''Pedestrians involved in personal injury traffic accidents are four times more likely to be killed than motorists.''[99] Most are ''relatively impaired for the task of walking in the presence of traffic. The very young[100] and the very old have impairment of judgment and mobility associated with their age.''[101] Decreased vision and intoxication also contribute to pedestrian deaths. In a pedestrian-auto collision, the pedestrian

[95] *The New York Times,* March 14, 1965, Sect. L, p. 85.

[96] Joseph Kelner, ''Highway Murder,'' *The New Republic,* Vol. 157 (September 2, 1967), p. 13.

[97] Julian Waller, ''High 'Accident' Risk Among Middle-Aged Drivers and Pedestrians,'' *Geriatrics,* Vol. 21, No. 12 (December 1966), p. 134.

[98] John H. Rosenow and Robert W. Watkins, ''What the Doctor Can Do to Cut the Traffic Toll,'' *Modern Medicine,* Vol. 35, No. 12 (June 5, 1967), p. 50.

[99] ''Researchers 'Rev Up' for Safer Driving,'' p. 990.

[100] The pedestrian accident risk is highest for children between five and ten years old. The first hour after school is dismissed on weekdays is the time of peak risk for these children. The spring months are particularly dangerous. (''Researchers 'Rev Up' for Safer Driving,'' p. 990, citing A. J. McLean, Department of Epidemiology, Harvard University School of Public Health.)

[101] Julian Waller, ''High 'Accident' Risk Among Middle-Aged Drivers and Pedestrians,'' p. 131.

is not usually "run over."[102] He is lifted up by the car. It runs under him. His head hits the hood, or, while sprawled on the hood, he travels briefly along with the fast-moving vehicle, striking his head on the windshield and car roof. Cars without sloping hoods inflict more severe head injuries to a pedestrian than those with longer hoods. Similarly, cars with "gingerbread" projections are more injurious. The benefits of safer auto design are apparent, not only for the driver, but also for the pedestrian.

motorcycle hazards

"Let go thy hold," counsels the Fool in *King Lear,* "when a great wheel runs down a hill, lest it break thy neck with following it" (II.iv.72–74). Good advice, but not easily followed by modern motorcyclists. Too often they have no chance to let go. They are jarred loose and thrown.

In 1972, there were 2,600 motorcycle deaths in the United States, a 16.2 percent increase over the preceding year. A motorcycle accident is far more likely to kill the driver than an automobile collision. Incomplete data from various states suggest the following general profile of a motorcycle accident: it involves an inexperienced and untrained young male, driving a rented or borrowed standard-sized motorcycle, in daylight, on a summer Saturday, on a dry road, at a speed too fast for conditions, who collides at right angles with a passenger car or truck, the driver of which will claim he never saw the motorcycle.[103]

Experience is of critical importance for safe motorcycle driving. In a British study, Ryan found that drivers with less than six months' experience had a considerably higher accident rate than those with more experience.[104] Training in motorcycle operation is essential. More than half of the motorcycle accident victims sustain head injuries. Not all helmets are adequate. Ryan recommends "that the minimal standards for motorcyclist helmets should be British Standard . . . This provides for an all-enveloping shell, completely lined with energy absorbing material." Protective clothing on the legs and compulsory installation of crash (roll) bars on motorcycles have also been urged.[105]

"be it ever so humble . . ."

"A child playing on the floor suddenly cries out in pain and immediately jumps to a standing position. Either the child or a nearby adult inspects the painful

[102] A tragic exception is the small child run over by a car backing out of a driveway. Every year three hundred children in this country are killed in this way. (National Safety Council, "Children in the Driveway: Family Safety," cited in Harvey Kravitz and Alvin Korach, "Deaths in Suburbia," *Clinical Pediatrics,* Vol. 5, No. 5 [May 1966], p. 266.)

[103] Data from the Statistics Division of the National Safety Council: "Motorcycle Facts—1971," published by the Greater Los Angeles Chapter of the National Safety Council.

[104] G. Anthony Ryan, "Injuries in Traffic Accidents," *New England Journal of Medicine,* Vol. 276, No. 19 (May 11, 1967), pp. 1069–72.

[105] "Helmets Can Cut the Death Rate in Half," an editorial in *California's Health,* Vol. 25, No. 1 (July 1967), p. 6.

area and discovers a sewing needle partially penetrating . . . the knee.''[106] This is a rare household mishap. But the fact that the writers of this report carefully collected twenty-one cases of needle-in-the-knee does reflect the growing interest by medical people in household accidents.

Of the 27,000 people killed in the home in this country during 1972, a major portion were very young (under five) or old (seventy-five or over). Falls and burns account for a high proportion of deaths from household accidents.

falls The astronaut John Glenn managed to travel out of this world and back again without getting so much as a scratch. It was his crash landing on a bathroom floor that gave him dizzy spells for months. That year, he was one of the 3 million citizens of this nation who were involved in accidents in the home.

In no age group are fatal falls more common than among the elderly. Arthritis, dizziness induced by poor blood supply to the brain, vision impairment—all commonly precipitate falls. Emotional stress or depression may be just as conducive to falling as a misplaced rug or a slippery floor. An elderly retiree may rise in the morning, out of sorts, still vaguely fatigued. He can think of no place to go. Not bothering to tie his shoelaces is but another sign of his discouragement. But if he stumbles down the stairs, he may lose his life. Railings, elastic shoelaces, night lights, luminous paint around light switches—these are among the devices wisely suggested to prevent falls by the elderly.[107]

Toddlers are a special problem. Only slowly do they learn to practice safety. While they are growing up, they must be protected—not frightened—from their normal curiosity. ''About fifteen children die daily as a result of needless accidents: this is more than die as a result of the five leading diseases combined (cancer, congenital malformations, pneumonia, gastroenteritis, and heart disease).''[108] Between 3 P.M. and 6 P.M. the preschooler is most tired and hungry and is most likely to have an accident. It is also the time when his mother is likely to feel that she is losing the footrace with her runabout child. The use of a babysitter for an hour or two—especially during the extra-busy early after-school hours—is often a surprisingly good investment.

fires When Longfellow wrote about a ''martyrdom of fire,'' he was being painfully autobiographical. Years before, his wife had been preparing to seal some locks of their children's hair with wax when her flimsy dress had caught fire. She died. The poet had tried to save her; his face was badly burned in the process. It was

[106] Robert H. Ramsey and Floyd G. Goodman, ''The Sewing Needle and the Knee,'' *Journal of the American Medical Association,* Vol. 199, No. 1 (January 2, 1967), p. 23. Another childhood household accident of unknown frequency is trauma to the penis of small boys caused by the dropping down of the elevated toilet seat. It has been referred to in a major medical journal as ''the Toilet Seat Syndrome'' or ''the Small Slam.'' Prevention presently ''consists of informing mothers with young boys to avoid putting covers on toilet seats. The ultimate cure may have to be legislation mandating thicker rubber cushions on the toilet seat which will protect the vulnerable penis should the seat fall onto the bowl top.'' (Howard C. Mofenson, ''Penile Trauma,'' *Journal of the American Medical Association,* Vol. 225, No. 11 [September 10, 1973], pp. 1388–89.)

[107] Dorothy M. Sharp, ''Safety in the Home,'' *Canadian Journal of Public Health,* Vol. 58, No. 1 (January 1967), p. 23.

[108] ''Pediatric Briefs,'' *Clinical Pediatrics,* Vol. 5, No. 12 (December 1966), p. 12A.

probably to hide the scars that he grew his famed full beard.[109] The tragedy that befell him is still common. Every year no fewer than 150,000 people in this country suffer burns because of clothing that catches fire. Thousands more are injured or killed by blazes in bedding or other household furnishings. Most of these terrifying experiences are preventable.

Wool is the most naturally fire-resistant of all fabrics. Cotton, viscose, and rayon burn quickly, but unless they are very sheer they can be made fire-resistant by the addition of chemicals without adverse changes in their texture. The Gemini space astronauts wore space-suits made of high-temperature–resistant nylon, as did all but one of the drivers in the 1966 Indianapolis "500" automobile race.[110] Glass textiles are permanently flame-retardant. Polyester can be made flame-retardant. Fiberglass Beta yarns are sheer and softly fine. They are now used in bedding, draperies, and home furnishings and soon will be added to some clothing. Saran is flame-retardant. Acrylic (which is better known by the trade names Orlon, Acrilan, Creslan, and Zafron) is very flammable. It can be combined with Modacrylic, a flame-retardant fiber. Mixed fibers may be dangerous. Clothing of a combination cotton and synthetic material can be most hazardous. Cotton and rayon support combustion. Some synthetic fibers, when afire, melt into sticky substances which cause grievous burns. Those who purchase play clothes for children should remember that denim burns slowly. Paper garments are best avoided.

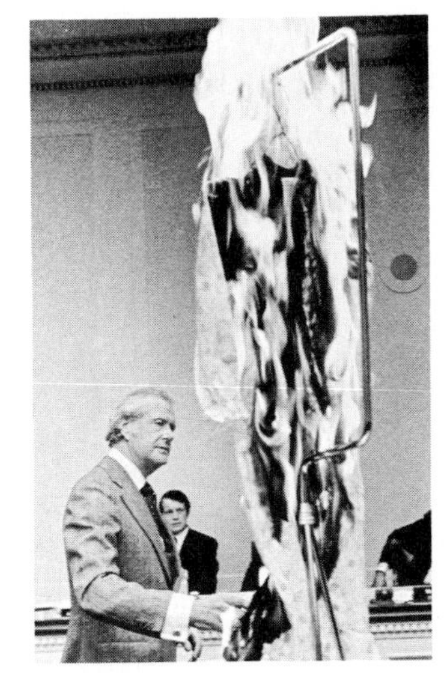

3-11 *A demonstration of the dangerous inadequacy of the standards set by the Flammable Fabrics Act. A match put to a nightgown causes it to burst instantly into flames.*

Little girls are particularly susceptible to clothing fires because most girls are attracted to such hazards as ruffles, flounces, and bell-type sleeves. Women preferring these styles must exercise special care. Indeed, women's clothing, in standing further out from the body than men's, is more susceptible to fire.[111]

suffocations and poisonings

In the home, suffocations and poisonings of children occur with tragic frequency. Some children suffocate from regurgitation of food; consequently, propping up a baby's bottle and leaving him to eat alone can be dangerous. Plastic bags and small metal objects constitute a distinct hazard. They fit into a toddler's eager mouth and may clog his windpipe.

The dimming vision of the elderly is responsible for many medication accidents. Clear labeling of bottles, adequate lighting in the bathroom, and corrected vision can combine to prevent many painful mistakes. But most accidental poisonings happen to children. Every year, in this country, about three hundred youngsters under the age of five die from ingested poisons. More poisonings occur between the ages of eighteen and twenty-four months than during any other six-month age-span. The most commonly ingested chemicals are aspirin, cleaning and polishing agents, and pesticides.[112] When a possibly poisoned child is being rushed to a physician for help, it is important to remember to bring along the poison container. A physician can telephone the nearest poison control center and be provided with immediate information about the poison and its antidote. Such centers exist in all major cities.

[109] *M.D., Medical Newsmagazine,* Vol. 1, No. 4 (April 1957), pp. 42–43.
[110] "Fabrics and Accidental Burns," an editorial in *Clinical Pediatrics,* Vol. 6, No. 8 (August 1967), p. 455.
[111] Manuel Castro, "Torch of Tragedy," *Michigan's Health,* Vol. 55, No. 3 (May–June 1967), pp. 6–9.
[112] Henry L. Verhulst and John J. Crotty, "Childhood Poisoning Accidents," *Journal of the American Medical Association,* Vol. 203, No. 12 (March 18, 1968), pp. 1049–50.

dangerous fun and games

Some sportsmen get their pleasure from daring death. In this country, some thirty thousand people taunt it by racing automobiles. During three years (1964–66), more than a hundred racing drivers were accidentally killed.[113] Skydiving is another daredevil sport that is gaining popularity.

Perhaps a million people skin dive and scuba dive. Those with a history of illness, particularly if it is related to the heart and the lungs, should do neither. The experience of some physicians has led them to also apply this restriction to those with minor colds and moderately high blood pressure. As basic as medical fitness is training; few well-trained divers are ever endangered. The minimum beginning age should be about seventeen. No diver should ever engage alone in the sport. A "buddy" should always accompany him. An important aspect of skin and scuba diving, rarely considered by amateur divers, is the quality of air. A few fly-by-night operators selling contaminated air can do much harm. The local health department is the best source of advice about air.

In 1972, about 7,400 people drowned in the U. S. Males drown six times as often as females. Moreover, many more males than females drown as a result of water transportation accidents. Many studies attest to the estimate that fully "half the people in the United States do not swim well enough to cope with emergencies in water."[114] Nor are near-drowning victims immediately out of danger merely because they return to consciousness. Death from oxygen-shortage may still occur. All near-drowning victims should promptly be hospitalized for further care. Adequate water safety programs are long overdue. Most drownings, however, occur in water not specifically set aside for recreation. The old swimming hole is not as safe as a public beach.

Experienced skiers among this nation's 5 million skiers know the importance of adequate ski equipment, physical conditioning, and training. Particularly important is the proper adjustment of the boot's release-bindings so that when undue stress occurs the boot will easily release from the ski. Muscles both steer and brake the skier. Their condition is critically important. Preseason exercise programs are valuable, as are warm-up periods before starting down a hill. Excessive fatigue should be avoided. Training in equipment use and skiing technique is essential, but such training does not supplant the wisdom of knowing one's limits on the slopes. About 225,000 skiers in this country are injured every year. Eighty percent of all injuries and 89 percent of all fractures involve a leg. For every 1,000 skiers, an average of 4.5 will be injured on any given day. The beginning skier has an injury rate about five times greater than an expert's. One week of instruction halves that rate.[115] The Ski Patrol, a splendid organization of experienced skiers devoted to first aid, should be supported by everyone interested in skiing, the most rapidly growing winter sport.

[113] "Fatalities in Hazardous Sports," *Statistical Bulletin* of the Metropolitan Life Insurance Company, Vol. 48 (May 1967), p. 7. Unfortunately, because of changes in record keeping, more recent reliable data on deaths of racing drivers is presently unavailable.

[114] *Statistical Bulletin* of the Metropolitan Life Insurance Company, Vol. 49 (March 1968), p. 5.

[115] Arthur E. Ellison, "Skiing Injuries," *Journal of the American Medical Association,* Vol. 223, No. 8 (February 19, 1973), pp. 917–19.

summary

Because humans are best able of all living creatures to control their environment, they are best able to pollute it. As humans have increased in numbers and needs, their relationship with their environment has deteriorated. They are now beset by numerous man-made environmental hazards, including:

1. *Water pollution.* U.S. waterways are threatened by wasteful use of water, inadequate sewage treatment, disposal of industrial chemical wastes in rivers and lakes, and thermal pollution (pages 45–48). The Water Quality Act of 1965 and the Water Pollution Control Act of 1966 are helping to protect surface waters—rivers, lakes, and streams—but pollution of deep wells remains a problem. The Great Lakes Water Quality Agreement signed in 1972 by the United States and Canada was one step toward the restoration of the vast and vital Great Lakes waterway. Programs have also been undertaken to halt the pollution of such other surface waters as Oregon's Willamette River and New York's Hudson River.

2. *Solid waste.* Solid waste (garbage and rubbish) is often disposed of by *open-dump burning* or *dumping into water* (page 51). Better disposal methods attempt to reuse solid wastes; such methods include *incineration* (which can produce a usable ash) and using garbage as *land fill* (page 51). Still more efficient methods are *pulverization, compaction, composting,* and *pyrolysis* (pages 51–52).

3. *Air pollution.* The two types of air pollution, *London-type smog* and *Los Angeles-type smog,* are caused by *temperature inversion* (page 53). Among the dangers of London-type smog is the suspension of sulfuric acid in fog (page 54). In Los Angeles-type smog (also called "oxidizing" or "photochemical" smog), pollutants are trapped near the ground by an inversion layer of warm air; the sun's ultraviolet light reacts with the pollutants, notably the *hydrocarbons* and the *oxides of nitrogen,* to produce poisonous *ozone* (page 55). Another deadly polluting gas is *carbon monoxide,* a product of the combustion of gasoline (pages 55 and 59). Major air pollution disasters have occurred in London in 1952 and in Donora, Pennsylvania, in 1948 (page 56). "Excess deaths" from respiratory ailments occurred during pollution episodes in New York City in 1953 and again in 1966 (pages 56–57). Air pollution may be associated with lung cancer (pages 58–59). Because the automobile is the major source of air pollution, stricter emission standards are being imposed and methods of transportation are being sought that are cleaner and more efficient than the internal combustion engine. The first worldwide effort to curb pollution was the United Nations Conference on the Human Environment, held in Stockholm in 1972.

4. *Traffic accidents.* Every year in the United States, traffic accidents kill thousands of people (56,600 in 1972) and injure millions of others (about 14,600 each day). These grim numbers can be reduced by the use of safety belts, air bags, and safe and well-cared-for tires, by safer vehicle design, and by construction, improvement, and maintenance of better roads.

5. *Other accidents.* Accidents in the home cause thousands of deaths each year. Many home accidents can be prevented, for example by using flame-retardant clothing, by ensuring that the home is adequately lighted, and by storing poisons and medicines out of the reach of children. Sports are another source of accidents, particularly automobile racing, skydiving, skin and scuba diving, swimming, and skiing.

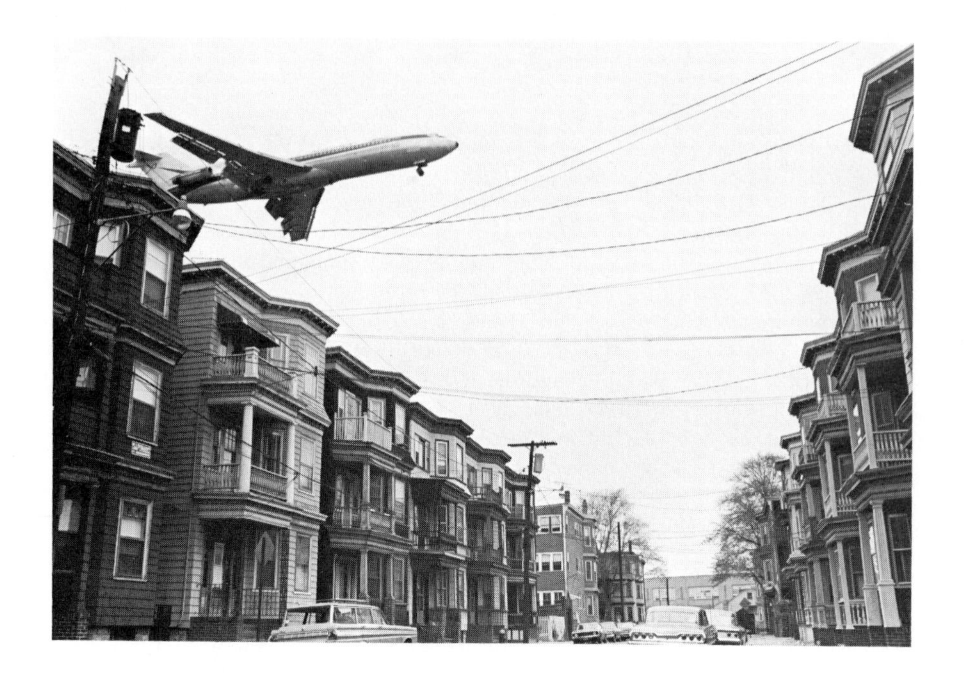

chemicals, radiation, and noise

4

pesticides

To insure health, a man's relation to Nature must come very near to a personal one; he must be conscious of a friendliness in her . . . I cannot conceive of any life which deserves the name, unless there is a certain tender relation to Nature.
(Henry David Thoreau, *Journal,* 1858)

Suddenly the Maharaja Palden Thondup Namgyal sat up. He leaned forward in his camp chair beside the roaring Teetsa River. His eyes lit up with pleasure. He pointed to an orange and silver butterfly, a dazzling ephemera, lightly hovering above a delicately scented clematis blossom. "Maybe they are coming back to Sikkim," he murmured hopefully. "That's the fifth butterfly I've seen in an hour's time."

Once Sikkim was a butterfly's paradise. Some native butterflies had a wing span of eight or nine inches. Now they are all gone. The Sikkim ecosystem had also included the malaria mosquito. DDT rid the tiny Indian protectorate of malaria, but the pesticide was unselective. The butterfly perished too.[1]

One day some years ago, in Cincinnati, Ohio, a great red cloud darkened the sky. In less than an hour the city lay in a shroud of red dust. Yet, nobody seemed to be harmed. Analysis proved the dust to be loaded with pesticides and other agricultural chemicals. Days, months, perhaps years before, they had been laid down on farms in Texas and Oklahoma. An unusual windstorm had lifted them high into the atmosphere and had carried them more than a thousand miles to be dumped on Cincinnati.[2]

the competing insect: harbinger of hunger, bearer of disease

These incidents are rooted in a deep crisis. They are the result of the inexorable war between man and those plants and animals that threaten his food supply. The wistful Maharaja of Sikkim and the dusty citizens of Cincinnati reflect the increasing chemicalization of the world's ecosystems. Why has this occurred? Why does man use pesticides?

Issa (1762–1826), perhaps the most beloved of all Japanese poets, wrote:

> Oh, don't mistreat
> the fly! He wrings his hands!
> He wrings his feet![3]

The kindly Issa notwithstanding, men everywhere seek to destroy insects. Implacably competitive, insects bring two calamities to man: starvation and sickness.

In *The Good Earth,* Pearl Buck told about the first of these calamities:

> Then the sky grew black and the air was filled with the deep still roar of many wings beating against each other, and upon the land the locusts fell, flying over this field and leaving it whole, and falling upon that field, and eating it as bare as winter. And men sighed and said "So Heaven wills," but Wang Lung was furious and he beat the locusts and trampled on them.

Experienced with hunger, Wang Lung feared it.

[1] *The New York Times,* July 10, 1966, Sect. L, p. 15.
[2] Gladwin Hill, *The New York Times,* February 25, 1965, p. 68.
[3] Quoted in Harold G. Henderson, *An Introduction to Haiku* (Garden City, N.Y., 1958), p. 126.

how pesticides serve mankind

From the nutritional standpoint alone, it would be idle to deny the benefits of pesticides. To the people of the United States, they have made possible a diet envied almost everywhere. Vitamin deficiency diseases (see Chapter 22) are not nearly as common as they were a generation ago. And other diseases indicating poor nutrition are disappearing. Partly because of iodized salt, but also because of adequate food iodine, goiter (a thyroid gland disease) is no longer common in this country. In other parts of the world goiter is so common that dolls are made with swollen necks. People there think the enlarged neck normal.

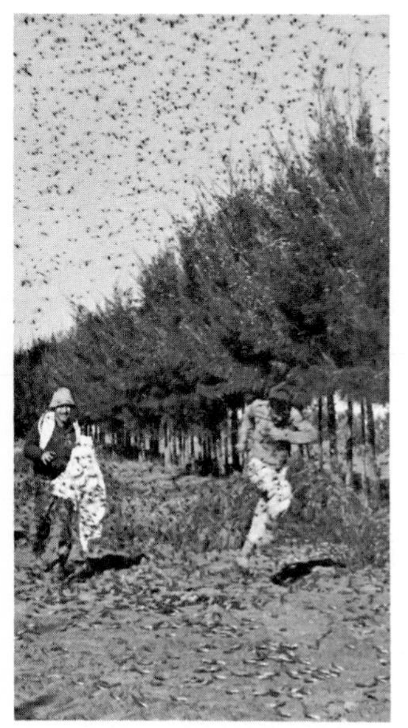

4-1 *The eternal battle between man and insect. Two farmers run from a swarm of locusts in Israel.*

But pesticides have done more than help provide an abundance of better foods for less cost. Countless lives have been saved by them. Typhus, yellow fever, and the river-blindness of Africa and Central America are but three of the insect-borne plagues of mankind that can be controlled by pesticides. But it is malaria that is most often cited as a classic example of the value of these insect-killing chemicals. Few diseases have so drained the strength and dwindled the numbers of man as malaria: "it has been accused of responsibility, directly or indirectly, for over one-half the world's mortality."[4] Since 1962, use of DDT has been intensified in many countries. In some previously malarial areas the consequent changes in the ecosystem have made the survival of the malarial mosquito impossible. The result: unparalleled prevention of sickness and great saving of life. Because of DDT, more than a billion people now live in malaria-free areas. Every year 3 million lives are spared. At last, entire countries have successfully brought malaria under control. Now they can hope for a better economy. Once it had been rightly said, "Whom malaria does not kill, it enslaves."[5] DDT changed all that. But what of the threat to the environment? Has mankind traded eventual catastrophe for temporary advantage?

[4] Louis L. Williams, "Pesticides: A Contribution to Public Health," in *Man—His Environment and Health,* a supplement to *American Journal of Public Health,* Vol. 54, No. 1 (January 1964), p. 34.
[5] Lewis Hackett, quoted in Louis L. Williams, "Pesticides: A Contribution to Public Health," p. 34.

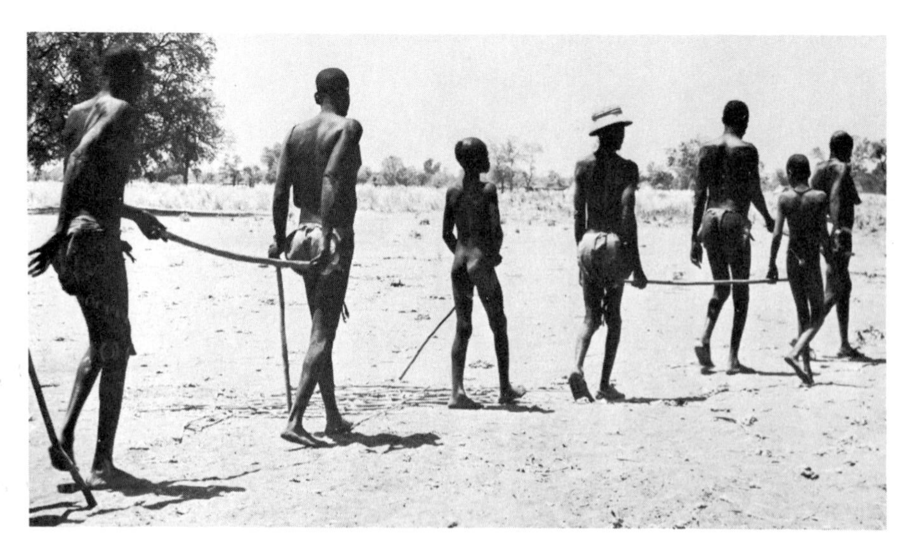

4-2 *A tiny fly that transmits river-blindness has brought tragedy to many West African villages. Many people have fled, leaving behind a population in which all the adults are blind and must be cared for by their children.*

pesticide problems

More than 56,000 trade name pesticides are marketed today. Designed to kill insects, rodents, fungi, and weeds, they also find their way into people. How? By inhalation of contaminated air, by absorption through the skin, and by oral ingestion. The people in the greatest danger are those whose occupations involve the use of these chemicals, such as workers in pest control operations in agriculture and in malarial areas. But one need not work with pesticides to be exposed to them. They are now part of man's diet; well over three-fourths of his intake is ingested with his food. The air he breathes and the water he drinks also provide him with added measurable doses. Because of the natural fats and oils in cosmetics, pesticides are a common, but generally harmless, contaminant of eye shadows, lipsticks, hair sprays, and hair dressings as well as creams and lotions. Asians (the people of India, for example) have much higher pesticide concentrations in their bodies than do Europeans (such as the English). This is because of the greater pesticide spraying programs in the developing countries. On the other hand, "in the past few years . . . concentrates of DDT in human fatty tissue are more than twice as great in the United States as they are in Britain."[6] And most of the damage to wildlife in this country is due to the inadequate supervision and regulation of DDT spraying here during the late 1950s and early 1960s.

Once absorbed, or during absorption, the pesticide may be broken down into simpler substances (which may then be rendered nontoxic by the liver), stored in various body tissues, or excreted in urine or bile. Fatty tissue is the major reservoir of pesticides. It has been found in such fat-containing tissues as the liver, brain, kidney, and gonads. People with severe kidney or liver diseases might be harmed by pesticide doses that are harmless to normal people. Thus, a man who works as a sprayer of one of these chemicals might become ill because his excretory processes are inefficient and the pesticide or its products pile up in his body.

By wind and water pesticides *spread;* today they are found in the strutting penguin of the Antarctic and the pheasant of California. Some pesticides are more persistent than others in that they are not quickly broken down in the environment; thus they *accumulate.* They also *concentrate* in living tissues. DDT, for example, is insoluble in water. Ingested by small marine animals called plankton, DDT is carried by them up the food chain. Along the way to the top, the pesticide concentrates and is harmful to birds and fish. That DDT can make eggshells thin and thus *interferes with bird reproduction* has been proven; but "it remains a sobering truth that more eagles have been shot by farmers than can possibly have been killed by DDT."[7] Perhaps the most sinister of the characteristics of pesticides is the development, by hundreds of species of insects, of a *genetic resistance* to them (pages 14–16). "The result is an escalating chemical warfare that is self-defeating."[8] Cotton crops are the world's major recipient of pesticide overloads. In California's Imperial Valley, overintensive

4-3 *A boll weevil sitting on a cotton plant.*

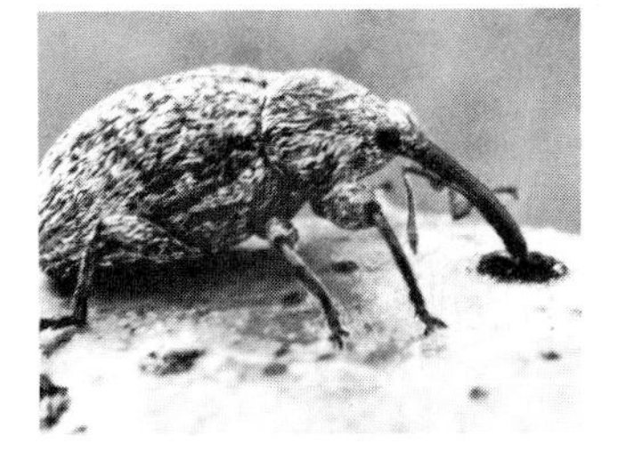

[6] "DDT May Be Good for People," *Nature,* Vol. 233, No. 5320 (October 15, 1971), p. 437.
[7] *Ibid.,* p. 438.
[8] George M. Woodwell, "Toxic Substances and Ecological Cycles," *Scientific American,* Vol. 216, No. 3 (March 1967), p. 31.

use of pesticides has resulted in a whole new breed of insecticide-resistant pests. In addition, the unwise application of pesticides has indiscriminately killed those harmless insects that kept harmful species in check; the destruction of tens of thousands of valuable honeybee colonies triggered a secondary pest invasion and brought the cotton industry in that area to the brink of ruin.[9]

are pesticides harmful to humans?

Unusually high doses of pesticides assuredly are harmful to humans. Twenty-five percent of the fatal poisonings of California children are due to careless storing of pesticides. Such data combined with the thousands of occupational poisonings due to mishandling are harsh testimony to the dangers inherent in these chemicals. But these instances are fortunately unusual. Is there too much pesticide in the average human ecosystem? Does the boy who eats too many apples in one day also eat too much pesticide? Does the woman applying lipstick also absorb and ingest a dangerous dose of an unwanted chemical? Certainly not according to any presently available evidence. DDT is one of the most persistent pesticides. Yet in the thirty years it has been used, there has never been a proved instance of death having resulted from its proper use. To control malaria in developing countries, DDT is not sprayed indiscriminately into the ecosystem; its use is confined to the walls inside homes. No toxic effects have been felt from DDT "in over 20 years of spraying by an estimated 200,000 spraymen working in campaigns around the world, nor, for that matter, by the billion people living in homes constantly sprayed."[10] Moreover, even persistent pesticides are destroyed in the soil, albeit slowly. They are also normally broken down in the body and excreted. They do not pile up indefinitely. Nevertheless, at present concentrations in the United States, does prolonged exposure to pesticides make people sick?

In hasty alarm, some observers have pointed to the effect of DDT on the ability of the hawk to successfully reproduce its kind. But is the observation of the hawk egg applicable to the human embryo? Hardly. The bird embryo has no afterbirth. In this sense it is isolated from the mother. Human maternal defense mechanisms that absorb, detoxify, and excrete pesticides are unavailable to the bird embryo. To produce adverse effects in the embryos of experimental mammals, very large doses, compared to human exposure levels, are necessary. In discussing the value of animal studies as determinants of the safety of pesticide levels for human beings, two experts write: "How reliable is extrapolation of animal data to man? The honest answer to this question is that we do not know."[11] A species that in every respect handles pesticides like man does not exist. However, various species do exist that provide pieces of information that can be extrapolated to man with some confidence. These applications are of a highly technical nature. So because pesticides affect the hawk in one way and a small mammal like the chipmunk in another, it does not necessarily follow

[9] Robert van den Bosch, "The Melancholy Addiction of Ol' King Cotton," *Natural History,* Vol. 80, No. 10 (December 1971), p. 89.

[10] "DDT: Pro and Con," *Gazette,* Pan American Health Organization, World Health Organization, Vol. 3, No. 2 (April–May–June 1971), p. 4.

[11] K. S. Khera and D. J. Clegg, "Perinatal Toxicity of Pesticides," *Canadian Medical Association Journal,* Vol. 100, No. 4 (January 25, 1969), p. 171.

that a human being would be affected in the same way. Without dismissing the potential danger of pesticides, the informed individual will nevertheless do well to understand the limitation of much of the available data and to question the ''scare'' statements that are often based upon them.

At present levels of pesticide pollution in this country, there are no available data to indicate a harmful effect to the general population. But what about the chronic effects of continued, and possibly increasing doses over a long period of time? Little is known. This is the basic challenge of the pesticide problem. As a result of a U.S. government order that went into effect after December 31, 1972, the agricultural use of DDT has been abolished except for a few minor crops, and then only if the need for it can be proved at hearings. However, concern is being expressed about highly toxic pesticides that may replace DDT.[12] The scientific community comprehends the problem of pesticides. What is it doing about it?

nonchemical pest controls

Considerable research is being conducted to find ways of controlling pests without the use of chemical pesticides. More than half the pesticides used in this country are directed against unwelcome insect visitors who come to stay. *Ship fumigation* and *restriction of incoming agricultural products* have reduced the number of these insect immigrants. And *controlled intentional introduction of foreign pests* provides natural enemies to those already present. Over 150 such predators have been imported for domestic insect control.

Many insects, susceptible to *physical attractants* such as light and sound, may be lured to certain death by poisons. *Chemical attractants,* however, offer more promise. The Mediterranean fruit fly, for example, finds it hard to resist proteins from ripening fruit. Even more irresistible to male insects are the *sex attractants.* Virgin insect females possess but a tiny amount of these chemical substances. But a little of this goes a long way in the insect world. Some insect sex attractants are now synthetically produced in the laboratory. Used as a lure, they entice the male to annihilation. *Sex ''repellents''* may also become useful. Female houseflies mate only once. During copulation the male fly transfers a substance to the female that causes her to reject advances by other males. Scientists are attempting to isolate this monogamy-inducing substance and then to create it in the laboratory. With an ample supply, the tremendous increase of rejecting females will surely decrease the housefly population.[13]

Sophisticated *genetic manipulations* enabled scientists to breed sterile male mosquitoes. It was reasoned that when they would mate with normal females, nothing would come of the union. But the totally sterile males turned out to be less amorous than their nonsterile wild cousins. Now partially sterile male mosquitoes are being bred. Remaining sexually competitive, they compete with normal males in the mating game. Not only are their progeny reduced, but their genetic aberration is bred into the mosquito population. Using such methods of insect birth control, the village of Notre Dame, in southern France, has re-

[12] Henry F. Howe, ''Tunnel Vision in Pesticide Control,'' *Journal of the American Medical Association,* Vol. 223, No. 5 (January 29, 1973), p. 552.
[13] ''Turning the Female House Fly Off Sex,'' *New Scientist,* Vol. 53, No. 786 (March 9, 1972), p. 527.

markably reduced its mosquito population,[14] and the little Burmese town of Okpo recently rid itself of the deadly, mosquito-borne disease filariasis.[15] More programs of this sort are in the offing.

Even an insect's own *hormones* have been turned against it. The development of most insects from larva to pupa is controlled by hormones. These must be secreted in exact amounts and at the proper time. If too much of a hormone is secreted or a hormone is secreted at the wrong time, the insect will not develop properly. Compounds that mimic the insect's own hormones can be turned into effective agents to disrupt insect life. Insects are also proving susceptible to various organisms not expected to be hazardous to other life. For a decade a bacillus has been successfully used against a particularly destructive leaf-eating caterpillar. The bacillus is harmless to the caterpillar's predators, so nature's help is not lost. Insect *viruses* also seem particularly promising, but much research needs to be done.[16]

some other dangerous substances

mercury: a metal named for the Roman god of commerce

The element mercury is familiar as the liquid, elusive "quicksilver" found in thermometers. It is the only metal that is liquid at room temperature. In its metallic form, as a liquid element, mercury is not ordinarily poisonous; "a person could swallow up to a pound or more of quicksilver with no significant adverse effects."[17] So if a child swallowed the mercury from a thermometer, he would not be harmed. Nor is the mercury in dental fillings harmful. However, scientists differentiate between *inorganic* and *organic* mercury. In unusual circumstances, poisoning from metallic mercury and inorganic mercury can occur, as it does among mercury miners who are exposed to the invisible and odorless mercury vapor for prolonged periods. They develop dizziness, headache, and hand tremors so severe that writing is impossible. In usual conditions of exposure, however, neither metallic nor inorganic mercury "remains in the body long enough to accumulate to serious levels."[18] It is the organic chemical methylmercury, and a variety of other organic mercury compounds, that are harmful because they remain in the body for longer periods of time and attack the central nervous system. Until recently, industries were permitted to dump

[14] "Making Mosquitos That Breed Themselves Away," *New Scientist,* Vol. 54, No. 794 (May 4, 1972), p. 248.

[15] "New Genetic Technique Turns Insects Against Themselves," *Newsletter,* a news release from the Public Information Office, Pan American Sanitary Bureau, Regional Office of the World Health Organization (Washington, D.C., August 1967).

[16] An excellent two-part review of recent research on the use of both hormones and viruses for insect control is Jean L. Marx, "Insect Control: Hormones and Viruses," *Science,* Vol. 181, No. 4101 (August 24, 1973), and No. 4102 (August 31, 1973), pp. 833–35. For an interesting review of the search for insect hormones as insecticides see Simon Maddrell, "Insect Hormones as Possible Insecticides," *New Scientist,* Vol. 54, No. 793 (April 27, 1972), pp. 203–05. This article explores the idea that ordinary insecticides may work by causing the release of large amounts of hormones; thus the use of the hormones themselves could avoid the serious disadvantages of pesticides.

[17] Leonard J. Goldwater, "Mercury in the Environment," *Scientific American,* Vol. 224, No. 5 (May 1971), p. 15.

[18] "Mercury in the Environment: Natural and Human Factors," *Science,* Vol. 171, No. 3973 (February 20, 1971), p. 171.

large amounts of inorganic mercury into lakes and rivers. Since mercury is thirteen times as heavy as water, it was assumed that it fell to the bottom, where it remained inert and harmless.

tragedy in Japan

Two Japanese mercury poisoning disasters did not change this belief. Both were due to methylmercury, an organic compound of mercury, and not to inorganic or metallic mercury.[19] The first, and the more serious, epidemic of organic methylmercury disease in Japan began in 1953. Two hundred and two people developed the disease as a result of eating fish taken from the industrially contaminated waters of Minamata Bay. Some signs and symptoms were: progressive blindness and deafness, inability to speak, muscle weakness and lack of coordination, paralysis, and mental retardation.[20] Fifty-two people died.

That methylmercury readily crosses the placental barrier, that it reaches a higher concentration in the red blood cells of an unborn child than it does in the red blood cells of the mother, that fetal nervous tissue seems to be particularly susceptible to injury by methylmercury, that it is possible for a pregnant woman to show no symptoms, yet give birth to a severely damaged child—these were among the bitter lessons learned from the Japanese experience. Organic methylmercury poisoning earned a dread name: *Minamata disease.* Why does methylmercury harm the child more than the mother? This is believed due to the differences in chemical structure between the embryonic and fetal hemoglobin in the red blood cells and that of the mother's. Moreover, a relatively moderate daily dose of the poison for a pregnant woman becomes a highly toxic dose for the much smaller child. A third reason that the unborn child is more likely to be damaged than the mother is that his nervous system is in the process of development. Only healthily dividing cells can result in healthy tissues and organs. Initial damage to dividing cells, then, results in accumulated damage. These factors are often forgotten by pregnant women who abuse drugs.

4-4 *A victim of Minamata disease stands as a silent reminder to the 1972 United Nations Conference on the Human Environment that "an individual cannot be replaced."*

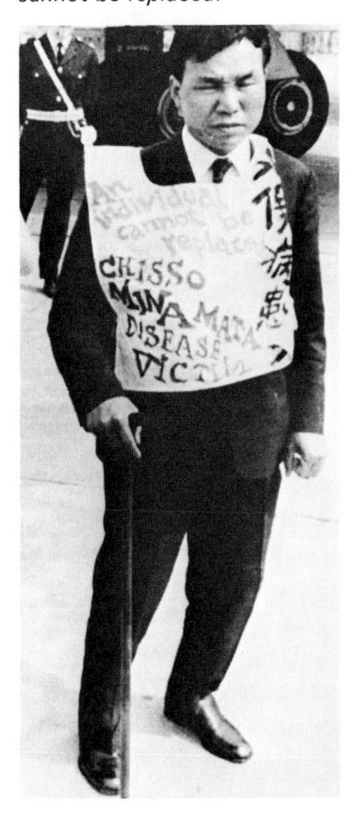

inorganic mercury may also become harmful

The belief that inorganic mercury was harmless was not disproved until 1970, when Swedish scientists reported that indiscriminate dumping of inorganic mercury into rivers and lakes could be dangerous. Relatively harmless inorganic mercury can be converted into poisonous organic methylmercury by microorganisms in the beds of these waters. The mercury can then leave the sediments at the bottoms of the waters and pass into the bodies of fish. Organic methylmercury in water is a natural phenomenon and so is its presence in fish. It becomes a poisonous hazard to man only when he consumes large amounts of fish from waters containing high levels of the chemical. So great was the amount of organic methylmercury in the waters of Minamata Bay that, despite

[19] "Mercury: A Modern Dilemma," *Michigan's Health,* Vol. 59, No. 2 (Summer 1971), p. 3.
[20] Willard A. Krehl, "Mercury, the Slippery Metal," *Nutrition Today,* Vol. 7, No. 6 (November–December 1972), p. 6.

their greater tolerance to the chemical, even the fish developed nerve-muscle disorders.[21] Moreover, microscopic examination of their nervous tissues revealed considerable damage. Fish lose their body methylmercury much more slowly than do terrestrial vertebrates that are higher on the evolutionary scale.[22] In Minamata Bay, the fish were simply taking in methylmercury more rapidly than they could rid themselves of it.

not all fish are unsafe

There is much public alarm that mercury pollution has made the consumption of all fish unsafe. This is not valid. Whether organic or inorganic, man's mercury pollutions are concentrated in one area, and they tend to remain restricted in that area. The contaminated fish of Minamata Bay cannot be compared to wide-ranging ocean fish, which have thrived in mercury-containing waters for millions of years. Organic mercury found in these fish is not generally due to man's pollutions. This is evident from the fact that mercury is present in preserved fish, found at archeological sites, that are hundreds, even thousands, of years old. Thus, for many centuries man has been consuming fish that contain varying amounts of natural organic mercury without apparent harm. In addition, recent evidence suggests that another widely distributed element, selenium (and its products), seems to protect organisms from the toxic effects of organic mercury. And there is authoritative opinion that mercury, like other trace elements, may be essential to health. Still another factor is of importance: people differ in their reactions to similar amounts of methylmercury. And, finally, it should be remembered that fish is not a popular food in some countries, including the United States, whereas in other countries, like Japan, fish may be eaten three times a day. Thus, it is not *whether* methylmercury is present in fish that is the basic factor in determining a threat to public health, but *how much.*

With these considerations in mind, the federal Food and Drug Administration has established standards for an acceptable level of the chemical in foods. It is worth noting that some experts consider these standards too conservative.

a young graduate student makes a contribution

As a result of the research of Norvald Fimreite, a Norwegian graduate student at the University of Western Ontario, the Canadian government, in March 1970, advised U.S. authorities of an unacceptably high level of organic methylmercury in fish in Lake St. Clair, downstream from a chemical plant in Sarnia, Canada.[23] The U.S. government swung into action. Several industrial

[21] Fish-eating cats were also dying of Minamata disease, and crows, also fish-eaters, were toppling from their perches. (John J. Putman, "Quicksilver and Slow Death," *National Geographic,* Vol. 142, No. 4 [October 1972], p. 516.)

[22] "Fish Retain Mercury for Long Periods," *Journal of the American Medical Association,* Vol. 220, No. 9 (May 29, 1972), p. 1180.

[23] Anthony C. Celeste and Clifford G. Shane, "Mercury in Fish," *FDA Papers,* Vol. 4, No. 9 (November 1970), p. 4. At about the same time as the discovery of the Lake St. Clair pollution, the nation was shocked to learn of the methylmercury poisoning of three children from a farm family in New Mexico. Every day for three months

plants were ordered to stop dumping mercury immediately. In April 1970, the U.S. Food and Drug Administration began an expanding effort to determine which U.S. bodies of water were being contaminated by mercury. Also begun was a program to test for mercury fish taken from both foreign and domestic waters. By mid-September 1970, fishing limitations had been imposed in eighteen states. Pollution of water by mercury has remained a continuing concern of both federal and state governments.[24]

PCBs: much use, too little knowledge

Still another example of widespread, inadequately regulated use of a chemical that results in possibly dangerous pollution is a group of highly toxic chemicals called polychlorinated biphenyls (PCBs). They are used in a wide variety of materials including adhesives, sealants, and paints. The major causes of pollution by PCBs are thought to be sewage outfalls and industrial disposal in waterways. High concentrations are being found in Long Island Sound and the Great Lakes. Are PCBs harmful? In high enough concentration they can be. Not long ago a thousand Japanese were accidentally poisoned by PCBs. PCBs easily cross the placenta, and babies believed sick from the pollutant have been born of apparently unaffected Japanese mothers.

The U.S. Food and Drug Administration has placed a safety limit on PCBs in human food. "Nevertheless, PCBs have been detected at concentrations far higher than the FDA's maximum."[25] Early in 1972 it was stated that "the biological actions of PCBs inside the body are . . . relatively unknown."[26] But subsequent research has been troubling. Birds given fatal doses of PCBs develop enlarged kidneys, leg paralysis, and trembling of the body and wings before dying. And high levels of PCBs given to rhesus monkeys for three months induced changes in their stomach linings that were strongly suggestive of cancer. Moreover, "The concentration of the biphenyl within the experimental diet was less than . . . that occurring in random food samples sold in the United States and less than levels which have occurred in food products as a result of industrial accidents."[27]

4-5 *A member of the farm family poisoned by methylmercury (footnote 23) learns to walk again at the age of twenty.*

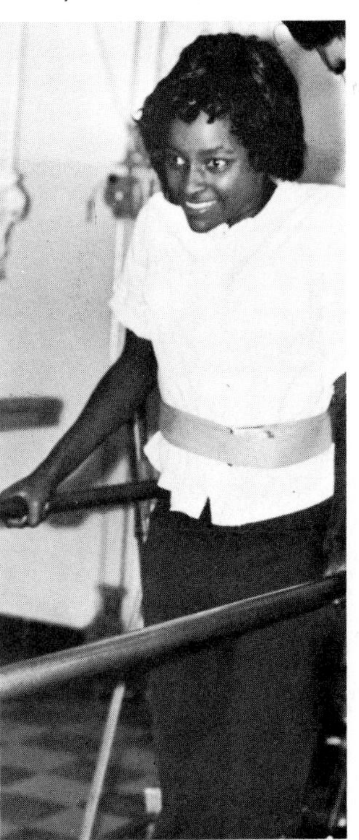

during the winter of 1969–70, they had eaten the meat of a boar that had been fed with a garbage mixture containing seeds that had been treated with a methylmercury pesticide. All the children survived. However, at the end of 1972, two were still severely handicapped. When the family started eating the meat, the mother was three months pregnant. Her baby is now blind and retarded. Had such contaminated pork reached the market, could an epidemic of methylmercury poisoning have resulted? No. A given consumer would receive only a small fraction of the carcass and, thus, too small a dose to cause concern. (Paul E. Pierce, Jon F. Thompson, William H. Likosky, Laurence N. Nickey, William F. Barthell, and Alan R. Hinman, "Alkyl Mercury Poisoning in Humans," *Journal of the American Medical Association,* Vol. 220, No. 11 [June 12, 1972], pp. 1439–41.) The federal government has taken steps to prevent a similar incident of this, the first known U.S. incident of methylmercury poisoning from contaminated food. The use of methylmercury compounds in such a way that they can enter the food chain is prohibited. This will prevent a repetition of a recent tragedy that occurred in Iraq. A large shipment of mercury-treated grain seed was distributed among villagers. They used it to make bread and to feed animals. Four hundred and fifty people died. Thousands more were stricken.

[24] Anthony C. Celeste and Clifford G. Shane, "Mercury in Fish," pp. 28–30. Since April 1970, thousands of samples of tuna, swordfish, and other fish have been examined in the laboratories of the U.S. Food and Drug Administration. Also carried out have been several nationwide tests of a wide variety of other foods. "The results of these studies indicate that mercury levels present in the bulk of the food supplies is very low; only in fish and fishery products were significant mercury residues detected." In these latter instances, all possibility of human consumption was prevented. (Albert C. Kolbye, "Mercury Residues," *Letters, Science,* Vol. 175, No. 4027 [March 17, 1972], p. 1192.)

[25] "PCB's Danger May Be Underestimated," *New Scientist,* Vol. 57, No. 832 (February 8, 1973), p. 284.

[26] "Chemical Pollution: Polychlorinated Biphenyls," *Science,* Vol. 175, No. 4018 (January 14, 1972), p. 156.

[27] J. R. Allen and D. H. Norback, "Polychlorinated Biphenyl- and Triphenyl-Induced Gastric Mucosal Hyperplasia in Primates," *Science,* Vol. 179, No. 4072 (February 2, 1973), p. 498.

Some PCBs are controllable, in that they are used in enclosed, sealed systems, making pollution unlikely. Others are noncontrollable, in that they come in direct contact with the environment. The chemical company that monopolizes the manufacture of PCBs in North America has already informed its customers that orders for noncontrollable PCBs would not be filled. Whether competing companies in Europe and Japan will follow suit remains to be seen.[28] However, it would seem wise to know the effect such chemicals have on people before permitting wide exposure to them.

lead poisoning: epidemic of childhood

Man has been digging lead out of the ground for five thousand years. Centuries of dismal experience have taught him caution with this highly useful metal. Not only did the ancient Roman aristocracy store wine in lead-containing earthenware pots, but they added lead oxide to the wine to reduce its acidity. It has been suggested that the consumption of lead-poisoned wine by the aristocratic women of Rome caused considerable sterility, stillbirths, and brain damage. Such widespread affliction among the ruling classes, it is theorized, deteriorated and diminished the following generations, thus contributing to the fall of the Roman Empire.[29] Today, lead-containing ceramic glazes used on clay pottery have caused lead poisoning and even death.[30] Large amounts of lead may be leached out of the glaze into acidic beverages or vegetables.[31]

Recent years have seen a growing concern about lead poisoning (*plumbism*) in small children. In 1970, the Surgeon General of the Public Health Service estimated that about 400,000 children in this nation have dangerously high lead levels in their blood.[32] One-fourth of those children treated for lead poisoning have suffered permanent damage, such as mental retardation and visual disorders. Most of the recognized cases have occurred in children between one and five years of age. Studies have revealed that 10 to 25 percent of this country's inner-city children have absorbed dangerous quantities of lead.[33]

[28] Jon Tinker, "The PCB Story: Seagulls Aren't Funny Any More," *New Scientist and Science Journal*, Vol. 50, No. 745 (April 1, 1971), pp. 16–18.

[29] Dale W. Jenkins, "The Toxic Metals in Your Future—and Your Past," *Smithsonian*, Vol. 3, No. 1 (April 1972), p. 65.

[30] Michael Klein, Rosalie Namer, Eleanor Harpur, and Richard Corbin, "Earthenware Containers as a Source of Fatal Lead Poisoning," *New England Journal of Medicine*, Vol. 283, No. 13 (September 24, 1970), pp. 4–7.

[31] Stephen K. Hall, "Pollution and Poisoning," *Environmental Science and Technology*, Vol. 6, No. 1 (January 1972), p. 31.

[32] "Lead Poisoning Can Cause Blindness," *The Sight-Saving Review*, Vol. 41, No. 2 (1971), p. 65, citing U.S. Congress, Senate Committee on Labor and Public Welfare, Hearings Before the Subcommittee on Health and Lead-Based Paint Poisoning, S.3216 and H.R.19172, 91st Congress, 2nd Session, U.S. Government Printing Office, Washington, D.C., November 23, 1970, pp. 45–46.

[33] *Ibid.*, citing U.S. Congress, House Committee on Banking and Currency, Hearings Before the Subcommittee on Housing, statement of the American Academy of Pediatrics, 91st Congress, 2nd Session, U.S. Government Printing Office, Washington, D.C., July 22–23, 1970, p. 257. The problem of lead poisoning is not new. "The child, at the turn of the century, lived in a world of lead . . . There was lead in the walls, woodwork and window sills, porch railings, furniture, play pens and cribs. Lead was used as a coloring for food. Toys were made of lead and painted with lead paint . . . lead was used in nipple shields . . . In Japan, lead salts were used in the manufacture of toilet powders, causing lead meningitis in hundreds of infants." (Vincent F. Guinee, "Lead Poisoning," *The American Journal of Medicine*, Vol. 52, No. 3 [March 1972], p. 284.) Despite the increase of lead in the U.S. atmosphere in the past twenty-five years, the amount of lead in the human body is less today than it was at the turn of the century. Rainwater is no longer collected from lead roofing and stored in leaded jugs, the use of lead in interior paints has been largely discontinued since 1950, and lead in stills, foods, and cosmetics is much more closely monitored than it was half a century ago. Thus the lead content of antique hair (1871–1923) is much greater than that found in the hair of modern (1971) popula-

How does the lead enter the child's body? Nose-high automobile exhausts have already been mentioned and are being investigated (page 58). But a better-known source is the paint of the houses in slum areas. Lead-based house paint was commonly used until the 1940s. (It has since been replaced by titanium-based paint.) Such paint contains sweet-tasting lead acetates. Unsupervised small children eat flakes of the lead paint. Some do so because they are afflicted with a condition known as *pica*—an abnormal appetite for unnatural articles of food, such as clay or chalk or paint. Some U.S. cities have "lead belts," in which most cases of childhood lead poisoning occur. "It is estimated that 450,000 apartment units in New York City are in such a state of disrepair that children living in them will be exposed to the hazard of lead poisoning. Approximately 120,000 children are living in these dwellings . . ."[34] In 1971, in that city, "More cases of lead poisoning occurred in black children than in all other children combined."[35] In New York's major "lead belts"—the South Bronx and Brooklyn—400 to 700 children were affected yearly by 1970. Of these, an average of 500 were hospitalized every year. And a considerable number of these small patients already had some brain damage. Those who survive must not be returned to dangerously leaded homes. If they are, they face a 25 to 100 percent increased chance of permanent brain damage.[36]

It should not be assumed that lead poisoning occurs only among the children of the poor. It has also been reported in children from well-to-do families. The poisoning may be due to sources of lead other than the paint and plaster of dilapidated housing. The levels of lead in the paint coating of pencils (the "lead" in the pencil is not lead, but graphite) used to be very high. In June 1971, an industry-led program was begun to reduce those levels. Still another source of lead poisoning: newspapers, comic books, magazines, children's books, and playing cards—particularly yellow, orange, and red inks. Children who habitually chew these paper products are in jeopardy.[37]

---

tions. (D. Weiss, B. Whitten, D. Leddy, "Lead Content of Human Hair [1871–1971]," *Science,* Vol. 178, No. 4056 [October 6, 1972], pp. 69–70.) It should be noted that the amount of lead absorbed through the lungs by breathing polluted air is small compared to the amount that reaches the blood through the stomach, as occurs when leaded paint is eaten. ("Lead Levels in Hair Lower Now Than in 1871," *Science News,* Vol. 102, No. 16 [October 14, 1972], p. 247.)

[34] Vincent F. Guinee, "Lead Poisoning," p. 285.

[35] *Ibid.,* p. 287.

[36] "Lead Poisoning: Price of Poverty," *The Sciences,* Vol. 9, No. 10 (October 1969), p. 13. New York is hardly the only city with a lead-poisoning problem. A 1971–72 federally sponsored survey of twenty-seven U.S. cities revealed that, of all the dwellings tested, 95 percent had at least one accessible surface containing hazardous amounts of lead. In all but four of the cities, some children were found to have blood levels indicating lead absorption. In Charleston, South Carolina, 41.6 percent of the children tested had demonstrable levels of lead. (Jane S. Lin-Fu, "Preventing Lead Poisoning in Children," *Children Today,* Vol. 2, No. 1 [January–February 1973], p. 5, citing "Childhood Lead Poisoning: A Summary Report of a Survey in 27 Cities," DHEW Publication No. 73-10002, 1972.)

[37] Jane S. Lin-Fu, "Preventing Lead Poisoning in Children," p. 6, citing M. M. Joselow, New Jersey College of Medicine and Surgery, personal communications, 1972. As recently as March 1973, a leading environmental publication stated that "the food product used almost solely in infant diets, canned milk, is also the only product still contaminated with lead, tin, and other metals, as a result of reliance on a century-old technology . . . There are no plans to introduce . . . newer canning techniques which would further reduce the contamination of milk and which are commonplace in the packaging of beer and soft drinks. In some respects, therefore, beer is now a safer diet for your infant than canned milk." (Kevin P. Shea, "Canned Milk," *Environment,* Vol. 15, No. 2 [March 1973], p. 11.) It is by no means certain that the observed lead levels in canned milk are indeed hazardous to children, the writer points out, but the chance is there. Why take it?

lead poisoning can be prevented

It takes about three months of steady lead ingestion before obvious symptoms of lead poisoning appear.[38] If the ingestion of lead is stopped before symptoms appear, the actual disease does not occur. Therefore, prevention is no less important than diagnosis and treatment. Recent studies have found that children who were thought to have only mild lead poisoning, without apparent brain involvement, did indeed have visual and other disturbances manifested by a variety of behavior problems. "Despite adequate intelligence, most of these children did not do well in school."[39]

To prevent severe childhood lead poisoning, the Public Health Service has recommended blood-testing all children between the ages of one and six who live in old, dilapidated homes. Testing must not be delayed until a child shows signs and symptoms of lead poisoning, such as loss of appetite, instability, vomiting, pallor (due to anemia), and, in the later stages, loss of consciousness and convulsions. By the time a diagnosis is made on the basis of signs and symptoms and a history of eating paint, the child may already have brain damage.[40] Immediate removal of the lead hazard from homes is essential. Parents of young children should look for chipped and peeling window sills, woodwork, doors, stairs, walls. Repainted cribs, furniture, toys, swings—all are potentially dangerous.[41]

Effective January 1, 1973, the Food and Drug Administration banned interstate shipment of paint containing dangerous lead levels. Early in 1971, moreover, the President signed a bill prohibiting the use of lead-based paint in federal or federally assisted construction. The bill also authorized money for research on lead poisoning and provided funds for community projects to detect, treat, and eliminate lead poisoning. In fiscal 1972, some forty such projects, costing $6.5 million, were funded. However, the funding provisions of the law expired on June 30, 1972. By the beginning of 1973 Congress had failed to authorize additional funds.[42] About $28 million are spent each year to treat lead-poisoned children.[43] For a discussion of the good-business aspects of preventive health care, see pages 751–52.

hexachlorophene

Patented in 1941, the antibacterial chemical hexachlorophene (HCP) had in thirty years become an ingredient of soap solutions, complexion creams, ointments, powders, cosmetics, toothpastes, antiperspirants, mouthwashes, and deodorant sprays. It was even used in furnace filters and plastic shower curtains. Then in 1971 three reports alerted the Food and Drug Administration to the possible hazards of HCP. The first report indicated that HCP fed to rats induced paralysis and brain lesions. The second study pointed out that babies

[38] *Ibid.*, p. 3.
[39] *Ibid.*, p. 4.
[40] "Lead Poisoning in Childhood," *American Family Physician*, Vol. 4, No. 6 (December 1971), p. 105, citing *Pediatrics* (May 1971), p. 950.
[41] "Lead Poisoning Can Cause Blindness," p. 65.
[42] Jane S. Lin-Fu, "Preventing Lead Poisoning in Children," p. 2.
[43] "Lead Poisoning Can Cause Blindness," p. 68, citing *The New York Times* (July 14, 1971), p. 71.

who were washed daily with diluted HCP absorbed the chemical through normal, unbroken skin into their blood streams at close to toxic levels. The third report was from the manufacturer of pHisoHex, the most widely used 3 percent HCP solution. Five newborn monkeys, washed daily for five minutes with pHisoHex for three months, showed brain damage similar to that observed in the experimental rats.[44] In December 1971, the Food and Drug Administration warned against daily, all-over bathing of infants and adults with products containing 2 and 3 percent HCP.[45] Then in February 1972, the FDA drastically reduced the amount of HCP that could be used in certain drugs, soaps, and cosmetics sold without prescription. In addition, new labeling regulations were put into effect.[46]

Within weeks after discontinuing use of HCP to bathe newborns, some hospitals reported outbreaks of staphylococcal infections in their nurseries. Representatives of the American Academy of Pediatrics and government experts emphasized that the transmission of staphylococci from one infant to another was due mostly to poor procedures regarding hand contact. Among their recommendations: strict enforcement of handwashing by nursery personnel with 3 percent HCP (or a similarly effective compound) before and after each contact with an infant. If nursery outbreaks of staph infection should occur, newborns could be bathed daily with an HCP solution,[47] provided they were rinsed thoroughly with water. Once an infant is taken home, the HCP bathing should be discontinued. Outbreaks of staph infection in hospital nurseries are being closely monitored by the nation's health departments.

radiation: the modern Janus

In Roman mythology, Janus was the two-faced god. Radiation has become the Janus of modern times. One of its faces views a limitless beginning for mankind. Is the other face turned to the end of man? What is radiation? What are the origins of so encompassing a power?

atoms and their behavior

Everything in nature is made up of elements, and elements are made up of atoms.[48] The core of each atom is its *nucleus.* Within it are positively charged particles called *protons* and particles that have no charge, *neutrons.*[49] Sur-

[44] Wayne L. Pines, "The Hexachlorophene Story," *FDA Papers,* Vol. 6, No. 3 (April 1972), pp. 11–14.
[45] "Hexachlorophene and Newborns," *FDA Drug Bulletin* (December 1971), p. 1.
[46] "Hexachlorophene in Drugs, Soaps, and Cosmetics," *FDA Drug Bulletin* (February 1972), p. 1.
[47] "Investigation of Hospital Use of Hexachlorophene and Nursery Staphylococcal Infections: United States," *Morbidity and Mortality, Center for Disease Control, Weekly Report for Week Ending February 5, 1972,* U.S. Dept. of Health, Education, and Welfare (February 11, 1972), p. 39.
[48] The following calculations have been made: if you weigh 150 pounds, you are made up of some 6,700,000,000,000,000,000,000,000,000 (6.7 octillion) atoms; and every time you lose or gain a pound you lose or gain this number divided by 150, or about 45,000,000,000,000,000,000,000,000 (45 septillion) atoms. If you gain a pound in a month, you have gained at an average rate of approximately 17,000,000,000,000,000,000 (17 quintillion) atoms per second. (George E. Davis, *Radiation and Life* [Ames, Iowa, 1967], p. 4.)
[49] The hydrogen atom is an exception in that most hydrogen atoms have no neutrons in the nucleus. It should also be noted that there are numerous additional transitory subatomic particles in the nucleus; however, they are not important to this discussion.

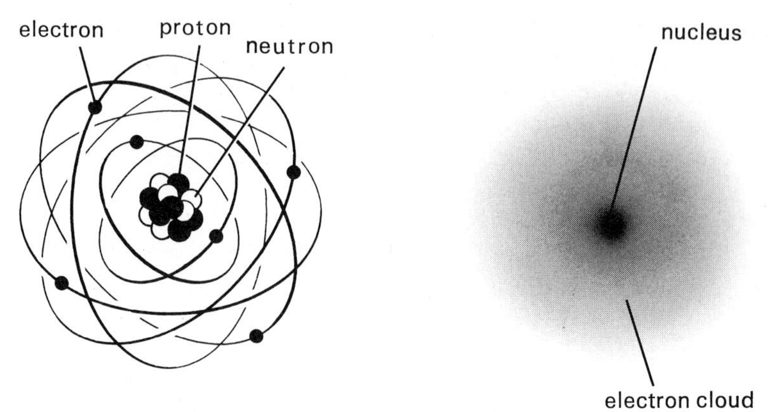

4-6 *Two models of an atom: an atom of carbon 12, which has six electrons, six protons, and six neutrons* (left), *and a generalized model schematizing an electron cloud* (right). *The left diagram is highly simplified in that all the orbitals shown there are elliptical; actually, orbital shapes vary.*

rounding the nucleus and dwarfing it like a star in space is a swirling cloud of negatively charged particles, *electrons.* Depending on where the electrons are whirling in their spacious orbitals, this cloud is more or less ball-shaped. Since the weight of this cloud of electrons is negligible, it is in the heavy nucleus that the protons and neutrons combine to give the atom almost all of its weight. For its size the atomic nucleus is the heaviest bit of matter on earth. In the cloud of each atom the number of negatively charged electrons cancels out or balances the electrical charge of an equal number of positively charged protons. Since the neutrons have no electrical charge, the electrically balanced atom is neutral. It has no charge.

The electrons whirling in the vast minispace of their thin orbital cloud determine the chemical behavior of an element. Food energy depends on these electrons, and so does the energy of fuel. But within the nucleus—the tiny, heavy nucleus—is leashed a source of energy unlike anything electrons provide. Although atoms of the same element have an equal number of protons and electrons, they can have an unequal number of neutrons. And because electrons determine chemical behavior and neutrons have weight (or mass), extra neutrons within an atom's nucleus will increase its weight but will not change its chemical properties. Atoms having the same number of electrons and protons (and thus the same chemical properties) but a different number of neutrons (and therefore different weights) are called *isotopes.* Almost all elements have more than one isotope.

Some isotopes are unstable. Their nuclei spontaneously disintegrate. Energy in the form of waves and particles is emitted from these unstable nuclei. This energy is called *ionizing radiation,* and the decaying isotope is a *radioactive isotope.*

sources of ionizing radiation

Ionizing radiation is a part of man's natural ecosystem. Radioactive materials in soil, rocks, air, food, and water, as well as in body and building materials, account for some 58 percent of the radiation to which man is exposed. From outer space comes cosmic radiation to bombard everything on earth. Most cosmic radiation is blocked from reaching earth by the atmosphere, else man would perish. Man is constantly riddled by natural ionizing radiation, but he has nevertheless flourished to make and use (as well as misuse) his own radiation. Man-made sources of exposure to ionizing radiation include X-rays, certain medical examinations, and some industrial processes. These account for 41 percent of man's ionizing radiation exposure. Fallout from nuclear weapons accounts for most of the remaining 1 percent.

one face of Janus: human radiation damage

At the turn of the century, the famous physicist Henri Becquerel carried around in his vest pocket a tube of the intriguing new element radium, in a compound of radium salts. Before long he noticed a burn on his belly. To check Becquerel's observation, Pierre Curie (who, with his wife Marie, discovered radium) deliberately applied radium to his arm. Again a burn developed. The little burn of Becquerel has left its mark on mankind. Suspicion of damaging effects of radiation dates from such observations.

Like all other matter, human tissue is made up of atoms. Their nuclei are also surrounded by clouds of negatively charged electrons. How can ionizing radiations damage human tissue atoms? When ionizing radiation collides with the various particles of tissue atoms or molecules, those tissue atoms or molecules are in turn ionized. Extensive damage can result. The radiation, causing the molecular disintegration of a cell's chemicals, interrupts cell function. Furthermore, the products of cellular destruction are believed to poison the cell. The general (somatic) body tissue cells and/or the specialized (gonadal) reproductive cells may be affected. Somatic cells may be grossly harmed or even killed by radiation. Damage to them may affect the lifetime of the individual exposed to the radiation, but damage to reproductive cells affects generations yet unborn—a cruel legacy for posterity. Radiation may change DNA structure directly or it may cause breaks in chromosomal structure that heal improperly. Here, too, toxic substances may be produced to poison the cell. Perhaps both chromosomal breaks and toxicity combine to violate the integrity of the DNA code and disrupt the cell. In a mutilated cell, ionized DNA sends improper messages. Abnormality is inevitable. (See Figure 18-11, page 538.)

How much damage will radiation cause? This varies according to individual susceptibility, cell susceptibility, the kind of ionizing radiation, the radiation dose, and the length of time of exposure. Just as people vary in their sensitivity to pollen or smog, so they differ in their sensitivity to equal doses of ionizing radiation. Also, tissue cells differ in their sensitivity and according to the type of ionizing radiation. Some kinds of ionizing radiation are more penetrating than others. Still other ionizing radiation has an affinity for specific structures because of its similarity to certain cellular constituents. Thus, the radioactive isotopes strontium 89 and 90 closely resemble (bone) calcium and concentrate in bone and its marrow; barium 140 also attacks the bone marrow; iodine 131, the thyroid gland; cesium 137 attacks the soft tissues, particularly the muscles and reproductive cells; the radioactive isotope carbon 14 assaults the whole body, including its reproductive cells. These poisons enter man in various ways. Iodine 131, barium 140, strontium 89 and 90, and cesium 137 may all be passed into man as he eats meats or dairy products provided by animals that have fed on contaminated plants. Or man can ingest them when he consumes contaminated grains or leafy vegetables. Carbon 14 can be ingested with food, inhaled with polluted air, or absorbed through the skin or mucous membranes. The cells most sensitive to radiation are those of the stomach and intestines, bone marrow and lymph nodes (concerned with immunity), spleen, and reproductive organs. Large doses of all types of radiation will kill cells. But they must be delivered over a short period of time. Spread over many years, a person's exposure to radiation may amount to a considerable total. He will show few if any noticeable effects. Concentrated into a brief time (a split second, for example), the same ordinary total lifetime dosage may be fatal. Why? Given time, the body repairs or replaces many cells. It was the overwhelming dose delivered over a short time that resulted in the terrible events at Hiroshima and Nagasaki.

atomic accidents happen

In March 1954, unexpected winds picked up radioactive products of a nuclear test explosion on the island of Bikini and showered them on twenty-three unlucky Japanese fishermen on their boat, *The Lucky Dragon,* as well as on various Pacific islanders. It was not until ten years later that some of the children on the Rongelap Atoll developed thyroid nodules,[50] abnormal thyroid function, and signs of growth retardation. Thus the absence of early organ changes after exposure does not necessarily mean that the exposed person has escaped serious harm. This tragic truth is emphasized by studies of Japanese who were ten years old or younger at the time of their exposure to the radiation of the Hiroshima and Nagasaki bombings. Between 1955 and 1969, among those individuals who were exposed to high doses of radiation, the incidence of carcinomas (cancers arising from the epithelial-cell linings of the body; see page 195) was seven times that expected in a normal population.[51]

Accidents involving atomic materials still occur too frequently. Nobody was hurt as a result of the nuclear plant accident at Windscale, England, some years ago. Nevertheless, an undue amount of radioactive iodine was released into this sparsely settled area. After the accident "authorities had to seize all milk and crops within 400 square miles of the plant."[52] No one was injured as a result of the seventeenth accident involving aircraft carrying nuclear weapons, in 1966. Nevertheless, the hazard exists and must be reduced to an absolute minimum.

An investigation into the worst fire in Atomic Energy Commission history at the Rocky Flats plutonium plant near Denver, Colorado, on May 11, 1969, did

[50] George M. Woodwell, "Toxic Substances and Ecological Cycles," p. 29.

[51] "New Wave of Cancer from Hiroshima Bomb," *New Scientist and Science Journal,* Vol. 50, No. 751 (May 13, 1971), p. 369.

[52] Roger Rapoport, "Secrecy and Safety at Rocky Flats," *Los Angeles Times* September 7, 1969, p. 18.

not help instill public confidence. Numerous smaller fires had preceded the May 11 holocaust at the Rocky Flats plant. Furthermore, over the years a considerable number of workers in the plant may have been overexposed to radiation. The plant at Rocky Flats is the only facility in the United States where plutonium triggers for nuclear weapons are made. Two years after the fire, the plant has "become one of the Atomic Energy Commission's most bitterly attacked facilities. The main charge has been offsite plutonium contamination."[53] There is considerable scientific opinion that the level of plutonium radiation considered acceptable is too high and, moreover, that pollution has occurred, at various times, at levels incompatible with human health. Also criticized is the inadequate method of studying the possible relationship of plutonium radiation and cancer among the workers at the plant. Because the state of health of workers who leave the plant is not rigorously followed, it is believed that the "claim that cancer incidence is low at Rocky Flats . . . is without a statistical base."[54] Denver suburbs are developing around the plant site; the residents are pollution-conscious. Unless security restrictions are relaxed enough to allow a more open approach to the problem, citizen pressures against the plant are certain to increase.

radioactive waste disposal

Nuclear fuel processing plants mean radioactive wastes. Finding a safe way to dispose of these wastes is a growing problem. Some radioactive wastes will remain hazardous for a million years. At some storage sites, a relatively small amount of liquid radioactive waste is leaking out of its containers into the ground. Other suggested methods, such as deep-sea burial and disposal in outer space, are either unsafe or prohibitively expensive. The Atomic Energy Commission has proposed that a national dump be established in salt mines northeast of Lyons, Kansas. It is believed that the very fact that the salt mines are still there is an indication that they have not come in contact with circulating ground water for some 250 million years. The geographic stability of the area and the absence of earthquakes would appear to make inconceivable any contact by stored radioactive wastes with any atmosphere containing life.[55] However, residents of Kansas (including state scientists) doubt that the salt mines guarantee safety. They have insisted on further studies.

the bomb

> I beheld the earth, and, lo, it was without form, and void; and the heavens, and they had no light.
> I beheld the mountains, and, lo, they trembled, and all the hills moved lightly.
> I beheld, and, lo, there was no man, and all the birds of the heavens were fled.
> I beheld, and, lo, the fruitful place was a wilderness, and all the cities thereof were broken down.

[53] Deborah Shapley, "Rocky Flats: Credibility Gap Widens on Plutonium Plant Safety," *Science*, Vol. 174, No. 4009 (November 5, 1971), p. 569.

[54] *Ibid.*, p. 570.

[55] Richard S. Lewis, "The Radioactive Salt Mine," *Science and Public Affairs: Bulletin of Atomic Scientists*, Vol. 27, No. 6 (June 1971), pp. 27–31, 33–34.

Thus does the prophecy of Jeremiah (4:23–26) tell of a destructive energy that suggests the most terrible of all inventions, the atomic bomb. Pressing the button of destruction at Alamogordo on the chill morning of July 16, 1945, men knew they had wrought the threat of their time. Almost twenty years later, J. Robert Oppenheimer, the director of the project that had developed the atomic bomb, repeated the haunting appraisal of a scared security guard: "The longhairs have let it get away from them."[56] For thousands of people, the threefold body assault by the bomb—burn, blast, and radiation—became agonizing reality. Until men live at peace, control of thermonuclear weapons will remain a consuming problem. The nuclear test ban is a step in the right direction. Not all nations have agreed to it.

radioactive fallout

When a nuclear bomb explodes, radioactive material is let loose into the atmosphere. This material, falling to earth by gravity, is "fallout." Within a few hours, some of the particles settle to the ground. Within several months, more descend. The lightest particles rise into the stratosphere and circulate around the world. Unless borne downward by rain or snow, they may not return to earth for months or years. Most fallout concentrates in the earth's Temperate Zone. In it lie the great cities of the world—London, Tokyo, New York, Moscow, Peking. And in this zone lives some 80 percent of the world's population.

epilogue: the St. Louis Baby Tooth Survey

"So well known has the BTS become that letters from children, addressed simply 'Tooth Fairy, St. Louis,' reach their destination at the CNI Office."[57] BTS means Baby Tooth Survey. CNI refers to the Greater St. Louis Citizens' Committee for Nuclear Information. The survey, started in 1958, is a splendid community-wide effort for measuring strontium 90 in baby teeth. It is just before and after birth that most strontium 90 is absorbed in the teeth of babies. So, baby teeth examined for strontium 90 reflect a situation seven to ten years old. The nuclear test ban occurred in 1963. If it could be extended and all nations would agree to abide by it, it could be hoped that someday there will be no need to do anything with baby teeth but tuck them under pillows.

the other face of Janus: radiation as man's benefactor

By means of nuclear reactors nuclear power can be converted to peaceful use on a worldwide scale.

Man-made radioisotopes may eventually replace natural fuels. The problems of the radiation hazards are being studied so that nuclear reactors will be safely controlled and shielded, and so that radioactive wastes can be disposed of without threatening future generations. Hopefully, in a world at peace, the problem of massive radiation will be confined to such projects as seeking new

[56] Told by J. Robert Oppenheimer in the 1962 Whidden Lectures, at McMaster University, and cited in Henry E. Duckworth, *Little Men in the Unseen World* (New York, 1963), p. 110.
[57] Yvonne Logan, "The Story of the Baby Tooth Survey," *Scientist and Citizen,* Vol. 6, Nos. 9–10 (September–October 1964), p. 39.

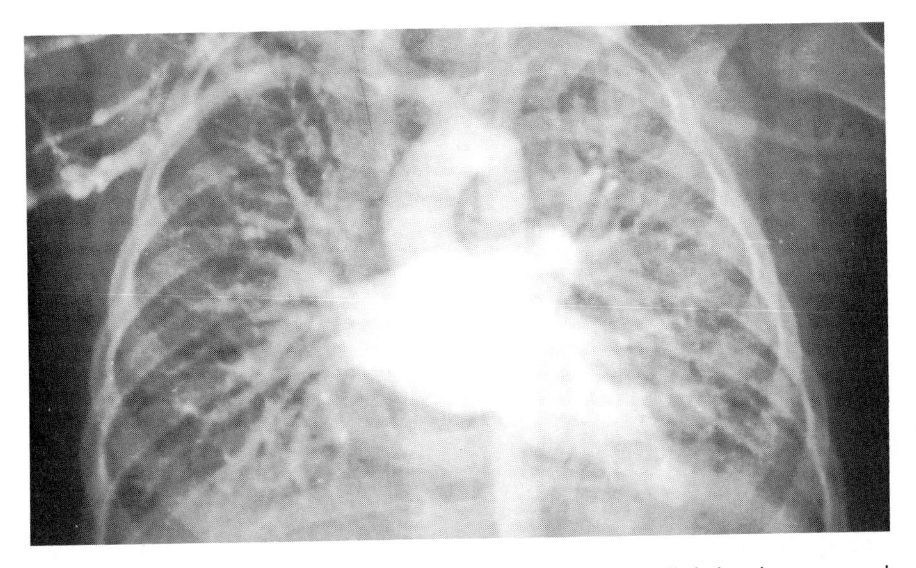

4-7 *An X-ray photograph of a normal heart. The large looped vessel coming from the heart is the aorta, the largest of all arteries.*

sources of energy for building dams, powering industry, lighting homes, and carrying technology forward. Unfortunately, agreement as to the best methods of accomplishing these benefits is not universal.

Perhaps more significant than the industrial potential of radiation are its medical uses. Radiation has provided new X-ray techniques for early diagnosis of cancer, and radiation has been used to treat cancers. For example, radiation has provided new X-ray techniques for early diagnosis of breast cancer. To women with this illness as well as to thousands afflicted with cancer of the uterine cervix, radiation has brought years of life. X-ray methods also provide ways of viewing the heart and blood vessels (see Figure 4-7).

In an auto accident a man's kidney is badly damaged. It would be best to remove it. Can the remaining kidney carry the load of two? There is no time for prolonged laboratory tests. Into the patient's vein is injected a compound containing certain radioactive atoms of iodine. Over the kidney area of the patient's back a radiation counter is placed. This measures the radioactivity of the hopefully normal kidney. By the way the kidney handles the radioactive material, the physician can, in minutes, determine whether the kidney will be reliable. Injected, the radioactive iodine material reveals its position. It can thus be traced and measured. Such radioisotopes are called *tracers*. Another example: a patient has a brain tumor. In order to remove it, one must know exactly where in the brain the tumor lies. The proper isotope is injected. Multiplying tumor cells will take it up more readily than normal surrounding tissue. Radioactive scanning techniques locate the tumor.

the need for strict controls

Just as there is a biological risk to human life from natural radiation, there is the same risk in man's use of radiation. In terms of human life and in no other terms, it has been seen that the benefits of radiation can far outweigh the costs. Under proper conditions, diagnostic and treatment radiations are proper risks. Nevertheless, problems, such as personnel shortages, hamper inspection of

X-ray equipment used in both medicine and industry. Not enough of this nation's medical X-ray installations meet state regulations or recommendations.[58] This is a dangerous loophole. For a considerable part of the population, X-rays and nuclear medicine have increased the average exposure to radiation as much as 100 percent above the former rate. Today, X-ray examinations account for about 90 percent of all exposure to man-made ionizing radiation in the United States. Slightly more than 60 percent of all X-rays are done in hospitals; the rest are done in physicians' offices (28 percent) and other health facilities (12 percent). From 1964 to 1970 there was a considerable increase in diagnostic X-ray use. Despite this, "The mean annual genetically significant dose of radiation received from diagnostic X-rays in the United States dropped about 35 percent."[59] Among the reasons for this improvement were better X-ray techniques and a decrease in the use of mobile X-ray units (such as were used in tuberculosis screening; see page 172).

Other recent man-made radiation sources need constant surveillance. Microwaves, used in a variety of ways ranging from military communications to food ovens, emit radiations that may be harmful, especially to the eye. The same is true of laser-maser concentrated light-energy systems, which are finding increasing use in industry and the military. So intense is the light energy of a laser that it can drill a hole through a diamond in moments—a process that, before lasers, took two days.

meeting energy problems: what is new? what is possible?

The need to find new sources of energy to eventually replace excessively polluting fossil fuels, such as coal, has already been emphasized (see pages 61–62). "The main new energy sources which sooner or later must take over are *fission energy, fusion energy,* and *solar energy.*"[60] Fission energy is now being obtained from nuclear power plants;[61] it is derived by splitting (fissioning) heavy isotopes. All fission reactors produce both plutonium and strontium 90. These are two of the most poisonous substances known; tiny amounts are lethal. Fission plant builders have been remarkably clever in developing safe operating conditions. However, some risk remains, and any risk is unacceptable because it is one that humanity has never faced before. "Normal" risks cannot include the slightest possibility of a nuclear catastrophe.[62]

[58] L. H. Fess and L. Seabron, "Preliminary Results of 5,263 X-ray Protection Surveys of Facilities with Medical X-ray Equipment (1962–1967)," cited in James T. Terrill, "Microwaves, Lasers, and X-rays," *Archives of Environmental Health,* Vol. 19, No. 2 (August 1969), p. 269. Moreover, few states regulate X-ray technicians. By early 1971, in only California, New York, and New Jersey were there legal requirements for training and licensing such technicians. ("Medical Uses of Radiation," *Journal of the American Medical Association,* Vol. 215, No. 12 [March 22, 1971], p. 1978.)

[59] "'Mean Genetic Radiation' Declines Despite Increased X-ray Use," *Journal of the American Medical Association,* Vol. 220, No. 4 (April 24, 1972), p. 469.

[60] Hannes Alfven, "Energy and Environment," *Science and Public Affairs: Bulletin of the Atomic Scientists,* Vol. 28, No. 5 (May 1972), p. 5.

[61] To describe the nuclear-powered industrial complex of the future a new term—"nuplex"—is being used.

[62] "In principle, nuclear reactors are dangerous," Edward Teller, the "father of the H-bomb," said in 1965. "By being careful, and also by good luck, we have so far avoided all serious nuclear accidents . . . In my mind, nuclear reactors do not belong on the surface of the earth. Nuclear reactors belong underground." (Edward Teller, "Energy from Oil and from the Nucleus," cited in Sheldon Novick, *The Careless Atom* [Boston, 1969], p. 38.)

Scientists are presently studying ways of obtaining energy by joining (fusing) the lighter isotopes instead of splitting those that are heavier. Within about five years it should be possible to tell whether a commitment to fusion energy is practical.[63] Fusion processes that release energy have a tremendous advantage over fission energy processes: their waste products (helium, hydrogen, and neutrons) are relatively harmless. The actual processes required to produce fusion energy, however, are not without considerable risk.

Energy from the sun (*solar energy*) is now available. In fact, the amount that arrives on 0.5 percent of the land area of the United States is more than the total energy needs of the entire country projected to the year 2000.[64] But solar energy is now about one hundred times more expensive than conventional energy. It may be collected on "solar energy farms" in sunny areas, preferably on deserts, in a variety of ways, such as in vast hothouses or by great mirrors. It is possible that collectors may be placed in orbit.[65] A concrete consequence of President Nixon's energy message to Congress on June 4, 1971, was the establishment of a Solar Energy Panel by the National Science Foundation and the National Aeronautics and Space Administration. Research and development programs will someday reduce the cost and solve some of the storage problems of solar energy.

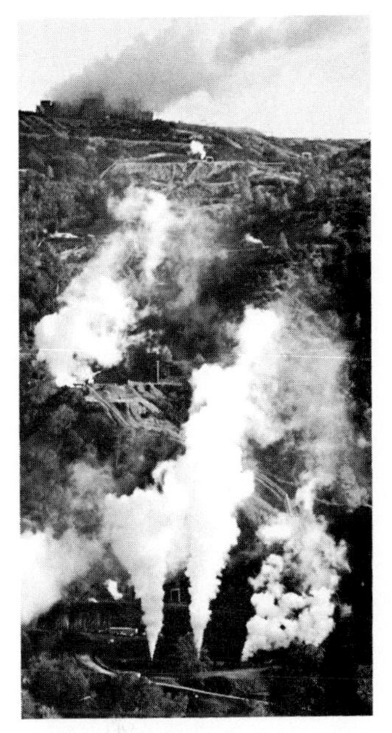

4-8 *"The Geysers," a geothermal steam field in northern California. Electrical energy is generated from underground steam.*

The day may also come when it will be possible to harness the solar energy collected by and stored in the seas (*"sea-thermal" energy*).

Geothermal energy is derived from the earth's internal heat. Both Russia and Iceland are already making use of this source. As a result of stupendous geological changes beneath the earth's crust, molten, plastic masses of rock called *magma* are released. The magma, congealing at high temperatures below the earth's surface, transmits its intense heat through solid rock to water captured in spongy porous rock above. Through breaks in this rock, the boiling water escapes upward. Some of the hot water escapes as steam. North of San Francisco is The Geysers. The largest dry steam field in the world, it provides electrical power to two northern California counties. By 1978, it is expected that The Geysers will produce enough energy for a city as large as San Francisco. Engineers are also seeking geothermal power in the form of steam or hot water in California's Imperial Valley. The United States is running out of natural gas; this is one reason the federal government has allocated $16 million for further exploration of geothermal energy.[66]

[63] Lawrence M. Lidsky, "The Quest for Fusion Power," *Technology Review,* Vol. 74, No. 3 (January 1972), p. 10.

[64] Allan L. Hammond, "Solar Energy: The Largest Resource," *Science,* Vol. 177, No. 4054, p. 1088. A recent study by the National Science Foundation/National Aeronautics and Space Administration projected that, by 1985, 10 percent of all buildings constructed will use solar climate control systems. (Peter E. Glaser and James C. Burke, "New Directions for Solar Energy," *Science and Public Affairs,* Vol. 29, No. 8 [October 1973], p. 42; also see Allen L. Hammond, "Solar Energy: Proposal for a Major Research Program," *Science,* Vol. 179, No. 4078 [March 16, 1973], p. 1116.)

[65] Dietrick E. Thompson, "Farming the Sun's Energy," *Science News,* Vol. 101, No. 15 (April 8, 1972), p. 237.

[66] John Henahan, "Full Steam Ahead for Geothermal Energy," *New Scientist,* Vol. 57, No. 827 (January 4, 1973), p. 16.

sound pollution: the modern earache

''Noise,'' wrote the nineteenth-century German philosopher Schopenhauer, not without his usual acrimony, ''is the most impertinent of all interruptions.''[67] Bitterly he railed against the ''wanton, cursed, brain-paralyzing whine of the coachman's whip.'' Were he alive today, he might well remember the coachman's whip with nostalgia. Over 90 million automobiles, 16 million trucks, and 2.5 million motorcycles roar through the streets of this nation. Inside the home, such appliances as dishwashers, garbage disposals, and food blenders raise enough racket to threaten human hearing. Above, the skies shake from over twelve hundred jet aircraft.

While most people are disturbed by noise not of their own making, noise affects different people variously. The thrumming voice of a cello relaxes one person and distracts another. An epileptic seizure was the response of one sensitive Wisconsin housewife to the voices of three different radio announcers. (The successful treatment was the repetitious playing of tapes of the announcers' voices until they no longer affected her.)[68] Noise is unwanted sound. But what is sound?

sound In a gust of wind, a heavy door swings. Its energy is expended in moving and in pushing air out of the way. The door slams shut. No longer can the moving door's energy be used in motion and pushing air. It is expended on the door frame and the walls. Immediately adjacent to the walls the air particles begin to vibrate. These, in turn, pass on their vibrations to the air particles next to them. This second group of particles cause a third group next to them to vibrate. So, starting from the vibrating air particles next to the shaking walls, vibrations are passed on from one group of particles to the next until the ear is reached. It is not the air particles that have moved from the wall to the ear. The air particles merely moved up and down, passing their vibrations along to their neighboring particles. It is the vibrations that have moved from the wall to the ear. The vibrations pass along in waves. Compare this phenomenon to a stone dropped in water. Ripples or waves spread out from the place where the stone fell. But the water itself merely moves up and down. A leaf in the water will move up and down with the disturbed water. It too will be disturbed but not moved along with the ripples or waves. In a like way, a slamming door will push air out of its way to make ripples or waves. These, combined with the air's vibrating particles, are the transmitted sound waves instigated by the energy of the slamming door. Over three hundred years ago, Galileo summed this up in his *Dialogues:* ''Waves are produced by the vibrations of a sonorous body, which spread through the air, bringing to the tympanum[69] of the ear a stimulus which the mind interprets as sound.'' Since sound depends on air particles to travel, there is no sound in a vacuum or on the moon.

[67] Arthur Schopenhauer, ''On Noise,'' *The Pessimist's Handbook, A Collection of Popular Essays,* tr. by T. Bailey Saunders (Lincoln, Neb., 1964), p. 217.
[68] *Science News,* Vol. 93, No. 23 (June 8, 1968), p. 549.
[69] The *tympanum* is the cavity of the middle ear.

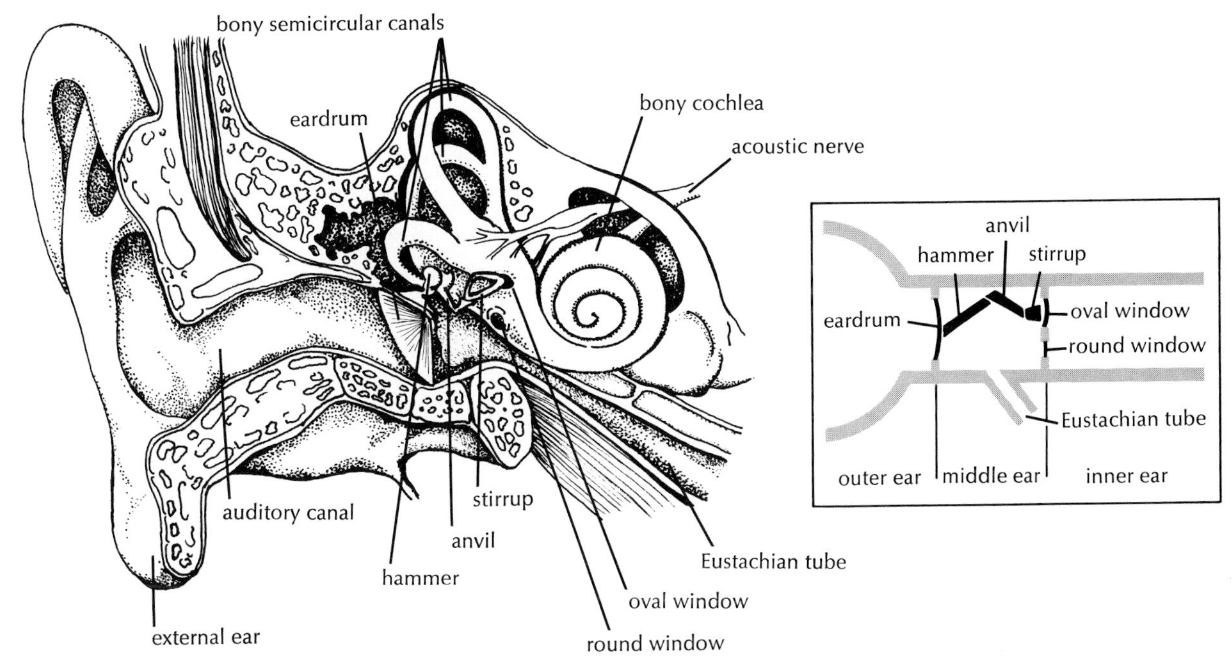

4-9 *The ear: detailed and schematic views. Not visible in the illustration at the left is the membranous cochlear duct, which is housed in the bony cochlea. It is the cochlear duct that, in turn, contains the organ of hearing—the spiral organ of Corti. And it is the organ of Corti whose stimulated hair cells will induce the impulses on the surrounding acoustic nerve fibers. These impulses will reach the brain as sound.*

the ear

For a sound to reach the brain for interpretation, each of the three main parts of the ear—*outer, middle,* and *inner*—must fulfill its purpose (see Figure 4-9).

The *outer ear* consists of the fleshy *external ear* (or *auricle*), which collects sound waves and directs them into the inch-long, funnel-shaped *auditory canal.* This canal ends blindly. It is closed off by the outer wall of the middle ear, the *eardrum* (or *tympanic membrane*).

Except for the membranous eardrum, the walls of the middle ear chamber are bone. The middle ear contains a connected chain of the three smallest bones in the body, named for their shape. The first is the *hammer* (or *malleus*). The handle of the hammer is attached to the inside of the eardrum. The second bone is the *anvil* (or *incus*), and the third is the *stirrup* (or *stapes*). Connecting the middle ear to the back of the nose is the *Eustachian tube,* named after a sixteenth-century anatomist, Eustacio. Ordinarily this tube is closed. With swallowing, however, it opens. Were it not for this tube, an increase in pressure in the auditory canal would force the eardrum into the middle ear; a decrease in pressure would draw it out. Air pressure changes within the auditory canal are small. For the eardrum to respond to such small changes, the average pressure on both sides of the eardrum must be kept the same. A loud noise, such as a cannon shot, can cause enough pressure within the auditory canal to rupture the eardrum. When the mouth is kept open, the pressure against the eardrum comes from both sides (auditory canal and Eustachian tube), which prevents this kind of damage. Those who fire cannon also often wear earplugs.

The inner wall of the middle ear is the outer wall of the inner ear. In this wall are two small openings—the *oval window* above and the *round window* below. The foot plate of the stirrup touches the thin membrane covering the oval window. As will be seen, the function of the tiny middle ear bones is to transmit the motion of the eardrum to the membrane of the oval window.

The *inner ear* is encased in bone. It consists of a series of minute and intricately tunneled bony canals, which contain membranous canals. Strands of connective tissue attach the membranous canals to their bony container. Within both the bony and membranous canals is a thin, limpid fluid. So the membranous canals are surrounded by this fluid and also contain it.

One part of the bony canals is molded into a pea-sized spiral passage making 2¾ turns; it is the *cochlea.* Its name is derived from the Latin word for "snail shell," which describes its shape. A second part of the bony canals are the *semicircular canals.* Within these bony semicircular canals fit the membranous *semicircular ducts.* The semicircular canals and their contained membranous ducts are concerned with balance. They have nothing to do with hearing.[70] It is the bony cochlea that is of present concern, for it houses the membranous *cochlear duct.* Within this duct, and attached to its floor, is a structure called the *spiral organ of Corti.* The organ of Corti contains sensory hair cells about which branch delicate fibers of the cranial nerve of hearing (the *acoustic nerve*). It is thus the organ of Corti that receives the stimuli of sound for transmission to the brain.

how hearing happens

Sound waves reaching the ear travel at about 1,100 feet a second. Compared to light waves they are very slow. That is why the puff of smoke of a distant train's steam whistle is visible long before the whistle is heard. Sound waves are caught by the external ear and are directed into the auditory canal. The waves strike the eardrum and set it to vibrating in time with the sound waves. The vibrations of the eardrum are conveyed by the bones of the middle ear to the oval window. The thin membrane of the oval window then vibrates. There the vibrations are converted into pressure waves in the fluid within the bony cochlea. These waves cause the membranous roof of the cochlear duct to vibrate. Waves are thereby set off in the fluid within the cochlear duct and these, in turn, set the membranous floor of the cochlear duct to vibrating. These vibrations stimulate the hair cells of the spiral organ of Corti attached to the floor of

[70] The membranous and fluid-filled organs of equilibratory sense are the semicircular ducts and the *utricle,* both of which are inside the semicircular canals. Reflexes, initiated by stimulated nerves of the semicircular ducts, cause appropriate body movements to maintain equilibrium. Disease (such as infection) of these ducts soon produces dizziness. However, it is the nerve receptors of the utricle that are responsible in sea, car, and other motion sickness. The utricle is also involved with gravity. The marvelous ability of a falling cat to land on its feet is due to the function of its utricle.

the cochlear duct. Finally, the stimulated hair cells of the organ of Corti induce impulses that are received by the surrounding fibers of the acoustic nerve and are carried to the brain for interpretation as sound. Thus is sound energy transmitted through air, bone, and fluid and converted, in the inner ear, into electrical nervous energy to be sent to the brain.

The round window is not directly involved in the transmission of sound energy. Located below the oval window, it is a membrane-covered window of adjustment. As the bones of the middle ear are stimulated by sound waves, the vibrating foot plate of the stirrup pushes the membrane of the oval window slightly inward. As was described above, this disturbs and displaces a small volume of the fluid within the bony cochlea. But fluid cannot be compressed. The displaced cochlear fluid must go somewhere. It is accommodated by the membrane of the round window. This membrane allows the fluid to push outward. When the foot plate moves outward, the fluid can move inward. So, the tiny membrane of the round window, by permitting the stirrup to move, permits hearing.

How sensitive is the hearing apparatus? The weakest sound that can be heard by the human ear causes its oval window to move no more than three-hundred-thousandths of a millionth of an inch. Comparing this amount of motion to the length of the ear canal is equivalent to comparing the thickness of a sheet of paper to the distance between London and New York. No less remarkable is the range of pressures to which the ear is sensitive. The eardrum can withstand, without damage, the pressure of a loud noise that is fourteen million times greater than the pressure of the softest sound the ear can normally hear.[71]

sound measured as a physical force

Sound waves traveling through the atmosphere cause changes of pressure within it. The smallest disturbance in air pressure that can be heard, under ideal conditions, by a young person is known as the *threshold of hearing.* It is from this threshold that sound levels in *decibels* are measured. What are decibels? They are the units of sound measurement—units of loudness. The "bel" in the word is named for the inventor of the telephone, Alexander Graham Bell. "Deci" is derived from the Latin *decem,* meaning "ten." Two sounds differ by one bel if their intensities are in the ratio 10 : 1. A decibel is thus one-tenth of a bel. As the number of decibels goes up from the threshold of hearing, the loudness increases as an exponent. One decibel is about the softest sound the human ear can usually hear. Ten decibels of sound is, thus, ten times louder, and a twenty-decibel sound is ten times louder than a ten-decibel sound. A thirty-decibel sound (a whisper) is ten times louder than a twenty-decibel sound. At one hundred feet a jet plane taking off is ten times louder than a pneumatic riveter, and the noise will hurt (see Figure 4-10). As decibels increase, sound energy multiplies in fantastic proportion. The greater this energy, the more the discomfort.

[71] Colin A. Ronan, *The Meaning of Sound* (New York, 1967), pp. 69, 71.

unwanted sound: noise as an air pollutant

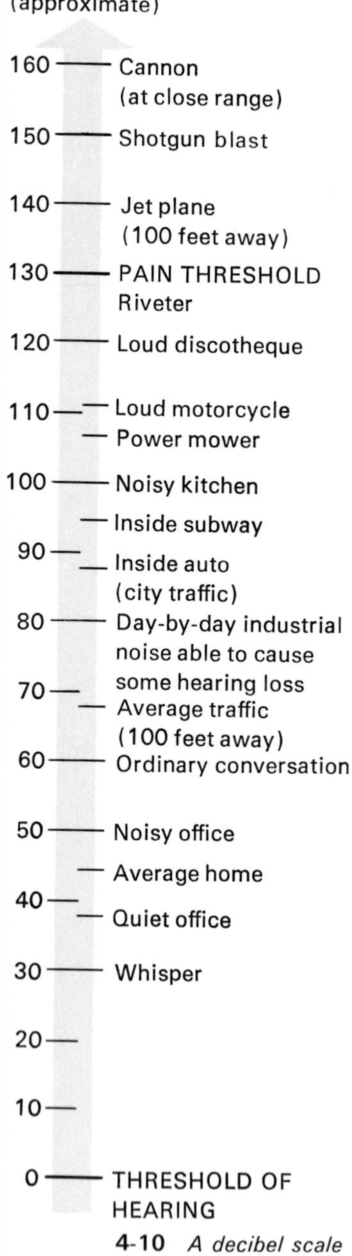

4-10 *A decibel scale of loudness.*

That noise, like all other sound, is a physical force has long been appreciated. The Bible says that the people led by Joshua at Jericho "shouted with a great shout, that the wall fell down flat . . . and they took the city" (Joshua 6:20). The heat released by the energy of focused sound vibrations at an intensity of 170 decibels can kill a small animal or start a fire. Relatively short exposure to noise in excess of 130 decibels may do permanent damage to the ears of normal persons. Long exposure to a noise level of 100 decibels may permanently harm hearing.

In this country, noise assaults the ear early in life, and escape is not always easy. Six months after conception, the human fetus can hear, and the uterus becomes a noisy abode. One researcher has suggested that "when a mother drinks champagne or beer, it sounds something like fireworks to the fetus inside her."[72] Although such occasional disturbances are surely more entertaining than harmful, studies do suggest that prolonged exposure to excessive noise before birth may have an adverse effect on hearing (see pages 552–53). Even the baby compartments of hospital incubators may be polluted by noise. One recent Chicago study found that "under the plastic hood of the incubators the noise spectrum fell well above the recommended acceptance level and, due to the prolonged exposure time, very close to the danger area."[73] And the incubator is not the only preserve of the child that is invaded by noise. In a downtown Boston school playground, a noise level of 78 decibels was recently recorded. In the Boston suburb of Wellesley, the noise level of a school playground was only 58 decibels. So the Boston city school children were exposed to noise a hundred times greater than were the suburban children.

As people grow, their exposure to noise often increases. In one study, five members of a musical combo were studied before, during, and after a two-and-one-half-hour rehearsal session. Three of the group were nineteen years old; two were twenty. After the rehearsal all five musicians reported "ringing" or a sensation of "fullness" in the ears. All demonstrated some reduced hearing ability, presumably temporary. During the loudest period of the rehearsal session, sound intensity levels ranged from 120 to 130 decibels.[74] At the press site of a departing Saturn moon rocket, the decibel noise level rises to 120 decibels. Noise levels at two San Francisco discothèques peaked at 120 decibels.

Investigators recently surveyed hearing ability of three thousand Knoxville, Tennessee, school-age children. Only 3.8 percent of the sixth-graders had some impaired hearing. Among ninth-graders the percentage rose to 11. Twelfth-graders showed a prevalence of 10.6 percent.

The same investigators sought to discover whether rock 'n' roll music caused permanent damage to the ear (see Figure 4-11). A guinea pig was subjected to rock 'n' roll music adjusted to sound levels approximating those found

[72] Theodore Berland, "Bbrrreeeeeeuuuuuaaaaaagggghhhh! Clatter, Rattle, Whirrr . . . Boom!" *Smithsonian,* Vol. 3, No. 4 (July 1972), p. 15.

[73] Frank L. Seleney and Michael Streczyn, "Noise Characteristics in the Baby Compartment of Incubators," *American Journal of Diseases of Children,* Vol. 117, No. 4 (April 1969), p. 450.

[74] Ralph R. Rupp and Larry J. Koch, "Effects of Too-Loud Music on Human Ears: But, Mother, Rock 'n' Roll HAS to Be Loud!" *Clinical Pediatrics,* Vol. 8, No. 2 (February 1969), pp. 60–62.

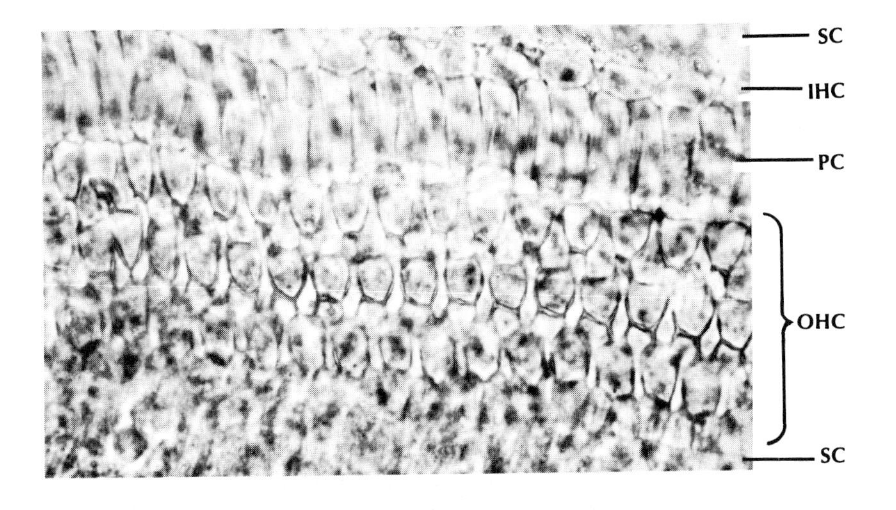

4-11 *Ear damage to a guinea pig from exposure to rock music. The animal's right ear was exposed; its left ear was protected by a plug.*

a. Normal-appearing tissues in the organ of Corti of the protected ear (X approx. 850), showing supporting cells (SC), inner sensory hair cells (IHC), pillars of Corti (PC), and outer sensory hair cells (OHC).

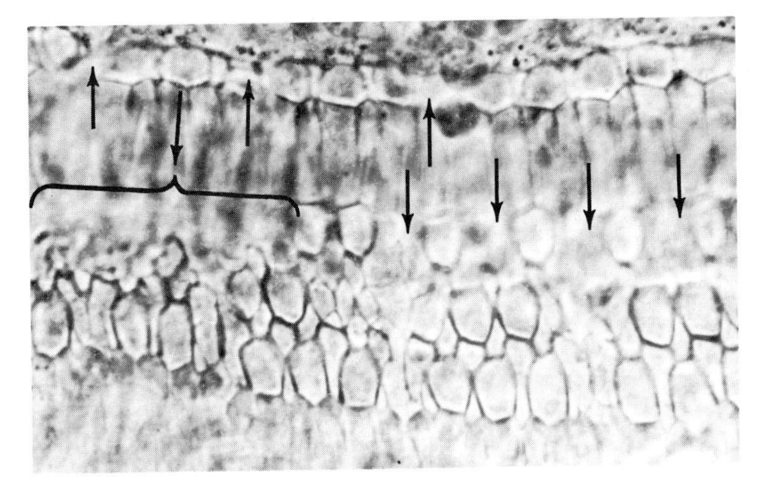

b. Damaged inner sensory hair cells (top arrows) and missing or collapsed outer sensory hair cells (bottom arrows) in the unprotected organ of Corti (X approx. 935). Other damaged cells can be noted in the second and third rows of outer sensory hair cells.

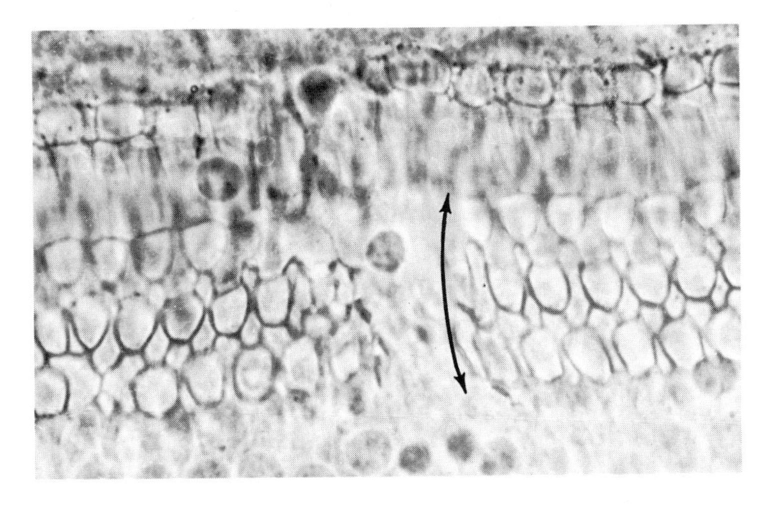

c. Torn segment of cochlear tissues from the unprotected ear. In this region of tissue, there was destruction across the entire breadth (arrow) of the organ of Corti (X approx. 935).

in dance halls (a peak of about 122 decibels). Only the right ear of the guinea pig was exposed. The left ear was protected by a plug. Stimulation periods were varied according to observed exposure by teen-agers to rock 'n' roll. Widespread irreversible damage to the hair cells in the cochlea of the exposed ear was noted.[75] Similar noise damage has been observed in experiments with other laboratory animals as well. Although care must be exercised in applying results of animal experiments to humans, it is apparent that such damage may be occurring among young persons similarly exposed.

There is yet an added danger. During ordinary conversation at 60 decibels, only the lower hearing acuity levels are required. But the constant pressure of excessively loud sounds may first wear out the small beginning area of the delicate hair cells. That is why the early stages of deafness so often go unnoticed. A person who, according to an audiometer test, has a hearing impairment in both ears of 40 percent may not even have noticed his deafness. Why? Because he can adequately hear speech. By the time a person is aware of his hearing problem—before he has trouble understanding speech—his hearing loss may already be considerable and permanent. So, insofar as hearing acuity is concerned, mere speech comprehension may be a cruelly deceptive measurement.

aged ears

"Aged ears play truant at his tales," wrote Shakespeare in *Love's Labor's Lost* (II.i.74). Indeed, deafness has long been considered an inevitable disability of old age. To some extent, it may be. But among the Mabaan tribe in the African Sudan the aged hear about as well as the young. And old Mabaans hear better than old people in this country. Why? The environment of the gentle Mabaans is quiet—the sound level averages about 40 decibels. The Mabaans even sing softly. Their hearing mechanism is undamaged by noise.

To the city dweller in the Western world, noise may well be a cumulative hazard. Though on a day-to-day basis it may seem to be only an annoying byproduct of city life, like any other air pollutant it may become a health hazard to people who suffer prolonged exposure. The cost of noise is widespread deafness among older people. But that is not all. Studies conducted among the Mabaans verified earlier German research. With the Mabaans, blood "pressures remain essentially the same throughout life . . . whereas in our culture the blood pressure rises in the aging in apparently healthy individuals."[76] Loud noise may cause constriction of small blood vessels and a reduced output of blood from the heart. Some researchers believe that, because of this diminished output, less nourishing blood reaches the hearing nerves and that this deprivation promotes nerve cell abnormality and deafness. The possibility of continuous noise causing high blood pressure (even peptic ulcer) cannot be dismissed. However, a direct cause and effect relationship has not been proved.

antinoise activity

Noise costs money. In lost production and accidents due to noise, the yearly cost to industry is estimated at $4 billion. Annual compensation claims from

[75] David M. Lipscomb, "High Intensity Sounds in the Recreational Environment: Hazard to Young Ears," *Clinical Pediatrics*, Vol. 8, No. 2 (February 1969), pp. 63–68.

[76] Donald F. Anthrop, "Environmental Noise Pollution: A New Threat to Sanity," *Bulletin of the Atomic Scientists*, Vol. 25, No. 5 (May 1969), p. 13.

deafness thought to be due to job noise in this country amount to millions of dollars. Merely by changing an assembly-line operation from an area next to a boiler room to a quiet section of the shop, one factory manager markedly reduced costly errors. Another large company found office soundproofing a sound investment. Typing errors dropped 29 percent, machine operator errors 52 percent, absenteeism and employee turnover 37 and 47 percent respectively.[77] The management of one large New York bank tried to solve their noise problem in a roundabout way. Plagued by high employee turnover due to the insufferable noise, they finally resorted to hiring deaf people.[78]

In noise control, the Old World may yet show the New World the way. In France, transistor radios are forbidden in public places. Plastic or rubber lids cover the garbage pails of Paris. TV or radio noise outside a West German home may prompt a summons. Construction noise (a massive problem in this country) is limited by law in West Germany. Britain is developing similar antinoise legislation. Muscovites may not indiscriminately blow auto horns. Antinoise building codes limit racket in the new apartments of Britain, Germany, Russia, and the Low Countries.

In this country it is hard to control construction noise through legal codes. Such codes are local matters, and the thousands of cities and towns in the United States are fiercely protective of their own prerogatives. Nor does all legislation adequately control the problem. A 1967 California law permits a 50-horsepower motorcycle to make as much noise as four 300-horsepower Cadillacs. Ways are being studied in which noise-controlled construction would be required for structures built under FHA mortgages.

the public gets involved

President Nixon signed the National Environmental Policy Act of 1969 as his first official act of the 1970s. Section 102 of that act has precipitated heated controversy. Among its requirements is that any federal agency proposing a major action or project must release to the public a detailed statement as to the impact of the project on the environment.[79] The *impact statement* must include a description of any adverse environmental effects and present possible alternatives. The act gives the public a mighty weapon in the battle to protect the environment. Administrators of federal projects can no longer proceed without

[77] *M.D., Medical Newsmagazine,* Vol. 10, No. 6 (June 1966), p. 122.

[78] "New York Employs Deaf," *Hearing and Speech News* (January 1967), p. 7, quoted in Robert Alex Baron, "Noise and Urban Man," *American Journal of Public Health,* Vol. 58, No. 11 (November 1968), p. 2061.

[79] Among its other requirements is that "all federal agencies must bring their own facilities in compliance with existing pollution regulations by 3 December, 1972, or show by that date that they are trying to do so." ("Pollution: Military's Cleanup Stresses Plumbing, Not R & D," *Science,* Vol. 175, No. 4017 [January 7, 1972], p. 45.) This has resulted in a massive Department of Defense effort to clean up its bases, installations, and ships. One of the Navy's biggest problems, for example, is shipboard sewage. Present practice is merely to dump it at sea. The Navy is going to have to find a way to store sewage on board (a procedure for which the thousands of Navy ships are not equipped) until it can be routed to shoreside sewage treatment plants.

first seeking and responding to public scrutiny.[80]

Irreconcilable disagreements between government administrators and environmentalists about the potential pollution of a government project have been taken to court. Federal judges have resolutely delayed a number of major projects—nuclear power plants, waterways, pipelines, and canals—until satisfactory impact statements have been submitted.[81] For example, the building of the trans-Alaska oil pipeline was held up for two years until a federal judge finally approved (in May 1972) the Department of the Interior's laboriously revised twenty-five-pound impact statement.[82]

The National Environmental Policy Act of 1970 applies only to federal projects and to projects that are funded and licensed by federal agencies. It does not regulate the activities of private, local land developers, who may place their own financial interests above ecological considerations. Some real estate developers make a sincere effort to enhance the land; others scar the land with quick-profit projects. In a historic decision in September 1972, the California Supreme Court ruled that the California Environment Quality Act applies not only to public, but also to any private developments for which any government body issues a permit. Environmental impact statements will now have to be prepared by California county officials. As on the federal level, these statements will be open to vigorous public discussion. Reinforcing the California decision, a U.S. Court of Appeals for the District of Columbia moved to extend the application of the National Environmental Policy Act to the District's private and local developments.[83]

Important as they are, federal and state laws to protect the environment are not the only legal recourse available to those struggling to prevent abuse of their surroundings. "Several [other] recognized legal remedies are available to the individual citizen or group wishing to combat specific acts of pollution or proposals deemed destructive of the environment."[84] Polluters use resources common to everyone, such as air and water, and may therefore be liable for the damage they cause. *Nuisance laws* give every landowner the right to use his property without unreasonable interference. *Trespass laws* prevent intentional entry into privately owned land without permission. In the case of pollution, such trespass may be hard to prove. However, "a recent Oregon case . . .

[80] "National Environmental Policy Act: How Well Is It Working?" *Science,* Vol. 176, No. 4031 (April 14, 1972), pp. 146–47. It is the National Environmental Policy Act which requires the president to transmit an annual Environmental Quality Report to Congress. The three-member Council on Environmental Quality, created by the act and selected by the president, assists the president in preparing the report and also has various other duties, such as developing policies to protect the environment and reporting to the president at least once yearly on national environmental conditions. The council's annual reports are a mine of information for those seeking detailed information about this subject. They can be ordered at minimal cost from the Superintendent of Documents, U.S. Government Printing Office, Washington, D.C. 20402. The Council on Environmental Quality should not be confused with the Environmental Protection Agency (EPA), which was created in 1970 to consolidate all major federal activities designed to control and abate pollution. (*Environmental Quality, The Third Annual Report of the Council on Environmental Quality, August 1972* [Washington, D.C.], p. 389.)

[81] Victor Cohn, "Cutting the Legs Off Section 102," *Technology Review,* Vol. 74, No. 6 (May 1972), pp. 7–8.

[82] "The Environment: A Week of Big Decisions," *Science News,* Vol. 101, No. 21 (May 20, 1972), p. 325.

[83] Richard H. Gilluly, "Are the Courts Shaping a New Environmental Ethic?" *Science News,* Vol. 102, No. 23 (December 2, 1972), p. 363.

[84] Donal R. Levi and Dale Colyer, "Legal Remedies for Pollution Abatement," *Science,* Vol. 175, No. 4026 (March 10, 1972), p. 1085.

awarded damages to a group of plaintiff farmers whose crop had been damaged by fluoride gases from an aluminum plant."[85]

Such active and responsible citizen participation in preventing pollution by existing legal means is spreading rapidly. In Washington, D.C., for example, the Emergency Committee on the Transportation Crisis, a group of militant citizens led by a commercial artist, has legally forced reappraisal of attempts to blight their living area.[86] Moreover, "environmentalist challenges before Atomic Safety and Licensing Boards and in the federal courts, along with criticism from scientists within its own ranks, have forced [the Atomic Energy Commission] to adopt new reactor design criteria that would reduce radiation emissions from power reactors a hundredfold . . . Thus, the intervention of citizens has created a new dimension of the new nuclear technology."[87]

What more can the individual do? Also in the nation's capital, a young lawyer, aided by several dozen willing professional and lay volunteers, has shown what one private citizen can do for public safety and against environmental pollution. His thorough understanding and adroit use of the U.S. legal system, technology, and public opinion, has been instrumental in congressional approval of the Wholesome Meat Act of 1967, the National Gas and Pipeline Safety Act of 1968, the Coal Mine Health and Safety Act of 1969, and the Occupational Health and Safety Act of 1970. His name: Ralph Nader.

summary

Other hazards resulting from man's abuse of his environment, in addition to those discussed in Chapter 3, are:

1. *Pesticides.* Chemical pest killers are of enormous benefit to humans. They improve health by helping to ensure an abundant food supply and by preventing insect-borne diseases such as malaria, typhus, yellow fever, and river-blindness. But pesticides, which are intended to kill insects, rodents, fungi, and weeds, also find their way into the human body by inhalation, absorption through the skin, or oral ingestion (page 79). Some pesticides—notably DDT—are *spread* by wind and water; they are not readily broken down and so they *accumulate;* they also *concentrate* in living tissue (page 79). Because knowledge about its very long-term effects is incomplete, the agricultural use of DDT has been partly abolished in the United States, and ways are being sought to control pests without using chemical pesticides.

2. *Other dangerous substances. Metallic mercury* and *inorganic mercury* may cause poisoning, but far more dangerous is *organic mercury,* especially *methylmercury* (pages 82–85). *PCBs* (polychlorinated biphenyls) are a group of highly toxic chemicals used in adhesives, sealants, and paints (pages 85–86). *Lead* is a very useful metal, but in high concentrations it is poisonous. *Plumbism* (lead poisoning) in young children is often caused by eating flakes of lead-based paint; brain damage can result (pages 86–88). *Hexachlorophene* has been found to cause brain damage in animals when present at high levels in the blood stream (pages 88–89).

3. *Radiation.* Everything in nature

[85] *Ibid.*
[86] Rice Odell, "To Stop Highways Some Citizens Take to the Streets," *Smithsonian,* Vol. 3, No. 1 (April 1972), pp. 24–29.
[87] Richard Lewis, "Citizens *v.* Atomic Power," *New Scientist,* Vol. 56, No. 821 (November 23, 1972), p. 450.

consists of *elements;* elements consist of *atoms;* and each atom consists of a *nucleus,* which contains positively charged *protons* and uncharged *neutrons* and which is surrounded by negatively charged *electrons.* Atoms of the same element that have the same chemical properties (that is, the same number of electrons and protons) but different weights (that is, a different number of neutrons) are *isotopes* of one another. Because some isotopes are unstable, their nuclei disintegrate, emitting energy known as *ionizing radiation* (page 90). In addition to natural ionizing radiation, humans are exposed to manmade radiation, as in X-rays; among these are some types of medical examinations, and certain industrial processes. Excessive ionizing radiation can damage tissues by causing the molecular disintegration of a cell's chemicals, thus interrupting cell function and perhaps poisoning the cell. Radiation damage to *somatic* (body) *cells* affects the individual, but radiation damage to *reproductive cells* affects future generations by changing DNA structure directly or by causing breaks in chromosomal structure (page 91). Major sources of concern are atomic accidents, disposal of radioactive wastes, thermonuclear weapons, and the effects of radioactive fallout (pages 92–94).

Despite its dangers, radiation has vast potential for benefit not only in medicine but also in industry, particularly as a source of energy. *Fission energy* is currently being obtained from nuclear power plants; other possibilities are *fusion energy, solar energy, "sea-thermal" energy,* and *geothermal energy* (pages 96–97). Development of such energy sources will help to avert future energy crises.

4. *Sound pollution.* Sound travels in waves from its source through vibrating air particles to the *outer, middle,* and *inner ear* (pages 98–100) and ultimately to the brain for interpretation. Sound waves cause changes in air pressure. The smallest disturbance in air pressure that can be heard under ideal conditions is the *threshold of hearing,* on the basis of which sound is measured in units called *decibels* (page 101). Long exposure to loud noise can permanently impair hearing or even cause deafness.

The public has recently become more involved in the struggle to protect the environment. Pressure from citizens' groups and individuals has resulted in environmental legislation on federal, state, and local levels.

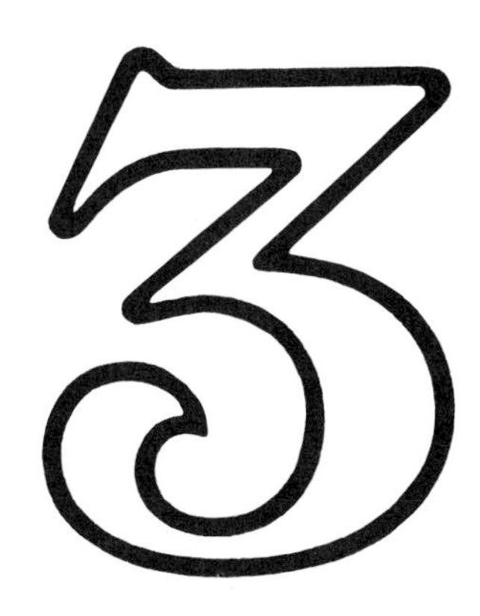

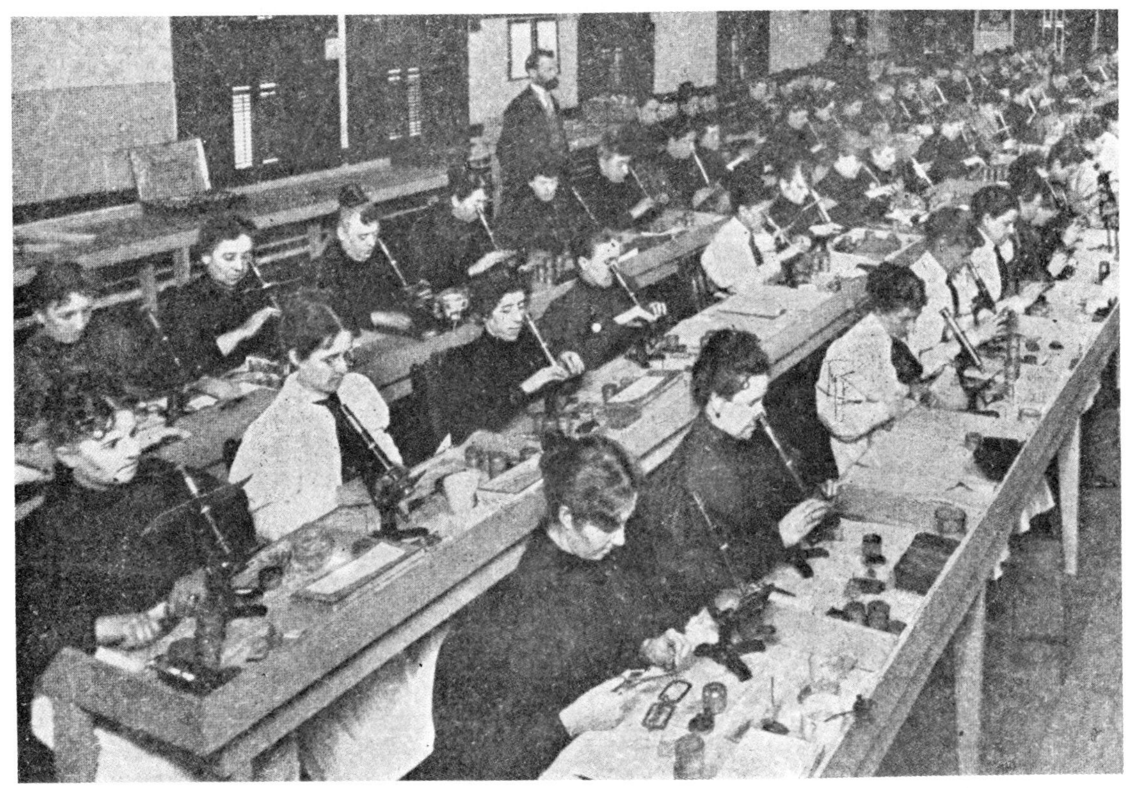

Microscopic examination of pork (1897) for trichinosis, "the garbage sickness" (see page 649, footnote 2).

man versus his smallest enemies

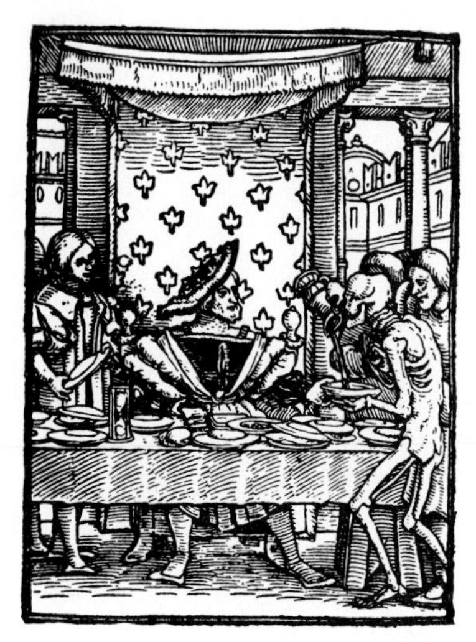
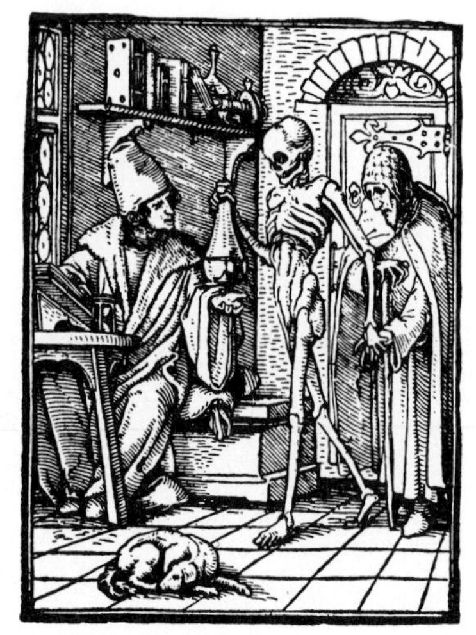
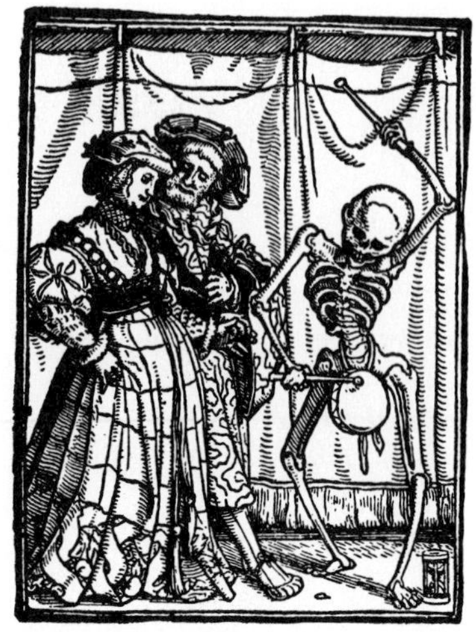

"The Dance of Death" (1538) by Hans Holbein the Younger (1497–1543). The dance of death was a major artistic theme, originating during the plagues and wars of the Middle Ages. Three of Holbein's forty-one woodcuts are reproduced here: "The King," "The Doctor," and "The Noblewoman."

disease and destiny

5

prologue

ALCIBIADES. *What is thy name? Is man so hateful to thee,
That art thyself a man?*[1]

Thirteen centuries ago (in 664) the Irish kings of Ulster and Munster called a meeting at Temora. Attending the council were the lay and clerical leaders of their kingdoms. The problem besetting them was famine. The poor earth could not supply their growing populations. The starving people were unable to work and growing restive. What could be done?

The two kings agreed on a plan of action. Through devout prayer and a fast, a direct appeal was to be made to God. In His infinite mercy, He would surely hear and help them.

Up to this point, there was harmony at the meeting. It was about the content of the prayer to the Lord that disagreement and debate arose. What the kings proposed to ask God for was a pestilence to kill the excess population, composed of ''inferior'' people. There would then be enough food for the ''superior'' and ''worthier'' survivors. As to who would be included among the survivors, there seemed to be no doubt.

One man dissented. Would it not be more in keeping with God's way, St. Gerald suggested, to pray, not for pestilence, but for more food? Certainly, it was just as easy. And the chances of being heard by a compassionate God would surely be greater. St. Gerald and a few supporters moved to ''supplicate the Almighty not to reduce the number of men till it answered the quantity of corn usually produced, but to increase the produce of the land, so that it might satisfy the wants of the people.''[2]

But this motion failed to carry. In opposing it, St. Fechin gained favor with the lords and most of the clergy. The motion he supported carried. God was to be implored for a plague to kill off the lesser people.

According to the records of the Church at Mayo, however, God punished this wickedness. A pestilence did indeed visit Ulster and Munster. But it was not so discriminating as some had hoped. The kings and at least one-third of the nobles who had beseeched the Lord for the visitation were carried off by it.

This immorality tale illustrates the grotesque vanity and indifference of those who enslave others. To the Irish tyrants, sickness and death were the expected due of their serfs. Sick societies are never free. Disease makes men susceptible to enslavement. Parents who see their babies die of hunger, who must prostitute their starving daughters for the family bread, who taste the dust of the land, will accept any promise, any hope. Modern leaders of free societies labor for the health of their people. A nation's vitality can come only from its people. In this age a nation prostrate with sickness can barely survive. Today, the world is small. The social convulsions of one nation are felt far beyond its borders. Whether in Biafra or Brazil, a sick man is the business of every man everywhere.

[1] William Shakespeare, *Timon of Athens,* IV.iii.51–52.
[2] Edward Bascome, *A History of Epidemic Pestilences* (London, 1851), p. 28.

The philosopher George Santayana said, "Those who cannot remember the past are condemned to repeat it." That is why this chapter will explore the effect of disease on past events. For the sake of continuity, one major disease has been chosen: plague. Many others could be used as examples—typhus, malaria, smallpox, leprosy, syphilis, cholera. In addition, the effect of individual illness on the course of history will be discussed, with Napoleon serving as the major subject. "God was bored with him," wrote Victor Hugo. But if any one man can be said to have brought agony to his age, it is surely he.

plague: what is it?

Throughout history, plague has killed an estimated 150 million people. It is primarily an affliction of rats and other rodents such as the squirrel and the chipmunk. In 1894 two men working separately, Shibasaburo Kitasato (a pupil of Koch) and Alexandre Yersin (a student of Pasteur), discovered its causative bacillus. This bacillus causes the several types of plague, of which the two most common are the *bubonic* and *pneumonic.*

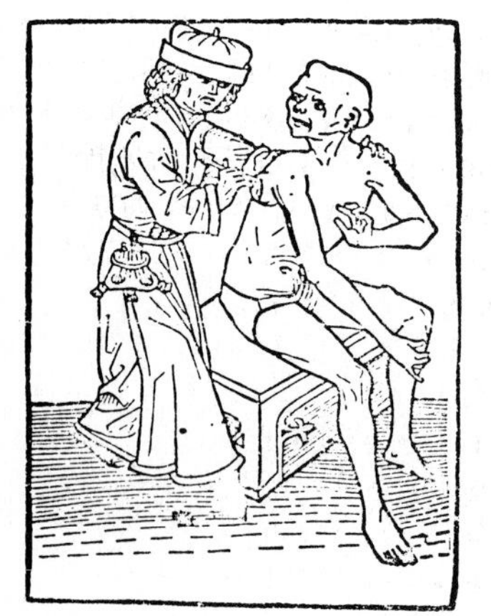

5-1 *Lancing a bubo.*

Fleas transmit the bacillus of plague, *Pasteurella pestis,* from rat to rat and from rat to man. However, the bacillus may, under certain conditions, be transmitted directly from the respiratory tract of one person to that of another person by airborne droplets. Epidemics of plague pneumonia (pneumonic plague) can thus occur.

A flea takes a blood meal from an infected rodent. Plague bacilli get into its alimentary tract. There they multiply. In feeding on another rat or a human, the infected flea vomits the bacteria into the bite, thus transmitting the disease.

Usually several days after being bitten by an infected flea, the infected person becomes desperately ill. He develops a raging fever. His blood pressure falls. His pulse becomes rapid and irregular. Within hours, the patient is prostrate and incoherent. The pain in his neck, groin, or armpit (or in all three) is excruciating. In any or all of these areas swellings rapidly develop. Soon these swellings, called buboes (bubonic plague), abscess. Upon rupturing they discharge great quantities of pus. Extensive hemorrhages under the skin are common. The skin may become blackish-purple. It is this dread characteristic that gave rise to the medieval designation "the Black Death."

plague in the Middle Ages

The Middle Ages began and ended with the plague. The best known of the early medieval epidemics occurred during the reign of Emperor Justinian the Great (527–565).

the plague of Justinian

The plague of Justinian was bubonic plague. Coming from the hinterlands of southwest Asia, it arrived in Constantinople, the capital of the Byzantine Empire, in about A.D. 532. Spreading west, it soon assaulted all Europe. A remarkable account of the epidemic at Constantinople was left by Procopius of Caesara. Plainly, he saw disease threatening civilization. ''During these times,'' he wrote with horror, ''there was a pestilence by which the whole human race came near to being annihilated.''[3]

So accurately did Procopius describe the symptoms of plague that there is little doubt as to the disease. Within a few days—at the most five—of the onset of sickness, death occurred. Soon the burial places were exhausted. The dead littered the streets. Instead of being buried, many bodies were collected and piled one on top of the other in unoccupied buildings. The rats infesting these buildings became infected. They carried their infection to the people. In this way the contagion spread.

The greatest city of the Eastern Roman Empire was paralyzed. ''The work of every description ceases . . . all the trades were abandoned by the artisans, and all other work as well.''[4] How similar this comment is to the report of a modern Peace Corps worker: ''They cannot work. They cannot learn. They can't do anything but be sick and die.''

In explaining a cause for the calamity, Procopius forsook classical reasoning in favor of the religious fatalism so characteristic of the Dark Ages: ''For this calamity it is quite impossible either to express in words or to conceive in thought any explanation except indeed to refer it to God.''[5]

With these words the intellectual night of the Dark Ages fell upon mankind.[6]

The seventh century ushered in a new era. The plague was not the only cause of the death of the old era, but its effect on administrations, plots and plans, campaigns and counter-campaigns, cannot be denied. *Pasteurella pestis* had twisted the course of history.

the Black Death

In 1333, a drought devastated China. Famine followed, then flood. In Kingsai, at that time the capital of China, some 400,000 people drowned. Deluge, locusts, earthquakes, famine—all followed one upon the other and spread across vast areas of the tormented land. Added to these sufferings was still another affliction—plague. Starting somewhere in central Asia, the scourge had spread rapidly to China and India. Finally the pestilence came to Europe. This is how.

In 1347, some Genoese businessmen were making their way from China back to Europe. Returning with luxury items such as furs and silks, the merchants met their ancient enemy—the Tartars. They barricaded themselves in Caffa, a small fort on the Crimean Straits. There they stayed to resist the Tartar seige. Weeks passed.

One summer day, the Tartars suddenly hurled new weapons of destruction

[3] Procopius of Caesara, *History of the Wars,* Book II, *The Persian War,* Vols. XXIV and XXIII, tr. by H. E. Dewing (New York, 1914), p. 451.
[4] *Ibid.,* p. 471.
[5] *Ibid.,* p. 453.
[6] During this period, even a sneeze was thought to herald certain death from plague. To mark this, there originated in sixth-century Italy the expression ''God bless you.'' (Raymond Crawfurd, *Plague and Pestilence in Literature and Art* [Oxford, Eng., 1914], pp. 93–94.)

over the city walls. These weapons were the dead bodies of their own men who had died of the plague. This early attempt at bacteriological warfare was successful. The Genoese merchants were terrified. Many fell sick and died. The survivors expected momentary capture. But the besieging Tartars did not attack. They panicked. Hundreds of their men were being killed by the plague. Tartar bodies lay rotting in the sun. The Tartars fled, leaving the small fortress to its misery.

Those Genoese still alive boarded four small ships and set sail for Constantinople—that great meeting place of Asia, Europe, and Africa. Along the route, they saw great ships drifting aimlessly; all on board were dead of plague. In Constantinople the Genoese merchants seeded the plague. The disease raced through Italy and then the rest of Europe.

In the constant competition between man and his parasites, it is the plague bacillus that came closest to wiping out the human race. Like a wind of death, the disease bereaved the world. Pope Clement VI (who kept the contagion from him by surrounding himself with two great fires) estimated the world loss of human life during this fourteenth-century pandemic at 43 million. The papal physicians considered the mortality in Europe to be between two-thirds and three-fourths of the population. Men thought the end of the world was at hand. Friar John Clyn, an Irish Franciscan, expecting death, left behind this touching note (1349):

> So have I reduced these things to writing; and lest the writing should perish with the writer, and the work fail together with the workman, I leave parchment for continuing the work, if haply any man survive, and any of the race of Adam escape this pestilence and continue the work which I have commenced . . .

Here the sentence trails off. The writer lived to add but two more words: "magna karistia"—great dearth. Another hand then briefly noted "here it seems that the author died."[7]

5-2 *Looting during the Black Death.*

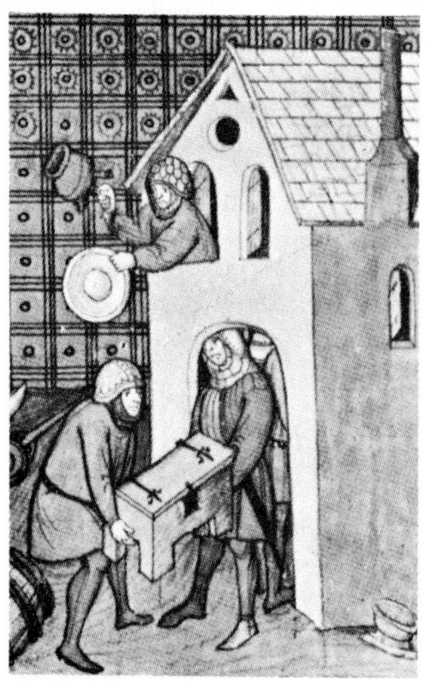

SOCIETAL CHANGES And so medieval Europe, terrorized by sickness, huddled under the repeated blows of the plague. As in the time of Justinian, the societal changes were incalculable. To the modern student, who sees whole populations in developing countries enslaved by disease, an understanding of these changes is essential.

First, *moral standards* were lowered. The plague had killed many policemen and judges. The courts were always closed. The process of law was stopped. Amorality became the rule. "Live today, tomorrow, death," was a way of existence. Debauchery and drunkenness were everywhere. Thievery was rampant. For a short time, stolen goods could be obtained at ridiculously low prices. But the time of low prices was short-lived. Disastrous *economic changes* followed. The surplus accumulated as a result of plague deaths was soon gone. The death of large numbers of men from the disease reduced the number of competent

[7] Friar John Clyn of the Convent of Friars Minor at Kilkenny, and Thady Dowling, Chancellor of Leighlin, edited from the manuscripts by R. Butler (Dublin, 1849), quoted in Charles Creighton, *A History of Epidemics in Britain,* 2nd ed., Vol. I (New York, 1965), p. 115.

hands to do the work. This shortage of labor resulted in higher prices. The twin economic spectres of diminished production and soaring prices pushed Europe to the brink of ruin.

The *societal character* of medieval life also changed. The *nouveaux riches* who were created by the plague did not result only from inheritance and thievery. New opportunities became legally available and were eagerly seized. Aristocratic holders of titles had died of the plague, many of them leaving no heirs. Their lands and titles were dispensed by the kings to newer favorites. But these new nobles were without tradition. "The decay in manners in the last half of the fourteenth century is an astonishing fact. The old fashioned gentility was gone; manners were uncouth, rude, brutal."[8]

In addition, there were *changes in government and the Church.* Both were to the detriment of the people. Again, excess death was the cause. It had taken centuries to develop a competent governing corps with a tradition of efficiency and service. In a short time, without warning, it was gone. Positions formerly held by able men were now filled by incompetents and opportunists. From every quarter rose cries for reform. The Church suffered even more severely than did the government, for the people had already begun to doubt. Had not prayer failed to stop the dying? There are those who hold the view that the Black Death led to such questioning of the authority of the Church that it helped bring on the Reformation and, indeed, the Renaissance.

Remarkable as the effects of the Black Death were on the economic, social, governmental, and religious structures, the effect on morals was even more astonishing. Insanity swept through Europe.

FLAGELLATION Whipping, as a religious activity, had been vigorously practiced by the ancient Egyptians, Romans, and Greeks. Every February 15, at the fertility festivals, the ancient Romans flogged their women. Ostensibly, this was to guard them against sterility. In the eleventh century, the Church recognized flogging as a form of penance. During the Black Death of the fourteenth century, it developed into mass mania.

Woe filled Europe. Everywhere were death and suffering. To punish man for his sins God had sent the plague. Man's only salvation lay in doing penance.

In Hungary first, then in Germany, arose the Brotherhood of the Flagellants. In long lines they wove through the cities of Europe. They were robed as if in mourning. Red crosses marked their breasts, backs, and caps. In their hands they clutched triple whips, tied in three or four knots. In each knot were fixed points of iron.

On arriving at a chosen place of penance, the flagellants stripped off all their clothes except for a linen dress that extended from the waist to the ankles. They then lay down in a circle. The position assumed varied according to the sin. The adulterer kept his face to the ground. The murderer lay on his back. The perjurer lay on one side holding up three fingers. They were then castigated by the master. After they had lain on the ground long enough to say five paternosters, they

5-3 *Flagellants in 1349. The cross on their hats earned these men and their fellow penitents the name Brothers of the Cross.*

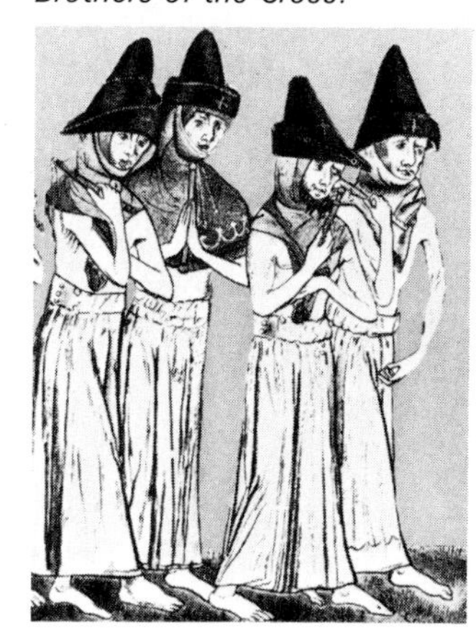

[8] James Westfall Thompson, "The Aftermath of the Black Death and the Aftermath of the Great War," *American Journal of Sociology,* Vol. 26, No. 7 (January 1921), p. 569.

rose and were whipped. All the while they sang psalms and prayed loudly for deliverance from the plague.

So powerful did the Brotherhood of the Flagellants become that it threatened the Church. However, the core of the movement had never been savory. Soon, crime and degeneracy crept in. Strict action by Pope Clement and the Holy Roman Emperor, Charles IV, curtailed this gloomy sect. Not only had it helped spread the plague, it also played a part in spreading throughout Europe the plague's vicious partners—suspicion and hatred.[9]

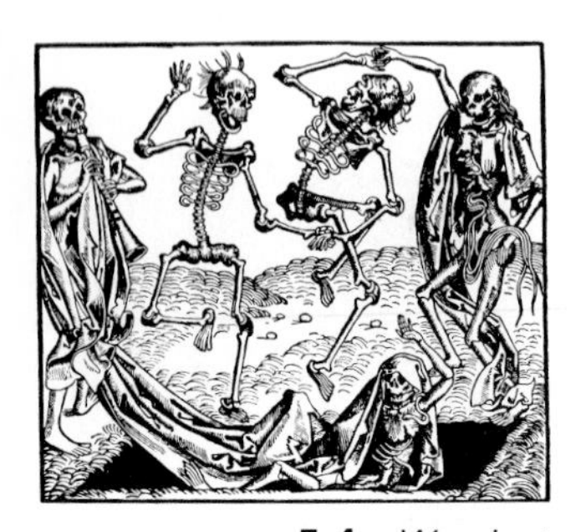

5-4 *Woodcut depicting the dance of death.*

THE DANCING MANIA Dancing and death have long been closely related. In primitive societies dances are often held to celebrate the death of a tribal member. Dancing was part of ancient Roman and Greek funeral rites. In his *Aeneid* Vergil depicted the joy of the dance in the land of the dead. The dance of death was a favorite subject of the medieval artist.

During the height of the Black Death, a dancing mania seized parts of Europe. Particularly in Germany, and to the northwest, strange assemblages of people behaved as if possessed. Holding hands at first, they formed circles. Then they would begin to dance. They danced with wild abandon, deliriously. Finally, exhausted, they collapsed. They lay and groaned as if in agony. This was a signal for swathing them in tight cloths, particularly around their waists. Apparently this relieved them. It is thought that their discomfort was due to the abdominal distension resulting from their exertions.

Sometimes the dancing mania (called the Dance of St. John or St. Vitus) began with a convulsion—with the afflicted falling to the ground and foaming at the mouth. Suddenly springing up, they would then begin to contort wildly.

THE PERSECUTION OF THE JEWS Among the most grievous consequences of the Black Death was the pitiless persecution of the Jews. Since the Jews of the fourteenth and fifteenth centuries contributed many physicians to southern Europe, the maddened public suspected them of bringing about the plague. Jews were "put to the question." Upon denying that they were poisoning the population, they were put to the rack. Long and detailed confessions were thus obtained. The tortured admitted, finally, that poisons from spiders and owls, some of which were colored red and black, had been provided by rabbis for the purpose of poisoning the wells. Other poison was smeared on the walls of buildings. Jews were accused of poisoning the very air. Hideous massacres took place. In Basel, Switzerland, all the Jews were enclosed in a wooden building, specially built for that purpose, and burned alive. Elsewhere, the Jews were handed over to the infuriated populace. So it was throughout Europe except in England, from which most of the Jews had already been banished.

ALAS, ALAS FOR HAMELIN! The sad legend of the Pied Piper of Hamelin was again brought to life at the time of the Black Death.[10] The incident of the Pied Piper is thought to have occurred in 1284, a year after a violent plague

[9] To this day, there is, among the Indians of New Mexico, a group of flagellants called the Penitentes.

[10] James Westfall Thompson, "The Aftermath of the Black Death and the Aftermath of the Great War," p. 571. Centuries later the story was immortalized by the English poet Robert Browning (1812–1889) in *The Pied Piper of Hamelin: A Child's Story.*

epidemic. But now, over sixty years later, the story was retold again and again. Rats were associated with plague. Some droll piper may, indeed, have appeared at Hamelin so long ago and offered to charm the rats away with his music. He would come again, it was now whispered. And, in those times of lunacy, there is no reason to consider that his offer would have been rejected. Was it not possible that the children would be swept away on the crest of mass hysteria, even as children had joined a Children's Crusade in 1237, and had been lured away by a piper in 1284?

It was a time of mass madness, public whippings, wild dancing. It was a period of debauchery, decay, deprivation, and death. Robert Browning's wistful lines fit too innocently into those terrible times:

> All the little boys and girls,
> With rosy cheeks and flaxen curls,
> And sparkling eyes and teeth like pearls,
> Tripping and skipping, ran merrily after
> The wonderful music with shouting and laughter.

plague in the early modern era

And now leave the Middle Ages. Enter into the early modern era. For the plague did just this. Like all communicable disease, it knew boundaries of neither nations nor time.

plague and the Bard of Avon

> O, when mine eyes did see Olivia first,
> Methought she purged the air of pestilence![11]

In the three centuries between the Black Death of the fourteenth century and the Great Plague of London of the seventeenth century, hardly a year went by without the winnowing of the population of some European area by the illness. In 1592, strict measures were taken to prevent the spread of plague in London. Upon such regulations William Shakespeare plotted some of *Romeo and Juliet.* The law read in part: "That in every howse infected, the Master, Mistris, governour, and the whole famulie and residentes therin at the time of such infeccon, shall remayne continuallie without departinge out of the same, and with the doores and windowes . . . shutt."[12]

Such an ordinance was used by the bard to set the tragedy of *Romeo and Juliet.* Friar Lawrence tells Juliet (IV.i.93–94):

> Take thou this vial, being then in bed,
> And this distilled liquor drink thou off.

The draught is to render her seemingly lifeless. Later she is to waken (IV.i.113–17):

[11] William Shakespeare, *Twelfth Night,* I.i. 19–20.
[12] R. R. Simpson, *Shakespeare and Medicine* (Baltimore, 1959), p. 208.

In the meantime, against thou shalt awake,
Shall Romeo by my letters know our drift,
And hither shall he come, and he and I
Will watch thy waking, and that very night
Shall Romeo bear thee hence to Mantua.

But the plot goes wrong. Juliet swallows the draught, and the good Friar Lawrence gives a letter to Friar John that is to be delivered to Romeo. But the letter never reaches him because of the plague regulation. The tragedy continues (V.ii.2–16):

FRIAR LAWRENCE. This same should be the voice of Friar John.
Welcome from Mantua. What says Romeo?
Or if his mind be writ, give me his letter.
FRIAR JOHN. Going to find a barefoot brother out,
One of our order, to associate me
Here in this city visiting the sick,
And finding him, the searchers of the town,
Suspecting that we both were in a house
Where the infectious pestilence did reign,
Sealed up the doors and would not let us forth,
So that my speed to Mantua there was stayed.
FRIAR LAWRENCE. Who bare my letter, then, to Romeo?
FRIAR JOHN. I could not send it—here it is again—
Nor get a messenger to bring it thee,
So fearful were they of infection.

Thus did a plague regulation prevent Romeo from knowing that the unconscious Juliet was still alive. Thinking she was dead, he killed himself.

Eyam

The year 1664 had been good to the people of the ancient English village of Eyam. The passing of summer had been celebrated by the annual feast on St. Helen's Day. On that day scores of visitors had been added to the usual population of about 380. There had been dancing in the alehouses. The men had toasted one another. If anyone knew of the plague raging in London, 150 miles away (which was unlikely in so remote a village), it did not dampen the enthusiasm of the celebration. The rural winds of Eyam, sheltered in the hollows of the Derbyshire hills, bore no breath of disease. That August Sunday was the last happy holiday the villagers were to know for a long time.

After the feast day, village life again became routine. It revolved around the church. The Reverend William Mompesson had recently come there, bringing his twenty-eight-year-old wife Catherine and their two children. The villagers respected him and liked his family.

Early in September a box of clothes arrived in Eyam from a London tailor. It was received by a village trader, Edward Cooper. George Vicars, a servant, opened the box. Remarking on the dampness of the tailor's samples, he hung them to the fire to dry.

This happened on the third of September. Three days later Vicars died in a delirium and with plague buboes swelling in his neck and groin. On September 22, Cooper's son was buried. The following day saw the funerals of Mary Thorpe and Sarah Lydall. Then two others died.

October began with two more funerals. That month twenty-two more villagers died. Like a slow stain, first apprehension, then terror spread in the village. "Pest families" were avoided on the street. The plague simmered. In November, only seven died of it. In December, nine. In January 1665, just four died. That month the villagers began to hope. Their hope was short-lived. In February, eight died; in March, six; in April, nine. In May, only three died. It was the best month in a long time and the villagers, desperate for some respite, again knew hope, barely spoken.

But, by the beginning of June, 74 of the 380 villagers of Eyam had died of the plague. Mrs. Mompesson implored her husband to send their children to Yorkshire. Reluctantly, he agreed. But he would not leave his people and she stayed with him.

It was in June that all the villagers began to think of flight. Some of the wealthiest had already left for other villages or the city. A few others had fled to the neighboring hills. Now the entire population wanted to run away.

At this point, the Reverend Mompesson spoke to his dwindling, stricken flock.

He told them this: In their hands lay the safety of the surrounding villages. Now they surely carried the disease. Spare the others, he implored them. He promised to seek help, to remain with them.

The villagers decided to stay.

An off-limits boundary, marked by stones and hills, was drawn, encircling all the land within half a mile of the village. Beyond this, nobody from Eyam would venture. North of Eyam was a rivulet. Today it is known as "Mompesson's Well" or "Mompesson's Brook." It was one of several places where articles were deposited for the villagers. From nearby villages people delivered provisions and placed them beside the brook and fled. Money for payment was left in the water in the hope of purifying it. On Mompesson's request the Earl of Devonshire also sent provisions.

Towards the end of June, the plague grew worse. Nineteen perished. Yet the living stayed.

July was a month of indescribable suffering. Each family began to bury its own dead or to hire Marshall Howe, who had apparently recovered from the disease and now seemed immune. His pay consisted of the possessions of the deceased. For many years after the plague, parents of Eyam stilled unruly children by threatening to send for Marshall Howe.

In July, fifty-seven were lost. Yet the ordeal was not over. August was an utter desolation. Every thought was of death. Seventy-eight perished. One woman dug graves for her husband and six children. On the twenty-second, Catherine Mompesson died. Towards the end of that harrowing summer month, 80 percent of the village had been killed by the plague. And still they stayed.

At last, by September, the plague began to abate. Only twenty-four per-

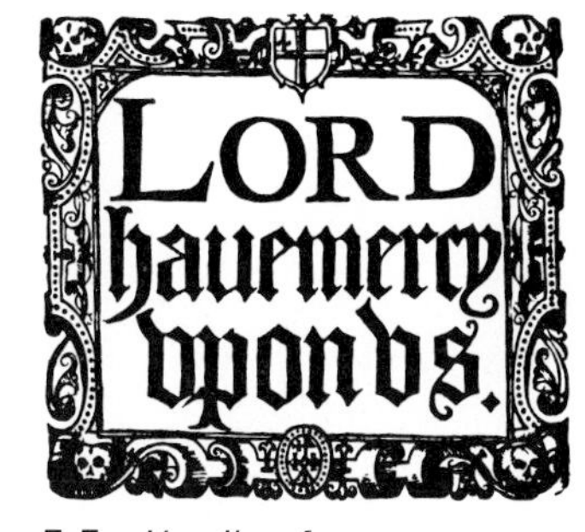

5-5 *Heading from a 1636 Death Bill, a list of plague victims and health measures.*

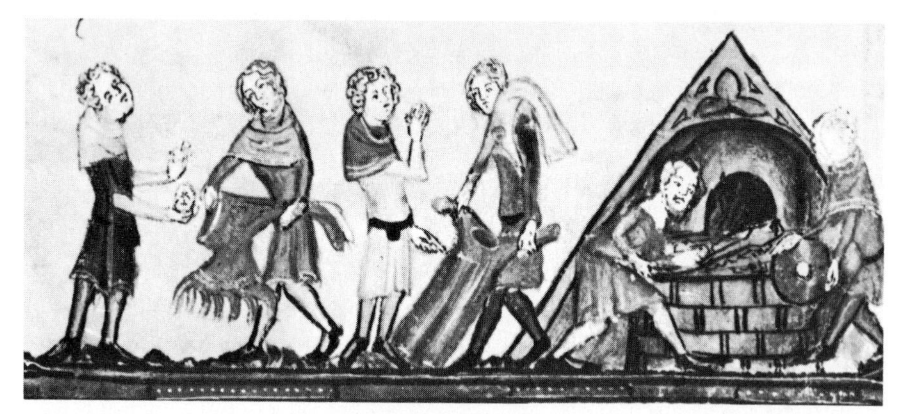

5-6 *Europeans burning infected clothes during the 14th-century plague.*

ished that month. With the death of fifteen more in October, the plague was finished with Eyam.

Thirty-three of the original 380 villagers of Eyam were left. (Mompesson did not die. Because he had walked among so much death, he lived to be ostracized by another village.)

What did the people of Eyam accomplish? Two things. First, they demonstrated rare fortitude. Second, they demonstrated the terrible price of medical ignorance.

By isolating themselves with their rats and fleas and bacilli, they condemned themselves. Had they all left Eyam soon after the appearance of the plague, leaving their possessions behind and submitting to isolation until dissemination of the illness was no longer possible, deaths would have been cut by 90 percent.[13] The error was as ancient as the ignorance. When, during the plague of Justinian, more than a thousand years before, the panic-stricken citizens of Constantinople piled their dead in buildings and locked the doors and windows, they guaranteed the spread of the disease.

Even as the villagers of Eyam doomed themselves, so was London shutting up infected people in their houses, thereby spreading the plague.

the Great Plague of London, 1665

> O let it be enough what Thou has done,
> When spotted death ran arm'd through every street.[14]

Of the numerous descriptions of the 1665 Great Plague of London, none is more celebrated or accurate than the *Diary and Correspondence* of Samuel Pepys. Pepys sallied forth into the midst of the Great Plague of 1665, noting

[13] W. G. Bell, *The Great Plague in London in 1665* (London, 1924), p. 297. As discussed on pages 123–25, a twentieth-century outbreak of plague in Los Angeles was partly handled by restricting the movement of people from an afflicted area. But modern public health procedures within the stricken area prevented a massive epidemic.

[14] John Dryden, *Annus Mirabilis,* verse 267, line 1065.

everything, truly touched by nothing. As his fellow Londoners suffered and perished, he worried about his wig. On September 3, 1665, he notes: "And it is a wonder what will be the fashion after the plague is done, as to periwigs, for nobody will dare buy any hair for fear of infection, that it had been cut off the heads of people dead of the plague."

When Pepys first saw two or three plague houses in Drury Lane "marked with a red cross upon the doors" and a notice, "Lord have mercy upon us," he was so distressed he "was forced to buy some roll-tobacco to smell and to chaw, which took away the apprehension."

But Pepys ends his review of the tragic desolation of the plague year in his diary in a more cheerful frame of mind:

> Thus ends this year, to my great joy in this manner. I have raised my estate . . . Pray God continue the plague's decrease! For that keeps the court away from the place of business, and so all goes to rack as to public matters, they at a distance not thinking of it.

How can one account for such destructive epidemics of plague during this time? Poor sanitation and poor personal hygiene combined with overcrowding always promote community infection. Rats seek garbage. The filth of both people and rats provided a fertile soil for pestilence. Both man and animal were the abode of vermin. They, and their surroundings, were unspeakably dirty. People bathed infrequently, if at all. The little available water was needed for drinking and cooking. Among the well-to-do, perfumes were used to mask body odors. Soap was a rare commodity. Seventeenth-century English judges wore wigs to cover their heads, shaved (as with the ancient Greeks) "as far as the louse." Throughout the centuries vermin and rats had continued to multiply appallingly. In 1170 monks recovered the body of the murdered Thomas à Becket to reverently prepare it for burial. As the brothers divested the body of its tight-fitting undergarment of coarse haircloth, this is what they saw:

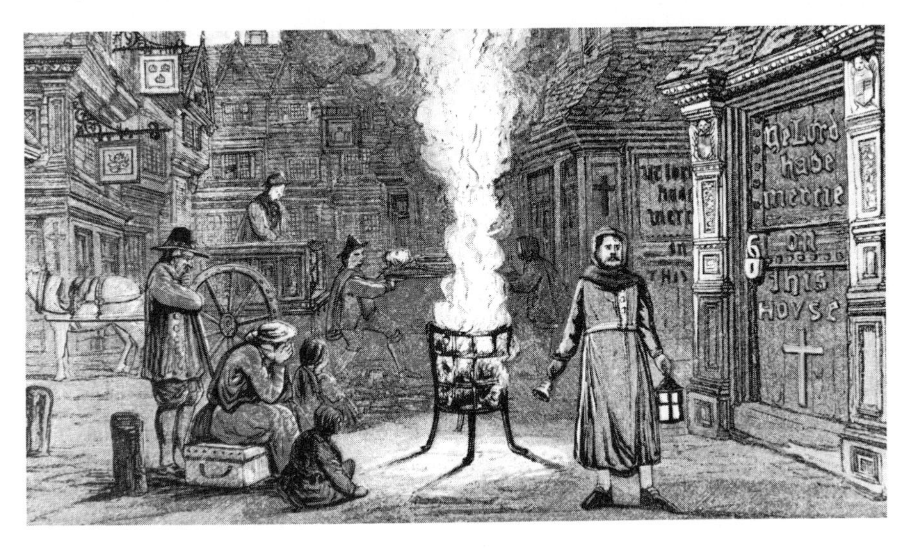

5-7 *London during the Great Plague, 1665. Fires were built in the streets; it was thought that the smoke might drive away the plague. More than a century later, such fires were built in the cities of the New World to drive off epidemics.*

> The innumerable vermin which had infested the dead prelate were stimulated to such activity by the cold that his hair-cloth, in the words of the chronicler, "boiled over with them like water in a simmering cauldron."[15]

Rats, it is known, will desert a sinking ship and vermin a cold dead body. This maxim explains, in one sense, how they spread disease.

The surroundings of the early modern era were no cleaner than their inhabitants. Erasmus (1466–1536), the celebrated Dutch scholar, wrote of the medieval English hovel in this way: "The floors are commonly of clay, strewn with rushes, which were occasionally removed, but underneath lies unmolested, an ancient collection of beer, grease, fragments of fish, spittle, the excrement of dogs, cats and everything that was nasty."[16] One can only imagine the filth that accumulated when plague patients were, according to the practice of the times, locked up in their houses.

Samuel Pepys may have had a good year in 1665, but few other Englishmen could say the same. In this, "the poor man's plague," over 100,000 Londoners lost their lives. The constant presence of death, always somehow unexpected because it was so quick, sapped the moral strength of the Englishman and drained his vitality. Trade, industry, and agriculture suffered. With the decrease in productive enterprise (which might have bolstered a flagging economy), expenditures on welfare and relief increased. Prices rose. Stores, offices, warehouses, ships—all were without workers. Because those with money feared to risk it, investment was at a low ebb. Although, as Pepys amply shows, English life continued, government administrative routines were either halted or greatly slowed. In times of war, societies plan for better times, meanwhile carrying on societal functions. But during the 1665 London plague, the machinery of society worked erratically. True, the social disorganizations that had accompanied the fourteenth-century plague did not now recur. The moral, political, economic, and religious convulsions of the earlier period were not characteristic of Pepys's time. Yet it is apparent that widespread sickness helped change the age and thus the course of human history.

Nonetheless, the plague was an ill wind that blew some good. From the enormous disorder came a degree of order. Dire need caused attention to improving sanitation. Hospitals were constructed. Straw for bedding and floors (in which vermin could breed) fell into disuse. Brick replaced rotting wood for buildings. Because planners could start anew, the Great Fire of London made possible a better-organized city. Crowding was diminished. As the eighteenth century approached, England took a long, deep breath of air. *Pasteurella pestis* was gone. But a new plague, air pollution, had replaced the old (Chapter 3).

plague in more recent times

Up to this point, the effect of plague on the course of history has been considered in relation to the distant past.

In this century, however, one finds that the plague bacillus still abounds in

[15] Sir William MacArthur, quoted in Arthur Swinson, *The History of Public Health* (Exeter, Eng., 1965), p. 19. During the medieval years of the Black Death, human cleanliness was not fostered. In some quarters it was a mortal sin to view one's own body. It became easier to whip it than to wash it.

[16] Quoted in Edward Bascome, *A History of Epidemic Pestilences,* p. 206.

India, Africa, and even in South America. And it still menaces this country. In the United States, as late as 1924, the threat became reality. That year, the same plague bacillus, the same flea, the same rat that combined to produce the epidemics that slew the innocents of Justinian's time, demoralized Europe in the fourteenth century and again in the sixteenth century, and depopulated little Eyam, were working together to kill people in Los Angeles, just as they had, around 1900, already killed in Oakland and San Francisco.

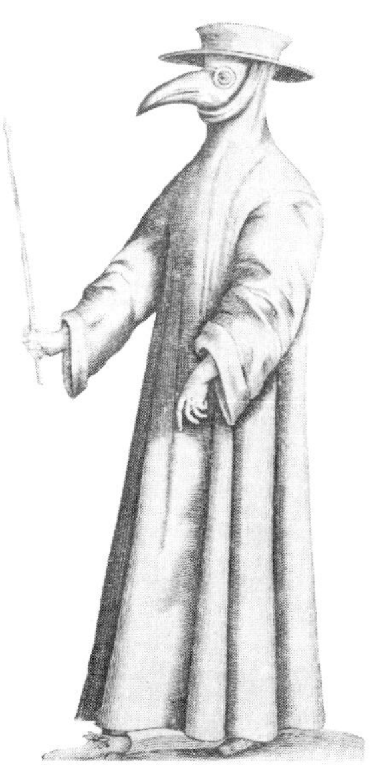

the plague infects Los Angeles

As certain diseases—smallpox, poliomyelitis, typhoid fever, diphtheria, and yellow fever, for example—disappear in developed countries such as the United States, increasing numbers of young physicians have only a textbook acquaintance with them. This situation is of some concern to health officers. For, despite every precaution, disease can be imported into this country. Every epidemic starts with a first case infecting an inadequately vaccinated person. That is why only one case of smallpox in this country would make national headlines.

In view of this limiting factor in medical education, one can hardly be critical of the physician who telephoned the communicable disease section of the County of Los Angeles General Hospital on an October day in 1924. He was puzzled and was glad to share his problem with the resident expert in communicable diseases.

5-8 Top: *A physician as a plague fighter in Marseilles, 1720. The beak contained herbs thought to prevent infection.* Bottom: *A public health nurse as a plague fighter in Los Angeles, 1924.*

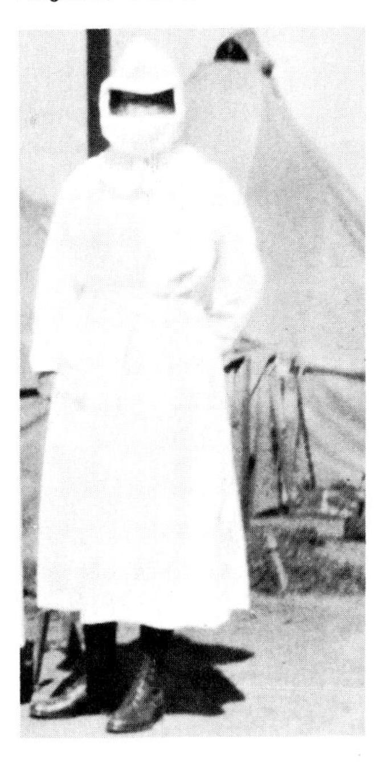

On Clara Street, in the Belvedere district of Los Angeles County, he had just examined an extremely sick elderly Mexican-American woman. The patient had a high fever and a severe pain in the back and chest. A young man in the house, as well as other neighborhood people, had similar symptoms. The illness could easily be contagious. Would it not be best to hospitalize the patients and then seek a definite diagnosis? The resident agreed. Ordering an ambulance, he went along to help.

Arriving at the address, the resident found the patient was feverish. She was coughing and crying. Lying on a couch along the wall was a young man, perhaps thirty, who also seemed to be very sick. Neither patient spoke English. A neighbor offered to act as interpreter.

The young man had been sick all day. First he had had a pain in his chest. Within a few hours he had a backache and a fever. Now there were red spots on his chest.

The old woman had been stricken a few days before the man and in about the same manner. For two days she had been coughing. Now she was breathing heavily and coughing up large amounts of bloody sputum.

As the two patients were being placed in the ambulance, the interpreter asked the hospital resident if he would be willing to look at some other people in the neighborhood who were sick in the same way. In another house, the doctor found a man in bed. He had a high fever and complained of a terrible pain in the back and chest. His young wife, in an adjoining bedroom, had similar symptoms. On a settee in the front room sat a young girl. She was holding her head in her hands. Her face was flushed, but she insisted that she was not sick. "I'm just tired," she said. "Awfully tired."

Three days later the man was dead and his young wife was dying. The young girl also lay dying in the hospital.

At this time, however, the resident made plans for their immediate hospitalization. Another ambulance would soon come, he told them. He turned to leave. Again the interpreter approached him. He thought the doctor should know that not more than two weeks before the mother and father of the young man who was being taken in the ambulance had died in the hospital. They had been sick the same way as their son now was. Someone had said they had died of pneumonia. Furthermore, the interpreter continued, there were four boys in the neighborhood—relatives of these sick people—who also had this sickness. The doctor went to see the boys and that night they were brought to the hospital. On the following day six more patients were admitted. Each of the six had severe pneumonia. They spat blood. Their skins turned blue. During the first day of hospitalization three died.

An autopsy of one of the patients who had so died was performed. Lung smears showed the presence of the plague bacillus. It was October 31.

On that day a nurse was admitted to the hospital. She had cared for the first patient during his few remaining hours of life in the pneumonia ward. She had plague. The next to be admitted to the hospital was the forty-eight-year-old priest, who had administered the last rites to a boy ill with the plague. He was followed by one of the ambulance drivers. Of the three, only the nurse survived.

In rapid succession thirty-three people died of the plague. Of the thirty-one people who had pneumonic plague, twenty-nine died; of the six with bubonic plague, four died.

And so, most people who got the plague in Los Angeles that autumn died. It has been seen that plague can become widespread, affecting whole cities, depopulating entire countries, sweeping across continents.

How was the plague stopped in Los Angeles? Known cases were immediately isolated in the hospital. They were seen only by those who were taking care of them. Seven blocks surrounding the Clara Street address were promptly quarantined. The entire area was roped off. Seventy-five officers were assigned to patrol its boundaries. Until the situation was under control, none of the sixteen hundred persons inside were allowed to leave the area. At one point, some of those quarantined attempted to break through the barriers. Sawed-off shotguns were provided to some of the quarantine guards. The residents stayed. To prevent gatherings of people, the theatre and dance hall were closed. After special instructions, selected health department nurses and inspectors entered the area. Street clothes were not worn. "The nurse has to wear cap, mask, gloves, and gown," ordered a health officer. "Also each nurse will please wear trousers and puttees provided, and high shoes if possible." This last was to protect against contact with rats. Day after day the nurses visited homes where they knew people had been exposed to see if any of them were sick. Those who were ill were promptly hospitalized. For those who were not, other necessary help was brought. In those days there was no known cure for the plague. It was dangerous work. Still another precaution was instituted. All undertakers were instructed not to embalm the body of a person from the plague-stricken area who had died suddenly or of undetermined causes until the body was examined by a health department physician.

Meanwhile, inside the lines and in the neighboring areas, health department workers were trying to stop the plague from spreading. A house-to-house canvass was begun. All lumber had to be elevated eighteen inches above the ground. Garbage and rubbish were collected and burned. The whole area was subjected to a general cleanup. Rats were killed by the thousands. Many rats were found to be infested with the flea that carries the plague bacillus. A direct attack on the flea was mounted by the use of chemical sprays and lime. Squirrels also carry plague. Three men were constantly occupied in shooting squirrels found in the city limits.

To this day the County of Los Angeles Department of Health Services maintains vector control specialists. It is their job to combat the rat. Such vigilance buys freedom from plague—and from all communicable disease.

some other pestilences

> So, naturalists observe, a flea
> Hath smaller fleas that on him prey;
> And these have smaller still to bite 'em;
> And so proceed *ad infinitum*[17]

This narrative has shown that one disease, plague, played a major role in the drama of human history. Soon after 1665, the disease disappeared from London. During the eighteenth century, it left Europe. It then lashed at this continent. Even today, it lurks in the wildlife of the West. In these pages, the broad review of its havoc has surely pointed to the international character of disease and its capacity to affect the course of human events. The rat that carries plague has found its way to every port. It has exerted as great an influence on history as any politician or general.

But plague is not the only pestilence that has affected man's destiny. Today, the defeat of epidemic disease holds great promise for the future of the world's developing nations. So it was with this country. For example, unless the mosquito that carried the *yellow fever* virus to man had been conquered, the Panama Canal could never have been built. This country had been hit early by the disease. In 1793, Philadelphia, at that time the nation's capital, became literally a ghost town because of the illness. Poor advice on how to control epidemics persisted and traveled long distances. In 1665, during the Great Plague of London, the boys at Eton had been forced to smoke or be whipped. A hundred and twenty-eight years later, cigar smoking was thought by Philadelphians to prevent yellow fever.

[17] Jonathan Swift, "On Poetry, A Rhapsody."

In the nineteenth century, *cholera* decimated the armies of the Crimean War, the American Civil War, and the Austro-Prussian War. In his 1866 campaign, Bismarck lost more men from cholera than from war wounds. More than a decade ago an epidemic of cholera began in Indonesia. It is still a menace to the Indian subcontinent and to Africa. Yet the disease is completely reversible by adequate sanitation and personal hygiene.

The scales of more than one war have been tipped by *typhus*—that disease of armies. Soldiers of the past were particularly prone to become victims of typhus. Sanitation was poor; personal hygiene, almost impossible. Crowding was inevitable. The microbe-carrying flea or louse could easily transmit the disease from rat to man. Coming and going, Napoleon's armies in Russia were tormented by typhus. During the 1845 potato famine in Ireland, it will be remembered, this disease added to the general misery. But perhaps the most devastating toll that typhus ever took of human life was in Russia following the Revolution of 1917. Disease has always spread with great population movements. After the revolution, masses of Russians were on the move in search of food. Their sufferings were piteous. In some areas even cannibalism was practiced. From the starving cities streamed the Mechotniki, or "sack carriers." They wandered from place to place hoping to find a crust of bread to put in their sacks. Instead they found typhus, and death. They also spread the disease. From 1917 through 1921, an estimated 25 million Russians developed typhus fever. Three million died.[18]

This chapter so far has been dealing with the historic consequences of epidemic diseases. Can individual health problems also affect the course of history?

individual illness and history

The steward and loyal follower of Joan of Arc testified that Joan never menstruated. Was this indeed true? If so, what relation did this simple physiologic fact (a not infrequent problem in the gynecologist's office) have to her hearing voices telling her that she was to remain a virgin? And does this help account for her chasing away the women who followed the men of her armies, smiting and actually killing one with her sword?[19] (On hearing of Joan's action King Charles is said to have asked, reasonably enough, "Would not a stick have done quite as well?") Did Henry VIII really have syphilis, and did he, indeed, transmit the disease to his various wives? If so, this could have been the reason that some of them were disposed to miscarry or to have stillborn babies. Frantically Henry

[18] In 1910, during a Mexican outbreak of typhus, two American doctors, Dr. Howard T. Ricketts and Dr. Russell Wilder, confirmed the transmission of the disease by the louse. They also described microscopic organisms, much smaller than ordinary bacteria, as a possible cause of the disease. During the outbreak Ricketts died. It remained for Von Prowazek, in Serbia, to identify the organisms as the cause of typhus. In 1915, Von Prowazek, too, died of the disease. The causative microorganism of typhus is named *Rickettsia prowazeki* in honor of these two investigators who died so far apart in distance, but not in purpose.

[19] It was customary for droves of women to accompany armies. During the seige of Troy, they were present in great numbers. The armies of Alexander tolerated a considerable female following, as did the Crusaders. These prostitutes frequently numbered into the thousands.

searched for a wife who could provide him with a male heir. When he thought that a wife would fail him, he divorced or executed her and manipulated still another marriage. His desire to divorce his first wife, Catherine of Aragon, led to his quarrel with the Church and to the establishment of the Anglican faith. Had Peter the Great perished of smallpox, in 1685, would his ambitious sister, Sophia, successfully have taken control of Russia? What effect did the emotional disorder of George III, first noted early in 1765, have on the restrictive English policies towards his angered American colonies?[20] Had Marat's inflamed skin itched less, would he have been more tolerant, and would the cruelties of the French Revolution have been eased and its bloody course changed? What effect did Robert E. Lee's diarrhea, disabling him for two critical weeks, have on the Civil War? What would have happened to the national economy if the news had leaked out of Grover Cleveland's two highly secret operations for mouth cancer? Had Woodrow Wilson not been crippled during his last presidential years, what would the era following the First World War have been like? It has been written that his stroke was followed by episodes of paranoia.[21] After also suffering terribly from delusions of persecution, the first U.S. Secretary of Defense, James Forrestal, committed suicide in 1949. This may have affected history.

But of all the aches and pains of the powerful, those of Napoleon Bonaparte most intrigue footnote historians. History is a culmination of events; it has many aspects of varying consequence. And the sickly Napoleon Bonaparte lends credence to this concept. Consider the effects of his illnesses on his Russian campaign.

Napoleon at Borodino

The Battle of Borodino was Napoleon's great opportunity to finally conquer Russia. Not only had a French Grande Armée been collected for the purpose, but also in the Corsican's ranks were unwilling Germans, Italians, Poles, Austrians, Swiss, and Hollanders. They wheeled through Prussia and Poland, a vast conglomeration of men and arms. Pillaging their way past Kovno, Vilna, Vitepsk, Smolensk, and Viasma, they came to Borodino, fifty miles from Moscow. Napoleon could taste victory. In all of Europe nobody had a more rapacious appetite for it.

At Borodino, on September 5, 1812, the Russian general, Kutuzov, turned to face Bonaparte. Here he would fight it out. He waited for the onslaught. But for two days Napoleon did nothing. Why?

It has been said that Napoleon did not attack either on the fifth or sixth of September because he had a cold. The truth is, he had more than a cold. He suffered from prostate trouble; thus he could not pass urine without great pain. (Some cynics claim that Napoleon's grim expression, as he rode his white steed in Russia, may well have been caused by this factor rather than by concern for his troops.) By the time Napoleon's prostate eased, he had developed a sore

[20] His particular symptoms are today thought to have been associated with a hereditary disease of body chemistry.

[21] Robert E. Kantor and William G. Herron, "Paranoia and High Office," *Mental Hygiene,* Vol. 52, No. 4 (October 1968), pp. 507–11.

throat and was so hoarse that he could not dictate his orders. His hand shook as he was forced to write them.

At Borodino Napoleon failed to destroy the Russian army. Later that army returned to hound him. Some historians lay this failure to his limited ability to make decisions at Borodino. The Russian army escaped to the east. In escaping, it battered the French army with its parting shots and retreated to return at a more opportune time. Always before, Napoleon had based his success on quickly conquering a country and then living off its wealth. Had he not successfully done this in his earlier Italian, German, and Austrian invasions? Had he not taken a ragged French army and, by quick victories, rewarded them with the wealth and women of the conquered?

The Russians provided neither him nor his army with these comforts. When the French Emperor and his army entered Moscow, they found a bleak, bitter, and burning capital. Was the course of history changed because Napoleon could not pass urine? Or because he had a cold?

In his novel *War and Peace,* Tolstoy rejects the notion that Napoleon's illness affected the outcome at Borodino:

> If it had depended on Napoleon's will to fight or not to fight the Battle of Borodino, and if this or that other arrangement depended on his will, then evidently a cold affecting the manifestation of his will might have saved Russia, and consequently the valet who omitted to bring Napoleon his waterproof boots . . . would have been the savior of Russia.

Tolstoy goes on to wisely emphasize the psychological state of the Napoleonic army at Borodino. "The way in which these people killed one another was not decided by Napoleon's will, but occurred independently of him, in accord with the will of hundreds of thousands of people who took part in the common action." Napoleon only thought "that it all took place by his will." True, Napoleon made the major decision in choosing to assail rather than to dislodge the Russian army. However, once that decision was made, the mood of his army was such that he could not have rescinded it under any circumstances. Men who must endure a leader's decisions may not long suffer his indecisions. Even if it were true that discomfort or sickness partly molded his decisions, sickness hardly explains the vast, cataclysmic events that had brought the sensitive inflamed prostate of the French dictator to the chilled winds of Borodino.

From the Tsar, who had fled to the east, came no word of surrender. In Moscow, Napoleon awaited evidence of peace overtures. None came. He offered an armistice. It was treated with cold contempt. Moscow was a black ruin. Morale was low, and so were supplies. In the streets, the men bickered among themselves or stood silently, longing for home. A Russian winter was coming. An apocalyptic air hung over them all. There was nothing to do but get out.

On October 19, Napoleon ordered his men to leave Moscow for home. In the long, sad annals of human conflict, there is no more ghastly story than that grim retreat. Men starved and froze. Napoleon's military genius never encompassed the notion of a medical corps. He failed to understand the importance of sanitation for an army. On the way to Moscow, and in the city too, typhus had plagued Napoleon's soldiers. Now it broke out with increased severity. The loss of life was appalling. And, meanwhile, in a sort of hit and run operation, the intact armies of Tsar Alexander kept hitting him, harassing him. With Napoleon trapped in the cold vastness of Russia, time and space became the enemies of the invaders, the allies of the Russians. Disease, hunger, and cold scourged the remnants of the Napoleonic army. The living robbed the dying. There were endless desertions. Men wandered aimlessly about the countryside. Starving, they gnawed on the bones of horses and the frozen roots of plants.

Some ended up in Polish Vilna. Conditions there were unspeakable. The living stumbled over the dead and dying, feebly beseeching help. Gangrene was prevalent. Typhus, and now an epidemic of typhoid, were killing Russian victors and French prisoners alike.

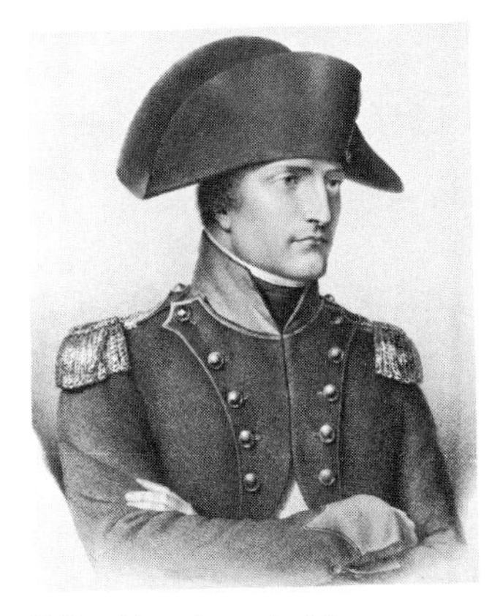

5-9 *Napoleon in his early thirties, when he was First Consul of France.*

The Tsar came to Vilna. To those men of Russian Poland who had sided with the invaders, he granted an amnesty. Every effort was made to relieve the agony. Hospitals were established. The remnant Napoleonic forces were well treated. It will be remembered that men of several countries served under Napoleon in Russia. The rulers of these countries sent money to help relieve the suffering. Only one man sent nothing—Napoleon.[22]

Napoleon at autopsy

''Look, Doctor,'' said Napoleon to his physician as he came naked out of his room after an alcohol rub. ''Look what lovely arms! What smooth white skin, without a single hair! What rounded breasts! Any beauty would be proud of a bosom like mine.''[23]

Joan of Arc had heard voices inspiring her to save France. Napoleon needed no voices to inspire his belief in himself as the savior of Europe. Until he turned forty, he was remarkably successful. At that age, however, Napoleon underwent a remarkable physical change. When he should have been at his peak, he was a has-been.

As a young man, Napoleon had been thin. His eyes were piercing. He had an eager look. His movements were quick, his manner imperious. Sleep was a waste of precious time.

5-10 *Napoleon as Emperor, between the ages of thirty-five and forty-five.*

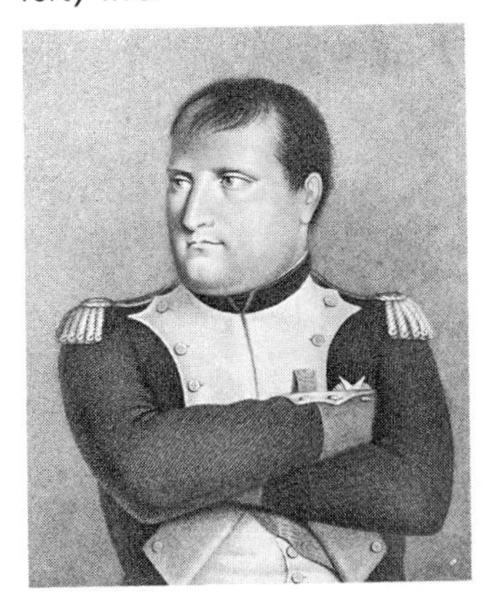

At forty, he was fat and slow. His eyes were dull, his expression placid. His hair, previously thick, became thin. It was curiously silken. He waddled a trifle. His body developed feminine tendencies. ''He has a roundness of figure not of our sex,'' Count Las Casas once remarked, perhaps nervously. Napoleon began to suffer from an overwhelming need for sleep.

On Saturday, May 5, 1821, Napoleon died. On the following afternoon, at 2 P.M., seventeen people, English and French, assembled on St. Helena for the autopsy. The dissection was performed by Dr. Antommarchi, Napoleon's personal physician. On removal of the heart and stomach, a wave of sentiment welled up in General Count Bertrand and General Montholon, members of the Emperor's staff at St. Helena. They begged for the heart. The English were not so sentimental. The heart was placed in a silver vessel. As a preservative, some

[22] Hereford B. George, *Napoleon's Invasion of Russia* (London, 1899), p. 398.
[23] W. R. Bett, ''An Hypothalamic Interpretation of History,'' *Bulletin of the History of Medicine,* Vol. 27, No. 2 (March–April 1953), pp. 128–32.

spirits of wine were added. Antommarchi, who had contributed little to Napoleon's health in life, requested the cancerous stomach. By it he could prove that nobody could have successfully treated the Emperor. The stomach, however, was deposited in another vessel. Both vessels were left in the sealed coffin. In later years, there was to be some disagreement between Dr. Antommarchi and an English doctor, Rutledge, as to who sealed the vessels and, indeed, how. Rutledge claimed to have sealed the vessel containing the heart with a shilling bearing the head of George III. Antommarchi heatedly denied this final victory over Napoleon. It might be interesting to have a look.

Scientific shenanigans aside, three separate autopsy reports were made. Part of one, by the English observer Dr. Henry, is singularly revealing:

> The whole surface of the body was deeply covered with fat . . . the skin was . . . particularly white and delicate as were the hands and arms. Indeed the whole body was slender and effeminate. There was scarcely any hair on the body and that of the head was thin, fine and silky. The pubis much resembled the Mons Veneris in women . . . the shoulders were narrow, the hips wide . . . the penis and testicles were very small, and the whole genital system seemed to exhibit a physical cause for the absence of sexual desire and the chastity which had been stated to have characterized the Deceased.[24]

So did the colossal Corsican conqueror appear in death.

Some think that Napoleon, at about forty, had developed Fröhlich's syndrome, or adiposogenital dystrophy. This is a disease of the hypothalamus, a small area at the base of the brain near the pituitary gland. Among its many functions is the regulation of many activities of the pituitary gland (see pages 254–58). It is, thus, intimately involved in growth, sexual activity, and reproduction. If Napoleon did indeed have this rather rare disease, it would surely be fair to wonder about its effect on world history. It is, however, important to indulge in such speculations only within their proper perspective.

concluding thoughts

The great medical historian Sigerist has written:

> History is made by individual human beings, to be sure, and whether they are healthy or sick, sane or insane, makes a difference. Yet the place an individual holds, the power with which he is invested, and the use he is permitted to make of his power are determined by a great variety of factors, by social and economic conditions first of all, but also by hopes and fears, ambitions and frustrations and other psychological factors . . . disease of an individual and even a deadly disease does not alter the course of history. A cause may collapse when the leader dies but not because of his collapse. It collapses only when the forces that carried the leader have lost their momentum. Otherwise, his death may activate the cause, as history has demonstrated more than once.[25]

Tolstoy and Sigerist agree on the relatively limited effect on history of individual sickness. Concerning past events this is indisputable. But it need not

[24] James Kemble, *Napoleon Immortal: The Medical History and Private Life of Napoleon Bonaparte* (London, 1959), p. 282.

[25] Henry E. Sigerist, *Civilization and Disease* (New York, 1944), pp. 127–28.

apply to the future. Neither Tolstoy nor Sigerist refers to tomorrow's risks. What can the illness of past leaders teach those who plan for the future?

Leadership is an exhausting ordeal. A Washington correspondent aptly wrote:

> It would be hard to overestimate the physical and nervous tension on the men at the top of this government.
>
> They are on the go 18 hours a day, and in the President's case, often longer: endless conferences, constant testimony on Capitol Hill, a succession of tedious ceremonial dinners, pressure for more bombing, pressure for less bombing—all this, and a constant drumfire of criticism at home and abroad. The Johnson system here is based on the assumption that men can do whatever they have to do . . . It is a dubious assumption.[26]

Leaders need help and health. It is not only their responsibility but also the obligation of those they lead, to make certain that they have both.

epilogue

> There is no national science, just as there is no national multiplication table; what is national is no longer science.[27]

Malaria, smallpox, influenza, typhoid fever—these and other enemies of man have killed him and taught him. But have they taught him enough?

> The surest safeguard against the spread of communicable disease, whether it be smallpox or Asian influenza, is control of the disease in the country of origin. In the absence of such internal control, a next safeguard is a worldwide communicable disease intelligence program geared to early detection of epidemics—and the attendant possibility of international transmissibility.[28]

This basic statement calls for a degree of international maturity more often seen in health than in other aspects of world politics. It is doubtful that man, by his own efforts, will ever completely eliminate communicable diseases. However, he is slowly conquering and controlling them. Constant vigilance is essential. Nonetheless, one cannot gainsay the virtual disappearance of malaria, smallpox, plague, yellow fever, cholera, and typhus from vast, formerly devastated areas. And the picture will improve. In many areas of the Western world, regular measles and poliomyelitis are also disappearing. The realization by developing societies that sickness grievously impedes their development—the sure knowledge that a community riddled by malaria, for example,

[26] James Reston, "A Tired, Tense Administration," quoted in Robert E. Kantor and William G. Herron, "Paranoia and High Office," pp. 507–11.

[27] From *The Personal Papers of Anton Chekhov,* tr. by S. S. Koteliansky and Leonard Woolf (New York, 1948), p. 29.

[28] Lenor S. Goerke, "Preface: Graduate Training for Responsibilities in International Health," in Lenor S. Goerke, ed., *Proceedings of the Los Angeles World Health Conference* (Los Angeles, 1962), pp. 2–3.

cannot take its place in the modern world—is a local stimulus for improvement. To those whose societies already benefit from disease control, helping to create such a stimulus in other countries is an opportunity. Those who seek a better world, who seek bridges, not walls, between nations, must understand the paramount necessity of controlling disease. This is the fundamental proposition of this chapter—a proposition whose meaning has been made abundantly clear by history.

The United States, through the Agency for International Development, the Peace Corps, the International Health Division of the Public Health Service, the World Health Organization, and the armed services, is combining with a massive effort by such voluntary agencies as the Ford and Rockefeller Foundations, in making an enormous health contribution to the world's developing areas. Whether it be through a technical health expert in Sierra Leone, a WHO worker in Asia, a child health project of the Ford Foundation, or a Peace Corps worker in northern Brazil, the contribution is palpable and important. Moreover, the World Health Organization is promoting medical research on an international level. Such an effort promises even more than new knowledge about such health enigmas as cancer. From such international undertakings there develops a dialogue between nations that surely promotes understanding and peace between war-weary peoples. Is it too much to hope that the health worker will yet show the way to the greatest health of all—peace?

Disease knows no boundaries. This is a harsh historical experience. Even in wartime, countries have cooperated in health matters. In 1800, France and England were at war. At that time, Jenner's vaccination against smallpox was being tested in England. French doctors wanted to learn about it. Special arrangements were made by the French Foreign Minister, Talleyrand. An English physician came to France, was treated with great regard, and vaccinated French children with English vaccine. Today, scientists are seeking proof that some viruses may be involved in the development of human cancers. Scientists from the United States and the Soviet Union are exchanging viruses for cooperative study, and plan to exchange personnel.[29] During a visit to Russia, President Nixon, on May 23, 1972, signed a joint agreement of cooperation in the fields of medicine and public health. Projects under this agreement were begun in the areas of cancer, cardiovascular disease, environmental health, and arthritis. In September 1973, instantaneous exchanges of vital scientific information between scientists of the two countries were made possible by a special teletype. It was the first direct communication link between the United States and the Soviet Union since the White House–Kremlin "hot line."[30] Is there better proof of hope for mankind?

Only a short time ago, a group of sixty eastern U.S. college students were asked to list the six largest (in population) cities of America. Only five included Mexico City. It is a long road from such parochialism to a sympathetic knowledge of the customs of other societies, but this kind of knowledge is being acquired. The good international health worker no longer tries to impose his

[29] "Russians, Americans Swap Viruses," *New Scientist*, Vol. 57, No. 829 (January 18, 1973), p. 148.
[30] "Medical Hotline," *Medical World News*, Vol. 14, No. 35 (September 28, 1973), p. 5.

culture on others. He understands that other cultures have developed other ways to handle problems than those to which he is accustomed.

To assist those of the less developed world to improve their health, one must first learn to appreciate their social edifice. This is one of the wise principles on which the Peace Corps is based. But there is a paradox in this. One may rightly ask: Is my world truly better? Is it really preferable to theirs? Do we not lose by needless heart attacks what we save by penicillin? Whose disease, whose destiny is better? Is it not best to leave them alone?

But no longer can anyone depend on being left alone. One can but work so that each culture will gain, and not suffer, from the others. For although the scientist can distinguish innumerable ecosystems, the world is one all-inclusive ecosystem that is shared by all men.

Failing to learn this, men fail to learn anything.

summary

Mankind may be his own worst enemy, but he is not his only enemy. His smallest enemies, the bearers of disease, have often twisted the course of human history. To illustrate this point, this chapter explores the history of one disease, plague. It also discusses the effect of individual illness on history, using Napoleon Bonaparte as a major example.

Plague is caused by a bacillus, *Pasteurella pestis,* which is transmitted by fleas to rats and humans (page 112). The two most common types of plague are the *bubonic* and *pneumonic* (page 112). During the Middle Ages, bubonic plague was called "the Black Death." A major medieval epidemic occurred in the sixth century A.D. during the reign of Emperor Justinian the Great (page 112). Another, in the mid-fourteenth century, spread from central Asia to China, India, and Europe (page 113). Such epidemics caused profound and undesirable changes in moral standards, social character, government, and the Church. The moral disintegration that swept through Europe was characterized by flagellation as a means of doing penance, the dancing mania, and persecution of Jews (pages 114–16).

In the early modern era, the 1665 Great Plague of London spread from London to remote villages like Eyam, where almost the entire population died. Poor sanitation, poor personal hygiene, and overcrowding encouraged the spread of infection (page 121). Misunderstanding of how plague spreads caused many of the deaths.

Plague has remained a threat in modern times in India, Africa, South America, and, as recently as 1924, the United States (pages 122–23). Constant vigilance against the plague-carrying rat will reduce the danger of an epidemic.

Besides plague, other pestilences that illustrate the international character of disease and its capacity to affect human history are *yellow fever, cholera,* and *typhus* (pages 125–26).

Individual illness may also indirectly affect the course of events. An example of this may be the link between the gradual deterioration of Napoleon's health and the eventual defeat of his troops by the Russian army. But no single person's health is decisive in determining the outcome of human events (pages 126–31).

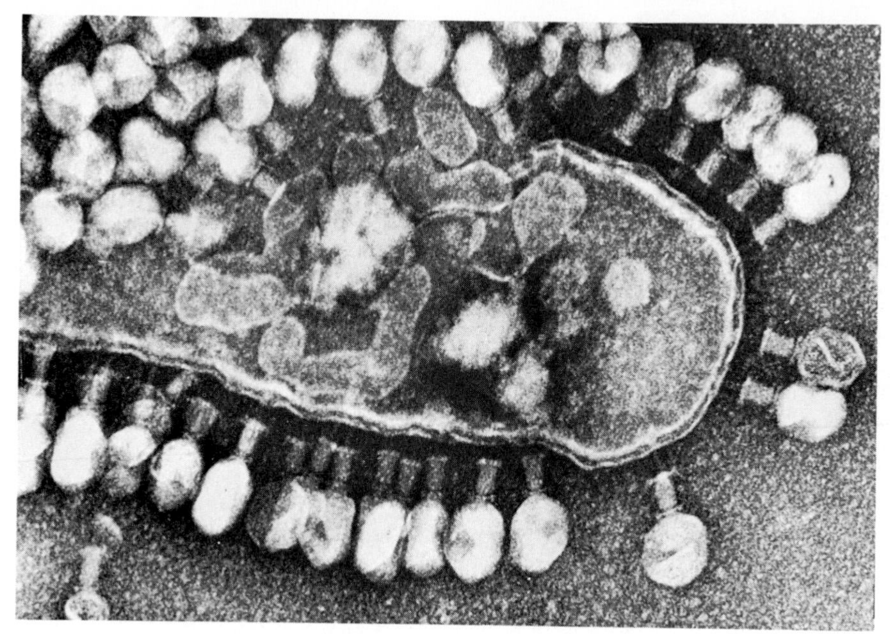

A biotic drama revealed by the electron microscope: viruses attacking a bacterium.

the agents of communicable sickness, part 1

6

the "animalcules" of van Leeuwenhoek

"Dear God," wrote Anton van Leeuwenhoek, "what marvels there are in so small a creature!" It was autumn of 1693. The Dutch cloth merchant and microscope maker had achieved a magnification of 270. With growing excitement, he explored a "wee" world, a new ecosystem. Under his lenses he placed his own blood, the saliva of friends, a cow's urine. In his own excrement he found "animalcules a-moving very prettily." Describing his own semen, he cautioned, "What I investigate is only what . . . remains as a residue after conjugal coitus." The first to completely describe red blood cells, to see protozoa and bacteria, the mild Dutchman made a path on which no proper signpost would be placed for another two hundred years. For not until 1870 did Robert Koch prove that bacteria could cause disease. Then Koch, joined by a host of other investigators (including his unfriendly rival Louis Pasteur), began a great search to find man's tiniest adversaries—disease-causing organisms.

A microorganism is a minute, usually microscopic, living organism. When such an organism invades the body, lives off it as a parasite, and may cause disease, *infection* results. For infection to occur, then, there must be a causative organism (the *parasite*) invading a receptive individual (the *host*) in an ecosystem, or *environment,* in which all interact. Some organisms are more likely to cause disease than others (*virulence*). Some individuals are better able to ward them off (*resistance*). With infection there may be active combat between the invading parasite and the host. Or the parasite and host might exist together in ecological balance; with imbalance, as occurs when the host loses resistance, disease results.

When the infection can be transferred from one person to another, it is *communicable.* Some infectious diseases are more communicable than others. For example, regular measles, which is spread via droplets in the air, is much more communicable than a form of leprosy that is usually spread by skin contact. With time, an infectious disease may even lose its ability to be communicable. Untreated, syphilitic infection may persist in the body for years, even a lifetime, silently attacking the circulatory and nervous systems. But two years after the initial infection, the period of active communicability is usually over. The microorganism causing the disease does not surface to the mucous membranes to be transferred. It remains deep in the body. There is no danger to anyone else.

Not all organisms causing infection are too small to be seen by the naked eye. Some *helminths* (parasitic worms) such as the tapeworm can be seen without a microscope (their eggs, however, are microscopic). The helminths are the largest of the organisms that may enter the body and cause infection. Other organisms, the *ectoparasites,* such as fleas, lice, and mites, may also be easily observed without aids. Smaller than these, and in the order of their decreasing size, are *fungi, protozoa, bacteria, rickettsia,* and *viruses.* These are the *etiological agents* (Greek *aitia,* cause + *ology*); these are the organisms that cause infectious disease.

6-1 *A three-inch-long Leeuwenhoek microscope (back view). The lens is in the small hole in the circular bulge.*

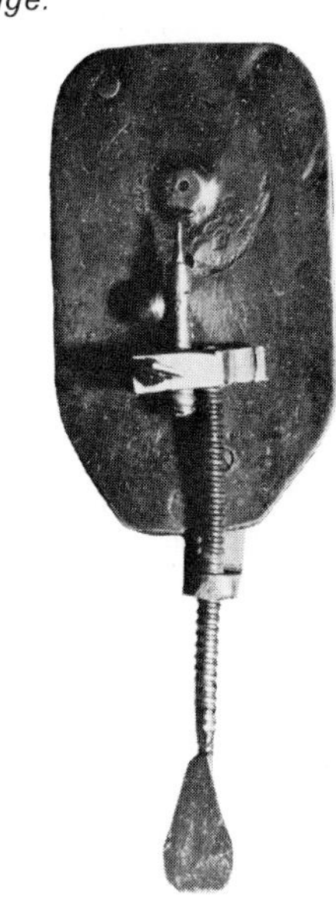

the variety of etiological agents

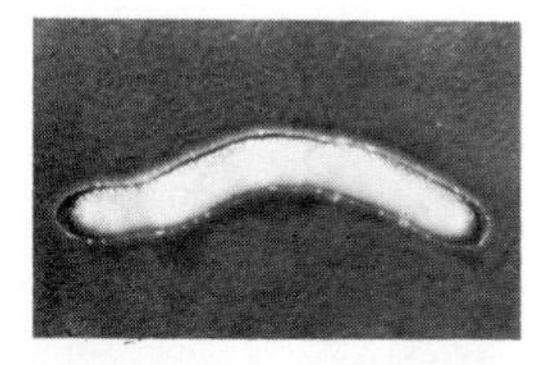

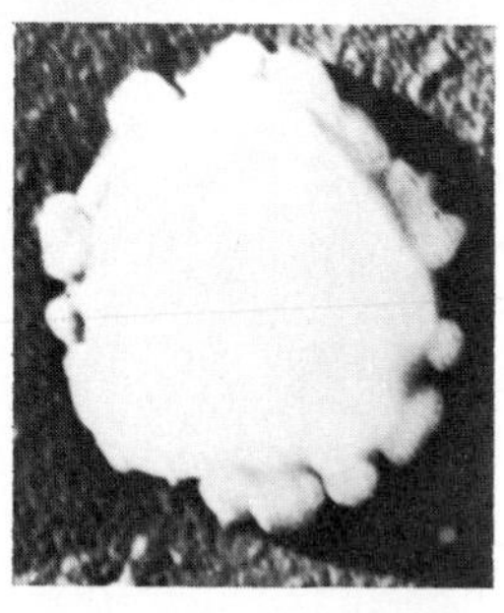

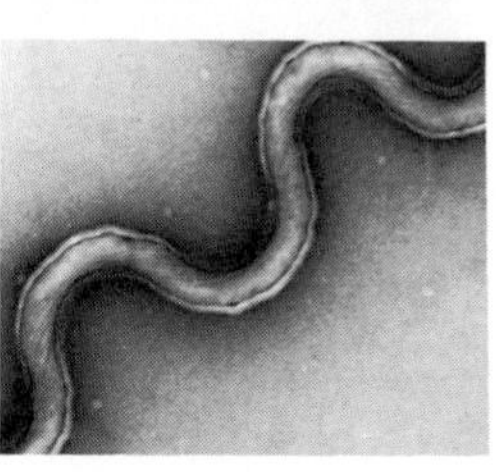

6-2 *Bacteria:* Mycobacterium tuberculosis, *a bacillus* (top); Neisseria gonorrhoeae, *a coccus* (center); Treponema pallidum, *a spiral-shaped microorganism* (bottom).

Helminths, the parasitic worms, are responsible for a wide variety of worldwide human infections, including tapeworm, hookworm, and pinworm.

The mite causing *scabies* ("the itch"), an example of an *ectoparasite,* invades only the outer skin. The male of the species causing this illness is hard to see, but the female is twice as large as the male and can be seen. The female burrows into the superficial skin to deposit her eggs.

Fungi are plants. They include the *molds* and the *yeasts.* Many of them cause disease. Molds, for example, cause ringworm and athlete's foot. One category of mold, *Penicillium,* produces penicillin. (Another mold, appropriately named *Penicillium roqueforti,* is responsible for Roquefort cheese.) Maladies caused by yeastlike fungi include a lung infection called *valley fever,* and *thrush,* a disease (usually of children) characterized by whitish spots in the mouth.

Protozoa are one-celled animals. Among the illnesses caused by protozoa are malaria and amebic dysentery.

Bacteria that are rod-shaped are called *bacilli* and spherical bacteria are *cocci.* There are also spiral-shaped organisms. Bacilli cause such illnesses as tuberculosis and diphtheria. The meningococcus and gonococcus, causing meningitis and gonorrhea, respectively, are perhaps the best-known spherical bacteria. The *Spirochaeta pallidum* (*Treponema pallidum*), the bacterium that causes syphilis, is an example of a spiral-shaped organism. Some bacteria (tetanus bacilli, for example) have the capacity to form spores—protective shells that shield them, for years if necessary, against a hostile environment such as soil. When these bacteria come in contact with a more agreeable ecosystem, such as human tissue, they revert to their active, disease-causing state.

Rickettsia, classified between viruses and bacteria, have characteristics of each. Like viruses, they are found within cells. Unlike viruses, but like bacteria, they are visible under an ordinary microscope. Their discoverer, Howard T. Ricketts (1871–1910), died of typhus fever, a rickettsial disease.

There are some two hundred *viruses* of importance to man. These smallest of all infectious agents cannot multiply outside a cell. They are responsible for a host of man's ailments ranging from the "cold sore" to poliomyelitis.

Because they are the most common causes of communicable disease in this country, the bacterial and viral disease agents will be the major concern of this chapter and Chapter 7.

how microbes leave one home and find another

> Contagion has this illness widely spread;
> And, I feel sure, will further spread it yet.[1]

Microbes have a number of ways of moving from one host to another. The material from an open lesion (perhaps the sore of syphilis or an open staphylococcic

[1] Juvenal, *Second Satire,* quoted in Heinrich Oppenheimer, *Medical and Allied Topics in Latin Poetry* (London, 1928), p. 78.

skin sore) may be directly transmitted from one person to another. The nineteenth-century Hungarian physician Ignaz Semmelweis proved that in his hospital, direct contact between the pus-stained hands of doctors who had just left the autopsy rooms and mothers laboring in childbirth meant infectious death to many a trusting woman.

Transmission of infection may be indirect. A child with measles coughs. Within the droplets forcibly expelled from the respiratory tract swarms the measles virus. The infected droplets hover suspended in the air, wafted about by its currents. Numerous susceptible persons may inhale them. Or, instead of air, some inanimate object may act as the transmitting agent. Examples are a handkerchief (contaminated, perhaps, with the hardy bacillus of tuberculosis) and food (such as milk, in which the typhoid bacillus thrives so well).

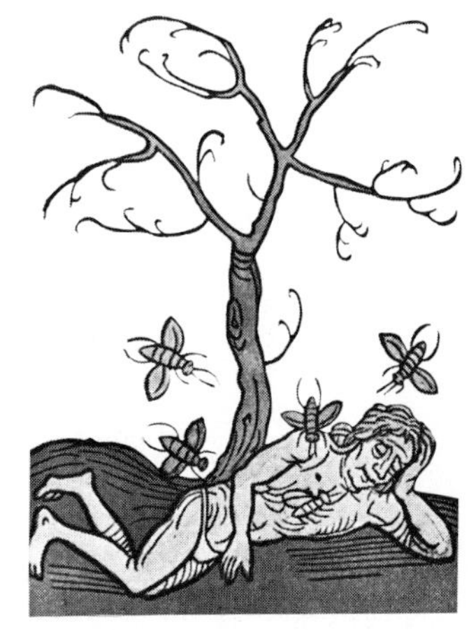

6-3 *Mosquitoes and man, from a 15th-century book on natural history.*

The indirect routes of spread may be still more circuitous. A person who has recovered from typhoid fever may continue to harbor its bacillus for a long time. He is, therefore, a *carrier* (see page 174). Occasionally, he excretes the typhoid bacillus in his stool. If he fails to wash his contaminated hands he may contaminate someone else's food. Scores of typhoid fever outbreaks have occurred in this way.

Insects and other animals may carry disease. A person shaking with malaria may infect stray female mosquitoes feeding on his blood. After an interval, the mosquitoes inoculate other people. A rabid animal may inoculate another animal or person by biting him.

The routes by which infection enters and leaves the body and the ways of its transmission are thus numerous and often devious. An outbreak of communicable disease often has all the elements of a mystery. The knowledge that gonorrhea is almost always directly spread through sexual intercourse or that an outbreak of typhoid fever may have been caused by water or food contaminated by human feces give the public health detective leads to the source of the disease and to its control. By charting the routes of communicable disease a microbial culprit may be found, the linked chain of spread broken, and a new chain of prevention forged.

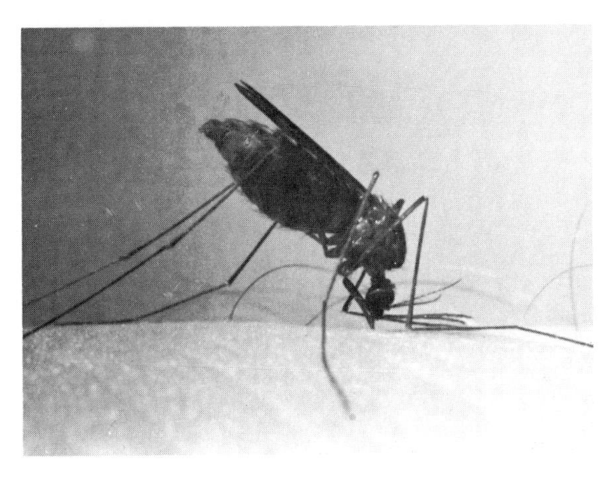

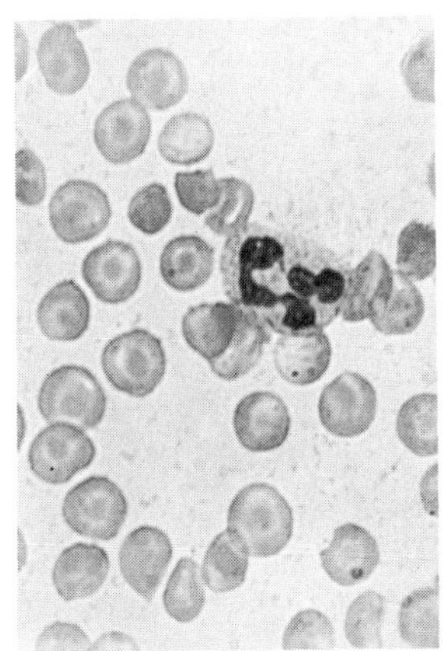

6-4 Left: Anopheles balabacensis, *an important transmitter of malaria in Southeast Asia. This mosquito is resting after a blood meal; note the greatly distended abdomen.* Right: *Red blood cells containing the malaria-causing organism.*

body resistance to microbial invasion

Broken skin will admit microbes to start an infection. Intact, the skin is a natural fortress against countless organisms. Nevertheless, hookworm larvae and the spirochete of syphilis may penetrate even the unbroken skin. The intact mucous membrane also resists infection. Yet, the mucous membrane of the respiratory tract may fail to resist and be overcome by the diphtheria bacillus; in the same manner the gonococcus may infect the urogenital system. If the mucous membrane of the mouth, pharynx, stomach, and intestine is intact, the tetanus organism may be swallowed harmlessly. Indeed the human intestine is a common habitat of this organism. It is when the tetanus organism finds an abrasion on the skin or on the mucous membrane of an unimmunized person that this serious disease can occur. Within the intestine, the colon bacillus usually (but not always) lives in ecological balance with man. But should it escape through a ruptured appendix into the abdominal cavity, it would be cause for concern. Saliva has some bacteria-killing power, and stomach acid has even more. So, despite some vulnerability, the body does possess mechanical and other barriers to fight infection.

Should invading microbes penetrate these first lines of defense, the body rushes certain white cells to attack, engulf, and destroy the invader. This white-blood-cell resistance to infection is called *phagocytosis* (Greek *phagein,* to eat + *kytos,* hollow vessel). Malnutrition, fatigue, poor general health (including other infections), anemia—all promote poor resistance. All favor infection. Even one's anatomy influences the struggle between invading microbe and body resistance. The short, straight Eustachian tube (see page 99) of the child provides an easier route for infection of the middle ear than does the curved and longer tube of the adult.

But these are *nonspecific* aspects of resistance. There is also *specific* resistance, a resistance resulting from the body's exact response to each separate specific invader. This is *immunity.*

Lady Montagu's harsh lesson about immunity in the community

Mary Pierrepont was only eight years old in 1697, but she was already so exquisite that the members of her father's literary club toasted her as the beauty of the year. Forming gracefully into womanhood, she did not disappoint them. A fine fair complexion and great eyes made her a striking English beauty. At twenty she married well, if impulsively, and settled down, as Lady Mary Wortley Montagu, to a life of taste and wit.

Then, at twenty-six, she contracted smallpox. Her long eyelashes were lost forever. Deep angry scars pitted her skin. In a poem, she mourned, "My beauty is no more!" Unable to hide her visible wounds, she nevertheless bore her invisible hurt well. She accompanied her husband to his new post as ambassador extraordinary to the distant Turkish port of Constantinople. To a friend, she sent an excited letter. "I am going to tell you a thing that I am sure will make you wish your selfe here," she wrote. "The Small Pox, so fatal and so general amongst us, is here entirely harmless by the invention of ingrafting."[2]

[2] Quoted in Hubert A. Lechevalier and Morris Solotorovsky. *Three Centuries of Microbiology* (New York, 1965), p. 9.

What was ''ingrafting''? From the pustular sores of a mild case of smallpox, old Turkish women would collect matter and place it in a walnut shell. They would then visit family parties, often held for smallpox ingrafting. The operation was simple. With a needle a vein was opened. A small amount of matter was then inserted into the vein. The wound was bound. The ingrafting was complete. In a week, the recipient was sick and feverish. At the inoculation site, running sores developed. On the face about twenty-five pustules appeared. But in about another week, there was complete recovery. There was no scarring. Best of all, resistance or *immunity* to the disease seemed complete.

how did the immunity come about?

Smallpox is caused by a virus (see pages 155–67). Like all other microorganisms and, indeed, all other life forms, viruses are basically composed of chemical substances. But each specific virus has its own chemical structure, its unique arrangement and number of chemicals. The chemical structure of the smallpox virus is different from that of the chickenpox virus, which in turn is different from that of the measles virus, and so on.

The old Turkish ingrafters had inoculated a small amount of smallpox virus into people susceptible to the disease. To the body cells of those recipients, the chemical structure of that virus was an unacceptable foreigner, an invading stranger. Unchallenged, it would continue to multiply, consume, overwhelm, and finally destroy the host. How could overwhelming invasion by the foreign virus be resisted? By deliberately giving a susceptible individual a mild case of the disease. The Turkish ingrafters did not know why a mild case of smallpox apparently prevented later severe smallpox; all they knew was that it did. (They were not the first to discover the value of this procedure. Thousands of years before, the Chinese had used powdered smallpox scabs as snuff to prevent smallpox.) Those eighteenth-century Turks who were inoculated with the smallpox virus did not even become sick during a smallpox epidemic. Those not inoculated frequently sickened and died. Why? For several reasons. The matter used by the ingrafters was taken from mild cases. Carried about in nutshells, some of the virus probably weakened in time and some died. So the inoculated dose was doubtless smaller and weaker than that inhaled. Also, local inoculation gave the body time to build resistance against the invaders.

Many years after Lady Montagu's letter about the Turkish ingrafters, a better way to protect against smallpox was found. As a teen-aged surgeon's assistant, Edward Jenner had heard a milkmaid's memorable answer to the suggestion that she might be developing smallpox. ''I cannot take that disease,'' she said, ''for I have had the cowpox.'' Jenner never forgot that remark, and on May 14, 1796, he inoculated a small boy, James Phipps, with material from a cowpox pustule taken from the wrist of Sarah Nelms, a cooperative milkmaid. Some six weeks later Jenner tested the ability of cowpox virus to prevent smallpox virus infection. He deliberately inoculated the boy with matter taken from a smallpox pustule on the body of a patient. The boy had no reaction; he was immune. In the years that followed, Jenner so tested ''poor Phipps''

VACCINATE

Yourself and your family with pure Vaccine Virus taken fresh from the Calf, uncorrupted with the impurities with which that taken from the Human Subject is frequently tainted. Quill Slips, enclosed in airtight packages, sent by mail to any address with full directions for use. Price 25c. per Quill Slip. If directions are faithfully followed, it is found to prove effective. This Virus is almost exclusively in use by the Boards of Health in this country. Address VACCINE DEPOT, Brooklyn City Dispensary, No. 11 Tillary Street, Brooklyn, New York.

6-5 *Smallpox prevention by mail order. This advertisement appeared in* Harper's Weekly *magazine in 1876.*

(as he called him) almost two dozen times. Nothing significant ever happened. The case was proved. Illness from cowpox resulted in prolonged immunity to smallpox. But how is this fact related to smallpox vaccination?

Cowpox is a viral disease of cattle. Smallpox is a viral disease of man. Cowpox virus and smallpox virus are, genetically speaking, extremely close cousins and belong to the same family, the *poxvirus* group. To humanity's good fortune, Jenner found that cowpox could be transmitted to man as an extremely mild infection and that this cowpox infection in humans would prevent infection by the smallpox virus. In the years following Jenner's discovery, the arm-to-arm transmission of (probably weakened) smallpox virus was replaced by arm-to-arm transmission of cowpox virus. As this was done, the cowpox virus doubtless became contaminated with smallpox and other viruses. Still it remained wonderfully useful. Today the material used for vaccination against smallpox is *vaccinia* virus (Latin *vacca,* cow), a laboratory-developed virus related to both the smallpox and cowpox viruses. Live vaccine virus stimulates the production of protein substances in humans that effectively render smallpox virus harmless. Although prolonged, this immunity is not lifelong. The vaccination must be repeated every several years.

To summarize: to be immune to smallpox virus infection, one must have circulating in the blood enough protein substances specific to that particular virus. These substances will neutralize the specific virus. In the case of smallpox, a person's capacity to do this may be stimulated in two ways:

1. *By having the disease.* This may be deliberately accomplished by inoculation with a weakened smallpox virus, the method of the Turkish ingrafters, or it may be achieved by accidental inhalation or ingestion, as occurs in outbreaks of the disease.

2. *By being vaccinated.* A second way of stimulating smallpox immunity is surely best—that is, by vaccination with the smallpox virus' laboratory-produced first cousin, vaccinia virus. A mild disease prevents a serious one. It is a good bargain. Not since 1949 has the United States reported a valid case, and that one occurred secondary to a case imported from Mexico (Mexico has been smallpox-free since 1955).[3] On September 30, 1971, the U.S. Public Health Service accepted the recommendation of its Advisory Committee on Immunization Practices to discontinue routine smallpox vaccination in this country in favor of a selective vaccination program limited to those population groups that may be exposed to smallpox.[4]

But what are the mechanisms of resistance? Why does mild smallpox infection prevent later smallpox reinfection? What body mechanism accounts for the

[3] In 1972, Yugoslavia experienced a serious smallpox epidemic. By April of that year, 140 cases and 20 deaths had been reported. (*Morbidity and Mortality Weekly Report,* U.S. Department of Health, Education, and Welfare, Vol. 21, No. 13 [April 1972], p. 1.) Travelers entering the United States from Yugoslavia and neighboring countries were carefully screened and followed, as were those entering from other known smallpox areas. When indicated, smallpox vaccinations were performed. The United States escaped importation of a single case.

[4] Among the factors leading to this decision were the twenty-five year absence of smallpox in this country, the rare but sometimes serious complications (and even deaths) resulting from smallpox vaccination, the improved methods of control in the event a case of smallpox did enter the country, and the success of the World Health Organization program promoting vaccination against smallpox in formerly afflicted countries.

success of the ancient Chinese powdered scab-sniffers and the Turkish ingrafters? In what ways does the body achieve immunity, not only to the smallpox virus but to a host of other viruses, as well as to many bacteria and fungi? There is some relatively recent, still incomplete, information.

the immune response: two lines of defense

Millions of years of evolution have provided the body with two ways of responding to invasion by microbes or other life-threatening foreigners. One is known as the *antibody response;* the other is the *cell-mediated response.* Together, these two systems are called the *immune response.* The activity of both depends on a type of white blood cell, the *lymphocyte.* During the early months of life within the uterus, primitive lymphocytes (called *stem cells*) are manufactured in the body's major factory for blood cells, the bone marrow. On reaching a proper stage, the lymphocytes leave the marrow to swarm into the blood stream. Their manufacture and emigration continue throughout the life of the individual. Once in the blood stream, the lymphocytes differentiate into two

6-6 *Chambon, a Brooklyn physician, uses his ready source of cowpox virus, while the patients in his parlor wait to be treated.*

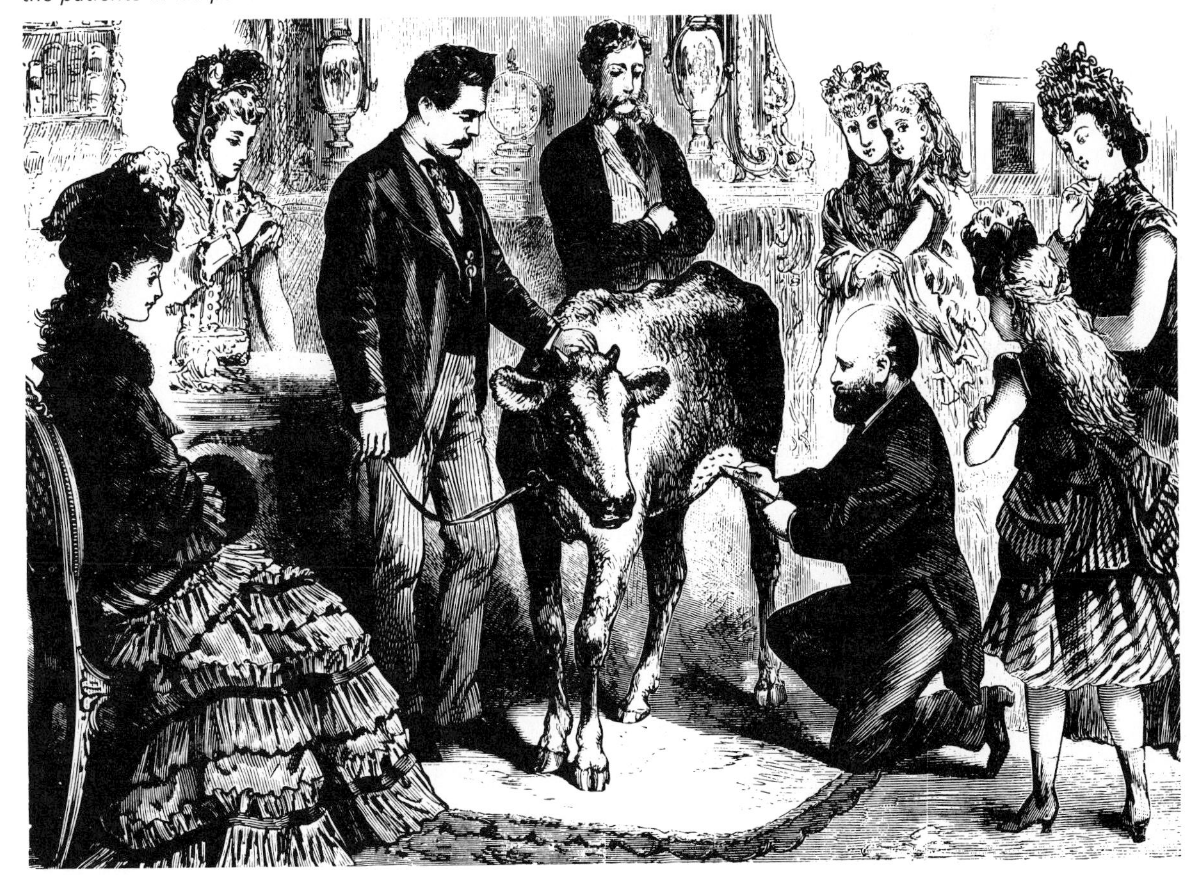

Thymus

T cells

"Killer" lymphocyte

CELL-MEDIATED IMMUNITY

T cell cooperation?

Bone marrow

B cells

Antigen

Stimulation of cell division to produce a large number of antibody-forming plasma cells

ANTIGEN-ANTIBODY IMMUNITY

6-7 *The two main types of immune response, and the likely mechanisms of their generation.*

types of cells—B lymphocytes and T lymphocytes.[5] If an individual's bone marrow cannot produce the primitive stem cells that become lymphocytes, or if the lymphocytes in his blood stream fail to differentiate into B and T cell types, he is at a serious disadvantage in combating the constant onslaught of infection. How do the two systems of immune response use B and T lymphocytes to fight infection?

6-8 *Most B lymphocytes* (top) *are rough and most T lymphocytes* (bottom) *are smooth. This may be because B lymphocytes have many more antigen receptors.*

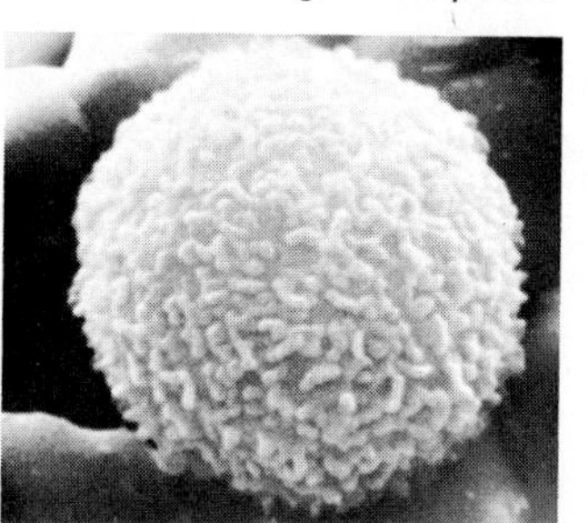

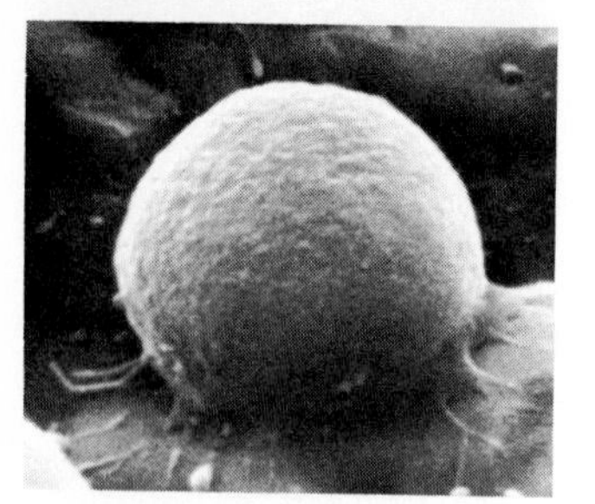

the antibody immune response[6]

Both B lymphocytes and T lymphocytes are involved in the antibody system of immune response, but the B lymphocytes play the major role. In the lymph nodes throughout the body, molecules of invading microbes stimulate the B lymphocytes to divide and proliferate into numerous *plasma cells.* These plasma cells then produce a protein called an *antibody.* The newly formed antibodies neutralize the microbial molecules that could cause sickness (Figures 6-2, 6-11, 6-12, 6-13, 6-16). Any substance—toxin, enzyme, protein—that stimulates B lymphocytes to differentiate into plasma cells, which then produce antibodies, is an *antibody generator,* or *antigen* (antibody + Greek *gennan,* to produce). On invading the body, parts of microorganisms act as antigens. So exact in chemical structure are the stimulating antigen and the generated anti-

[5] These lymphocytes are called "T" and "B" because of their origins and destinations after leaving the bone marrow. Some lymphocytes migrate via the blood stream to the small *thymus gland* located in the chest behind the breastbone. While in the thymus gland, they mature into T lymphocytes. From the thymus gland, the T lymphocytes continue their journey into the circulation to fight microbial and other body invaders as needed. B lymphocytes, on the other hand, derive their initial "B" from the fact that in the experimental chicken, after leaving the bone marrow, they pass through a sac-like structure called the *bursa of Fabricius.* Both birds and mammals (including man) have a thymus gland, but mammals have no bursa of Fabricius. However, it is believed that all mammals, including man, do have a site (or sites) equivalent to the bursa of Fabricius where lymphocytes mature into B lymphocytes. What that site is remains unknown. B lymphocytes are located primarily in the lymph nodes, where, upon stimulation by an antigen, they become antibody-producing plasma cells.

[6] Also known as the *humoral antibody response.* The word "humor" is from the Latin *humor,* meaning "a liquid." Humors, then, designate certain fluid materials in the body.

body, so specific is one to the other, that their protein building blocks are arranged to fit exactly into one another. They actually have combining sites. As a key fits a lock, specific antibody molecules "lock into" the very type of antigen molecules that generated them.[7] The plasma cells are able to produce any one of thousands of different antibodies, each one of which is specifically made to neutralize a specific invading antigen.

What role do T lymphocytes play in this system of antibody production? T lymphocytes do not produce antibodies. However, it is believed that B lymphocytes often cannot differentiate into antibody-producing plasma cells without the aid of nearby T lymphocytes. What is the mechanism of this help? That remains unclear; research suggests only that a chemical reaction is involved.

the cell-mediated immune response

The neutralizing antibodies manufactured in the antibody response are the infantry, the foot soldiers of immunity. They are effective against most microbes. But some microorganisms stubbornly resist the antibody mechanism of immunity. For them the body has an alternative battle plan, using heavy artillery. This battle plan is the cell-mediated immune response. The heavy artillery is the T lymphocyte.[8] The T lymphocyte is called a "killer" cell, meaning that it directly attacks and destroys many organisms that invade the body. No cell-produced antibody is involved; the cell itself is directly responsible for the protective immunological work—hence the term "cell-mediated." While B lymphocytes seem to be confined to the lymph nodes, T lymphocytes roam throughout the blood stream. But the T lymphocyte is not a lonely scavenger. In some way as yet unclear (again possibly by means of a chemical mediator), it acts upon still another type of white blood cell called a *macrophage*. Together, T lymphocytes and macrophage cells attack, ingest, and digest microbial invaders, destroying them in the process. It is believed that they also gobble up and destroy the linked antigen–antibody combinations.

Clearly, the body's two immunological responses, antibody and cell-mediated, are related to each other. Which mechanism predominates when infection occurs may depend largely on the type of invader and the body's needs. When the measles virus enters the body, for example, the antibody–antigen mechanism becomes active; however, the T lymphocyte is also important. When the invader is a fungus or the tuberculosis bacillus, the cell-mediated immune response is paramount. With smallpox virus infection the antibody–antigen mechanism operates, but the cell-mediated process of immunity is also active.

[7] Immunologically speaking, this extreme antigen–antibody specificity is a two-edged sword. It helps man to fight infection, but it may also harm him. It explains why influenza antibodies formed in one year are so ineffective against a slightly changed influenza virus a few years later (page 150). In addition, this extreme specificity and efficiency in antibody formation can apply not only to harmful protein microbes but also to ordinarily harmless proteins that enter the body. Because of this the body becomes sensitized to foreign proteins, such as eggs. Upon a subsequent exposure, a formerly harmless protein can cause an allergic reaction (pages 249–50).

[8] Graham Chedd, "Immunological Engineers," *New Scientist and Science Journal,* Vol. 50, No. 751 (May 13, 1971), p. 396.

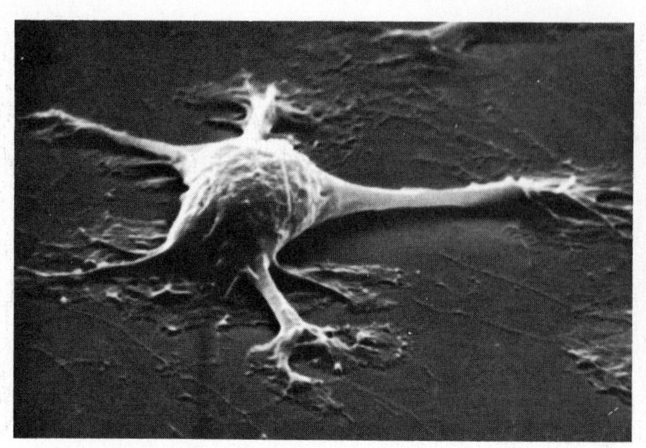
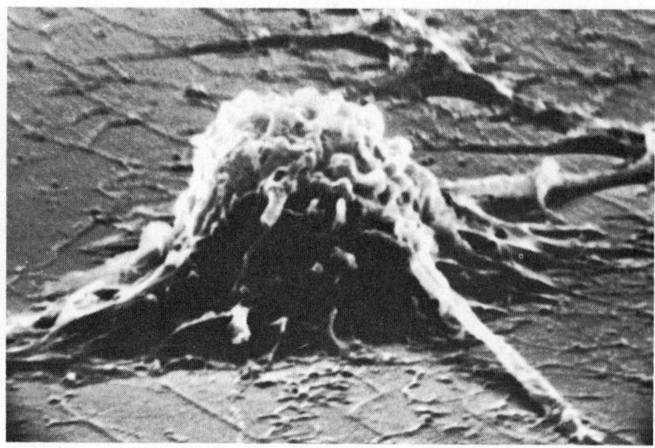

6-9 *A macrophage in action. At left, the macrophage is dormant (× 6,000). At right, it has been stimulated into activity by the presence of an antigen (× 7,000).*

Both mechanisms of immunity enabled the ancient Chinese and the Turkish ingrafters to achieve resistance to smallpox. Antibodies, generated by the deliberately induced mild smallpox infection (the antigen), ''locked into'' and thus neutralized some of the smallpox virus antigen that was later inhaled.

immunological memory

But how did this come about? What happens when a person who has been exposed to an antigen, and who has made antibodies to neutralize it, is reexposed to the same antigen? The first exposure leaves the individual with immature or precursor plasma cells, which upon stimulation by the second invasion of the antigen become mature plasma cells. These manufacture a second massive number of antibodies to meet the antigenic threat. The precursor cells are called *memory cells* and the entire process is called *immunological memory.* Now this question must be asked: How are the proper precursor cells chosen for each specific antigen? It is believed that during the initial infection, the precursor cells develop distinctive mechanisms that later enable them to be stimulated by the antigen and selected out by it from all the other lymphocytes. And how is cell-mediated immunity involved? Coming to the aid of the antibody mechanism, T lymphocytes and macrophages together attack and destroy the antigen.

A host of questions remain unanswered. What is the manner and extent of the cooperation between B lymphocytes, T lymphocytes, and macrophage cells? What precisely are the differences between them? Are the T lymphocytes that help B lymphocytes exactly the same as the T lymphocytes that behave as ''killer'' cells? Such questions are more than academic. For example, a transplanted organ is foreign tissue to its recipient; killer T lymphocytes attack and kill the transplanted cells. Thus, they interfere with life-saving efforts to transplant an organ, such as a kidney, from one person to another. If it were possible to selectively rid the body of killer T lymphocytes, would the remainder of the patient's immunological system be ruined? Cancer cells are also foreign to the body; why are they not rejected like tissue grafts? Is it not possible that some cancers produce an antigen that combines with its antibody, and that this reaction results in the release of some sort of chemical blocking factor in the blood that protects the cancer from attack by killer T lymphocytes? And if this is so, could not a substance be found that would nullify the blocking factor, thus releasing the body's immunological system to fight the cancer?[9] Throughout the world, scientists are eagerly seeking the answers to these and other vital questions.

the active immunity of individual effort

No matter how a virus (or any other infectious agent) enters the body, B lymphocytes must themselves actively react to the intruder. They must produce their own protective antibody. The body actively produces its own immunity. This way of reacting to the invader is called *active immunity.* The B lymphocytes do not borrow. Stimulated by the foreign microbial antigen and according to their own genetic instruction, they actively work for and earn their immunity. And, like money that is earned and banked, active immunity lasts a long time.

A vaccine contains living or dead organisms, and it is these organisms that act as antigens to stimulate antibody formation. All vaccine antigens stimulate active immunity. Table 6-1 shows those immunizing agents most commonly used in the United States. With the exception of diphtheria, whooping cough, and tetanus, all the diseases they prevent are caused by viruses. Few benefits of science have so successfully prevented sickness and death as have vaccines. Table 6-2 shows, for selected years, the number of reported cases in the United States of certain previously common communicable illnesses. For all of them, effective vaccines are available. Much progress has been made. More work needs to be done.

Vaccination with live vaccinia virus to prevent smallpox has already been discussed. Now consider the other vaccines that are now most commonly used in this country.

some viral vaccines

In 1885, Pasteur developed a rabies virus vaccine. Until the 1930s, vaccines to protect against smallpox and rabies were the only two virus vaccines in use. Modern scientists are not so handicapped. Increasing knowledge about viruses has led to more vaccines to prevent the diseases some of them cause.

It has been seen that the injection of a virus, even weakened (attenuated), causes specific antibody production and, consequently, immunity. The injection of dead viruses may have the same effect. A weakened virus vaccine causes a mild infection but no significant sickness. A vaccine in which the microbe is killed causes no infection.

TWO VACCINES TO PREVENT POLIOMYELITIS AND ONE AGAINST MUMPS Salk's *killed poliomyelitis virus vaccine* contains virus that, although killed by a chemical (formalin), retains the ability to generate antibodies. Sabin's *attenuated poliomyelitis virus vaccine* contains live poliovirus weakened

[9] For a discussion of the immune system as it relates to treatment of cancer, see pages 208–09.

TABLE 6-1

Immunization Becomes More Acceptable . . .

DISEASE[a]	VACCINE TYPE	AGE AT WHICH IMMUNIZATION MAY BEGIN	NUMBER OF BASIC DOSES	BOOSTERS
Regular[b] measles (rubeola)	Viral (infective attenuated)	1 year	1 injection	None
German[b] measles (rubella)	Viral (infective attenuated)	1 year	1 injection	None
Poliomyelitis	Viral (infective attenuated —Sabin vaccine	6 weeks	Under age 18[c]: 2 oral doses 6–8 weeks apart; 3rd oral dose 8–12 months after second[d]	One oral dose on entry into school.
Influenza	Viral (noninfective, killed)	Considered at any age with chronic debilitating conditions	Adults: one dose Infants: as determined by physician[e]	Yearly, in the fall. Must contain the current strains of virus.
Mumps[b]	Viral (infective attenuated)	1 year	1 injection	Need for booster not established.
Diptheria Tetanus Pertussis (whooping cough)	Toxoid Toxoid Bacterial (noninfective) } DTP	6–8 weeks	3 injections 1 month apart; 4th injection 1 year later.	On entry into school. Thereafter, a booster every 10 years.[f]

[a] Smallpox is not included here because routine vaccination against smallpox has been discontinued in the United States (see page 140).

[b] By midsummer of 1971, several combination live virus vaccines had been licensed. These were combined to prevent measles-mumps-rubella, measles-rubella, and rubella-mumps.

[c] Routine immunization for adults residing in the continental United States is usually unnecessary except in epidemic situations.

[d] It has been recommended that regular measles and German measles virus vaccines may be given simultaneously with the third dose of oral poliomyelitis vaccine during the second year of life. Moreover, there is evidence that when the licensed combination of regular measles, German measles, and mumps vaccine is given simultaneously with the oral poliomyelitis vaccine, a satisfactory level of immunity against all four diseases is obtained. (''Simultaneous Administration of Certain Live Virus Vaccines, Supplementary Recommendation,'' Recommendations of the Public Health Service Advisory Committee on Immunization Practices, *Physician's Bulletin,* Orange County Health Department, Vol. 23, No. 3 [January 29, 1973], p. 1.)

[e] Influenza virus vaccine is not routinely given during childhood. Moreover, in 1973, the single dose of vaccine that supplanted the two doses formerly given protected primarily against some type A influenza viruses and a type B virus strain. However, in December 1972, new strains of type B influenza virus appeared in Hong Kong and later in Australia and England. Thus, the 1973 recommendations included the additional administration of a second type B influenza virus vaccine to be given two weeks after the first. (''Influenza Vaccine: Recommendations of the Public Health Service Advisory Committee on Immunization Practices,'' *Physician's Bulletin,* Orange County Health Department, Vol. 23, No. 12 [June 4, 1973], p. 2.)

[f] Pertussis vaccine is not included in the booster given after age seven because of undue reactions. The diphtheria fraction of the booster is, moreover, much lessened in amount.

Source: ''Supplement: Collected Recommendations of the Public Health Service Advisory Committee on Immunization Practices, 1972,'' *Morbidity and Mortality Weekly Report,* U.S. Department of Health, Education, and Welfare, Vol. 21, No. 25 (June 24, 1972).

TABLE 6-2

. . . and History Records the Changes

Reported cases for selected years in the United States of some diseases preventable by immunization*

YEAR	SMALLPOX	REGULAR MEASLES	POLIOMYELITIS (ACUTE)	DIPHTHERIA	PERTUSSIS (WHOOPING COUGH)	TETANUS
1945	346	146,013	13,624	18,675	133,792	Figures not available.
1950	0	319,214	33,300	5,796	120,718	486
1955	2†	555,156	28,985	1,984	62,786	462
1960	0	441,703	3,190	918	14,809	368
1965	0	261,904	61	164	6,799	300
1967	0	62,705	40	219	9,718	263
1968	0	22,231	53	260	4,810	178
1969	0	25,826	18	241	3,285	185
1970	0	47,351	28	435	4,249	148
1971	0	75,290	21	215	3,036	116
1972	0	32,275	31	152	3,287	128

*Figures include Alaska from 1959, Hawaii from 1960.
†These cases did not fulfill the generally accepted criteria for diagnosis of smallpox.
Sources: For 1945 and 1950, *Weekly Morbidity Report,* Public Health Service, National Office of Vital Statistics, Vol. 2, No. 53 (February 17, 1953). For 1955 and 1960, *Morbidity and Mortality Weekly Report,* U.S. Department of Health, Education, and Welfare, Vol. 9, No. 53 (October 30, 1961). For 1965 and 1967, *Morbidity and Mortality Weekly Report,* Annual Supplement/Summary, 1967, Vol. 16, No. 53 (November 1968). For 1968 and 1969, *Morbidity and Mortality Weekly Report,* Annual Supplement/Summary, 1970, Vol. 19, No. 53 (August 1971), p. 4. For 1970, 1971, and 1972, *Morbidity and Mortality Weekly Report,* Vol. 21, No. 53 (July 1973).

6-10 *A polio victim in ancient Egypt.*

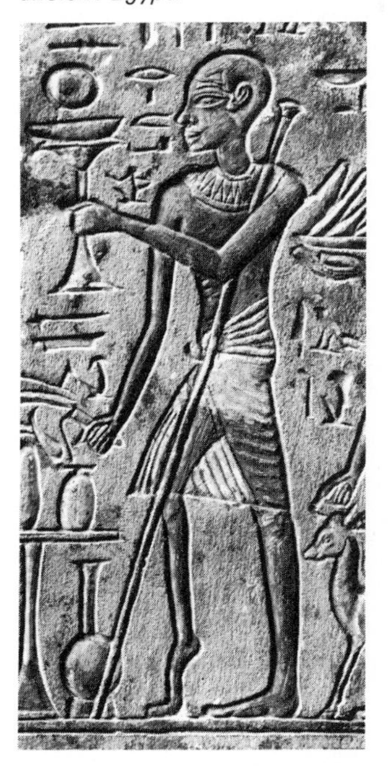

in the laboratory.[10] The mild poliomyelitis infection it produces is so unaccompanied by paralysis or symptoms that it is one of mankind's safest vaccines. Although serious permanent complications from mumps are uncommon, the illness does cause considerable discomfort and disability. A safe and effective *attenuated live mumps virus vaccine* is available. It may be administered after one year of age. Children approaching puberty, adolescents, and young adults (especially males) who have never had mumps are particularly benefited.

TWO VACCINES TO PREVENT TWO DIFFERENT KINDS OF MEASLES Two different kinds of measles, caused by distinctly different viruses, are regular measles (*rubeola*) and German measles (*rubella*). The *live attenuated regular*

[10] These vaccines are named after two contemporary scientists who pioneered in their development—Jonas Salk and Albert Sabin.

measles (*rubeola*) *virus vaccine* is so weakened by laboratory procedures that it can no longer cause significant illness. It does, however, cause a relatively minor infection followed by a durable immunity. Vaccination against regular measles has brought about a resistant population in which the virus is not able to survive. It was hoped that in the 1970s regular measles would become a relatively rare disease. Unfortunately, partly because of parental laxity in seeing that their children are vaccinated, this has not been the case (see Table 6-2).

German measles (rubella) presents special problems, and so does the presently available *attenuated live German measles virus vaccine.* For both school children and adults, German measles is usually a brief, mild, and uncomplicated disease. It is to the unborn child that German measles is a serious threat (see page 164). The main objective of German measles vaccination, therefore, is indirect; it is to prevent infection in pregnant women and thereby avoid damage to the embryo and fetus. Hoping to accomplish this, mass-vaccination programs of school children who have not yet reached puberty have been carried out in this country for several years. It was reasoned that such mass vaccinations would diminish the pool of the German measles virus in the community. The school child would no longer be the major source of infection of the pregnant woman. The vaccinated child would be her shield against the virus. By August 1972, almost 29,200,000 doses of rubella vaccine had been distributed through public programs (the vaccine had been licensed in 1969). This was sufficient to immunize over half the U.S. population between the ages of one and nine. In 1964, almost 500,000 cases of German measles had occurred in the United States. During the first thirty-nine weeks of 1972, there were only 21,424. And, since 1964, there has not been a single nationwide epidemic of German measles.[11] Pregnant women have not received the vaccine; it is known that, as a live virus, it might damage both the placenta and the fetus.[12]

So great a number of vaccinations would seem to be abundant cause for elation. It is not. First, the duration of immunity provided by the vaccine is shorter than desired: antirubella antibodies tend to decrease within a few months. Second, the vaccine does not provide complete protection: when successfully vaccinated individuals are later exposed to the virus, most of them become reinfected. This does not mean that they all show evidence of German measles; their infection is *subclinical*—that is, without symptoms. It is possible, although not proven, that they can carry the virus and infect others. Such reinfection upon exposure occurs in 50 to 84 percent of vaccinated individuals. In people who are naturally immune (who have had the disease), reinfection occurs in only 3.4 percent of cases. Thus, immunity that results from having the disease is fifteen to twenty-five times more efficient than that induced by artificial vaccination. Does a pregnant woman who was vaccinated in childhood, and who is reinfected by the German measles virus, run the risk of damaging her child? Although this is unlikely, she cannot be certain.

[11] "Rubella—United States, First 39 Weeks, 1972," *Morbidity and Mortality Weekly Report,* U.S. Department of Health, Education, and Welfare, Vol. 21, No. 49 (December 9, 1972), p. 417.
[12] "Rubella Vaccination of Women," *The Medical Letter,* Vol. 14, No. 13 (June 23, 1972), p. 45.

A third shortcoming of mass vaccination programs against German measles is that they have apparently not always succeeded in checking severe outbreaks of the disease in highly immunized populations.[13] In Casper, Wyoming, for example, over one thousand cases of German measles occurred between January 8 and May 20, 1971. Eighty-four percent of these were persons twelve to eighteen years old; twenty-seven cases occurred in women, of whom seven were pregnant. Nine months before, 83 percent of Casper's elementary-school children and 52 percent of its preschoolers had been vaccinated against German measles. In Casper, as elsewhere, mass vaccination against German measles of a high percentage of prepubertal children failed to accomplish the primary aim of the program—protection of pregnant women and their unborn children.[14]

For these reasons, direct vaccination of adolescent girls who are known not to be pregnant, and also of adult women known to be nonimmune, immediately after delivery of a child, is being increasingly recommended.[15] Recently delivered women who are vaccinated would need to avoid becoming pregnant again for at least two months and preferably three. The determination of susceptibility (nonimmunity) to German measles can be made by a complex laboratory test. It is believed that women of childbearing age should be tested for susceptibility to rubella before being immunized against it. It should be understood that the vaccine destroys the value of laboratory tests that might be helpful in deciding whether an abortion should be done after exposure. In addition, arthritic symptoms, ranging from mild stiffness to severe arthritis, are not infrequent after vaccination against German measles. The frequency of this varies with different preparations of the vaccine, and increases as the age of the vaccinee increases.[16] In some parts of the United States, laws have made vaccination against German measles compulsory. Immunization of children should not be discontinued; vaccine-induced protection is better than none. Nevertheless, some physicians consider such laws indefensible.[17] Research is being conducted for a better vaccine against German measles.[18]

THE INFLUENZA VIRUS VACCINE In this vaccine, as in Salk's, the virus is killed and so cannot cause infection and disease. The killed virus nevertheless retains the ability to stimulate antibody production and, therefore, to produce a resistance. Occasionally people who have received the influenza vaccine in-

[13] Te-Wen Chang, "Strategy of Rubella Vaccination," *The Journal of Infectious Diseases,* Vol. 123, No. 2 (February 1971), p. 224.

[14] Lawrence E. Klock and Gary S. Rachelefsky, "Failure of Rubella Herd Immunity During an Epidemic," *New England Journal of Medicine,* Vol. 288, No. 2 (January 11, 1973), pp. 69–72.

[15] "Rubella Vaccination of Women," *The Medical Letter,* p. 46.

[16] *Ibid.*

[17] Louis Weinstein and Te-Wen Chang, "Rubella Immunization," *New England Journal of Medicine,* Vol. 228, No. 2 (January 11, 1973), pp. 100–01.

[18] Why does attenuated live oral poliomyelitis vaccine provide enough immunity to prevent outbreaks, while the present German measles vaccine does not? The basic reason is that, when the weakened polio virus vaccine is given orally, it causes an intestinal infection. It is then difficult for the "wild" (or natural) virus to infect the same intestinal sites. Another reason is that poor personal hygiene (such as inadequate handwashing after a bowel movement) may result in the spread of the virus in the vaccine to close contacts; immunization of these contacts then occurs. Why does regular measles (rubeola) vaccination prevent outbreaks while German measles (rubella) vaccination does not? Nobody knows.

jection complain of aftereffects—fever, backache, and sore arm. These mostly result from vaccine impurities, not from the killed virus. Improved procedures have produced a new influenza vaccine with very few side effects. Killed influenza virus vaccines will prevent influenza for six months to a year in 70 to 90 percent of those who receive them.[19]

Influenza virus vaccine presents a special problem. Genetically speaking, the virus does not stand still. Influenza virus contains RNA.[20] From generation to generation, the RNA carries the genetic chemical structure. But, too often, a "genetic mishap" occurs. In such instances, when new influenza virus is made in the invaded cell, the chemical arrangement of the protein overcoat of a succeeding generation is not the same as the one that preceded it. Antibodies built up in the body against the preceding generations of influenza viruses are relatively helpless against the new influenzal viral antigen. What has occurred is an antigenic *shift* or *drift.* Many virologists use these terms interchangeably. Others prefer to call major antigenic changes "shifts" and minor ones "drifts." When the antigenic change is major, the immunological system is caught unprepared. Major antigenic shifts accounted for a type A0 virus in 1933, an A1 subtype in 1947, and an A2 subtype in 1957. Within each of these major antigenic subtypes are numerous variants; these result from relatively minor changes in the chemical arrangement of the protein overcoat. These are the antigenic drifts. Clearly, type A influenza viruses go through a process of continuous minor antigenic drifting, punctuated every ten to fifteen years by a major antigenic shift, against which a population has little or no resistance.[21]

In mid-July 1968, a variant of the A2 subtype of influenza virus suddenly broke out in Hong Kong (footnote 24). The antigenic drift was considerable. It was not great enough for this variant to be designated a new subtype A3, but it was certainly enough to make hundreds of thousands of people in Hong Kong sick. Implacably, the virus continued on to the Philippines. By the end of August, Taiwan, Malaysia, and Singapore had been affected. In September came similar reports from Vietnam and Bombay. In that month, at Teheran, one-third of over a thousand delegates to the International Congress on Tropical Medicine and Malaria fell sick with influenza. They had come from all parts of the world to share information about communicable diseases. In this country, there was growing concern. Why? A mutation had occurred. The antigenic components of the 1968 influenza virus were different from any previous influenza A2 virus (1957, 1961, or 1966). Previous vaccines, containing earlier variants of the influenza A2 virus, were relatively ineffective. A new vaccine was needed. But it takes time to manufacture a new vaccine that meets scrupulous scientific requirements. Feverishly, U.S. drug companies labored to produce enough vaccine. Meanwhile, travelers carried the virus to this country, seeding

[19] "The Hunt for Live-Virus Flu Vaccine," *Medical World News,* Vol. 14, No. 7 (February 16, 1973), p. 22.

[20] For a discussion of viral genetics, see pages 156–60.

[21] Theodore C. Eickhoff, "Immunization Against Influenza: Rationale and Recommendations," *The Journal of Infectious Diseases,* Vol. 123, No. 4 (April 1971), p. 446. There is a type B influenza virus with its own host of variants, but these are much less important in the production of epidemics than the A subtypes and variants. A type C influenza virus has also been classified.

it in the population. Between the virus and man a race developed. Could sufficient vaccine be made in time to avert an epidemic?

Man lost.

He lost again in 1971 and 1972. From such influenza listening posts as the World Influenza Center in London and the WHO International Influenza Center for the Americas in Atlanta, Georgia, came reports of influenza A2 outbreaks that were caused by a variant of the Hong Kong virus. Few areas in the world were spared. How effective was the available vaccine? Aboard one U.S. naval vessel in the South Pacific, 15 percent of those vaccinated less than six months previously became ill.[22] In 1972–73 an influenza A2 virus again attacked people all over the world. Again the illness was caused by a close relative of the Hong Kong virus. Although the new viral mutant had first appeared in south India about mid-1971, the fact that it was isolated from a few cases of influenza in England in January 1973 prompted scientists to name it A/England/42/72. The illness was then dubbed "London flu." By February 1973, some fifty-two strains of influenza A2 virus had been isolated in Germany alone; most of them were antigenically close to A/England/42/72. For the 1973–74 U.S. influenza season, an influenza vaccine was prepared that contained this variant as well as an influenza B variant that had been minimally reported in the country. It was hoped that this combination would provide adequate protection. But, during 1973, new mutant strains of B viruses were recovered from people in Hong Kong, Australia, and Britain. Fearful lest these would invade the United States, every effort was made to prepare a supplementary influenza vaccine that would protect those people most likely endangered by the new type B influenza virus. But not enough could be produced. Again, the antigenic shifts had outwitted man.[23] By early 1974, influenza B was being reported in the United States.

The scientific servants of mankind have good reasons to seek methods of making a better influenza vaccine. An estimated 20 million people throughout the world died of the disease and its complications during the 1918–20 epidemics. In the United States, the 1957 influenza A2 epidemic sent some 22 million people to bed. In the winter of 1963, an estimated 57,000 more deaths occurred in this country than would have been expected in the absence of an influenza epidemic. During a 1967–68 winter influenza epidemic in the United States, excess deaths were reported in all parts of the country except on the West Coast. So it was during a 1972–73 epidemic, except that the West Coast did not escape. During such epidemics, most deaths occur among the elderly or chronically ill (especially people with heart disease, hypertension, diabetes, and tuberculosis).[24]

[22] *Influenza-Respiratory Disease Surveillance,* Center for Disease Control, Public Health Service, U.S. Department of Health, Education, and Welfare, Report No. 88 (January 1973), p. 15.

[23] *Morbidity and Mortality Weekly Report,* U.S. Department of Health, Education, and Welfare, Vol. 22, No. 5 (February 9, 1973), p. 37, and Phil Gumby, "New B-type Influenza Virus Strains May Reach U.S. This Winter," *Journal of the American Medical Association,* Vol. 226, No. 9 (November 26, 1973), pp. 1063–65.

[24] Recent years have seen much activity in influenza virus vaccine research. One recent experimental vaccine is attenuated and is composed of two influenza virus strains. One strain is a genetically defective 1965 Asian influenza virus. The genetic material within it is purposely made defective by cultivating it in a media containing a chemical called 5-flourouacil. The changed 1965 Asian influenza virus is thus a mutant. It will not grow in the lungs; it will, however, grow in the cooler temperatures of the upper respiratory passages. In so doing,

some bacterial vaccines

Not all antigens are viral. There are *bacterial antigens,* which may be used to prepare *bacterial vaccines.* Like the viruses in viral vaccines, the bacteria in bacterial vaccines may be weakened or killed in the laboratory. In both cases the ability to stimulate antibodies is retained. There is still another special type of vaccine, which prevents diphtheria and tetanus. This type is made not from the bacterium itself but from the toxic products resulting from bacterial multiplication.

A VACCINE OF LIVING ATTENUATED BACTERIA The BCG[25] vaccine is useful in preventing tuberculosis, but it has found less favor in this country than abroad. Why? Because it causes a positive skin test (*Mantoux test*) for tuberculosis. A positive Mantoux test may mean either active tuberculosis or a former tuberculosis that has healed. In either case, it is a signal that the person has been infected by someone else. The infectious source must be sought, found, and treated. The Mantoux test has great value in finding possible cases and screening suspected sources. But if everyone were given the BCG vaccine, almost everyone would have a positive Mantoux test, and the test would lose its detection value. Still another advantage of the Mantoux test that would be lost is that the test could no longer be used as an indicator for treatment of selected individuals who react positively to it. People without active tuberculosis who have not received BCG and who show a positive Mantoux test have a markedly greater chance of developing active disease. These risks are much reduced by preventive treatment. Without a way of separating those infected by ordinary routes and those infected by BCG vaccination, a large program of

---

it stimulates the reproduction of antibodies. In the laboratory, this mutant strain is cultivated with a second, more recent (1968) Hong Kong influenza virus strain (page 150 and footnote 7). Together, the mutant strain of the 1965 Asian influenza virus and the strain of the 1968 Hong Kong influenza virus broaden the immunological possibilities of the new experimental vaccine. This attenuated vaccine is sprayed into the nose. Experimental trials with human volunteers are encouraging. The attenuated virus does not spread from vaccinees to unvaccinated volunteers. (''Switch in Viral Genes Leads to New Flu Vaccine,'' *Journal of the American Medical Association,* Vol. 221, No. 11 [September 11, 1972], pp. 1217–18; also, ''Defective Flu Virus Looks Like Effective Vaccine,'' *Medical World News,* Vol. 13, No. 31 [August 18, 1972], p. 18.) Also being studied is a ''five-year influenza virus vaccine.'' It is hoped that this vaccine will protect against influenza virus mutations that might occur until 1978. Influenza viruses are known to mutate when they are attacked by antibodies that are specific to them. As was stated on page 150, the mutation is the result of a change in the chemical structure of the coat of the virus. Every ten or fifteen years that change results in a new major subtype of the influenza virus. However, in intervening years there occur minor changes in the viral coating. These result in numerous variants of the major subtypes of the influenza virus. The theory (which is open to question) is that these minor changes into variants progress in an orderly fashion. As each new antigenic variant arises, it is presumed to be the senior of all its predecessors. This means that the antibodies raised against any one particular senior variant are effective against all the variants that led up to it, but not against those variant viruses that will develop after it. Now, the theory continues, new influenza virus variants will spring up until no new antigenic changes are possible. The notion that the final variant subtype—the dominant senior—can stimulate antibodies against all the subtypes that occurred before it, has led scientists into an interesting procedure. They have incubated virus variants in serum containing hostile antibodies. Eventually, a viral mutant results that is not neutralized by the antibodies. Using this senior viral variant, antibodies are developed that are effective against it. It is hoped that such a repeated process of incubating and selecting will result in a mutant influenza virus variant that can then be killed to provide a vaccine against future influenza epidemics caused by minor antigenic shifts. It is questionable whether this forcing of the evolution of a virus, by bombarding it with antibodies it would have to face in the future, mimics the natural evolution of the virus. In addition, a major problem is that of determining which mutant virus is the dominant senior. (''Can the Pasteur Institute Predict the Future?'' *New Scientist,* Vol. 57, No. 833 [February 15, 1973], p. 351.)

[25] Bacille (bacillus) Calmette Guérin, named after the French scientists Albert Léon Charles Calmette (1863–1933) and Alphonse François Marie Guérin (1816–95).

prophylactic therapy against tuberculosis would be impossible (see page 172). Tuberculosis specialists in this country have accomplished as much without widespread BCG vaccination as have specialists in other countries where such vaccination is routine practice. In this country, however, some physicians strongly recommend BCG vaccination, particularly for unduly exposed groups: doctors and nurses,[26] slum residents, and people who live with a tuberculosis patient.[27]

VACCINES OF NONLIVING BACTERIA Another way of using bacterial antigens is to kill them with heat or chemicals. Thus rendered noninfectious yet retaining their ability to stimulate antibodies, they are used as vaccines. The *whooping cough* (*pertussis*) and *typhoid fever vaccines* are prepared from dead bacterial cells that retain their power to generate antibodies.

ON THE USES OF BACTERIAL POISONS The principle that certain body cells produce a substance to combat poisons is hardly modern. Clearly the idea had occurred to the first-century Roman epic poet Lucan. In writing of the resistance of some Africans to snake poison he says:

> Them not the serpent's tooth nor poison harms.
> Nor do they thus in arts alone excel,
> But nature too their blood has tempered well,
> And taught with vital force the venom to repel.[28]

That the repeated injection of small doses of snake venom by bite or by needle into an individual (or an animal) produced immunity to the poison (or *toxin*) was known by Emil A. Von Behring (1854–1917). The venom, or toxin antigen, stimulated the body to produce protective antibody antitoxin. This knowledge helped the German Nobel Prize winner to develop concepts of diphtheria prevention and treatment that have saved generations of children.

As snakes produce poisons, so do some bacteria produce toxins as they multiply. As microbial agents stimulate the body to produce antibodies, so do toxins enter the body as foreign proteins to stimulate plasma cell production of antitoxins. When certain toxin-producing bacteria invade the body, it is not they per se, but rather their toxin liberated into the body tissues as they multiply, that causes sickness. The diphtheria bacillus multiplies in the respiratory tract; the bacillus of tetanus in a wound. Locally, each produces a toxin. Carried by the blood, the diphtheria toxin may affect distant organs. With tetanus, the toxin travels to peripheral nerves and the central nervous system is irritated. Fatal diphtheria often results from an affected heart, although several other factors may cause or contribute to death, such as airway obstruction or nerve affliction with paralysis. In both cases, the toxin is the antibody generator, the antigen. How can it be used to prevent disease?

[26] "BCG Vaccination," a letter to the editor drafted by W. H. Oatway, Jr., and cosigned by twenty other physicians, in *American Review of Respiratory Disease,* Vol. 96, No. 4 (October 1967), pp. 830–31.

[27] David T. Smith, "Diagnostic and Prognostic Significance of the Quantitative Tuberculin Tests," quoted in *Modern Medicine,* Vol. 36, No. 5 (February 26, 1968), p. 110.

[28] Lucan, *Pharsalia,* quoted in Heinrich Oppenheimer, *Medical and Allied Topics in Latin Poetry* (London, 1928), pp. 285–86.

Toxoid: active immunity from modified toxin antigens. Grow the tetanus or diphtheria bacterium on a rich culture medium and it produces toxin. Filter the laboratory culture. The fluid portion passing through the filter contains the toxin. The toxin can do two things: cause sickness and produce antitoxin. How can one reduce the first effect and conserve the second? Add formalin, which is a 40 percent solution of gaseous formaldehyde. The toxin antigen is modified. Its toxic properties are destroyed, but injected into the body, it can stimulate the production of antibody antitoxin. It is now called *toxoid.* Diphtheria toxoid and tetanus toxoid can be added to killed pertussis (whooping cough) bacterial cells. A triple antigen is produced—the *diphtheria, tetanus,* and *pertussis* (*DTP*) *vaccine* (Table 6-1). Injected, it stimulates active immunity against all three diseases.

Antitoxin. Inject a small measured amount of diphtheria or tetanus toxin antigen into a horse. Each day, for some days, slowly increase the injected dose of toxin antigen. The horse obligingly responds to the foreign protein toxin antigen by producing antibody antitoxin. The horse produces his own (active) immunity. Bleed the horse. In the laboratory, isolate the antibody antitoxin from the blood. The antibody antitoxin can be used to neutralize toxin antigen—to render it harmless. How?

Circulating in the blood of a child desperately sick with diphtheria or tetanus is the killing toxin antigen specific for the disease. The toxin stimulates the child's cells to produce antitoxin. But the process is too slow. An emergency exists. Antitoxin is needed immediately. Can borrowed horse antibody antitoxin be used to neutralize the toxin antigen? Yes. Injected into the child's vein, the horse antibody antitoxin neutralizes the child's circulating toxin antigen. Used in time, the injection will save the child's life. Horse tetanus antitoxin, once so useful, has been replaced by a human blood product—*tetanus immune globulin* (*TIG*). Since it is not so foreign, it causes few of the disagreeable and even serious side effects so common with the horse product. The immunity achieved by using another person's or an animal's antibodies is called *passive immunity.* What does that term really mean?

passive immunity: the temporary resistance provided by borrowed antibody

Passive immunity is borrowed immunity. Through vaccination or disease, another creature (man or animal) must first earn active immunity—must first be stimulated actively to make his own antibodies. Then that creature is bled. From the blood the actual antibody is obtained. It has been seen that horse blood containing antibody antitoxin can be borrowed to treat diphtheria and tetanus. But sometimes human blood, containing antibodies, can similarly be borrowed. *Gamma globulin* is the part of the human blood that is the antibody.

Human gamma globulin may be used to prevent rubeola and infectious hepatitis. For example, an individual susceptible to rubeola is exposed to the disease. If given within six days of the exposure, the injection of enough gamma globulin (somebody else's earned antibodies) will prevent the disease. Another person is exposed to a case of infectious hepatitis. He has shared the same home, the same meals, and may have ingested the virus. An injection of gamma globulin within about a month of the time of exposure may prevent jaundice in the contact. Although the gamma globulin is merely borrowed antibody, it is enough to meet the circulating virus antigen, to "lock into" it, and to render it harmless before visible sickness can occur.[29] Within about two to six weeks, the used borrowed antibodies are excreted. So borrowed immunity is like borrowed money. It lasts but a short time.

Passive immunity that passes through the placenta, from mother to baby, is also temporary. A newborn will lose his mother's polio antibodies in about six weeks. The mother's measles and mumps antibodies remain with the baby for only a year (or slightly less) after birth. The family physician does not vaccinate a child against polio until he is six weeks old. And he waits until the first year before vaccinating against measles and mumps. Otherwise the mother's antibodies in the child interfere with the injected antigen (vaccine).

viral competitors in the human ecosystem

how may viruses be known?

Most viruses (the smallest microorganisms) are visible only under the electron microscope.[30] The simplest viruses are chemically composed of a tightly packed central core of nucleic acids within a protein overcoat (see Figure 6-11). The central core of nucleic acids (the genes of the virus) is responsible for the infection. The protein overcoat determines the specificity of the virus as an antigen; its structure decides which specific antibody the virus will cause to be produced.

The central core of viral genes is of two types: RNA (ribonucleic acid) or DNA (deoxyribonucleic acid). Viruses contain either RNA or DNA but never both. (Cells of higher organisms, whether bacteria or people, do contain both.) Viruses differ from one another in their *size.* The influenza virus, for example, is ten times bigger than poliovirus. Viruses also vary in *shape.* The "cold sore" (herpes simplex) virus is spherical. Other viruses are shaped like bricks, still others like threads. Moreover, the length of time that elapses between an infection by a virus and the onset of symptoms (the incubation period) varies with the disease. For example, the average incubation period of regular measles (rubeola) is about ten days; of German measles (rubella), about a week longer.

In one major respect all viruses are identical. They cannot multiply outside a cell. As obligatory parasites, they may cause disease. But this feature also makes it possible, in the laboratory, to grow and study some of them in a culture of cells.

6-11 *Asian influenza virus* (×*250,000*).

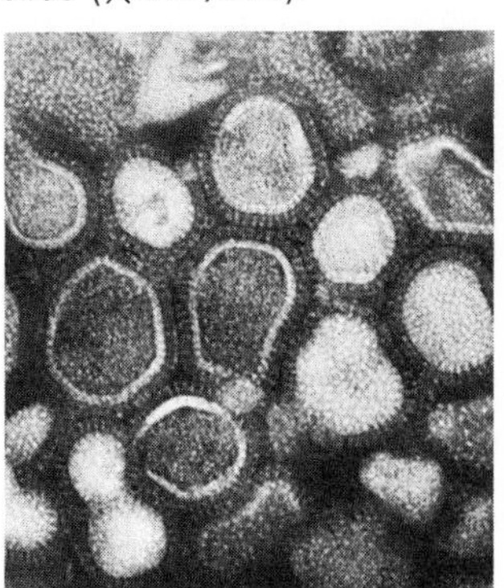

cell culturing

This process is a modern scientific achievement of paramount importance. Sick cells are placed in a container of specially prepared "soup." There they are

[29] Chickenpox and shingles are caused by exactly the same virus, and, if given in time, a special gamma globulin (shingles antibodies) can prevent severe chickenpox in those exposed. It is in very short supply.

[30] To give an idea of their size, the virus of tobacco-mosaic diseases is "300 millimicrons long by 15 wide, or 60/5,000,000 of an inch by 3/5,000,000," according to Greer Williams, *Virus Hunters* (New York, 1959), p. 104.

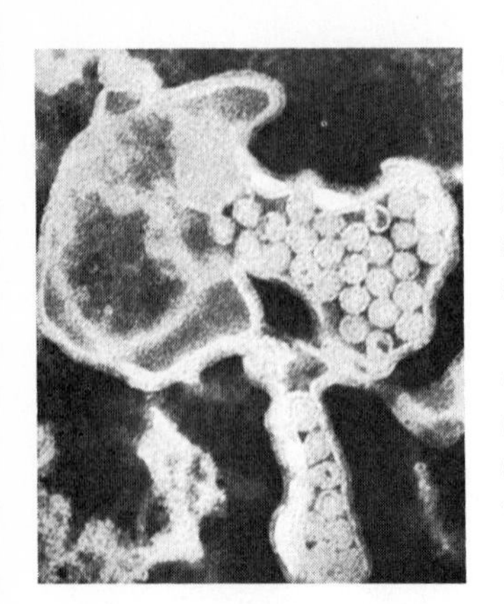

6-12 *Poliovirus particles (the clustered round objects) inside a fragment of a cell (×320,000).*

nourished and multiply. Waste collects. So some of the cellular growth is transferred to another container of fresh nourishment. These transferred cells multiply in turn. Another transfer is made and then still another. Only abnormal, and not healthy, cells can do this. Healthy cells treated in this fashion will die within about a year even with the best of methods. Some years ago, cancer cells from a patient's uterine cervix were obtained and, by transfer, repeatedly cultured. Literally tons of cells, originating from this one person's original cervical cancer cells, have been distributed to virus laboratories throughout the world. There are many other sources of cells in which to grow viruses. Among them are surgically excised human and monkey tissues. Healthy, they survive usefully for a limited time. When viruses gain entrance into a cell, whether it be of a plant or a laboratory animal or a human being, they may cause it to sicken (see Figure 6-12).[31] How? By interfering with the manner in which a normal cell uses nutrients to live.

normal cellular protein manufacture: a brief account

The manner in which a normal cell makes protein is described in Chapter 18, pages 532–35. Briefly, the process is as follows. The nuclear DNA bears the master plan of genetic characteristics for protein manufacture. But that DNA may not leave the nucleus. So a molecule of messenger RNA, by apposing itself to the nuclear DNA, incorporates within itself the proper message for protein manufacture. It becomes a working copy. Then the messenger RNA leaves the nucleus and enters the surrounding territory, the cellular cytoplasm. Throughout this cytoplasm are located the ribosomes—the workbenches at which protein will be manufactured. Ribosomal structure also depends on the DNA. As a form of RNA, it had left the nucleus to be established in the cytoplasm. Messenger RNA, carrying from the nucleus the DNA instructions, associates itself with a ribosome. At the ribosome, the RNA instructions for making protein are then followed. How does protein building material get to the ribosome? A third RNA, transfer RNA, leaves the nucleus. Its job is to bring cytoplasmic amino-acid building blocks to the ribosome for protein construction. (Thus, three kinds of RNA originate in the cell's nucleus to be governed by DNA—ribosomal, messenger, and transfer.)

viral infection A virus invades a bacterial cell in one way, an animal cell in another. When a virus invades a bacterium, it first attaches itself to the bacterium and then erodes the covering cell membrane. Then, through a tiny hole in its tail, the virus ejects its nucleic acid core, or genes, into the bacterium. In this case, the protein overcoat, left outside the bacterial cell, is washed away. Viruses that infect bacteria and destroy them are called *bacteriophage* (bacteria + Greek *phagein,* to eat). (See Figure 6-13.)

The complex animal cell reacts differently to viral infection than does the simple bacterium. But, like a bacterium, an animal cell infected with a virus is sick. In its sickness it can be affected in four ways and with four results:

[31] This is called the *cytopathogenic* effect (Greek *kyto,* hollow vessel [cell] + *pathos,* disease + *genesis,* production).

I. *The invading virus uses the animal cell to make more viruses.* First, virus particles attach themselves to a cell, and then they penetrate it (see Figure 6-12). The virus enters the cell, protein overcoat and all. A cell with virus in it is infected. Once in the cell, the virus undergoes an ''uncoating phenomenon''; that is, the protein coat opens, the virus disrobes (or is disrobed, it is not known which), and the nucleic acid molecules are released ''naked'' into the cell. When they are thus freed in the cell, the viral nucleic acids interrupt the cell's

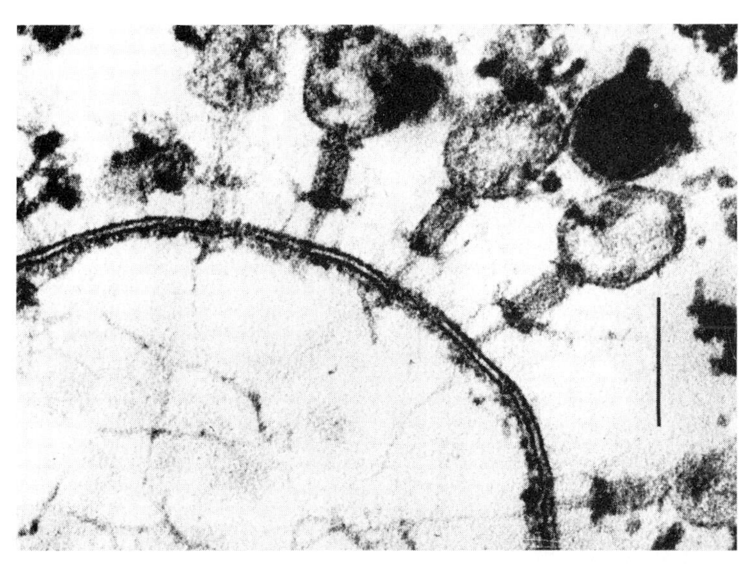

6-13 Left: *The electron microscope reveals that each virus is bound directly to the bacterial cell wall by its short tail fibers. The tail cores have just penetrated through the bacterial wall* (arrow), *and dark fibers of DNA extend from the tail tips within the cell.* Bottom left: *An ''untriggered'' T2 virus* (×*450,000*). *Within its six-sided head lie coiled its genes—its infective DNA (not shown).The virus' tail is surrounded by a screw-shaped sheath.* Bottom right: *The virus has met with a bacterium (not shown; see the photograph on page 134). A bacterial substance caused the sheath to contract, releasing its tail fibers. The ''triggered'' virus* (×*450,000*) *has injected its DNA into the bacterium.* (*See also Figure 1-2, on page 10.*)

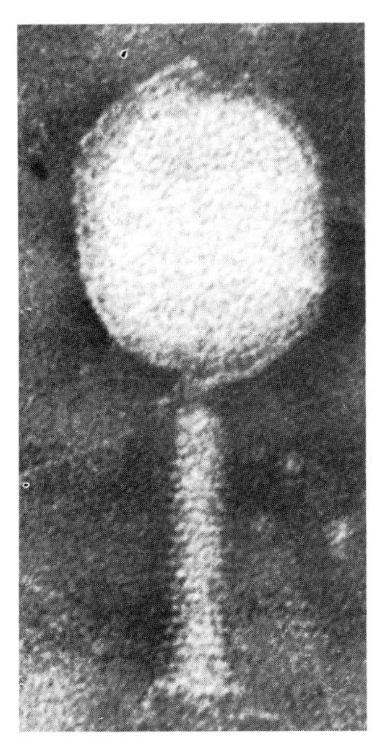

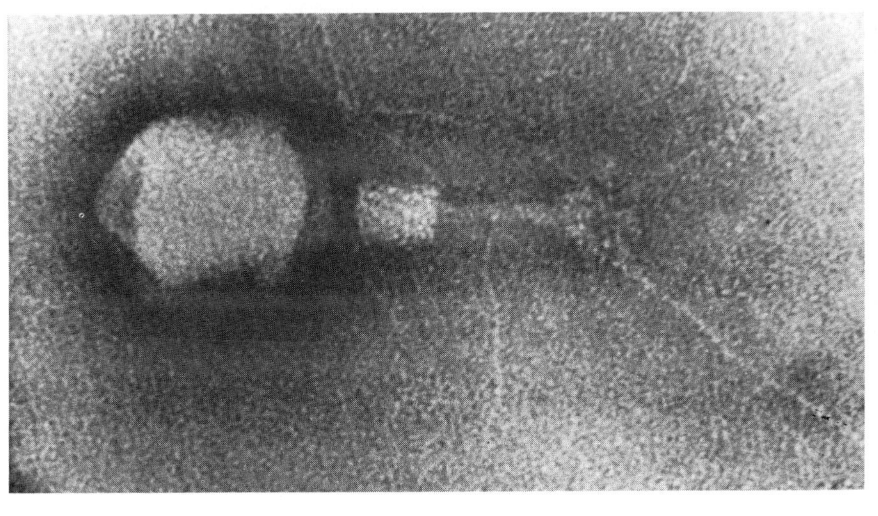

normal DNA mechanism. How the invading virus accomplishes this is not yet completely clear. However, what happens to the different kinds of infected cells depends on whether the invading virus contains DNA or RNA.

A. *If it is viral DNA that is released into the cell* after the uncoating phenomenon, it follows that the cell is burdened. Normally it is geared to contain only cellular DNA. Now it contains two kinds of DNA—cellular DNA, which is designed to make protein for more cells, and viral DNA, which is designed to make more virus. For a while they may exist together without harm to the cell. Usually, they compete promptly. The viral DNA does not tell the cell's DNA what to do. Viral DNA merely uses the available servants and the housekeeping equipment normally used by the cell's DNA. For example: to operate normally for protein production, the cell's DNA must use ribosomes. Viral DNA also uses the ribosomes but to make more virus. To make protein, the cell's DNA must use cytoplasmic amino acids. Viral DNA also uses the cell's amino acids. In normal cell protein production, cellular DNA directs the synthesis of cellular enzymes and messenger RNA, and both participate in the manufacture of cell proteins. In viral production, viral DNA directs the cell to synthesize enzymes and messenger RNA that will participate in the manufacture of viral proteins and more viral DNA. The intruding viral DNA "crowds" the cell's normal DNA. Within the cell there is a "chemical overpopulation." The usurped cell sickens and dies. But not before viral nucleic acids, exactly like those that were within the original invaders, have been assembled at its ribosomes and clothed in new overcoats. Dying, the cell ruptures and the new virus escapes to seek other cells.[32]

B. What happens *when the invading virus contains RNA* instead of DNA molecules? There are two possibilities:

1. *The viral RNA can act as its own messenger.* Carrying its own coded message to the ribosome, it seduces the cell into making enzymes that, in turn, favor the production of viral RNA and viral protein instead of cellular RNA and cellular protein. Where do the amino acids that are destined to become viral protein come from? They are picked out of the cytoplasmic pool. How do they reach the ribosome at which the viral RNA waits with its instructions? Whether a form of viral RNA is created to accomplish this or the regular cellular RNA works for the creation of virus protein is not known. But the viral RNA can itself

[32] In the summer of 1973, two New York virologists announced findings about one DNA virus that created a considerable stir in the scientific world. The smallpox virus is a member of a group of viruses called *poxviruses;* these contain DNA as their genetic material. It has been known for several years that the smallpox virus makes several enzymes, two of which are called *DNases*. (The suffix "ase" designates an enzyme.) The recent discovery had to do with the function of one of these enzymes. It will be remembered that an enzyme has the power to initiate or accelerate a chemical reaction. When a smallpox virus enters a cell, one of the DNases is released. The DNase then switches off the synthesis of the invaded cell's DNA. In this way the smallpox virus is able to fashion a weapon with which to destroy any cell it infects. Thus, the smallpox poxvirus can direct a cell to make more virus, but the death of the cell is caused by an enzyme made by the poxvirus in the cell. Poxviruses kill the cells they infect, but, as will be seen, this is not true of all viruses that enter a cell. Cancer viruses, for example, may kill a cell or encourage it to give rise to future generations of cancer cells (see pages 198–99). Moreover, it is of interest that most effective anticancer drugs work by turning off the DNA in cancer cells (see pages 199–200). The possibility of someday using a viral enzyme to accomplish the same effect will need research, as will a host of questions raised by the new discovery. Among them: Do other DNA viruses produce enzyme weaponry? Can RNA viruses do the same thing, and, if so, which ones? ("Virus Enzymes: Weapons of Destruction," *Science News,* Vol. 104, No. 1 [July 7, 1973], p. 3.)

act as a template and use the cell's servants and housekeeping equipment to make more RNA like itself. Some normal cellular RNA continues to be made. However, viral RNA soon overwhelms the cell. As in the case of DNA viral infection, the cell breaks open. The newly created virus is released. But the virus cannot tolerate freedom. Away from the cell its ecosystem is utterly inadequate. It must quickly find more cells in which to multiply and prosper. The irony is this: if the virus kills enough cells, the host dies. Then the virus, trapped in a host of dead cells, must find a new host or also die.

2. *Instead of acting as its own messenger, the viral RNA can direct the production of DNA.* This it accomplishes by virtue of the recently discovered enzyme associated with some RNA viruses called *reverse transcriptase.* The discovery of this enzyme ranks as a major scientific event of the early 1970s. It was known that DNA, helped by an enzyme, could direct the production of RNA, and that this RNA was a copy (or transcript) of part of the DNA. The formula for the genetic process, DNA $\rightarrow$ RNA, was believed to be always a one-way street. Now it was found that this genetic process could be reversed. Helped by reverse transcriptase, RNA could direct the production of DNA, and this DNA was a copy (or transcript) of part of the RNA. Thus, when some RNA viruses invaded a cell, the genetic process could be RNA $\rightarrow$ DNA. An RNA virus containing reverse transcriptase, then, could enter an animal cell, could undergo the uncoating phenomenon, and, instead of acting as its own messenger (as described above), could direct the production of DNA. And, for this reversal, the enzyme reverse transcriptase was necessary.[33]

The RNA-dependent DNA can behave in several ways. Like a DNA virus, it can compete with the cell's DNA. In this way it can direct the cell to make more virus. Or the DNA, made under the direction of viral RNA and helped by reverse transcriptase, can be incorporated in the cell's DNA. The usurped DNA of the cell may then be directed to lose its control and become cancer. As will be seen below, this last refers to the fourth major possible ill effect of a virus upon a cell. The cancer-causing ability of some viruses is discussed in more detail on pages 197–201.

II. *A second consequence of viral infection is that the cell may be instructed to decrease its speed of multiplication and growth.* This is the "reverse cancer effect." An unborn baby, up to three or four months after conception, can be secondarily infected by the mother's infection with the German measles (rubella) virus (see pages 148 and 164). The virus takes over the genetic mechanism directing the fetus' rapidly multiplying cells. The rate of cellular multiplication is slowed down. Fewer cells are formed. Twenty percent of such children are born with an inadequate number of cells; these children may be blind, deaf, or retarded, or they may have heart and other defects.

III. *Upon entering a cell, the virus may become temporarily inactive.* This is

[33] Reverse transcriptase is also called *RNA-dependent polymerase.* How did this enzyme get its formidable name? The word "polymerase" is a combination of "polymer" and the enzyme suffix "ase." A polymer is a substance that consists of large molecules that are formed by the combination of smaller molecules of the same substance. The polymerase in question makes DNA; thus it is a DNA polymerase. And DNA polymerase is indeed "RNA-dependent": without RNA transcription it could not exist.

not the straightforward infection described in I and II above. This is a *latent* viral infection; that is, it is not immediately apparent, but is capable of being expressed. For many years, even for a lifetime, the viral nucleic acids (its genes) remain dormant in the cell. It is believed that they are tucked away in the genes of the cell that they have infected. In a sense, then, the invading virus remains in ecological balance with the host cell. During this time there is no apparent harm to the cell. The genes of the latent virus remain in a ''switched-off'' state and are passed on, during cell division (*mitosis;* see page 529), from parent to daughter cells. Often, however, stimulated by another infection or by some other stress, such as severe emotional upset, serious sunburn, or exposure to radiation or to chemicals, some genes of the virus are ''switched on,'' and viral multiplication is initiated. Cells fall ill. They may be inflamed. Some die. One example of this is the common ''cold sore'' (herpes simplex), caused by herpesvirus 1. Another is the genital sores caused by herpesvirus 2. Both of these will infect people for a lifetime, flare up as sores following some stress, and apparently remain in a latent state in people's cells for long periods (see pages 185–86).

IV. *The invading virus can cause animal cancer.* In nonhuman animals, the DNA or viral RNA captured in the cell may send messages of malignancy. There is a ''cancer effect.'' The capacity for controlled growth (previously so inherent a part of the normal cell's DNA or RNA function) is lost. Tumor results. As of early 1974, it had yet to be proved that viruses cause cancer in humans. An increasing number of researchers are taking the view that some human cancers are caused by the above-described latent viral infection. But this is merely a first step. The cancer results, they believe, not from the activity of all the genes of the virus, but from a ''switching on'' of only a few of its genes. The whole virus itself, they theorize, never is manufactured. (This is more fully discussed on pages 197–201).

interferon

The time: 1960. The place: a capsule hurtling through space. It is all very dramatic. Four of Flash Gordon's members lie dead. Then another falls sick. He sinks into a coma. Then still another crew member succumbs. But then, in the nick of time, enter interferon!

It works. The rest of the crew is saved.

Interferon is not, however, the product of cartoonist Dan Barry's imagination. It is the product of the labor of British scientists Alick Issac and Jean Lindenmann. What is interferon?

It is a protein. As was just noted, virus-infected cells may be instructed to produce more virus. In some way, as yet not clearly revealed, the viral nucleic acid is responsible for the production of interferon within infected cells. Interferon does not protect the cell that is already infected and that, indeed, is producing it. It is thought to prevent the infection of as yet uninvolved adjacent cells. Moreover, interferon does not itself inhibit viral replication. The interferon interacts with the animal cell membrane. The cell membrane then produces a

FLASH!
FOUR DEAD... THE OTHERS IN COMA! AND NOTHING WE CAN DO BUT WATCH THEM GO... ONE BY ONE!

THIS COULD BE IT! INTERFERON! IT KNOCKED OUT THE VIRUS IN THE LAB ANIMALS!
HURRY!

WELL, DOCTOR...?
THE INTERFERON WORKS! THE FEVER IS GOING DOWN!

NURSE — CHECK THEIR TEMPERATURE EVERY THIRTY MINUTES! WE'LL TRY INJECTIONS AGAIN IN THREE HOURS!

WE MADE IT, DALE! THERE'S GOING TO BE A WEDDING AFTER ALL! HAPPY, DARLING?
Y-YES, STEVE! OF COURSE!

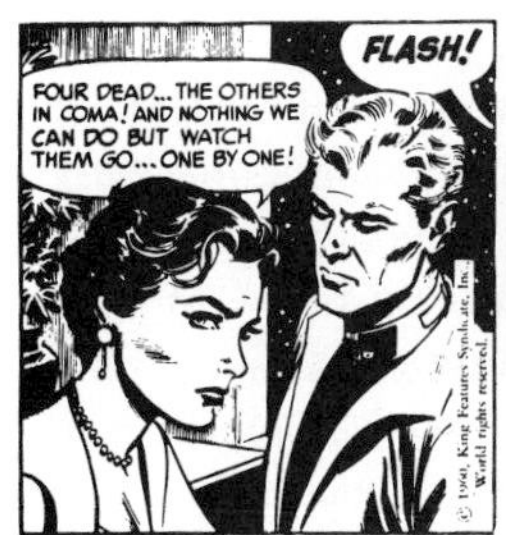

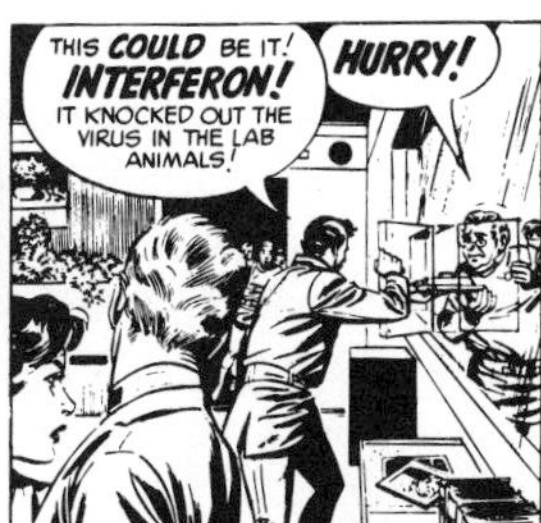

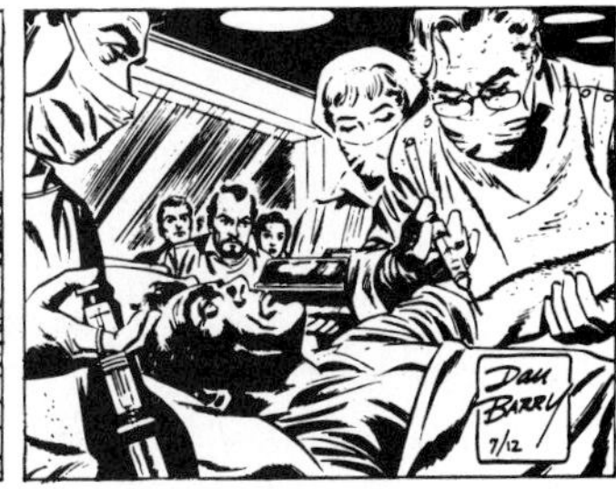

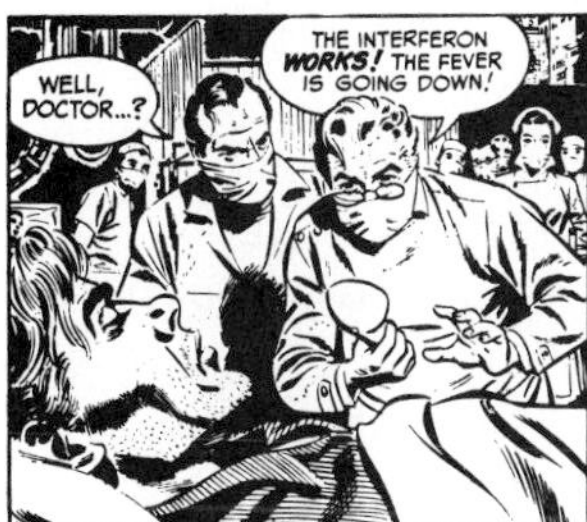

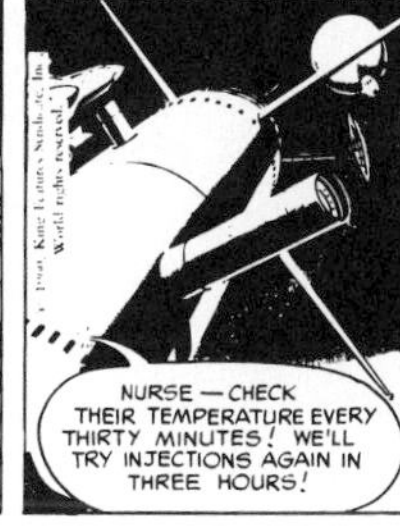

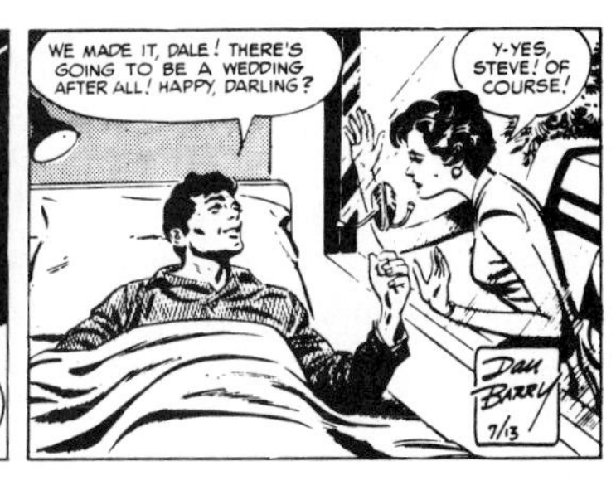

6-14 *Enter interferon!*

substance which blocks further viral development. Thus, strangely, the virus not only corrupts the cell into making more virus, but also provides a way, via interferon, of preventing exactly that from happening in adjacent cells. Interferon so produced may be involved in preventing infection by many other viruses attacking the host. Growth of microscopic agents other than viruses is also inhibited. Indeed, interferon has recently been shown to be involved in inhibiting the growth of a malarial parasite of rats and the microorganism of parrot fever (psittacosis), both of which grow only in the host's cells.

Viruses are not essential to cells for interferon production. The production of interferon is stimulated by some bacteria, as well as by some bacterial toxins. Among the synthetic chemicals inducing interferon, one called poly I:C is of special interest because it is not so toxic. This drug has already stimulated interferon that cures rabbits of a serious viral eye disease. If a way is found to produce interferon in large amounts and if interferon does indeed play a role in impeding virus production, perhaps man will have a new way of preventing viral disease.

6-15 *Virus-infected chick embryo cells in a Petri dish. Interferon applied in the center diffused outward. The clear area shows where infected cells were destroyed.*

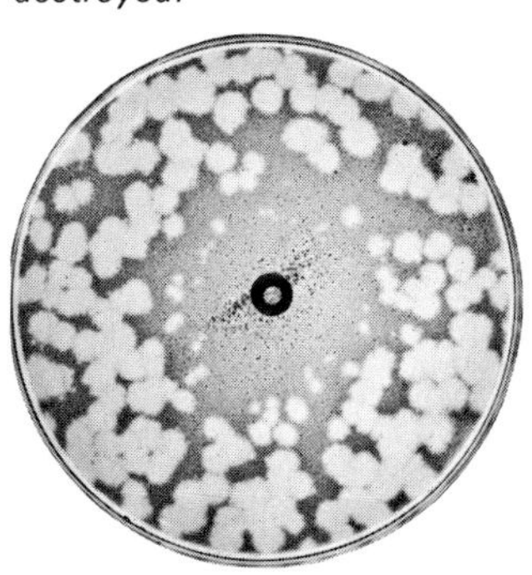

drugs versus viruses

Because viruses multiply in cells, most known drugs are generally helpless against them. Most drugs that kill viruses kill cells too. The problem then is to kill the virus without harming the cell. Bacteria do not enter the animal cell. They attack it from the outside. That is why drugs that are able to differentiate between bacterial and animal cells are effective against bacterial diseases. By early 1974, only a few drugs were known to be effective against human viral disease without serious harm to the human host: a compound called *IUdR* is effective against a viral infection of the cornea of the eye; Symmetrel (or amantadine) seems to prevent influenza A2 (British and Russian studies suggest it is effective against the Hong Kong strain too); rimantadine also apparently prevents (and perhaps treats) influenza A2; and Marboran (methisazone) seems to prevent smallpox if taken during the incubation period of the disease. Most (not all) of these drugs enter the cell to interfere with viral multiplication. Amantadine prevents the influenza A2 virus from entering the cell. Mankind's future attack against the virus world will probably be by a combination of vaccines, interferon, and drugs.

the common cold: the vagrant viruses

A cold is not, in the traditional sense, a disease. It is a collection of signs and relatively mild symptoms. Sometimes these lead the way to more severe symptoms and serious disease. Symptoms of a cold may be caused by a wide variety of microorganisms ranging from viruses to fungi.

An example: an unvaccinated person who has never been infected with poliovirus is susceptible to it. Assume such an individual is invaded by the virus. If his resistance is adequate, he will show no symptoms. This is usual. With less resistance he will have cold symptoms. This is occasional. Rarely he will develop paralysis and even die. In such an instance, resistance was indeed poor. This is unusual. These stages are caused by the same poliovirus. At any stage the body resistance may overcome the poliovirus. The body is then immune to that specific virus. Later, another virus attacks. This time it may be a rubeola virus. Then a person with inadequate resistance and without previous vaccination may develop cold symptoms (respiratory symptoms usually involve the lower as well as the upper respiratory tract), a velvety, itching rash, and, once in a thousand cases, serious brain inflammation (measles encephalitis). With infection, therefore, the forces of resistance are in combat with the forces of the infecting agent. The stage of disease called the cold may or may not occur, depending on the powers of the host's resistance.

With scores of other viral infections (perhaps a hundred or more) the same spectrum of stages occurs. Influenza virus may cause no symptoms, or cold symptoms, or pneumonia, or even death. But viruses are not alone in causing cold symptoms. A serious bacterial disease, such as tuberculosis, may also be heralded by mild symptoms of a cold. The same may be said for some fungus diseases, such as ''valley fever.''

THE PREVENTION AND TREATMENT OF COLDS A cold vaccine that would include all the microorganisms that can cause the signs and symptoms of a common cold may never be developed. Vaccines are, however, available for some illnesses for which a cold is introductory or in which it is a transient phase (see page 147). Vaccination against measles or mumps, for example, will protect not only against these diseases, but also against the colds that are an early stage of them. An *adenovirus*[34] *vaccine* (developed in 1958) effectively pre-

[34] A group of viruses found in adenoid tissue. Colds are but one of a variety of disease syndromes produced by adenoviruses; discussed in Greer Williams, *Virus Hunters,* p. 373.

vented the colds that, between 1942 and 1945, had sent many thousands of soldiers-in-training to the hospital. And hope for a drug that is effective against colds has hardly been abandoned. Late in 1973, a drug was discovered that inhibited the synthesis of twenty-five different cold viruses in human lung cells.[35]

Present-day antibiotics, such as penicillin, are helpless against viruses. (They can often, however, destroy secondarily invading bacteria, such as staphylococci or pneumococci. This explains their occasional use in some severe respiratory infections.) Fever-reducing aspirin (or its numerous associated compounds) should be used only with the family doctor's advice. Alcohol, by causing nasal and pharyngeal congestion, may prolong and worsen a cold. To ease the symptoms and shorten the siege of an ordinary cold, one should drink enough fluids, eat what is desired, but moderately, and get extra rest. Four centuries ago a physician wrote this advice for the treatment of colds: "The beste and moste sure help in this case is not to meddle with anye kynde of medicines, but to let nature worke her operacio."[36] That advice may soon be proven inapplicable. A recent study suggests that for some people, vitamin C may prevent colds and lessen the days of disability caused by these infections.[37]

[35] "New Cold Drug," *Science News,* Vol. 104, No. 22 (December 1, 1973), p. 347.

[36] Thomas Phaire, *The Boke of Chyldren* (The Book of Children), quoted in John M. Adams, *Viruses and Colds: The Modern Plague* (New York, 1967), p. 135.

[37] In 1970, the eminent chemist Linus Pauling urged massive doses of vitamin C to prevent and treat colds (Linus Pauling, *Vitamin C and the Common Cold* [San Francisco, 1970]). Among his many critics was a panel of physicians writing for the authoritative publication, *The Medical Letter.* Pointing out that Pauling's conclusions were based on inadequate studies and mere personal experience, the panel warned that vitamin C, in doses as large as those recommended by Pauling, could result in stones in the urinary tract. ("Vitamin C and the Common Cold," *The Medical Letter,* Vol. 12, No. 26 [December 25, 1970], p. 106.) Consumption of such large doses of vitamin C by anyone with a tendency to gout or to kidney and bladder stones was particularly inadvisable. Also, the ingestion of large amounts of vitamin C could make certain urine tests for diabetes inaccurate.

Nevertheless, Pauling's claims did stimulate needed (and recommended) research. (G. H. Beaton and S. Whalen, "Vitamin C and the Common Cold," *Canadian Medical Association Journal,* Vol. 105, No. 4 [August 21, 1971], p. 357.) Investigators at the University of Toronto performed a trial in which 407 volunteers received vitamin C and 411 controls received an inactive substance. (T. W. Anderson, D. B. W. Reid, and G. H. Beaton, "Vitamin C and the Common Cold: A Double-Blind Trial," *Canadian Medical Association Journal,* Vol. 107, No. 6 [September 23, 1972], pp. 503–08.) No volunteer knew which he was taking; nor could the investigators themselves determine this until the results were ready for comparison. In addition, in the event they began to come down with a cold, the volunteers were instructed to increase the dose of whichever substance they were taking so as to approximate the preventive dose recommended by Pauling. The trial was conducted from January through March; only individuals who ordinarily experienced at least one cold during these months were admitted to the study. The members of the two groups were closely matched as to age, sex, and other characteristics. The results of the study were as follows:

1. Compared with the controls, the vitamin C group showed a slight decrease, *per person,* in both the average number of colds and the average number of days of sickness. However, these differences were too small to be statistically significant.

2. On the other hand, the *number of people* who were free of illness throughout the study was greater in the vitamin C group. Moreover, those in the vitamin C group who did become ill were less disabled and stayed away from work fewer days. Both of these results were statistically significant. The vitamin C group experienced less generalized discomfort, chills, and fever. However, local symptoms, referable to the nose, throat, and chest, were less markedly different in the two groups.

Although this research was carefully conducted, and several verifying studies have subsequently been done, certain questions must be answered. How does vitamin C affect the course of an infection that is caused by numerous viruses? What about the safety of prolonged high doses of vitamin C? What is the effect of various dosages? These are among the problems of continued interest to the Toronto researchers. Until there are complete answers, they do not firmly recommend vitamin C for the prevention or treatment of the common cold.

German measles (rubella)

In most of the United States except the West, winter and spring of 1963–64 were marked by widespread rubella. The same seasons of the following year saw a similar epidemic in the Pacific states. As a result of these infections, many malformed babies were born.

Women of childbearing age who have not had rubella are susceptible to this highly infectious disease. A laboratory test is available to determine whether rubella infection has occurred. Should a woman contract the disease just before or during the first twelve weeks of her pregnancy, the risk of bearing a malformed child is about 20 percent. Abnormality of the child has, however, occasionally been reported with maternal infection in the second three months of pregnancy.

A wide range of abnormalities has been described, including defects of hearing and vision, cardiac problems, and mental retardation. In addition, the affected child (as well as an apparently normal child exposed in the uterus) remains contagious for months after delivery. Such a child must be isolated, especially from pregnant women and susceptible babies.

The effectiveness of gamma globulin in preventing rubella infection, and resultant infant disability, is not proven. Many physicians feel that, if desired by the parents, abortion is indicated if maternal rubella has occurred in the first fourteen to sixteen weeks of pregnancy. Factors of consummate importance include religious belief, the age of the parents, and the number of children they already have.

The rubella vaccine is discussed on pages 147–49.

other viruses affecting the unborn

Various other viral diseases occasionally threaten a pregnancy. In this country, smallpox is at present nonexistent. Some evidence indicates that vaccination of a pregnant woman against the disease may harm the child within her. Except under unusual circumstances, therefore, smallpox vaccination is best deferred until after delivery. Although maternal chickenpox may terminate a pregnancy, there is no evidence that its virus causes malformations. Children of women who develop chickenpox in the last week or two of pregnancy may be born with the disease or develop it soon after birth. This is rarely serious. For an adult, the "cold sore" virus produces a common and mild infection. Fortunately, it rarely infects the unborn child. When it does, it may end the pregnancy.

In this country, the menace of the regular measles virus to children should disappear in the wake of the effective vaccine (see pages 147–48). Before the vaccine was available, regular measles killed between four hundred and five hundred children every year. Every epidemic, moreover, left an army of the physically and mentally retarded. Recent studies absolve the regular measles virus of responsibility for infection and malformation of unborn children.

Cytomegalic inclusion disease is an illness whose name is descriptive of some of its aspects. *Kyto* (Greek, a hollow vessel) denotes relationship with a cell. *Megalic* is derived from the Greek *megaleios* (meaning magnificent) and refers to the unique large cells associated with the disease. The word "inclusion" describes the unusual inclusion bodies found within those cells. This illness, usually noted in the first month of life, is due to cytomegalovirus infection. In the adult the disease is usually so mild that it is not detected. When transmitted from pregnant woman to fetus, it often manifests itself by a wide variety of malformations in the newborn child. As with German measles, children with the disease may be contagious for months after delivery. They should be isolated, particularly from pregnant women.

A relationship between mumps and birth defects has been disproved. Nor do infectious hepatitis and chickenpox have a deleterious effect on the unborn child. But a growing suspicion that many other viruses may affect the child within the uterus indicates the need for more research in this field.[38]

mumps

Although, during mumps infection, virus is carried by the blood to all body tissues, several organs most frequently show manifestations. When the parotid glands swell, their ducts may be occluded. In such cases, giving the patient a pickle or other sour food stimulates the gland and there is pain. But this "home diagnosis" of mumps is not reliable because the salivary glands do not always swell. Mumps is milder when it occurs before puberty. With adolescents and adults the disease can be more troublesome. At a maximum, about 20 percent of all male mumps patients thirteen years of age or over develop swelling (as a result of inflammation) of the testicle (*orchitis*). Young soldiers are frequently attacked. Inflammation of the ovary (*oophoritis*) does occur, but is much less frequently reported than orchitis, perhaps because the ovaries are not visible nor as easily palpated as the testicles.

The incidence of male sterility from testicular swelling is in dispute. It most certainly is rare. Public apprehension on this account is understandable, but unjustified. Nor is a case of female sterility from mumps known.

The third most common mumps complication is an inflammation of the lining of the brain (*meningitis*) or of the brain itself (*encephalitis*). Ninety-nine percent of all victims of mumps meningitis recover, and almost an equal percentage show no aftereffects. Fortunately, mumps encephalitis is rare; it is much less frequent than mumps meningitis, but it is much more serious. It is fatal in about 20 percent of cases.

Despite the usual mildness of mumps and most of its complications, many old wives' tales have been spun around the horrid effects of mumps, particularly on the testes, ovaries, and meninges. The infection is not known to cause impotence, although parents' distress with an adolescent son's swollen testicles may leave the child with psychological problems. Although death from mumps is extremely rare and serious complications are quite uncommon, the illness may cause considerable temporary discomfort and disability. The attenuated live mumps virus vaccine (see page 147) is effective and safe.

[38] "Babies: Measles and Malformations . . . Four Viruses Vindicated from Causing Birth Defects," *Science News*, Vol. 105, No. 2 (January 12, 1974), p. 20.

infectious mononucleosis

This is a viral disease[39] manifested by fever, fatigue, swollen neck lymph nodes (lymph nodes throughout the body may be involved), and sore throat. There is a marked increase in the number of lymphocytes (see pages 141–42) in the blood. Enlargement of the spleen and liver is common. Very occasionally the sick person may have a rash or be jaundiced. Serious complications, such as brain and heart inflammation, are rare. Some individuals may become easily fatigued for months. Recent work suggests a relationship between the virus causing infectious mononucleosis and other illnesses, but this is as yet unclear.

Unless abetted by direct and intimate contact, the disease is not readily transmitted. The illness is not uncommonly diagnosed in (but hardly limited to) college students. For this reason it has been variously called the ''college'' or ''student's'' or ''kissing'' disease.

Infectious mononucleosis lasts from one to three weeks. However, it can be prolonged for months. The incubation period is usually between one and two weeks, sometimes longer. It is probably communicable before symptoms begin. It may remain communicable until the fever and sore throat are gone. Recovery is the rule. A vaccine to prevent infectious mononucleosis is presently being tested and shows considerable promise.[40]

6-16 Top: *The first visualization of the viruslike particles believed to cause infectious hepatitis* (×225,000). Bottom: *The three types of viral particles associated with serum hepatitis. The largest—called the Dane particle—is thought to be the agent causing serum hepatitis* (×280,000).

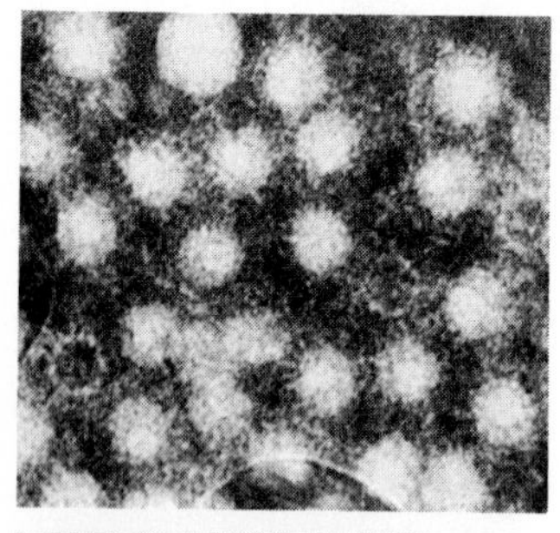

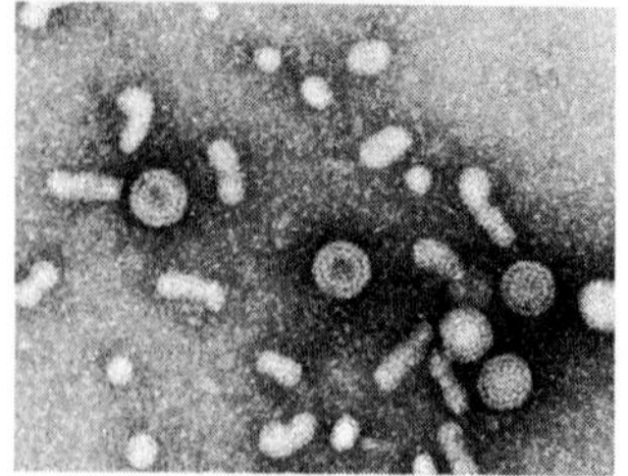

viral hepatitis A and B

The symptoms of the most common viral hepatitis (inflammation of the liver) are caused by two distinct types of infection. *Hepatitis A* is also called *infectious hepatitis.* It is usually incidental to overcrowding, inadequate sanitation, and poor personal hygiene. It is generally transmitted by fecal contamination of food or water. An individual who is careless about hand-washing may, therefore, spread the infection. *Hepatitis B* is also called *serum hepatitis;* it is usually transmitted by the blood of an infected individual entering the blood stream of a susceptible person. This may be accomplished by transfusion of infected blood or by the sharing of infected needles, syringes, or other intravenous paraphernalia. The sharing of dirty needles is common among drug abusers and people who get tattooed; serum hepatitis is common among them too. Serum hepatitis has also been increasingly related to hospital blood transfusions.[41] And there is an association between viral hepatitis and ear piercing.[42]

Recent years have seen a marked increase, particularly among young people, of both infectious hepatitis and serum hepatitis. The symptoms of the two diseases may be indistinguishable. They include loss of appetite, fever, head-

[39] Werner Henle and Gertrude Henle, ''Epstein-Barr Virus and Infectious Mononucleosis,'' *New England Journal of Medicine,* Vol. 288, No. 5 (February 1, 1973), pp. 263–64.

[40] ''Vaccine for Infectious Mononucleosis,'' in ''Medigrams,'' *American Family Physician,* Vol. 6, No. 2 (August 1972), p. 101, citing George F. Springer, Martin Seifert, and James C. Adye of the Northwestern University Medical School, Chicago, Illinois.

[41] ''Prevention of Viral Hepatitis,'' *Journal of the American Medical Association,* Vol. 218, No. 11 (December 13, 1971), p. 1693, citing R. Katz, J. Rodriguez, and R. Ward, ''Post-transfusion Hepatitis: Effect of Modified Gamma Globulin Added to Blood in Vitro,'' *New England Journal of Medicine,* Vol. 285 (1971), pp. 925–32.

[42] ''Viral Hepatitis in Young Women After Ear Piercing,'' *Morbidity and Mortality Weekly Report,* U.S. Department of Health, Education, and Welfare, Vol. 22, No. 47 (November 24, 1973), pp. 390, 395.

ache, nausea, weakness, muscle pain and joint stiffness, and pain in the upper right abdomen. As either disease progresses, the urine becomes dark and the stool light. With the occurrence of jaundice, the individual may become severely depressed. The jaundice may persist for about six weeks. As long as three months may be required for recovery. Chronic liver problems sometimes result from viral hepatitis. About 90 percent of the approximately 74,000 hepatitis cases reported annually in this country are of the infectious type. Nevertheless, serum hepatitis is a far more dangerous disease than is infectious hepatitis. This may be because people who are infected by the serum hepatitis virus through medically necessary injections or transfusions are already weakened by illness.

It is now known that serum hepatitis and infectious hepatitis are caused by separate viral agents. In recent years, the viral cause of serum hepatitis has received most of the research attention. The increasing knowledge about the cause of serum hepatitis, combined with its recently successful laboratory transmission to nonhuman primates, holds promise for the development of a vaccine. Laboratory methods of identifying the hepatitis B antigen have made possible the exclusion of some of the infected blood that might otherwise have been used for transfusion. It is possible for people to carry the virus antigen in the blood without being sick. By laboratory detection, some of these individuals may now be eliminated as would-be blood donors.[43]

Passive immunity (borrowed antibodies) by means of gamma globulin inoculation has long been available for preventing infectious hepatitis; no active immunization has yet been discovered for this disease. In the case of serum hepatitis, matters are more promising; some progress in the development of both active[44] and passive[45] immunizations have recently been announced. However, the likelihood of generally available effective vaccines against either type of viral hepatitis seems remote.[46] As yet, the best tool for the prevention of either type of hepatitis is cleanliness. This is not always easy. The infectious hepatitis fostered by the unavoidably difficult conditions of some army installations is an example of such a circumstance. Armies on the move often suffer epidemics of infectious hepatitis. To prevent the disease, vast amounts of gamma globulin were used among U.S. personnel in Vietnam. Sterilization of needles, syringes, and other equipment used in blood or intravenous work is essential to the prevention of viral hepatitis of either type.

The next chapter will be concerned with other major communicable diseases: tuberculosis, certain illnesses spread via foods, meningococcic meningitis, tetanus, and diseases that are usually or often sexually transmitted.

[43] "The Public Health Implications of the Presence of Hepatitis B Antigen in Human Serum," *A Statement by the Committee on Viral Hepatitis of the Division of Medical Sciences, National Academy of Sciences–National Research Council, Morbidity and Mortality Weekly Report,* U.S. Department of Health, Education, and Welfare, Vol. 21, No. 16 (April 22, 1972), pp. 133–34.

[44] Saul Krugman, Joan P. Giles, and Jack Hammond, "Viral Hepatitis, Type B (MS-2 Strain): Studies on Active Immunization," *Journal of the American Medical Association,* Vol. 217, No. 1 (July 5, 1971), pp. 41–45.

[45] Saul Krugman, Joan P. Giles, and Jack Hammond, "Viral Hepatitis, Type B (MS-2 Strain): Prevention with Specific Hepatitis B Immune Serum Globulin," *Journal of the American Medical Association,* Vol. 218, No. 11 (December 13, 1971), pp. 1665–70.

[46] James Chin and Florence R. Morrison, "Epidemiology of Viral Hepatitis in California, 1950–1970," *California Medicine,* Vol. 118, No. 2 (February 1973), p. 27.

summary

Infection is the result of invasion by a causative organism, which lives off its *host* as a *parasite* (page 135). When the ecological balance between host and parasite is upset, disease results (page 135). Two major kinds of *etiological agents* (organisms that cause infectious diseases) are *bacteria* and *viruses.*

The human body has *nonspecific* ways of resisting infection (page 138). There is also *specific* resistance, or *immunity,* which results from the body's response to each infecting agent (page 138). Two ways of achieving immunity from a specific disease are *by having the infection* or *by vaccination* (page 140). Two systems are involved in the bodily mechanism that yields immunity: the *antibody immune response* and the *cell-mediated immune response* (page 141). Both depend on a kind of white blood cell called a *lymphocyte.* The marrow-derived lymphocytes eventually differentiate into *T lymphocytes* and *B lymphocytes* (pages 141–42).

1. In the *antibody immune response,* the B lymphocytes play the major role. Molecules of microbes that invade the body act as *antigens*—that is, they stimulate the B lymphocytes to proliferate into *plasma cells,* which produce an *antibody,* a protein that is specifically structured to neutralize the antigen that generated it (pages 142–43).

2. In the *cell-mediated immune response,* the T lymphocytes act as "killer" cells, directly destroying the invading organisms rather than producing antibody to do so. They are assisted by *macrophages,* another type of white blood cell (page 143).

There are two kinds of immunity. 1. In *active immunity,* the lymphocytes actively respond to microbial invaders, producing their own antibody. Active immunity is long-lasting. Vaccines contain killed or weakened but living organisms that act as antigens, stimulating antibody formation that provides active immunity. Vaccines are available to combat a number of viral and bacterial diseases (pages 145–53).

2. *Passive immunity* is achieved by using another person's or an animal's antibodies, rather than the individual's own. For example, human gamma globulin containing antibodies against rubeola or infectious hepatitis can be injected to prevent those diseases in another person (page 154). Passive immunity does not last long.

Viruses are a major group of disease-causing agents. Each virus has a *core* of nucleic acids, which causes infection, surrounded by a protein *overcoat,* which determines the specific antibody that the virus will cause to be produced (page 155). When an animal cell is invaded by a virus, any of four effects may occur:

1. The virus may shed its protein coat, disrupt the animal cell's DNA mechanism, and use the cell to make more viruses. If *viral DNA* is released into the cell after uncoating, it encroaches on the functions of normal cellular DNA until eventually the usurped cell dies, rupturing to release new virus that seeks other cells (page 158). If *viral RNA* is released, either it directs the cell to produce viral instead of cellular RNA and protein (pages 158–59), or with the enzyme *reverse transcriptase* it directs the production of DNA, which usurps the cell's DNA (page 159).

2. The cell may slow its division and growth—the "reverse cancer effect" (page 159).

3. The virus may become inactive, remaining *latent* until some stimulus "switches on" the infection (pages 159–60).

4. The virus may cause cancer in animals (page 160).

Among the viral infectious diseases are the common cold (pages 162–63), German measles, or rubella (page 164), mumps (page 165), infectious mononucleosis (page 166), and hepatitis A (infectious hepatitis) and B (serum hepatitis) (pages 166–67).

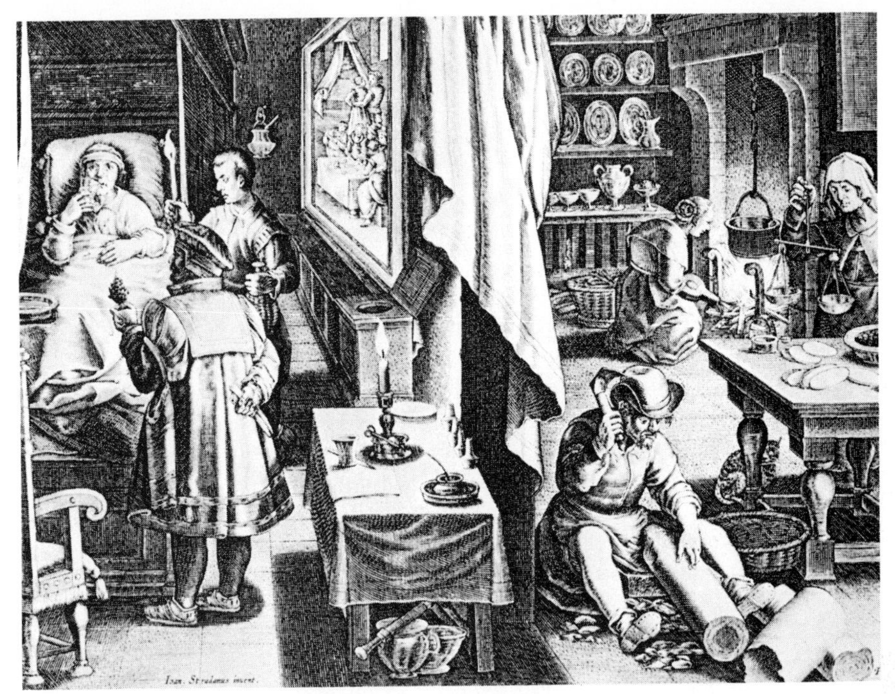

Treatment of syphilis in the Middle Ages. Note the medicaments being prepared nearby and the pitiful pallor of the patient.

the agents of communicable sickness, part 2

7

bacterial competitors in the human ecosystem

tuberculosis

''Mounting the stairs made her breathe very quick . . . she coughed troublesomely sometimes.'' Thus does Emily Brontë describe a character who is soon to die of tuberculosis. Emily's sister Charlotte also knew only too well what she described in *Jane Eyre* as ''the sound of a hollow cough.'' Pitifully, all the Brontës knew tuberculosis intimately. Charlotte, Emily, Anne, Maria, Elizabeth, Bramwell—all six Brontë children died of the disease. Maria and Elizabeth did not even live to teen age.

Tuberculosis infection may involve almost any part of the body but it is far most common in the lung. When the bacillus causing tuberculosis first invades the lung, the inflammation that occurs in that organ is called a primary infection. Within about two to eight weeks from the time of infection, the person will show a positive reaction to the Mantoux (tuberculin) skin test for tuberculosis (see page 152). Many such primary cases of tuberculosis heal without treatment and may never again recur actively. Some, however, do recur. Such *reinfection* tuberculosis may occur under two circumstances. Because of a reduced resistance, an original lesion may break down and thus become activated, or the person may be exposed to another dose of bacilli. Even such reinfections may heal without treatment. However, many progress until the lesion breaks into a bronchus (see page 388). It is then that the case of tuberculosis is ''open.'' For with coughing or sneezing, indeed with a forced expulsion of air, myriad infecting bacilli escape into the air. The symptoms of early chronic tuberculosis may be so mild as to be hardly noticeable—perhaps no more severe than a cold. Among the more common symptoms are loss of weight, night-sweats, and chronic cough. It is the unknown case of tuberculosis that is the greatest danger both to the affected individual and to his community. Early modern drug treatment heals the tuberculosis lesion rapidly and decreases the cough and the number of bacilli in his sputum so quickly that the illness soon becomes noncommunicable.

Today, the Mantoux test is a routine part of medical examination of young children. The physician will first do this allergy test when the child is about six months of age. Infection with the bacillus of tuberculosis causes an individual to be allergic to its growth products, *tuberculin.* A positive tuberculin test means that infection has occurred, although the disease may be self-healed and thus not active. Should the child's Mantoux test be negative, it would be regularly repeated. A positive Mantoux test may indicate the need for treatment. For the individual, the Mantoux test is a diagnostic tool. For the community, it is a tool for surveillance. Why? If positive, it raises a question that the physician and health department must seek to answer: where did the child get the infection? To find and treat the case, to find and treat the source, to seek out all possible close contacts, and thus prevent further spread—these are among the essential concepts of tuberculosis control (see BCG vaccine, pages 152–53).

In the past few years the Mantoux test has taken on added importance. In this country, more than 25 million people are Mantoux positive. The vast majority of them do not have active tuberculosis. They have been infected and presumably have recovered from the disease. Nevertheless, recent studies prove that every positive reactor has a greatly increased risk of developing active tuberculosis. Ideally, everyone with a markedly positive Mantoux test should take the preventive drug isoniazid. The tablets would be taken daily for a year. People who take them must have regular check-ups to make certain that they do not react adversely to the drug, although such reactions are rare. To provide isoniazid tablets to all positive tuberculin reactors is beyond the resources of health departments. Therefore, priorities have been established. These are largely based on the relative risk of developing tuberculosis and infecting others. Family physicians and local health officers cooperate closely in selecting priorities for preventive treatment.[1]

In these ways repetitions of the Brontë tragedy can be avoided. Slowly, tuberculosis has diminished remarkably in this nation. At the turn of this century the U.S. death rate from tuberculosis was 194.4 per 100,000 population. By

[1] Gordon M. Meade, "Chemoprophylaxis of Tuberculosis," *GP*, Vol. 38, No. 3 (September 1968), pp. 113–19.

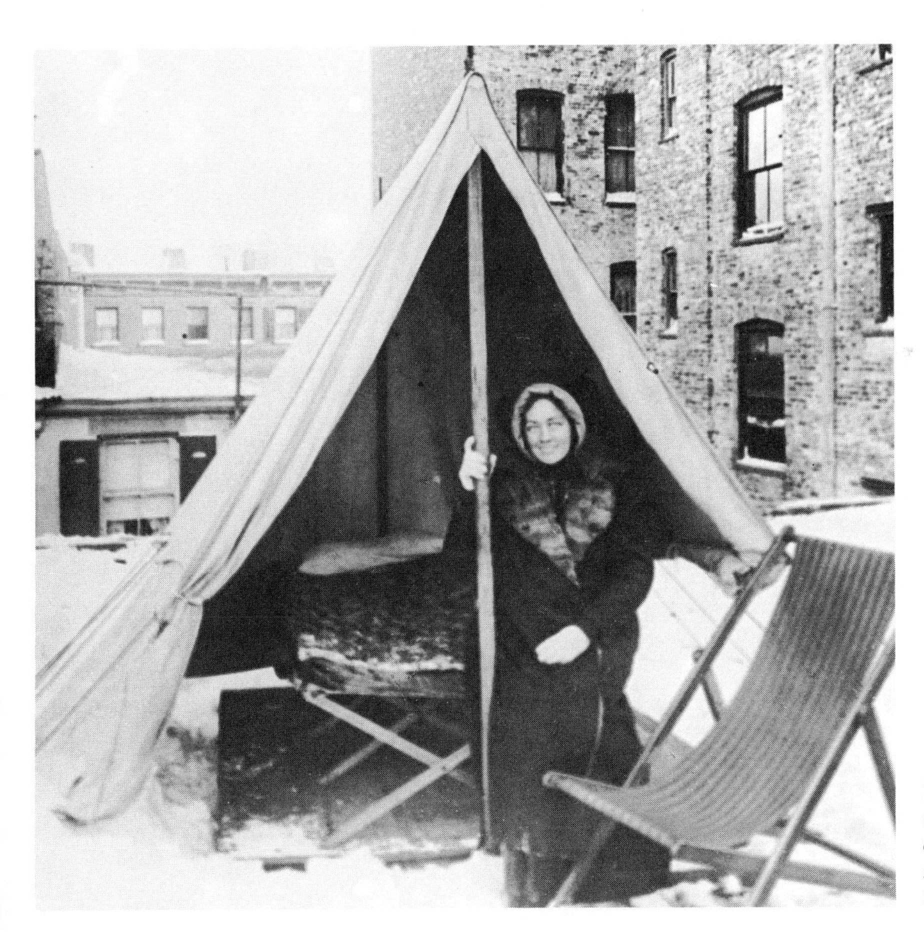

7-1 *A rooftop tuberculosis sanitarium on New York's Lower East Side at the turn of the century.*

1972, it had decreased to 2.2. Other countries are less fortunate. Worldwide, it is estimated that more than 100 million people harbor, and are spreading, virulent tuberculosis bacilli. Every year, more than 2 million of the world's people die of the disease. "Tuberculosis is a disease of poverty," Robert Koch said. The discoverer of the tuberculosis bacillus, he knew that wherever there was the stress of grinding poverty, of malnutrition, and of overcrowding, there people perished in great numbers from tuberculosis.

Antituberculosis tools are available—drugs, such as isoniazid, rifampin, and streptomycin, tuberculin tests, X-rays, BCG, programs of treatment and prophylaxis, and methods of case finding.[2] These, plus constant effort and, above all, a better standard of living, will someday bring mankind relative freedom from "the white plague."

sickness from food contamination

Many microorganisms can cause illness using food as a convenient medium. As many as 10 million illnesses are caused every year in this country by these microorganisms. Only the common cold occurs with more frequency. However, food-borne infections are usually much more severe.[3] Salmonellosis, caused by a group of microorganisms called *Salmonella,* can live and grow in the intestinal tract. A continuous infecting cycle is thus established. The organism may be spread from animal to man, man to man, and man to animal.[4] There are more than twelve hundred species of the genus *Salmonella.* Many cause disease in man. (The *typhoid* bacillus is but one of the salmonellae.) Some years ago, fifty-three hospitals in thirteen states experienced a serious outbreak of salmonellosis of one species. In each hospital the causative salmonellae were isolated from patients, staff, and contaminated raw and undercooked eggs. The outbreak ended when raw and undercooked eggs were no longer used in meal preparation. The infection was being transmitted both by the eggs and by hospital personnel handling the food and careless about personal hygiene. Since salmonellae in no way affect the taste, smell, or appearance of food, their presence was not betrayed until sick people got sicker.[5]

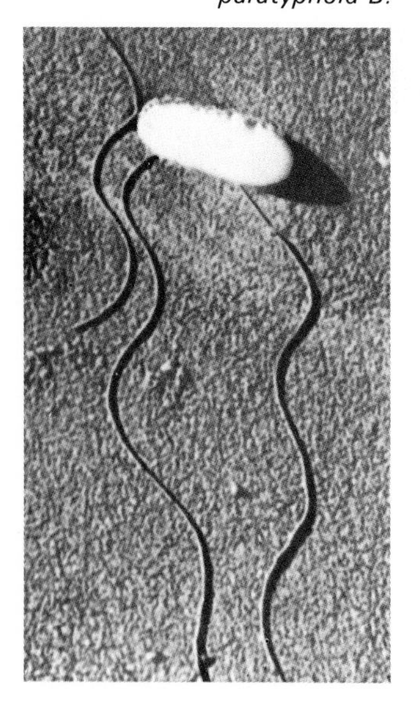

7-2 *A type of salmonella unusual in the United States (×25,000). It causes paratyphoid B.*

[2] In 1970, the familiar Chestmobiles uncovered only 2.5 percent of all new cases of active tuberculosis in the United States. In Denver, for example, between 1965 and 1970, each Chestmobile-discovered case cost $8,115 to find. The high cost, for so low a yield, has resulted in the abandonment of the Chestmobile as a tuberculosis case-finding vehicle in many areas. In Brooklyn, however, the Cancermobile has taken its place. It is designed to screen for breast cancer. (*Medical World News,* Vol. 12, No. 44 [November 26, 1971], p. 4.)

[3] "How Serious a Problem Is Food Poisoning?" *Medical World News,* Vol. 12, No. 42 (November 12, 1971), p. 53.

[4] Considered to be the most widespread animal-borne microorganisms in the world, salmonellae infect between 1 and 2 million people in this country every year. About 1 in every 1000 people affected die. And, although salmonellae infect more infants than people in any other age group, most deaths occur in individuals forty years old or over. In the United States, poultry are the most common source of infection; however, infection of household pets is frequent. About 1 in 5 household dogs carry salmonellae; cats carry these microbes somewhat less frequently. Other commonly infected pets are chicks, ducklings, and especially turtles. (James M. Steele, "Salmonellosis: Its Potential for Harm Grows with Our Population," *Consultant* [September–October 1969], pp. 41–48.) So serious has turtle-associated salmonellosis become in the United States that federal action is being taken to prohibit the importation of turtles except those proven to be free of infectious disease. ("Restrictions on Sale of Turtles Sought by CDC and FDA," *California Morbidity,* No. 16 [April 28, 1972], p. 1.)

[5] Another important genus of microbes found in contaminated food is called *Shigella.* Now under study is a vaccine to prevent infection against one type of shigellosis. In recent years, still another microorganism called *Clostridium perfringens* has been causing an increasing amount of food-borne sickness.

TABLE 7-1

Two Ingredients of Food-Borne Illness: Staphylococcus and Salmonella

TYPE OF ORGANISM INVOLVED	MODE OF ACTION	INCUBATION PERIOD	COMMON SYMPTOMS	COMMON FOOD SOURCES	FOOD-HANDLING CAUTIONS
Staphylococcus	Toxin	Under 6 hours (usually 2–4 hours)	Vomiting (in almost all cases) Cramps Diarrhea No fever (temperature may be below normal)	Pastries Custards Salads, salad dressings Sliced meats	Cook food thoroughly. Refrigerate food. (Staphylococci grow rapidly at room temperature, producing toxin. Salmonellae grow rapidly at temperatures between 60°F and 120°F.) Be scrupulous about personal hygiene (especially handwashing). Protect food from animal excreta. Clean the cutting wheel of the kitchen can opener regularly.
Salmonella	Bacterial infection	6–48 hours or more (usually 12–24 hours)	Abdominal pain Diarrhea (in almost all cases) Vomiting Fever	Poultry Raw eggs Egg products Raw milk Meats, meat pies Fish Lightly cooked foods	

Staphylococcal food poisoning is a true poisoning. Why? Because while growing in food, the staphylococcus produces a toxin. It is the toxin, not the staphylococcus, that, upon ingestion, causes the illness. This is not the case with most bacterial illness associated with food. In the hospital-salmonella infections, it was the bacteria, not the toxin liberated in the food, that caused the symptoms. Table 7-1 presents some basic differences between staphylococcic *intoxication*[6] and salmonella *infection*. One can readily see how judicious interrogation about such points as what time the symptoms began and what foods the victim had eaten can lead an investigator to the cause of an outbreak of food poisoning.[7]

[6] *Botulism* is also caused by a toxin which is produced by the growth of its microbe in improperly canned or preserved foods. Fortunately, it is rare. Its toxin, and that of tetanus, are perhaps the most poisonous known.

[7] Low doses of atomic radiation slow the rate of food spoilage by microorganisms, and higher doses stop spoilage completely. Radiation also kills grain insects. Canada, Israel, the Netherlands, Spain, the United States, and the Soviet Union have all cleared certain radiated food products for human consumption. Intensive research is being conducted in this method of preserving the wholesomeness of foods and thus preventing disease and waste. Since early 1971, studies on the wholesomeness of irradiated foods have been jointly sponsored by nineteen nations. (Kevin G. Shea, "Radiation for Fresher Food," *New Scientist and Science Journal,* Vol. 49, No. 735 [January 21, 1971], pp. 108–10.)

one type of meningitis, its "carrier state," and the closing of schools

A *carrier* of a communicable disease is a person who harbors the specific organisms of that disease without himself having the symptoms. Probably unaware of this, he innocently spreads his infection. The carrier state of no disease is more misunderstood than that of *meningococcic meningitis* ("spinal meningitis"). In this disease, the meningococcus causes an inflammation of the membrane covering the brain and spinal cord (page 265). A few years ago, a seventeen-year-old southern California high school senior was diagnosed as having the illness. Not twenty-four hours before, he had complained of only a headache and a mild cold. Now he lay desperately ill. Panic swept through the school. Almost everybody seemed to remember some "close contact" with him the day before. Frantic parents besieged private physicians and health department officials demanding "a shot of penicillin." A delegation of mothers excoriated school officials for not closing the schools. Then, suddenly, came a numbing blow. The young patient died. In front of the health department building the lines were three blocks long. One reporter seized a shoddy opportunity. "As many as five percent, and even more, of the people in this town can carry this killer bug," his newsy article proclaimed.

Together, medical men and school officials joined with the health department to bring the truth to the community. What are some of the facts?

1. Outside of its host, man, the extremely fragile meningococcus dies speedily. Common germicides, cold, drying, sunlight—all rapidly kill it. Contracting the disease indirectly, as from an infected mattress, is hardly likely.

2. The microbe is transmitted from person to person by intimate contact. So close must this contact be that infected nose and throat secretions of one person must ordinarily reach, quite directly, the nose and throat of another individual. That is why outbreaks occur in crowded quarters, such as army barracks.

3. It is quite true that, at any time and even between epidemics, between 5 and 20 percent of the healthy persons in a given population might be harboring the organism in the nose and throat.[8] But that by no means suggests that all of these carriers will get the disease. In years of higher incidence of the disease, not one in ten thousand individuals, in that part of the general population carrying the microbe, will become ill. During years of ordinary incidence, the risk is often closer to one in twenty thousand, even less. Why do so many individuals harbor the microbe without developing the disease? Nobody knows for sure. Some people may harbor just a few of the microbes and so may be able to resist them. Other people may have slowly built up resistance as a result of having been exposed to the microbe in small numbers over a period of time. Los Angeles County health officials have noted a relationship between several influenza epidemics and a subsequent increase in reported cases of this type of meningitis. With some people it is possible that influenza diminishes resistance to the meningococcus. The ecological balance between the microbe and the host may be upset by the host's previous infection.

4. In view of the enormous number of normal carriers, it would be both foolish and dangerous to attempt to provide penicillin or sulfadiazine prophy-

[8] The carrier state is true of many host-microbe relationships.

laxis to the casual contacts of a case of meningococcic meningitis. The hazard from adverse reactions to either drug is, for the ordinary contact, doubtless greater than the danger of coming down with the disease. Preventive drugs should be considered for extraordinarily close contacts (such as barracks mates) of this type of meningitis victim.

5. Those who demand closing of schools should consider this: no urban epidemic (or outbreak) has ever been controlled in this manner. Worse, closed schools disperse students from the watchful eye of the school health workers (and these include teachers) to the unsupervised corner drug store and movie house. Consideration should be given to closing schools only when (a) there is an inadequate number of teachers, nurses, and physicians to observe the students and exclude the sick, and (b) well students will strictly isolate themselves one from the other. These conditions are likely only in very rural communities.

A safe and effective vaccine against one type of the meningococcus is being used by the military services. Use of this vaccine has virtually eliminated this type of meningococcal disease among military recruits.[9] Trials among civilians with this vaccine are difficult to appraise, but encouraging. Experimental vaccines against two other important strains of meningococci have been developed. Their ability to induce antibodies in recipients is over 90 percent. As of spring 1973, the efficiency of a vaccine against a fourth group of meningococci remained unknown.[10]

tetanus

On a vacant lot in a suburban town two boys scuffle. One pokes at the other's arm with a stick. He succeeds in hitting him, causing a small, penetrating wound. There is hardly any bleeding. In a day or two the wound is healed, forgotten. Yet ten days later, the scratched boy lies critically sick. His back is arched. His hands are clenched. His face is fixed in a ghastly grin of agony. Utterly exhausted, he cannot rest. He cannot move normally. For every muscle contracting one way, another contracts in the opposite way. As one observer has remarked, "He is pitted against himself." Worried doctors work to relieve his contractions and racking pain. They know that his chances of survival are a tossup. The stick had been contaminated with soil containing the tetanus organism. Tetanus (lockjaw) is a completely preventable disease (see pages 153–54).

The symptoms of tetanus are caused not by the bacterium but by the deadly toxin liberated by it. Indeed, so unaffected is the original wound that it is often hard to find. In this country, tetanus still occurs with disturbing frequency (see Table 6-2). In the past fifteen years, almost three-fourths of all tetanus in New York has occurred among heroin abusers, who doubtless inject themselves with the tetanus organism via dirty needles. In developing countries, where immunization levels are low and sanitation is poor, tetanus is common. Tetanus of the newborn is a frequent baby-killer in many of these countries. Immunization of mothers might prevent this tragedy.

[9] "Meningococcal Disease Trends," *Physician's Bulletin, Orange County Health Department,* Vol. 22, No. 21 (October 9, 1972), p. 1, from *California Morbidity* (October 6, 1972).

[10] "Eradicating Meningococcal Disease," quoting Dr. Ronald Gold at the American Academy of Pediatrics, Boston, April 9, 1973, in "Medigrams," *American Family Physician,* Vol. 7, No. 6 (June 1973), p. 140.

the two most common sexually transmitted diseases

historical notes

Syphilis gives still more evidence that microbes know no borders. Two years after Columbus discovered America, Charles VIII of France (1470–98), seeking a Byzantine Empire, invaded Italy and laid siege to Naples. At that time the port city was being defended by Spaniards. Like all armies of that era, the Spanish army was accompanied by a host of harlots. Many of these women, it was thought, had been infected by sailors formerly with Columbus. If the account of the sixteenth-century anatomist Fallopius is to be believed (and it is not by everyone), the Spanish deliberately sent their debauched women to meet the French army. This unmilitary maneuver succeeded. The soldiers of the French army lost no time in meeting the harlots. They caught syphilis.[11]

Too diseased to fight, the French army retreated. In dispersing, they spread their disease throughout Europe. The Italians and Spanish called the affliction the "French disease." To the French, it was, at first, the "Neapolitan disease" and then the "Spanish sickness." The Germans named the malady the "Polish pocks." The Poles retaliated with "German pox." Bitterly remembering the Crusades, the unforgiving Turks called it the "disease of the Christians." To others, it could only be the "Persian fire." Finally, in 1530, an Italian medical man and poet, Girolamo Fracastorius, wrote of a shepherd, Syphilus, who aroused the ire of the sun god by worshiping at an altar of his king. In jealous anger, the sun god sent a plague to earth. Syphilus was its first victim. The disease was thus named, if not claimed.

Often contracted together, syphilis and gonorrhea were, at first, incorrectly thought to be different manifestations of one disease. An eccentric eighteenth-century Scottish surgeon, John Hunter, did not help matters. Deliberately, he infected himself. "Two punctures were made on the penis with a lancet dipped in venereal matter from a gonorrhea."[12] Apparently he got more than he experimented for. Developing both gonorrhea and syphilis, he carefully and wrongly described them as one disease. Another—less heroic—Scottish physician, Benjamin Bell, inoculated his students and learned that the diseases were clinically different. In Dublin, William Wallace inoculated healthy patients to prove that the rash of syphilis was contagious.[13] Not until the gonococcus was identified (in 1879) and the *Treponema pallidum* discovered (in 1905) were gonorrhea and syphilis proved to be caused by different microorganisms.

the V.D. problem: extent and causes

There are five different venereal diseases. In this country, the most important are syphilis and gonorrhea. They are described in Tables 7-2 and 7-3. The other three—chancroid, lymphogranuloma venereum, and granuloma inguinale—are infrequently seen in this country. Worldwide, about 50 million people have infectious syphilis, 150 million gonorrhea—a total almost equal to the popula-

[11] Gabriel Fallopius, *On Gallic Disease,* quoted in Herbert Silvette, *The Doctor on the Stage* (Knoxville, Tenn., 1967), p. 196.
[12] Greer Williams, *Virus Hunters* (New York, 1959), p. 18.
[13] R. S. Morton, *Venereal Diseases* (Harmondsworth, Eng., 1966), p. 21.

tion of the United States. In 1943 it was demonstrated that a single massive dose of penicillin cured most early syphilis as well as gonorrhea. This led to a de-emphasis on previously energetic venereal disease control programs. Contact tracing, the search for those people who were a source of new infections, was no longer considered of paramount importance. This policy turned out to be a grievous error. But the damage was done; people wrongly came to believe that penicillin had solved the V.D. problem. For some years in the United States there was a downward trend in syphilis cases, but in 1970 the number of cases began to rise. A downward trend in the rate of gonorrhea reversed itself in 1959; since that time the rates have risen steadily. A 1968 survey indicated that private physicians were treating 80 percent of all syphilis and gonorrhea diagnosed, but were reporting less than one-fifth of their infectious cases.[14]

Venereal disease is particularly frequent among the young. In 1972, by far the greatest majority of infectious cases in the U.S. were in persons between twenty and twenty-four years of age. In the County of Los Angeles, for example, where gonorrhea is increasing at a rate some four and a half times that of the population, gonorrhea is increasing among teen-agers at twice the rate of other age groups. The repeat-rate of gonorrheal infection is striking. Two, three, four, and even more gonorrheal infections per year in one person are not uncommon.

Several interrelated changes seem to be responsible for the current epidemic of venereal diseases. Changes in individual sexual behavior, such as in-

[14] "International Venereal Disease Symposium," *Modern Medicine,* Vol. 39, No. 12 (June 14, 1971), p. 61. A basic reason for the physicians' reluctance to report their V.D. cases to health departments for contact tracing, is their concern that the traditional confidential relationship between patient and physician will be violated. Those who cooperate closely with health departments find that this fear is unjustified.

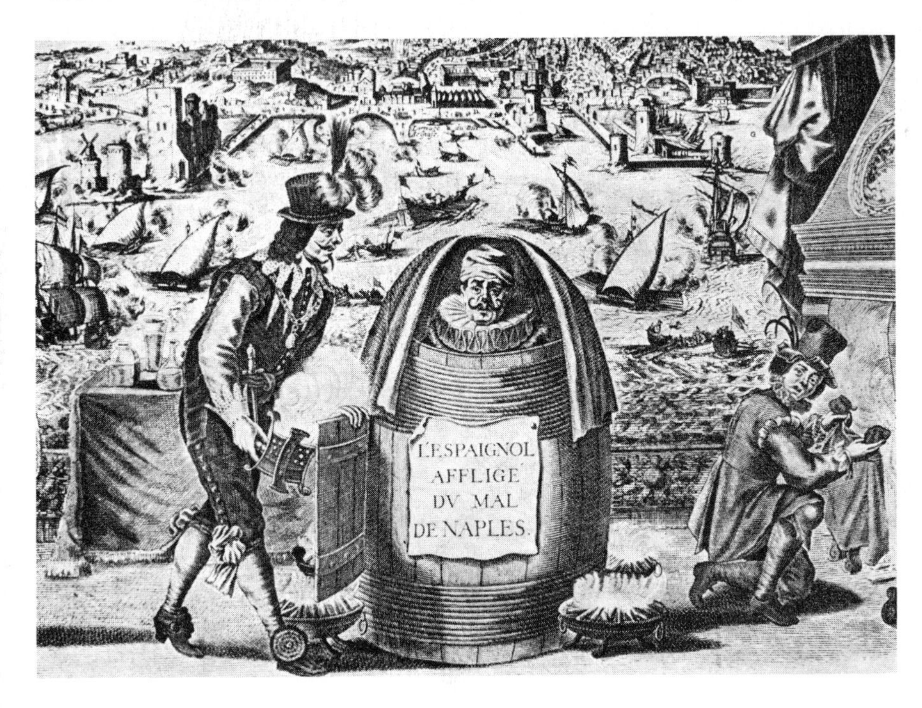

7-3 *A Spaniard afflicted with Neapolitan disease: a French satire of 1647, showing one treatment for syphilis in those days—sweating in a hot box.*

creased sexual activity among people whose orientation is homosexual and the greater availability of contraceptives, have contributed to the spread of the venereal diseases. The environment has also changed; societal factors influencing the rise of V.D. are increased population mobility, increased financial and sexual independence of women, the drug subculture, and increased sexual permissiveness as evidenced by the relaxation of restraints formerly imposed by religion, the family, and public opinion. Added to these is a change from public clinics as the major treatment centers of V.D. to private physicians who do not have adequate facilities for contact tracing. One of the agents of V.D. has also changed; the microbe that causes gonorrhea is increasingly resistant to antibiotics, especially penicillin.[15]

the silent epidemic

Both syphilis and gonorrhea are more commonly reported in males. Although the primary sore, or chancre, of syphilis neither hurts nor usually itches, the man can usually see it. Very often, however, the primary chancre may be absent or be so insignificant as to be missed. The male can, moreover, most often see a gonorrheal discharge, and his pain on urination may drive him to a physician. By no means, however, is this always true. In one study of 124 males brought to treatment by contact tracing, 61 percent had symptoms but had not sought medical advice.[16] Nor do all males with gonorrhea have symptoms; various investigators report asymptomatic gonorrhea in 12 to 30 percent of men examined.[17] Not only do these men spread their disease, but they risk serious complications such as inflammation of the joints, heart, and meninges.

For the woman, syphilis and gonorrhea are a special risk. Because of her anatomy, she may not as easily see or feel the warning signs. Her external genitalia are not as visible to her; moreover, the entire surface of the cervix (where most gonorrheal infections are located) and much of the vagina are without a nerve supply. A painless, invisible syphilitic lesion can hardly give her any warning of a syphilitic infection. Gonorrheal infection gives her even less warning. Usually the female urinary system is not severely involved, so painful urinary symptoms are uncommon. Between 70 and 90 percent[18] of women who have gonorrhea do not know it. In May 1971, it was estimated that 640,000 women in the United States had gonorrhea without knowing it. In 1969, 1970, and 1971, routine screening for gonorrhea was conducted among 740,446 women in thirty-six towns and cities in twenty-two states; 8.9 percent had gonorrhea. Eighty percent of those who had gonorrhea had no symptoms.[19] Unless found and treated, such women may remain a reservoir of infection for months.

7-4 Top: *The spirochete is the corkscrew-shaped microorganism that causes syphilis.* Bottom: *The gonococcus, which appears in pairs, is the bacterium that causes gonorrhea.*

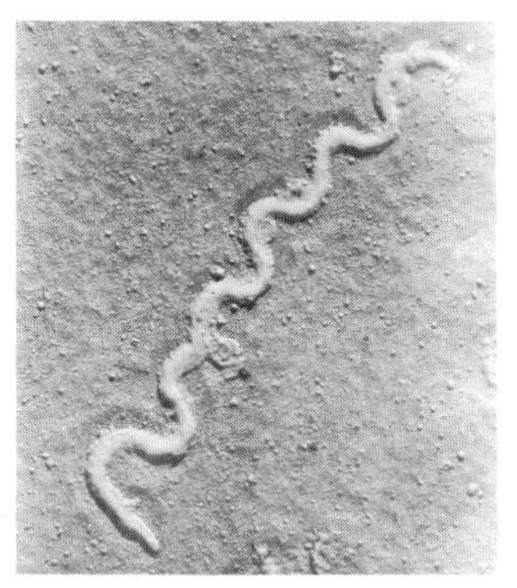

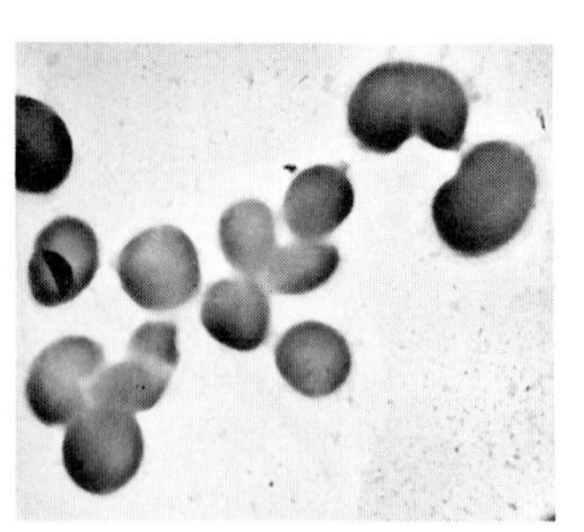

[15] Nicholas J. Fiumara, "Factors in VD Increase," *Medical Aspects of Human Sexuality,* Vol. 5, No. 3 (March 1971), pp. 216, 220.

[16] "Many Males with Symptoms of GC Do Not Seek Therapy, CDC States." *VD Clinical News,* Vol. 2, No. 1 (January–February 1972), p. 4.

[17] *Ibid.,* and "Beware Male Asymptomatic Gonorrhea," *Medical World News,* Vol. 13, No. 16 (April 21, 1972), pp. 4 and 5.

[18] "In the Norfolk Venereal Disease Clinic, 90% of the Women Found to Have Gonorrhea Were Asymptomatic," "International Venereal Disease Symposium," *Modern Medicine,* Vol. 39, No. 12 (June 14, 1971), p. 64.

[19] "Gonorrhea Culture—Screening Summary, United States Fiscal Years 1969–71," *Morbidity and Mortality Weekly Report,* U.S. Department of Health, Education, and Welfare, Vol. 20, No. 49 (December 11, 1972), pp. 1–2.

About 10 to 15 percent of women who have gonorrheal organisms within the opening of the cervix develop serious complications. These may be manifested as gonorrheal blood-poisoning, arthritis, dermatitis, or inflammation of one or both Fallopian tubes and ovaries.[20] Because joint destruction from gonorrheal arthritis can be so swift, delay in treatment can be exceedingly hazardous.[21] Without early treatment of Fallopian tube infection, sterility often results. The need for surgery to cure illness due to an old gonorrheal infection is not uncommon. It is believed that about half the hospital cases of Fallopian tube infections are due to the gonococcus.[22]

One clinician emphasizes that "in terms of frequencies and consequences of gonorrheal complications the most important is pelvic inflammatory disease (PID) or salpingitis [inflammation of the Fallopian tube]. Eighty percent of patients with gonococcal arthritis and other forms of disseminated gonococcal infection are women." He estimates that almost 12 percent of asymptomatic patients with gonorrhea develop pelvic inflammatory disease. The symptoms are acute lower abdominal pain, fever, and occasionally a gastrointestinal disturbance. "Abscesses," he continues

> may occur as early as five to ten days after infection in the untreated or inadequately treated cases. Scarring of the inner walls may lead to sterility. Damage from previous gonococcal salpingitis is considered the No. 1 predisposing factor in the occurrence of ectopic or tubal pregnancy. Probably the most important of all sequelae of acute PID is chronic or recurrent infection. Often, less virulent organisms invade the pelvic tissue previously devitalized by gonococcal infection . . . Rupture of an ectopic pregnancy is a surgical emergency that always necessitates the removal of the Fallopian tube that is involved . . . 6% to 7% of maternal deaths are due to rupture of ectopic pregnancy . . . the fetus can never survive.

He reports the case of a twenty-three-year-old woman with a gonorrheal peritonitis whose pelvic abscess was adherent to the bowel. Only hysterectomy and surgical castration helped save her life.[23] Had she been found, diagnosed, and treated early, this could have been avoided.

"It's no worse than a cold," one young man was heard to scoff.

There are an increasing number of young people who are finding it difficult to believe him.

For women the problem is complicated by yet another factor. Birth control pills reduce the acidity of the vaginal environment, thus encouraging the growth of the gonorrhea-causing microbes. It has been estimated that women who are taking oral contraceptives are about 100 percent vulnerable to gonorrheal infection; women not on oral contraceptives, about 40 percent.[24]

[20] R. H. Kampmeier, "The Matter of Venereal Diseases in 1971," *Annals of Internal Medicine,* Vol. 75, No. 5 (November 1971), p. 794, and "What to Do About Rampant Gonorrhea," *Medical World News,* Vol. 12, No. 24 (June 18, 1971), p. 20.

[21] "Gonococcal Arthritis: A Medical Emergency," *AMA Health Education Service,* Vol. 13, No. 1 (January 1973), p. 3, citing "Arthritis and VD: A Medical Emergency," *Arthritis News* (December 7, 1972).

[22] "Systemic GC Lesions Found Not Limited to Common Sites," *VD Clinical News,* Vol. 2, No. 5 (June 1972), p. 3.

[23] "You Pay and Pay for 'Hidden' Gonorrhea," *Medical World News,* Vol. 13, No. 23 (June 9, 1972), pp. 15–16.

[24] "The Doctor's Role in Gonorrhea Control," *Medical World News,* Vol. 13, No. 8 (February 25, 1972), p. 20.

venereal disease transmitted from mother to child

In passing through the cervix and vagina of a gonorrhea-infected woman, a newborn child may pick up the disease. His eyes may become infected. For this reason, most states make it mandatory to apply a silver nitrate solution to every newborn infant's eyes. Moreover, it has recently been discovered that the gonococcus may pass up into a pregnant woman's uterus, causing the *gonococcal amniotic infection syndrome.*[25] Premature birth, premature rupture of the membranes (twenty-four hours or more before delivery), inflammation of the umbilical cord, and maternal fever are among the complications of this syndrome. It has not been proved that the gonorrhea-causing microbe is the exclusive cause of this condition; other organisms may be involved.

A syphilitic woman can also transmit her infection to her child. Infection of the unborn child can take place any time after the seventeenth week of pregnancy; before then the woman's spirochetes cannot pass through the insufficiently developed placenta. After a few years, a person with untreated syphilis usually no longer spreads the disease because the microbes have settled deep into the tissues. Occasionally, however, spirochetes do appear in the blood stream. Should a woman contract syphilis and remain untreated, she will be able to transmit the disease to her unborn child during the late stages of pregnancy throughout the first six to eight years of her infection. However, even late in pregnancy, adequate treatment of the woman can prevent syphilitic infection of the fetus. It is wise to have blood tests done several times during pregnancy.

about oral-genital transmission of venereal disease[26]

The oral area is much more resistant to gonorrheal infection than to syphilitic infection. By far the greatest number of gonococcal infections are of the urinary tract. Nevertheless, gonococcal infection of the mucous membrane of the mouth and the tongue are occasionally seen[27] and a gonococcal sore throat (pharyngitis) is now being increasingly diagnosed. Gonococcal pharyngitis is rarely reported to result from mouth-kissing or from contact between the mouth and external female genitalia. It is usually diagnosed following penile-oral contact. A person with gonococcal pharyngitis will not usually spread the infection to the genitals of a male or female partner. This is because the gonococci that enter the body via the mouth can survive best in the tonsillar area, where some lymphoid tissue is present even in individuals who have had a tonsillectomy. The patient with gonococcal pharyngitis develops a sore throat a day or two after oral exposure; there may be some redness and swelling of the tonsillar area and some fever. Lymph nodes in the neck may be enlarged. People with gonococcal pharyngitis usually have gonorrheal signs and symptoms in other areas such as the rectum, urethra, or cervix.[28] The gonococcal pharyngitis may be part of a picture in which there is invasion of the blood stream by the gonococci.

[25] "Gonococcal Infection Can Blight Newborn," *Medical World News,* Vol. 13, No. 8 (February 25, 1972), p. 19.

[26] Much of this discussion is based on Nicholas J. Fiumara, "Gonococcal Pharyngitis," *Medical Aspects of Human Sexuality,* Vol. 5, No. 5 (May 1971), pp. 195, 199, 204, 209.

[27] "Clinicians Advised Oral Lesions May Be Signs of Gonorrhea," *VD Clinical News,* Vol. 3, No. 1 (January–February 1973), pp. 1, 3.

[28] Nicholas J. Fiumara, "Gonococcal Pharyngitis," p. 177.

TABLE 7-2

Natural History of Acquired Syphilis

DISEASE	RESERVOIR FOR AGENT	CAUSATIVE AGENT	INCUBATION PERIOD	MODE OF TRANSMISSION	IMMUNITY
Syphilis	Man	*Treponema pallidum* (a spirochete)	10–90 days, usually 21 days following exposure.	Direct physical contact, usually during sexual relations.	A vaccine to prevent syphilis recently proved successful in rabbits. Hopes are high that a successful vaccine to prevent human syphilis will soon be available.

the disease process

The first sign of *primary syphilis* is usually a single, painless sore called a *chancre*. Most often it appears at the place where the germs enter the body—the genital area. Sometimes this chancre does not appear or is overlooked, especially in women. If it does appear, it disappears without treatment in about two weeks. In a short time, which may vary from a few weeks to six months, *secondary syphilis* signs appear. The disease is then no longer local. The entire body is infected. Although different people have different symptoms, the most common are lesions, which may be few or many, large or small, and which may appear on various body areas. There may be a widespread rash. This is not common; frequently it is absent. This rash, and the chancre that preceded it, teems with spirochetes. Whitish patches in the mouth or throat, "moth-eaten" or "patchy" falling hair, low fever, painless swelling of lymph glands, and pain in bones and joints may all be signs of secondary syphilis. While the *primary* and *secondary* manifestations persist, the disease is highly contagious. Lesions in moist body areas, such as the mouth, anus, or genitals are most contagious. Without treatment, the secondary symptoms often disappear in less than a month, although they may persist for a longer period.* The disease then enters a period of *early latency*. The degree of communicability associated with *early latent syphilis* is governed by the recurrence of secondary lesions. Because of such a possibility, the disease is considered communicable for approximately two years following initial infection. The final category, *noncommunicable late latent syphilis*, may eventually cause heart disease, insanity, paralysis, blindness, or death. These end results of untreated syphilis may not take place until ten to thirty years after the primary infection. Most often they do not occur.

*The chancre of primary syphilis and the signs and symptoms of secondary syphilis disappear by themselves without treatment. This accounts for the "success" of the quack. His phony treatments "cure" these signs and symptoms. But the patient is left with the destructive living spirochetes in his body.

Source: Gerald A. Heidbreder, retired Deputy Director, Community Health Services; Department of Health Services of the County of Los Angeles.

Several cases of gonococcal pharyngitis have involved the skin and the joints.[29]

Syphilis of the oral area is not rare. It may be transmitted directly by mouth-kissing, or oral-genital contact. A common manifestation of secondary infectious syphilis is a mouth lesion, or patch. Since they teem with *Spirocheta pallida,* these patches are ready sources of infection.

[29] Paul J. Wiesner, Evelyn Tronca, Paul Bonin, Alf F. B. Pederson, and King K. Holmes, "Clinical Spectrum of Pharyngeal Gonococcal Infection," *New England Journal of Medicine,* Vol. 288, No. 4 (January 25, 1973), p. 181, citing A. Bro-Jorgensen, T. Jensen, "Gonococcal Tonsillar Infections," *British Medical Journal,* Vol. 4 (1971), pp. 660–61; A. L. Metzger, "Gonococcal Arthritis Complicating Gonococcal Pharyngitis," *Annals of Internal Medicine,* Vol. 73 (1970), pp. 267–69; and F. La Luna and B. Agus, "Gonococcal Pharyngitis and Arthritis," *Annals of Internal Medicine,* Vol. 75 (1971), p. 649.

TABLE 7-3

Natural History of Acquired Gonorrhea

DISEASE	RESERVOIR FOR AGENT	CAUSATIVE AGENT	INCUBATION PERIOD	MODE OF TRANSMISSION	IMMUNITY
Gonorrhea	Man	*Neisseria gonorrheae,* the gonococcus (a bacterium)	Within 3–8 days (often less) following exposure for 85% of males; 2–8 days for females when symptoms occur.	Usually sexual intercourse. Practically never from toilet seats, towels, or other objects.	Recent results of field trials of a vaccine against gonorrhea have been disappointing.

the disease process

Gonorrhea is a local disease of the body parts affected. Unlike syphilis, it is usually not a body-wide or systemic disease. A blood test for gonorrhea is available and being evaluated.

In the male, the disease manifests itself as a burning on urination and a discharge of pus. The disease is quite painful. Discomfort may force the male patient to seek medical attention. A man may have gonorrhea without symptoms. Although not very common, *chronic* male gonorrhea may lead to involvement of other portions of the body, particularly the urinary or generative system, and may, if not treated early, produce sterility.

In the female, the early symptoms of gonorrhea are usually absent or very mild. For this reason, the infected female rarely seeks early treatment. Progression of the disease often leads to infection of the Fallopian tubes, ovaries, and lower abdomen. In this event, pain is severe. Due to scarring and closure of the tubes, or to emergency surgery, sterility often results. Rectal infection can occur in both sexes. This occurs more commonly among men whose behavior is homosexual. It is seldom recognized because its symptoms consist only of a sensation of wetness or itching around the anus.

Source: Gerald A. Heidbreder, retired Deputy Director, Community Health Services; Department of Health Services of the County of Los Angeles.

prevention of syphilis and gonorrhea

Properly used, the condom can be an effective mechanical barrier to the organisms that cause both syphilis and gonorrhea. Although the condom can hardly prevent the occasional adult gonococcal infection of the eye, it can prevent gonorrheal infection of the penile urethra, and thus prevent further transmission of the disease by that organ. The condom prevents gonorrhea more efficiently than it does syphilis. The infectious primary chancre of syphilis is most frequently found on the genitalia, but it may be on the lip, anus, finger, or elsewhere. Both the secondary skin lesions and mucous patches of syphilis also teem with infection. For a man, after exposure, thorough washing of the genital area with soapy water may help to prevent infection. Although douching following coitus has been suggested, there is much doubt that it is effective. ''Repeated douching usually accomplishes only the untoward result of washing protective levels of residual acidity from the vagina. Thereafter, secondary infection frequently develops.''[30] Some physicians recommend the use of large doses of antibiotics, such as penicillin, several hours before, or immediately after, an exposure. This would undoubtedly reduce the risk of infection, but it presents problems, such as the development of allergic drug reactions and the growing resistance to antibiotics by the gonococcus.

In Nevada, an old drug called Progonasyl was recently tried. This iodine

[30] William H. Masters and Virginia E. Johnson, *Human Sexual Inadequacy* (Boston, 1970), p. 274.

preparation has been used in the effective treatment of vaginal inflammations and as a killer of spermatozoa. It was used on a trial basis by a group of Nevada's legal prostitutes; they were checked each week for syphilis and gonorrhea.[31] Initial reports indicated that a daily vaginal instillation of Progonasyl reduced the rate of gonococci found by laboratory examinations of the Nevada prostitutes. Since blood tests for syphilis had been negative for two years before the study, the negative blood tests during the study could not be considered significant.[32] Some women experienced a drying of the vaginal mucous membrane after using Progonasyl; there were no serious side effects.

A copper-containing intrauterine device (IUD), used for birth control (see page 631), may possibly prevent gonorrhea. Unlike some microorganisms, the gonococcus is killed by tiny amounts of copper. The copper that is contained in some IUDs is slowly released over a period of two years. Half of it is absorbed through the wall of the uterus; the rest is carried out of the body by secretions from the cervix and uterus. It is theorized that the copper concentration in these secretions is enough to be lethal to the gonococcus. Studies of the possible prophylactic effect of copper-containing IUDs are underway.[33]

Studies are now being conducted on the V.D.-preventive action of the now lesser-used contraceptives, such as the jellies, foams, and powders. Unlike the contraceptive pill, these produce an acid vaginal environment; this is believed to inhibit the survival of several V.D.-causing bacteria. Furthermore, some vaginal contraceptives contain chemicals that may be effective against venereal disease.[34]

a word of caution for the man treated for gonorrhea

Some male patients recovering from gonorrhea strip or "milk" the penis to see if there is still a discharge. This is inadvisable; the inflamed mucous membrane will not tolerate rough handling. The practice may delay healing and worsen the inflammation of the urethra.[35] For the same reason, the patient should not masturbate while he has or is recovering from gonorrhea.

on helping to find those who need help

People who have a venereal disease almost always got it from someone. And frequently they give it to others. The sick must be immediately and adequately treated. In addition, public protection demands a thorough investigation of the source and spread of every new case. Without active contact tracing, the reservoir of the venereally infected in a community grows; and with it, a spreading sea of chronic sickness and despair. The venereally infected individual who refuses to name his contacts is not being chivalrous. He is refusing information (held, by both law and practice, in absolute confidence) that will spare others

31 "Progonasyl Study Gets Red . . . Er . . . Green Light," *Medical World News,* Vol. 12, No. 31 (August 20, 1971), pp. 4–5.
32 "Venereal Disease Symposium," *M.D.,* Vol. 16, No. 5 (May 1972), p. 92.
33 "IUDs May Wipe Out Gonorrhea," *New Scientist,* Vol. 57, No. 829 (January 18, 1973), p. 118.
34 "Vaginal Contraceptives Declared Anti-VD," *VD Clinical News,* Vol. 2, No. 1 (January–February 1972), pp. 1–2.
35 Walter H. Smartt, "Aggravating Urethritis," *Medical Aspects of Human Sexuality,* Vol. 6, No. 4 (April 1972), p. 10.

endless pain. "Fools alone their ulcered ills conceal," wrote Horace. This ancient thought of the Roman poet might well be applied to modern venereal disease control. One recent study investigated sixty-nine venereal disease outbreaks eventually involving almost 10,000 people in twenty-eight states. "One man infected with syphilis initiated the ultimate exposure of 274 other persons resulting in 42 additional cases of infectious syphilis within a relatively short period."[36]

It pays to investigate. And to cooperate.

other common sexually transmitted diseases

trichomoniasis Trichomoniasis is a very common infestation of the female genitourinary tract; it is caused by a unicellular member of the lowest division of the animal kingdom—the protozoa. The protozoon that causes trichomoniasis, the *Trichomonas vaginalis,* is readily visible under the microscope. In females it may live in great numbers on the vaginal surface as well as on the cervix; in about 20 percent of the cases the urinary tract is also affected. The Bartholin's glands and Skene's ducts may also become involved (pages 482–83). However, it rarely spreads to the upper female tract. In males, trichomonads usually inhabit the urethra, bladder, and seminal vesicles; rarely, the prostate and upper urinary tract are involved (see page 469). Trichomoniasis is most commonly spread as a result of heterosexual intercourse.[37] There are two other types of trichomonads that inhabit the human body; one lives in the mouth, the other in the pouch situated between the small and large intestines. Neither inhabits the genital tract. Treatment of both sexual partners is mandatory. Otherwise one partner is treated only to be reinfected by the untreated partner (a situation that is also common in gonorrheal infections). Sometimes the woman is accidentally infected as a result of using borrowed clothing or towels.

Trichomonads may inhabit the vagina for years without producing any symptoms. In some women the infection may be so mild as to cause only minor itching. This annoyance is often aggravated by the soiling of underclothes due to vaginal discharge. Frequently symptoms are exacerbated during pregnancy and before and after menstruation. Many women develop more severe symptoms. Itching, burning, and soreness of the vulva and even the thighs plague the more severely infected women. The profuse and frothy yellowish-white vaginal discharge has a musty, foul odor. Pain during sexual intercourse (*dyspareunia;* see pages 513–14) and urination are common symptoms.

In the male the signs and symptoms are much milder. Often they are absent. The male may feel a mild itching and a burning sensation while urinating, and

[36] The Association of State and Territorial Health Officers, the American Public Health Association, the American Venereal Disease Association, and the American Social Health Association: A Joint Statement, *Today's VD Control Problems,* cited in Walter H. Smartt, "Venereal Disease," in Lenor S. Goerke, Ernest L. Stebbins, *et al.,* eds., *Mustard's Introduction to Public Health,* 5th ed. (New York, 1968), p. 290.

[37] Warren A. Ketterer, "Homosexual Transmission of Trichomonas and Monilia," *Medical Aspects of Human Sexuality,* Vol. 5, No. 6 (June 1971), p. 144.

there may be a mild or profuse discharge. During the period of treatment, sexual intercourse should be avoided. Recently developed drugs that are taken by mouth have proved effective in the great majority of cases. These are curative for both sexes.

moniliasis

Another infection that may be sexually transmitted is variously known as moniliasis, candidiasis, thrush, and candidosis. This condition is usually caused by the fungus *Monilia albicans* (*Candida albicans*). Most often the disease has a nonsexual basis. Oral and skin moniliasis may occur in babies and debilitated elderly people. Sometimes ill-fitting dentures promote the disease.

The fungus can live in the female genital tract without causing symptoms. But there are conditions under which the monilia may increase in number to produce symptoms.[38] Among these are pregnancy, an excess of sugar in the urine, and the prolonged use of antibiotics. An antibiotic may kill the microbes that check the growth of the fungus; the resultant overgrowth of the fungus causes illness. Oral, penile, and anal monilial infection may occur in the male; there is thus the possibility of spread among homosexually oriented males.

Since vaginal moniliasis in the pregnant woman can be transmitted to the newborn, it is particularly important to treat it early in the pregnancy. The principal symptoms in the woman are vulval itching associated with a white vaginal discharge. The anus may also itch. The skin of the external genitalia may become red and fissured. In the male, discomfort may be due to inflammation of the urethra, penis, scrotum, or thighs. Moniliasis and trichomoniasis often exist together in the same individual. Both can be successfully treated.

genital herpes[39]

The herpes viruses affect man almost universally.[40] One member of this group is the herpes simplex virus. As will be discussed further in Chapter 8, it is of two types, designated 1 and 2. Type 1 is usually associated with nongenital infections, such as those of the lip (the common "fever blister" or "cold sore"), certain eye, gum, and mouth infections, and even brain inflammations, as well as skin eruptions above the waist. Only about 5 percent of genital herpetic infections are caused by Type 1 virus. Type 2 herpesvirus, however, is primarily associated with disease of the genital organs and other sites below the waist, such as the thighs and buttocks; it is also the cause of an increasing number of infections of newborn babies. Type 1 herpesvirus is usually spread by non-

7-5 *Electromicrograph showing two clusters of herpes simplex particles in a human cell (×20,000).*

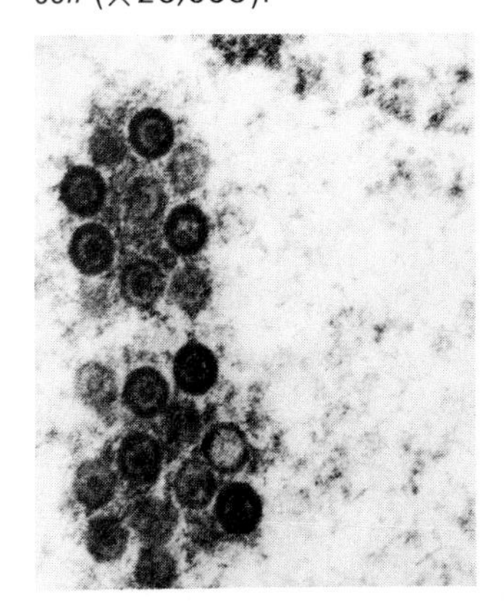

[38] Investigators have recently discounted the belief that the incidence of moniliasis (candidiasis) is increased among users of either sequential or combined oral contraceptives." (George E. Tagatz and Richard B. McHugh, "Oral Contraceptives—A Continuing Appraisal," *Postgraduate Medicine,* Vol. 50, No. 2 [August 1971], p. 124, citing B. Lapan, "Is 'The Pill' a Cause of Vaginal Candidiasis? Culture Study," *New York State Journal of Medicine,* Vol. 70 [1970], p. 949; B. A. Davis, "Vaginal Moniliasis in Private Practice," *Obstetrics and Gynecology,* Vol. 34 [1969], p. 40; and C. A Morris and D. F. Morris, "'Normal' Vaginal Microbiology of Women of Childbearing Age in Relation to the Use of Oral Contraceptives and Vaginal Tampons," *Journal of Clinical Pathology,* Vol. 20 [1967], p. 636.)

[39] For an excellent review, bibliography, and commentaries on this important venereal disease, see William E. Josey, André J. Nahmias, and Zuher M. Naib, "Genital Herpes Simplex Virus Infection," *Medical Aspects of Human Sexuality,* Vol. 7, No. 2 (February 1973), pp. 114, 118–19, 122–23, 126, 131, 133–34, 136.

[40] One virus of this group—the herpes zoster virus—causes chicken pox in children, reappears as shingles (herpes zoster) in adults, and may cause shingles in either adults or children (although usually in the former).

sexual contact; type 2 herpesvirus infection is a specific venereal disease, although nonvenereal transmission is possible. Type 2 herpesvirus infection is particularly common among sexually promiscuous persons such as prostitutes; it is prevalent among exposed teen-agers and young adults. There is a significant association between herpesvirus 2 and other venereal infections. It has been estimated that, for every five to fourteen cases of gonorrhea detected among women attending venereal disease clinics, there is one case of genital herpes.

Like gonorrhea, herpesvirus 2 infection in women may be unnoticed and the principal site is in the cervix. Thus, the beginning of the disease, except for an occasional mild discharge, is relatively without symptoms. This is also true when the infection affects the vaginal walls. With involvement of the external genitalia, single or multiple blisterlike lesions are observed. It has been found that prior infection with herpesvirus 1 lessens the signs and symptoms of herpesvirus 2 infection. Indeed, the most severe herpesvirus 2 infections occur in those individuals who have never had prior exposure to either type. In such people, not only is the spread of the lesions more extensive (to the thighs, buttocks, and even the lower legs), but there may be fever, pain, and swelling of the local lymph nodes. Moreover, the inner mucosal lesions of the outer female genitalia are more likely to ulcerate. They then become secondarily infected with other microorganisms and cause an odorous discharge. In the male, the lesions affect the head of the penis, the prepuce, or the space between the two. The shaft may also be involved and, less commonly, the scrotum, thighs, and buttocks. In either sex the urethra and urinary bladder (see page 469) may be involved, and in the male, infection of the prostate has occurred.

Scarring strictures of the urethra which may interfere with urination have been reported. Occasionally, severe infections by secondary microorganisms complicate the picture. Rarely, meningitis occurs. Perhaps the most serious aspect of herpesvirus 2 infection is its possible relationship to cancer of the cervix (see pages 198–99).[41]

Although active infection is self-limited, in that the lesions will disappear spontaneously, recurrence is common. At present, no treatment has been proved to permanently cure the primary disease. Smallpox vaccinations are not effective and may have serious side effects (see page 140, footnote 4). A herpesvirus 1 vaccine may be effective in treating recurrent type 1 infections; it appears useless with recurrent type 2 infections. A herpesvirus 2 vaccine is being tested in West Germany.

Genital herpes during pregnancy is hazardous to the fetus and the newborn. Should a pregnant woman have an active infection at or near the time of delivery, a cesarean section should be considered. This is true even though the unborn child would have received antibodies via the placenta.[42]

[41] For a recent discussion of this relationship, see Keen A. Rafferty, Jr., "Herpes Virus and Cancer," *Scientific American,* Vol. 229, No. 4 (October 1973), pp. 26–33.

[42] André J. Nahmias, "Herpes Genitalis: Treatment, Effect on Pregnancy," and "Herpes Genitalis: Risk to Newborn," *Journal of the American Medical Association,* Vol. 217, No. 9 (August 30, 1971), p. 1250.

venereal tumors

The *wart* and *molluscum contagiosum* are the only human tumors known to be caused by viruses. Both affect the skin; both may or may not be transmitted by genital contact. Neither is malignant. *Genital warts* are not caused by the same virus as those that are seen in other areas of the body, such as the fingers. With the female, genital warts usually begin their growth on the mucous membrane of the vulva. They can extend to the vaginal walls, the cervix, and about the anus. A profuse vaginal discharge, as from trichomoniasis or, less frequently, gonorrhea, may worsen genital warts. In the male, genital warts usually begin about the base of the glans penis and may also become extensive. The condition is curable.

The beginning skin tumor of molluscum contagiosum[43] is usually a small, solid skin elevation (*papule*) that may be skin-colored or pink. Sometimes it looks more like a blister, and then some people call it a "water wart." A white curdlike material may be squeezed from the lesion; this contains the infective virus particles within epithelial cells. It is believed that the virus is transmitted by this material. One to eight weeks after exposure to molluscum contagiosum, five to twenty papules appear on the lower abdomen, pubis, genitals, or inner thighs. As the weeks go by, the lesions slowly enlarge and develop a characteristic central pit or depression. One or more of these lesions may become painfully inflamed, prompting the person to seek medical attention. Often, when left untreated, individual lesions disappear within a year and a half. However, during this time new lesions may appear. Untreated, the disease may persist for years.

scabies

The mite causing scabies ("the itch") invades only the outer skin. It may be distributed over most of the body or, less commonly, may be somewhat limited to the genital area. In both instances sexual intercourse is one way in which the mite is transmitted from one person to another. As the female mite burrows into the superficial skin to deposit her eggs, severe itching results which is worse at night than in the daytime. Treatment involves the use of an ointment or lotion that contains a chemical that kills the mite. Scrupulous body cleanliness and attention to linens, which are also infested, are essential. All close contacts of the patient, both sexual and nonsexual, must also be treated to avoid reinfection.

The cause of scabies has been known since 1687; indeed, it was the first disease of man for which the cause was known.[44] Present-day treatments are effective, yet, since 1963, the prevalence of the disease has been increasing in many parts of the world. It is now being seen with greater frequency in venereal disease clinics in London and San Francisco. Occasionally the chancre of syphilis is seen in a skin lesion of scabies.[45]

[43] Peter J. Lynch, "Molluscum Contagiosum: Recognition and Therapy of Venereally Transmitted Lesions," *Medical Aspects of Human Sexuality,* Vol. 7, No. 5 (May 1973), p. 33. This article is an excellent discussion of the subject, containing valuable references and commentaries by two other experts.

[44] Milton Orkin, "Resurgence of Scabies," *Journal of the American Medical Association,* Vol. 217, No. 5 (August 2, 1971), p. 593, citing R. Friedman, *The Story of Scabies,* Vol. 1 (New York, 1947).

[45] *Ibid.,* p. 595, citing C. H. Beek and K. Mellanby, "Scabies," in R. D. G. P. Simon, ed., *Handbook of Tropical Dermatology and Medical Mycology* (Amsterdam, 1953), pp. 875–88.

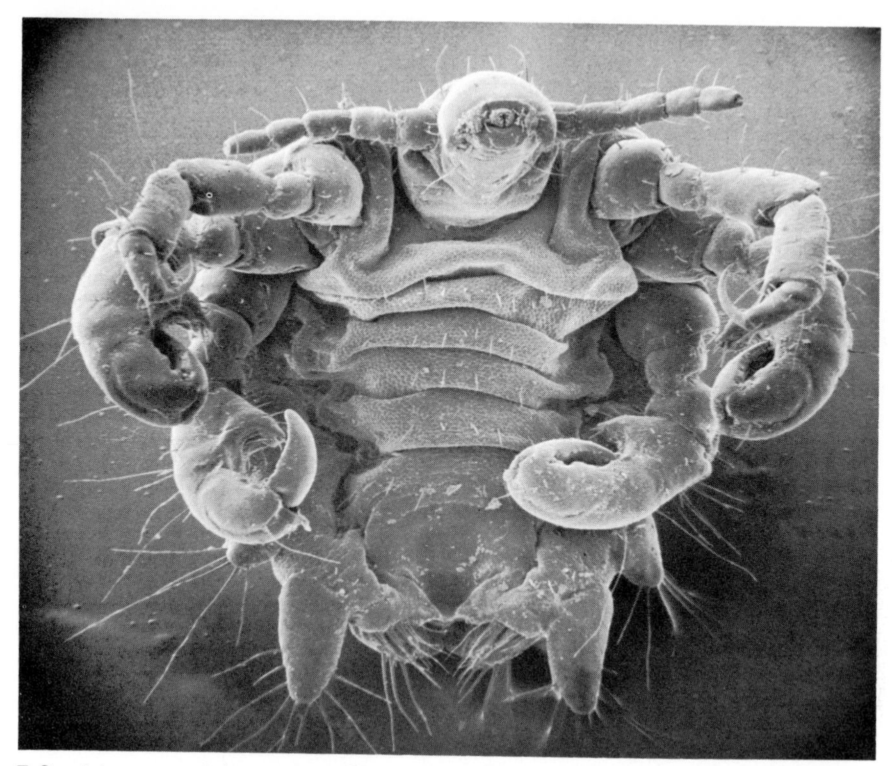

7-6 *A human crab louse, seen from underneath (× 150). The thick legs and large claws are used to grasp hair shafts on the host.*

genital lice

In his "To a Louse" the great eighteenth-century Scottish poet Robert Burns wrote indignantly:

Ye ugly, creepin', blastit wonner,
Detested, shunn'd by saunt an' sinner!
How dare ye set your fit upon her,
Sae fine a lady?
Gae somewhere else, and seek your dinner
On some poor body.

Shakespeare had been more tolerant. In *The Merry Wives of Windsor* the Welsh parson refers to the louse as "a familiar beast to man, and signifies love."[46] Inadvertently, he differentiated between the head louse, the body louse, and the crab (genital) louse. The crab louse is a distant relative of the other two; it is the one that is most often transmitted as a result of sexual intercourse. From the pubic region in which they multiply these stubborn travelers

[46]William Shakespeare, *The Merry Wives of Windsor,* I.i.21.

spread to the other hairy parts of the body except the scalp. The lice can be seen anchored at the hair roots and can be removed for examination. The nits (eggs) can also be removed for examination. Treatment is easy, but, again, all close contacts must be found and treated. Without early treatment the itching and skin irritation may become most distressing. Genital lice may also be contracted from unclean beds or toilet seats.[47]

nonspecific venereal disease

There have been recent reports of a common, sexually communicable disease caused by an as yet unspecified microbe. A variety of organisms, among them staphylococci and streptococci, have been incriminated, but the cause remains uncertain. More than one microbe may be involved. Symptoms begin seven to twenty-one days after exposure; there may be a mild mucous discharge, although some cases resemble gonorrhea or an infection with trichomonas. The disease has a tendency to persist and recur. An antibiotic is the most effective treatment of what may be a stubborn condition.[48]

In industrial countries, progress against communicable diseases has removed ancient terrors. In developing nations, health workers still labor to provide their people with proven methods of prevention and cure. But no matter what the stage of success, the greatest enemy is laxity. A single case of plague in New Mexico, an outbreak of typhoid in New York, an epidemic of gonorrhea in Los Angeles—these warn against a false sense of security. Only constant vigilance buys freedom from the communicable diseases.

[47] To breed properly, lice must drink human blood about every three hours. During the Second World War, the infestation rate of head lice among women in the British army was about 30 percent. This was primarily due to the protection of the lice by acetone-fixed hairdos. (However, the problem could not be compared to the situation of the seventeenth- and eighteenth-century English noblewoman, whose wigs were a veritable haven for vermin.) Today, the head louse is resistant to all known insecticides except Malathion and Carbaryl. Head lice are equally at home in long or short hair; they are undisturbed by vigorous hair washing, although repeated combing might dislodge a few. Head lice seem to prefer the hair of little boys and girls (between the ages of four and six), although anybody will do. The body louse and the pubic (crab) louse are not so choosy. *Garden malathion is an extremely dangerous poison and must not be used on the human head. The pure malathion prescribed by the physician is safe.* So far, both body and pubic lice seem to be susceptible to most insecticides. How long this merciful situation will continue cannot be estimated. (Adrian Hope, "The Lice Explosion," *New Scientist,* Vol. 57, No. 836 [March 8, 1973], p. 562.) In this country, considerable concern has been expressed about the spread of all human lice. Two million human cases are estimated to occur annually—an increase of more than 800 percent between 1963 and 1973. The body louse is a particular threat because it carries to man a variety of serious illnesses, such as a form of typhus fever. ("Spread of Human Lice Worries Experts," *Journal of the American Medical Association,* Vol. 226, No. 1 [October 1, 1973], pp. 21–22).
[48] "Venereal Disease Symposium," p. 92.

summary

Another major group of agents that cause infectious diseases, in addition to viruses (discussed in Chapter 6), are the *bacteria.* These microbes are responsible for such diseases as:

1. *tuberculosis* (pages 170–72). This infection most commonly occurs in the lung. A positive *Mantoux skin test* indicates sensitivity to the products of the growth of the tubercle bacillus, which causes tuberculosis; the test does not necessarily indicate active disease.
2. *sickness from food contamination* (pages 172–73), caused by either infection (as in salmonellosis) or intoxication (as in staphylococcal food poisoning, in which illness is caused by toxin released by the bacteria, not by the bacteria themselves).
3. *meningococcic meningitis* (pages 174–75), or spinal meningitis, is one of a number of diseases that can be spread by *carriers*—persons who harbor the organisms of the disease without themselves displaying the symptoms.
4. *tetanus* (page 175), or lockjaw, another disease caused by bacterial toxin.

An important group of communicable illnesses are the sexually transmitted, or venereal, diseases. Bacteria are the agents of the two most common venereal diseases, *syphilis* and *gonnorhea.* Incidence of venereal disease has reached epidemic proportions (pages 176–77). Many people, especially women, have syphilis or gonnorhea but do not know it (page 178). Venereal disease can be transmitted from mother to unborn or newborn child (page 180). It can also be transmitted through oral-genital contact (pages 180–81). The spread of syphilis and gonorrhea may be prevented by the use of condoms (page 182), by antibiotics such as penicillin (page 182), and by tracing of sexual contacts (page 183). In addition, the V.D.-preventive action is now being investigated of Progonasyl (page 182), of a copper-containing intrauterine device (page 183), and of lesser-used contraceptives such as jellies, foams, and powders (page 183).

Other diseases that can be sexually transmitted are *trichomoniasis* (page 184); *moniliasis* (page 185); *genital herpes* (pages 185–86); *venereal tumors*—genital warts and molluscum contagiosum, which are the only human tumors known to be caused by viruses (page 187); *scabies* (page 187); *genital lice* (page 188); and *nonspecific venereal disease* (page 189).

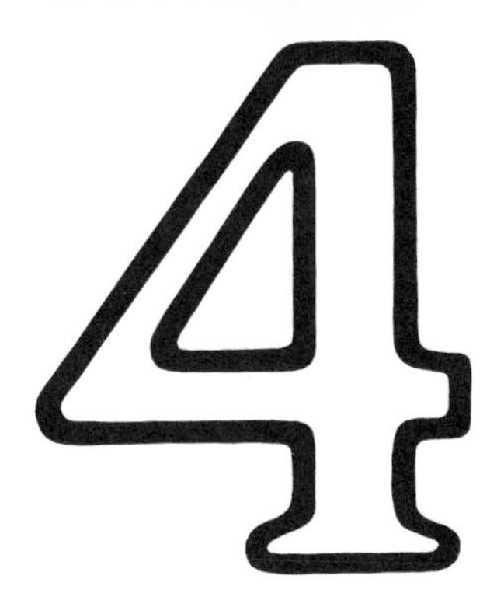

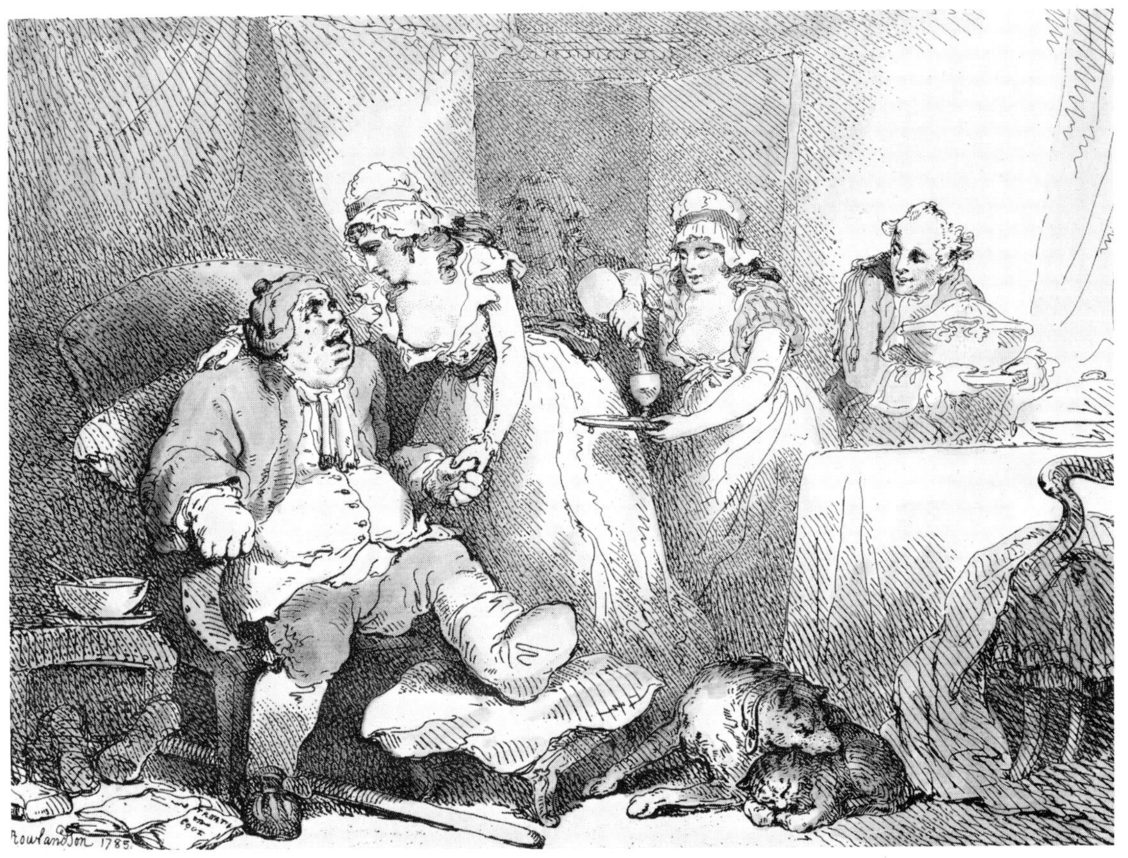

"Comfort in the Gout," Thomas Rowlandson (1756–1827).

# of structure, function, and chronic impairments thereof

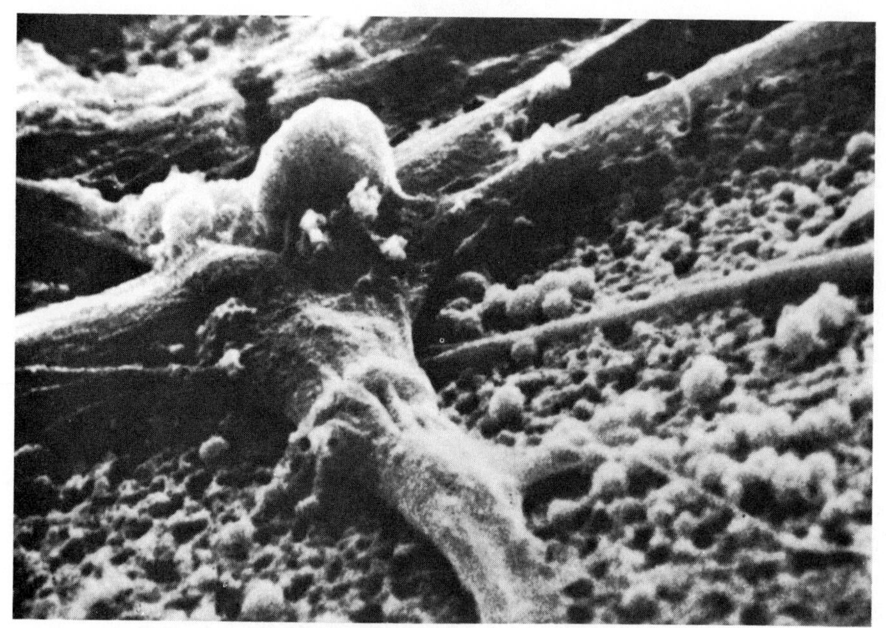

A cancer cell (magnified more than 3,500 times) spreads like the roots of a tree and can invade normal tissue.

cancer

8

chronic disease: the price of success

At the turn of this century, infectious diseases were the primary health menace to this nation. Acute respiratory conditions such as pneumonia and influenza were the major killers. Tuberculosis, too, drained the nation's vitality. Gastrointestinal infections decimated the child population. A great era of environmental control helped change all this. Water and milk supplies were made safe. Engineers constructed systems to handle and treat perilous human wastes and to render them safe. Food sanitation and personal hygiene became a way of life. True, new environmental hazards replaced the old (Chapters 3 and 4). But people survived to suffer them. Moreover, continual labors of public health workers diminished death rates of mothers and their infants. Countless children were vaccinated. Tuberculosis was increasingly brought under control. In 1900, the average person in the United States barely eked out fifty years of life. Some twenty years have since been added to this life expectancy.

But each generation is saddled on the last. Yesterday's success often brings tomorrow's challenge. The longer life span—a mark of progress—intensified another group of health problems and made them predominant, the *chronic degenerative diseases:* ''chronic,'' because they linger; ''degenerative,'' because they may cause progressive deterioration of tissues. As a group they share certain characteristics: their causes are frequently unclear; often, they are a long time developing; the disability they bring may be relatively prolonged; usually they leave some residual impairment; and their treatments, because they are long-term, are costly.

That the chronic diseases have become the nation's major health problem is apparent from a few statistics: at the turn of this century, one in seven deaths was due to heart disease and stroke; today, that ratio is one in every two. Cancer has joined heart disease and stroke in a destructive assault on the middle and advanced years. But chronic illness is also a major concern of youth. For most chronic diseases, cure, as it is generally understood, remains unlikely. But suffering stimulates research, and the search into the unknown begets knowledge.

Cancer will be discussed in this chapter. The next chapter will deal with the structure and disorders of the circulatory system and the kidneys. Allergies, joint disorders, and the structure and some of the disorders of the nervous system and the endocrine and exocrine glands will be discussed in Chapter 10.

cancer: the lawless cells

''Anarchy, anarchy! Show me a greater evil!'' cries Creon, King of Thebes, in Sophocles' great tragedy *Antigone.* Cancer is cellular anarchy. Its microscopic, greedy lawlessness, contemptuous of body government, ''destroys man in a

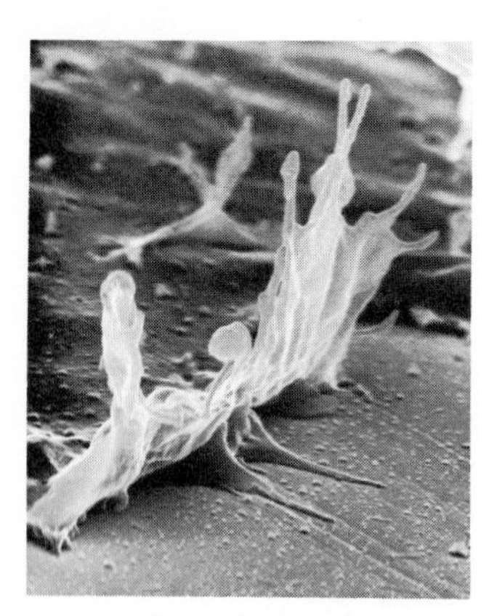

8-1 *Cell migration. A normal hamster cell putting out vertical "ruffles," which will drop and adhere to the surface. The rest of the cell will then slowly flow into and over this leading edge* ($\times$ *15,000*).

unique and appalling way, as flesh of his own flesh, which has somehow been rendered proliferative, rampant, predatory, and ungovernable."[1]

In Chapter 18, the momentous destiny of the fertilized egg—the *zygote*—is described. Under genetic direction, it divides. There are then two cells, and these divide to produce four cells. Each of these divides, and so on. As cells grow in number, they migrate. Some divide here, others there. All the while their DNA is active. To obedient RNA molecules, DNA imparts codes to construct proteins. The proteins are destined to play their vital part in the structure of various tissue, whether brain or liver or skin or any other. So cells differentiate. Nourished in the womb's wall, the disciplined cluster of cells is alive. But now is it held together? Cells lay down nonliving substances between one another. They spare salts, for example, long ago borrowed from the seas, for bone construction. This cellular division, migration, and differentiation, this laying down of framework, is not haphazard. A rhythmic miracle, rivaling the movements of the celestial bodies, it is a directed plan for growth. This is body government. When this government is usurped, there is anarchy, chaos, cancer.

At birth all organs are differentiated. But growth continues, and so does cell division. With adolescence a special spurt of cell division occurs in the sexual organs. At twenty the average person is full-grown. Normally, he is a harmonious ecosystem of cells, and each of his trillions of cells is an ecosystem too.

Some cells stop dividing, but not all. The neurons in the adult brain and spinal cord no longer divide, but the cells of their supporting tissue do. Some cells divide only when necessary. Bone, liver, kidney, and endocrine gland cells divide to replace those killed by infection or other injury. (There are cells that do not divide but grow. In this way a woman's uterus and breasts respond to pregnancy.) Still other cells divide throughout life. One reason blood cells continually need to be replaced is that they are buffeted about and destroyed during their extensive travels. So blood cell division continually goes on in bone marrow and lymph nodes. Surface skin cells and those of the linings of the respiratory, gastrointestinal, and urinary tracts also undergo harsh treatment. Hence, the destroyed cells are constantly replaced. It is estimated that the entire mucous lining of the gastrointestinal tract is replaced about twice a week.[2]

The basic difference between normal cells and tumor cells is that normal cells are controlled. Tumor cells have escaped normal body controls. They are instructed by the genetic material to divide. But, as will be seen, the management has been taken over. Tumor cells are in ecological imbalance with the body that feeds them. Thus, they are doomed, as, too often, is their host. How this occurs is described below.

tumors are benign or malignant

Tumors, as indicated above, are masses of cells resulting from uncontrolled growth.[3] *Benign tumors* are not cancers. Of themselves, they do not kill. Only by incidentally interfering with function (for example, by obstructing the bowel)

[1] Peyton Rous, "The Challenge to Man of Neoplastic Disease," Nobel Prize acceptance speech delivered in Stockholm, December 13, 1966.

[2] Most susceptible to becoming tumors are the cells that constantly divide. Cells dividing when needed for repair or for a new function also go out of control, but less frequently.

[3] The late distinguished U.S. physician James Ewing called tumors "an uncontrolled new growth of tissue."

can they cause death. Such tumors are regularly defined and encapsulated. They are a localized cellular overgrowth. A surrounding capsule keeps them within bounds. As they grow, they do not penetrate tissues; they push them. Surgically, they can be shelled out of their capsule; cure results.

Malignant tumors are the cancers. By the very nature of their behavior, they can kill. Crab-shaped (Greek *karkinos,* crab), they behave like crabs. Not withheld by a capsule, they project into normal tissue, clawing their way, destroying all cells in their path.

cancer: a "solid" or a "generalized" malignant tumor

Cancer is a disease of the cell. That is, the initial event leading to a cancer is an abnormal change in a single cell. As the changed cell divides, and cell division continues, the abnormal change is perpetuated in succeeding generations of cells. The malignant cells may ultimately form a mass—a "solid" tumor—or they may at once become "generalized"—widespread throughout the body. For the sake of simplicity, therefore, cancers are often considered to be of two basic types: *"solid"* or *"generalized."* More specifically, "solid" tumors come from one source; "generalized" tumors occur simultaneously at many sites. These two types are, in turn, classified according to the tissues from which they arise.

the "solid" tumors

> Carcinomas are the most common form of cancer. They arise from epithelial cells, important as a covering or lining tissue, which exists in numerous forms. Skin is composed of one kind of epithelium; when it becomes cancerous, it is designated as skin carcinoma. Other carcinomas arise from the glandular organs, such as the breast, which are composed of different epithelial tissue, as are the smooth, shiny mucous membranes such as those that line the mouth, stomach, and lungs.
>
> Sarcomas occur less frequently. They are a more heterogeneous group of cancers, arising from fibrous (connective) tissue and from muscle, bone, and cartilage. Together, the carcinomas and sarcomas have been classified as "solid" tumors.[4]

HOW "SOLID" TUMORS TRAVEL The destructive capacities of carcinomas and sarcomas are not limited to adjacent tissues. "Solid" tumors often *metastasize.* Breaking loose from their original sites, some cancer cells travel to other body locations, near and far. Once there, the migrant cells seed new and secondary malignant growths. There are three routes by which they travel. (1) By penetrating the delicate lymph channel walls, they set up secondary cancer depots in nearby and distant lymph nodes (see page 224). Eventually, they might reach the blood stream via the lymphatic circulation from these sites (pages 223–24), and thereby endanger other organs. (2) In addition, cancer cells may invade the veins, which are less resistant than the arteries. Following the circulatory routes, they then set up secondary tumors in remote places. That is why cigarette smoker's cancer is so often fatal. Deluded that his cough is a "cigarette cough," that the pain in his chest is temporary, the smoker may not

[4] *Progress Against Cancer 1969: A Report by the National Advisory Cancer Council,* National Cancer Institute, U.S. Department of Health, Education, and Welfare, pp. 52–53.

see a physician until his lung cancer has been long dispersed to the body's vital centers.[5] (3) Cancer cells may break off from an original location and migrate to the fibrous sacs enclosing the intestines, the lungs, or the heart. Then, after penetrating the sac, they may float in its enclosed fluid, finally settling down on an organ. They may then start a secondary cancerous growth.

Not all metastases cause early death. The traveling cells of some tumors end in the lung, for example, and there they die. Others go to some distant bone (as do cells of some breast cancers). They may stay there without causing disease for many years. Nobody knows why.

the ''generalized'' tumors

The ''generalized'' tumors include the *leukemias* and the *lymphomas.* Leukemias are cancers of the blood-forming tissues. Usually generalized from their onset, they are characterized by an uncontrolled multiplication and accumulation of abnormal white cells. Lymphomas are cancers of some of the infection-fighting structures of the body, such as the lymph nodes. They may begin as a localized disease, but often quickly become widespread.

the causes of cancer

physical causes

There are four basic groups of cancer causes: *physical, chemical, genetic, and viral.*

As was discussed in Chapter 4, some substances emit cancer-causing radiations as they degenerate. Such irradiation may produce a chemical change in the genetic structure within the cell. The genetically altered cell may then progress to cancer. Examples of radiation-produced cancers are the lung cancer of Colorado uranium miners, the increased leukemia rates among Hiroshima and Nagasaki survivors (the incidence of leukemia among them is five times that of the rest of the Japanese population[6]), the increased incidence of female breast cancer (two to four times) among these same survivors,[7] and the higher leukemia rates among X-ray workers. The sun's ultraviolet light radiation is responsible for most skin cancers[8] (see page 204).

[5] It was recently estimated that of 61,000 people in the United States who contracted lung cancer in 1968, close to 75 percent would be dead within one year, 93 percent within five years. Of 100 lung cancer patients medically examined, 50 to 60 would be beyond chance for cure. Of the remaining 40 to 50, only half are operable. ''Of the 20 to 25 with operable growths, only 5 to 8 live 5 years after surgery.'' Of these, almost one-fourth recur. (Bernard Roswit, cited in ''Medical Science Notes,'' *Science News,* Vol. 94, No. 3 [August 1968], p. 112.) From 1936 through 1973, there has been a 1,400 percent increase in lung cancer among men. (''US Cancer Deaths Continue to Rise,'' *Journal of the American Medical Association,* Vol. 226, No. 8 [November 1973], p. 850.) These figures are not included in cigarette advertising.

[6] R. J. C. Harris, *Cancer* (Baltimore, 1962), p. 50.

[7] C. K. Wanebo *et al.,* ''Breast Cancer After Exposure to the Atomic Bombings of Hiroshima and Nagasaki,'' *New England Journal of Medicine,* Vol. 279, No. 13 (September 26, 1968), pp. 667–71.

[8] Robert G. Freeman and John M. Knox, ''Skin Cancer and the Sun,'' *CA—A Cancer Journal for Clinicians,* Vol. 17, No. 5 (September–October 1967), p. 235.

chemical causes

That chemicals can cause cancer was first reported in 1775 by an English surgeon, Percival Potts. He correctly attributed the frequent scrotal cancer of chimney sweeps to prolonged exposure to coal soot. In this association, he was certainly helped by the chimney sweeps themselves, who called their scrotal sores "soot warts." Only too often did an orphaned six-year-old, recruited to work in the chimneys, also sleep in them. Many grew to manhood remaining chimney sweeps, laboring long hours, constantly exposed to soot, rarely changing clothes or washing.

Sometimes chemicals combine with injuries, particularly burns, to cause cancer. In Panama, washerwomen smoke cigarettes with the lit end inside their mouths. Among them, mouth cancers are frequent.

Today, man is surrounded by potential chemical *carcinogens* (cancer-producing substances). Although "no final conclusion about the effect of atmospheric pollution is yet possible,"[9] recent research indicates that smog may be one of the causes of cancer (see pages 58–59). Industries that use coal tar and its derivatives are too often dangerous; they account for the largest single group of occupational cancers. Also implicated as cancer agents are the chemicals used in the rubber and cable industries. Alcohol can also be a carcinogen; deaths from cancers of the mouth, pharynx, larynx, esophagus, and liver have been associated with heavy drinking.[10]

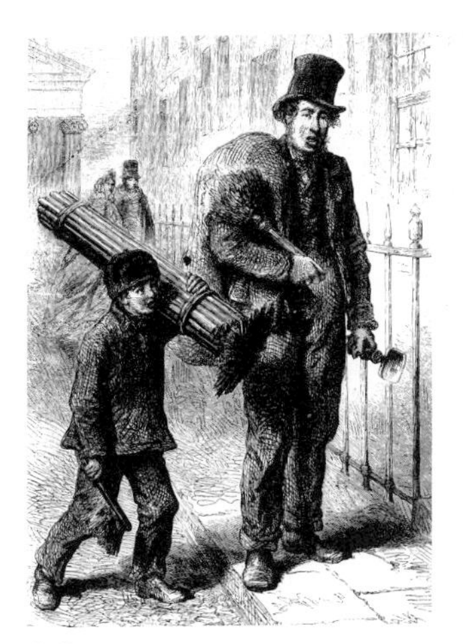

8-2 *A French engraving of 19th-century London chimneysweeps.*

genetic causes

Laboratory animals are of enormous importance to cancer research. Mice have been bred that invariably develop a particular cancer. Such genetically dependable pure strains, produced by brother-sister matings of twenty or more generations, have provided an indispensable laboratory creature. These mice help man, for heredity plays a role in human cancer. Exactly what that role is remains, as yet, unclear. Exceedingly few cancers are strictly genetic or hereditary. Among the ones that are hereditary are an uncommon tumor of the retina and another of the nervous system, each of which is determined by a specific gene. The familial aspects of female breast cancer are discussed later in this chapter (page 205).

viral causes

In 1911, Peyton Rous showed that chickens developed connective tissue tumors from viruses. But scant attention was paid to his work. Years later, a virus that was recovered from a mouse produced cancers in rats, guinea pigs, hamsters, and other species. A new research race was on. And perhaps to mark it, fifty-five years after his original work, Rous was awarded the Nobel Prize.

how infecting viruses cause animal cancers

It is understandable that the solution to the cancer riddle is being sought in the laboratories of the virologists. It has been seen that cancer is a disease of the cell. And in Chapter 6 it was pointed out that viruses are obliged to multiply in living cells. The viruses that can cause animal cancers, like all viruses, consist

[9] Richard Doll, *Prevention of Cancer: Pointers in Epidemiology* (London, 1967), p. 62.
[10] *Ibid.*, p. 81.

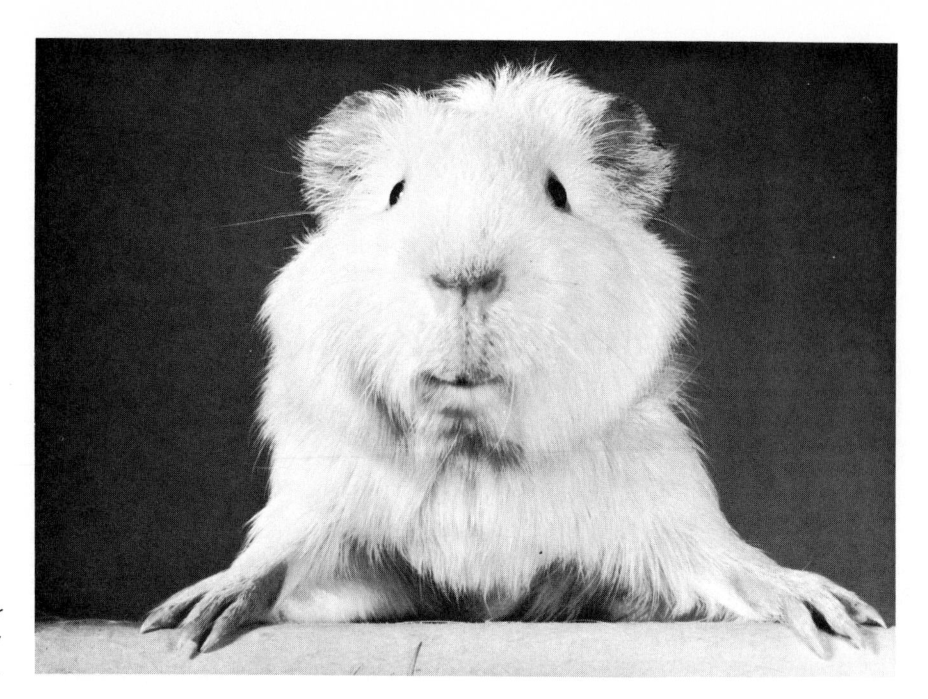

8-3 *A hero of cancer research: the guinea pig.*

of a protein overcoat and a core of nucleic acid. The protein overcoat is the part of the virus that gives it specificity as an antigen. It is the core, however, that causes cellular infection. That core of the virus is composed of either RNA or DNA, but never both types of nucleic acid. Thus it is the core of the virus that contains its genes. Within the nucleus of the animal cell, comprising its genes, there is also DNA, and it is DNA that directs the formation of RNA. So the core of the virus contains the same basic genetic chemicals as the nuclear core of animal cells.

It will be recalled (Chapter 6) that a virus attaches itself to an animal cell, penetrates it, and undergoes uncoating to free its nucleic acid molecules—its genes. Theoretically, four things may then occur to the animal cell. (1) The viral nucleic acid may subvert the cell into making more virus. (2) The speed of cellular multiplication may be retarded by the viral nucleic acids (a ''reverse cancer effect''). (3) Nothing that is apparent may happen for some time. Having entered the cell, the viral genes lurk latent within the cellular genes. In this dormant state, the complete viral genes are passed on from parent to daughter cells during cell division (*mitosis;* see page 529). At some point, the entire genetic structure of the virus (its *genome*) is stimulated into action. The latent virus is now ''switched on''; *all* its genes participate in producing the delayed infection. Examples of such happenings are believed to be herpesvirus 1 and 2, which cause common ''cold sores'' (*herpes simplex*) and genital sores respectively (see page 160).

(4) The fourth result of viral invasion includes the occurrences of the third, but with a major alteration. After the viral invasion and subsequent period of latency, not all, but only a few of the viral genes are ''switched on.'' The com-

plete virus does not get manufactured. It is thought that the virus alone is not enough to cause a tumor. What might stimulate those few viral genes into action? Chemicals, perhaps another virus, some nonviral disease—these may be the triggers. Considerable support has been given this theory by studies of the Epstein-Barr virus (EBV). This virus has been found in association with two diseases—one relatively mild, the other deadly. There is no longer much doubt that EBV causes infectious mononucleosis.[11] And EBV "remains probably the leading candidate . . . for a human cancer virus."[12] That cancer occurs among East African children; it is called *Burkitt's lymphoma.* Many scientists agree that EBV invades the lymph nodes of the neck and jaw. They also believe that in infectious mononucleosis, there is no period of latency, while in Burkitt's lymphoma, the virus does remain latent among the genes of the host's cells. If these assumptions are valid, this is one of the questions that must be answered: Why is the virus cancerous in East African children, yet relatively mild among U.S. young people? It is suggested that only part of the invading EB virus is activated in the cells of the East African child, while in this country the entire virus replicates in the cells to produce a comparatively benign infection. What, however, stimulates only a few genes of the virus within the cells of the East African child? Nobody knows. (Fortunately, Burkitt's lymphoma can be treated with considerable success.)

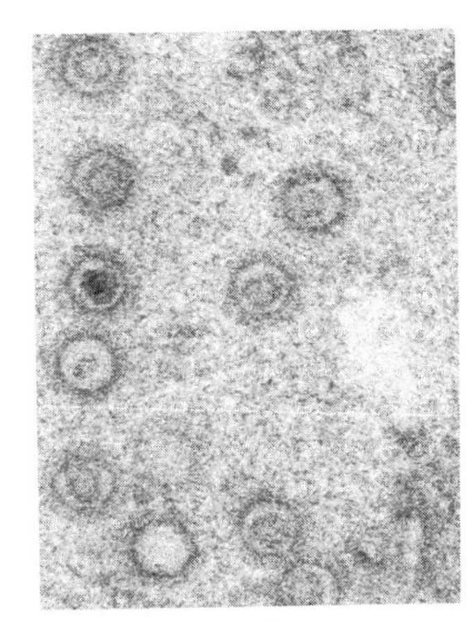

8-4 *Epstein-Barr virus particles in a human lymphoblast* (*a developing lymphocyte; see page 141*).

So, for a cancer to develop in a human being, it is believed that only a few of the viral genes are "switched on," and the complete virus is never replicated. But this raises problems. If this concept is correct, searching a human cell for a newly made complete virus, or even virus particles, would no longer appear to be as fruitful as was originally thought. Indeed, finding a virus, or a virus particle, in a cancer cell never was conclusive evidence that it was a cancer-causing agent. One could not be sure that it was not just another virus or particle in the cell causally unassociated with cancer. Scientists are pursuing other leads to indicate a viral cause of human cancer. Research is being directed at more subtle, indirect evidence of the presence of a cancer-causing virus in an afflicted cell. Their reasoning is this: viruses produce substances in the cell that are not part of the virus itself. These viral substances are foreign to the cell and should act as antigens (see page 142). Thus they should produce specific antibodies. Examining cancer cells (of the cervix, for example) for the antibodies produced by substances of a theoretical cancer virus, and noting whether this specific antibody level correlates with the state of the disease, might be helpful in indirectly tagging a viral cause of human cancer. It is like looking for the partial footprints of a possible cancer virus in a cell. There has been some success in this direction with the herpesviruses and cancers of the lip and cervix.

Clearly, animal studies have revealed much about the virus–cancer relationship. Clearly, much is theoretical. But it does appear that the beginnings of the virus–cancer effect depend, in part, on which viral genetic structure, RNA or DNA, invades the cell. Consider them separately. *If the cancer-causing virus*

[11] Werner Henle and Gertrude Henle, "Epstein-Barr Virus and Infectious Mononucleosis," *New England Journal of Medicine,* Vol. 288, No. 5 (February 1, 1973), pp. 263–64.
[12] Graham Chedd, "Herpesvirus: Wolf in Sheep's Clothing?" *New Scientist,* Vol. 58, No. 852 (June 28, 1973), p. 809.

contains DNA, the virus invades the cell and sheds its coat. Then the viral DNA is free to actually become incorporated into the cellular DNA. Then it is assumed that the above-described period of latency begins. As the cell divides, the incorporated viral DNA is passed along with the cell's normal hereditary material to the daughter cells. But the daughter cells are now irrevocably altered, and so are the genetic instructions they carry.

What happens *when the invading cancer-causing virus contains not DNA, but RNA?* There are various theories. It is believed that nature provides the RNA virus with a powerful means of surviving in the cell: It is in the form of the enzyme *reverse transcriptase* (pages 159 and 530–35). Normally, when no virus is present, the cell's genetic information, encoded in its DNA, is transcribed into messenger RNA, and that message is then translated into the sequence of amino acids appropriate for a normal specific protein. All this is made possible by the enzyme *DNA polymerase* (footnote 33 on page 159). However, when an RNA virus enters a cell, the virus's reverse transcriptase (an RNA-dependent DNA polymerase; see pages 530–35 and footnote 33 on page 159) makes it possible for the virus to direct the production of DNA that is coded for the production of substances useful to the virus. The normal DNA ⟶ RNA transcription continues; but the infected cell now contains, and must support, an additional DNA. As is the case with a DNA virus, the DNA made under the direction of viral RNA carries a message very different from that of the cell's own DNA: a message of disease. And to enforce that message, it (like the DNA in a DNA virus) also incorporates itself into the cell's DNA. As was explained above (pages 198–99), not all, but only some of the genes of the DNA or RNA virus are involved in producing tumors.

And so, cancer-causing viruses, whether DNA or RNA, move into an animal cell, plunder it, become a part of it, and then, after lying dormant within its genes for a while, are "switched on" by some stimulus to direct it to disaster. This usurpation of some of the functions of the cell's DNA by viral RNA or viral DNA robs the cell of its ability to direct the making of healthy cellular protein. The ability of healthy cells to stick to one another is also lost. In short, viral DNA or viral RNA disrupts all the life processes of the cell. The cellular DNA can now send only messages of malignancy. Malignant cells divide into daughter cells that carry and transmit the deadly instructions of their parent cells, including the capacity for uncontrolled growth. A cancer is born.

are cancers communicable?

Some one hundred different viruses (both DNA and RNA) are now known to cause cancer in various species of amphibians, birds, and mammals. Some RNA cancer viruses give rise to lymphomas and sarcomas in mammals; others cause breast cancers in certain strains of mice. Some RNA virus particles may be passed to offspring via maternal milk. But are these cancer viruses contagious? Studies suggest that chickens spread leukemia virus to other chickens and cats transmit cat leukemia virus to other cats but not to humans.[13] Do cancer viruses

[13] "Cat Virus Indicates Cancer Is Contagious," *Science News,* Vol. 104, Nos. 7 and 8 (August 18 and 25, 1973), p. 104.

spread among human beings? As of early 1974, no virus had been proven to cause human cancers. But recent work by a Columbia University group has shown that some human breast cancers and leukemia cells do contain RNA molecules that are remarkably similar to the genetic material of RNA viruses known to cause the similar cancers in animals. Only the most pronounced skeptic would now deny a role for viruses in at least some human cancers. In 1966, a distinguished researcher, who died of cancer that year, wrote of "the sly and indirect processes" of some animal tumor viruses.[14] He emphasized, however, that it is no longer realistic to contend that human cells are different from the cells of other species of animals in their capacity to react to cancer-causing viruses.[15] Nevertheless, the concept outlined above—that the genetic substance of cancer viruses is incorporated into the chromosomes of normal cells—militates against the possibility that cancer is communicable in the customary way.

One theory carries the notion of a viral cause of cancer a step further. It holds that during the evolutionary process, the genetic material of certain types of RNA tumor viruses, aided by reverse transcriptase, became integrated (possibly as virus-specific DNA) into the chromosomal structure of most or all vertebrates, including man. It is suggested that these potentially cancer-causing molecules are transmitted in the genes from parent to child. They remain inactive unless some of them are "switched on"—that is, prompted into cancerous activity by some stimulus, such as irradiation or a chemical. A particularly significant finding in support of this theory is the discovery of *fetal antigens* that are associated with cancer. These antigens are normally present in the tissue of embryos and fetuses; they disappear after birth, only to reappear with the occurrence of a cancer. This would tend to corroborate the possibility that a cancer gene (perhaps of viral origin) is switched on during fetal life, switched off after birth, and switched on again when cancer occurs. Even if this theory were to be proven one day, it would lend no credence to the notion that human cancer is generally communicable. There is too little that is proven about the pattern of occurrence and distribution of human cancers to indicate that they are commonly communicable, as that term is understood today.

the extent of the cancer problem

For thirty years cancer has ranked second only to heart disease as the cause of death in the United States. At present rates, more than 53 million people in this country—one person in four—will develop cancer. In early 1974 the

[14] Richard E. Shope, "Evolutionary Episodes in the Concept of Viral Oncogenesis," *Perspectives in Biology and Medicine,* Vol. 9, No. 3 (Winter 1966), p. 273. How indirect the viral role is in cancer is amply illustrated by a recent massive study of the ten-year past patterns of the occurrence and distribution of Hodgkin's disease (see page 207) among the students and teachers of several schools. It suggested that the disease might be contagious. (Nicholas J. Vianna and Adele K. Polan, "Epidemiologic Evidence for Transmission of Hodgkin's Disease," *New England Journal of Medicine,* Vol. 289, No. 10 [September 6, 1973], pp. 499–502.) This possibility needs more investigation. If, indeed, there is a risk of contagion, it is certainly very low. "At ages 15 to 24 the general risk of development of Hodgkin's disease during a 10-year period is about 0.4 percent per thousand persons." (Brian MacMahon, "Is Hodgkin's Disease Contagious?" *New England Journal of Medicine,* Vol. 289, No. 10 [September 6, 1973], pp. 532–33.

[15] *Ibid.,* p. 270.

TABLE 8-1

Cancer: Estimated Casualty Figures for 1974, Warning Signals, and Safeguards

SITE	ESTIMATED NEW CASES 1974	ESTIMATED DEATHS 1974	WARNING SIGNALS (IF YOU HAVE ONE, SEE YOUR DOCTOR)	SAFEGUARDS	COMMENT
Breast	90,000	33,000	**Lump or thickening in the breast.**	Annual checkup; monthly breast self-examination.	The leading cause of cancer death in women.
Colon and rectum	99,000	48,000	**Change in bowel habits; bleeding.**	Annual checkup including proctoscopy, especially for those over 40.	Considered a highly curable disease when digital and proctoscopic examinations are included in routine checkups.
Lung	83,000	75,000	**Persistent cough or lingering respiratory ailment.**	Prevention: heed facts about smoking; annual checkup; chest X-ray.	The leading cause of cancer death among men, this form of cancer is largely preventable.
Oral (including pharynx)	24,000	8,000	**Sore that does not heal; difficulty in swallowing.**	Annual checkup.	Many more lives should be saved because the mouth is easily accessible to visual examination by physicians and dentists.
Skin	300,000	5,000	**Sore that does not heal, or change in wart or mole.**	Annual checkup; avoidance of overexposure to sun.	Skin cancer is readily detected by observation, and diagnosed by simple biopsy.
Uterus	46,000	11,000	**Unusual bleeding or discharge.**	Annual checkup; including pelvic examination with Pap test.	Uterine cancer mortality has declined 65% during the last 35 years. With wider application of the Pap test, many thousands more lives can be saved.
Kidney and bladder	43,000	16,000	**Urinary difficulty; bleeding, in which case consult your doctor at once.**	Annual checkup with urinalysis.	Protective measures for workers in high-risk industries are helping to eliminate one of the important causes of these cancers.
Larynx	10,000	3,000	**Hoarseness; difficulty in swallowing.**	Annual checkup, including mirror laryngoscopy.	Readily curable if caught early.
Prostate	54,000	18,000	**Urinary difficulty.**	Annual checkup, including palpation.	Occurs mainly in men over 60; can be detected by palpation and urinalysis at annual checkup.
Stomach	23,000	14,000	**Indigestion.**	Annual checkup.	A 40% decline in mortality in 20 years, for reasons yet unknown.
Leukemia	21,000	15,000	Leukemia is a cancer of blood-forming tissues and is characterized by the abnormal production of immature white blood cells. Acute leukemia strikes mainly children and is treated by drugs which have extended life from a few months to as much as ten years. Chronic leukemia strikes usually after age 25 and progresses less rapidly. Cancer experts believe that if drugs or vaccines are found which can cure or prevent any cancers, they will be successful first for leukemia and the lymphomas.		
Lymphomas	28,000	20,000	These diseases arise in the lymph system and include Hodgkin's disease and lymphosarcoma. Some patients with lymphatic cancers can lead normal lives for many years.		

Source: American Cancer Society, *'74 Cancer Facts & Figures,* p. 11.

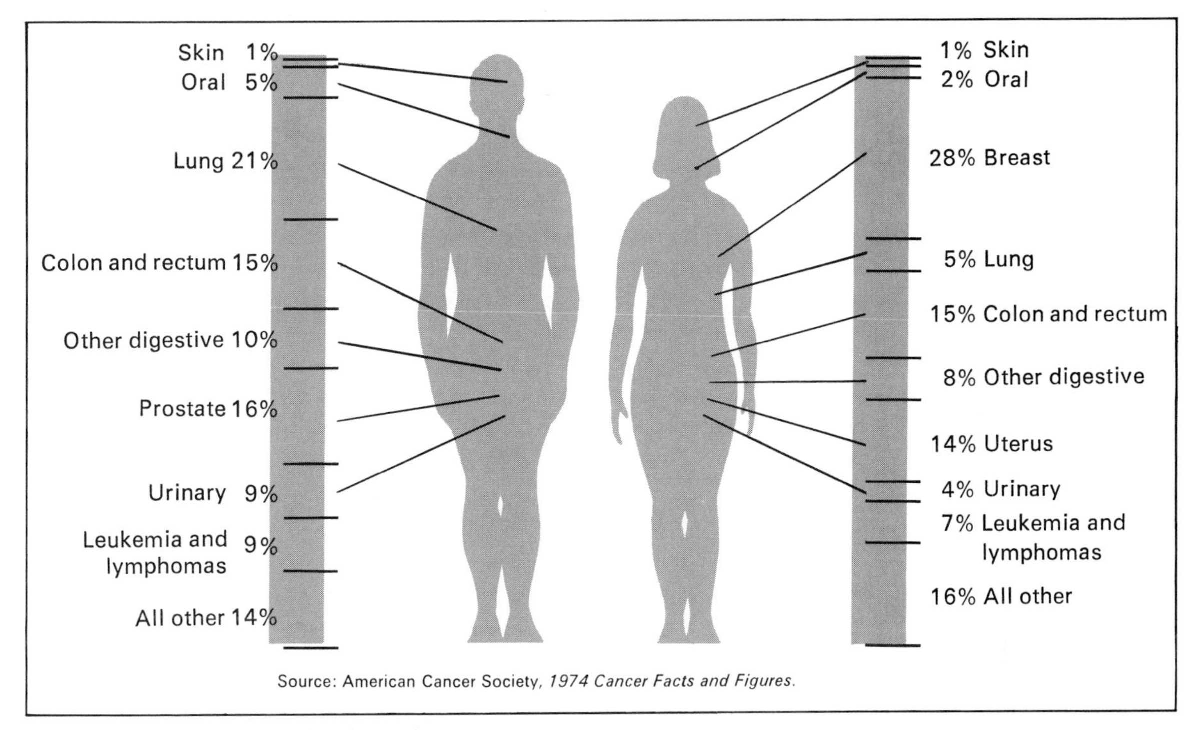

8-5 *Cancer: the incidence by site and sex.*

American Cancer Society made its annual—and usually devastatingly accurate—predictions of cancer casualties (Table 8-1). For 1974, the estimated number of U.S. cancer deaths was 355,000, and the estimated number of newly diagnosed cancer cases was 655,000. Every year cancer kills more than 3,200 children under fifteen years of age.[16]

Recent studies have revealed a startling increase in cancer among blacks. During the eighteen years from 1950 to 1967, the death rate from cancer among black males jumped 50 percent; for blacks of both sexes the increase in cancer mortality was 20 percent. During that time there was no comparable increase for whites of both sexes. U.S. blacks have the world's highest known mortality rates for cancer of the pancreas and prostate. Why the sharp increase in cancer mortality among U.S. blacks? It is not due to genetic differences nor to more accurate reporting on death certificates. One reason may be increased exposure in the past twenty years to urban pollutants and to industrial carcinogens. Interestingly, cancer of the cervix has declined faster among black women than white women in the past few years; this has been attributed to increased access to running water and better opportunities to practice personal hygiene.[17]

[16]American Cancer Society, *1974 Cancer Facts and Figures,* pp. 3, 13.

[17]"In Blacks, More Deaths from Cancer," *Medical World News,* Vol. 13, No. 23 (June 9, 1972), p. 52. Not only are the cancer death rates for blacks higher than those for whites in the United States, but cancer claims the lives of more men than women. The 1974 predicted male–female death ratio was 54:46. This is due to the sharp decrease in cancer of the uterine cervix and, despite some isolated encouraging experience, the tremendous increase since 1936 in lung cancer (see footnote 5). ("US Cancer Deaths Continue to Rise," *Journal of the American Medical Association,* Vol. 226, No. 8 [November 1973], p. 849.)

Another study of data extending as far back as three decades indicated that in the first year of treatment for cancer, poor patients apparently have lower survival rates than do the comparatively well-to-do. This may be due, in part, to the tendency of poor patients to seek treatment later in the course of their disease than do private patients. However, after the first year of treatment, the survival rates of nonpaying patients are not markedly different from those of patients who can afford to pay. Such data emphasize once again the critical need for better health education and for easily available health services for the nation's poor.[18]

prevention and early detection of cancer

Using health education techniques as a common denominator, any disease prevention program is concerned with the *prevention of its occurrence* and, failing in this, *prevention of its progression.* Three basic ways are available to prevent the occurrence of cancer: (1) avoidance of those ecological factors associated with a high incidence of certain malignancies; (2) the removal of lesions that, although not yet malignant, may become cancers; (3) discouragement of marriages that would produce children with a high risk of developing cancers (as is emphasized below, such strictly "hereditary" cancers are very rare).

Consider the *ecological factors.* Excessive exposure to sunlight is a major cause of *skin cancer,* especially among fair people.[19] Although it has a 95 percent cure rate, it is the most common cancer and still causes about five thousand deaths a year in this country. It usually occurs in people over fifty. However, one-third to one-half of the total lifetime exposure to the sun occurs in the first twenty years of life. The family physician can suggest the most effective sunscreen preparations.

Two factors associated with a still high incidence of *cancer of the uterine cervix* are continued sexual activity at an early age and poor hygiene of the external genitalia.[20] Promiscuity or too-early marriage accounts for the first of these. Poor personal hygiene, particularly in the uncircumcised male, results in the collection under the covering penile skin fold (the prepuce) of a thick, creamy, ill-smelling secretion called *smegma.* With the female it may collect around the clitoris. Smegma has been shown to cause cancer in animals.[21] Some (but not all) cancer experts agree that women whose husbands are circumcised (and are, therefore, able to practice more thorough personal hygiene) have a much lower incidence of cervical cancer than women whose husbands

[18] "Is High Cancer Death Rate a Matter of Too Little Care or Too Late?" *Medical World News,* Vol. 13, No. 25 (June 23, 1972), pp. 16–17.

[19] Robert G. Freeman and John M. Knox, "Skin Cancer and the Sun," pp. 231–37.

[20] K. S. Moghissi and H. C. Mack, "Epidemiology of Cervical Cancer," *American Journal of Obstetrics and Gynecology,* Vol. 100, No. 5 (March 1, 1968), pp. 607–14; I. D. Rotkin, "Sexual Patterns and Cervical Cancer," *American Journal of Public Health,* Vol. 57, No. 5 (May 1967), p. 815; Clyde E. Martin, "Marital and Coital Factors in Cervical Cancer," *ibid.,* p. 803.

[21] William M. Christopherson, "Sex Activity and Cancer of the Cervix," *CA—A Cancer Journal for Clinicians,* Vol. 15, No. 6 (November–December 1965), pp. 278–82.

are not circumcised. A simple, painless examination of vaginal fluid, the Papanicolaou (Pap) test—named after its originator, Dr. George Papanicolaou—provides excellent diagnostic information about cervical cancer. The Pap test has become a routine part of a physical examination (see Figure 8-6). Women can easily obtain their own cervical cells without going to a physician.[22] Though not as reliable as those obtained by the physician, these cells can be examined by laboratory specialists recommended by him and can be of great diagnostic value.

Cigarette smoking is a cause of *lung cancer.* It is, moreover, associated with an increased incidence of other malignancies, such as those of the mouth and urinary bladder. Cigarette smoking is killing people, and it should be condemned (Chapter 13). Much has been accomplished in *removing cancer-causing agents from industrial environments,* but much remains to be done. For example, workers occupationally exposed to asbestos fibers and uranium miners exposed to ionizing radiation still have higher than average lung cancer rates.

Precancerous lesions always indicate an immediate, often lifesaving visit to the family physician. The warning signals listed in Table 8-1 may indicate not cancer, but a cellular change that may become malignant if neglected.

The extremely rare precancerous and cancerous tumors that are caused by *gene abnormalities* have been mentioned on page 197. Is *cancer of the female breast* solely hereditary? No. It is true that a genetically determined predisposition to a particular cancer may occur in some families. But this genetic predisposition is complicated by many other factors. Studies of cancer incidence in identical twins (that is, with identical genetic constitutions) have shown that the same cancer rarely occurs in both twins.[23] It is true, however, that there are a number of instances of breast cancer in identical twins. Moreover, there is evidence of an inherited susceptibility to breast cancer. Statistically, female relatives, particularly sisters, of breast cancer patients have two to three times the average tendency to the disease. But the statistical high-risk group also includes (among other factors) those who started menstruating early, have been menstruating for more than thirty years, have never been married, have done little or no breast feeding, have had few or no pregnancies, and have had some previous breast disease.[24] Thus, a host of variables are involved. This is not to suggest that a woman to whom one or more of these variables applies will inevitably develop breast cancer. All women must ever be on guard against this scourge. At the end of each menstrual period (but continuing after the menopause), self-examination of the breast is an essential part of every woman's health regimen. This is the procedure:

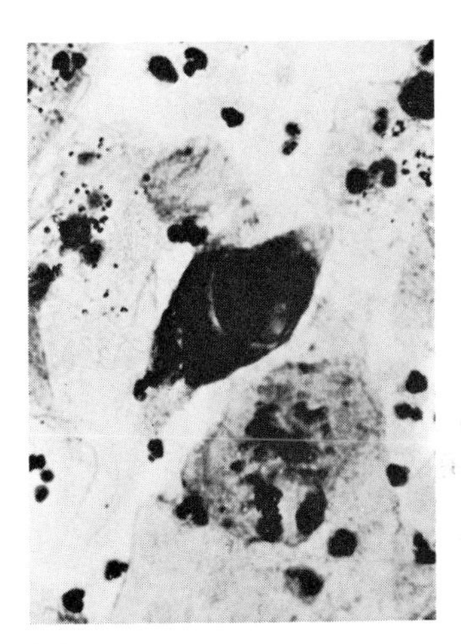

8-6 *Slides of Pap smears for microscopic detection of cancer of the uterine cervix: normal cervical cells* (top) *and cervical cancer cells* (bottom).

[22] W. A. D. Anderson and Samuel A. Gunn, "Cancer of the Cervix. Further Studies of Patient-Obtained Vaginal Irrigation Smear," *CA—A Cancer Journal for Clinicians,* Vol. 17, No. 3 (May–June 1967), p. 102. Recent years have seen a sharp reduction in deaths from cancer of the uterine cervix; part of the reason is that it has become readily detectable. (US Cancer Deaths Continue to Rise," *Journal of the American Medical Association,* Vol. 226, No. 8 (November 1973), p. 850.)

[23] P. C. Koller, "Chromosomes: The Genetic Component of the Tumor Cell," in E. J. Ambrose and F. J. C. Rose, eds., *The Biology of Cancer* (London, 1966), p. 48.

[24] Catherine B. Hess, "Some Epidemiological Aspects of Breast Cancer in Need of Further Investigation," *CA—A Cancer Journal for Clinicians,* Vol. 18, No. 1 (January–February 1968), p. 28.

Step 1: Sit straight before a mirror, with the arms first relaxed at the sides and then raised high above the head. In each position, observe whether any change has occurred in the size or shape of the breasts, especially any abnormal puckering or dimpling of the skin.

Step 2: Lie down, place a folded towel under the left shoulder, raise the left arm and place the hand under the head. With the flat of the fingers of the right hand feel gently the inner half of the left breast, from nipple line to breast bone, and from top to botton. Less than 20 percent of cancers occur here.

Step 3: Bring the arm down to the side and feel gently the outer half of the breast. Since this is the area of maximum danger, it should be examined with special care. Give particular attention to the upper outer section where most cancers of the breast—some 47 percent—occur.

Follow steps 2 and 3 for the right breast.[25]

Any lump or thickening merits immediate consultation with the family physician. Early breast cancer is usually painless. These routine self-examinations supplement, but do not replace, the periodic physical examinations by the family physician. New X-ray techniques are available which can detect breast tumors that are not ordinarily palpable.

The major element preventing the progression of any cancer is early diagnosis. The most common internal cancers are those of the *rectum* and *colon.* Delay may mean death. Early diagnosis means cure. Using a recently improved appliance for visualizing the affected area with little or no discomfort to the patients, doctors can now diagnose almost three-fourths of these conditions early.

In the race for life, cancer always has a head start. It need not win. It is delay that so often ends in despair. "Through early diagnosis and prompt treatment of cancer, the present survival ratio could be one in two."[26]

The above-mentioned warning signals listed in Table 8-1 do not necessarily mean cancer. They do require an immediate visit to the family doctor. Every physician has a high index of suspicion. He often needs to embark on a time-consuming but always worthwhile investigation. If a cancer is localized, he can hold out hope. If it has escaped from its origin, if there is regional involvement, hope diminishes. For example, if cancer of the breast is localized, the five-year survival rate is 85–90 percent; but only 40–45 percent of the women with regional involvement are alive at the end of five years.[27]

Should one unconcernedly await signs and symptoms? No. If cancer is found in a symptomless individual, the outlook for a five-year cure is brightest. For example, a woman whose breast cancer is diagnosed before symptoms appear has as much as a 34 percent better chance of cure; when a symptomless cancer of the colon is diagnosed, the chances of cure are more than 35 percent higher than they would have been if the diagnosis had been made after symp-

[25] These directions are provided by the National Cancer Institute, in *Breast Self-Examination,* Public Health Publication No. 48 (Washington, D.C.).

[26] *CA—A Cancer Journal for Clinicians,* Vol. 18, No. 1 (January–February 1968), p. 13.

[27] For patients with other cancers the data are just as emphatic. For cancer of the uterus they are 81 percent compared to 48 percent; of the urinary bladder, 71 to 26 percent; for the colon and rectum, 70 to 37 percent; 68 percent of patients with localized ovarian cancers are alive in five years; with regional spread, only 31 percent. For cancer of the prostate the figures are 67 versus 47 percent; for stomach cancer, 40 versus 13 percent; for lung cancer, 27 versus 5 percent.

toms had appeared. Every family doctor's office is a cancer detection center. His physical examinations save lives. Moreover, numerous communities sponsor cancer detection programs. These provide routine cancer examinations for those without symptoms. A cancer detection program, provided for all, could save approximately eighty thousand lives a year in this country.[28]

"Many cancers run their course from 'early operable, easily removable and highly curable' to 'advanced stage . . . , inoperable and incurable' in the course of less than a year."[29] The tumor may have been present for many years, but the changes in it from curable to incurable may occur in less than one. So crucial is the thorough annual physical examination.

the treatment of cancer

current methods of treatment

Today, cancers are treated by *surgical removal, radiation,* or *drugs.* Sometimes all three are combined. The usefulness of radiation is limited because often the amount needed to destroy all the cancer cells may also destroy normal tissue. However, radiation specialists are today achieving results that would have been considered miraculous a few years ago. Cancer of the prostate, when it has not spread beyond the gland, has responded remarkably well to radiation; one group of physicians reports a five-year cure rate of 73 percent.[30] In one type of leukemia, a combination of drugs and intensive central nervous system irradiation has resulted in a large number of children who have remained free of the disease for five years or more.[31] One group of children, who are considered by some specialists to be cured, had not received any additional therapy for as long as three and a half years.[32] Hodgkin's disease, a progressive and painful enlargement of lymph nodes, spleen, and other lymphoid tissue, used to be invariably fatal. Today, early diagnosis and irradiation, plus surgical removal of the spleen, have brought prolonged life, even apparent cure, to numerous victims.[33] From Dublin came a report that a drug called warfarin has doubled the survival rate of patients suffering from a variety of recurrent cancers.[34] Another example of success: a considerable percentage of persons treated with a salve containing a substance called 5-FU have been cured of skin cancer.[35] Some 15 percent of all human cancers have proved to be highly amenable to drug therapy.[36]

[28] Emerson Day, "Value of Regular Medical Examinations," in Ronald W. Raven and J. C. Roe, eds., *The Prevention of Cancer* (London, 1967), p. 367.
[29] Francis D. Moore, "Hesitation and Delay as a Social Phenomenon," *New England Journal of Medicine,* Vol. 289, No. 1 (July 5, 1973), p. 41.
[30] "Success Against Prostatic Cancer," *Medical World News,* Vol. 12, No. 43 (November 19, 1971), p. 80.
[31] "We Believe We Can Cure Childhood Leukemia," *Medical World News,* Vol. 13, No. 23 (June 9, 1972), pp. 48–50.
[32] Donald Pinkel, "Five Year Follow-Up of 'Total Therapy' of Childhood Lymphocytic Leukemia," *Journal of the American Medical Association,* Vol. 216, No. 4 (April 26, 1971), p. 648.
[33] "Early Hodgkin's Yields to Irradiation Blitz," *Medical World News,* Vol. 12, No. 2 (January 15, 1971), pp. 23–24.
[34] "Warfarin Said to Double Survival in Ca Patients," *Hospital Tribune,* Vol. 7, No. 5 (February 5, 1973), pp. 1, 8.
[35] Donald Robinson, "Anti-Cancer Drugs," *Family Health,* Vol. 4, No. 12 (December 12, 1972), pp. 28–29, and "Skin Ca Needs More 5-FU—for Longer," *Medical World News,* Vol. 14, No. 28 (July 20, 1973), p. 39.
[36] Carl G. Baker, "Opportunities for Progress Against Cancer," *Medical Annals of the District of Columbia,* Vol. 40, No. 7 (July 1971), p. 426, citing C. G. Zubrod, personal communication.

The critical importance of the team approach to cancer treatment is being increasingly emphasized.[37] As was seen above, cancer is not one disease with one cause; it is many diseases and has many causes.[38] The proper combination of surgery, radiation therapy, and drug treatment for each patient must be decided on by a variety of readily available, highly trained specialists.

the immune response and cancer treatment

Treatment that involves the principles of the *immune* response (see pages 141–45) may soon benefit some cancer patients.[39] This new development is a dividend from experience with organ transplant failures. Organ transplants are foreign invaders; they are rejected because the "killer" white blood cells (certain lymphocytes of the recipient; see pages 143–44) attack the antigens that are on their surfaces. (It is now known that such antigens are on the surface of many kinds of cancer cells.) A transplant recipient must take drugs to depress his natural immune response. Only by doing so can he prevent his white blood cells from attacking and rejecting his desperately needed donated organ. But such a patient is more prone to develop cancer possibly because the immune response that would control a cancer has been suppressed. Treatment of cancer, therefore, could conceivably entail the enhancement of the patient's natural immune response.[40] One way to stimulate the immune response is by antigen injections of the patient's own cancer cells or those of another patient with the same kind of cancer.

This knowledge, that a lowered level of immunity results in a diminished resistance to cancer, is one reason that scientists suspect that the immunological response may suppress cancer. There are other reasons. First, some cancers regress spontaneously, without treatment. Second, autopsies of people who died from causes other than cancer reveal that the incidence of symptomless and thus unknown or "silent" cancers is greater than was ever suspected. But the immunological mechanism that accounts for the body's all too frequent failure to destroy its own cancer cells was recently discovered by a Swedish husband-and-wife team, Karl Erik and Ingegard Hellstrom. Blood was drawn from a patient suffering with a lethal type of skin cancer called a *malignant melanoma.* From the liquid serum of this blood they separated the lymphocyte "killer cells" (see page 143). These "killer cells" were then added to a test tube containing cells of the patient's malignant melanoma. The melanoma cancer cells were killed. This proved that the patient's blood serum contained killer cells capable of destroying the cancer. Then the Hellstroms repeated the experiment, but this time they added the patient's serum to the mixture of killer and cancer cells. The cancer cells were not killed. This proved that some substance in the patient's serum prevented his killer cells from destroying his cancer cells. This substance has been named a "blocking factor." Further research revealed

[37] Denman Hammond, "Multidisciplinary Teamwork in the Management of Childhood Cancer," *California Medicine,* Vol. 116, No. 3 (March 1972), pp. 74–75.

[38] Peter C. Nowell, "Genetic Causes in Cancer: Cause or Effect?" *Human Pathology,* Vol. 2, No. 3 (September 1971), pp. 347–48.

[39] Loren J. Humphrey, "Tumor Immunity," *Journal of Surgical Research,* Vol. 10, No. 10 (October 1970), p. 506.

[40] George W. Santos, "Immunological Concepts and Their Potential Role in Cancer Therapy," *Postgraduate Medicine,* Vol. 48, No. 5 (November 1970), pp. 194–98.

not only that the blocking factor was an antibody-generating antigen (see pages 142–43) released by the cancer cells, but that the killer cells behaved specifically—that is, those from a patient with malignant melanoma killed the cells of only that tumor and none other. More than this, it is now known that normal cells also shed antigen into the blood. However, cancer cells release so massive a flow of blocking antigen that the body's immune system is overwhelmed.[41] Indeed, as a cancer spreads, an increasing amount of antigen is detectable in the blood.[42]

The fact that cancers can be antigens, which may stimulate the body to produce antibodies against them, has raised hopes "for a battery of tests which will allow the early detection of tumors and possibly even their identification."[43] Indeed, an antigen that is apparently tumor-specific for human breast cancer has been used in immunological tests that correctly identified breast cancer in all but one of fifty-one patients.[44] Such early diagnosis makes cure more likely.

Since it has been proved that viruses can cause animal cancers, and vaccines have proved effective in preventing some of these, is there hope that a preventive vaccine may someday be developed for some human cancers? Yes. Viruses—or virus-like particles—have been found to be associated with human leukemias, breast cancers, and certain tumors of connective tissue. These viruses are, at present, structurally indistinguishable from viruses known to cause cancer in some animals. This could suggest that effective vaccines may also be developed for humans. But first, as has been noted, it must be proved that viruses do cause human cancers.[45] And vaccines against animal cancers are by no means easy to prepare.[46]

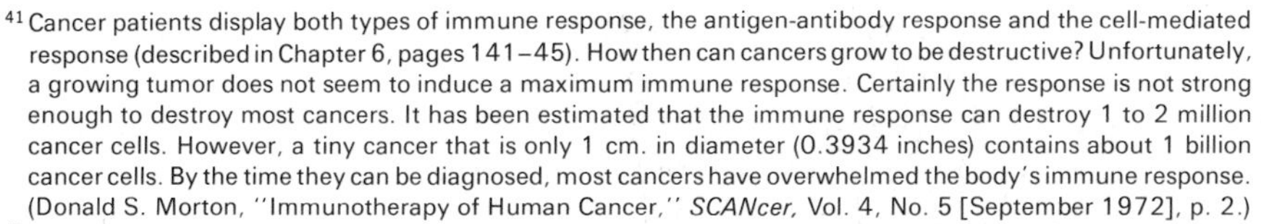

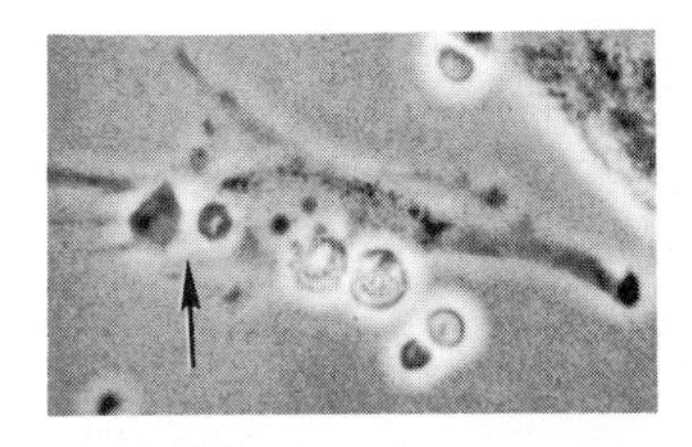

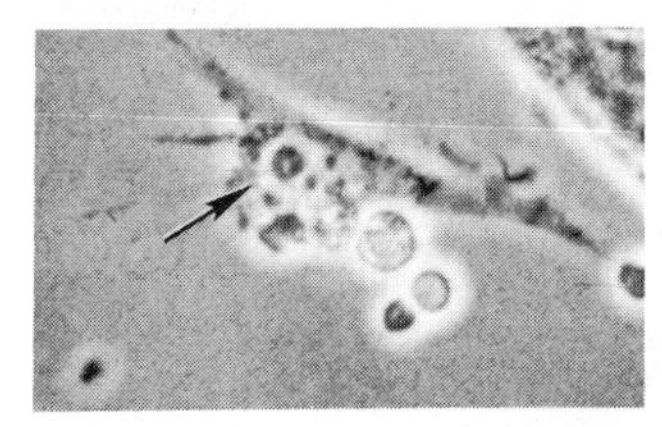

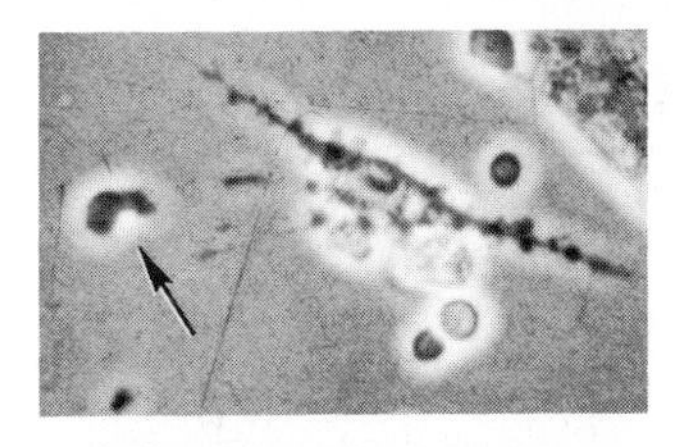

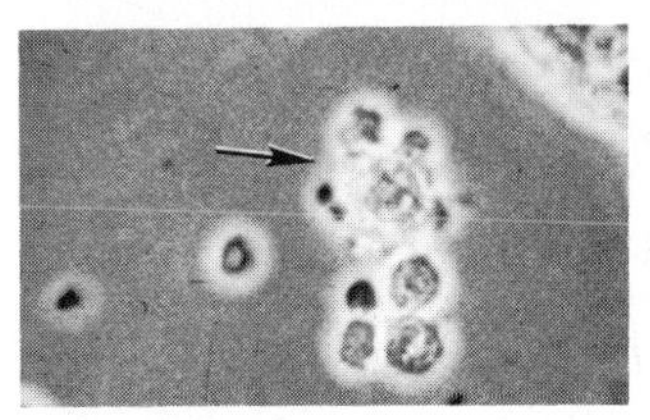

8-7 *B lymphocytes destroy a cancer cell.* Top photograph: *A B lymphocyte* (arrow) *attacks a cancer cell flattened on a microscope slide.* Second photograph: *The B lymphocyte has penetrated the cancer cell membrane; other B lymphocytes are moving toward the cell.* Third photograph: *The B lymphocytes retreat from the cell; the "kill" now begins.* Bottom photograph: *The dead cancer cell* (arrow), *now just a mass of protoplasm.*

[41] Cancer patients display both types of immune response, the antigen-antibody response and the cell-mediated response (described in Chapter 6, pages 141–45). How then can cancers grow to be destructive? Unfortunately, a growing tumor does not seem to induce a maximum immune response. Certainly the response is not strong enough to destroy most cancers. It has been estimated that the immune response can destroy 1 to 2 million cancer cells. However, a tiny cancer that is only 1 cm. in diameter (0.3934 inches) contains about 1 billion cancer cells. By the time they can be diagnosed, most cancers have overwhelmed the body's immune response. (Donald S. Morton, "Immunotherapy of Human Cancer," *SCANcer,* Vol. 4, No. 5 [September 1972], p. 2.)

[42] Roger Lewin, "New Assaults on Cancer," *World,* Vol. 2, No. 4 (February 13, 1973), pp. 32, 34, 55. More help may come from yet another source. Beginning research suggests that in some acute leukemia, the BCG vaccine used against tuberculosis (page 152) may prolong remission periods, during which all signs and symptoms temporarily disappear. (George N. Santos, "Immunological Concepts and Their Potential Role in Cancer Therapy," p. 197, citing G. Mathe *et al.,* "Active Immunotherapy for Acute Lymphoblastic Leukaemia," *Lancet,* Vol. 1, No. 7597 [April 5, 1969], pp. 697–99.) A specially prepared BCG vaccine is now being tried as a nonspecific booster to the immune response. ("A Better Antitumor Mix," *Medical World News,* Vol. 13, No. 19 [May 12, 1972], p. 61.) However, to claim it successful at this time would be highly premature.

[43] B. Cinader, "Immunodiagnostic Tests for Cancer," *Canadian Medical Journal,* Vol. 107, No. 7 (July 8, 1972), p. 7.

[44] "An Antigen Test Detects 50 of 51 Tumors of Breast," *Hospital Tribune,* Vol. 6, No. 5 (March 6, 1972), pp. 1 and 16.

[45] "Cancer Vaccine Outlook: Hopeful, but Not Soon," *Journal of the American Medical Association,* Vol. 219, No. 12 (March 20, 1972), pp. 1555–56.

[46] This is partly because of the varying kinds of antigens produced by the different cancers of different animals. To be effective, a cancer vaccine must be made with antigens that are similar for each cancer. Even here, however, there is hope. It is possible that some animal cancers are caused by the same or a similar virus. Should this be the case, immunization against this virus is not beyond the scope of possibility. Such immunization would make it feasible for a patient to make his own antibodies against a cancer. Is passive, borrowed immunity (see pages 154–55) a possibility? Can specific antibodies, made in another animal, be injected into human beings, for both the diagnosis and treatment of cancers? Recent work in this area is encouraging. ("Specific Antibodies—Next Aid in Cancer Diagnosis, Treatment?" *Journal of the American Medical Association,* Vol. 224, No. 11 [June 11, 1973], pp. 1473–74.)

other possibilities for detection, treatment, and cure

From laboratories throughout the world come new methods of detection and treatment, and new pieces of information that will someday add up to a cancer cure. A vaccine, prepared with mouse leukemia virus (see Figure 8-8), has been found to prevent the disease in certain laboratory animals. In mice, interferon (page 160) inhibits viruses known to cause animal cancers, delays the progression of some forms of mouse leukemia, and produces regression not only of some mouse leukemias but also of mammary gland tumors that have been transplanted from one mouse to another. Moreover, it has been shown that interferon destroys only the cancer cells, not normal cells. In the western United States, an investigator extracted a chemical from the wings of the Taiwanese yellow cabbage butterfly that was effective against a tumor in an experimental rat.[47] In a midwestern laboratory, another researcher has developed a "dip-stick" urine test for one of the most common and lethal cancers of childhood.[48] From an eastern laboratory a simplified test for solid tumors has been announced.[49] At three major U.S. laboratories, a platinum compound is being tested for its ability to dissipate a wide variety of tumors.[50] At the National Cancer Institute a chemical from a rare Chinese tree is said to be effective against some cancers. It holds so much promise for the treatment of cancer of the colon that the U.S. Department of Agriculture has planted some 50,000 seedlings of it.[51] *Vinca rosea,* the West Indian periwinkle, has yielded two valuable antitumor drugs, and a derivative of the American May apple may be useful in treating advanced Hodgkin's disease.[52] From Japan, where stomach cancer is a shocking national tragedy,[53] comes the gastrocamera, which provides unrivaled pictures of the stomach's interior.[54] New X-ray techniques provide a means of early diagnosis of breast tumors long before they can be felt.[55] In Canada, an antigen has been isolated from certain bowel tumors that does not appear in normal tissue; a test has been developed that detects as little as one billionth of a part of this antigen in the blood.

8-8 *The virus that causes mouse leukemia* ($\times$ *150,000*).

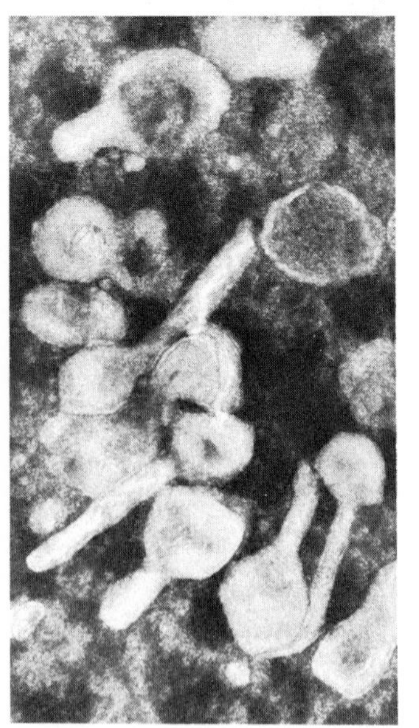

The Annual of Czechoslovak Medical Literature has recently noted that 2,200 works on cancer are published yearly in thirty languages.[56] More than twenty-five years ago the famous German surgeon August Bier remarked, "There is a tremendous literature on cancer, but what we know for sure about it can be printed on a calling card."[57] No longer is that true.

The search for a solution will yield no single cure for so very complicated a

[47] "Waiting in the Wings?" *Medical World News,* Vol. 12, No. 36 (October 1, 1971), pp. 6–7.
[48] "A Dip-Stick to Find a Cancer," *Medical World News,* Vol. 13, No. 15 (April 14, 1972), p. 49.
[49] "A Test That Spots 90% of Carcinomas," *Medical World News,* Vol. 13, No. 22 (June 2, 1972), pp. 16–17.
[50] "Platinum Compound Possesses Tumor-Dissipating Activity," *Journal of the American Medical Association,* Vol. 216, No. 4 (April 26, 1971), pp. 597–98.
[51] "Chinese Tree Yields Drug Effective Against Cancer," *Journal of the American Medical Association,* Vol. 212, No. 4 (April 27, 1970), pp. 555–56.
[52] "Cancer Chemotherapy," *MD, Medical Newsmagazine,* Vol. 15, No. 7 (July 1972), p. 70.
[53] "Epidemiology of Gastric Cancer," *The New England Journal of Medicine,* Vol. 286, No. 6 (February 10, 1972), pp. 316–17.
[54] Philip J. Hodes, "Advances in Diagnostic Radiology," *Postgraduate Medicine,* Vol. 48, No. 5 (November 1970), pp. 79–83.
[55] *Ibid.*
[56] "Miscellaneous Intelligence," *Nature,* Vol. 225, No. 5233 (February 14, 1970), p. 581.
[57] Quoted in "Cancer Moonshot, Part II: The Researchers Speak," *Medical World News,* Vol. 12, No. 12 (March 26, 1971), p. 27.

disease. Despite the dolorous data about many cancers, the U.S. picture is by no means all gloom. The Pap smear and better personal hygiene are together responsible for a remarkable decline in the death rate from cancer of the cervix and uterus. In forty years the death rate from uterine cancer has dropped about 65 percent.[58] Since the 1930s the incidence of cancer of the stomach in both men and women has declined almost 70 percent; some investigators suggest that the trace element selenium and vitamin E found in breakfast cereals may be responsible for the decline.[59] Treatment with drugs "is now the key factor responsible for long-term survival in at least ten types of widespread cancer occurring largely in children, adolescents, and young adults."[60] The incidence of one form of leukemia in children under the age of five has dropped remarkably during recent years, and, for those who do develop the disease, new treatments have given years of life.[61] Various agencies of the U.S. government have ordered many industrial cancer-causers out of use; the use of some possibly cancer-causing pesticides and food additives is being sharply limited. The Atomic Energy Commission has repeatedly lowered allowable levels of radiation exposure, and there is even evidence that the number of "former smokers" in the nation is increasing—raising hopes for a decline in lung cancer.[62] And even that major killer is now being treated more successfully, especially when detected in its early stages. Some physicians report almost 50 percent of their lung cancer patients to be alive and well three years after diagnosis.[63] U.S. government support of research and service programs for cancer is enormous; a particularly meaningful act was the change, in 1971, of Fort Detrick, Maryland, from a vast laboratory devoted to research on bacteriological warfare to one devoted to warfare against cancer. In 1972, an agreement was reached between the United States and the Soviet Union to exchange cancer research information,[64] and the World Health Organization has long played a significant role in cancer research.

summary

In this century, the longer life span enjoyed by humans has increased their chances of developing *chronic degenerative diseases* (page 193). One chronic degenerative disease, cancer, is the subject of this chapter.

Cancer may be described as cellular anarchy (page 193). Normal cell growth or

[58] Clifton R. Read, "The Cancer Women Can Defeat," *Family Health,* Vol. 5, No. 3 (March 1973), p. 26.

[59] Thomas H. Maugh II, "Trace Elements: A Growing Appreciation of Their Effects on Man," *Science,* Vol. 181, No. 4096 (July 20, 1973), p. 253.

[60] C. Gordon Zubrod, "The Basis for Progress in Chemotherapy," *CA—A Cancer Journal for Clinicians,* Vol. 23, No. 4 (July–August 1973), p. 203.

[61] Marvin A. Schneiderman and James A. Peters, "Cancer Prevention," Letters, *Science,* Vol. 178, No. 4062 (November 17, 1972), pp. 697–98.

[62] *Ibid.*

[63] " 'Incurable' Tag for All Lung Ca Seen as Much Too Pessimistic," *Internal Medicine News,* Vol. 6, No. 1 (January 1, 1973), pp. 3 and 14.

[64] "1972: Year of the Quest," AMA Health Education Service for Schools and Colleges, Vol. 13, No. 3 (March 1973), p. 1, citing "Medicine in Review—1972," *AMA News Release,* December 25, 1972.

division is controlled by the body's genetic material. But tumor cells escape normal body controls and continue to divide (page 194). *Tumors* are masses of cells that result from the uncontrolled division (page 194). *Benign tumors* are localized, encapsulated cellular overgrowths. They are not cancers, but may cause harm by interfering with bodily function (pages 194–95). *Malignant tumors* are the cancers. They are not contained within a capsule, so they can penetrate normal tissue, destroy normal cells, and, ultimately, kill (page 195).

Cancer begins with an abnormal change in a single cell, a change that is passed on to succeeding generations of cells (page 195). The malignant cells either eventually form a mass—a *"solid" tumor*—or immediately become widespread throughout the body—a *"generalized" tumor* (page 195). These two types of tumors are classified according to the tissue from which they arise:

"Solid" tumors are (1) the *carcinomas,* the most common form of cancer, which arise from the epithelial cells of the skin, of glandular organs (such as the breast), and of mucous membranes lining the mouth, stomach, and lungs (page 195); and (2) the *sarcomas,* which arise from connective tissue, muscle, bone, and cartilage (page 195). "Solid" tumors *metastasize;* that is, some cancer cells break loose from their original sites and travel to other body locations, where they seed new and secondary malignant growths (page 195).

"Generalized" tumors are (1) the *leukemias,* which arise in the blood-forming tissues and are characterized by uncontrolled multiplication and accumulation of white blood cells (page 196); and (2) the *lymphomas,* which arise from some of the body's infection-fighting structures, such as the lymph nodes (page 196).

There are four basic groups of cancer causes:

1. *physical.* Some substances—for example, uranium—emit cancer-causing radiations as they degenerate (page 196).

2. *chemical.* Cancer has been known to result from prolonged exposure to some chemical *carcinogens* (cancer-producing substances) (page 197).

3. *genetic.* It is known that heredity plays a role in human cancer, though the exact nature of that role remains unclear (page 197).

4. *viral.* Cancer can be caused in animals by viruses, containing either DNA or RNA (pages 199–200). They move into an animal cell and then, after lying dormant within its genes for a while, may be "switched on" by some stimulus—chemicals, another virus, some nonviral disease—to start the cellular changes that result in cancer (page 200). Some animal cancers (cat and chicken) may be contagious. No virus has yet been proved to cause human cancer (pages 200–01).

At present rates, one U.S. citizen in four will develop cancer. There has recently been an increase of some cancers among U.S. blacks (page 203). The survival rates of poor cancer patients are apparently lower than those of people who can afford to pay, but only in the first year of treatment (page 203).

There are three basic methods for preventing cancer: (1) *avoiding ecological factors* associated with a high incidence of cancer (pages 203–04); (2) *removal of lesions* that may become malignant (page 203); (3) *discouraging marriages that might produce children with a high risk of developing cancer* (page 203).

Knowledge of the warning signals of cancer and a thorough annual physical examination are crucial to the cure of cancer. There is evidence of a familial susceptibility to breast cancer. All women should examine their breasts every month (page 205). At present, cancers are treated by *surgical removal, radiation, drugs,* or a combination of the three (page 207). Treatment involving the body's own *immune response* may also prove to be of value (pages 208–09).

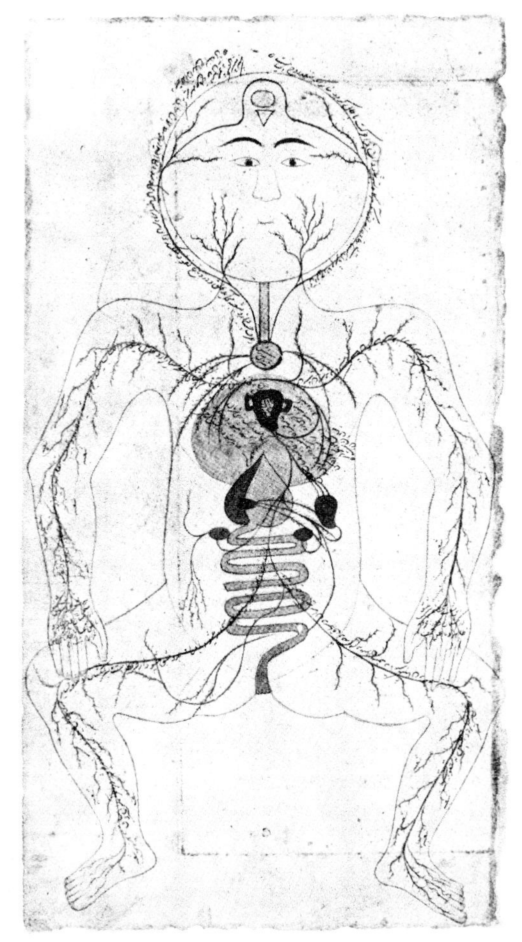

A 16th-century Persian drawing of the body's system of arteries.

circulation and filtration

9

the body's circulatory system

Two hundred years ago an autopsy was being carried out by the English physician Edward Jenner. Jenner's friend Caleb Parry recorded his words:

> I was making a . . . section of the heart . . . when my knife struck something so hard and gritty, as to notch it. I well remember looking up to the ceiling, which was old and crumbling, conceiving that some plaster had fallen down. But on a further scrutiny the real cause appeared: the coronaries [the blood vessels supplying the heart] were become bony canals.[1]

The man Jenner examined had succumbed to a degenerative process of the circulatory system that kills more people in this country today than any other condition—*atherosclerosis.* To understand this and other circulatory problems, one must know something about the circulatory system and how it functions.

In its broadest meaning, the term *circulatory system* refers to the channels through which flow the nutrient and other vital needs of the body. As will be seen below, this is a more inclusive term than the word *cardiovascular,* which pertains only to that part of the body's circulatory system composed of the heart and blood vessels. In this section, the cardiovascular apparatus—the heart, the blood vessels, and the blood within them—will be discussed first. Then the discussion of the circulation will be expanded to include the ''trade routes'' of the blood. As these routes of the circulatory system are traced, it will become apparent how the necessities of life are brought to each cell and how that cell is relieved of its wastes so that it can remain vital. Then will follow a brief description of the circulation not of blood, but of a body fluid called *lymph.* The rest of this section on the circulatory system will be concerned with impairments of the cardiovascular apparatus.

the cardiovascular apparatus

The cardiovascular apparatus is the body's inner transportation system. By means of the circulation of blood within it, (1) oxygen, nutrients, hormones, and other vital materials are delivered to cells of all the body tissues and organs, and (2) wastes (carbon dioxide and other products) are transported from these cells to points of elimination such as the kidneys or liver. The circulating blood is also involved in (3) fighting infection, and the blood vessels help in (4) regulating body temperature. When skin blood vessels are dilated (widened), body heat is dissipated; when they are constricted (narrowed), heat is conserved.

the heart of a sprightly gentleman

England has had few monarchs so graceful as the ill-starred Charles I (he was executed in 1649). Devoted to ceremony (Charles was the only European monarch of his time who was served on bended knee), he loved good living. But

[1] Caleb Hillier Parry, *An Inquiry Into the Symptoms and Causes of the Syncope Angiosa, Commonly called Angina Pectoris,* quoted in Henry J. Speedby, *The 20th Century and Your Heart* (London, 1960), p. 84.

he also appreciated science. This led him to permit his friend and family physician, William Harvey, to dissect deer in the royal park. Such royal empathy helped Harvey to discover the circulation of the blood.

When King Charles heard of the astonishing case of the young Irish Viscount Montgomery, he dispatched Harvey to investigate. As a child, the Viscount had endured an accidental chest wound, leaving, in Harvey's words, "a vast hole in his breast, into which I could easily put my three Fore-fingers and my Thumb: . . . I perceived a certain fleshy part sticking out, which was driven in and out by a reciprocal motion, whereupon I gently handled it in my hand." The wound had "miraculously healed and skinned over with a membrane on the Inside, and guarded with flesh all about the brimmes." The Viscount's man servant daily cleansed the wound. Harvey brought "the young and sprightly gentleman" to the king. Thus, more than three hundred years ago, patron king and physician friend together felt the pulsing heart and, through the wound, noted also the "motion of his Heart; . . . in . . . Diastole it was drawn in and retracted, and in the Systole came forth, and was thrust out."[2]

Such dynamic observations helped to make modern heart surgery possible.

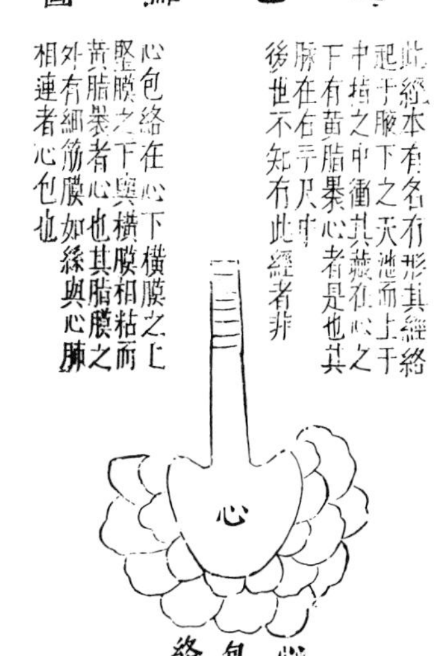

9-1 *The heart, from an early 17th-century Chinese book.*

the heart as a double pump

The adult heart (Figure 9-2) is a fist-sized, $12\frac{1}{2}$-ounce muscular organ located beneath the breastbone, in the left center of the chest (see body chart 9 in the color section). It is above the diaphragm and between the lungs and is enveloped and suspended in a loose *pericardial* sac containing lubricating (pericardial) fluid.

Each of the two sides of the heart has an upper chamber, the *atrium* (Latin for hall), and a lower chamber, the *ventricle* (Latin for belly, so named because ventricles are the large cavities of the heart). The two sides of the heart are separated by a wall, or *septum,* in which there is normally no opening. Each atrium is a very temporary storage chamber, holding the blood for less than a second. And each atrium is separated from the ventricle below it by a valve. To permit blood to flow through it, the valve opens. To prevent blood from flowing backwards, it closes. The valve between the right atrium and the right ventricle is called the *tricuspid valve* (Latin *tricuspis,* having three flaps or cusps). The two-pointed or *biscuspid valve,* between the left atrium and left ventricle, is also called the *mitral valve.* It is shaped somewhat like a bishop's mitre.

Although the heart is a single organ, it circulates blood in two separate circuits. For each circuit the heart has a separate pump. In the smaller *pulmonary circuit* (Latin *pulmo,* lung), blood is pumped by the right ventricle to the lungs (via the pulmonary artery) and returns to the left atrium (via the pulmonary veins). In passing through the lungs, the blood gives up carbon dioxide and takes on oxygen (see Figure 9-4). The pump of the larger *systemic circuit* is the

[2] From *Anatomical Exercitations,* quoted in George Keynes, *The Life of William Harvey* (Oxford, 1966), p. 156. *Systole* (the contraction of the heart) and *diastole* (the dilatation and relaxation of the heart) are discussed on page 217.

From the pacemaker—the sinoatrial (S-A) node—rhythmic impulses fan out over the atria. The atria then contract. The impulses then continue to the atrioventricular (A-V) node, where specialized fibers begin—the atrioventricular bundle of His. This conducts impulses to right and left atrioventricular bundles, which go on to Purkinje fibers. These distribute impulses to the ventricles and the papillary muscles. As the ventricles contract, the papillary muscles stabilize the tricuspid and bicuspid valves via their fine tendinous cords (chordae tendineae).

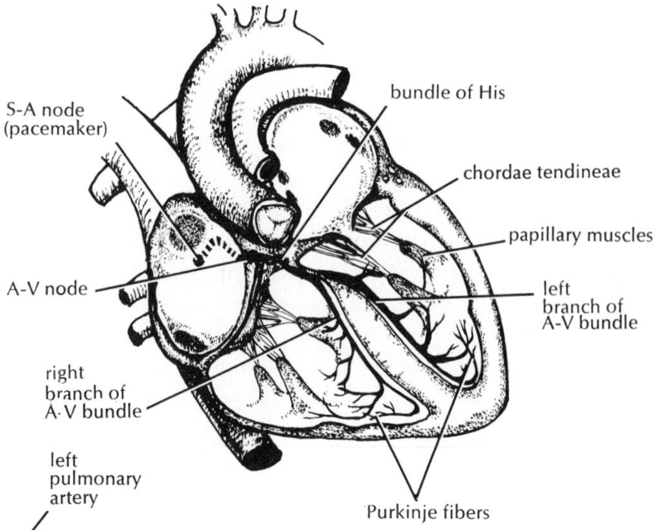

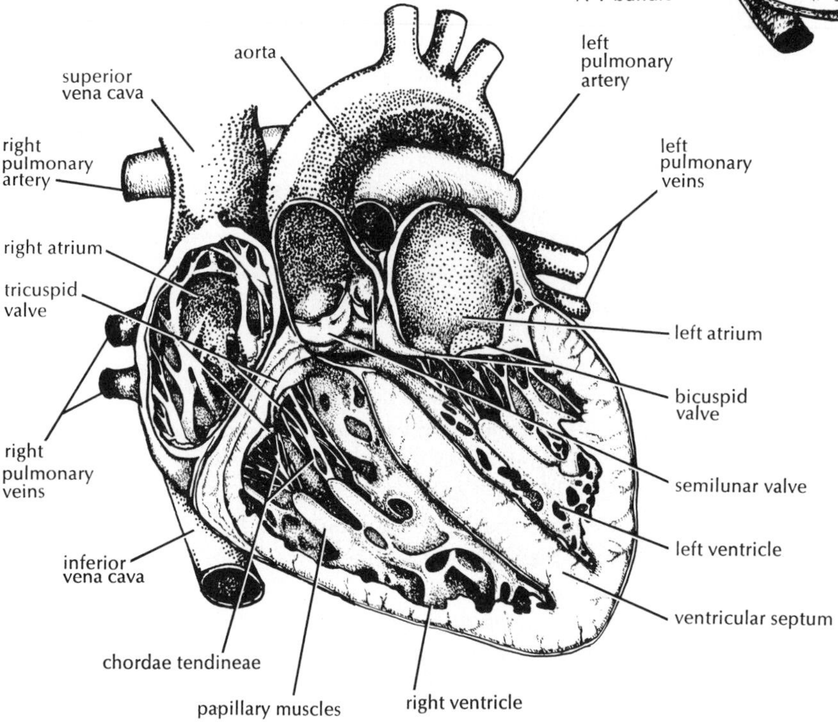

9-2 *The heart: general anatomy* (left) *and electrical pathways* (above).

left ventricle, which sends blood, via the *aorta,* to the rest of the body. The superior vena cava and the inferior vena cava return the venous blood from the body to the right atrium.

the heart as an electrical mechanism

The sheer labor of the human heart is wondrous. In a seventy-year lifetime, it will beat 2.5 billion times and pump some 600,000 tons of blood. Every minute every drop of blood travels the distance from the heart to the tissues and back again. What keeps the heart beating rhythmically? Specialized cells in the heart known as the *conducting system* are responsible. Within the right atrial wall is one group of such cells called the *pacemaker,* located in the *sinoatrial node* (Figure 9-2). Located in the septal wall dividing the atria is another group of specialized cells. This second group of conducting cells is the *atrioventricular node.* Inherent within the pacemaker is the remarkable ability to emit rhythmic bursts of electrical impulses. The pacemaker discharges its impulses and then recharges itself about seventy times a minute. With each electrical impulse, both atria are directly stimulated to contract almost simultaneously. The stimulus then quickly spreads to the atrioventricular node. This node then sends stimuli to the ventricles. The ventricles also contract almost simultaneously. The contraction phase, during which blood is squeezed out of the heart into the systemic and pulmonary circulation, is called *systole.* Between beats the heart rests. This period is *diastole.* During diastole the chambers of the heart fill with blood entering from the veins.

In addition to the intrinsic electrical cardiac mechanism described above, the heart can also be greatly influenced by sympathetic nerves, which increase its action, and by parasympathetic nerves, which decrease its activity. Thus, parasympathetic nerves affect the heart during rest. During stress, such as exercise and heat, sympathetic nerves increase the heart rate (see page 242).

the blood vessels

ARTERIES AND VEINS Blood is carried from the heart to the tissues by a closed system of *arteries;* it is carried from the tissues to the heart by a closed system of *veins.* Within these veins, one-way valves prevent the back-flow (see body chart 10 in the color section). The thick elastic walls of the arteries serve to withstand the heart's pumping pressure of blood. Vein walls are thin. In veins, the blood flows under less pressure, although this flow may be speeded by body muscle contraction.

ARTERIOLES, CAPILLARIES, AND VENULES Between the arterial and venous circulations are microscopic canals called *capillaries.* They are so narrow that, in some, red blood cells can only pass through in single file. So numerous are the capillaries that, in volume, they make up most of the circulatory system.

The smallest *endings* of the arteries, the *arterioles,* end in the capillaries. The smallest *beginnings* of the veins, the *venules,* begin from capillaries (see Figure 9-3).

9-3 *The relationship of arterioles, capillaries, and venules.*

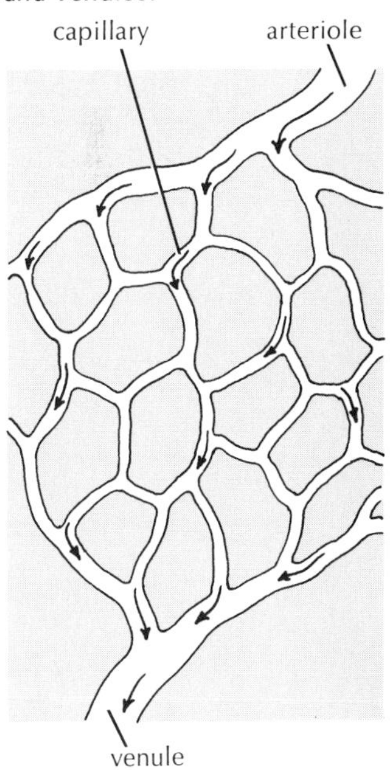

THE CORONARY CIRCULATION How does the heart itself receive its blood supply? From seepage of the blood that constantly courses through it? No. The heart has its own blood supply. Like all other organs, arteries lead to it, and veins lead away from it. But the heart receives first choice of the blood that, fresh from the lungs, is newly oxygenated (see Figure 9-4). Even before the great aorta branches off to carry blood to the head, trunk, or limbs, it gives off two crucial branches, the *coronary arteries.* Like an inverted crown or corona, these embrace the heart. After supplying the heart muscle with blood, the coro-

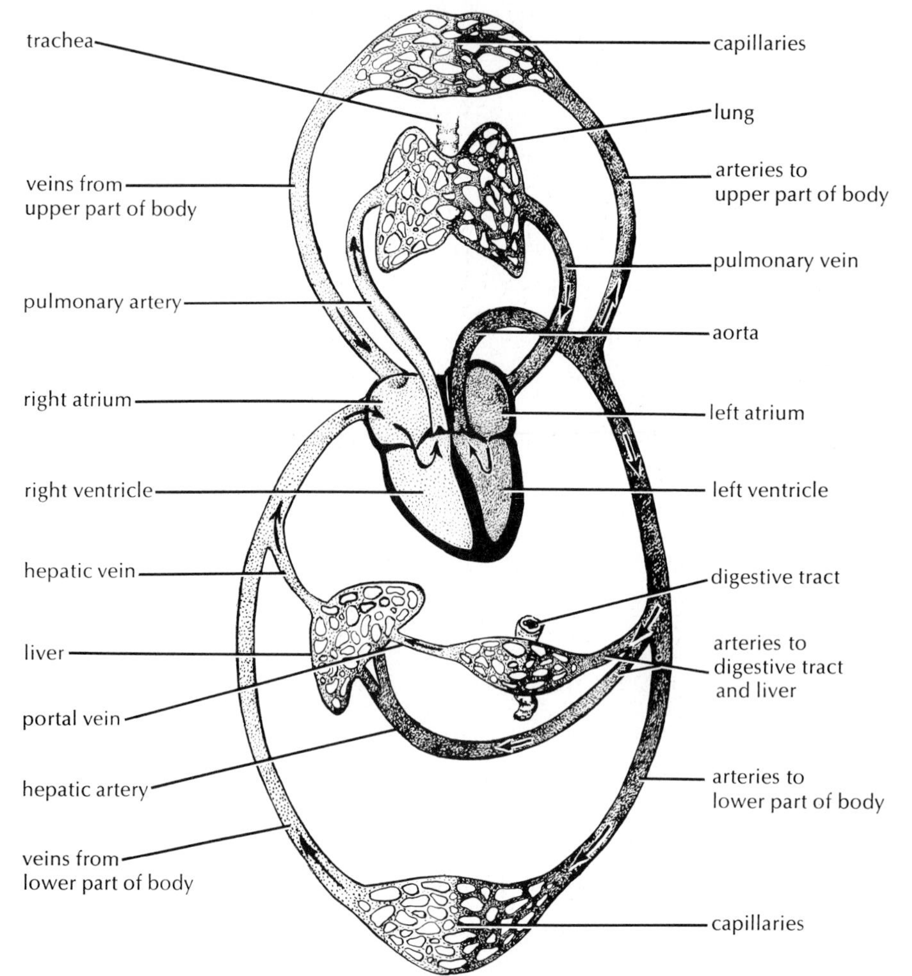

9-4 *The two circuits of blood circulation: the* pulmonary, *in which blood is pumped by the right ventricle to the lungs and back to the left atrium, and the* systemic, *in which blood is pumped by the left ventricle to the rest of the body. Oxygenated blood is shown here in darker gray.*

nary arteries eventually terminate in a capillary bed, which empties into veins ultimately discharging venous blood into the right atrium.

Like capillaries elsewhere in the body, the capillaries of the heart have an important characteristic. Unless they are needed because of unusual activity, many lie empty and unused. There is no nerve control of capillaries to make them dilate. Carbon dioxide accumulation in tissue, as well as nerve controls, causes dilation of arterioles. The capillaries respond passively to the arteriolar dilation, thus regulating the volume and flow of blood within them. If a segment of the heart has been damaged, the capillary reserve in heart muscle tissue can be lifesaving.

Now follows a discussion of the blood "that swift as quicksilver . . . courses through the natural gates and alleys of the body."[3]

[3] William Shakespeare, *Hamlet,* I.v.66–67.

the blood: fluid tissue of transport

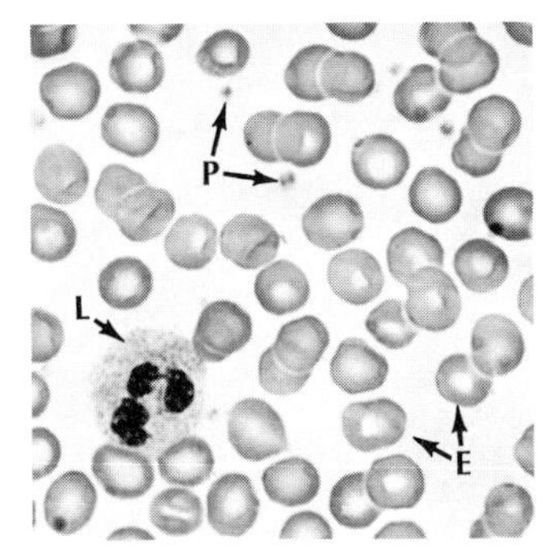

9-5 *Human blood cells: red cells, or erythrocytes (E), white cells, or leukocytes (L), and platelets (P).*

The nine liquid pints of blood in the body of the average human being teem with floating, suspended cells. The liquid, called *plasma,* is largely (80 percent) sea water. Man's evolution from sea life involved taking the sea water characteristic of that geological time with him. Sea water and plasma share the same salts but in different concentrations. The precise concentration of the plasma salts must be maintained within narrow limits. Otherwise cells die. With excess sweating, for example, body fluid and salt (sodium chloride) are lost. In some circumstances, the family physician might suggest salt tablets to prevent the salt concentration in the plasma from falling below the proper level.

The cells suspended in the blood plasma are as follows (Figure 9-5):

1. *Erythrocytes* (Greek *erythros,* red + *kytos,* hollow vessel). In the blood of the average adult male are some 25 trillion (1 trillion is a million million) red cells. The average adult female's blood contains about 17 trillion. These comprise 99.9 percent of the total blood cells. They have no nuclei. The average red blood cell circulates for about 120 days before it disintegrates and is replaced. Other red blood cells are constantly being manufactured in the bone marrow. For this manufacture, vitamin B_{12} and folic acid are essential.

A complex protein called *hemoglobin* is formed in the cytoplasm of the red blood cells. The iron it contains gives the hemoglobin molecule the ability to combine with and release both oxygen and carbon dioxide. A diet deficient in iron leads to *anemia* (Greek *an,* negative + *haima,* blood + *ia*). Normally, there is a balance between the number of red blood cells produced and the number lost. Health depends upon this ecological balance in the blood's ecosystem. When this equilibrium is disturbed, the concentration of red blood cells in the blood is diminished and anemia results.[4] Added to iron deficiency as a cause of anemia is blood loss. This may be gradual or sudden. Sometimes red blood cells are destroyed, as occurs in *erythroblastosis fetalis,* which is due to problems involving the Rh blood factor (see page 553). Inadequate production of red blood cells can result in *pernicious anemia;* this occurs because of a vitamin B_{12} deficiency. Rarer causes of anemia are poisons or excessive ionizing radiation.

Symptoms of anemia can vary from the mild but extremely distressing headache, weakness, and shortness of breath occurring with moderate iron deficiencies, to the far more serious consequences of severe hemorrhage. With anemia the blood cannot carry enough oxygen to the cells. Oxygen starvation ensues. Also, the heart tries to compensate for a decreased number of red blood cells bringing an inadequate amount of oxygen to the tissues. It works harder, trying to increase the speed of the circulating blood. In doing this, the heart is overworked. In severe and prolonged anemia the heart may enlarge and even fail.

2. *Leukocytes* (Greek *leukos,* white + *kytos*). Since leukocytes contain no hemoglobin to color them, they are also called *white blood cells.* About 75 billion of them defend the body against such stresses as infection. With most

[4] Rarely, an excess number of red blood cells is produced in the marrow, and this may lead to illness.

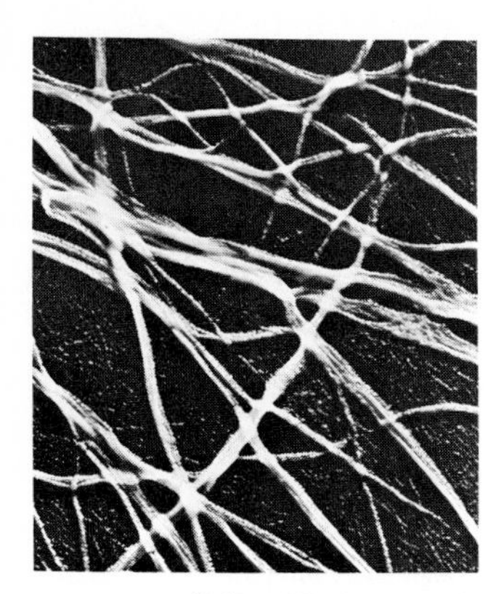

9-6 *Fibrin strands* (×*45,000*).

bacterial infections, leukocytes increase from a normal quantity of about seven thousand per cubic millimeter of blood to twelve thousand, twenty-five thousand, or even more. This increase is called *leukocytosis.* Pus is partly made of dead and dying leukocytes. Leukocytes consume bacteria by *phagocytosis* (see page 138). Most leukocytes are manufactured in the bone marrow. As has been seen (pages 141–43), certain leukocytes, such as *lymphocytes* and *macrophages,* are essential to immunity, the body's system of resistance to infection.

With cancer of leukocyte-producing tissue, white cells are overproduced. Moreover, they are usually abnormal cell types and unlike normal leukocytes, fight infection poorly. This is *leukemia* (see page 196). The number of leukocytes per cubic millimeter of blood may increase to a quarter of a million. This enormous overproduction interferes with erythrocyte manufacture. Anemia results. The invading white blood cells of leukemia overwhelm other tissues, interfering with their normal functions.

3. The third type of blood cells produced in the bone marrow are the *platelets.* By their involvement in clotting, they help to stop bleeding. Also important to clotting are proteins called *fibrinogen* and *fibrin* (Figure 9-6). Plasma from which fibrinogen has been separated in the process of clotting is *serum.*

BLOOD GROUPS Before the turn of this century, transfusion was often followed by severe reactions and even death. It was discovered that this occurred because a donor's blood was often incompatible with that of the recipient. This meant that the recipient was immune to certain proteins in the donor's blood cells. As a result, the antibodies in the recipient's serum caused clumping and disintegration of the donor's red blood cells. Thus, incompatibility depends on the absence or the presence of antigens in the red blood cells and of antibodies in the serum. A person's red blood cells could contain A or B antigens, both, or neither. His serum could contain anti-A or anti-B antibodies, both, or neither. When a donor's blood, containing one or more antigens, is transfused into a recipient's blood containing incompatible antibodies, the clumping of the recipient's red blood cells that occurs is called *agglutination.* The antigens are called *agglutinogens* and the antibodies, *agglutinins.* Four main blood groups are differentiated (see Table 9-1).

A *universal donor* is a person with group O blood. Since group O red blood cells contain no A or B antigen, group O blood can usually be used for anyone.

TABLE 9-1
The Basic Blood Groups

BLOOD GROUP	ANTIGENS (AGGLUTINOGENS) IN THE RED CELLS	ANTIBODIES (AGGLUTININS) IN THE SERUM
O	None	Anti-A and anti-B
A	A	Anti-B
B	B	Anti-A
AB	A and B	None

It is sometimes used in great emergencies when blood-typing of a recipient would be too time-consuming. People with group AB blood are *universal recipients.* Since their blood contains no anti-A or anti-B antibody, they can usually receive any blood with relative safety.

THE TRADE ROUTES OF THE BLOOD To trace human blood circulation one may begin at the tissue-cell–capillary level (see Figure 9-7). These billions of body depots are basic chemical communities. Within them occurs an alchemy of exchange. Tissue cells are wet. They are surrounded by sealike salt water, and the water is within them too. Through this bathing wetness, the oxygen diffuses into the hungry tissue cell. And, through this same wetness, the tissue cell rids itself of its waste gas—carbon dioxide. Then this waste gas seeps through the capillary wall. Some of it attaches itself to a red blood cell. The rest of it is dissolved in the plasma. At its capillary level each tissue cell breathes. What has occurred? An exchange of gases. And, as a gas, the carbon dioxide waste is eventually capable of being vaporized through the distant lung capillaries.

But much more than an exchange of oxygen and carbon dioxide gas occurs at the tissue-cell–capillary level. Also transferred from capillary blood to the tissue cell are nutrients and hormones, as well as other vital materials. Fluid from the plasma, not red cells, carries these necessities of life to the tissue cell.

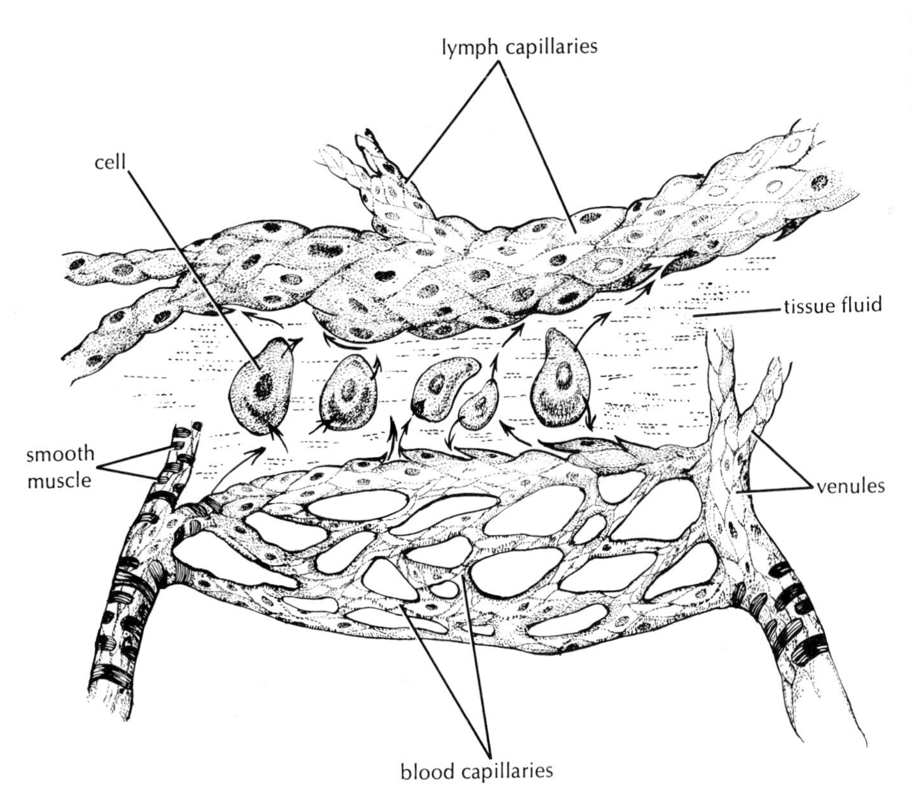

9-7 *Oxygen, nutrients, and other vital substances in the blood seep through the blood capillary walls into the fluid space surrounding the tissue cell. If there is then a higher concentration of a needed substance outside the cell than inside it, the cell membrane will admit it. Similarly, wastes traverse the cell membrane and reach the fluid spaces between the cells. The wastes may then be carried off with lymph (page 223) to eventually enter the venous blood, or they may enter venous blood by seeping directly into a blood capillary. The kidneys, liver, and lungs clear wastes from venous blood.*

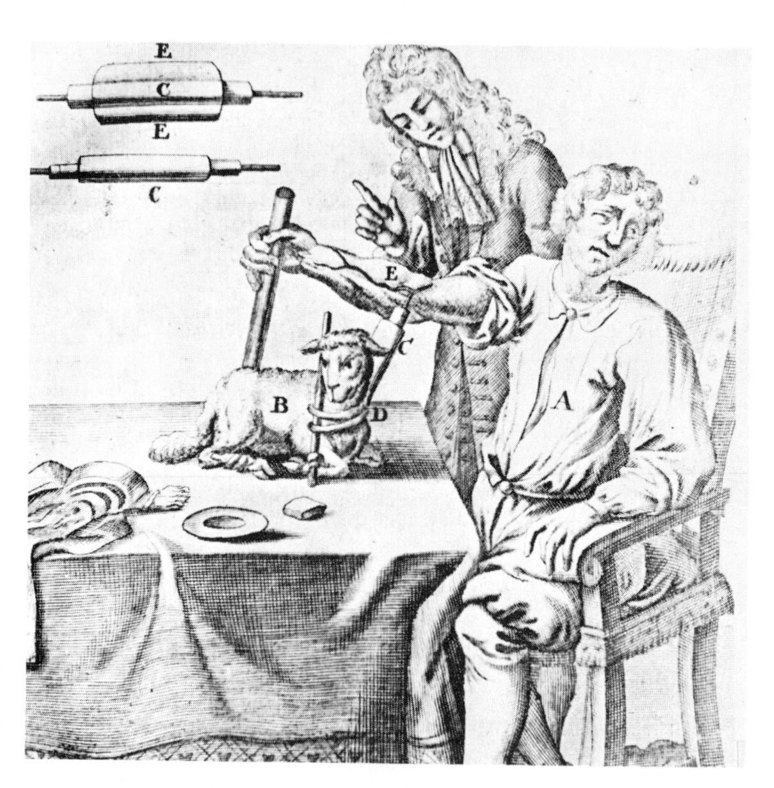

9-8 *An animal-to-man blood transfusion. First performed in 1667, such transfusions were usually intended as therapy for emotional disturbances rather than for replacement of lost blood.*

To survive, the tissue cell utilizes them. But, just as the tissue cell produces carbon dioxide from the use of oxygen, it produces additional wastes from the use of these other materials. Unlike carbon dioxide, this second type of waste is not gaseous. It cannot be vaporized through the lungs. Only with the help of the kidney and liver can it leave the body. Whether or not arterial blood reaching capillaries contains these wastes depends on whether or not the blood has yet passed through the liver and kidneys.

The blood, having provided the cells with their needs, and loaded with carbon dioxide and nonvaporescent wastes, continues along its route. It leaves the capillaries for the venules. Propelled by the contraction of muscles through which the veins course, the waste-laden blood proceeds toward the right heart. On the way it picks up blood from the liver, via the *portal vein* (see Figure 9-4). This blood contains nutrients that have been acted upon by the liver. Now containing nonvaporescent wastes, carbon dioxide, and food for the cells, the ''mixed'' blood reaches the right heart. It cannot reverse its flow because of the one-way valves of the veins. By way of two large veins—the *superior vena cava* (draining the upper body) and the *inferior vena cava* (draining the lower body)—the blood enters the heart's right atrium (see Figure 9-2).

As soon as the right atrium is filled with mixed blood, it contracts. The tricuspid valve is forced open. Blood pours into the right ventricle. The moment the right ventricle is filled, the tricuspid valve closes (thus blood cannot seep back into the atrium). Immediately the filled right ventricle contracts. Blood enters the pulmonary artery and is propelled to the lungs. It continues on into branching, spreading arteries of diminishing size (arterioles) until it reaches the maze of lung capillaries. Single file, the red blood cells course through the capillaries, ridding themselves of poisonous carbon dioxide and of water vapor (but not of other wastes), while taking on life-giving oxygen. From the lung's capillaries, newly oxygenated blood, still containing nonvaporescent wastes and nutrients, continues on into tiny lung veins (venules) and then to increasingly larger veins until it reaches the four large pulmonary veins. These enter the heart's left atrium.

The blood that enters the left atrium contains life-giving oxygen and nutrients and some potentially death-dealing wastes. The first two must be delivered to the waiting cells. The wastes must be eliminated by the kidneys and the liver. How?

When the left atrium is filled, it contracts. The bicuspid (mitral) valve is forced open. Blood pours into the left ventricle. As soon as the left ventricle is filled, the mitral valve closes to prevent back-flow. At once the left ventricle contracts. (Its muscle is thicker than that of the right ventricle because its circuit is longer. The right ventricle needs to pump blood only through the pulmonary circuit. The left ventricle must pump blood a much greater distance.) It pumps blood into that greatest of all arteries, the *aorta.* From the aorta, large arteries carry cellular wastes as well as oxygen and cellular nourishment to the liver and the kidneys. It is the liver and the kidneys that will finally rid the body of all the remaining cellular wastes. As with all other body cells, nourishing food and oxygen are brought to the liver and kidney cells. The liver and kidneys, then, must deal with two different wastes. One is produced by their own cells. The other is the remaining waste not vaporized in the lung. Both kinds of nonvaporescent wastes ultimately end in the urine and the bile, to be eliminated via the kidney and intestine, respectively. Blood, rid of wastes, continues on through progressively larger veins. Eventually, the right heart is reached. After circulating through the lung and left heart, cleansed, newly oxygenated blood is ready for distribution to the cells.

The circle is complete.

the lymphatic system

Like the blood capillaries, the terminal vessels of the lymphatic system begin at the cellular level (see Figure 9-7). (Figure 22-12, page 690, shows the lymphatic blood vessels in the villi of the small intestine.) Unlike the blood capillaries, the lymphatic capillaries do not act as tiny connecting canals between two larger vessels. Originating as blind-ended, microscopic vessels, the lymphatic capillaries, moreover, do not communicate with the blood capillaries, although they may intermingle with them. At the level of the cells, the fluid within the lymphatic capillaries is exactly like the fluid in the extracellular spaces. Within the lymphatic system, that fluid is called *lymph* (Latin *lympha,* water). The lymphatic capillaries coalesce, blending to form larger vessels, and these, in turn, coalesce to form even larger vessels. An accessory circulatory system containing lymph is thus formed (see Figure 9-10). In their course the

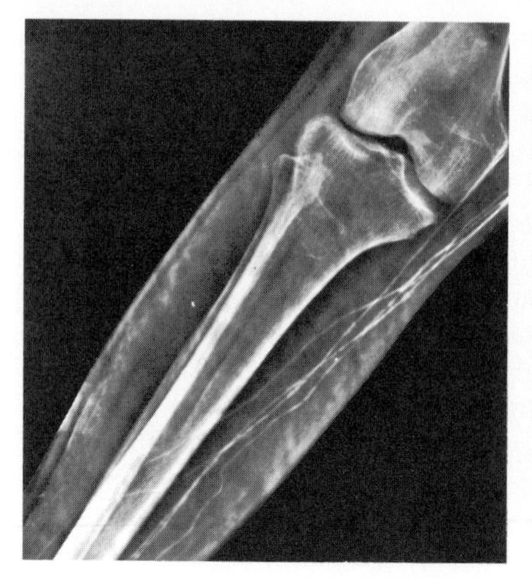

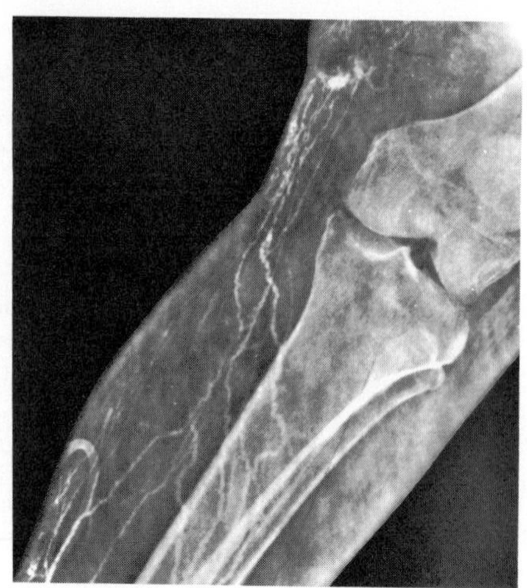

9-9 *Lymphangiograms—X-ray photographs of lymphatic vessels, which are made visible by injecting a radiopaque dye into them. In the normal leg* (left), *the lymphatics appear as thin, straight vessels. In the swollen leg* (right), *the lymphatics are both more numerous and widely distributed; they are also tortuous, beaded, and dilated. An obstruction to the lymph flow in the groin caused this condition.*

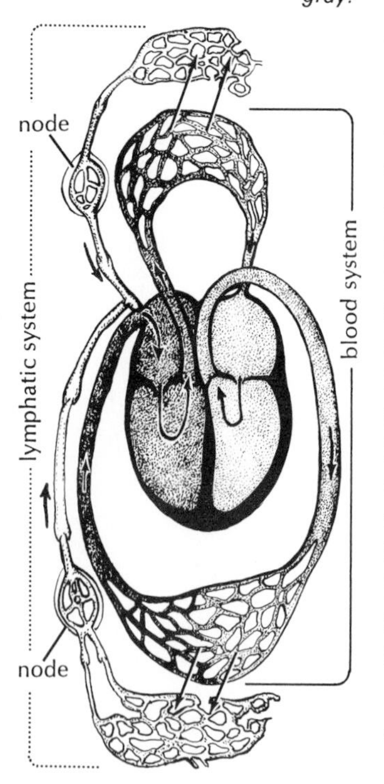

9-10 *A schematic diagram of the blood and lymphatic circulatory systems. Oxygenated blood is shown here in lighter gray.*

vessels of the lymphatic system never connect with the blood vessels until they finally empty, as two large lymphatic trunks, into veins in the neck. By the lymphatic channels, large protein molecules, which had originally left the blood plasma to seep through blood capillaries into the extracellular spaces, are returned to the blood, and so a critical factor in the body's ecosystem is kept in balance. But lymph also contains white cells loaded with cellular debris, toxins, and other wastes (even bacteria) that must be kept out of the blood. This service is provided by the *lymph nodes.* Lymphatic vessels lead to these discrete organizations of specialized lymphoid tissue. Lymph nodes are not "lymph glands," for they do not secrete anything. Before lymph reaches the circulation, it is filtered in the lymph nodes. By special cells within the nodes, cellular debris and other wastes are digested and made harmless. It is in the lymph nodes that lymphocytes proliferate and plasma cells make antibodies (page 141). In some parts of the body, lymph node tissue groups to form organs. The best known are the *tonsils* and *adenoids.* They can become diseased and may need to be removed.[5] The largest lymphoid organ, the fist-sized *spleen* (see Figure 22-7, page 675), is situated in front of the left kidney and to the left of the stomach. It plays a role in the process of immunity and helps remove used blood cells. The spleen also filters some lymph and blood. It is, moreover, one of the sites for the manufacture of a protein-clotting factor that prevents normal people from having hemophilia, a rare hereditary disease in which blood clots slowly or not at all. Many of its functions are not clearly delineated. Its removal, a common operation, is not met by serious problems. With removal of the spleen the clotting factor is not lost; other body parts are believed to make this important substance, among them probably the liver.

[5] Infection can acutely inflame the lymphatics, causing *lymphangitis.* When this occurs a red line can often be observed extending from the source of infection to enlarged and tender local lymph nodes.

terms describing impediments to the flow of the vital stream

The circulating blood is life's vital stream. And as all parts of the system in which the blood circulates are connected, so are the disorders that affect these parts related. A clot that plugs an artery deprives a portion of the cerebrum of nourishing blood. This condition is called *cerebral ischemia* (Greek *ischein,* to suppress + *haima,* blood), pronounced is-keé-me-ah. Cerebral ischemia can also occur from prolonged spasm of a cerebral artery. Portentous symptoms, such as dizziness and unsteady gait, may occur. The term covering the ailments that result from an inadequate blood circulation in the cerebrum is *cerebrovascular disease.*[6] When a coronary artery leading to the heart is obstructed, the resulting condition is *heart* or *cardiac ischemia* (see page 229). With severe ischemic heart disease, a portion of the heart muscle dies from lack of blood. Since the heart muscle is also known as the *myocardium* and the dead tissue is called an *infarct,* the term for a sudden heart attack is *acute myocardial infarction.* This condition, often called, simply, "heart attack," is a major and epidemic cause of death in this country. Another example of the interrelatedness of circulatory disease can be found in the instance of an increased blood pressure in the arteries. Such *hypertension* may result in heart disease. This is because the heart is forced to pump against the increased pressure. The heart may enlarge, even fail. Hence the term *hypertensive heart disease* (see page 242). Sometimes disease of the arteries leading to the kidneys (the *renal* arteries) decreases their lumen, so that less blood can flow through them. The *ischemic kidneys,* inadequately nourished, respond by producing a general hypertension—and *hypertensive heart disease.* Or, hypertension from other (sometimes unknown) causes can secondarily affect the kidneys. How? The kidney arterioles narrow. Kidney tissue is starved for blood. It deteriorates. This, in turn, promotes hypertension. The afflicted individual is caught in a destructive cycle of disease. Table 9-2 presents the 1972 picture of death from cardiovascular diseases in this country. The basic cause of the majority of these deaths is *atherosclerosis.* Consider it now.

atherosclerosis

Atherosclerosis is a prolonged destructive process of the major and minor arteries of the cardiovascular system. As a degenerative condition of these arteries, atherosclerosis affects them in such a way as to impede the flow of blood within them. It can be so widespread in the body, is so common, and causes so much sickness and death that it will be dealt with as a separate subject. However, atherosclerosis is not a disease but a disease process primarily causing many ailments of the circulatory system but secondarily affecting the organs dependent upon that system. Thus, one cannot, for example, consider atherosclerosis without being concerned about its effect on the heart or brain or legs. Moreover, the circulatory system may be affected by adversities other than atherosclerosis. Hence, following the discussion of atherosclerosis of the coronary arteries supplying the heart (leading to heart disease) will be a consid-

[6] The word "vascular" can refer to a vessel or mean "full of vessels." The above context refers to the former. Cerebrovascular diseases cause signs and symptoms referrable to the central nervous system, such as paralysis and the inability to speak. For that reason they are discussed in the section of Chapter 10 dealing with the nervous system (see pages 269–73).

TABLE 9-2
Deaths in the United States Due to Major Cardiovascular Diseases, 1972*

	CAUSE OF DEATH	NUMBER	RATE (per 100,000 population)
	Active rheumatic fever and chronic rheumatic heart disease	14,130	6.8
	Hypertensive heart disease (with and without renal disease)	13,160	6.3
DISEASES OF THE HEART	Ischemic heart disease	685,190	328.4
	Chronic disease of the endocardium and other myocardial insufficiency	5,330	2.6
	All other forms of heart disease	36,910	17.7
	TOTAL	754,720	361.8
HYPERTENSION		7,700	3.7
CEREBROVASCULAR DISEASE		210,690	101.0
ARTERIOSCLEROSIS		32,910	15.8
OTHER DISEASES OF ARTERIES, ARTERIOLES, AND CAPILLARIES		25,620	12.3
TOTAL		1,031,640	494.6

*Total deaths in the United States, from all causes, were 1,966,120; the overall death rate was 942.4 per 100,000 population.
Source: National Center for Health Statistics, *Monthly Vital Statistics Report,* Provisional Statistics, Births, Marriages, Divorces, and Deaths for January 1973, Vol. 22, No. 1 (March 29, 1973), p. 6.

eration of other afflictions causing heart disease—such as infections. Atherosclerosis may also result in the already mentioned hypertension, but much hypertension is apparently unrelated to arterial degeneration. And so, although atherosclerosis as a disease process will predominate in this consideration of the ailments of the blood's circulatory system, some of the other problems of that system will also be discussed.

international cooperation with a major health problem

Two centuries ago a Frenchman, Pouletier de la Salle, isolated a waxy substance in the bile (a fluid secreted by the liver and poured into the intestine). Fifty years later, another Frenchman, Chevreul, named it *cholesterol* (Greek *chole,* bile + *stereos,* solid). A German, in 1847, noted its presence in lesions (or plaques)[7] of certain arteries. And another German, Rudolf Virchow, noting the changing consistency of the lesions, named them *atherosclerosis* (Greek *athero,* soft, gruel + *skleros,* hard.)[8] So atherosclerosis is a lesion primarily in larger and

[7] A *plaque* is a patch or flat area.
[8] *Arteriosclerosis* is a more inclusive term referring to loss of elasticity, thickening, and hardening of the arteries from any cause.

middle arteries, with deposits of yellow plaques containing cholesterol and fatty substances. The plaque itself or a loose, broken-off piece of a plaque or a clot forming around a plaque can occlude an artery and impede the flow of blood. In 1909, a Russian medical officer, A. Ignatowski, observed that army officers had more heart attacks than did peasants. Officers could afford meat. Peasants had to be satisfied with vegetables. Could the difference be dietary? Ignatowski then produced arterial disease in rabbits by feeding them animal products. Another Russian, N. Anitschkow, fed egg yolk to rabbits. This high-cholesterol diet produced atherosclerosis.

So Russian, German, and French scientists were united in seeking truths for all men. Like pieces of a jigsaw, accumulated evidence fit together to make a picture: atherosclerosis was associated with high-fat, high-cholesterol diets (see pages 237–39).

Comparative international studies have supported this conclusion. During the semistarvation years of the German occupation, the Danes experienced less atherosclerosis and heart attacks than in later years, when food became plentiful. Relatively rich countries, such as the United States, West Germany, and Australia, have reported more atherosclerosis and heart attacks than poor countries, such as India and Korea, whose inhabitants have lower blood levels of cholesterol and fat. The Bantu of South Africa were found to have little atherosclerosis or heart disease. Only 17 percent of their calories came from fats. White South Africans were less fortunate. Over one-third (37 percent) of their total calories came from fats (mostly animal). They were plagued by atherosclerotic heart ailments.[9] Similarly, the U.S. government appointed Inter-Society Commission for Heart Disease Resources recently noted that in Japan, 3 percent of calories come from saturated fats, and the coronary disease death rate is 20 per 10,000 men, while in eastern Finland, 22 percent of calories come from saturated fats and the coronary disease death rate is 220 per 10,000 men.[10] Another five-year study of thousands of men in seven countries, concluded that "the outstanding risk factor, both within and between the various national groups, proved to be the concentration of cholesterol in the blood."[11]

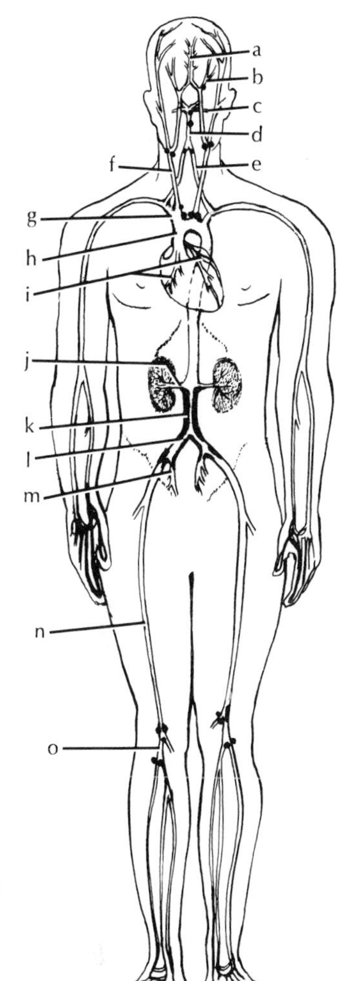

9-11 *Common arterial sites of atherosclerosis: cerebral (a–c), basilar (d), vertebral (e), common carotid (f), innominate (g), aorta (h), coronary (i), renal (j), abdominal aorta (k), iliac (l, m), femoral (n), popliteal (o).*

how atherosclerosis begins and progresses

That modern magnifier, the electron microscope, combined with other tools, has added much to the knowledge of the atherosclerotic process. The early invasion of the inner arterial lining by fatty substances can now be seen. Small amounts of cholesterol are also detectable. Fatty red streaks and spots, ominous precursors of atherosclerotic lesions, can be stained so as to become visible to the naked eye.

[9] Alton L. Blakeslee and Jeremiah Stamler, *Your Heart Has Nine Lives* (Englewood Cliffs, N.J., 1963), pp. 42–48.
[10] Jean Mayer, "Nutrition and Heart Disease: National Commission Report," *Postgraduate Medicine*, Vol. 49, No. 2 (February 1971), p. 257.
[11] Walter Alvarez, "Coronary Disease in Seven Countries," *Geriatrics*, Vol. 27, No. 5 (May 1972), p. 67.

How does atherosclerosis begin and progress? One must begin with the anatomy of the artery. In the young child, the healthy artery consists of a one-celled inner layer called the *intima* and a layer of elastic tissue. As the child grows older, smooth-muscle cells accumulate to thicken the intima, and more smooth-muscle cells form a third layer. The thickened intima is more permeable where the arteries branch, and these branching places are the most likely sites for the formation of atherosclerotic lesions, or plaques (see Figure 9-11). Now, within the blood *plasma* (the fluid portion of the blood in which the corpuscles are suspended; see pages 219–20) are a group of chemicals called *lipoprotein complexes.* The lipid portions of these complexes are a large class of substances, having a greasy feel; they include fats and waxes. It is theorized that these lipoproteins are kept from the middle layer of smooth-muscle cells by the arteries' internal lining of cells. With damage, this protection fails and the lipoproteins irritate the smooth-muscle cells to contribute to plaques. Since cholesterol can be a component of lipoprotein, this hypothesis fits in well with the observed relationship between a high cholesterol level in the blood and the formation of atherosclerotic plaques.[12]

The process is not yet completely explained. What actually triggers the severe changes of the smooth-muscle cells of the artery walls (the cells that are the major cellular component of atherosclerotic plaques)? Is the artery wall penetrated by fatty acids and cholesterol? Does a clot form on the inner surface of the wall? Recent research suggests that there is a transformation—a mutation (see page 537)—in a smooth-muscle cell of the artery, and, moreover, all the cells of a single atherosclerotic plaque are derived from that same mutated or changed cell. In short, the plaque itself is believed to be like a benign tumor (see page 194) of the arterial muscle. It has been caused, the theory continues, by a chemical (or even a virus) in the blood. Perhaps both chemicals and viruses are involved. It has been suggested that the likelihood of cellular mutations is enhanced by factors, such as an increased level of blood fat from the diet or high blood pressure, that stimulate cell proliferation. Also, it may be that rapidly proliferating cells are more susceptible to mutations.[13]

That changes do occur to the intima and smooth-muscle cells of arteries destined to have atherosclerotic plaques is indisputable. As the damage progresses, the body does what it can to repair. Tiny capillaries grow into the lesion. They may rupture and bleed. The lesion worsens; it may ulcerate. Eventually, however, it heals. Calcium is deposited. The artery stiffens, hardens, is partly or wholly occluded. No longer can it adequately supply blood to a needy body area. When such an artery is cut at autopsy, an inexperienced surgeon might be forgiven for sharing Jenner's impression of falling plaster.

As has been pointed out above, the arteries of some body sites are particularly prone to atherosclerosis. The atherosclerotic process tends to begin at a

[12] Colin Tudge, "Pulling Together Theories on Atherosclerosis," *New Scientist,* Vol. 59, No. 854 (July 12, 1973), p. 65. Blood cholesterol levels are increased not only by diet but by several other factors. Among these are cigarette smoking, stress, and lack of exercise.

[13] "Mutation and Atherosclerosis," *Scientific American,* Vol. 229, No. 2 (August 1973), p. 44.

point where an artery branches. Figure 9-11 is a simplified diagram showing some locations of arterial branching that are common sites of atherosclerosis. For example: note that the popliteal artery, a continuation of the femoral artery, divides into branches. At the point of branching, atherosclerosis may occur and impede blood circulation to the leg. Complete obstruction would lead to *gangrene.*

When the average middle-aged person has a heart attack or a stroke, it has been a long time coming. The symptoms may be agonizingly acute, but the disease has been brewing for a long time. Few diseases have so prolonged an incubation period—so long a period between the first body changes and the onset of symptoms.

the four basic ways in which heart disease is manifested

The four basic categories into which heart disease may be classified are:

1. cardiac ischemia;
2. congenital defects;
3. infection;
4. metabolic and endocrine disorders.

1. Consider the first of these, *cardiac ischemia,* which results from the *inability of a coronary artery to deliver enough blood to the heart.* Any of four conditions may cause cardiac ischemia:

a. A *coronary occlusion* takes place when the artery is suddenly closed off by a clot forming at the site of an atherosclerotic plaque or by a plaque swollen by a hemorrhage within it. A *thrombus* (Greek *thrombos,* clot) may be the plug (*coronary thrombosis*). At times, a piece of a clot, an *embolus* (Greek *emballo,* to throw in), may break off and occlude a smaller coronary artery. Although that part of the heart bereft of blood dies, the patient may survive. In that fortunate event, a circuitous blood supply develops around the dead heart tissue. The dead heart tissue is a *myocardial infarct.* So susceptible to occlusion is that part of the coronary artery supplying the front of the heart that it is called "the artery of sudden death."[14]

[14] Heart surgery for patients who have suffered coronary artery disease has become relatively commonplace. Remarkable new X-ray techniques indicate heart muscle areas receiving an inadequate blood supply due to an occluded coronary artery. Corrective surgery involves a "jump" or "bypass" graft, in which a vein from

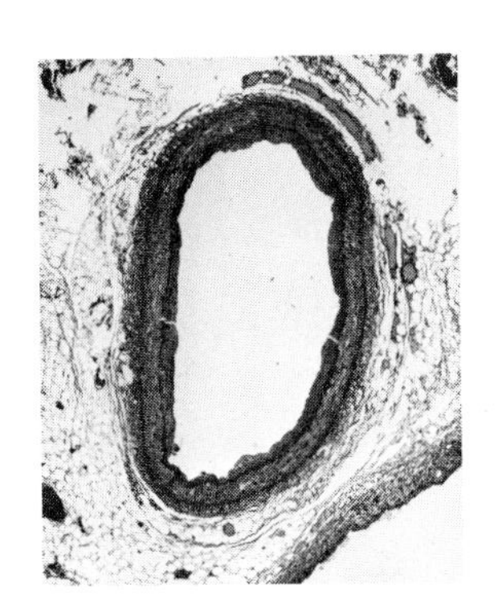
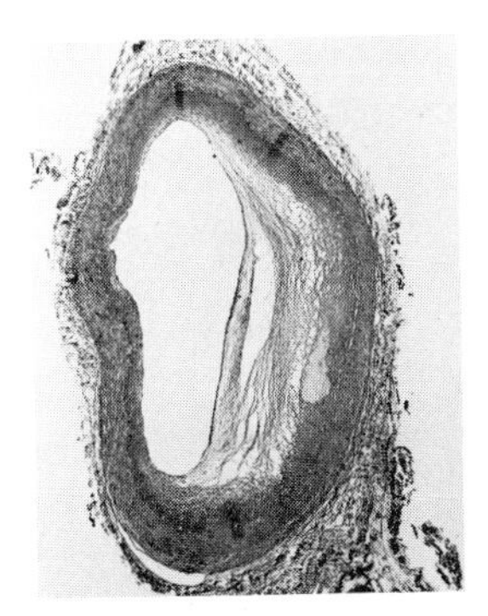
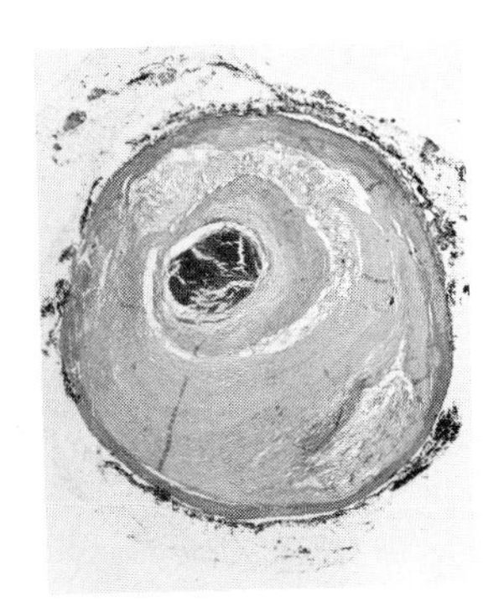

9-12 *A normal artery* (left), *an artery with atherosclerotic deposits in the inner lining* (center), *and an artery narrowed by atherosclerotic deposits and now blocked by a blood clot, the dark inner circle* (right).

b. The basic symptom of *angina pectoris* (Latin, a choking in the chest) may vary from a mild sense of pressure to a crushing, viselike chest pain. Often it heralds an occlusion. For an individual with diseased coronary arteries, excitement, exertion, or excessive eating may precipitate an attack of angina pectoris. Often the pain radiates up into the neck or down the left arm, usually into the fourth and little fingers.

c. *Rhythm disturbances* often result from myocardial damage. The infarct may include the conduction pathways from the specialized pacemaking cells responsible for a regular heartbeat. This infarction interrupts the normal pathways of conduction. Many varying disturbances of heart rate and rhythm may result. Should the ventricles twitch (fibrillate), blood cannot reach the body. Death may occur. For those with faulty natural pacemakers of their hearts, implantation of artificial pacemakers is lifesaving.[15]

d. When *congestive heart failure* has occurred, the heart has been considerably weakened by disease. This type of heart failure may occur immediately following a severe heart attack, or it may happen years after damage to the

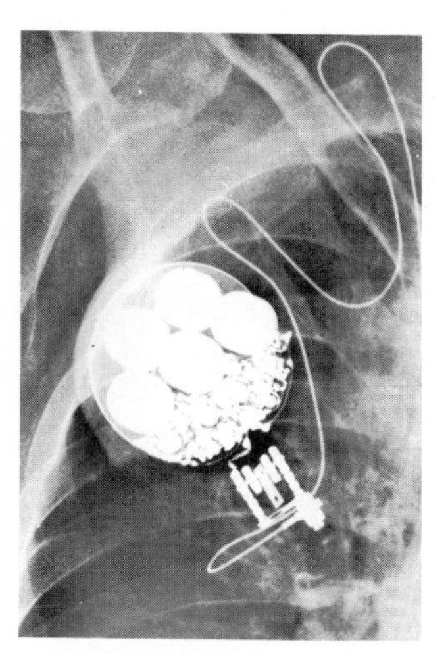

9-13 *This X-ray shows an electrical pacemaker placed just under the skin of the chest. It will help to continue and control the heart beat.*

---

the patient's thigh or internal artery of the breast is grafted to the heart muscle in order to bypass the coronary blockage to the heart and thus restore circulation. By early 1973, some 25,000 bypass operations had been performed in this country. Such vein grafts are being performed in order to prevent actual heart attacks. Candidates for this procedure are patients with severe angina pectoris who would be likely to have a heart attack because of advanced atherosclerosis of the coronary arteries. In carefully selected patients, such vein grafts have a low mortality rate, immediately eliminate angina, strengthen the contraction of the heart muscle, and improve the quality of life. (Irvine H. Page, "How Good Is the Coronary Bypass?" *Modern Medicine,* Vol. 41, No. 1 [January 8, 1973], p. 36.) Although further research is needed, one study comparing patients who had bypass surgery with patients who did not, indicated that after five years, "the bypass group has a 15 percent greater chance of survival." ("Hard Evidence That Bypass Grafts Buy Longer Life," *Medical World News,* Vol. 13, No. 43, p. 15.) Sometimes an acute coronary thrombosis results in enough heart damage to cause rupture of the septum between the ventricles or rupture of the papillary muscles (Figure 9-2, page 216). In the case of such cardiac catastrophes, surgical intervention can give good results. (Donald C. Harrison, "Advance in the Study and Treatment of Acute Myocardial Infarction," *California Medicine,* Vol. 114, No. 5 [May 1971], p. 83.)

[15] In this country, more than five thousand artificial cardiac pacemakers are being implanted each month. One person in five thousand is kept alive by a pacemaker. ("Pacemakers for Heart Block," *British Medical Journal,* Vol. 4, No. 5785 [November 20, 1971], p. 442.) Having a pacemaker involves certain risks. Pacemaker activity may be subject to interference not only by radio and television broadcasting, but also by radio frequency transmission from radar and microwave ovens, carrier current or power transmission lines, electrical currents in certain power tools, and the ignition systems of aircraft, automobiles, motorcycles, and lawnmowers. One woman "became pulseless in her automobile while the motor was running." Her pacemaker had failed. It was found that "the car's ignition system . . . producing broad-band radio frequency signals, also inhibited five additional pacemakers of the same model up to distances of 15 feet." ("Convention Report, American Heart Association," *Modern Medicine,* Vol. 35, No. 19 [November 6, 1967], p. 24.) Research is underway to redesign pacemakers so as to suppress such interference. ("Environmental Influences on Implanted Cardiac Pacemakers," *Journal of the American Medical Association,* Vol. 216, No. 12 [June 21, 1971], pp. 2006–07.) The external electromagnetic field equipment that is used as a weapon detector at airports to forestall hijacking has been found to be safe for pacemaker wearers. (Oliver C. Hood, John M. Keshishian, Nicholas P. D. Smith, Edward Podolak, Archie A. Hoffman, and Normal R. Baker, "Anti-Hijacking Efforts and Cardiac Pacemakers—Report of a Clinical Study," *Aerospace Medicine,* Vol. 43, No. 3 [March 1972], pp. 314–22.) A method has been developed to recharge nickel-cadmium batteries in pacemakers; this promises to do away with the repeated surgery necessary to replace run-down batteries in ordinary pacemakers. ("Pacemaker Recharges Without Surgery," *Medical World News,* Vol. 13, No. 2 [January 14, 1972], pp. 4–5.) In addition, nuclear-powered cardiac pacemakers are now being used in both Europe and the United States. (John C. Norman, Glenn W. Sandberg, and Fred N. Huffman, "Implantable Nuclear-Powered Cardiac Pacemakers," *New England Journal of Medicine,* Vol. 283 [November 26, 1970], pp. 1203–06.) By the beginning of 1973, plutonium-powered pacemakers, having a life expectancy of more than ten years, had been implanted in more than 130 patients throughout the world. By that time hospitals in thirteen countries, including the United States, had been licensed to implant nuclear-powered pacemakers. ("Plutonium Powered Pacemakers Prove Out," *Medical World News,* Vol. 14, No. 2 [January 12, 1973], p. 76.)

heart muscle. Coronary artery disease is but one of the heart ailments that can result in this condition. It is, therefore, discussed separately (see page 232).

2. With improper development of the embryo heart, inborn or *congenital defects* occur. Every year some forty thousand babies in this country (less than one percent) are born with such a malformation. The heart of such a child cannot pump sufficient blood to the lungs for oxygenation. Some of these affected children have a bluish discoloration of skin and mucous membrane. This is called *cyanosis* (Greek *kyaneos,* dark blue) and is responsible for the term "blue baby."

Inborn heart defects vary in severity. A defect may remain unnoticed until late in life or may not be noticed at all. With mild cases, cyanosis might occur only upon exertion and then is noticeable on the lips and fingertips. In some instances cyanosis does not occur. In many cases, growth is slowed. The child is handicapped. With exceedingly severe heart defects, death may occur soon after birth.

The cause of most inborn heart defects is unknown. A small percentage are due to German measles or other viral infections of the pregnant woman (see below). Many of the more than thirty-five kinds of inborn heart defects are amenable to surgery. The heart-lung machine has been a surgical boon. By shunting the blood from the heart, it temporarily takes over the heart's blood-circulating function as well as the function of the lung in ridding the blood of carbon dioxide and taking on oxygen. The heart is thus "dry." While the machine substitues for the heart and lungs, the heart can be operated upon.

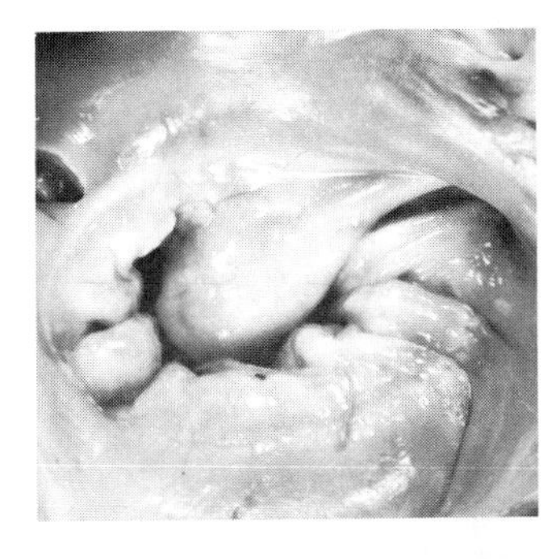

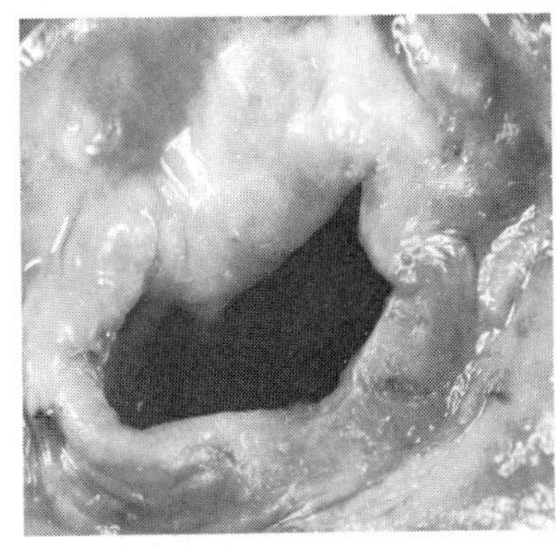

9-14 *Normal mitral valve, left atrial side* (top), *and a mitral valve thickened and scarred as a result of rheumatic fever* (bottom). *The scarred valve cannot open or close completely.*

3. *Infection* can harm the heart at any time, even before birth. Should a woman develop German measles (rubella) in the first three months of pregnancy, she has a 20 percent chance of having a child with the *congenital rubella syndrome* (see page 164). Such children commonly have heart malformations and other defects. Only a small percentage of congenital heart defects, however, are due to German measles. Surgery has dramatically improved the outlook for many of these small patients.

Rheumatic heart disease is no longer the scourge of childhood. This disease is a secondary reaction to a particular streptococcus. Why do some persons develop rheumatic fever after streptococcal infection, while others escape the disease? This is not known. Most often the streptococcal infection is of the throat, nose, and tonsil. The child may have a sore throat or joint pains. He may just feel unwell. Diagnosis is not easy. A good physician may need to watch the child carefully for some time. He is only too aware that, should disease involve the heart valves, eventual healing will result in valve scarring and distortion (see Figure 9-14). In consequence of such scars and distortion, the leaflets of the affected heart valves fail to appose one another properly. The valves try to close tightly but cannot. Blood leaks. Or a valve may fail to open completely. Blood flow is impeded. The physician will hear significant heart murmurs. (Not all murmurs, however, signify disease. Some are quite normal.)

Penicillin and other antibiotics can usually prevent rheumatic fever. One attack of rheumatic fever predisposes a child to another. For a child with a previous attack, penicillin pills are usually given daily until well into adulthood. In this way subsequent attacks are prevented. Surgical repair and replacement of valves scarred by rheumatic disease are now almost commonplace.

Medical advice for children with previous rheumatic fever is to be carefully followed. But the child should not be smothered with overattention. ''The living of strictly by Rule, '' wrote the seventeenth-century observer La Rochefoucauld, ''for the preservation of *Health* is one of the most troublesome Diseases that can be.''[16]

4. *Metabolic and endocrine disorders* may adversely affect the heart. An overactive thyroid gland (see page 259) may add to the stress of the heart muscle, as does the excess epinephrine produced by a tumor of the adrenal gland (see pages 258–59), albeit by a different mechanism.

about congestive heart failure

Any illness causing impairment of the heart's action as a pump can result in congestive heart failure. (*Congestion* refers to the abnormal accumulation of blood in a body part.) Normal effectiveness may be seriously reduced by the valvular scarring and distortion of rheumatic fever. A long-standing hypertension may, at last, by its excessive work demands, seriously weaken the heart muscle. A heart frittering away its energy in the wild muscular twitchings caused by a damaged conducting system will result in congestive failure. Or the heart, long ago having endured damage from a coronary thrombosis, at last fails. An acute myocardial infarction may precipitate cardiac muscle incompetence. So congestive heart failure is not itself a disease. It is a complex of signs and symptoms that may result from various types of heart disease.

Either or both of the two heart pumps may fail. If the left heart pump fails, the fluid of the blood backs up into the lungs. There is a ''rattling'' in the patient's chest. His congestion causes him to cough and to be grievously short of breath. Sitting up relieves him a little. He seeks comfort from the support of several pillows as a back rest. Should the right pump fail, fluid backs up into the abdomen and legs. *Edema* (Greek *oidos,* swelling) results. Press a finger into the leg edema. For a while, the pressure point remains depressed. If both pumps fail, edema may be quite generalized. The kidneys cannot help. The weakened heart muscle cannot pump enough blood to the kidney. Salt that would ordinarily be excreted with the urine is reabsorbed by the kidney. Water is retained with the salt in the body's tissue spaces. Fluid collects. The treatment may include a diet low in sodium (which is most commonly found in table salt) and the use of *diuretics* (Greek *diouretikos,* promoting urine) to remove sodium, and thus water, from the body.

But it is the flowering *foxglove* plant that provides the classic medicine for congestive heart failure. When its flowers die, its dull green leaves are finger-shaped. So the Scots call the foxglove ''bloody fingers,'' and Welshmen call it ''elf's gloves.'' A sixteenth-century German botanist named the plant *digitalis,* which is Latin for ''like a finger.'' For centuries the practical peasant

[16] From George F. Powell, ed., *The Moral Maxims and Reflections of the Duke de La Rochefoucauld* (New York, n.d.), p. 86.

women of Shropshire, England, had been preparing a foxglove powder with which to treat dropsy. In 1776, Dr. William Withering tried a recipe of herbals he had heard "had long been kept a secret by an old woman in Shropshire."[17] The patient was a woman "nearly in a state of suffocation . . . her breath very short . . . her countenance sunk . . . She could not lye down in bed . . . her stomach, legs, and thighs were greatly swollen; her urine very small in quantity, not more than a spoonful at a time, and that very seldom." His fears of censure by fellow medical men unacquainted with digitalis "soon gave way to desire of preserving the life of this valuable woman . . . five . . . draughts . . . acted very powerfully upon the kidneys, for within the first twenty-four hours she made upward of eight quarts of water . . . our patient being thus snatched from impending destruction."[18] Withering's *An Account of the Foxglove and Some of Its Medical Uses* (1785) is a treasured medical classic.

the Framingham Study

In 1949, perhaps the most significant prospective study of heart disease ever conducted in this country was begun in the Framingham, Massachusetts, area. The study comprised a population of 5,127 adults (2,282 men and 2,845 women) forty-nine to seventy years of age, all of whom were initially free of any manifestations of coronary artery disease. After fourteen (in some cases sixteen) years of careful follow-up of these individuals, it was reported that:

1. 151 men and 37 women showed evidence of coronary artery disease that would account for a heart attack.[19]
2. 102 men and 18 women died of coronary heart disease before they were sixty-five years old.[20]
3. Fifty-eight percent of the male deaths and 39 percent of the female deaths occurred within an hour of the attack.
4. For both men and women sudden death was more likely if they were less than fifty-five years old at the time of the attack.[21]
5. Not all heart attacks produced symptoms. Routine examinations during the fourteen-year period revealed an astonishing fact: a considerable number of men and women sustained myocardial infarcts without knowing it. Of those who suffered such heart muscle damage, 22 percent of the men and 35 percent of the women were unaware that it had occurred. Either these individuals had no symptoms during the episode of heart muscle damage, or their symptoms were too atypical to warn them or their doctors. These are known as "silent coronaries."[22]

[17] William Withering, *An Account of the Foxglove and Some of Its Medical Uses* (London, 1785), p. 3.
[18] *Ibid.*, pp.13–14.
[19] "The Silent Coronaries," *Journal of the American Medical Association*, Vol. 213, No. 8 (August 24, 1970), p. 1327.
[20] "The American Way of Death," *Scientific American*, Vol. 224, No. 5 (May 1971), p. 44.
[21] *Ibid.*, p. 45.
[22] "The Silent Coronaries," *Journal of the American Medical Association*, p. 1327, citing W. B. Kannel, P. M. McNamara, M. Feinleib, *et al.*, "The Unrecognized Myocardial Infarction: Fourteen-Year Follow-Up Experience in the Framingham Study," *Geriatrics*, Vol. 25, No. 1 (January 1970), pp. 75–87. As much as 70 percent of a coronary artery may be occluded without producing any symptoms whatsoever. Nobody knows why. ("Coronary Heart Disease Discovered in Asymptomatic Men," *Journal of the American Medical Association*, Vol. 221, No. 3 [July 17, 1972], pp. 241–42.)

6. 303 patients developed angina pectoris. The investigators were surprised to find that the continuous cardiac ischemia (lack of blood to the heart; see page 229) which caused the angina was about as fatal as coronary thrombosis.[23] Such ischemia seems to cause constant heart muscle irritability.

7. The data on congestive heart failure were no more encouraging. Congestive heart failure occurred in every age group studied; its most common precursors were high blood pressure, coronary artery disease, and rheumatic fever. "Despite modern management, congestive heart failure proved to be extremely lethal. The probability of dying within five years from onset of congestive failure was 62 percent for men and 42 percent for women."[24]

8. The risk of heart disease resulting from cardiac ischemia (failure of the coronary arteries to bring sufficient blood to the heart) is increased by such factors as high blood pressure, overweight, increased blood cholesterol, and cigarette smoking.[25] Moreover, people who do not exercise not only have three times as many heart attacks[26] as people who do but also are more likely to die from them.

plan to live: know the "coronary profile"

Who is most likely to have a heart attack? What elements compound the risk? There is not complete agreement on the answers to these questions. A high-fat, high-cholesterol diet, kidney disease, high blood pressure, heredity, excessive smoking, diabetes, thyroid insufficiency, physical inactivity, obesity, even previous arterial damage—any or all of these may well be involved. Some of the most frequently associated factors are these:

1. *A familial history of coronary heart disease;* the presence of diabetes mellitus, hypertension, obesity, and certain personality characteristics.
2. *Sex and age.* Men are generally more susceptible than women and both become increasingly susceptible with advancing years.
3. *Environmental factors* such as a diet rich in saturated fat and cholesterol, cigarette smoking, and habitual physical inactivity.[27]

Consider some of these factors of the "coronary profile" individually.

genetic factors and heart disease

There is a familial tendency to heart attacks. So long as other risks are reduced to a minimum, this hereditary factor need not be alarming. True, the risk of

[23] "More Data Reported on Angina Patients in Framingham Study," *Journal of the American Medical Association,* Vol. 215, No. 11 (March 15, 1971), p. 1739.

[24] Patrick A. McKee, William P. Castelli, Patricia M. McNamara, and William B. Kannel, "The Natural History of Congestive Heart Failure: The Framingham Study," *The New England Journal of Medicine,* Vol. 285, No. 26 (December 23, 1971), p. 1441.

[25] "The American Way of Death," *Scientific American,* pp. 44–45.

[26] William B. Kannel, "The Disease of Living," *Nutrition Today,* Vol. 6, No. 3 (May–June 1971), p. 6.

[27] American Heart Association, *Diet and Disease* (October 1968), p. 6. Recent studies have indicated an increase in coronary heart disease in U.S. and Canadian soft-water areas as compared to hard-water areas. As early as 1957, Japanese scientists linked some quality of drinking water with cerebral hemorrhage—the number one cause of death in Japan. What the relationship (if any) is between water softness and coronary heart disease is now being investigated. ("Soft Water and Heart Disease," *Science News,* Vol. 95, No. 20 [May 17, 1969], p. 471.)

heart attacks is statistically greatest among short men with a heavy, rectangularly outlined, hard physique. Moreover, people whose blood group is A have higher cholesterol levels than those in other blood groups,[28] and there is a genetically caused lipid disorder manifested by high fat and protein levels in the blood; people with these conditions are particularly prone to coronary artery disease. Family histories of diabetes, gout, high blood pressure, atherosclerosis, and coronary artery disease also increase the risk of heart disease. But such genetically influenced characteristics do not, as factors in heart disease, exist alone. Like health, disease exists in an ecosystem. A personal preventive program may add the normal years to the life span. To sensibly exercise, to avoid smoking,[29] to avoid excessive stress, and to control one's diet, substantially reduce the risk.

gender and heart disease

The fragility of the male is discussed in Chapter 18. In no other part of his body does the male more abundantly demonstrate that he is the weaker sex than in his coronary arteries. In the United States in 1969, of the deaths due to all diseases of the heart, 57.1 percent were male, 42.9 percent female. For coronary artery disease deaths, the ratios that year were 60.2 percent male compared to 39.8 percent female.[30] These data do not tell the whole story. The internal lining of a baby boy's coronary arteries is thicker than a girl's. In this respect the male gets a relatively poor start. His already narrower coronary passage is more susceptible to occlusion. In 1965 a leading U.S. statistician wrote, "Up to the age of 40, twenty-four men to one woman will experience a heart attack." Not until age fifty was the ratio reduced to 15 to 1. At sixty years it was 8 to 1. By age seventy, the ratio was equal.[31]

Today these ratios may be changing. A report from Brookdale Hospital Medical Center in Brooklyn and the Westchester County Medical Examiner's Office in Valhalla, New York, attributes the striking increase of sudden deaths among women to cigarette smoking.[32] In the 1950s, the ratio of sudden deaths from coronary artery disease was 12 men to 1 woman. By the late 1960s, that ratio had dropped to 4 to 1. Sixty-two percent of the women who died suddenly from coronary heart disease were heavy smokers; only 28 percent of those who died from other causes smoked heavily. The mean age of the nonsmoking woman who died suddenly of a heart attack was sixty-seven; for the light smoker it was fifty-five; for the heavy smoker, forty-eight. Thus, heavy smoking could cut a woman's life short by almost twenty years. In triggering fatal heart attacks, heavy smoking was more lethal for women than for men. Among men the ratio

[28] "Genetic Correlation," *Nature,* Vol. 224, No. 5217 (October 25, 1969), p. 310.
[29] For a discussion of heart disease and smoking, see pages 393–95.
[30] National Center for Health Statistics, *Monthly Vital Statistics Report,* Final Mortality Statistics, 1969.
[31] Louis I. Dublin, *Factbook on Man from Birth to Death* (New York, 1965), pp. 94–95.
[32] David M. Spain, Henry Siegel, and Victoria A. Bradess, "Women Smokers and Sudden Death," *Journal of the American Medical Association,* Vol. 224, No. 7 (May 14, 1973), pp. 1005–07.

of smokers to nonsmokers in sudden death from coronary heart disease was 3 to 1; in women, the ratio was 9 to 1.

Although coronary heart disease remains more common in men than in women, the condition among women is a major killer and, tragically, getting worse. In this country, more than 200,000 women die of the disease every year.[33] (For a further consideration of smoking, see pages 386–400.)

age and heart disease

Among the young, circulatory disease is not a major cause of death. It rarely kills babies; indeed of those who die of heart disease only 3 percent are under forty-five. Between the ages of forty-five and sixty-five the percentage climbs rapidly to almost 25. Most people (about three-quarters) who die of heart disease are over sixty-five years old. Stroke is even more an elderly person's nemesis. More than four out of five people who die of stroke are over sixty-five.

But does atherosclerosis afflict only the aged? Has it now come to prominence only because more people live to be old? Decidely not. Infant autopsies reveal atherosclerosis shortly after birth. Its telltale fatty streaks have been plainly visible in three-year old arteries. In many thirty-five-year-old males, studies show as much as 50 percent arterial narrowing.[34] An astonishing majority of autopsied U.S. soldiers killed in Korea (at an average age of twenty-three) revealed atherosclerotic plaques.[35] Autopsies of 114 U.S. soldiers killed in Vietnam, however, revealed that only 45 percent had some degree of atherosclerosis, as compared to 77.3 percent of the Korean battle casualties.[36] Among the possible reasons for this difference is the hot and humid climate of Vietnam, resulting in changed fat metabolism and decreased blood pressure, which would not be conducive to atherosclerosis.[37]

exercise and heart disease

The errors of great men often outlive their wisdom. So it was with the brilliant Canadian-born physician Sir William Osler (1849–1919). For many years, medical students studied his description of "athlete's heart," supposedly a condition resulting from prolonged, excessive exercise. Recent studies, however, have "failed to reveal cardiac enlargement, even in men who had engaged in the most vigorous physical effort for many years. . . . It has become

[33] Eve Weinblatt, Sam Shapiro, and Charles Frank, "Prognosis of Women with Newly Diagnosed Coronary Heart Disease—A Comparison with Course of Disease Among Men," *American Journal of Public Health,* Vol. 63, No. 7 (July 1973), p. 577.

[34] William F. Enos *et al.*, "Coronary Disease Among U.S. Soldiers in Korea Killed in Action," *Journal of the American Medical Association,* Vol. 152, No. 12 (July 18, 1953), p. 109.

[35] David M. Spain, "Atherosclerosis," *Scientific American,* Vol. 215, No. 2 (August 1966), p. 49.

[36] J. Judson McNamara, Mark A. Molot, John F. Stremple, and Robert T. Cutting, "Coronary Artery Disease in Combat Casualties in Vietnam," *Journal of the American Medical Association,* Vol. 216, No. 7 (May 17, 1971), p. 1185.

[37] Frank B. Macomber, "Coronary Artery Disease in Vietnam Casualties," *Journal of the American Medical Association,* Vol. 217, No. 4 (July 26, 1971), p. 478.

a nondisease and disappeared from the medical scene."[38] Today, a sensible program of regular exercise is widely recognized to be helpful in both prevention of and recovery from heart attacks. Even heart transplant patients begin walking the second day after surgery, lift dumbbells on the third day, and, as outpatients, are encouraged to engage in golf, tennis, and bicycling.[39] Carefully programmed exercise under medical supervision has been shown to improve heart function in patients with coronary artery disease and angina pectoris.[40] Resumption of customary sexual activity is also not contraindicated for recovered heart attack patients once they are able to resume brisk walking or climbing stairs without discomfort.

For further discussion of exercise and heart disease, see Chapter 23.

diet: "taking the dying out of eating"[41]

As has been pointed out on pages 226–27, diet is an important factor in heart disease. Obesity materially increases the risk. "Mortality from circulatory conditions among males 20 percent overweight is 25 percent higher and for those 30 percent overweight 42 percent higher than for those with normal weight. For women 20 percent overweight, the mortality is 21 percent higher, and for those 30 percent overweight 30 percent higher."[42] Those who are overweight for their body build should, with the aid of their physician, lose weight.

The type of food commonly eaten is also involved. Many students in this area believe fats to be the food villain in heart disease.

Saturated ("hard") *fats* usually solidify at room temperature. As a rule, they come from animals. Foods high in saturated (but low in unsaturated) fats include cheeses, butter, cream, lard, and meats, particularly pork, beef, and lamb. "Marbled" meats may be as streaked with fat as an atherosclerotic artery. Pretenderized meat is as tasty, less expensive, and more healthful.

Polyunsaturated fats usually remain liquid at room temperature and, generally, come from vegetable or fish oil. Both safflower oil and peanut oil are high in polyunsaturated and low in saturated fats.[43] However, it is a mistake to think that they lessen the risk of atherosclerosis to an equal degree. It is the chemical structure of the fat that is important; two fatty acids unique to peanut oil make

[38] Bernard Straus, "Defunct and Dying Diseases," *Bulletin of the New York Academy of Medicine,* Vol. 46, No. 9 (September 1970), pp. 695.

[39] "Heart Transplant Patients Tolerate Exercise Well," *Journal of the American Medical Association,* Vol. 215, No. 4 (January 25, 1971), pp. 555–56.

[40] David R. Redwood, Douglas R. Rosing, and Stephen E. Epstein, "Circulatory and Symptomatic Effects of Physical Training in Patients with Coronary Artery Disease and Angina Pectoris," *New England Journal of Medicine,* Vol. 286, No. 18 (May 4, 1972), pp. 959–66.

[41] Alexander Comfort, "The World Diet Revolution," *Center Report,* Vol. 6, No. 3 (August 1973), p. 36. Dr. Comfort "would bring out a soy and mold protein called Kindheart or Concern (takes the dying out of eating) and promote it with commercials of a slaughterhouse in action, and an unwidowmaking butter, knowing that the future mothers now in college will program the healthy food habits of future husbands and sons."

[42] Louis I. Dublin, *Factbook on Man from Birth to Death,* p. 177.

[43] Fats are carbohydrates; that is, they are made up of only three chemical elements—carbon, hydrogen, and oxygen. Saturated fats have the maximum possible number of hydrogen atoms attached to the chains of carbon atoms in their chemical structures. Unsaturated fats have fewer hydrogen atoms in proportion to carbon atoms.

it much more likely to produce atherosclerosis in rats than corn, safflower, cottonseed, or olive oils. Experimentally, coconut oil is also a "bad fat."[44]

> In October 1968, experts of the American Heart Association stated that in general, a diet designed to decrease the risk of coronary heart disease involves the following three recommendations:
>
> 1. *A caloric intake adjusted to achieve and maintain proper weight . . .*
> 2. *A decrease in the intake of saturated fats, and an increase in the intake of polyunsaturated fats . . .* an intake of less than 40% of calories from fat is considered desirable. Of this total, polyunsaturated fats should probably comprise twice the quantity of saturated fats . . . margarines that are high in polyunsaturates usually can be identified by the listing of "liquid oil" first among the ingredients . . .
> 3. *A substantial reduction of cholesterol in the diet . . .* Careful planning is necessary to lower the intake of cholesterol without impairing the intake of foods high in proteins.[45]

In December 1972, the Council on Foods and Nutrition of the American Medical Association published similar recommendations.[46] Studies consistently support them. A massive, twelve-year study in Norway recently revealed that a cholesterol-lowering diet halved heart disease deaths among men.[47] In addition, research at the University of Chicago[48] has shown that, in Rhesus monkeys, advanced stages of atherosclerosis can, to some degree, be reversed if low serum cholesterol levels are sustained for prolonged periods.[49]

Radical dietary changes should not be made without the physician's advice. To restrict one's diet may not seem easy, but "the world's most difficult undertakings," wrote Lao-Tzu (604?–531? B.C.) in the *Teh Ching* (Classic of Virtue),

[44] "A New View of Lipids and Atheromas," *Medical World News,* Vol. 12, No. 38 (October 15, 1971), p. 64.

[45] Other fatty materials, in addition to cholesterol, are involved in the problem of atherosclerosis. Fat molecules containing phosphoric acid and organic chemicals (*phospholipids*), and *triglycerides* (glycerine combined with three fatty acids) surely participate in the problem. But, for many people, it remains basically true that the intake of saturated fats and high-cholesterol foods should be reduced. (American Heart Association, *Diet and Heart Disease* [October 1968], 4 pages.)

[46] "Diet and Coronary Heart Disease," *Joint Policy Statement of the AMA Council on Foods and Nutrition and the Food and Nutrition Board of the National Academy of Sciences–National Research Council, Journal of the American Medical Association,* Vol. 222, No. 13 (December 25, 1972), p. 1647.

[47] "Diet Halves Heart-Disease Deaths," *New Scientist,* Vol. 56, No. 817 (October 26, 1972), p. 190.

[48] The University of Chicago Office of Public Information, February 21, 1973.

[49] Recent research has pointed to other relationships between diet and heart disease. Unlike most mammals, neither men nor guinea pigs can manufacture their own vitamin C; they must get it from their food. It has been demonstrated that a low vitamin C intake by guinea pigs leads to elevated blood cholesterol levels. Although such laboratory results are not applicable to human beings, it may be that an adequate intake of vitamin C is essential for the prevention of human atherosclerosis. (Emil Ginter, "Cholesterol: Vitamin C Controls Its Transformation to Bile Acids," *Science,* Vol. 179, No. 4074, pp. 702–04.) Still other research, carried out by the Boston Collaborative Drug Surveillance Program, indicated that drinking more than five cups of coffee daily carried twice the risk of developing coronary artery disease as drinking no coffee at all. Both sugar consumption and cigarette smoking were ruled out as explanations for these data. So was caffeine; tea drinkers were unaffected. The data are most likely due to the probability that heavy coffee drinkers lead more stressful lives. However, some workers suggest that coffee may alter blood fats; a positive correlation was found between serum cholesterol levels and daily coffee ingestion. ("Even De-Caffeinated Coffee May Be Bad for the Heart," *New Scientist,* Vol. 56, No. 826 [December 28, 1972], p. 734, citing "The Boston Collaborative Drug Surveillance Program," *Lancet,* Vol. 2 (December 16, 1972), pp. 1278–81.) Nevertheless, "more evidence is needed before we can confidently add coffee to the growing list of faulty living habits that must be curtailed in the quest for a lower coronary incidence." (William B. Kannel and Thomas R. Dawber, "Coffee and Coronary Disease," *New England Journal of Medicine,* Vol. 289, No. 2 [July 12, 1973], pp. 100–01.)

"necessarily originate while easy . . . Treat things before they exist. Regulate things before disorder begins . . . Only by becoming sick of sickness can we be without sickness."[50]

SHOULD THE CHILD'S DIET BE CHANGED? Such recommendations, as well as the considerable incidence of atherosclerosis among young people in this country (see page 236), have prompted an increasing number of parents to ask pediatricians whether the diet of young children should be changed. The unborn child is nourished on a low-fat diet. The placental transfer of cholesterol and triglycerides from mother to child is minimal. Consequently, the cholesterol concentration in the newborn's blood serum is only about one-third that of the mother's.[51] After birth, however, most children are fed a diet high in calories, cholesterol, and saturated fats. When this is combined with a genetic tendency to heart disease (see page 234), dietary intervention may be warranted, according to a 1972 statement of the Committee on Nutrition of the American Academy of Pediatrics. A family history of coronary artery disease before the age of fifty in first cousins and closer relatives would justify analysis of a child's level of serum cholesterol, triglycerides, and lipoproteins. Children of diabetic parents also merit special attention. It has been found that abnormal metabolism of fats may precede the onset of diabetes by ten years or more. Therefore, it has been suggested that the accelerated atherosclerosis often seen with diabetes might be retarded by a program concerned not only with sugar metabolism but also with blood lipids, body weight, and blood pressure. Generally, pediatricians urge the prevention and correction of childhood obesity through careful attention to diet and programs of adequate exercise. It has also been recommended that "The pediatrician should discourage the common habit of adding salt to childhood diets."[52]

The Committee on Nutrition recommended against radical dietary changes for all children, noting only that "dietary intervention may be warranted in special circumstances, but not before 1 year of age." The committee emphasized that the claimed relationship between dietary cholesterol and coronary heart disease would be more persuasive "if restriction of dietary cholesterol in the population at large could be shown to reduce the frequency of coronary heart disease."[53] In search of such evidence, a federally funded project is studying thousands of school children in Muscatine, Iowa, in order to learn whether there is a relationship between future coronary artery disease and obesity, high blood pressure, and elevated serum cholesterol-triglyceride levels during childhood.[54]

[50] Quoted in Paul Carus, *The Canon of Reason and Virtue: Being Lao-tzu's Tao Teh Ching* (Chicago, 1913), pp. 118–19, 124.

[51] Allen Drash, "Atherosclerosis, Cholesterol, and the Pediatrician," *Pediatrics,* Vol. 80, No. 4 (April 1972), p. 694.

[52] William B. Kannel and Thomas R. Dawber, "Atherosclerosis as a Pediatric Problem," *Pediatrics,* Vol. 80, No. 4, part I (April 1972), p. 550.

[53] "Pediatrics and Heart Disease," *Dairy Council Digest,* Vol. 43, No. 2 (March–April 1972), pp. 11, 12, citing the Committee on Nutrition, American Academy of Pediatrics, *Pediatrics,* Vol. 49, No. 2 (February 1972), pp. 305–07.

[54] "Tracking Heart Disease to Its Roots," *Medical World News,* Vol. 13, No. 32 (September 1, 1972), pp. 54–55.

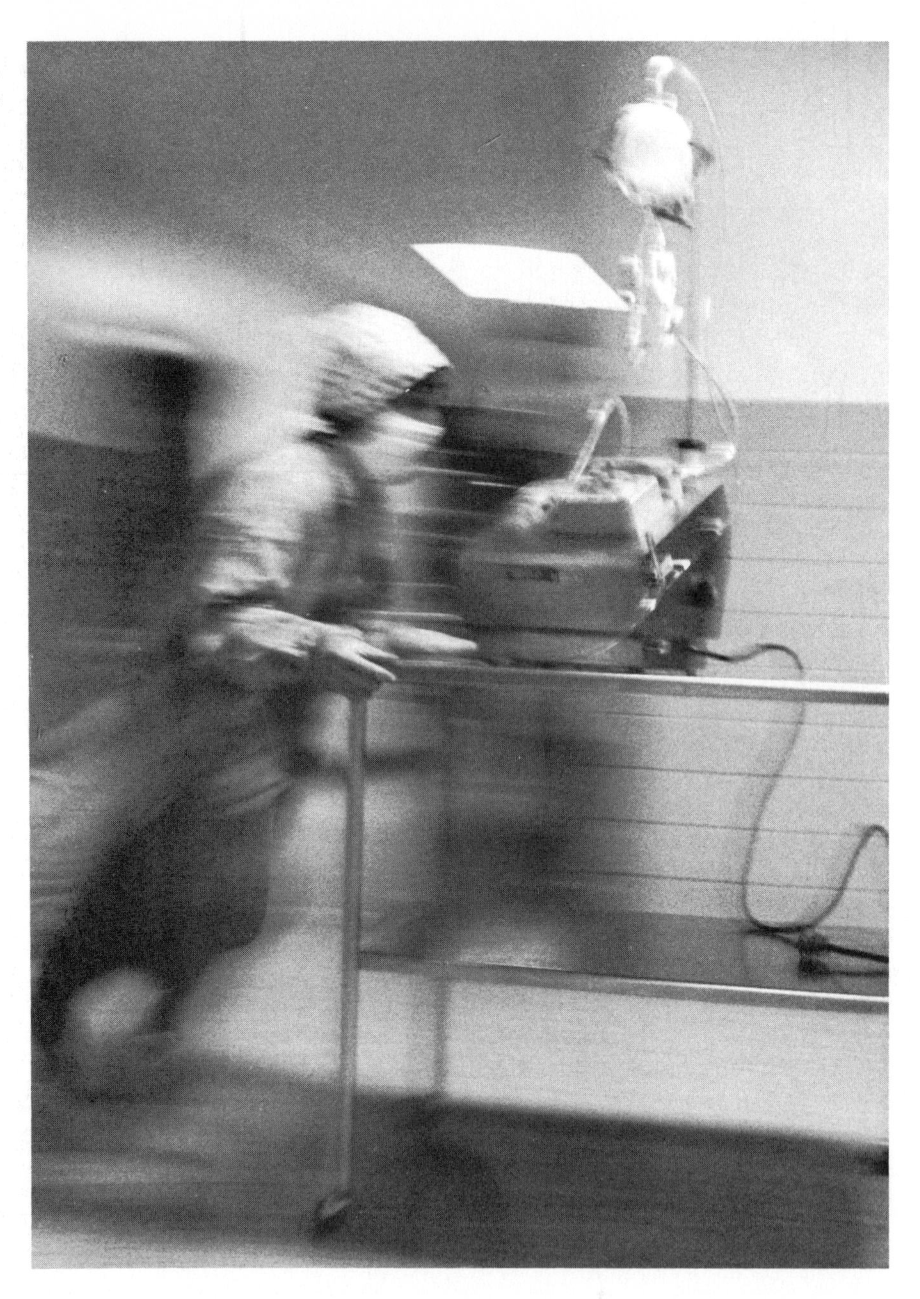

9-15 *A nurse rushes to an operating room with emergency apparatus.*

heart attack: emergency!

Studies like those conducted in Framingham have shown that about half the deaths from acute coronary disease in the United States occur in the first hour. Every year, more than 300,000 heart attack victims die before they reach a hospital. Emergency coronary care programs are aimed at reducing three time-consuming factors: (1) the *victim's decision time* that elapses between the onset of illness and the seeking of help; (2) the *transportation time* to a coronary care unit; (3) the *hospital time* that passes before adequate emergency treatment is begun. The first of these can be shortened only partly by education. Denial by the patient of the coronary event (often based on fear of death) frequently results in a fatal delay. Knowledge of the symptoms of a heart attack can, however, be life saving. Often, a victim will agree to examination only at the insistence of someone else. To reduce the second cause of delay, use of specially equipped cardiac ambulances is becoming widespread. Transportation of the victim to a hospital is carried out by specially trained ambulance personnel. Today, 75 percent of all hospitals with one hundred beds or more have coronary care units that provide emergency attention to heart attack victims.[55]

But every study of coronary heart disease leads to a basic conclusion: the best and most difficult objective is to prevent the attack.

about a poet's woeful physiology

In 1867, Walt Whitman wrote:

> Of physiology from top to toe I sing . . .
> Of Life immense in passion, pulse, and power,
> Cheerful-for freest action form'd.[56]

On the morning of January 24, 1873, he awoke to find his left arm and leg paralyzed. He had suffered a stroke. Later he wrote such lines as these:

> A batter'd, wreck'd old man . . .
> I am too full of woe!
> Haply I may not live another day;
> I cannot rest O God, I cannot eat or drink or sleep . . .
> My hands, my limbs grow nerveless,
> My brain feels rack'd, bewildered.[57]

For almost twenty years Whitman was ill. His seventh stroke was his last. What manner of disease destroyed him?

[55] Lawrence M. Herman, "The Critical First Hour in Acute Coronary Attacks," *The Los Angeles County Medical Association Bulletin,* Vol. 102, No. 13 (July 20, 1972), pp. 9, 11. Another innovation designed to reduce the heart attack deaths that occur before victims can reach a hospital is the "Patient Technology Packet." Although not yet approved by the Federal government as of early 1973, this survival kit holds great promise as a life-saver. It consists of three elements: (1) an automatic injector containing a drug called *atropine.* It is the fibrillation of the ventricle (see page 215) that is responsible for most deaths that occur within the first hour of a heart attack. In a hospital, a suitably applied electric shock can usually arrest the ventricular fibrillation. Heart-attack victims whose heart rates are abnormally slow can inject themselves with atropine, which increases the heart rate and diminishes ventricular fibrillation. Atropine also increases the blood pressure, which drops dangerously in victims with slow heart rates. (2) *Lidocaine,* a drug that has no effect on the heart rate. Suppresses fibrillation of the ventricle, which makes it useful for heart-attack victims whose heart rates are normal or faster than normal. (3) A "Cardio Beeper"; this element of the survival kit is a small electronic device that enables the heart-attack victim to transmit his heartbeat and electrocardiogram, by telephone, to his physician or to a central emergency heart service. The patient can then be advised which drug to inject. ("Survival Kit," *Scientific American,* Vol. 227, No. 2 [August 1972], pp. 45, 46.) In March 1972, a patient from Manila transmitted his electrocardiogram via telephone to the Stanford University Medical Center in California. "As the call went by satellite, the electrocardiogram travelled some 51,000 miles without serious distortion," ("Doctor, My Ticker's Bleeping," *New Scientist,* Vol. 53, No. 788 [March 23, 1972], p. 647.)

[56] Walt Whitman, "One's Self I Sing," in Mark Van Doren, ed., *Walt Whitman* (New York, 1945), p. 311.

[57] Walt Whitman, "Prayer of Columbus," in Hugh I'Ansom Faussett, ed., *Walt Whitman, Poet of Democracy* (New Haven, Conn., 1942), pp. 248–49.

normal blood pressure

Turn on a water faucet. For water to flow, a steady water pressure must be maintained within, and thus against, the water pipes. A second propulsive pressure, augmenting the first maintenance pressure, must keep the water flowing. In a similar fashion, the heart maintains blood pressure. But healthy arteries are muscular and elastic, not rigid like pipes. They are well able to adjust to the pulsating flow of blood, which may constantly vary in velocity, volume, and pressure. The propulsive pressure of the blood in the arteries is the *systolic pressure.* The maintenance pressure is the *diastolic pressure.* Fundamentally, the basic regulation of the blood pressure is normally under kidney control. The kidneys respond to arterial pressure changes by altering their secretion of a chemical substance called rennin, which in turn precipitates other body chemical changes leading to blood pressure control.

abnormal blood pressure (arterial hypertension)

With abnormal narrowing of the terminal twigs of the arteries (the arterioles), blood cannot easily pass through them to the capillaries. The pressure within the arteries increases. This excessive pressure within the arteries is *hypertension.* To overcome it, the heart must work harder. A vicious cycle begins. Artery walls toughen and lose elasticity. To compensate, the heart muscle (the myocardium) thickens. This is particularly true of the wall of the left ventricle. *Hypertensive heart disease* develops. Increased pressure of long duration may damage the kidney and other vital organs. Occasionally, a hardened, weakened, small artery in the brain, under prolonged tension, ruptures. A small amount of blood escapes. The individual thus experiences a "little stroke"—a minor, transient paralysis (see page 270). It is a warning. Treatment and rest may delay a more severe hemorrhage for many years, and it may never occur. Sometimes, a more severe hemorrhage does happen. Paralysis, as occurred after the First World War in the case of Woodrow Wilson, may result. A massive cerebral hemorrhage, as in the case of Franklin D. Roosevelt, kills.

The resting heart rates of warm-blooded animals vary. The mouse heart flutters about five hundred times a minute. A man's heart beats seventy times a minute; an elephant's thirty-five. But for both man and elephant, the blood pressure is about the same. For a twenty-year-old human, the average systolic pressure is about 115 to 120 millimeters of mercury. The average diastolic pressure is about 75. Normal blood pressures vary greatly. For days, even weeks, many individuals have an elevated blood pressure without harm. Exercise, tension, and excitement raise the blood pressure. So does age. At sixty-five, a blood pressure of 135 systolic and 85 diastolic would hardly be considered abnormal. Only when the blood pressure is unduly high, over a prolonged period of time, is disease likely. Many physicians consider a consistent systolic pressure of 150 questionable, and a diastolic of over 90 high. Of the two, the diastolic signifies the lowest constant blood pressure in the arteries. It, therefore, means more.

Partial blocking of a main kidney artery may cause hypertension. Sometimes, kidney inflammation (*nephritis*) or other kidney damage may result in high blood pressure; the exact mechanisms are unknown. By liberating adrenalin, adrenal tumors may raise the blood pressure. This is rare. But most hypertension is unrelated to any other disease, nor is the cause for it known. This type is called *essential hypertension*—not, however, because it is necessary. "Essential" here means "self-existing" or "having no obvious, external cause."

The headache, dizziness, even the shortness of breath of some hypertension may occur with many other impairments. Treatment of hypertension includes drugs, diet, and surgery. Side effects from drugs have, in recent years, been greatly reduced. Diets designed to reduce weight may be helpful. Restriction of sodium (which is most commonly found in table salt) sometimes helps to lower the blood pressure. For hypertensives smoking is especially harmful since it further constricts the arteries. The unduly distressed may be helped by psychotherapy. Of most importance is moderation in all things. By attention to rest and weight and by avoidance of tensions, years of useful living can be added to the life of the hypertensive individual. Today, a case such as Whitman's should be extraordinary. With tragic frequency it is not.

RESEARCH ABOUT HYPERTENSION: ABOUT A GRAIN OF SALT AND MORE The often inaccurate ancient Roman scholar Pliny (A.D. 23–79), in his *Natural History,* wrote that Mithridates VI (d. 63 B.C.), king of the then Roman province Pontus, had a mortal fear of being poisoned. Thus, he always took a grain of salt as part of an antidote to avert poisoning. When the Roman general Pompey (106–48 B.C.) seized Mithridates' palace, wrote Pliny, he found the formula for the antidote and doubted its value. The skeptical phrase "to take with a grain of salt" may have originated then, or from the observation that salt makes some unpalatable foods easier to swallow. In any event, history has seen many bitter international conflicts over salt. People need some salt; for some, even a slight excess may be harmful.

Years of painstaking research at the Brookhaven (N. Y.) National Laboratory has helped to unravel part of the hypertension enigma.[58] It has been learned that salt (NaCl) can induce permanent and finally fatal hypertension in rats. Moreover, there is a definite correlation between the average salt intake of various population groups and the incidence of hypertension among them. Third, it appears that some people have a greater genetic tendency than others to respond to salt with hypertension. Salt is not the only variable causing the illness; also to be considered are other nongenetic factors, such as glomerulonephritis, pyelonephritis, even the emotional stress referred to in Shakespeare's *Henry IV, Part 2* (I. II. 127–32): "This apoplexy [crippling by a stroke] . . . hath its original from much grief, . . . from perturbation of the brain."

the body's filtering system

kidney structure and function

Every twenty minutes all the body's blood filters through the kidneys. They are not alone in clearing the body of wastes. But the liver, lungs, and skin, important to excretion as they are, do not compare to the excretory activity of the kidney.

[58] "Dr. Dahl on: Predisposition + NaCl = Hypertension," *Hospital Tribune Hypertension Bulletin* (March 12, 1973), pp. 11–18.

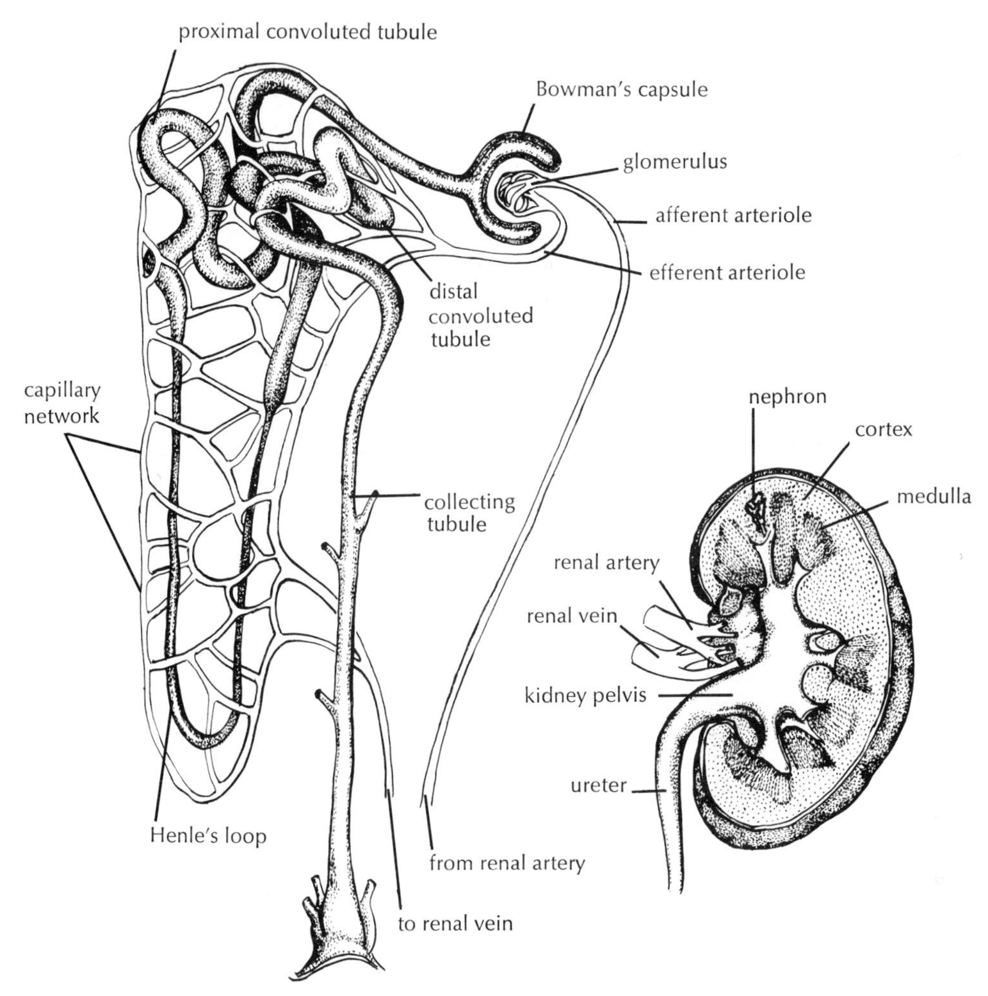

9-16 *A nephron* (left) *and its relation to the kidney as a whole* (right). *The nephron in the illustration of the kidney has been drawn disproportionately large so as to be visible.*

The kidneys lie at the back of the abdomen at the level of the lower ribs. A large branch of the great aorta enters each kidney as the *renal artery.* Like all other arteries, it progressively divides to become arterioles. But these arterioles (the *afferent arterioles*) do not, like all others, immediately end in capillaries, which, in turn, become venules. Instead, each afferent arteriole first leads into a tiny tuft of daintily coiled capillaries, a *glomerulus* (see Figures 9-16 and 9-17). Each tubule (Figure 9-16) in the kidney is associated with such a glomerulus. A tiny vessel (an *efferent arteriole*) leads away from each glomerulus to drain it and then branches into a unique second capillary network around the tubule. Other branches of this efferent arteriole end in capillaries that, after feeding the kidney tissue itself, become larger veins leading to the heart.

The capillary tuft fits into the hollow of a *Bowman's capsule,* which is at one end of the tubule (see Figure 9-16). In this way the cavity of Bowman's capsule surrounds the glomerulus. The epithelium of the inner wall of Bowman's capsule that covers the capillaries of the glomerulus is made of specialized cells. These cells have tiny structures (visible only under the electron microscope) resting directly on the capillaries of the glomerulus. These structures can take up material from the blood in the capillaries, and they control not only the amount of fluid leaving the glomerulus but also the content of that fluid.[59]

Each tubule plus its capillaries is called a *nephron* (Figure 9-16). This is the unit of excretion. As the heart pressures blood into the renal arteries, fluid and salt pass through the glomerulus into the hollow tubule. The fluid traverses the entire length of the tubule—down the proximal convoluted tubule, around Henle's loop, up the distal convoluted tubule, and out the collecting tubule. It then drips into the kidney pelvis (see Figure 9-16). There are some 2 million nephrons in each kidney; each nephron has its own glomerulus and tubule. So fluid from some 2 million collecting tubules drips into each kidney's pelvis.

But the fluid that drips into the kidney pelvis is a mere 1 percent of the fluid that passed into the beginning of the tubule. The other 99 percent is reabsorbed along the way by the capillary net surrounding the tubule. It thus seeps back into the circulation.

kidney dysfunction

Kidney disease costs this country 100,000 lives a year. It is estimated that over 3,300,000 people in the United States have undiagnosed kidney disease. Some kidney diseases give immediate warning. Others do not. Once kidney disease has developed, its progression must be stubbornly resisted.

Pyelonephritis is inflammation of the kidney and its pelvis. At all ages, it is the most common kidney disease. In its early stages, it need not interfere with kidney function. As a chronic disease, pyelonephritis plays havoc with kidney function.

The *nephrotic syndrome* (*nephrosis*) is not a single inflammatory disease of the kidney. It is a group of kidney ailments with a variety of causes. When it occurs, large amounts of protein molecules escape from the blood into the urine. Body water accumulates (*edema*). The syndrome may affect children. The cause is unknown, yet there is adequate treatment. In some cases, depending on the underlying cause, the drug cortisone is helpful.

Acute glomerulonephritis is not a direct inflammation of the kidneys. Their inflammation results from an infection elsewhere in the body, usually caused by a type of streptococcus. It is rarely fatal. (It will be recalled that rheumatic heart disease is also associated with a streptococcal infection.) During episodes of acute glomerulonephritis many nephrons may be destroyed. Kidney function is diminished. A prominent sign may be blood in the urine. In a few weeks the patient usually recovers from the acute attack. However, repeated attacks of acute glomerulonephritis will destroy an increasing number of nephrons.

9-17 *A glomerulus. Blood enters and leaves at A. After filtering through the glomerular capillaries, fluid enters Bowman's space (B), which drains into the convoluted tubule.*

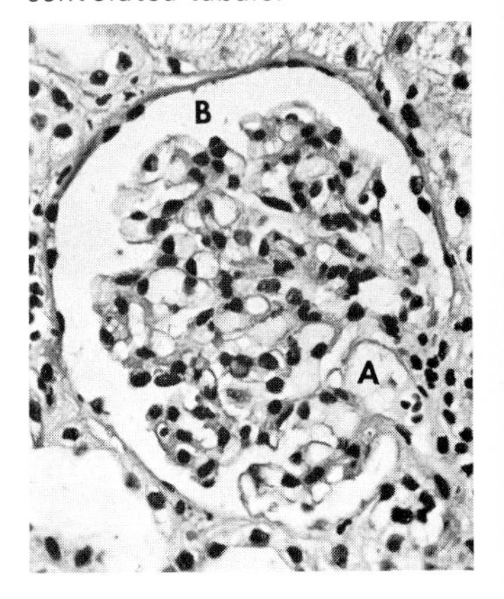

[59] Two common chemicals, caffeine (in coffee) and theophylline (in tea), cause dilatation of the afferent arterioles. This results in an increased pressure in the glomerulus. The rate of its filtration increases and, therefore, so does the urine output.

Chronic glomerulonephritis may result from repeated attacks of acute glomerulonephritis. However, many people with chronic glomerulonephritis give no history of such previous repeated episodes. Chronic glomerulonephritis results in progressive damage to the glomeruli; uremia (see below) is inevitable. There is no cure. However, much can be done to delay the ravages of the illness.

Polycystic kidneys occur as a result of improper embryological development of the nephron. This condition may be diagnosed at birth or during early infancy. The kidneys may be filled with fluid-filled cysts or cavities of varying size. When there are too many large cysts, the kidney will not function properly. Fortunately, most people with polycystic kidneys have the condition only mildly. They lead normal lives.

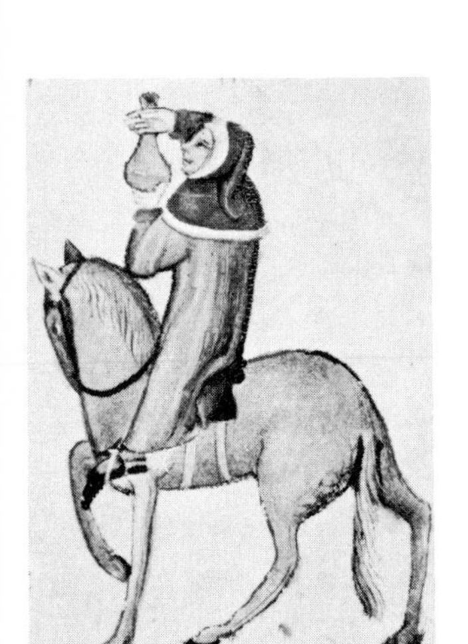

9-18 *". . . Thine urinals, God bless them, and our Lady Saint Marie!" A medieval physician examines a flask of urine.*

Unchecked chronic kidney disease results in a wide variety of symptoms. There may be a burning sensation upon urination, or the affected person may have to urinate frequently. The urine may turn a dark coffee color or appear bloody. In severe cases, widespread swelling of body tissues occurs. Thus the feet, legs, face, or abdomen may swell. Failure of the kidney to excrete waste results in a virtual accumulation of such waste in the blood. This is *uremia* (Greek *ouron,* urine + *haima,* blood), a most serious condition.

Modern miracles have prolonged the life of many kidney disease sufferers. Antibiotics fight infection. *Diuretic* drugs (page 232) help the kidney eliminate salt and water, thus relieving edema. As already noted, *cortisone* is helpful in the treatment of nephrosis; as yet, nobody knows why. *Artificial kidneys* are wonderfully complex mechanical devices that purify polluted uremic blood by filtration. Tragically, the procedure, which saves lives, is very expensive, and there are not nearly enough artificial kidney machines attended by trained personnel to keep alive all those who could benefit from the treatment. A new, smaller, and less expensive artificial kidney has been developed and is being tested.[60] *Kidney transplants* are today quite common. A transplant from a living donor is possible because a person can function with just one kidney. A recipient's body is not as likely to reject a transplanted kidney donated by a blood relative as one donated by a nonrelative; the former has a 75 percent chance of surviving for a year or more in the recipient's body; the latter has but a 25 to 40 percent chance. Failure of a kidney transplant need not be fatal. Second and third transplants have been successful. The transplant procedure, like all other successful methods of treatment of kidney disease, is the happy result of long years of scientific labor. How important is this achievement? As one writer has put it: "Bones can break, muscles can atrophy, glands can loaf, even the brain can go to sleep, without immediately endangering our survival; but should the kidneys fail to manufacture the proper kind of blood, neither bone, muscle, gland nor brain could carry on."[61]

[60] A capsule has recently been developed that serves as a tiny kidney dialysis unit. It has already been shown to be effective with animals with impaired kidney function. Swallowed, the capsule absorbs uremic wastes directly from the gastrointestinal tract. When filled with waste, it is excreted intact from the gastrointestinal tract. ("'Future Is Now' in Research to Aid Renal Patients," *Journal of the American Medical Association,* Vol. 218, No. 12 [December 20, 1971], pp. 1777–78.)

[61] Homer W. Smith, *From Fish to Philosopher* (Boston, 1953), p. 4.

summary

Another major group of chronic diseases (in addition to cancer, discussed in Chapter 8) afflict the body's systems of circulation and filtration.

The *cardiovascular* apparatus of the circulatory system consists of:

1. the *heart.* The two sides of the heart are separated by a *septum*. Each side has an upper chamber, or *atrium,* and a lower chamber, or *ventricle*. The flow of blood through these four chambers is controlled by the *tricuspid* and *bicuspid* (or *mitral*) valves (page 215). The heart circulates blood to the lungs in the *pulmonary circuit* and to the rest of the body (via the *aorta*) in the *systemic circuit* (pages 215–16). The heart is kept beating rhythmically by the emission of electrical impulses from its *pacemaker* (the *sinoatrial node* (page 217).

2. the *blood vessels.* These are the *arteries* and *veins,* the *arterioles, capillaries,* and *venules,* and the *coronary circulation* within the heart itself, particularly the *coronary arteries* of the aorta (page 217).

3. the *blood.* The blood consists of fluid *plasma,* in which are suspended different kinds of cells: *erythrocytes,* or red blood cells, in which *hemoglobin* is formed (page 219); *leukocytes,* or white blood cells (pages 219–20); and *platelets* (page 220).

By means of the circulatory system, oxygen, nutrients, hormones, and other vital materials are carried to the body's tissue cells, and carbon dioxide and other wastes are carried away (pages 221–22)—carbon dioxide to be vaporized through the lungs, nongaseous wastes to be filtered out by the liver and kidneys (page 223). An accessory circulatory system, the *lymphatic system,* consists of the lymphatic vessels (filled with a fluid called *lymph*) and lymph nodes. This system returns protein to the blood and keeps cellular debris, toxins, and other wastes out of the blood. These wastes are digested by the *lymph nodes,* in which lymphocytes proliferate and in which plasma cells make antibodies (page 224). Lymph node tissue forms lymphoid organs—the *tonsils, adenoids,* and *spleen.*

The basic cause of most deaths from circulatory ailments is *atherosclerosis* (page 225), a condition that begins with damage to the internal lining of arteries, with deposits of *plaques* containing *cholesterol* and other fatty substances (pages 226–29).

The four basic manifestations of heart disease are:

1. *cardiac ischemia,* the inability of a coronary artery to deliver enough blood to the heart (page 229). This may result in any of four conditions: *coronary occlusion* (page 229), *angina pectoris* (page 230), *rhythm disturbances* (page 230), or *congestive heart failure* (pages 230–31).

2. *congenital defects* (page 231).

3. *infection* (pages 231–32).

4. *metabolic and endocrine disorders* (page 232).

Investigations such as the *Framingham Study* (pages 233–34) have indicated that the "coronary profile" of factors frequently associated with heart disease includes *heredity* (pages 234–35), *gender* (pages 235–36), *age* (page 236), *inactivity* (pages 236–37), and *improper diet* (pages 237–39).

Hypertensive heart disease, associated with abnormally high *blood pressure,* is a major killer in the United States (pages 241–43).

The body's circulating blood filters through the *kidneys,* the major organs of excretion of wastes (pages 243–46).

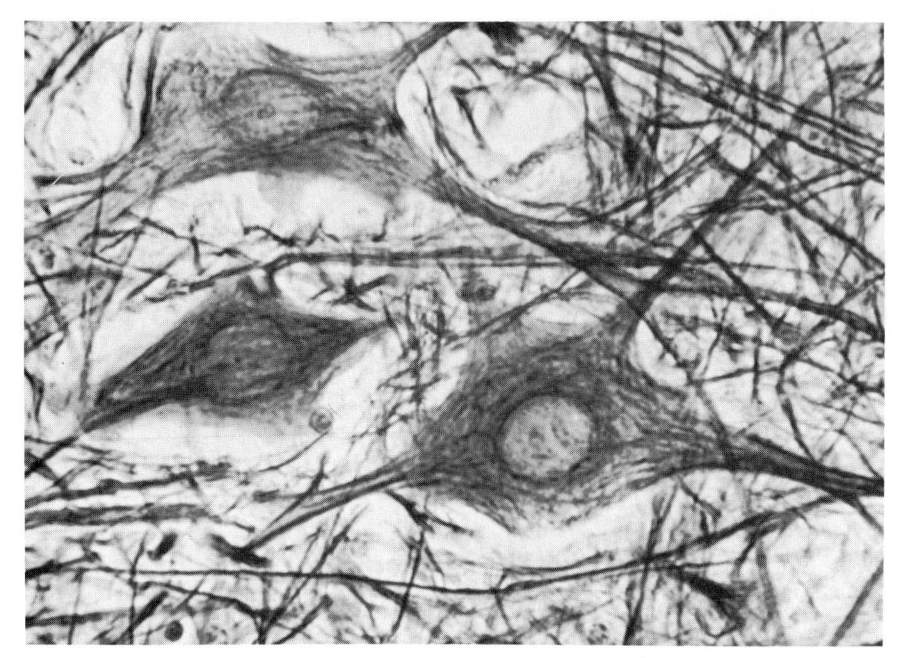

A human motor nerve cell, greatly magnified.

allergies, the bones and joints, certain glands, and the nervous system

10

allergy: a swelling

how allergy occurs

Whatever turns your skin to scum,
Or turns your blood to glue,
Why that's the what, the special what,
That you're allergic to.[1]

To be allergic to a causative substance, a susceptible individual must encounter it at least twice. The initial time he is sensitized to it. Later he reacts to it. At the first encounter, the foreign substance—the antigen—stimulates the body cells to generate specific antibodies to it (see Chapter 6, pages 142–43). The individual shows no symptoms. At the second encounter, the antigen reacts with the very antibodies it had previously caused to be formed. Thus has the reaction of an individual to a specific stimulus been altered. This altered reaction is allergy.

An antigen-antibody reaction on a cell injures the cell. This injury causes the release of histamine and histaminelike substances. When liberated, they cause the dilation of local capillaries and arterioles. More blood rushes to the scene. The injured cells are fed more oxygen, more nourishment, more of life's healing alchemy. With allergy there is an excess influence of histamine and an abnormal dilation of capillaries and arterioles. In overabundance, blood fluid leaks into the tissue spaces. There is swelling. This may occur in a small body organ, or the entire respiratory tree may be involved. In this latter instance, excessive swelling of the lining of the bronchioles (one of the smaller subdivisions of the branched bronchial tree) results in narrowed airways and difficult breathing. In the skin, it is swelling that produces hives. It is swelling that is responsible for all the manifestations of allergy.

the kinds of allergic reactions

The various types of allergy are legion and are endured by legions of sufferers. There are the nasal allergies manifested by sneezing, runny stuffed nose, itching, tearing eyes, and dulled hearing, taste, and smell. The sneezing season varies in different areas. In some parts of the East, for example, the sources of hay fever are trees in March, grasses in May, and weeds in August. Some peo-

[1] Ogden Nash, "Allergy Met a Bear," in *I'm a Stranger Here Myself* (Boston, 1938), p. 125.

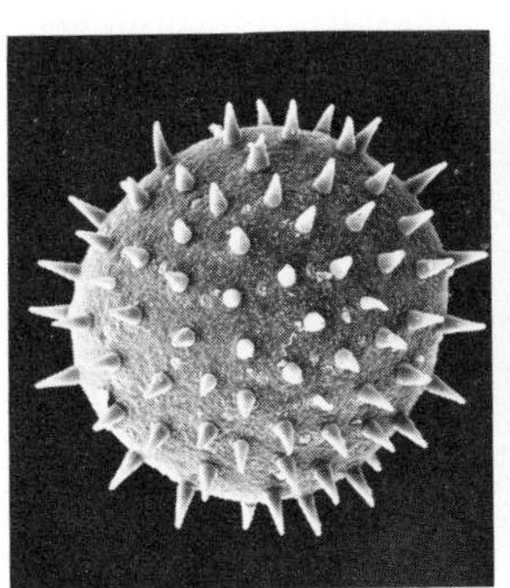
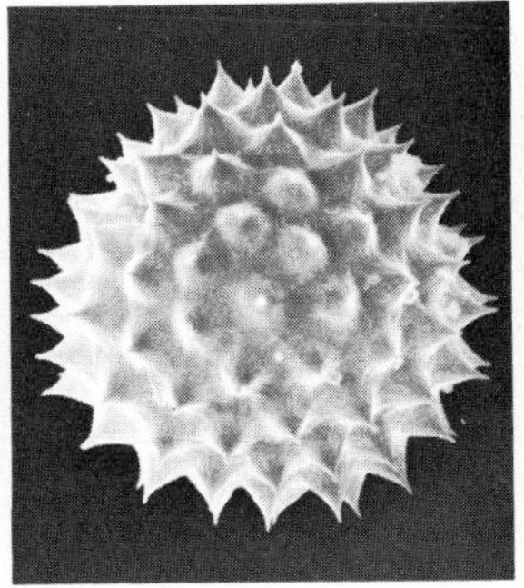
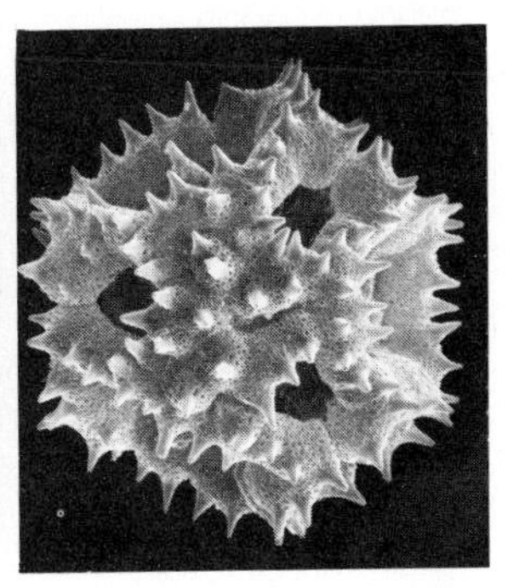

10-1 *Pollen grains: hibiscus* (left, ×*380*), *giant ragweed* (center, ×*2,380*), *and dandelion* (right, ×*2,340*). *A pollen grain, one of the most durable structures found in nature, is the male sex cell of a flowering plant, encased in a tough wall to protect it on its wind-carried fertilizing journey.*

ple, often children, are troubled all year.[2] Commonly, secondary superimposed infections plague them. *Asthma* is an evil manifestation of bronchial allergy. In chronic cases, the constantly irritated, thickened muscle fibers of the smaller breathing tubes go into constricting spasm. The channels of the breathing tubes, already decreased by swollen linings and plugged by thick secretions, are further narrowed. The sufferer coughs, wheezes, struggles for breath. There are two types of asthma: *extrinsic* asthma develops when the individual is sensitized, and thus made allergic, to a substance in his environment; in *intrinsic* asthma it is impossible to find any external cause of sensitization. Some physicians feel that intrinsic asthma results from an infection within the patient's respiratory system. Asthma can debilitate and it can kill.

The itching raised areas of *hives* may be a skin manifestation of food or drug allergy. *Eczema,* a chronic skin disease, is now considered an allergic illness. A common manifestation of skin allergy is termed *contact dermatitis.* The classic example is poison ivy. However, perfumes, hair bleaches, and similar products are frequent offenders. Some physicians consider the dreadful headache of *migraine* to be caused by an allergy to various foods or inhalants. There is frequently a strong emotional component to these episodes.

the treatment of some types of allergies

The treatment of hay fever or allergic inflammation of the nasal mucous membranes depends largely on *avoidance of the cause* and, perhaps, *hyposensitization.* In this latter procedure, small, but increasing, doses of the offending agent (antigen) are injected into the susceptible individual. As a result, the patient slowly builds a tolerance to the antigen. Thus, he becomes able to endure higher doses of exposure before symptoms are precipitated: he becomes less sensitive, or *hyposensitive.* Some physicians question the effectiveness of hyposensitization for all forms of allergic asthma. Although used for years, and seemingly often helpful, this method still needs further study.

Treatment with antihistamines is effective with some hay fever patients. (They are of little or no apparent value in eczema or asthma.) They do neutralize histamine and relieve symptoms. But they do not prevent cellular injury. Thus, although treatment of hay fever patients with antihistamines alone is temporarily effective, without added treatment it may be dangerous. Why? Such inadequately treated individuals may develop asthma or bronchitis. Individuals with hay fever should, therefore, seek total treatment from their physicians. Self-medication with over-the-counter antihistamines gives only transient relief.

some chronic muscle and joint disorders

gout

Gout may be considered a contributing cause of the American Revolution. More than once, William Pitt rose on his swollen foot in the House of Commons to defend the colonists. ''The Americans,'' he declared, ''are entitled to the common rights of representation and cannot be bound to pay taxes without their

[2] It is a grievous irony that ragweed, an herb tormenting innumerable asthmatics, is of the genus *Ambrosia*—a word that may also refer to a delicious, fragrant food or drink.

consent."[3] A particularly violent attack of gout, forcing the English statesman to be absent from the House, made it possible to pass a colonial duty on tea. The Boston Tea Party of 1773 resulted.

The painful, hot, swollen, blue-red joint of the gout sufferer has long and wrongly been attributed to overindulgence in food and drink. In the blood and other body fluids of gout victims there collects an excess of uric acid. This is deposited, as crystals, in the joints and other tissues. The disease runs in families, is uncommon in children and premenopausal women,[4] and is most common in people thirty years of age and older. In this country some 350,000 people are afflicted with it. Elevation of the extremity, rest, drugs, and diet are the best treatment. Gout is but one of almost fifty *rheumatic diseases.* All have one common denominator: connective tissue is involved. This includes not only the delicate scaffolding between cells, but also the tendons, ligaments, cartilage, and fat that, along with bone, provide support and shape for the body. In the rheumatic diseases it is usually the muscles and joints that are involved. *Arthritis* (Greek *arthron,* joint + *-itis,* a word ending denoting inflammation) is not a specific disease. It is a joint inflammation causing pain, swelling, and stiffness.

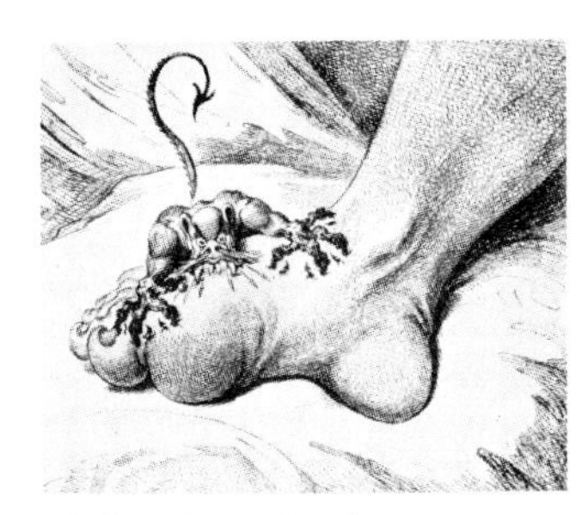

10-2 *The pain of gout: a fanciful rendition.*

About three-fourths of people with rheumatism have one of two conditions: *rheumatoid arthritis* or *osteoarthritis.*

rheumatoid arthritis

The use of the word "arthritis" should not mislead one into considering rheumatoid arthritis a mere joint inflammation. The connective tissue throughout the whole body is involved. An infectious agent has not been proven; the disease is not communicable. A wide variety of circumstances seem to trigger it. These include exposure, infection, cold, and emotional distress. It attacks women more often than men. No other chronic disease disables more people during the working years. Although even infants have the disease, about 80 percent of the cases occur between those vital years, twenty and fifty. The Arthritis Foundation estimates that about 5 million people in this country have the disease. The joints hurt most, the smaller hand joints (particularly the knuckles) most often. If the joints of one hand are affected, the corresponding opposite joints are usually soon involved. In early stages, the individual may experience periods of temporary improvement. It is then that he is most susceptible to quackery.

Recent research has revealed much about this widespread ailment. In Chapter 6 (pages 141–45), the role of the white blood cells in the immune response was shown to be essential to health, even to survival. But the normal immune response can turn against body function and cause tissue inflammation. This is the *autoimmune theory of rheumatoid arthritis.* Also, scientists now suspect that *prostaglandins* are responsible for triggering the inflammation. (These hormonelike substances act locally in many body tissues; see pages 630–31.) This notion was strengthened when it was discovered that aspirin can

[3] W. S. C. Copeman, *A Short History of the Gout and the Rheumatic Diseases* (Berkeley, 1964), p. 96.
[4] "Juvenile Gout," *British Medical Journal,* Vol. 1, No. 5793 (January 15, 1972), p. 129.

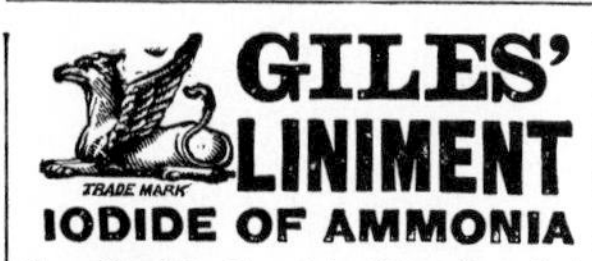

Cures **Neuralgia, Face Ache, Rheumatism, Gout, Frosted Feet, Chilblains, Sore Throat, Erysipelas, Bruises,** or **Wounds** of every kind in man or animal.

We sell more of GILES' LINIMENT IODIDE OF AMMONIA; it gives better satisfaction than any Liniment we ever saw. It is a pleasure to have something that a druggist can conscientiously recommend.

F. & E. BAILEY & CO.,
Apothecaries, Lowell, Mass.

Sold by all Druggists. Depot 451 Sixth Ave., N. Y. Only 50 cents and $1 per bottle.

10-3 *Quackery to cure rheumatism. This advertisement appeared in* Harper's Weekly *magazine in 1876.*

prevent the manufacture of prostaglandins in the body. For example, eight aspirins a day markedly reduced the amount of prostaglandins in the seminal fluid of male volunteers. This seemed to explain why aspirin is so helpful in the treatment of rheumatoid arthritis: it inhibits the manufacture of prostaglandins.

But it has also been found that prostaglandins not only can turn on inflammation but also can curtail it. It is theorized that this is due to their ability to stop the release of inflammation-causing enzymes from the white blood cells. How can this paradoxical action be explained? One possible answer: via a rather common body function—the negative feedback mechanism (see pages 255–58). When chemicals reach certain levels in the body, those very levels signal the body to discontinue the production or release of the chemical until it is again needed.[5]

A more complete understanding of this and other arthritic processes is gained by an understanding of the role of *collagen* (see page 684), which is the main supportive protein of skin, tendon, bone, cartilage, and connective tissue. Without collagen the body would indeed "come unglued."[6] Recently, an enzyme, *collagenase,* has been discovered, which can degrade collagen. Now, the smooth inner lining of a joint cavity—the synovial membrane, or *synovium*—encloses *synovia,* a fluid resembling egg white. Collagenase, when produced and released by the rheumatoid synovium, destroys cartilage and other supportive connective tissue. In the laboratory the destructive action of collagenase can be inhibited; this knowledge points the way to research for possible treatments. Using penicillamine, a close relative of the antibiotic penicillin, English researchers in 1973 reported dramatic success in providing arthritics with relief.[7]

Thus, the outlook is hopeful. The total crippling of another day is now rare. Rest is an important aspect of treatment. Splints, proper exercise, and physical therapy help to prevent deformity. About one-fourth of the cases of rheumatoid arthritis seem to recover completely. Another half have considerable periods of freedom from the disease. Surgical excision of the synovial membrane, such as that lining an affected knee joint, can alleviate pain and swelling for at least five years. Eventually, however, the membrane regenerates and again becomes diseased.[8]

osteoarthritis

Osteoarthritis is a degenerative joint disease, not an inflammation (see Figures 10-4 and 10-5). The *-itis* is thus unjustified. It is surely the most common of all joint ailments. After forty, almost everyone has it to some degree. Most people, diagnosing their own "arthritis," most likely have degenerative joint disease. Animals are also susceptible. Because of it, more than one racehorse has been put to pasture.

In this chronic condition, cartilage, a specialized fibrous connective tissue,

[5] "Prostaglandin Complicity in Rheumatoid Arthritis," *Science News,* Vol. 102, No. 12 (September 12, 1972), pp. 181–82.

[6] "Learning How Man May Come Unglued," *Medical World News* (January 14, 1972), pp. 15–18.

[7] "Good News for Arthritics," *Medical World News,* Vol. 5, No. 5 (May 1973), p. 8.

[8] Dugald Gardner, "Antirheumatism Battle Progressing but Not Won," *Hospital Tribune,* Vol. 5, No. 21 (November 1, 1971), p. 14.

gradually deteriorates. So does bone. This occurs because of the constantly repeated small injuries of weight-bearing. Chronic joint irritation due to obesity, poor posture, old damage from infection, dislocation, or fracture—all these promote osteoarthritis. Unlike rheumatoid arthritis, with osteoarthritis the damage is local. Healing is slow (cartilage is the slowest-healing body tissue). Orthopedic appliances (when necessary), weight reduction, physical therapy, and mild drugs to mitigate discomfort all help. The surgical treatment of advanced osteoarthritis has progressed greatly in recent years. In selected cases, hip joints, for example, can be replaced with a combination of plastic and metal.[9]

[9] *Ibid.*

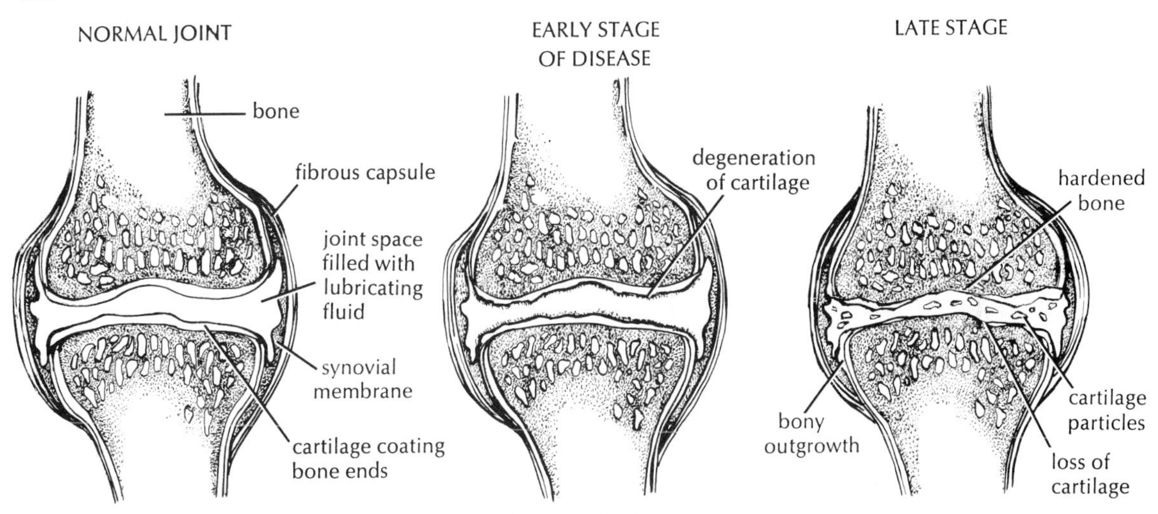

10-4 *A normal joint and early and late stages of osteoarthritis.*

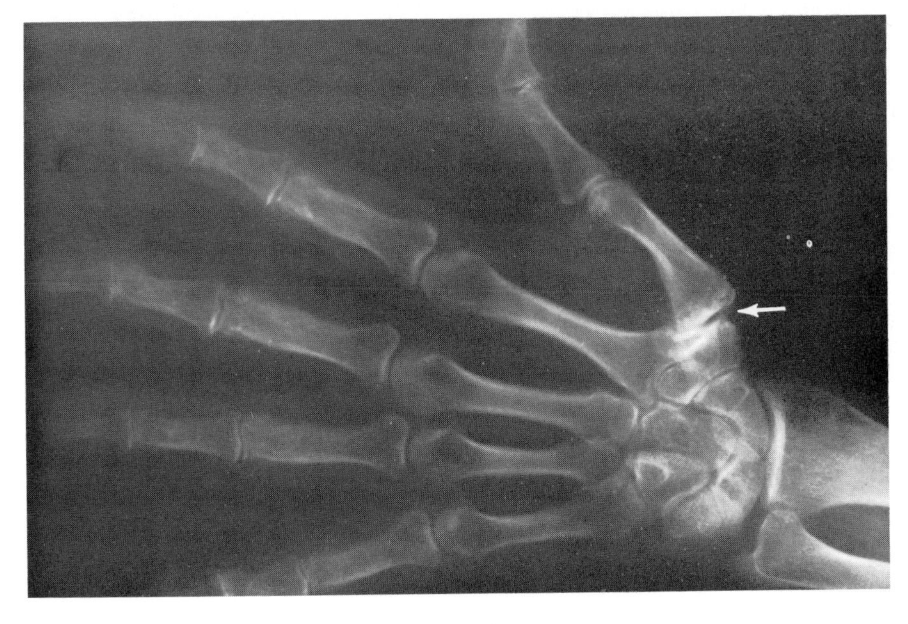

10-5 *An X-ray of a hand diseased by osteoarthritis. The light areas on either side of the arrow represent increased bone formation, which is partly in response to loss of cartilage in the joint. This joint—the junction of the thumb and wrist—is the most common site of osteoarthritis in the hand.*

rheumatism not involving a joint

A wide variety of rheumatic disorders, involving various body parts other than joints, come under the heading *nonarticular* (Latin *articularis,* of a joint) *rheumatism.* One of these is *fibrositis,* an inflammation of the body's white fibrous tissue, particularly the tissue sheathing muscles. Muscle soreness and stiffness are major symptoms. However, neither joint swelling nor bone damage occurs. Fibrositis can be precipitated by emotional and physical strain, cold, and fatigue. *Lumbago* means back pain. It may be a local fibrositis or it may be due to the much more serious rupture of one of the discs between the bones of the spinal column. Each disc is made of *fibrocartilage* (a specialized connective tissue with a considerable groundwork of fibrous tissue). These *intervertebral discs* act as shock absorbers. When damage occurs to the ligaments holding them in place, they slip and bulge. This condition requires expert care. Surgery may be indicated. The pain of *sciatica,* extending along the large branching nerve to the leg, may be caused by a ''slipped disc.''

Aspirin, injections of anesthetics, heat, massage, light exercise, and hot baths are all useful in treating most of these conditions. If the patient cooperates, the outlook is excellent.

the exocrine and endocrine glands

their pervasive role in body government

The secretions of some glands are carried through outlet tubes, or *ducts.* These glands secrete externally or into hollow organs. Among these are the breasts or mammary glands (page 483) and the sweat, tear, and salivary glands (page 483). These are *exocrine* glands (Greek *exo,* outside + *krinein,* to separate).

Unlike these, the *endocrine* glands are ductless (see body chart 15 in the color section and Table 10-1). *Endocrine* is Greek for ''I separate within.'' From the many chemicals carried in the blood of the arteries, the endocrine glands manufacture their own potent secretions or *hormones* (Greek ''I arouse'' or ''I stimulate''). Releasing their finished hormonal products into the veins over a long time and in perfectly accurate doses, the endocrine system of glands governs various body processes. Endocrine glands profoundly influence personality. They are supervised by the central nervous system. (There is growing evidence that hormones affect the activity of genes.)

The endocrine glands are the *pituitary* (pages 254–58), *thyroid* (page 259), *thymus* (page 142, footnote 5), *parathyroid,* part of the *pancreas* (page 687), *adrenal* (pages 258–59), and tissue within the *gonads* (ovaries and testes). Some functions of the endocrine glands are listed in Table 10-1. Consider some of them separately.

the pituitary gland

Attached to the base of the brain by its short stem, and snugly encased in its bony fortress, is the pituitary gland. It is no larger than a cherry and weighs no more than two baby-dose aspirins. It has a front (anterior) lobe and a back (posterior) lobe. So profoundly influenced are both lobes of the pituitary gland by that part of the brain that is nearest to them—the *hypothalamus*—that this relationship must here be examined.[10]

THE HYPOTHALAMUS AND THE POSTERIOR LOBE OF THE PITUITARY GLAND It has long been believed that the two hormones of the posterior lobe of the pituitary gland are actually synthesized by secreting nerve cells in the brain's hypothalamus. Then these two hormones are believed to be transported to nerve endings of the pituitary gland's posterior lobe via axons (see page 262) that extend between it and the hypothalamus. The posterior lobe itself manufactures nothing; it merely acts as the storage and releasing center of its two contained hormones. Thus it is not true endocrine gland tissue. The major action of one of its hormones, *oxytocin,* is the stimulation of uterine contractions and the contractions of the muscle-epithelial cells surrounding the outer walls of the alveoli (small sacs) of the breasts, which in turn expresses milk into the lobules and ducts (see page 843). *Vasopressin,* the second hormone of the pituitary gland's posterior lobe, includes among its functions the stimulation of the contraction of the muscular tissue of the arterioles and the capillaries; this raises the blood pressure. It also stimulates the intestinal muscles, promoting peristalsis (see page 685). However, its major function is in greatly limiting the excretion of water by the kidneys, thus permitting its reabsorption for reuse by the body (see pages 243–45).

THE HYPOTHALAMUS AND THE ANTERIOR LOBE OF THE PITUITARY GLAND Because of its relationship with other glands in the body, the anterior lobe of the pituitary gland has been called "the master gland." It is not. In the first place, its relationship to the other glands is as much reciprocal as it is controlling. Second, recent research has shown it to be largely dependent on the hypothalamus. Unlike the posterior lobe, the control of the anterior lobe is not mediated by nerve fibers. All known chemical exchanges between it and the hypothalamus are made through a unique network of tiny blood vessels (capillaries; see page 217). Thus, different kinds of hypothalamic nerve fibers liberate hormones from their endings into nearby capillaries. These hormones are then carried by slightly larger vessels to the anterior lobe of the pituitary gland. There they, in turn, either stimulate or inhibit the release of the various anterior pituitary hormones.

Although the anterior lobe of the pituitary is a single structure, it is composed of a variety of cells; and each variety is ready to respond to the specific bidding of the brain's hypothalamus. Once the anterior lobe of the pituitary has been influenced to manufacture and release one of its hormones, that hormone enters the blood to reach target organs. The amount of hormone must be controlled with exquisite accuracy. How is this accomplished? Through a subtly responding feedback mechanism, by which the target organ sends a chemical message back to the anterior lobe of the pituitary, and thus on to the hypothalamus, to halt stimulation.

[10] An excellent review of recent research in this area is Andrew V. Schally, Akira Arimura, and Abba J. Kastin, "Hypothalamic Regulatory Hormones," *Science,* Vol. 179, No. 4071 (January 26, 1973), pp. 341–50.

TABLE 10-1

Some Human Endocrine Glands and Hormones and Some of Their Effects

ENDOCRINE GLAND	HORMONE	SOME OF THE PROCESSES AFFECTED OR CONTROLLED	RESULTS OF EXCESS	RESULTS OF DEFICIENCY
Thyroid	Thyroxin	Level of metabolism, oxidation rate, etc.	Irritability, nervous activity, exophthalmos	Cretinism when severe in infancy; lethargy, myxedema
Parathyroids	Parathyroid hormone	Calcium balance	Bone deformation	Spasms; death if severe[a]
Adrenal medulla[b]	Epinephrine	Stimulation similar to that of sympathetic nervous system	Increased blood pressure, pulse rate, blood glucose[c]	None
Adrenal cortex	Aldosterone	Salt balance	Accumulation of body fluid[d]	Addison's disease[e]
	Hydrocortisone	Carbohydrate metabolism	Abnormality of sugar metabolism	
Pancreas[f]	Insulin	Glucose metabolism	Shock, coma	Diabetes
Ovary[g]	Estrogen	Female sex development and menstrual cycle		Interference with menstrual cycle and sexual activity
	Progesterone	Control of ovary and uterus during pregnancy		Sterility or miscarriage
Testis[h]	Testosterone	Male sex development and activity		Lessened development of male characteristics and lessened sexual activity

But not all these hormones are controlled by target feedback. For some, the hypothalamus makes hormones that inhibit pituitary overproduction. Thus, the hypothalamus produces hormones (also called *factors*) that (1) cause the anterior pituitary to make and release hormones destined for target organs and (2) inhibit the anterior pituitary from producing too much.

Hypothalamic hormones that induce anterior pituitary target hormones are:

1. Thyrotropin-releasing hormone (TRH), which causes the anterior lobe of the pituitary gland to both manufacture and release thyrotropin. By way of the blood circulation, thyrotropin reaches the thyroid gland to stimulate it to produce the iodine-containing hormone thyroxin.

2. Luteinizing-hormone–releasing hormone (LH-RH). When released by the anterior lobe of the pituitary, luteinizing hormones cause a mature follicle in the ovary to rupture, releasing the ovum. In the male, luteinizing hormone has various functions, of which a major one is the production of testosterone.

3. Follicle-stimulating-hormone–releasing hormone (FSH-RH). Follicle-

TABLE 10-1 (*continued*)

ENDOCRINE GLAND	HORMONE	SOME OF THE PROCESSES AFFECTED OR CONTROLLED	RESULTS OF EXCESS	RESULTS OF DEFICIENCY
Pituitary				
Anterior lobe	Adrenocorticotropic hormone (ACTH)	Control of adrenal cortex	Symptoms related to glands controlled.	
	Thyrotropic hormone	Control of thyroid		
	Gonadotropic hormones	Control of sex glands		
	Growth hormone	Growth	Gigantism	Dwarfism
Posterior lobe	Vasopressin	Kidney action	Excessive water in body	Excessive loss of water
	Oxytocin	Contraction of uterine muscle		Lessened or no milk production

[a]Parathyroid deficiency used to follow the surgical removal of thyroid tissue when part or all of the parathyroids were accidentally removed at the same time. Surgeons are now aware of this danger and avoid it.
[b]The medulla is the inner part of the adrenal gland. The hormone epinephrine is also known as adrenalin.
[c]The symptoms noted are apparently normal results of increased adrenal secretion, but they may result from other causes not involving excessive epinephrine secretion.
[d]Aldosterone causes the kidney to retain sodium. Excessive sodium retention causes the retention of an osmotically equivalent amount of water.
[e]Addison's disease, fortunately rare, has among its symptoms coloration (bronzing) of the skin, low blood pressure, general weakness, loss of water from the body, and upset carbohydrate metabolism.
[f]The pancreas as a whole is not an endocrine gland, but it contains clusters of cells, the islets of Langerhans, that have an endocrine function and secrete insulin.
[g]The ovary as a whole is not an endocrine gland, but some of the cells around the developing eggs produce estrogen. After an egg leaves the ovary, *corpus luteum* develops, and this secretes progesterone.
[h]Like the ovary, the testis is not exclusively an endocrine gland but does contain hormone-producing tissue.
Source: Adapted from George Gaylord Simpson and William S. Beck, *Life: An Introduction to Biology,* 2nd ed. (New York, 1965), pp. 342–43.

stimulating hormone promotes the growth and maturation of the Graafian follicle in the ovary of the female, and the production of spermatozoa in the testes of the male (see page 474).

4. Growth-hormone–releasing hormone (GH-RH). Growth hormone has a widespread effect on the body at different stages of life. Produced in excess during the growth period, *gigantism* may occur (see Figure 10-6); produced in excess in the mature adult, the hormone may cause bone thickening of the face and extremities (*acromegaly*). A genetically based shortage of growth hormone is responsible for *dwarfism.*

5. Prolactin-releasing hormone (PRH). Upon its release from the anterior lobe of the pituitary, the hormone prolactin induces lactation (the production of milk) in mammals.

6. Melanocyte-stimulating-hormone–releasing hormone (MRH), which stimulates the pituitary's melanocyte-stimulating-hormone (MSH) to, in turn, stimulate melanocytes, skin cells, to make their dark pigment—*melanin.*

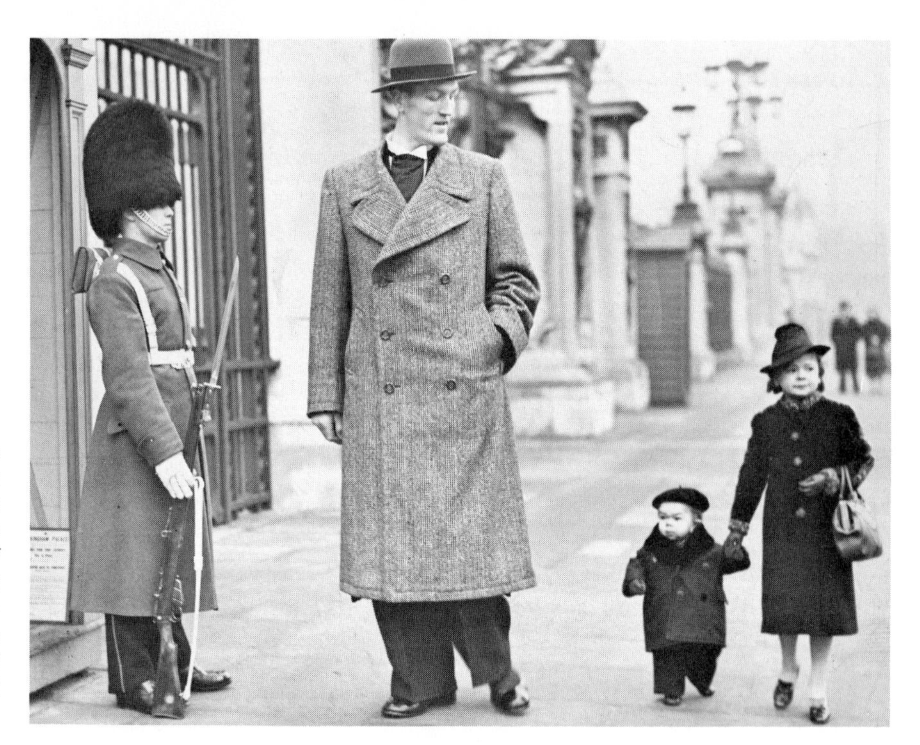

10-6 *Three adults with pituitary dysfunction walk past a sentry at Buckingham Palace some years ago. Olaf Petursson, 25, is 8 feet 6 inches tall; Prince Daumling, 33, is eighteen inches; and Helga, 29, is 3 feet 6 inches.*

7. Corticotropin-releasing hormone (CRH), which stimulates the anterior pituitary to release corticotropin (also called *adrenocorticotropic hormone,* or ACTH). ACTH stimulates the outer rind, or cortex, of the adrenal gland (see below).

Hypothalamic hormones that directly inhibit the anterior pituitary are:

1. Growth-hormone-release–inhibiting hormone (GHR-IH), which is produced by the hypothalamus to make up for the lack of a limiting *feedback mechanism* from target organs (see above).
2. Prolactin-release–inhibiting hormone (PRIH).
3. Melanocyte-stimulating-hormone-release–inhibiting hormone (MRIH).

the adrenal gland

The *medulla* (central portion) of the adrenal gland secretes both epinephrine and norepinephrine. In concert with the sympathetic nervous system, epinephrine produces the rapid heart rate, increased blood pressure, and increased blood sugar associated with stress. There is evidence that chronic excitement can cause adrenal damage.

The adrenal *cortex* (outer portion) provides chemicals called *adrenocortical steroids,* which regulate sugar and salt metabolism. Steroids, such as *cortisone,* are sometimes useful in treating severe asthma and arthritis.

Three groups of steroid hormones are produced by the adrenal cortex. *Hydrocortisone* aids in forming sugar from protein. It also has a widespread anti-inflammatory action throughout the body. It is, moreover, called forth in times of stress such as emotion (anger, fear), excessive muscular exercise, severe infection or trauma, and extreme heat and cold. There is a pituitary-adrenal axis in the sense that the pituitary gland releases a special hormone stimulating the adrenal cortex to make and release enough hydrocortisone in the blood. By its direct action on the kidneys, a second steroid hormone, *aldosterone,* maintains the sodium–potassium balance in the body. The third of the steroid hormones is a group called the *androgens.* In the male most of the androgen is produced by the testes. Only a small amount is normally produced by the adrenal cortex. Rarely, a tumor of the adrenal cortex will produce excess androgen. This can cause serious masculinizing effects even of the female. A normal amount of adrenal androgen in the female does not make her masculine and is, indeed, necessary for her health.

the thyroid gland

The thyroid gland straddles the trachea (windpipe) and larynx. It governs the rate of body metabolism. Severely diminished thyroid function resulting in insufficient production of the iron-containing hormone thyroxine causes *cretinism* and *infantile myxedema.* A child with cretinism grows poorly and is sexually and mentally retarded. Infantile myxedema is characterized by diminished physical and mental vigor, hair loss, weight increase, and a thickening of the skin. *Hyperthyroidism,* resulting from an overactive thyroid, produces severe nervousness and weight loss. Sometimes the hyperthyroid person has protruding eyeballs (*exophthalmos*). Surgical removal of part of the thyroid gland often corrects this condition. *Goiter,* an enlargement of the thyroid, is discussed on page 656, footnote 24.

two major glandular dysfunctions

cystic fibrosis: an exocrine dysfunction

Cystic fibrosis is this country's greatest genetic killer of white children. If both the mother and father are carriers of the cystic fibrosis gene, each child they have stands one chance in four of having the disease. About one of 1,500 U.S. newborns has the disease. Cystic fibrosis seems nonexistent in Oriental children and rare in blacks.

Affected are the sweat glands and those ductal glands emptying into organs leading to the outside of the body. Either or both may be involved. The clear, usable fluid usually produced by these glands is replaced, in cystic fibrosis, with a sticky, thick material. There is widespread clogging of the ducts. Complicating these secretory impediments is an excessive salt secretion by the sweat, salivary, and tear glands. On hot summer days, the excessive salt loss of heavy perspiring can lead to serious heat exhaustion.

Not all afflicted children have all or even the same symptoms. Clogging of the pancreatic duct deprives the child of digestive enzymes. The hungry child eats well yet loses weight. His bulky stools are fatty and foul-smelling. The chronic plugging of the air passages leads to a nagging cough. The breathing is labored. The child tires easily.

The future of these little patients depends on constant alertness to possible lung infection. This affliction needs and is getting much research. Early in 1973, a cystic fibrosis factor had been found not only in the blood of its victims, but also in the serum of their carrier parents. This discovery will hopefully lead to a screening procedure. It is also possible to detect the factor before birth by examining the amniotic fluid by a process called amniocentesis (see page 565).[11]

diabetes mellitus: an endocrine dysfunction

Diabetes has been known for thirty-five centuries. That oldest of all medical texts, the Ebers papyrus (1550 B.C.), mentions a treatment for one of its prominent symptoms—frequent urination. To trace the disease to the pancreas required millennia.

Pancreatic tissue is both exocrine and endocrine. By way of a duct, enzymatic digestive juice is delivered to the small intestine. Ductlessly, its insulin, produced by certain of the specialized pancreatic cells in the *islets of Langerhans,*[12] is released directly into the blood. Normally, insulin regulates sugar metabolism. The dramatic effects of too much blood sugar (*diabetes mellitus*) result from the failure of the pancreas to either produce or release insulin. Many other factors may be involved. Diabetic people have disorders of fat metabolism and also of connective tissue which predispose them to atherosclerosis. But how do the major symptoms of untreated diabetes develop?

By combining carbohydrates and oxygen, cells produce life-sustaining heat and energy. Without insulin from the pancreas, this cannot happen. Insulin controls the entry of carbohydrate (glucose) into the cell. Without insulin very little glucose can enter the cell. Cellular (and body) use of glucose is slowed. Production of energy by the cell is slowed. The inability to use enough glucose for energy is a basic abnormality of diabetes mellitus. Unused, sugar (glucose) collects uselessly in the blood. It spills over into the urine. In the midst of plenty, the cells starve.

The body has no alternative but to seek other sources of heat and energy. Proteins and fats are other sources. But the overutilization of protein results in a shortage of amino acids for tissue-building. For these reasons, the untreated diabetic grows poorly, infects easily, and heals slowly. Fats, called upon to perform an unexpected duty, are also used to excess, so they respond by producing an excess of "ketone bodies." Should the concentration of these "keto acids" rise to a high enough level within and between the cells, cells will be poisoned. The diabetic will sink into a coma and die. A multitude of signs and symptoms besets the diabetic. Because of the excess use of fat and protein, he loses weight, yet he eats voraciously to relieve his constant hunger. Because of the excess glucose in his urine, he loses vast amounts of water via the kidney. He tries to slake his thirst by drinking equally great quantities of water. Fatigue,

[11] "Isolation of Cystic Fibrosis Factor May Lead to Test for Carriers," *Journal of the American Medical Association,* Vol. 224, No. 4 (April 23, 1973), pp. 455–56.

[12] Discovered in 1869 by Paul Langerhans, then a University of Berlin medical student.

weakness, blurring of the vision—all these, and more, plague him. What is even worse, prolonged, untreated diabetes promotes atherosclerosis (pages 225–29), and with it a host of circulatory disorders varying from heart disease to stroke. Without insulin the diabetic is doomed. But insulin is readily available.

In 1922, two Canadian doctors, Frederick G. Banting and Charles H. Best, announced an epochal discovery:[13] purified animal insulin could replace the natural insulin lacking in the human diabetic. Their finding brought a normal life span to millions. Since then, natural animal insulin has always been used. True, many diabetics now do very well with an oral medicine that stimulates a flagging pancreas to yield more insulin. Other chemical products relieve diabetes differently, but their mechanism is unknown. Ordinary insulin and diet are usually satisfactory for a great number of diabetics. The future will see constant improvements in the treatment of diabetes. But it is to the basic work of Banting and Best that diabetics will always owe their gratitude.

the nervous system: ease and disease

By means of his nervous system man perceives his ecosystems, relates to them, and communicates with other people within them. To deprive him experimentally of almost all environmental stimuli leads to hallucinations, space-time disorientations, even panic. It is perhaps not entirely coincidental that the brain's cerebral cells "are the most sensitive to arrest of circulation, beginning to die within five minutes. The whole brain may be considered dead in 15 minutes."[14] So, although the peripheral nerves live longer, the brain can no longer receive and perceive their messages. That is one reason why victims of threatened heart stoppage or near-drowning need extremely rapid emergency treatment.

the complexity of the nervous system

A mother leans to her baby. Lightly she strokes his cheek, tickling him. His pleasure is intense. No less gently, a stranger tickles the child. The reaction: fear. The tickler, then, must be a familiar person. To enjoy the caress, the infant must associate it with a giver of pleasure, must know that the tickler means no harm, must sense the difference between being tickled pink and tickled to death. So the tickle is more than a pressure stimulus to local skin nerves. Higher brain centers are involved.

Since a tickle is but "an itch that moves,"[15] consider the itch. Only in its immediate relief is there pleasure. Yet first there is pain. A severe itch (as occurs with some skin disorders) insists on virtual violence. The scratch must be enough to tear off the whole upper layer of itching skin, including some of the network of tormenting nerves. So the itch, the tickle, and skin pain are related. Indeed, all three are thought to be mediated by the same group of nerve cells.

[13] Banting and John James Macleod, a Scottish physiologist, shared the 1923 Nobel Prize for medicine and physiology. Macleod was also associated with the discovery. Best did not receive the Nobel Prize.

[14] "The Moment of Death," an editorial in *World Medical Journal,* Vol. 14, No. 5 (May 1967), p. 133.

[15] Thomas Mintz, "Tickle—The Itch That Moves," *Psychosomatic Medicine,* Vol. 29, No. 6 (November–December 1967), pp. 606–11.

They are differentiated high in the brain. But the itch, the tickle, and the skin pain all originate peripherally, as variously intense skin pressures. How do the stimuli reach the brain? By means of the basic working unit of the nervous system, the *neuron.*

the neuron: basic unit of the nervous system

Many billions of neurons coordinate man's body. Yet the structure of one is typical of them all. Figure 10-7 is a diagram of a neuron. Like other cells, its *cell body* contains a nucleus and other structures. Unlike other cells, its cellular material extends at each end into nerve *fibers* (see body chart 8 in the color section). It is these fine, threadlike extensions of the cell bodies that transmit information from one part of the nervous system to another. A bundle of thousands of nerve fibers constitutes a *nerve.* At one end of the cell body the nerve fiber extensions are the many-twigged *dendrites.* They pick up sensory impulses and transmit them *toward* the cell bodies. From the other pole of the cell body extends the longer, single *axon,* which carries impulses *away* from the cell bodies. Most (but not all) axons are sheathed in a whitish substance called *myelin,* which probably acts as an insulator. The degeneration of this myelin sheath results in *multiple sclerosis* (page 272). *Nodes* are constrictions of the myelin sheath at regular intervals. They behave as relay stations to improve conduction of a nerve impulse. The axon terminates in many branching filaments or *nerve terminals.* However, the myelin sheath disappears just before these branches occur.

the transmission of a nerve impulse

What happens when a stimulus—such as a tickle, an itch, or a skin pain—is received by a sensory nerve terminal? At that point the energy of the stimulus is converted into an electrochemical process. The electrochemical change then progresses along the nerve fiber, causing a small but measurable electric current—a *nerve impulse.* The impulse is usually transmitted in one direction—from the dendrites of one neuron, through its cell body, along the axon, to the dendrites or cell body of a second neuron or to a muscle or gland.

When the process of nerve impulse transmission is considered, several concepts should be kept in mind.

1. The place where the nerve terminals of an axon meet the dendrites or cell body of a second neuron is called a *synapse* (Figure 10-8). A synapse is a

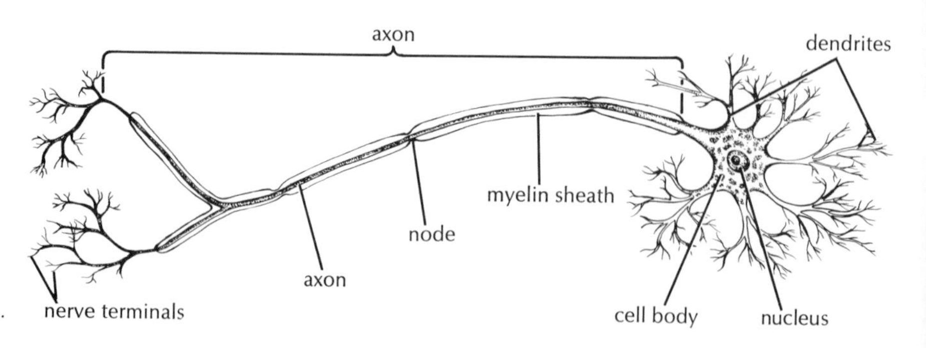

10-7 *A neuron.*

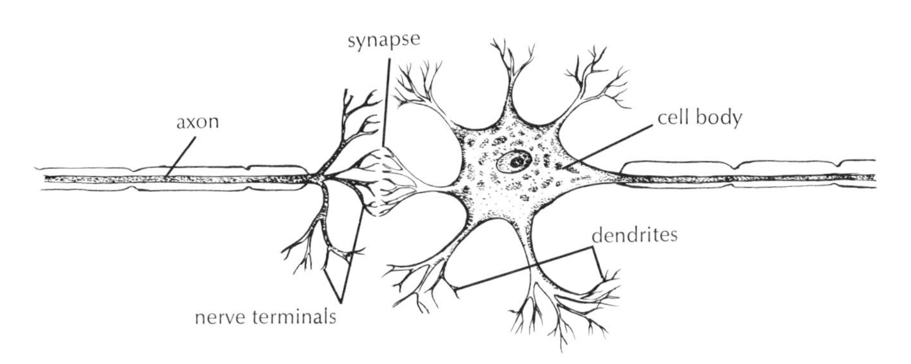

10-8 *Two views of the synapse: a diagram* (left) *and one of the first photographs of nerve fibers and synaptic knobs* (right). *It is believed the knobs pass nerve impulses from one cell to another.*

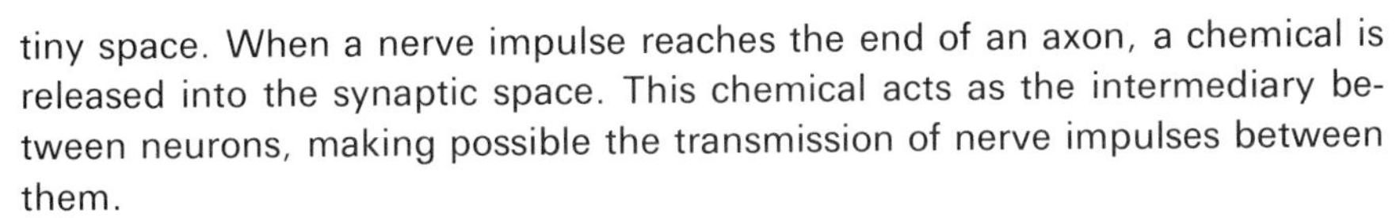

tiny space. When a nerve impulse reaches the end of an axon, a chemical is released into the synaptic space. This chemical acts as the intermediary between neurons, making possible the transmission of nerve impulses between them.

2. Neurons do not necessarily have a simple one-to-one relationship. The axons of hundreds of neurons can make synaptic junctions with the dendrites and cell body of a single neuron.

3. Neurons vary enormously in length. Remarkably, a single neuron may extend from the tip of the finger to the spinal cord. Or, in the brain, a single neuron may be but a microscopic fraction of an inch in length.

the three types of neurons

1. The *afferent* or *sensory neurons* (Latin *ad,* to or toward + *ferre,* to carry) conduct messages *toward* the brain and spinal cord from the sensory *receptor organs* of the body (see Figure 10-9). A receptor organ is a sensory nerve ending that responds to stimuli of various kinds. The five senses, of course, are sight, hearing, taste, smell, and variations of touch. In the *skin* there are five general kinds of receptors: those sensitive to touch, pressure, pain, cold, and heat. When stimulated, these are activated to relay information to the spinal cord and brain. Various skin receptors combine to give more complex skin sensations

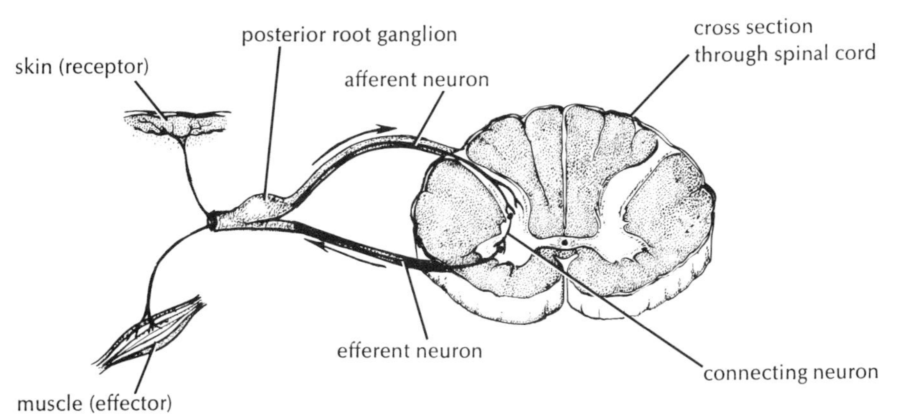

10-9 *Transmission of a nerve impulse. Illustrated here is the path of a stimulus received by skin and carried to muscle.*

such as burning or tickling. Receptors of messages that stimulate nerves are also found in the muscles, tendons, and joints. These are involved with the sense of body position and with muscle movements. Many sources may stimulate man at the same time. He must react with coordinated and integrated harmony. He touches a pot of percolating coffee. Not only are most of the receptors of the five primary skin senses stimulated, but those of hunger are stimulated as well.

2. *Efferent* or *motor neurons* (Latin *ex,* out + *ferre,* to carry) conduct impulses *from* the central nervous system to the muscles, glands, or blood vessels. Organs functioning as a result of such nerve impulses are called *effector organs.* They include the muscles and glands.

3. The *connecting neurons* are those between other neurons. Most of them are in the brain and spinal cord.

During evolution, as neurons increased in man's brain and their interconnections became more complex, man became less a creature of instinct and more a creature of reflection. He began to associate, to differentiate, to question his instincts. It is by using these neurons that he thinks to pick up a stone on the moon and to learn about it rather than to kick it out of the way. Rigidly inherited neuron patterns send birds on their migrations. But in man these have evolved into unique complex cerebral neurons used in thought. They compel him to think: "Here I will stay. This I will do. It is my duty." Even as a child, man had neurons associating, differentiating. For that is how the baby "decides" that the mother's caress is pleasant and the stranger's tickle frightening.

new explorations of the brain

Not long ago, a Yale scientist reported the case of an eleven-year-old boy institutionalized because of uncontrollable epilepsy and destructive behavior. Drugs were inadequate. To direct the brain surgery that was contemplated, electrodes were implanted in the boy's brain for several days. It was found that electrical stimulation of a certain brain convolution made the boy friendly and more communicative. In the past, the outlook for this young patient would have been dim. But today there is hope:

> In human beings, implanted electrodes are now used in major hospitals for the diagnosis and treatment of difficult cases of epilepsy, involuntary movements, organic pain, anxiety, and other illnesses. The presence of electrodes in the brain is not harmful or even uncomfortable, and patients lead normal lives in their own homes, going to work and returning to the hospital from time to time for ambulatory therapy.[16]

Such benefits for human beings have resulted from continuing animal experiments. Stimulation of specific brain centers by radio signals has brought about reactions ranging from halting a charging bull (see Figure 10-10) to inducing a mother monkey to ignore her infant. So modern science is reaching into

[16] José M. R. Delgado, "Radio-Controlled Behavior," *New York State Journal of Medicine,* Vol. 69, No. 3 (February 1, 1969), pp. 413–14. An interesting book on this subject is Delgado's *Physical Control of the Mind* (New York, 1969).

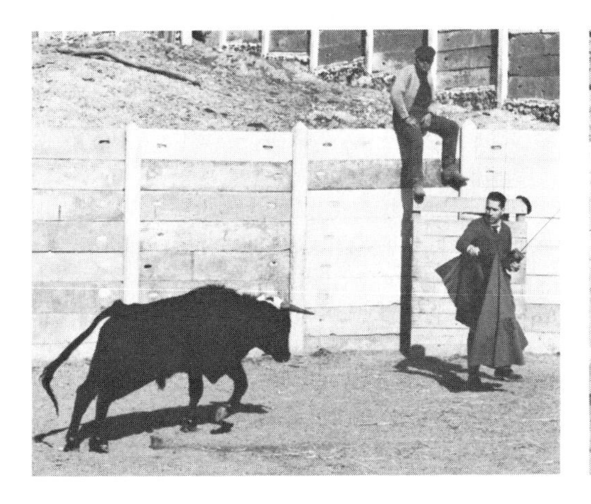
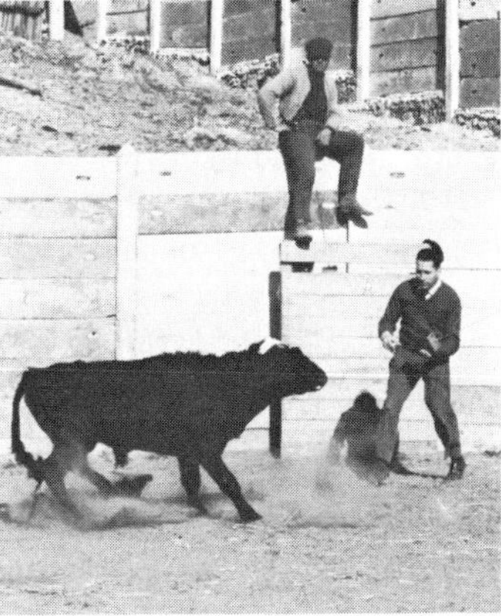

10-10 *A radio-controlled "bullfight." The charging bull* (left) *is stopped short* (right) *when the experimenter presses a button on the radio transmitter he is holding. The transmitter sends a mild current to electrodes that were planted in specific places in the bull's brain.*

the complexities of the nervous system to help mankind. What is the gross structure of this system? What are some of its afflictions?

a general view of nervous system structure

The entire nervous system has been seen to be a complex arrangement of neurons designed to bring about appropriate responses to internal and external environmental stimuli. The stimuli are picked up by the body's far-flung sensory receptor organs. The impulses are then conducted, via sensory nerve pathways, to the brain and spinal cord, where they are sorted. They are then transmitted by efferent nerves to responding effector organs. The main divisions of the nervous system are the *central nervous system* and the *peripheral nervous system.* The central nervous system consists of the *brain* and *spinal cord.* The remainder of the nervous system is peripheral. It includes the *cranial* and *spinal nerves* as well as the *autonomic nervous system.* (See Figure 10-12 and body charts 7 and 8 in the color section.)

the central nervous system

The brain and spinal cord act as a clearing house for receiving, classifying, and appraising information from the environment. Having done this, they instruct the more than six hundred muscles and the glands how to respond.[17] Bathed by a protective cushion of clear fluid, enveloped by three membranes (*meninges*), and encased in bone (the skull's *cranium* and the spine's *vertebral column*), the brain and spinal cord directly or indirectly affect every one of the trillions of body cells.

Not all stimuli reach the brain for decision. Some simple, local reflexes, such as the knee-jerk, are handled in the cord. But the brain is the body's ruling organ. At birth the human brain weighs about one pound, approximately one-

[17] Research on malnutrition has conclusively shown that "brains of animals deprived at critical stages of infancy and childhood never fully recover in spite of good nutrition in later life. There is a permanent loss of brain weight, of number of cells, and of fatty insulation between cells. The electrical activity does not mature properly and the amount of DNA is permanently reduced. Mental development is impaired, and the deprived animals never fulfill their earlier potentialities." ("Starved Brains Fail to Make the Right Connections," *New Scientist,* Vol. 54, No. 792 [April 20, 1972], p. 121.)

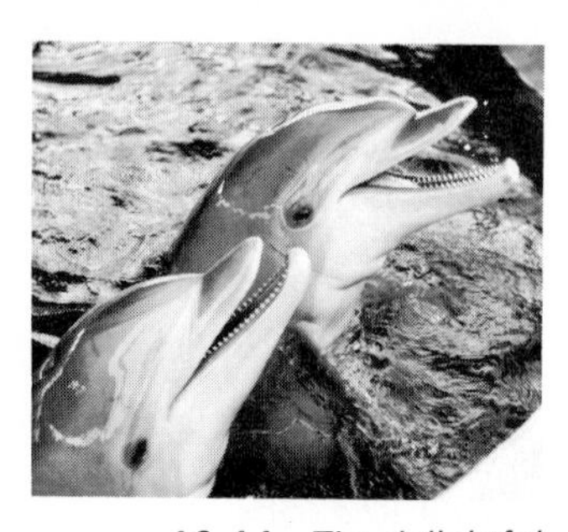

10-11 *The delightful dolphin—one of the brainiest of nonhuman creatures.*

seventh of the baby's total body weight. The average adult male brain, which weighs about three pounds, is some five and one-half ounces heavier than that of the female. Within the same species, there is no relation between brain weight and intelligence. One of the largest brains ever recorded belonged to an imbecile. There is, however, a relation between species and brain-to-body-weight ratios. The delightful dolphin (the large species) has a brain that weighs more (3.5 pounds) than man's, but its body weight is twice as great as man's. Man has the highest brain-to-body-weight ratio of all creatures.

Body chart 7 in the color section shows a cross section of the human brain and a portion of the spinal cord. The brain consists of a *cerebrum, cerebellum,* and *brain stem.* The cerebrum is divided into left and right cerebral *hemispheres.* The wrinkled surface of these hemispheres is the *cerebral cortex.* In it are the complexities of humanness, for it is responsible for the distinction that is man.[18] The *cerebellum* is a coordinator, being responsible for muscle tone, body balance, and the rhythms of body movements.[19] The *brain stem* supports the cerebral hemispheres. It contains pathways to and from the cerebral cortex as well as nerve centers controlling a wide variety of body functions including heartbeat, breathing, digestion, body temperature, and blood pressure.

Electrical energy is constantly produced in the normal brain. This electrical activity can be traced in definite patterns, or waves, on an *electroencephalogram* (EEG). People with head injuries, tumors, infections, and hemorrhages may show electroencephalographic changes. Epileptics usually reveal abnormal EEGs. The electroencephalogram is a valuable, painless diagnostic tool. However, emotional disorders are generally not detected by the EEG.

The *spinal cord* is continuous with the brain stem and is that part of the nervous system enclosed in the bony vertebral column. It is, however, much shorter than its bony protector and ends in a group of tail-like nerves that go to the organs within the pelvis and to the lower extremities.

The *cerebrospinal fluid* circulates not only around the outside surfaces of the brain and spinal cord but also around their internal surfaces. By inserting a needle through a space between two vertebral bodies of the vertebral column, a small amount of this cerebrospinal fluid may be withdrawn for examination (*spinal tap*). In this examination the needle does not touch spinal cord tissue. Spinal taps are important in the diagnosis of certain neurologic diseases. For spinal anesthesia, an anesthetic is introduced into a specific space filled with cerebrospinal fluid.

[18] It has been found that experimentally malnourished young rats suffer as much as a 41 percent reduction in the number of axon terminals put out by each neuron in the frontal cortex. "Since the axon terminals are the sites where synapses form, this means that the number of neuronal circuits that can be formed in the cortex is enormously reduced, and all aspects of nervous and mental development are severely and permanently impaired." ("Starved Brains Fail to Make the Right Connections," p. 121.) See "The Hurt of Hunger" in this text, pages 670–71.

[19] Studies of the cerebellums of malnourished newborn rats have shown a loss in both the weight and DNA content of this part of the brain. Even when the rats were given free access to food, the cerebellar damage was not completely reversed. ("Starved Brains Fail to Make the Right Connection," p. 121.) Studies of malnourished monkeys show significant adverse changes in the distribution and activity of various enzymes in the central nervous system. There is a decrease in the amount of RNA in certain cells of both the cerebellum and the spinal cord. ("Pinpointing Effect of Low Protein Diet," *Medical World News,* Vol. 13, No. 11 [March 17, 1972], p. 77.)

the peripheral nervous system

The *peripheral nervous system* is composed of all nervous structures not included in the brain and spinal cord. It brings environmental stimuli to the central nervous system and relays instructions from it to the body's effector organs.

Twelve pairs of peripheral nerves issue directly from the brain. They are called *cranial nerves* and chiefly supply the head and neck. However, one of the pairs of cranial nerves (the *vagus* nerve) extends to the heart, blood vessels, and other internal organs (see body chart 7 in the color section). Other cranial nerves include the *acoustic* (hearing), *optic* (seeing), and *olfactory* (smelling) nerves. There are cranial nerves controlling balance, eye motion, speech, taste, and other functions. The thirty-one pairs of *spinal nerves* carry impulses between the spinal cord and the skin and muscle below the brain level.

Part of the peripheral nervous system, the *autonomic* ("self-governing") *nervous system,* is so named because it has the specialized task of regulating body activities over which an individual usually exercises no conscious control. It connects the central nervous system with the glands and with the heart and the smooth muscle that lines the other internal organs, such as the stomach and intestines. Heart rate, circulation, digestion, respiration, and glandular function are among the body activities that are not ordinarily governed by the will but are controlled by the autonomic nervous system. Only recently has it been discovered, however, that some autonomic functions are not as much beyond individual control as had been thought. Experiments have demonstrated that rats can learn to increase or decrease their heart rates, stomach and intestinal contractions, blood pressures, kidney filtration rates, and the amount of blood flowing through their tails and stomach walls. They can even learn to increase the blood flow to one ear while maintaining the usual blood flow in the other. By experimental manipulation of the psychological environment, the development of duodenal ulcers (page 686) in rats has been controlled.[20] Can these findings be applied to relieving human psychosomatic illnesses? Possibly. Asthma without apparent cause, insomnia, irregular and rapid heart rates, a form of (essential) hypertension—these and other ailments may someday be helped by "visceral learning."[21] Meanwhile, some entrepreneurs have been quick to make money out of these findings. Do-it-yourself electroencephalographic kits are being sold that enable one to monitor one's own brain waves in order to train oneself to produce alpha waves. Most people can produce alpha waves merely by closing their eyes. (For a further discussion of quackery, see Chapter 24, pages 753–57.)

The autonomic nervous system has two divisions, the *sympathetic* and *parasympathetic* (Figure 10-12). The sympathetic division is composed of nerve fibers and masses of cell bodies called *ganglia,* which are located on either side

[20] Graham Chedd, "The Psychology of Ulcers," *New Scientist and Science Journal,* Vol. 51, No. 768 (September 9, 1971), p. 562.

[21] Graham Chedd, "Mental Medicine: Self-Help for Your Insides?" *New Scientist and Science Journal,* Vol. 51, No. 768 (September 1971), p. 561. There is much human experimentation on visceral learning. A recommended recent book on this subject is an annual compendium of articles, *Biofeedback and Self-Control 1972,* ed. by David Shapiro, T. X. Barber, Leo V. DiCara, Joe Kamiya, Neal E. Miller. and Johann Stoyva (Chicago, 1973). This volume is appropriate for the more advanced student.

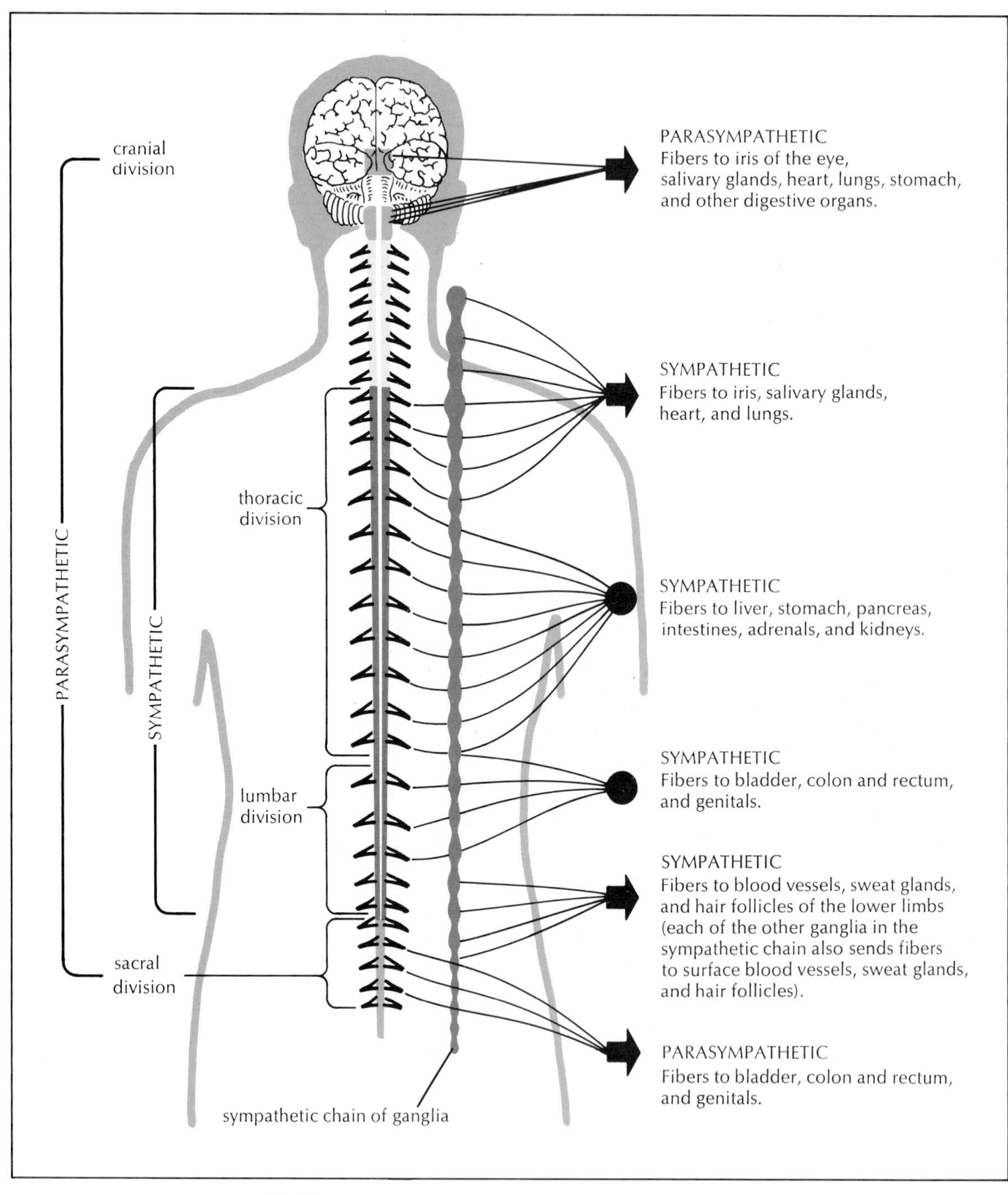

10-12 *The autonomic nervous system. The sympathetic system is characterized by chains of ganglia on either side of the spinal cord as well as by other large ganglia (represented here by large circles). The parasympathetic system has its ganglia (not shown) nearer the organs stimulated. Only half the autonomic nervous system is shown here; it is duplicated on the other side of the spinal cord.*

of the spinal column (see body chart 7 in the color section). Sympathetic nerves are concerned with emotions. When a person is under stress, the sympathetic division takes over from the parasympathetic division, which predominates when the person is relaxed. Sometimes the two autonomic divisions work together. In the sexual act, male erection is parasympathetic in origin, and ejaculation is sympathetic.

the Boston arm

The electrochemical nature of nerve impulses has afforded help to the disabled. By 1961 the Russians were using electrical signals from muscles to operate an open-and-close artificial hand. In this country, a motor-driven elbow has been invented that uses electrical signals stemming from muscle tension. From this has been developed the artificial "Boston arm" (Figure 10-13). An amputee who has lost an arm can, nonetheless, cerebrally will it into action. The enervated stump muscle discharges the same signal as an arm would discharge. In the Boston arm, this electrical signal is amplified. The amplified electric current controls a battery-powered electric motor in the arm. (The battery is worn in a belt around the waist.) The motor sends the arm into action. Ten pounds can be lifted with the Boston arm. Fifty pounds can be held back. And, to repeat, its control is *willed* by the user, through neurons high in the brain.[22]

some disorders of the central nervous system

It has long been thought that the adult central nervous system is capable of little or no regeneration after injury. Recent research has challenged this concept.

[22] *Hospital Tribune,* October 7, 1968, p. 8.

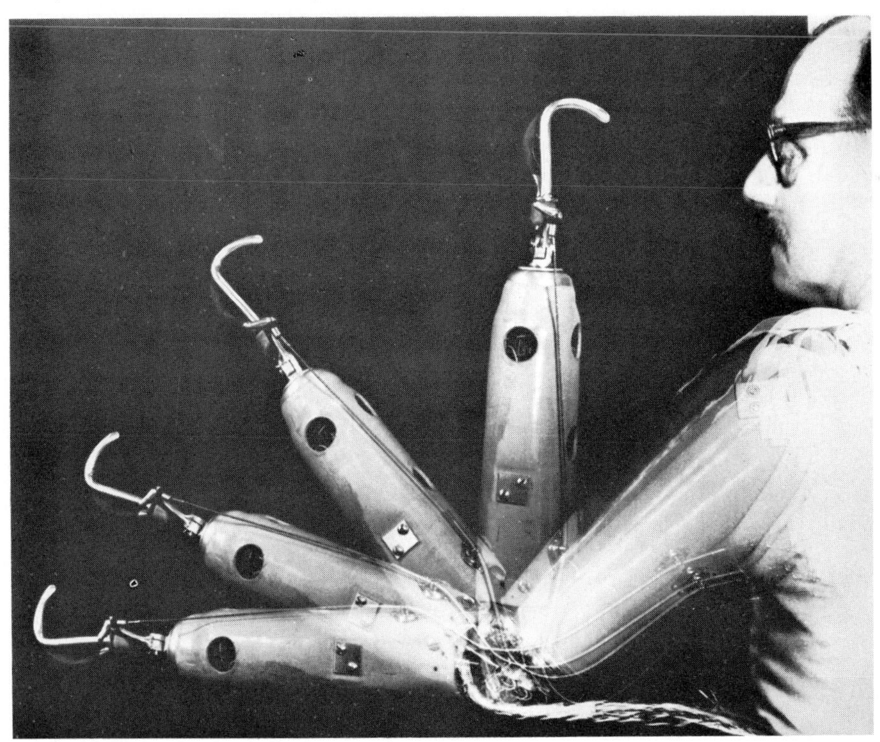

10-13 *A stop-action photograph of the "Boston arm." This is the first above-the-elbow artificial arm that an amputee can literally will into action.*

It has been found that at least one group of neurons in the adult mammalian brain and spinal cord does have a significant capacity for growth.[23] Nevertheless, early treatment is extremely important in central nervous system diseases. Early removal of a brain tumor, for example, can prevent widespread, hopeless dysfunction. Early treatment of syphilis infection precludes irreversible nervous (and other) damage. So it is with other assaults to the nervous system, such as those occurring from poisoning (alcoholism, for example) and malnourishment (beriberi, for example).

The loss of function from a central nervous system disease—such as a tumor or infection—depends on where the lesion is and how severe it is. One brain tumor will produce only a pressure headache; another may advance to a withering affliction in which few functions are spared. A few of the more common central nervous system diseases are briefly discussed here.

stroke

When the blood supply to the brain is impeded, the resultant lack of oxygen causes death of tissue. This *cerebrovascular disease* is called *stroke* (see page 242). It may be precipitated either by the formation of a clot in a cerebral vessel or by the rupture of such a vessel that has been weakened by disease. Paralysis and anesthesia (loss of feeling) result. Since each cerebral hemisphere controls the opposite part of the body, right-sided paralysis indicates left cerebral involvement and vice versa. With most people the left side of the brain is the area that controls the learning of speech. Damage to that side may deprive a person of the ability to talk. If there has been bleeding, some of the clot may be absorbed. The pressure on the brain is then relieved, and there is some recovery. Unlike the nerve fibers of the peripheral nervous system, most of the fibers of the adult central nervous system do not repair, and some permanent damage is not uncommon.

Strokes may be considered from both preventive and rehabilitative aspects. About three-fourths of stroke patients have warning signs and symptoms. Weakness of one or more extremities, speech difficulties, dizziness—these may herald an impending stroke. They are "little strokes." By early treatment of little strokes, big strokes can often be prevented. The great majority of stroke sufferers survive their first major episode. The stroke victim can learn to use undamaged nerve pathways and to strengthen weak muscles. Early and intensive rehabilitative treatment can do much to return stroke victims to useful lives.

epilepsy

The ancients considered those who suffered seizures (Greek *epilepsis,* seizure) divine. But the description of epilepsy by the Roman poet Lucretius (96?–55 B.C.) was hardly spiritual: "Ofttimes with vi'lent fits a patient falls, / As if with thunder struck; and foams and bawls."[24]

[23] "Regeneration of Nerves," *Science News,* Vol. 102, No. 17 (October 21, 1972), p. 264.
[24] From *On the Nature of Things,* quoted in Heinrich Oppenheimer, *Medical and Allied Topics in Latin Poetry* (London, 1928), p. 302.

Today, "at least 1 percent of the [U.S.] population suffers from seizures."[25] It is a mark neither of unusual intelligence nor of mental retardation. Nor is it a disease as such. It is but a sign of a disorder of brain electrical activity. Thus, it can often be diagnosed with the electroencephalogram (see page 266). Even between seizures many persons with epilepsy will show abnormal EEG patterns. The causes of the seizures (such as trauma or infection) are known in less than half the cases. An increasing number of seizures are precipitated by flashing lights of a suitable frequency, such as those emanating from a flickering television picture, fluorescent lighting, or home movies.

The most common types of epilepsy are *petit mal* (French, "little illness"), *grand mal*, and *psychomotor*. *Petit mal* episodes are manifested by momentary blackouts of consciousness and muscular twitchings. They may occur dozens of times a day. *Grand mal* seizures are more severe. Usually the affected person falls and is unconscious for some time. He may froth at the mouth or bite his tongue or lose control of bowel and bladder. *Psychomotor epilepsy* is manifested by unusual behavior. The individual smacks his lips or picks at his clothes. Often, he is confused and restless. A nameless terror may accompany such a seizure. Following all this, there is apparently no memory of the attack. Two out of three epileptics suffer from more than one type of seizure. A carefully calculated combination of drugs can control many of these. Brain surgery in selected cases may provide the best control of seizures.[26] (See page 316.)

Many absurd superstitions still surround epilepsy. For the vast majority of epileptics, research has made possible employability and a useful life. It has been claimed that to more than 50 percent of all epileptics, various combinations of modern medications have brought literally complete convulsion control. Another 30 percent, it is said, lead almost normal lives; their convulsions are relatively infrequent. This has been questioned. One specialist's studies revealed that when the term "seizure control" was strictly applied, the attack rate was considerably increased.[27] There is a genetic predisposition to most forms of epilepsy. Those concerned about marrying a person with epilepsy will find genetic counseling helpful (see page 562). However, the great majority of epileptics are just as dependable parents as anyone else.

cerebral palsy

Well over half a million people in this country have cerebral palsy. Every year, ten thousand more are born with the condition. The brain lesion causing cerebral palsy may occur before birth as a developmental failure. It may follow such infections as whooping cough and measles. It may be rooted in a blood incompatibility involving the Rh blood factor (see page 553). Head injury may be the

[25] "Epilepsy." *Medical World News*, Vol. 11, No. 10 (March 6, 1970), p. 29.

[26] "Environmental Epilepsy Rises," *Medical World News*, Vol. 12, No. 29 (August 6, 1971), pp. 30–31. There have been isolated reports that the use of certain drugs that effectively prevent convulsions of pregnant women can produce a greater than expected frequency of malformations in the child, such as cleft lips and cleft palate. However, although further studies are being urged, experts in the field believe that they must continue to weigh the risks: the prevention of possibly serious convulsions of a pregnant woman against the possible increase in treatable malformations. ("Weighing Evidence That Links Epilepsy Drugs to Fetal Defects," *Medical World News*, Vol. 14, No. 15 [April 13, 1973], pp. 22, 27.)

[27] *Ibid.*, p. 34.

cause. Thus, not all cerebral palsy results from birth injury. Moreover, brain damage can vary from mild involvement, with few, hardly discernible symptoms, to a widespread spastic paralysis (associated with severe tremor) and poor coordination.

Usually, there is more than one handicap. In half the cases speech defects occur. So do visual defects. About 25 percent have hearing problems. Another 25 percent have convulsions. About half of those with cerebral palsy are retarded.

It is a tragic truth that many thousands suffering cerebral palsy are unable to put to use the abilities they do have. Shortages of community facilities combine with indifference, even hostility, to deprive them of opportunity. Early diagnosis, combined with active treatment, rehabilitation, and education, can provide the willing community with many useful citizens.

multiple sclerosis

In *multiple sclerosis* (Greek *skleros,* hard) hardening of nerve tissue is distributed throughout the brain or spinal cord or both. Neither the cause nor the cure of this disease is known. Nor is present treatment adequate. However, modern physical therapy and other rehabilitative efforts today hold out the promise of years of productive life to these patients.

In this country an estimated quarter-million people have this progressive disease. For reasons unknown, it occurs more often in cold climates than it does in warm climates. The rate and degree of progression vary with individuals. The onset age is during the prime years—twenty to forty. The basic lesion is a patchy loss of *myelin,* the fatty covering that protects and insulates the nerve fibers of the brain and spinal cord. The myelin is replaced by scar tissue. One area may lose its myelin, unaccountably seem to improve, and then degenerate further. (It is just before and during such periods of remission that the patient, believing himself to be improving, may fall prey to a quack.) Eventually, widespread patchy degeneration results in a host of distressing symptoms such as weakness, numbness, double vision, tremor, and slurring of the speech. There may be loss of bowel and bladder control. Paralysis slowly develops. Occasionally the disease will progress rapidly.

Present research offers hope for this difficult disease. Sophisticated studies, aimed at a better understanding of the myelin mystery, have led to incidental information about other previously unknown factors of this nerve disease. Knowledge of the cause of the degenerative change will yet lead to its prevention and cure.

"the shaking palsy": Parkinson's syndrome

In 1915, the war-harassed Romanians reported an alarming sleeping sickness epidemic. By 1918, the epidemic had left much of Europe reeling. (That unhappy continent was still suffering from the war and influenza.) It then reached American shores.

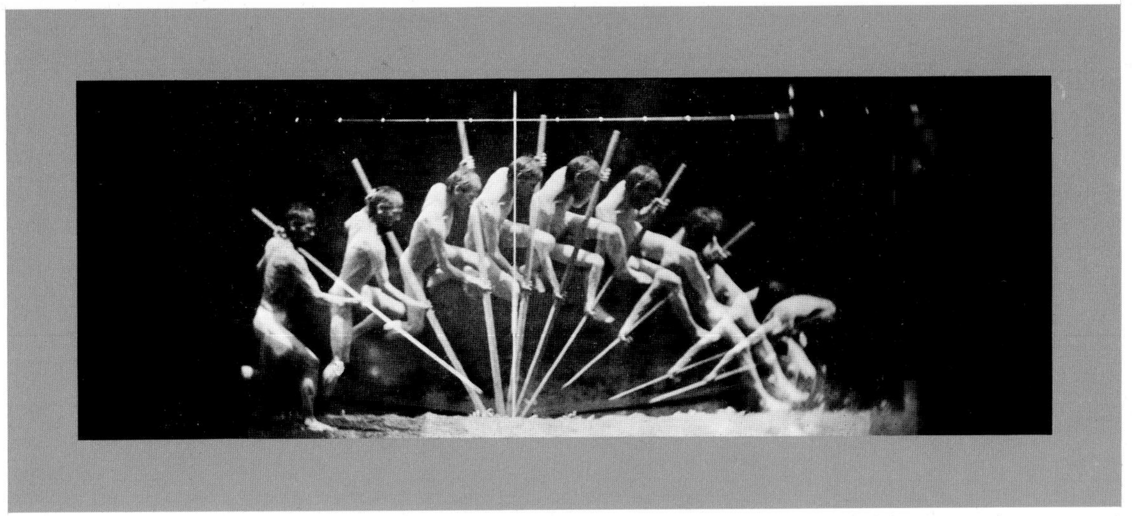

Multiple-exposure photograph by Thomas Eakins (1844–1916).

the human body

Photomicrographs courtesy CCM: General Biological, Inc., Chicago. Eakins photograph: The Metropolitan Museum of Art, gift of Charles Bregler, 1941.
Printed in the United States of America.

GUIDE TO CONTENTS

The numbers are the numbers of the body charts.

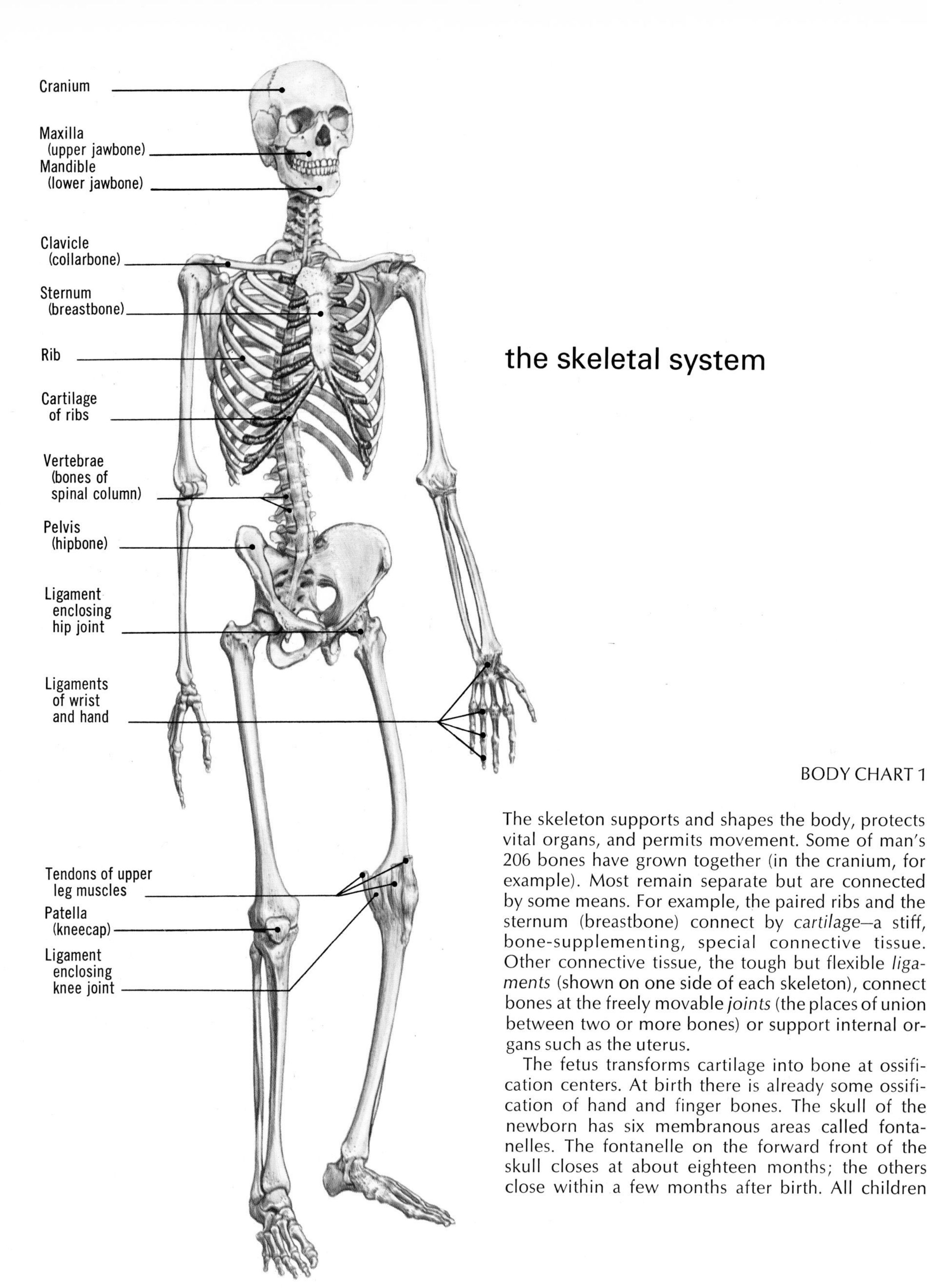

the skeletal system

BODY CHART 1

The skeleton supports and shapes the body, protects vital organs, and permits movement. Some of man's 206 bones have grown together (in the cranium, for example). Most remain separate but are connected by some means. For example, the paired ribs and the sternum (breastbone) connect by *cartilage*—a stiff, bone-supplementing, special connective tissue. Other connective tissue, the tough but flexible *ligaments* (shown on one side of each skeleton), connect bones at the freely movable *joints* (the places of union between two or more bones) or support internal organs such as the uterus.

The fetus transforms cartilage into bone at ossification centers. At birth there is already some ossification of hand and finger bones. The skull of the newborn has six membranous areas called fontanelles. The fontanelle on the forward front of the skull closes at about eighteen months; the others close within a few months after birth. All children

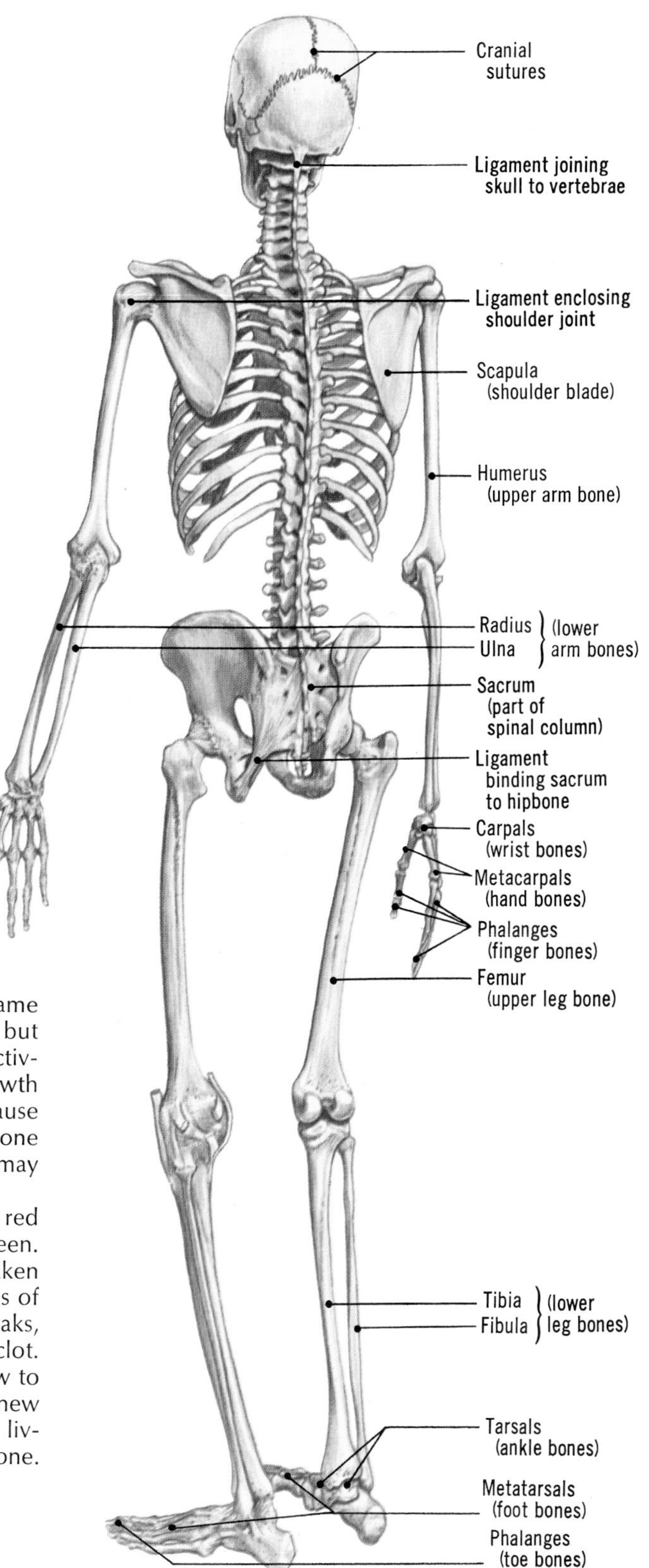

BODY CHART 2

ossify bones in the same order but not at the same rate. Order and rate are genetically established, but rate is influenced by nutrition, endocrine gland activity, and disease. Adverse effects on cartilage growth from pituitary or thyroid gland disease can cause dwarfism. Insufficient vitamin D may retard bone formation and development in children and may promote rickets.

Before bone structure appears in the fetus, red blood cells are formed mostly in the liver and spleen. As bone develops, red blood cell formation is taken over by marrow, the soft tissue filling the cavities of the bones (see body chart 6). When a bone breaks, the gap between the fragments fills with a blood clot. From unimpaired blood vessels, new vessels grow to bring the clot food. From surrounding tissue, new cells invade the clot. The nonliving clot becomes living tissue and the groundwork for repair of the bone.

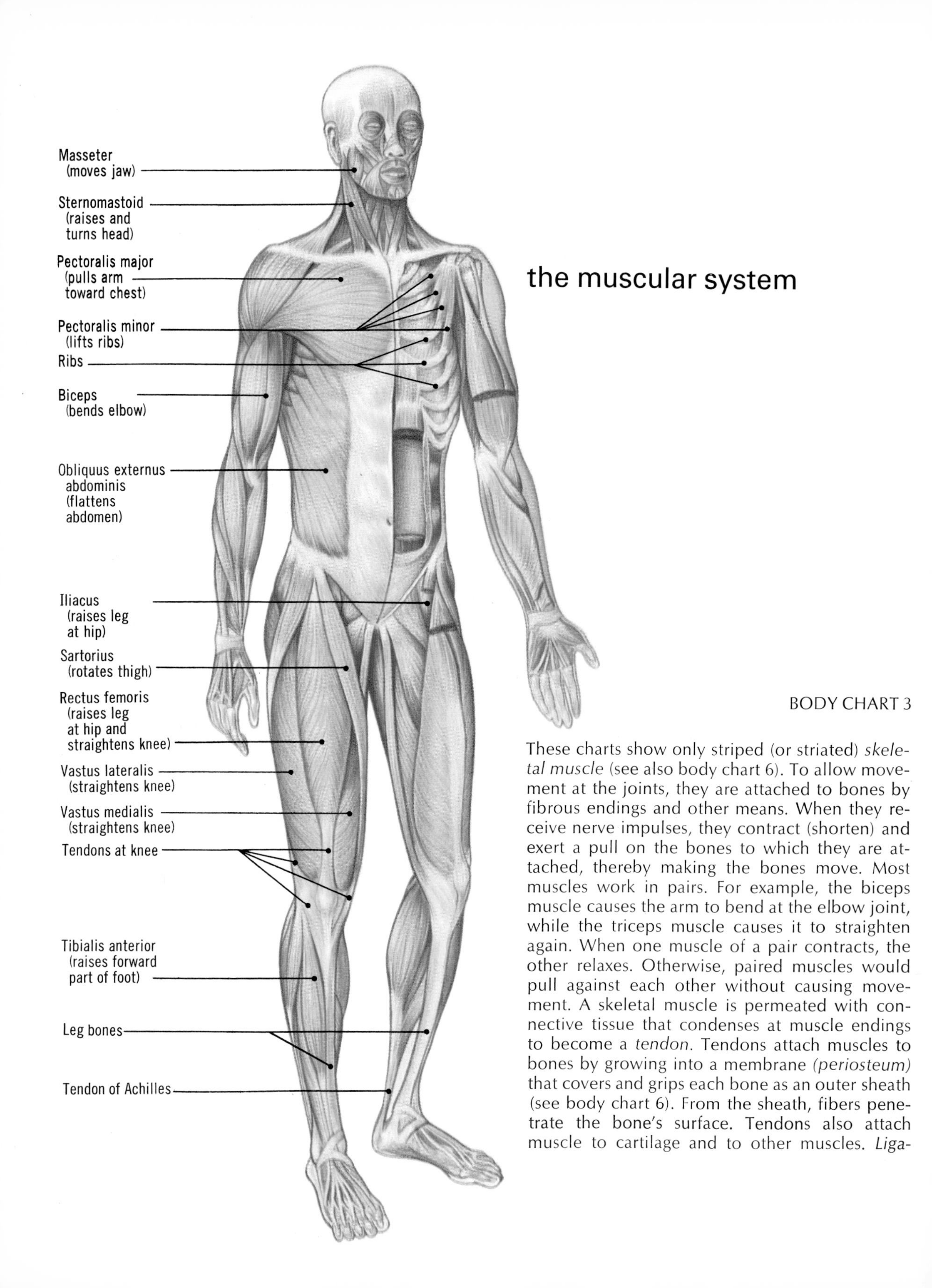

the muscular system

BODY CHART 3

These charts show only striped (or striated) *skeletal muscle* (see also body chart 6). To allow movement at the joints, they are attached to bones by fibrous endings and other means. When they receive nerve impulses, they contract (shorten) and exert a pull on the bones to which they are attached, thereby making the bones move. Most muscles work in pairs. For example, the biceps muscle causes the arm to bend at the elbow joint, while the triceps muscle causes it to straighten again. When one muscle of a pair contracts, the other relaxes. Otherwise, paired muscles would pull against each other without causing movement. A skeletal muscle is permeated with connective tissue that condenses at muscle endings to become a *tendon*. Tendons attach muscles to bones by growing into a membrane *(periosteum)* that covers and grips each bone as an outer sheath (see body chart 6). From the sheath, fibers penetrate the bone's surface. Tendons also attach muscle to cartilage and to other muscles. *Liga-*

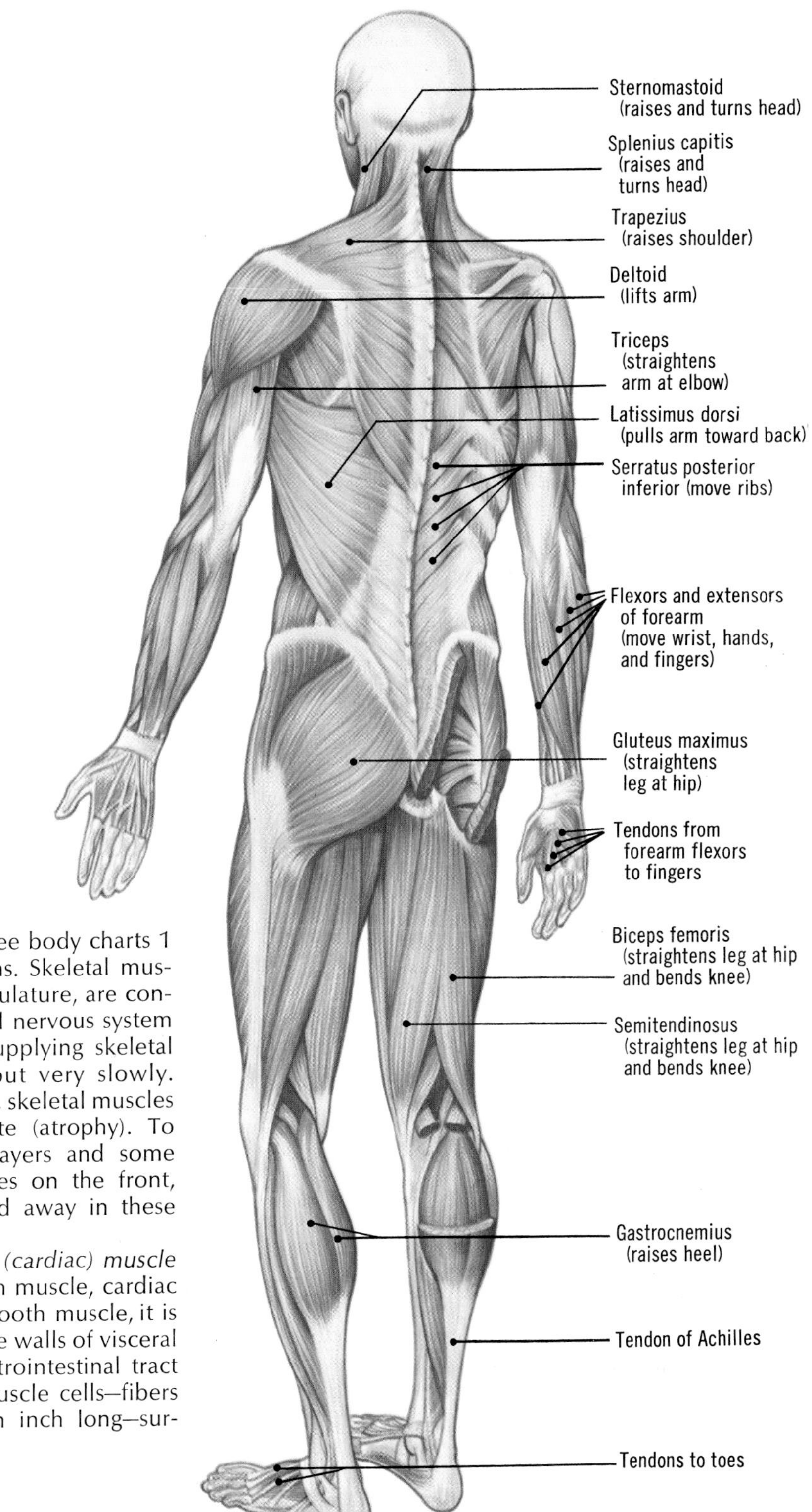

BODY CHART 4

ments connect bones at joints (see body charts 1 and 2) or support internal organs. Skeletal muscles, the bulk of the body's musculature, are controlled by the will. Unlike central nervous system fibers, peripheral nerve fibers supplying skeletal muscles tend to regenerate—but very slowly. Without adequate physiotherapy, skeletal muscles awaiting nerve repair will waste (atrophy). To show deeper skeletal muscle layers and some bone attachments, some muscles on the front, back, and one side are stripped away in these charts.

Not illustrated here are *heart (cardiac) muscle* and *smooth muscle*. Like smooth muscle, cardiac muscle is involuntary; unlike smooth muscle, it is striped. Smooth muscle forms the walls of visceral organs such as those in the gastrointestinal tract and urinary bladder. Smooth muscle cells—fibers less than one-thousandth of an inch long—surround capillaries.

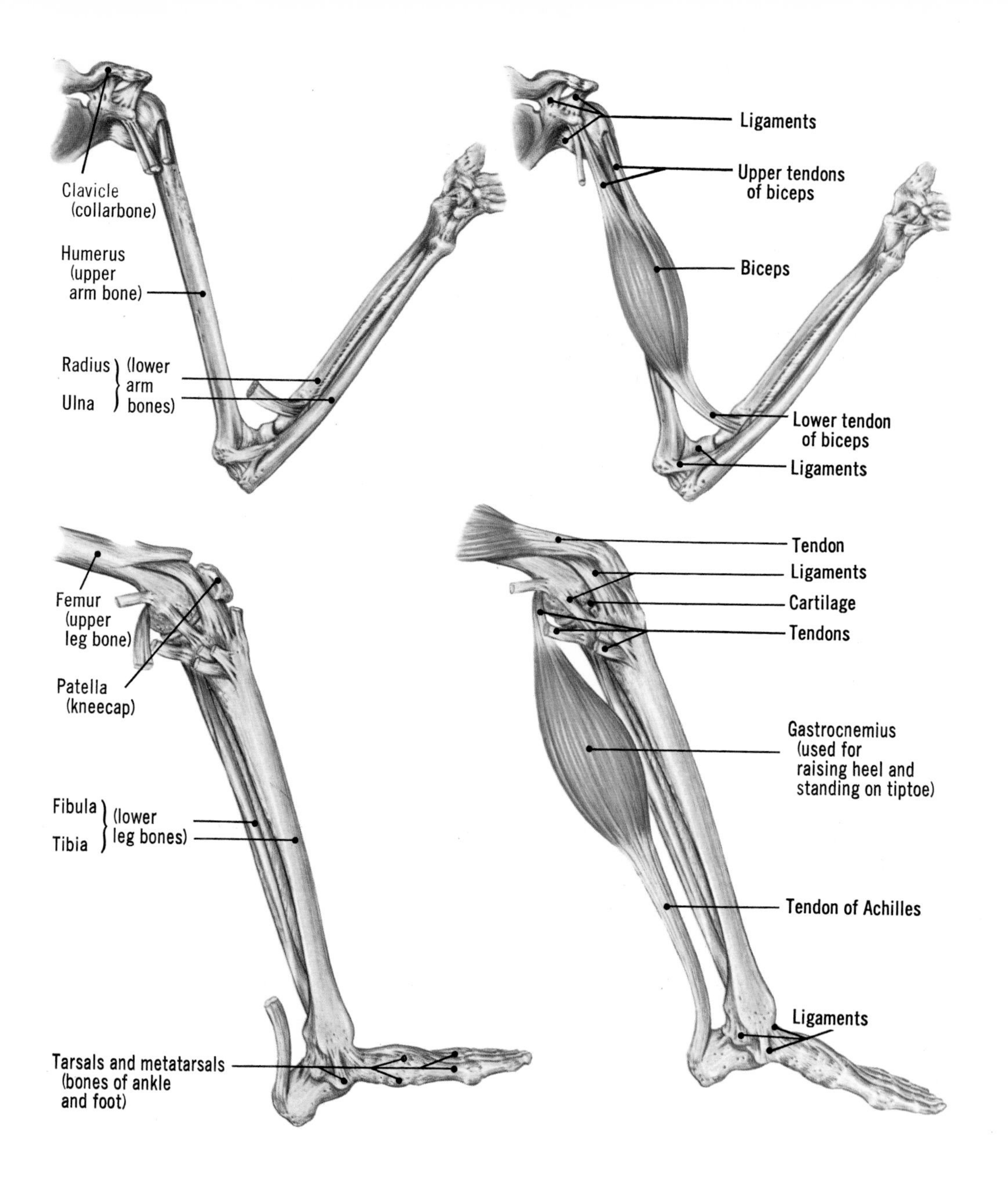

the bone-muscle relationship

The structure of an arm and leg clarifies the bone-muscle relationship. Muscles bending a limb at a joint (elbow, knee) are called *flexor* muscles; those that straighten the limb are *extensor* muscles. For movement to occur, bones must be joined at joints, and muscles must pull upon bones by contracting (shortening). Furthermore, the tendons at the opposite ends of each muscle must be attached to different bones. For example, the lower tendon of the biceps is attached to a bone of the forearm. Since the elbow is a freely movable joint, contraction of the biceps will cause the arm to bend. (Muscle fibers of the biceps are six to seven inches long and are among the body's longest cells.)

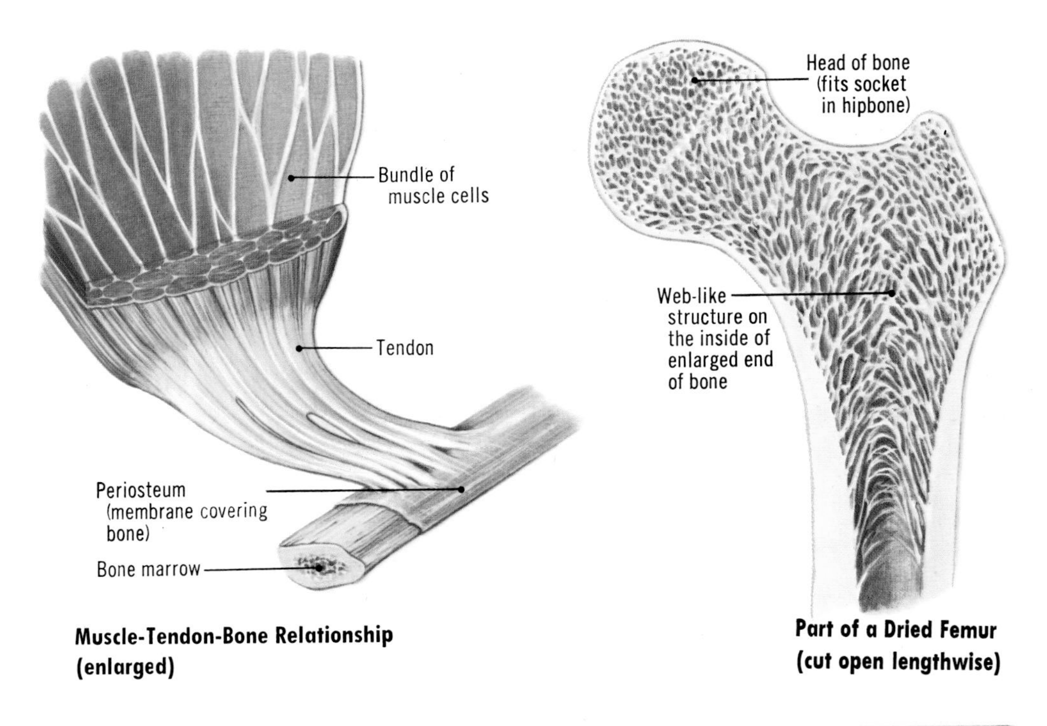

Muscle-Tendon-Bone Relationship (enlarged)

Part of a Dried Femur (cut open lengthwise)

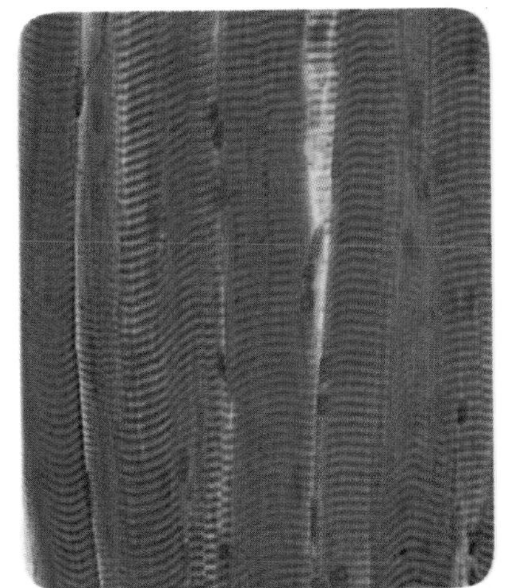

Small Parts of Several Stained Skeletal Muscle Cells (as seen under the microscope)

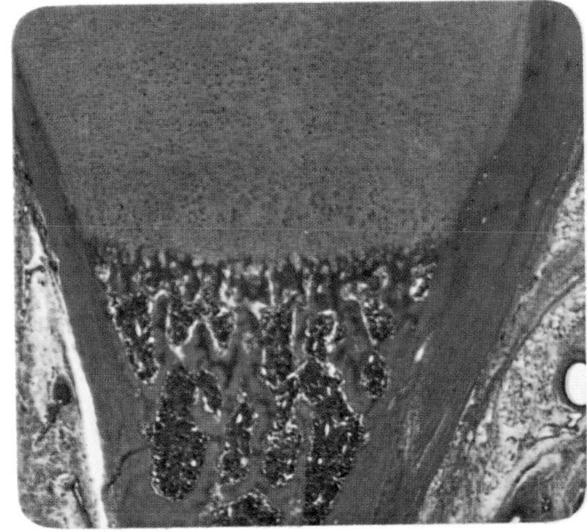

Cartilage (above) and Young Bone Cells (below) in Stained Fresh Bone (as seen under the microscope)

BODY CHART 6

The most versatile joint is that of the shoulder; it has the greatest range of movement. The knee is both the largest and weakest joint of the body. When a tendon rides over a bony surface, a small sac (a bursa) containing fluid protects it. These bursae are found at such places as about the elbow and knee joints and at the back of the heel. Between the kneecap (patella) and the skin is a bursa. Like other bursae, it may become inflamed (bursitis).

The muscles of adult men are stronger than those of women both because the muscles are larger and because men have a higher rate of oxygen consumption per pound of body weight than do women.

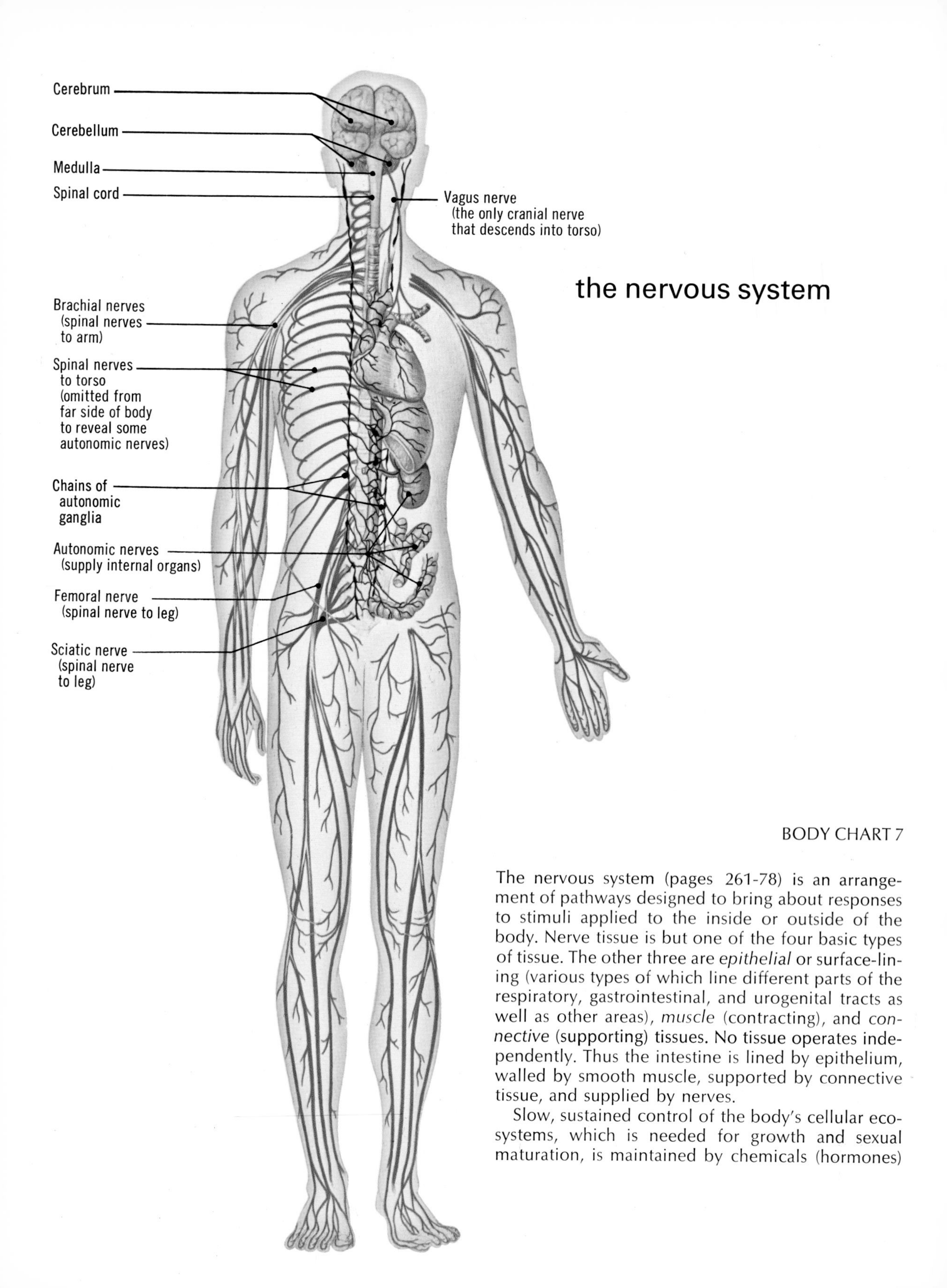

the nervous system

BODY CHART 7

The nervous system (pages 261-78) is an arrangement of pathways designed to bring about responses to stimuli applied to the inside or outside of the body. Nerve tissue is but one of the four basic types of tissue. The other three are *epithelial* or surface-lining (various types of which line different parts of the respiratory, gastrointestinal, and urogenital tracts as well as other areas), *muscle* (contracting), and *connective* (supporting) tissues. No tissue operates independently. Thus the intestine is lined by epithelium, walled by smooth muscle, supported by connective tissue, and supplied by nerves.

Slow, sustained control of the body's cellular ecosystems, which is needed for growth and sexual maturation, is maintained by chemicals (hormones)

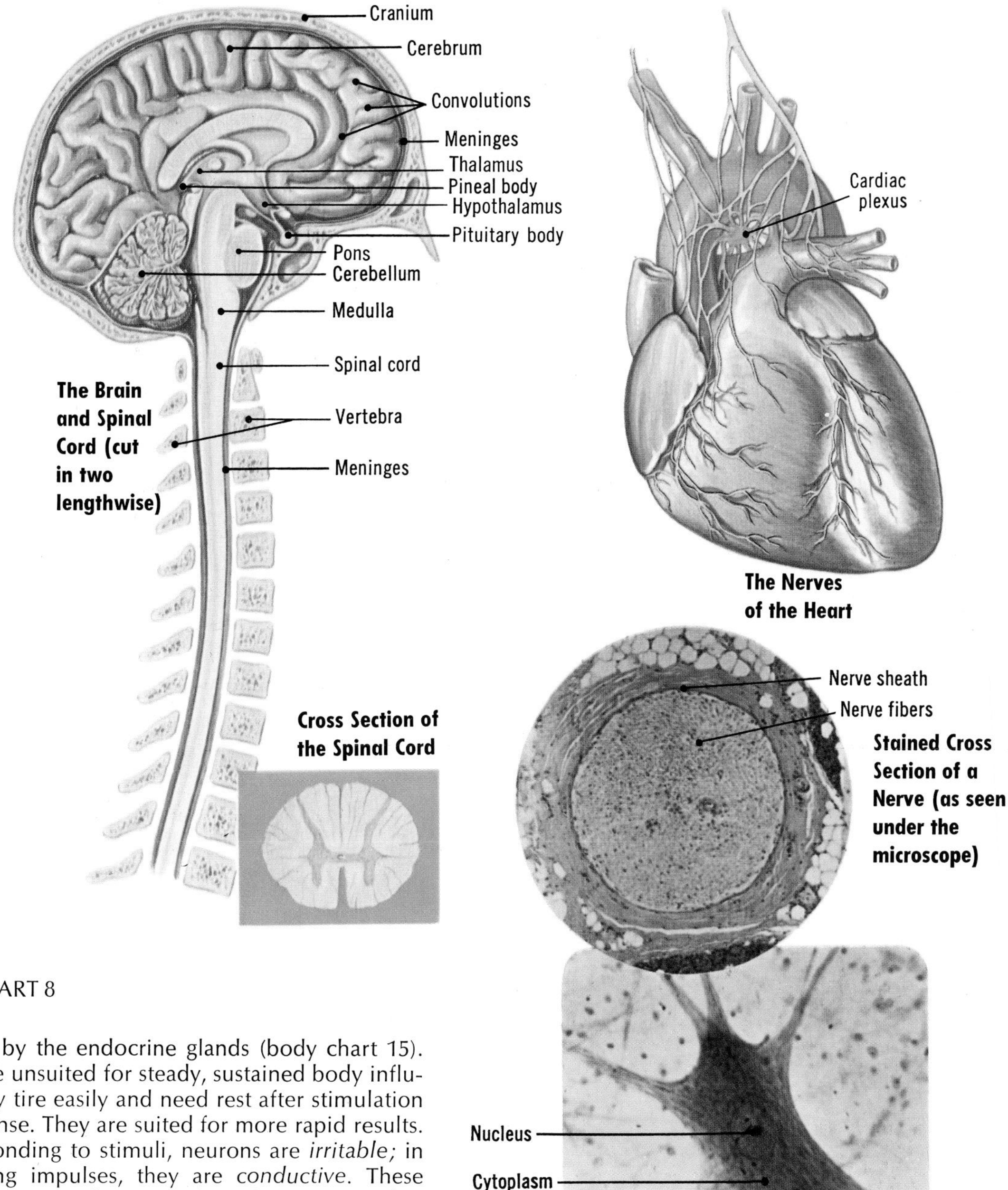

The Brain and Spinal Cord (cut in two lengthwise)

Cross Section of the Spinal Cord

The Nerves of the Heart

Stained Cross Section of a Nerve (as seen under the microscope)

Stained Cell Body of an Efferent (Motor) Neuron (as seen under the microscope)

BODY CHART 8

produced by the endocrine glands (body chart 15). Nerves are unsuited for steady, sustained body influence. They tire easily and need rest after stimulation and response. They are suited for more rapid results.

In responding to stimuli, neurons are *irritable;* in transmitting impulses, they are *conductive*. These two properties combine with their ability to *correlate* and *evaluate* on the basis of memory to make nerve tissue the most specialized of the four basic tissue types. It has been written that the hand without a thumb is but a hook, for it can no longer grasp. But a hand that loses its nerve function loses more than its ability to participate in creation; it loses the more primitive ability to warn its owner of surrounding dangers.

the circulatory system

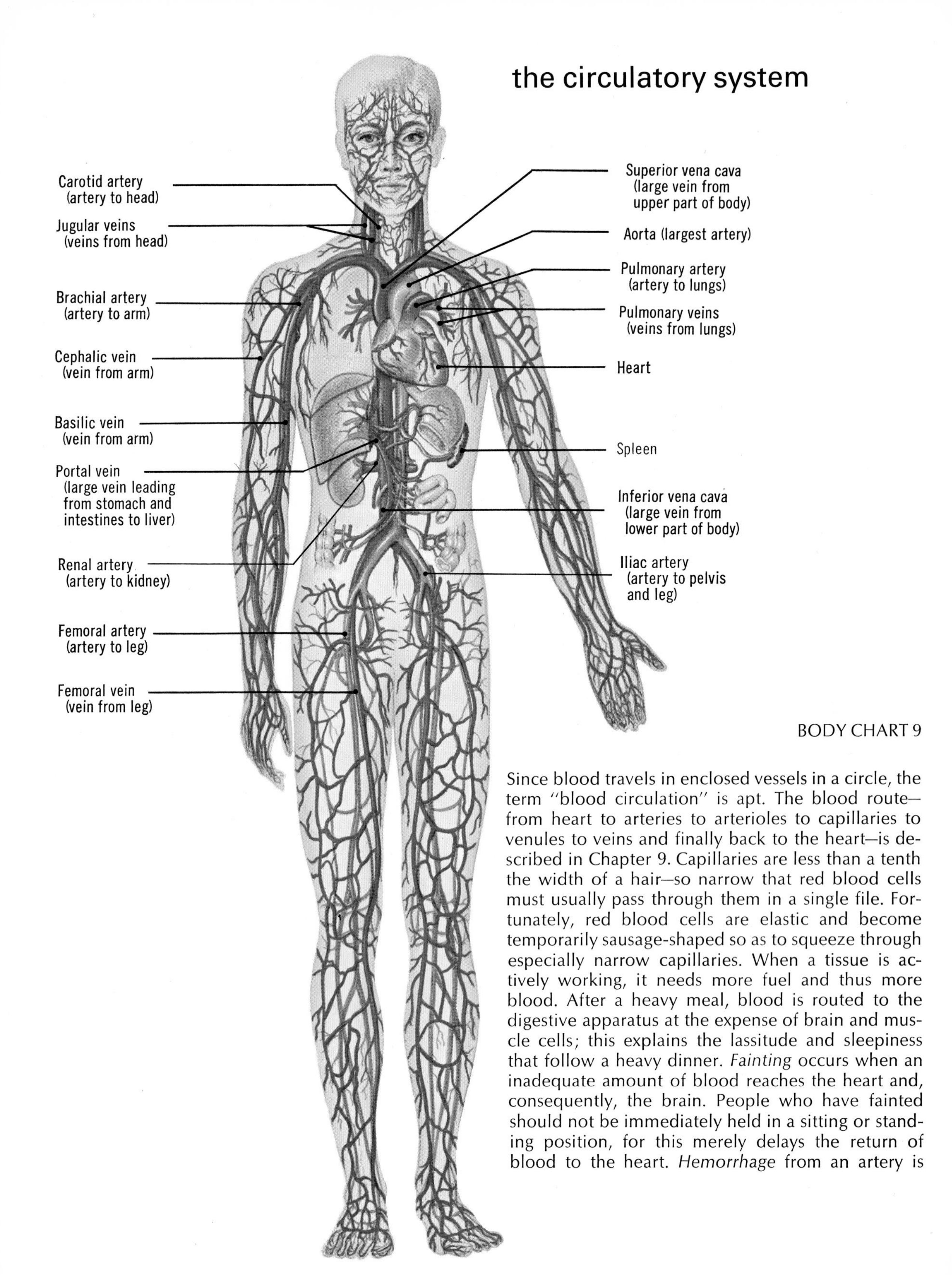

BODY CHART 9

Since blood travels in enclosed vessels in a circle, the term "blood circulation" is apt. The blood route—from heart to arteries to arterioles to capillaries to venules to veins and finally back to the heart—is described in Chapter 9. Capillaries are less than a tenth the width of a hair—so narrow that red blood cells must usually pass through them in a single file. Fortunately, red blood cells are elastic and become temporarily sausage-shaped so as to squeeze through especially narrow capillaries. When a tissue is actively working, it needs more fuel and thus more blood. After a heavy meal, blood is routed to the digestive apparatus at the expense of brain and muscle cells; this explains the lassitude and sleepiness that follow a heavy dinner. *Fainting* occurs when an inadequate amount of blood reaches the heart and, consequently, the brain. People who have fainted should not be immediately held in a sitting or standing position, for this merely delays the return of blood to the heart. *Hemorrhage* from an artery is

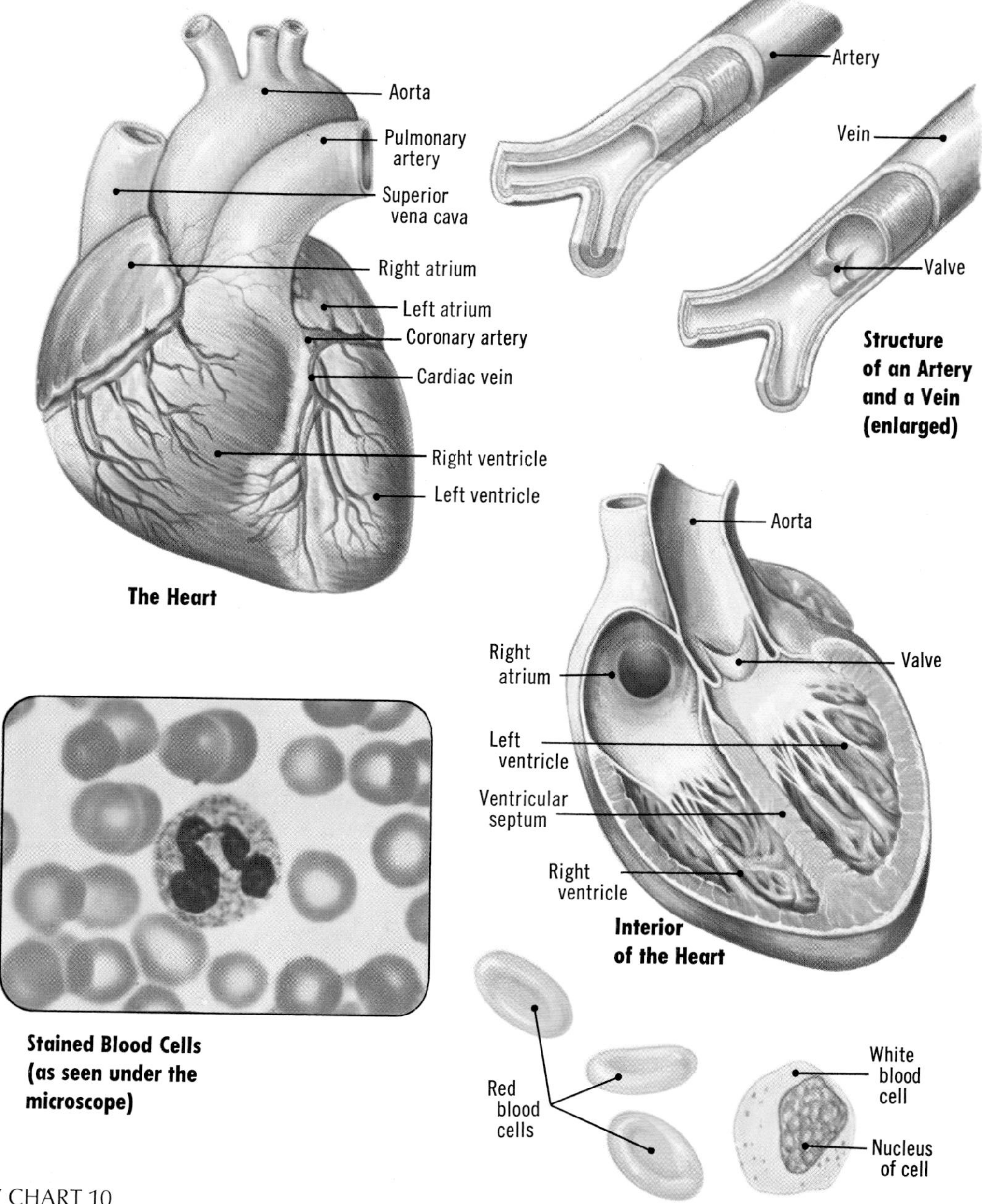

BODY CHART 10

bright red because the blood has been oxygenated. Arterial blood spurts because it escapes under pressure. The spurt may be stopped by the application of pressure between the point of bleeding and the heart. Most venous blood is bluish-red. With hemorrhage, it seeps or wells up into a wound. This bleeding can be stopped only by applying pressure beyond the bleeding point. Escaping capillary blood merely oozes and clots quickly. When serious hemorrhage occurs, rest is important. Alcohol should not be given. By increasing the force of the heartbeat and raising the blood pressure, both activity and alcohol increase bleeding. Moreover, by dilating the blood vessels, alcohol is certain to facilitate the escape of blood.

the respiratory system

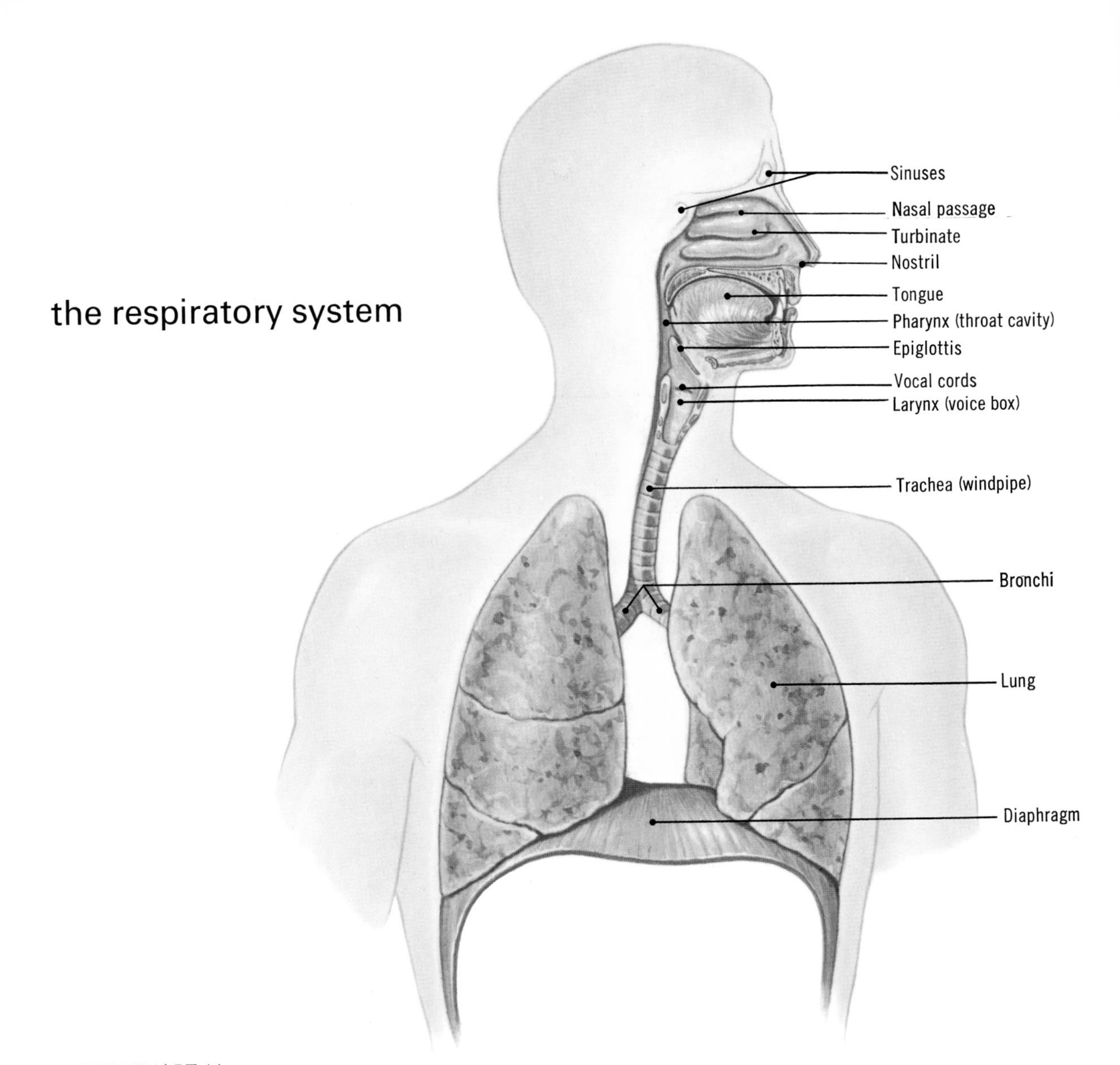

BODY CHART 11

The nasal cavity extends deep into the skull and is separated into right and left by a septum. Rarely, the septum deviates so much that only surgery permits proper breathing. Each side wall of the nasal cavity supports three shell-like projections called *turbinates,* and the furrowlike *nasal passages* run between these small mounds. The duct carrying tears empties into the lowest of these furrows. Also emptying into the nose are various sinus spaces.

The nose is an efficent filtering and air-conditioning system. Larger particles are trapped by coarse hairs in the nostril. The entire nasal cavity, including the sinuses, is covered with mucous membrane, which is kept moist by mucus. Mucus also picks up foreign particles and, aided by the sweeping motion of hairlike cilia, moves the particles toward the pharynx to be swallowed. In the upper part of the nasal cavity, the ciliated cells are replaced by specialized receptor nerve cells. This is the olfactory "organ"; bundles of axons run from neurons in this area through the bony roof of the nose and on to the brain. The mucous membrane covering the septum and that of the middle and lower turbinates is thick and full of blood vessels. When inflamed, this mu-

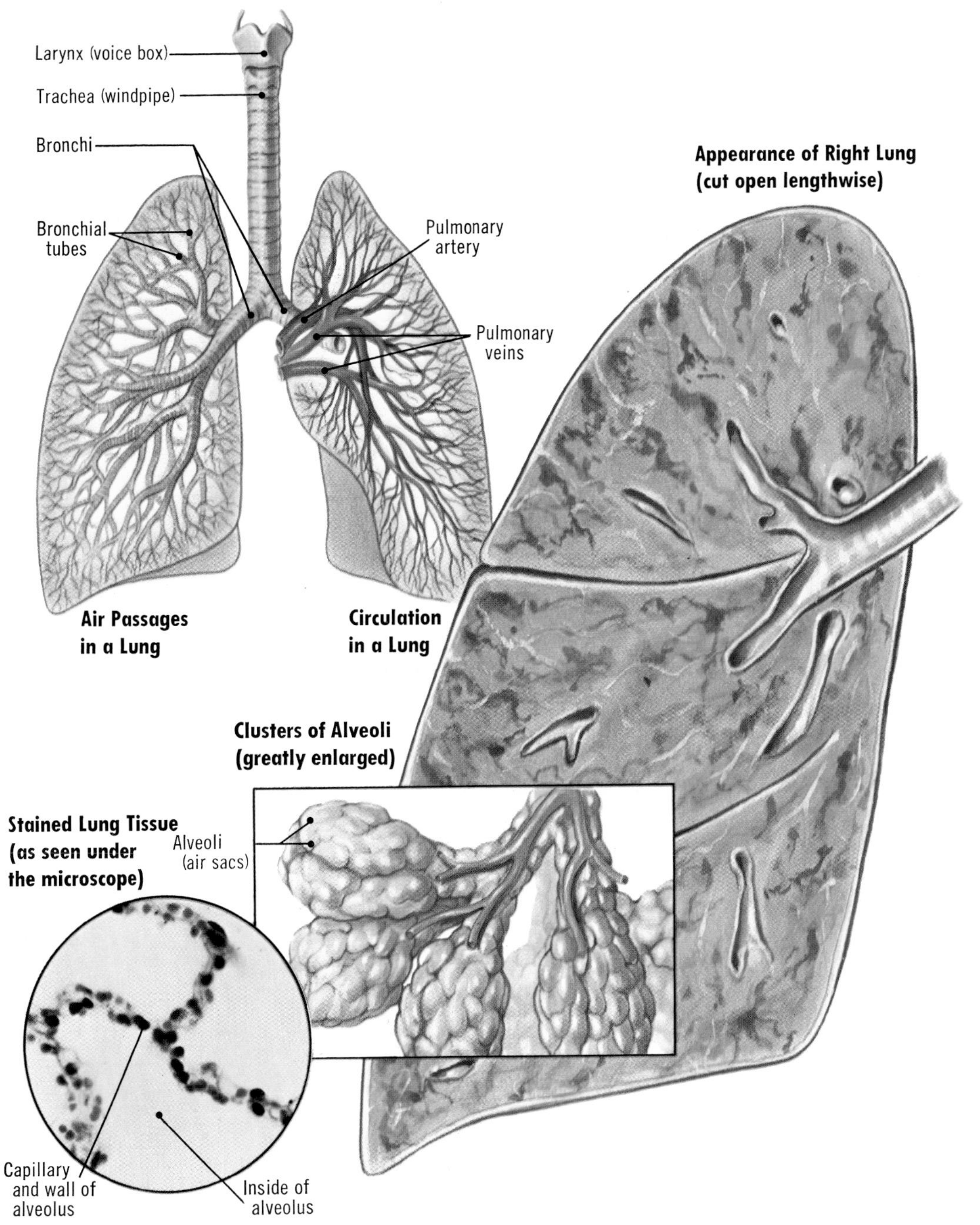

BODY CHART 12

cous membrane swells and blocks the nasal passages. Swollen mucous membrane in the sinuses may also block drainage. The veins in the mucous membrane of the middle and lower turbinates dilate to become venous spaces. With sexual excitement these venous spaces become engorged with blood in much the same way as does erectile tissue of the genital organs. Because of its great vascularity, this area bleeds easily. This very vascularity also makes the nose an excellent ventilating system, for cold air about the capillaries is warmed before entering the lungs. The respiratory tract is further discussed on pages 388-91.

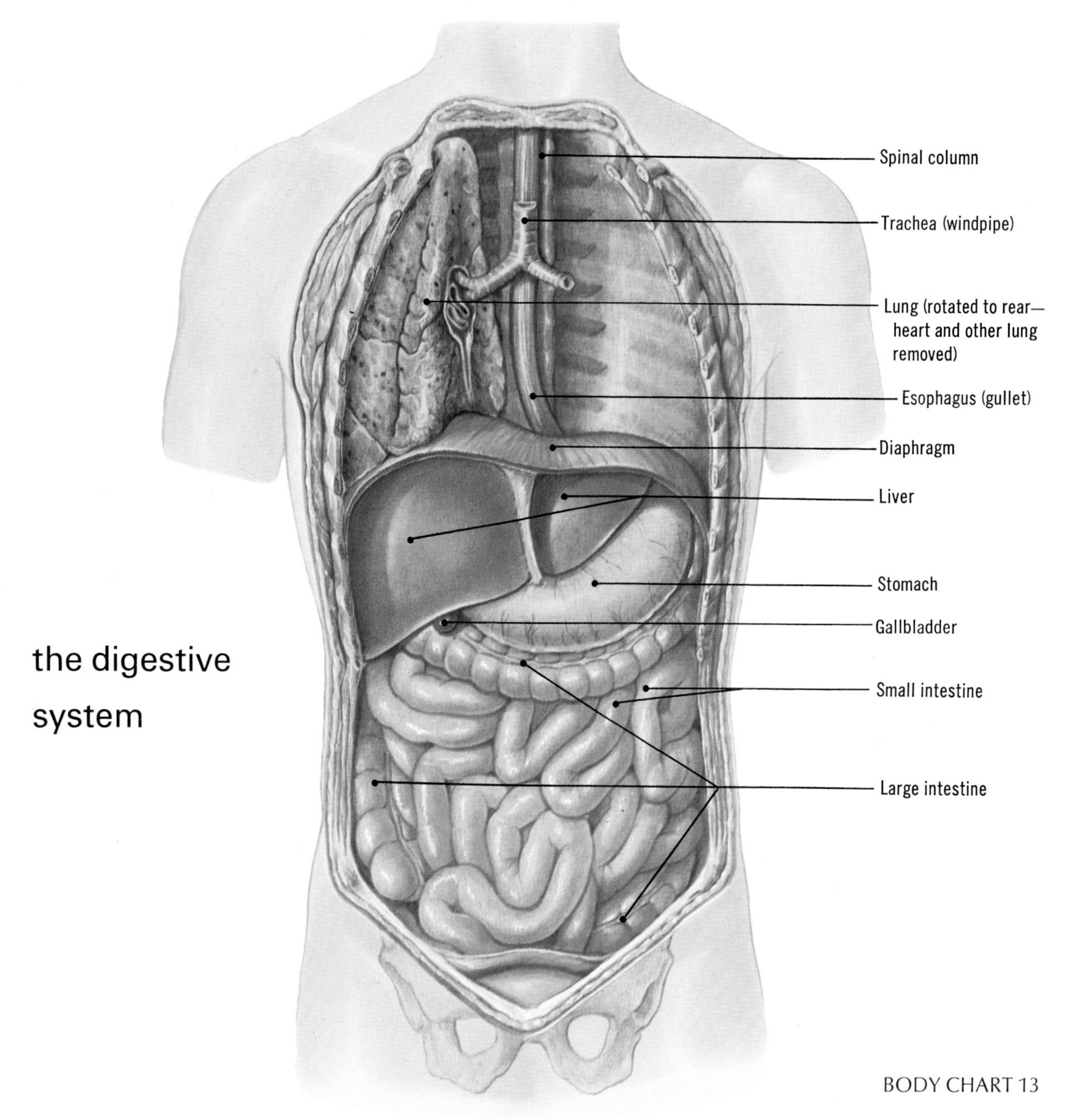

the digestive system

BODY CHART 13

The seventeenth-century English satirist Samuel Butler sardonically described the human body as "a pair of pincers set over a bellows and a stewpan and the whole fixed upon stilts"; he doubtless saw the teeth as pincers and the remaining digestive system as a stewpan. This system is somewhat more comprehensively described in Chapter 22.

From the lips to the anus the adult digestive tract is about 30 to 32 feet long. Two basic kinds of tissue contribute to the wall of the digestive tract from the lower part of the esophagus to the lower end of the small intestine—involuntary *smooth muscle* and the *mucous membrane* lining the muscle. This muscle contracts more slowly than skeletal muscle, and it is able to sustain rhythmic contraction without tiring. The mucosal lining of the digestive tract protects and lubricates. In the small intestine, its absorptive inner surface is unique.

The digestive tract provides the excretory apparatus for food residue; it also excretes other body

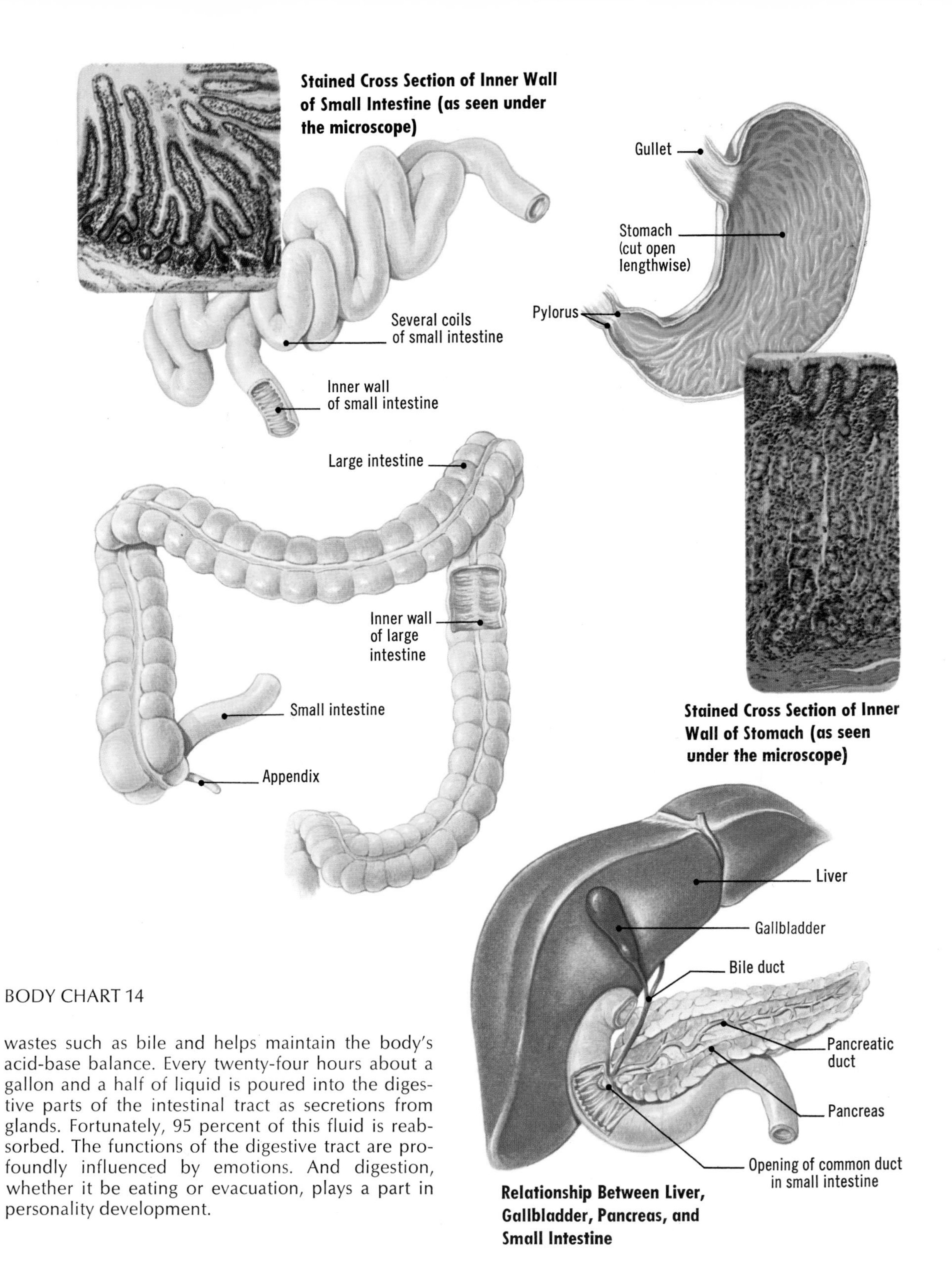

Stained Cross Section of Inner Wall of Small Intestine (as seen under the microscope)

Stained Cross Section of Inner Wall of Stomach (as seen under the microscope)

Relationship Between Liver, Gallbladder, Pancreas, and Small Intestine

BODY CHART 14

wastes such as bile and helps maintain the body's acid-base balance. Every twenty-four hours about a gallon and a half of liquid is poured into the digestive parts of the intestinal tract as secretions from glands. Fortunately, 95 percent of this fluid is reabsorbed. The functions of the digestive tract are profoundly influenced by emotions. And digestion, whether it be eating or evacuation, plays a part in personality development.

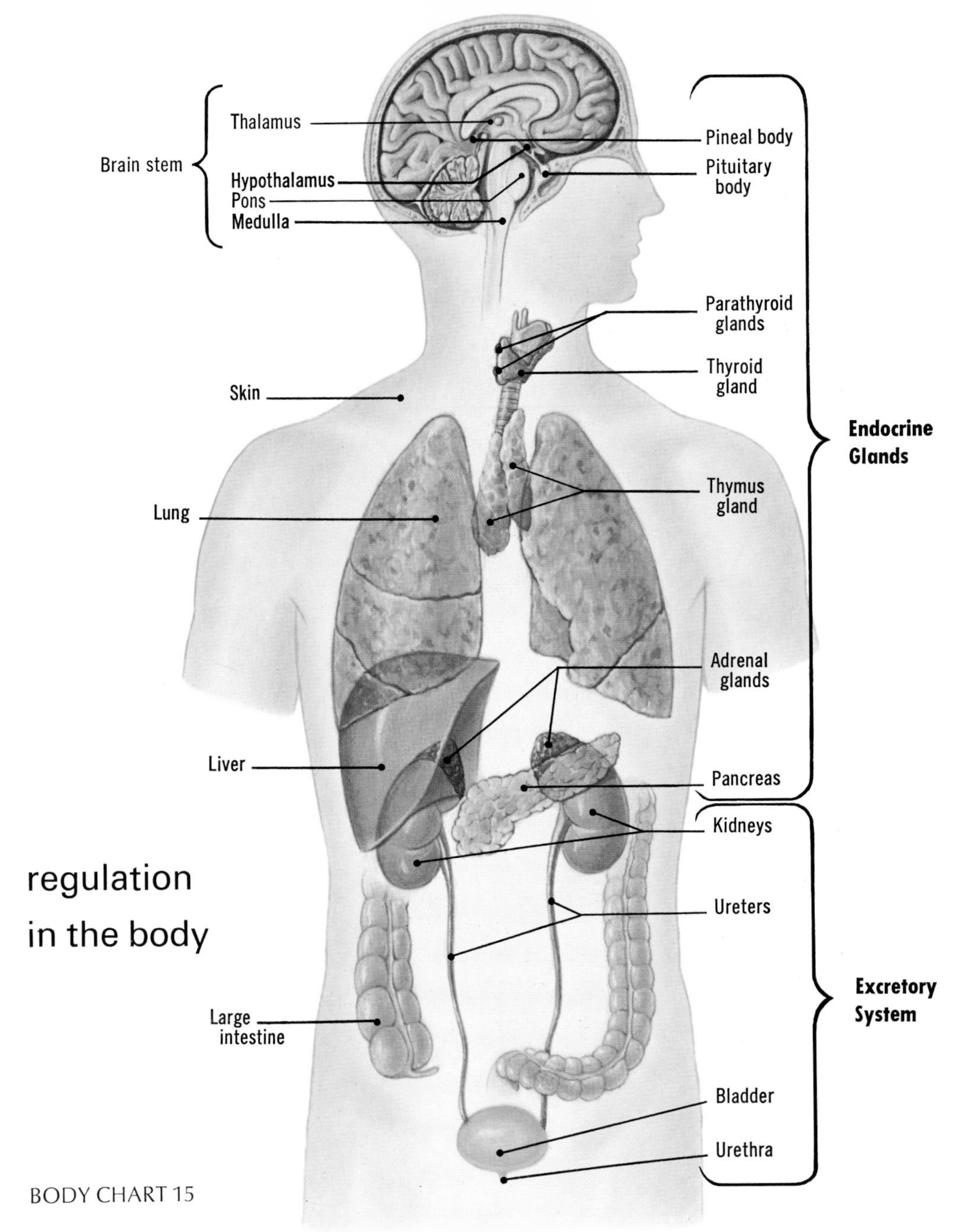

regulation in the body

BODY CHART 15

"The stability of the interior environment," wrote the nineteenth-century French physiologist Claude Bernard, "is the essential condition of free and independent life...all vital mechanisms, however varied they may be, have only one object: that of preserving constant the conditions of life in the interior environment." This chart illustrates some of the most important body regulators involved in maintaining a harmonious balance among the internal human ecosystems. But one can consider these inner ecosystems of man only as they relate to his outer ecosystems. An unhealthy external environment interferes with the ecological health of the internal environment. Man cannot long safely subject the sensitive organs regulating his "interior environment" to the gross pollutions with which he surrounds himself.

It is thought that this inflammation of the brain (believed to be viral) left many with the residual lesions of *Parkinson's syndrome.* Note the word "syndrome"—a complex of symptoms. Described a century and a half ago by a London doctor, James Parkinson, the disease is associated with the lack of a body chemical called dopamine. The lesion is deep in the brain. The limbs and trunk become rigid, the face masklike. The patient, usually elderly, may, to his embarrassment, drool. At rest, he has a four-to-six-per-second shaking tremor of the hands. When he moves, the tremor improves. He may well be depressed. But his mental ability is unaffected.

A new drug, L-dopa, seems to be helping many of these patients. This drug is changed by the brain cells to yield the lacking chemical, dopamine. Also, in selected cases, a unique surgery may relieve those whose tremor is worse on one side of the body. A lesion is purposely placed on the side of the brain supplying the more affected side. The patient may notice the dramatic diminution in tremor on the operating table. Physical therapy also helps.

sight, a special sense: order and disorder

"The light of the body is the eye" (Matthew 6:22).

The blind poet John Milton wrote these poignant lines:

> Why was the sight
> To such a tender ball as th' eye confin'd?
> So obvious and so easy to be quench't,
> And not as feeling through all parts diffus'd,
> That she might look at will through every pore?[28]

To substitute for the lost vision, the blind do indeed learn skillful use of other body parts. The dependence of actual seeing, however, on "such a tender ball" starkly emphasizes the constant need of preventive protection. The anatomic delicacy of the eye lends to its inordinate vulnerability. Some vision disorders develop stealthily, insidiously. Before one is aware enough to act, the damage is done and, often, permanent. Hence, the importance, at all ages, of routine, frequent eye examinations. With a five-year-old, for example, even mild nearsightedness (see Figure 10-17) is important. Like other eye conditions, this has a tendency to worsen with time. Early attention can prevent much vision loss.

Eye problems are rampant among school children. One survey[29] of some 200,000 Philadelphia school children from kindergarten through the twelfth grade revealed almost one in five with defective vision or eye strain. Older people suffer an even more appalling vision loss.

eye structure and function

The fluid of the eyeball is contained by a three-layered wall. These three layers, or coats, are the *sclera, choroid,* and *retina.* The tough *sclera,* the outer layer,

[28] Quoted in Kester Svendsen, *Milton and Science* (Cambridge, Mass., 1956), p. 185.
[29] Walter H. Fink, "Ocular Defects in Preschool Children," *The Sight-Saving Review,* Vol. 24, No. 4 (1954), pp. 196–200.

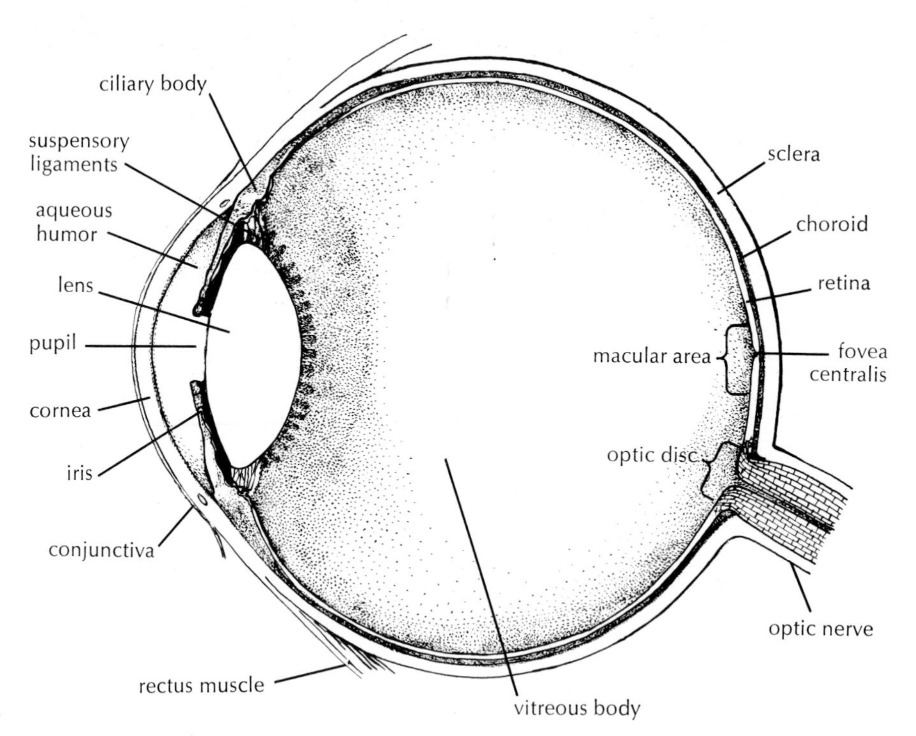

10-14 *The eye.*

sheaths the whole eyeball except the *cornea.* The sclera helps maintain the shape of the eyeball. It is the white of the eye and it protects the eye's delicate inner structure.

It is this fluid under pressure, regulated by a tiny system of canals, that keeps the ball of the eye normally tensed. Behind the lens, the jellylike *vitreous body* (99 percent water) fills the rear of the eyeball (see Figure 10-14). The *aqueous fluid* (*aqueous humor*), smaller in amount, fills the space in front of the lens. The aqueous fluid is constantly provided by filtration from, and through, capillaries. Normally it is drained off into the blood through a canal around the cornea.

Only the front center of the eye, the transparent cornea, which is a continuation of the sclera, is the true "window of the eye." It is so clear that it seems to be without structure. Actually it is composed of at least five layers of flat cells. Each layer is cemented on the next, like sheets of plate glass. Damage to the cornea may scar it. A severe scar may cause blindness. In a majority of carefully selected cases, corneal transplants are successful. Eye banks now preserve donor corneas for long periods.

Most of the blood supply to the eye is contained in the pigmented, middle *choroid* layer. Except for its opening in front, which is the *pupil* (seen as the darkest center spot of the eye), the middle choroid layer surrounds the entire eyeball. The choroid layer continues around the pupil as an encircling band, the *iris* (Greek *iris,* rainbow). The iris lends the eye its color. Expanding in front, the choroid is also continuous with the *ciliary body,* which is mostly the *ciliary mus-*

cle. The iris, lying between the cornea and the lens, is attached to the ciliary body. Suspended behind the iris is the crystalline, elastic *lens.* It is attached to the ciliary body by a *suspensory ligament.* The function of the lens is to send light rays to focus an image on the retina. By contracting, the ciliary muscle controls the shape of the lens and helps to adjust the eye to see near objects. Moreover, the iris itself is made up of tiny, exquisitely arranged, radiating and circular muscle fibers. Light waves are collected by the transparent cornea and then pass through the pupil. The muscle fibers controlling the size of the pupil are supplied by the sympathetic and parasympathetic nerve fibers of the autonomic nervous system. By their contraction or dilation, the iris muscle fibers regulate pupil size and, therefore, the amount of light entering the eye (see Figure 10-15).

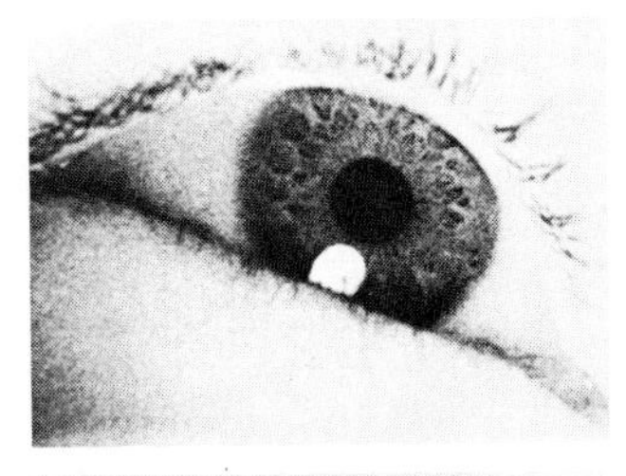

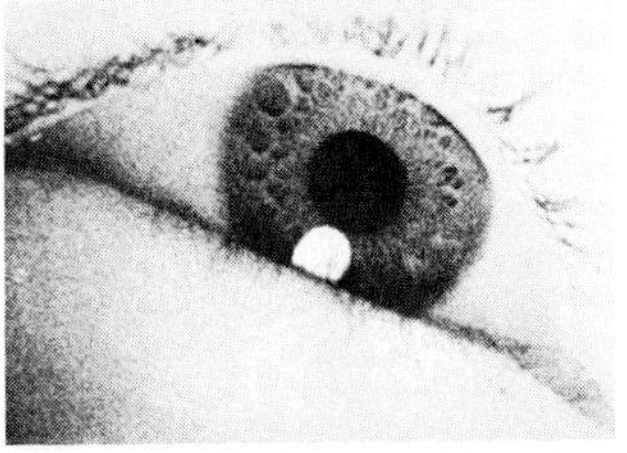

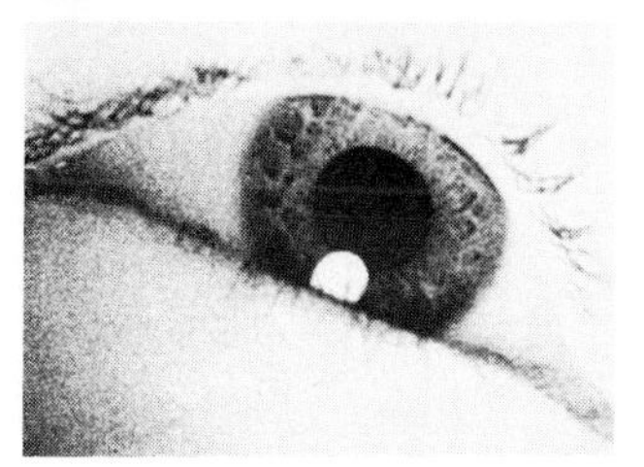

10-15 *Pupil response of a man looking at a picture of a pretty woman. These three photographs show (from top to bottom) a 30 percent increase in pupil size over a period of $2\frac{1}{2}$ seconds. Pupils dilate with pleasant stimuli and constrict with unpleasant stimuli.*

The innermost layer of the eyeball, the *retina,* is an extension of the optic nerve leading to the brain. It lines the back two-thirds of the choroid of the inner eye chamber. The retina contains ten layers, one of which consists of specialized visual receptor cells called *rods* and *cones.* These cells convert light rays into nerve impulses. Tiny nerve fibers, collecting these impulses, combine to form the *optic nerve,* which is the single nerve bundle leaving the orbit for the brain.[30] (The orbit is the bony cavity containing the eyeball.)

The point of exit of the optic nerve from the eyeball is a blind spot, the *optic disc.* The *fovea* of the retina, a tiny pit about one degree wide, and the area surrounding it, the *macular area,* is the region of clearest vision. Using an instrument called an ophthalmoscope (Greek *ophthalmos,* eye + *skopein,* to examine), the physician can examine the retina. A brain tumor, for example, may push the optic disc into the eyeball or, from injury or inflammation, the retina may become detached. A variety of conditions, such as diabetes and arteriosclerosis, are reflected by retinal changes.

disorders of vision

GLAUCOMA When the canal draining the aqueous fluid is clogged, drainage cannot occur. Pressure within the whole eyeball increases. The delicate nerve cells and fibers are damaged. This condition is *glaucoma.* Chronic infections and poor general health aggravate this disorder. It may be associated with defective circulation. The individual complains of blurred vision, halos, and rainbows around lights. In a darkened room, his eyes may hurt. Frequent changes of glasses do not help. Side vision is the first to go. There is only tunnel vision (see Figure 10-16). Slowly, the nerves of sight are crushed. Delay is disastrous. A painless, quick test measures pressure within the eyeball. With early diagnosis, eye drops usually prevent further blindness. To relieve the pressure, surgery may be necessary.

[30] Animal experimental evidence indicates that the nerve connections between the eyes and the visual centers of the brain are organized during a critical period early in life. It has been suggested that, in the human, this critical period is during the first six years of life. This emphasizes the need of eye examinations and correction of defects as early as possible. Otherwise, a permanent defect may result. ("Poor Eyesight Can Upset the Brain's Wiring," *New Scientist,* Vol. 54, No. 790 [April 6, 1972], p. 4.)

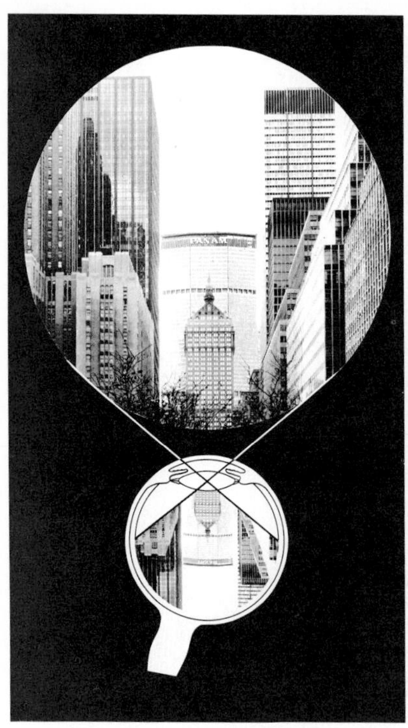

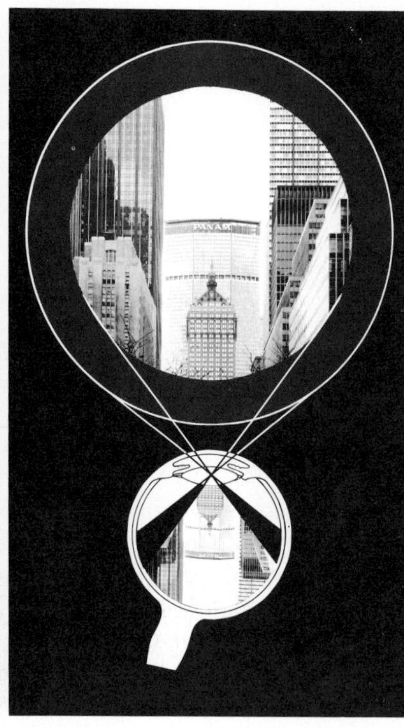

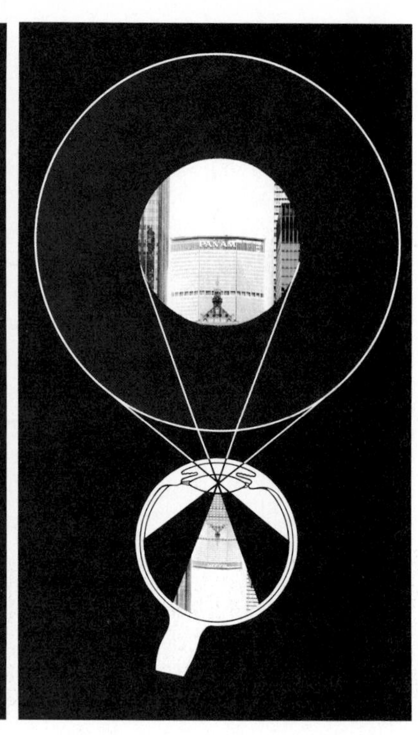

10-16 *Glaucoma narrows vision: normal vision* (left), *early glaucoma* (center), *and advanced glaucoma* (right). *Without adequate treatment, the person may eventually lose all sight.*

CATARACT *Cataract* (Greek *katarregnumi,* to break down) is a cloudiness in the lens. Therefore, light cannot pass through the lens. Cataract can occur at any age. A newborn, infected by the mother's German measles, may be born with cataracts. If no other eye damage is present, surgery is helpful. The cloudy lens is removed and eyeglasses are worn to properly focus images on the retina.

PROBLEMS OF FOCUS As one ages, the lens dries. It loses elasticity and becomes denser. Its ability to bend light is diminished. Thus images fall in back

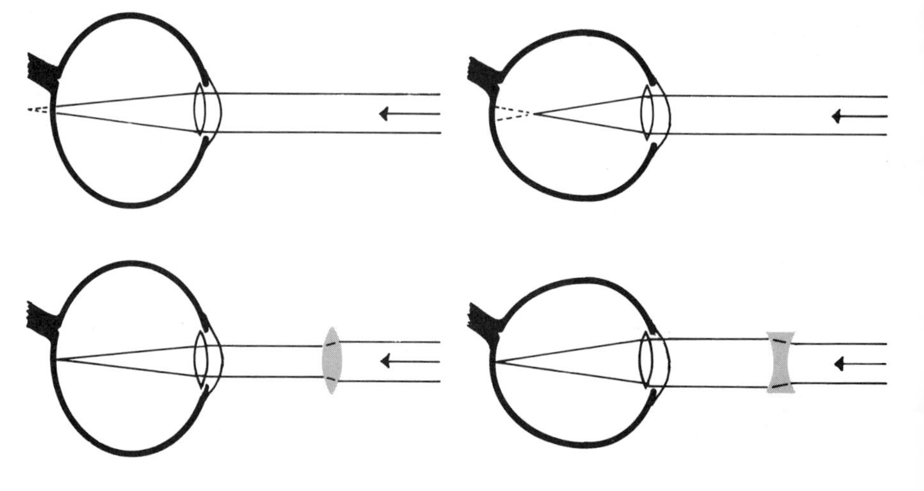

10-17 *Farsightedness* (top left) *and its correction with a convex lens* (bottom left), *and nearsightedness* (top right) *and its correction with a concave lens* (bottom right). *In both cases, the corrective lens makes images fall on the retina.*

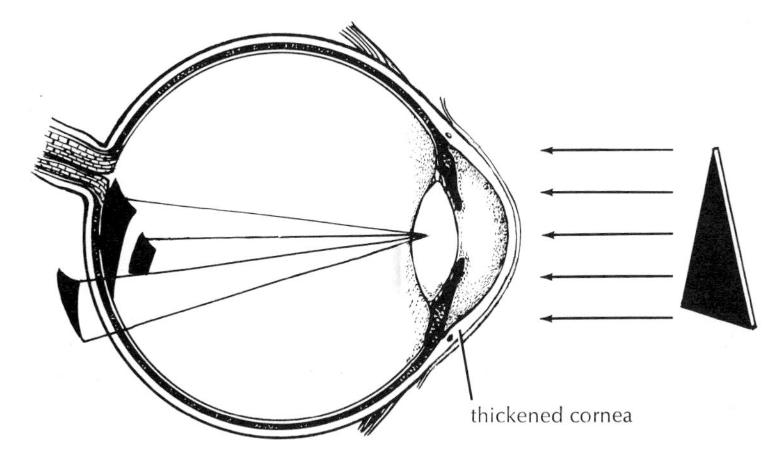

10-18 *Astigmatism. Because two adjacent portions of the cornea have different curvatures, light rays focus improperly.*

of the retina. This condition is *farsightedness,* or *hyperopia. Nearsightedness,* or *myopia,* is a disorder in which the images fall in front of the retina. Figure 10-17 illustrates both disorders and also the effect of corrective lenses on each. *Astigmatism* (Figure 10-18) occurs because two adjacent portions of the cornea have different curvatures. Some light rays focus on the retina, other rays focus in front of it, and still others focus behind it. Part of the image is blurred. A lens that bends only the nonfocusing light rays is corrective.

TWO DISSIMILAR BUT COMMON MINOR EYE PROBLEMS The *conjunctiva* is the transparent, delicate membrane covering the inside of the eyelid and the

10-19 *The severe astigmatism of two great Renaissance artists, Hans Holbein (1497?–1543) and El Greco (1541?–1614?), is believed by some to account for the distortion of their painted figures. For centuries these distortions, in themselves so beautiful and so characteristic of the artists' respective styles, have been widely and rightly admired.* Left: *Holbein's "Henry VIII."* Right: *El Greco's "St. Paul."*

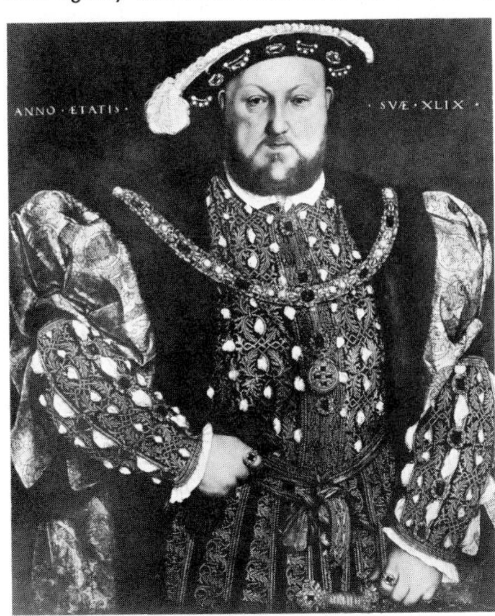

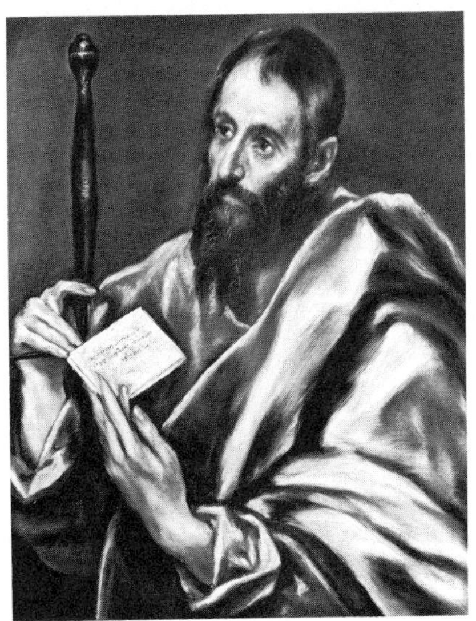

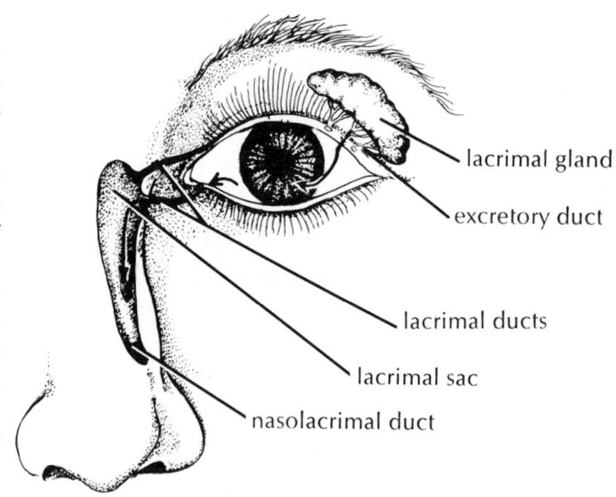

10-20 *The tear apparatus. Secreted by the lacrimal glands and spread by the blinking eyelids, tears reach the inner corner of each eye. Here they are collected by tiny holes at the inner end of each lid. Each hole leads to a lacrimal sac by way of a minute canal. From the sac, tears reach the nose via a nasolacrimal duct. Hairs in the nose move the tears back to be swallowed. With excessive tearing, the lacrimal apparatus is overwhelmed and tears spill down on the cheek.*

exposed surface of the eyeball (see Figure 10-14). Epidemic infection of this membrane (acute bacterial conjunctivitis, or "pinkeye") is particularly common in school and preschool children. It is caused by a variety of microorganisms. Eye drops containing an appropriate antibiotic are curative. The surfaces of the conjunctiva are kept lubricated by tear fluid which is continuously secreted by the *lacrimal gland* (see Figure 10-20). Like saliva, tears contain an antibacterial enzyme. Were it not for this constant slight flow of tears the conjunctiva would dry and become inflamed, and vision would be lost.

Color blindness is an inherited condition resulting from the mutation of a gene involving color vision in an X-chromosome. Since males possess but one X-chromosome in their body cells, color blindness is more common among them (8 percent of the population) than it is among females (0.4 percent), who have two X-chromosomes. The genes for color blindness are recessive (a recessive gene will usually produce an effect only when it is transmitted by both parents). For a female to be color blind, therefore, the genes of both X-chromosomes must be affected. Most color-blind people are unable to fully see either red or green.

hearing, a special sense: disorders

The apparatus for hearing was described in Chapter 4 and diagramed in Figure 4-9 (page 99). Its consummate workmanship, its very fragility, requires its deep encasement in protective bone. Before he sees danger, man usually hears it. Deafness, like blindness, is a harsh handicap. Yet, millions in this nation are chronically deaf to some degree. In older age groups, hearing defects occur in astronomical numbers.

Conductive deafness involves interference of sound transmission through the outer or middle ear. As simple a matter as excessive ear wax may cause deafness. Its removal by a physician is curative. Its removal by an amateur with a hairpin, or some other dangerous instrument, may lead to a pierced eardrum. "He has not so much brain as earwax," wrote Shakespeare in *Troilus and Cres-*

sida (V.i.58). This description might be applied to one who, in this manner, senselessly risks deafness. *Infection* of the middle ear, which sometimes accompanies or follows a childhood communicable disease, is a frequent cause of conductive deafness.

Hearing loss by way of the *Eustachian tube* is not uncommon. As was mentioned on page 99, the Eustachian tube is open only during swallowing. In this way an equal pressure on both sides of the eardrum is maintained. During an airplane descent, the passenger should repeatedly swallow. Otherwise, the high-altitude air pressure, trapped in the middle ear, will fail to correspond to the increasing atmospheric pressure on the outside of the eardrum. The eardrum may then rupture. An *upper respiratory infection* may, moreover, cause swelling around the opening and within the Eustachian tube. Sometimes this causes temporary deafness. An attempt to open the tube by vigorously blowing the nose may force infectious material into the middle ear. Children are more prone to middle ear infection than adults because infection travels more easily via their shorter, straighter Eustachian tubes. Indiscriminate use of nose drops or nasal sprays may promote such infection. The consequences may be serious and chronic.

Sometimes infection will cause stiffening of the joints between the three little bones in the middle ear. The bones become rigid. Their normal ability to vibrate is limited. Sound waves cannot be transmitted through them to the fluid of the inner ear. Hearing is diminished, even lost. But sound waves can be transmitted through the skull to the fluid, and it is on this principle that the hearing aid works.

However, the hearing aid does not help with *nerve deafness.* Here, the problem is in the cochlea of the inner ear, the auditory nerve, or even in the cerebral cortex. By injuring the nerve cells in the inner ear, excessive noise can cause deafness. This problem was discussed in Chapter 4. For a variety of reasons, many children are born deaf. Such deafness may occur when a pregnant woman's infection with German measles virus also infects her unborn child. A vaccine against German measles is now available (pages 147–49). A recent study suggests that the developing child may lose some hearing while in the uterus if the mother is exposed to prolonged excessive noise (see pages 552–53). Children born deaf will not speak unless taught through some pathway other than the ear. A deaf child need not be a dumb child. Schools for the deaf are an important societal service. So are those people trained to communicate with the hard-of-hearing.

summary

In addition to cancer (Chapter 8) and heart disease (Chapter 9), major groups of chronic diseases are allergies, diseases of the bones and joints, glandular disorders, and diseases of the nervous system.

The manifestations of *allergy* are caused by swelling produced by exposure to a substance to which the individual has become sensitized (page 249). Common allergic conditions are *hay fever, asthma, hives, eczema, contact dermatitis,* and possibly *migraine* (pages 249–50).

Rheumatic diseases, such as *gout,* affect connective tissue, usually involving the muscles and joints (pages 250–51). *Arthritis* is not a specific disease, but a joint inflammation (page 251). Most people afflicted with rheumatism have either *rheumatoid arthritis* (pages 251–52), which is not just a joint inflammation but involves connective tissue throughout the body, or *osteoarthritis* (pages 252–53), which is not a joint inflammation but a degenerative joint disease. *Nonarticular rheumatism* refers to rheumatic diseases that afflict body parts other than joints (page 254).

The *exocrine glands,* such as the mammary glands and the sweat, tear, and salivary glands, release their secretions through *ducts* (page 254). The *endocrine glands* are ductless, releasing their secretions—*hormones*—directly into the blood stream (page 254). The endocrine glands are the *thymus,* the *parathyroid glands,* part of the *pancreas,* the *gonads,* and

1. the *pituitary gland,* which is profoundly influenced by the *hypothalamus* of the brain. The hypothalamus is itself believed to manufacture the two hormones, *oxytocin* and *vasopressin,* that are merely stored in and released by the *posterior lobe* of the pituitary (page 255). The hypothalamus secretes some hormones, which stimulate the *anterior lobe* to make and release hormones going to target organs. The amount is controlled by a feedback mechanism. When this mechanism is absent, hypothalamic hormones control the amount (pages 255–58).

2. the *adrenal gland.* The *medulla,* or inner part, of this gland secretes *epinephrine* and *norepinephrine* (page 258). The *cortex,* or outer part, secretes three groups of *adrenocortical steroids: hydrocortisone, aldosterone,* and *androgens* (page 258).

3. the *thyroid gland,* which governs the rate of body metabolism (page 259).

Two serious and common glandular disorders are *cystic fibrosis,* an exocrine dysfunction (pages 259–60), and *diabetes mellitus,* an endocrine dysfunction (pages 260–61).

The basic unit of the *nervous system* is the *neuron,* of which there are three types: *afferent* or *sensory, efferent* or *motor,* and *connecting* (pages 263–64). The main divisions of the nervous system are the *central nervous system*—the *brain* and *spinal cord* (pages 265–66)—and the *peripheral nervous system*—the *cranial* and *spinal nerves* and the *autonomic nervous system,* which has two divisions, the *sympathetic* and *parasympathetic* (pages 267–69). Disorders in the central nervous system include *stroke* (page 270), *epilepsy* (pages 270–71), *cerebral palsy* (pages 271–72), *multiple sclerosis* (page 272), and *Parkinson's syndrome* (pages 272–73). Serious dysfunctions afflict *sight* (pages 273–75)—such as *glaucoma* (page 275) and *cataract* (page 276). Problems of focus include *farsightedness, nearsightedness,* and *astigmatism* (pages 276–77). *Conjunctivitis* (pages 277–78) and *color blindness* (page 278) also occur. *Hearing* may be impeded by *conductive deafness* (pages 278–79) and *nerve deafness* (page 279).

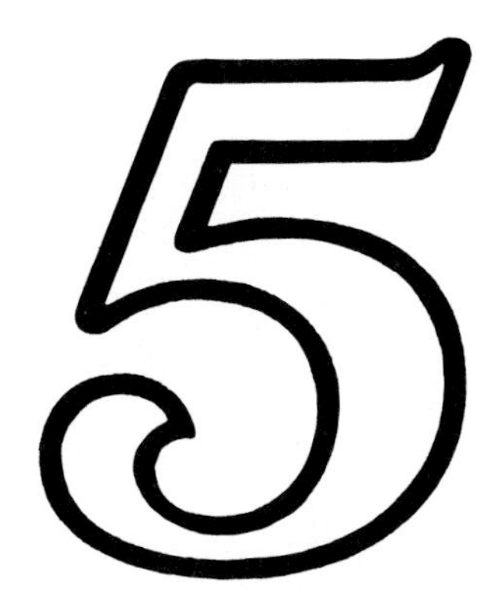

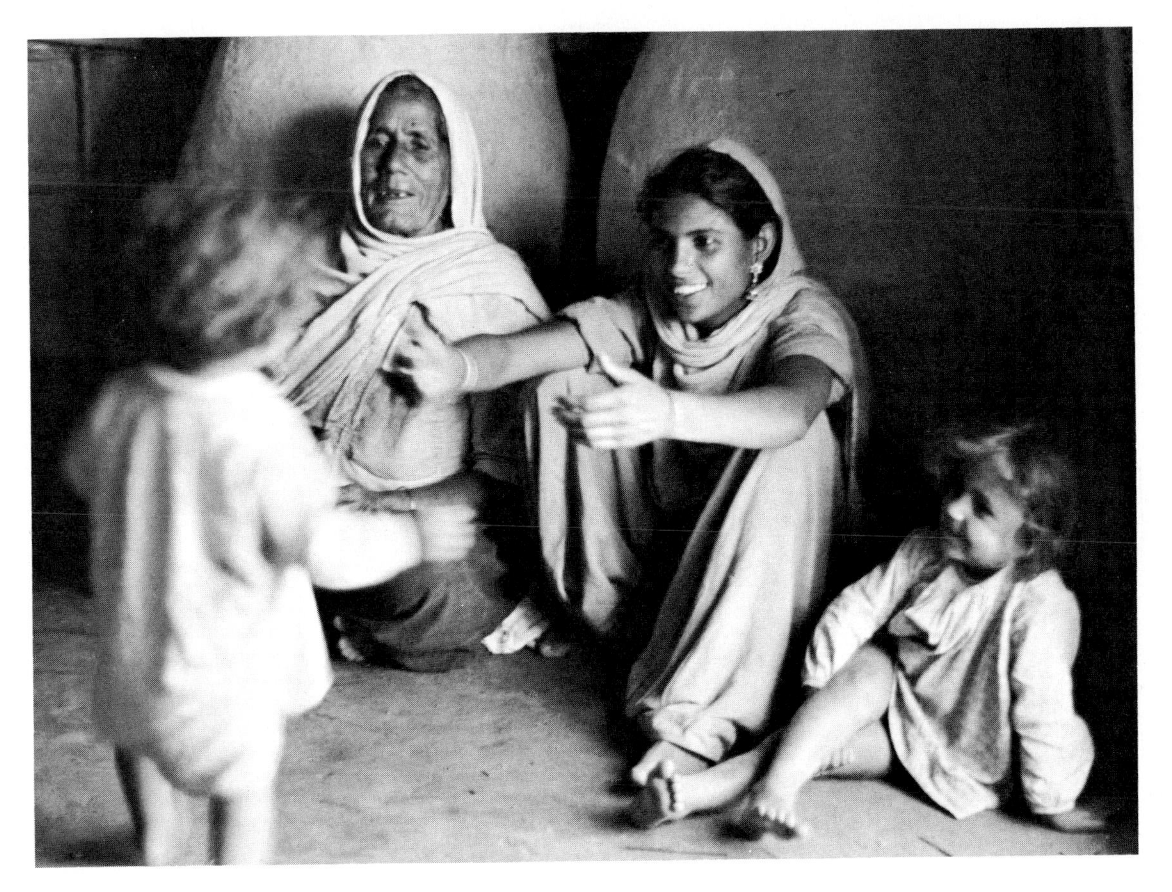

the emotional life

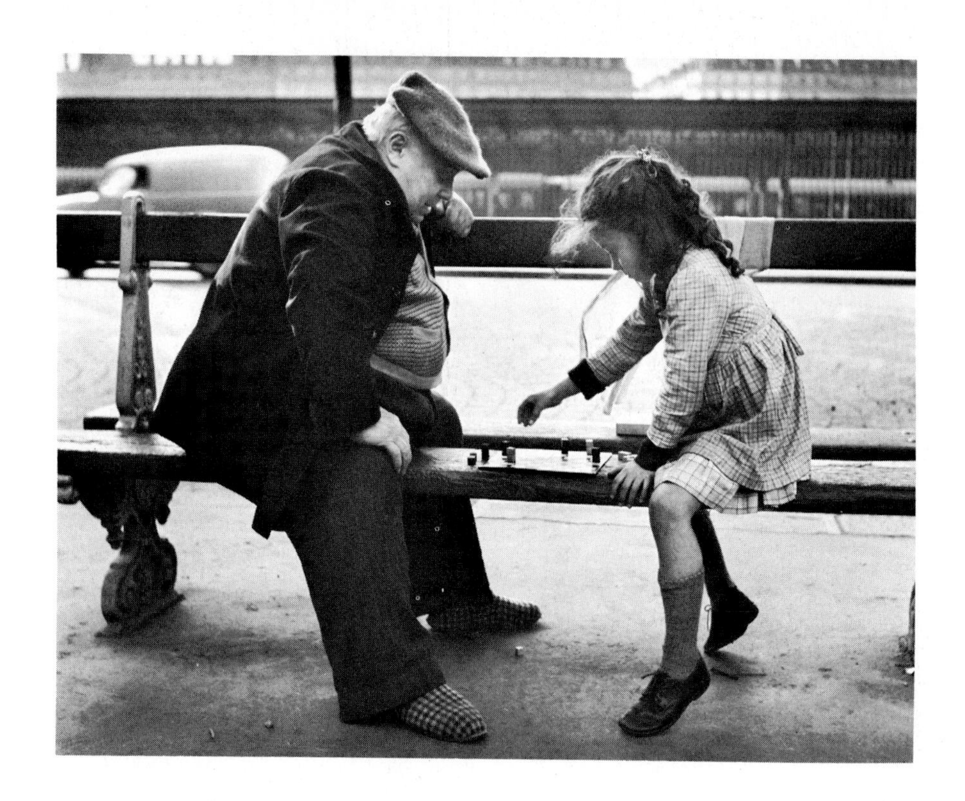

personality development

11

And if the soul
is to know itself
it must look
into a soul:
the stranger and enemy, we've seen him in the mirror.[1]

personality development

Begin at the beginning. Begin with the birth of the baby. He can suck and he can look, but not at the same time. Through eyes vacant like tiny unwashed windows, he can see only peripherally. He is aware of light and dark. He can cry and perhaps raise his head a trifle. Although six months will pass before his teeth can be seen, he has an immediate sweet tooth. He dislikes bitters. He can smell, and even before he was born he could hear. Three to ten minutes after he is born, he will turn his eyes toward a sound. He can feel pressure and warmth and cold. He can cough and sneeze. For a day or two, he will eliminate a blackish-green material called meconium from his rectum. This was formed during intrauterine life, when trial secretions of his digestive glands mixed with swallowed fluid. In a few days he will eat. Most of the time his gut will be able to push the food down. Sometimes he will spit it up. It will be months before he can suck and look at the same time.

During his first day, he will pass between one-half and one and one-half ounces of urine. This amount will increase. His heart beats about 150 times a minute, and he breathes 30 to 50 times a minute. If his head was born first, as is ordinarily the case, he probably breathed before all of him was delivered. At about six weeks of age the newborn can smile, not because of a gas pain but from pleasure.[2] Yet there is an old saying that man is expected to grieve. If he does not weep at birth, he is spanked until he does. Be that as it may, the child's first staccato cry heralds the change from aquatic to terrestrial life—an evolutionary change that required millions of years. After his first crying spell, the infant sleeps. When he awakens, he cries again. At this tender age, no other creature can howl so mightily. It is this second episode of weeping that is the concern of this chapter, for it tells that the infant can suffer. And, collecting stress and distress, often he reaches adulthood only to feel like Shakespeare's Antonio in *The Merchant of Venice:*

In sooth, I know not why I am so sad.
It wearies me, you say it wearies you;
But how I caught it, found it, or came by it,
What stuff 'tis made of, whereof it is born,
I am to learn.
And such a want-wit sadness makes of me
That I have much ado to know myself.[3]

[1] George Seferis, *Collected Poems, 1924–1955* (Princeton, N.J., 1967), p. 9.
[2] *M.D., Medical Newsmagazine,* Vol. 12, No. 3 (March 1968), p. 154.
[3] William Shakespeare, *The Merchant of Venice,* I.i.1–7.

What sadness makes Antonio feel a "want-wit"? What is the root of his anguish? In every time, in every tongue, in every lonely troubled corner on earth, this bewilderment has been uttered. Why is this so? Before the work of Sigmund Freud there were few answers.

some historical notes

The history of the investigation of human emotion may well be divided into before and after Freud. Thirty-four centuries before Freud, in 1550 B.C., the Egyptians wrote, in the Ebers Papyrus, that hysteria was caused by a wandering womb. About seventeen hundred years later, the ancient Greek physician Galen, "hoping to lure the vagrant uterus back to its normal position,"[4] recommended actual fumigation of the vagina to cure hysteria. In numerous passages, the Bible mentions emotional illness. Often it was thought a punishment from the Lord (Deuteronomy 6:5). In a fit of depression, Saul commits suicide (I Samuel 31:4). The delusion of Nebuchadnezzar, that he was a wolf, is famous.[5] Doubtless such references had a profound effect on later philosophers of religion. The original introspections of St. Augustine (d. 604), the first archbishop of Canterbury, had a penetrating effect on psychology. Spinoza (1632–77), whose philosophy emphasized insight into oneself as an ethical goal, was an authentic precursor of Freud. "What Freud calls mental health Spinoza calls the freedom of the mind."[6]

In the medieval era the emotionally sick were treated like animals. It remained for the physician-reformer Philippe Pinel to unchain the insane of France. Because of him, many nineteenth-century Europeans became convinced of the need for medical treatment of the emotionally ill (see Figure 11-1).

About the middle of the nineteenth century, the modern era of medicine began. Great discoveries in the natural sciences by Darwin, Pasteur, and others

[4] Franz G. Alexander and Sheldon T. Selesnick, *The History of Psychiatry* (New York, 1966), p. 21.
[5] *Ibid.*, p. 23.
[6] *Ibid.*, p. 100.

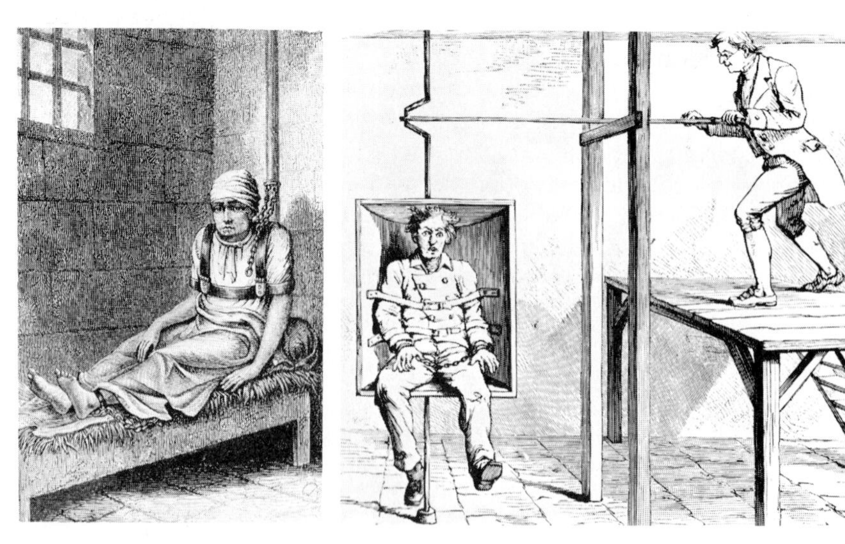

11-1 *Two early 19th-century methods of "treating" the emotionally ill: chains* (left) *and a circulating swing* (right).

formed the backdrop for the Freudian stage. Freud began his career with significant discoveries about the anatomy of the nervous system. Before his death, in 1939, he had become one of the most influential thinkers in history.

Freud's concepts were ecological. He began by calling attention to the child. Within each child were basic unconscious instinctual drives. Between these drives and the surrounding environment occurred constant and inexorable negotiations. From this interplay human personality resulted. In childhood, basic personality traits were established. With severe emotional trauma and crises, childhood personality development lagged. The resultant adult behaved like a child. The adult personality, then, was molded by the stress responses of childhood. "Pubescence," Freud wrote, "is an act of nature; adolescence is an act of man." In this way Freud emphasized the difference between merely growing and growing up. Moreover, Freud taught that the stresses of childhood could be changed. Therefore, patterns of behavior that were based on reactions to stresses could be changed. Early responses to stress, lying deeply buried in the subconscious for long periods of time, often caused eventual emotional problems. If these could be uncovered, confronted, and resolved by an individual who suffered them, cure could result.

Among the most influential of the psychologists who built on Freud's theoretical ideas is Erik Erikson. Like Freud, Erikson is aware that human behavior is created by and helps to create its own environment. His schema of personality development provides a useful and coherent concept of the flow of psychological happenings through which people must live to grow to emotional maturity. "How does a healthy person grow or, as it were, accrue from the successive stages of increasing capacity to master life's outer and inner tasks and dangers?"[7] This is the basic question that Erikson sets out to answer.

Erikson's eight stages of personality development

For Erikson, every human being's personality develops in eight stages, each of which takes place during a particular age. In each stage the developing individual is faced with a task. If the task is satisfactorily resolved, the individual enters healthily into the next stage. If it is not, the individual is ill-equipped to solve the task of the next stage. Future attempts to solve tasks are hampered by the emotional impedimenta caused by past failures. To heal these wounds to the personality, the individual needs help. Adequate help at critical times stabilizes the individual. Preparation for the next stage and the transition into it are then accomplished with a greater sense of personal competence and security. Better emotional health results. Without help, the person's inadequately resolved tasks turn into cumulative emotional scars—and personality disorders.

Each of Erikson's eight stages is named according to the task that is confronted. The name identifies both the desirable resolution of the task and the contrary development that takes place if the task is not resolved. The desirable resolution of the task of the first of the eight stages, for example, is *basic trust.* Its contrary development is *basic mistrust.* Thus the first stage is named *basic trust versus basic mistrust.* But there are no sharp dividing lines between Erik-

[7] Erik H. Erikson, "Growth and Crises of the Healthy Personality," in Clyde Kluckhohn, Henry A. Murray, and David Schneider, eds., *Personality in Nature, Society, and Culture* (New York, 1953), p. 186.

son's stages. During the later stages the resolution (or lack of resolution) of the tasks of earlier stages continues to develop.

As a result of continuous interactions with his environment during these stages, man develops a feeling of self-identity. This feeling, which Erikson calls *ego-identity,* is central to human personality development. Man's ego-identity is his awareness of himself as a distinct person with an influential past, an active present, and a controllable future. What must man live through to achieve this feeling of identity?

the infant

Basic trust versus basic mistrust is the first stage. In the first year, the infant will make a decision, based on the quality of his maternal care, as to whether the world is dependable and safe or fraught with frustration and fear. It is not a decision reached as the result of one incident or a few. Erikson does not mean that this stage (or any other) is like an obstacle race in which a few missteps forever doom the participant to emotional illness. The infant decision is the product of the ripening relationship between him and his mother. Completely self-centered, yet utterly dependent, he will inevitably be disappointed. No mother can always immediately meet all her baby's needs. And so, as a part of normal development, the child must learn to cope with a degree of frustration. His ability to do this will depend on his overall sense of security or insecurity. If his frustrations are not excessive in amount or in frequency, he will learn that, although things are not always to his liking, most of the time they are fine. A baby can adjust to that. Indeed, this lesson will help him face situations that will arise as he reaches his first year—situations that involve some degree of separation from his mother. If all that has preceded has been characterized by anxiety, he will approach this and future problems with fear and basic mistrust. But if the preponderance of his experience has taught him basic trust, he will have gained a sense of self-esteem that will stand him in good stead.

A CASE OF SEVERE BASIC MISTRUST What happens to a baby without an opportunity to develop a degree of basic trust? The story of Joey, the "mechanical boy,"[8] provides an instructive, though dramatically extreme, example. "He wanted to be rid of his unbearable humanity," Bettelheim wrote, "to become completely automatic."

> "I never knew I was pregnant," his mother said, meaning that she had already excluded Joey from her consciousness. His birth, she said, "did not make any difference." Joey's father, a rootless draftee in the wartime civilian army, was equally unready for parenthood. So, of course, are many young couples. Fortunately most such parents lose their indifference upon the baby's birth. But not Joey's parents. "I did not want to see or nurse him," his mother declared. "I had no feeling of actual dislike—I simply didn't want to take care of him." For the first three months of his life Joey "cried most of the time." A colicky baby, he was kept on a rigid four-hour feeding schedule, was not touched unless neces-

[8]The discussion of Joey is drawn from "Joey: A 'Mechanical Boy,'" a classic article by Bruno Bettelheim in *Scientific American,* Vol. 200, No. 3 (March 1959), pp. 117–27.

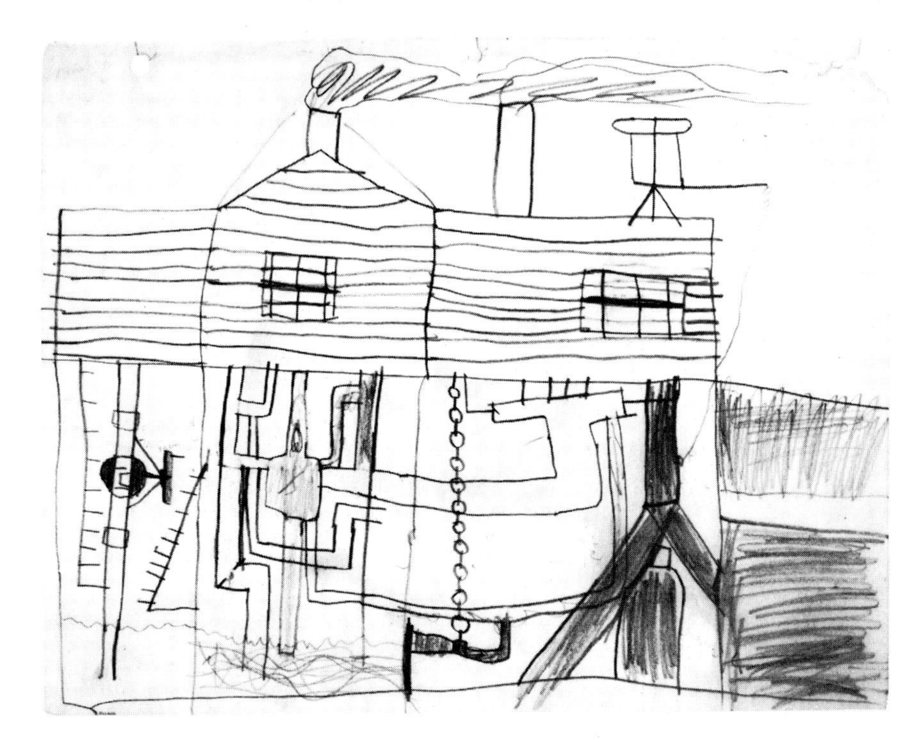

11-2 *One of Joey's early drawings. The house is small and simple. The mechanical sewer system is large and complex. Joey's impersonal and rigid toilet training is reflected in his obsessive interest in sewage disposal.*

sary and was never cuddled or played with. The mother, preoccupied with herself, usually left Joey alone in the crib or playpen during the day. The father discharged his frustrations by punishing Joey when the child cried at night.

Joey's existence never registered with his mother . . . When she told us about his birth and infancy, it was as if she were talking about some vague acquaintance.[9]

This parental indifference taught Joey little but basic mistrust. Only mechanical devices could be relied on to satisfy his greatest needs. Years later Bettelheim described Joey's bizarre behavior:

Entering the dining room, for example, he would string an imaginary wire from his "energy source"—an imaginary electric outlet—to the table. There he "insulated" himself with paper napkins and finally plugged himself in. Only then could Joey eat, for he firmly believed that the "current" ran his ingestive apparatus . . .

Many times a day he would turn himself on and shift noisily through a sequence of higher and higher gears until he "exploded," screaming "Crash, crash!" and hurling items from his ever present apparatus—radio tubes, light bulbs, even motors or, lacking these, any handy breakable object. (Joey had an astonishing knack for snatching bulbs and tubes unobserved.) As soon as the object thrown had shattered, he would cease his screaming and wild jumping and retire to mute, motionless nonexistence.[10]

[9] *Ibid.,* p. 118.
[10] *Ibid.,* p. 117.

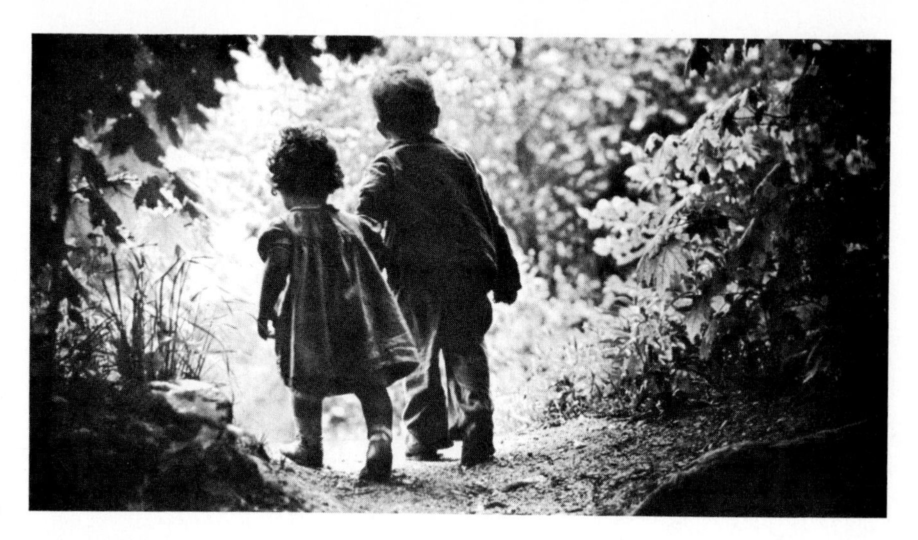

11-3 *Early childhood.*

the toddler

Autonomy versus shame and doubt characterizes Erikson's second stage of the developing personality. This stage is marked by growing individual muscle controls. As the toddler learns to consciously control his bowel and bladder, he also learns that he can get attention by withholding. If a baby competitor seems to have replaced him, he may use this method of regaining attention. His parents must learn patience. Rigidity and shaming are to be avoided. "From a sense of *self-control without loss of self-esteem* comes a lasting sense of autonomy and pride. From a sense of muscular and anal impotence, of loss of self-control, and of parental over-control comes a lasting sense of doubt and shame."[11]

At this stage what happened to Joey? He was toilet-trained rigidly. And the rigidity was rooted in indifference, not love:

> Going to the toilet, like everything else in Joey's life, was surrounded by elaborate preventions. We had to accompany him; he had to take off all his clothes; he could only squat, not sit, on the toilet seat; he had to touch the wall with one hand, in which he also clutched frantically the vacuum tubes that powered his elimination. He was terrified lest his whole body be sucked down.
>
> To counteract this fear we gave him a metal wastebasket in lieu of a toilet. Eventually, when eliminating into the wastebasket, he no longer needed to take off all his clothes, nor to hold on to the wall . . .
>
> It was not simply that his parents had subjected him to rigid, early training. Many children are so trained. But in most cases the parents have a deep emotional investment in the child's performance. The child's response in turn makes training an occasion for interaction between them and for the building of genuine relationships. Joey's parents had no emotional investment in him. His obedience gave them no satisfaction and won him no affection or approval. As a toilet-trained child he saved his mother labor, just as household machines saved her labor. As a machine he was not loved for his performance, nor could he love himself . . . By treating him mechanically his parents made him a machine.[12]

[11] Erik H. Erikson, "Growth and Crises of the Healthy Personality," p. 199.
[12] Bruno Bettelheim, "Joey: A 'Mechanical Boy,'" pp. 122, 124.

the preschooler

During the preschool years, the child, armed with the accumulated security of the first stage and the independent body control of the second, seeks to discover more about himself. Erikson calls this stage *initiative versus guilt.*

> Being firmly convinced that he is a person, the child must now find out *what* kind of person he is going to be. And here he hitches his wagon to nothing less than a star: he wants to be like his parents, who to him appear very powerful and very beautiful, although quite unreasonably dangerous.[13]

It is perhaps in this stage that the crushing tragedy of Joey's indifferent parents became most poignantly apparent. For the child, needing love, can endure impatience and even passing anger. He knows that even anger means caring. But indifference is too much to bear.

The preschooler knows his gender and is curious about sex. He examines himself and, when possible, others. He learns that handling his genitals is pleasurable (Freud's "phallic phase"). A shocked, forbidding parent will convince a child that he is basically dirty, unworthy. A relaxed, accepting parent teaches the child that he is worthy and that his worthiness includes the genitalia. Strongly disapproving parents at this phase create guilt and fear of punishment in the child. And untold numbers of children think of the same punishment—that the genitalia will be (with boys) or have been (with girls) cut off. (Figure 11-5 and its accompanying verse illustrate how a closely related fear is manufactured from a normal human activity. Parents need not be concerned about thumb-sucking until the child is about four. Past that age, teeth may be displaced, and the family dentist should be consulted.)

Expressions of the Oedipus[14] complex (which is associated primarily with the work of Freud) are also likely to appear during this stage. With childhood's devastating logic, the four- or five-year-old boy reaches two irreducible conclusions. First, his genitals cannot compare with his father's. Second, no matter how much he loves his mother, he cannot replace his father in her affections. Frequently, a male child may express a desire to marry his mother. The little girl may endure a similar experience (Electra complex). Mother had been her ideal; she now prefers her father. Only he can put her to bed, dress her, and care for her. The mother is rejected. But the girl still needs her mother, just as the boy still needs his father, no matter how much he wishes to be rid of him. It will not be their last entrapment in emotional ambivalence. Three hundred years ago, the philosopher Spinoza clearly defined emotional ambivalence as a "vacillation of the soul."[15]

Parental maturity and skill in handling these emotions, in preventing the

11-4 *"Feelings are more important than anything under the sun"—Joey's slogan upon entering the human condition (see footnote 17).*

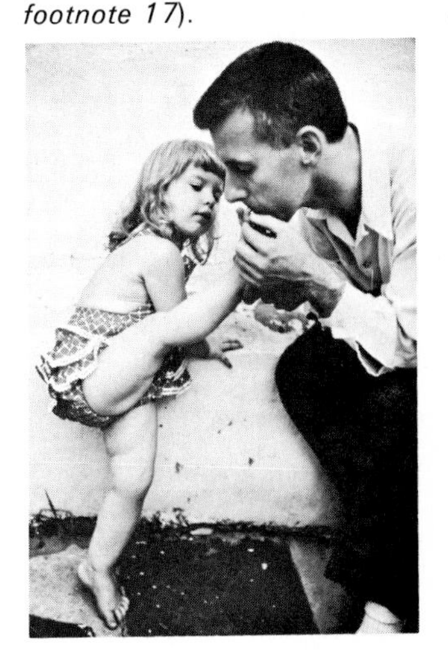

[13] Erik H. Erikson, "Growth and Crises of the Healthy Personality," p. 205.

[14] Oedipus, in the Sophoclean tragedy *Oedipus Rex,* kills his father and marries his mother. Later, on discovering the true relationship, he blinds himself. In females, the Oedipus complex is called the Electra complex. In Greek mythology, Electra is supposed to have urged her brother, Orestes, to kill their mother, Clytemnestra, who had murdered their father, Agamemnon.

[15] Quoted in Franz G. Alexander and Sheldon T. Selesnick, *The History of Psychiatry,* p. 97.

the story of little suck-a-thumb

One day, mamma said: "Conrad dear,
I must go out and leave you here.
But mind now, Conrad, what I say,
Don't suck your thumb while I'm away.
The great tall tailor always comes
To little boys that suck their thumbs;
And ere they dream what he's about,
He takes his great sharp scissors out
And cuts their thumbs clean off—and then,
You know, they never grow again."

Heinrich Hoffman, quoted in Burton Egbert Stevenson, ed., *The Home Book of Verse* (New York, 1922), p. 123.

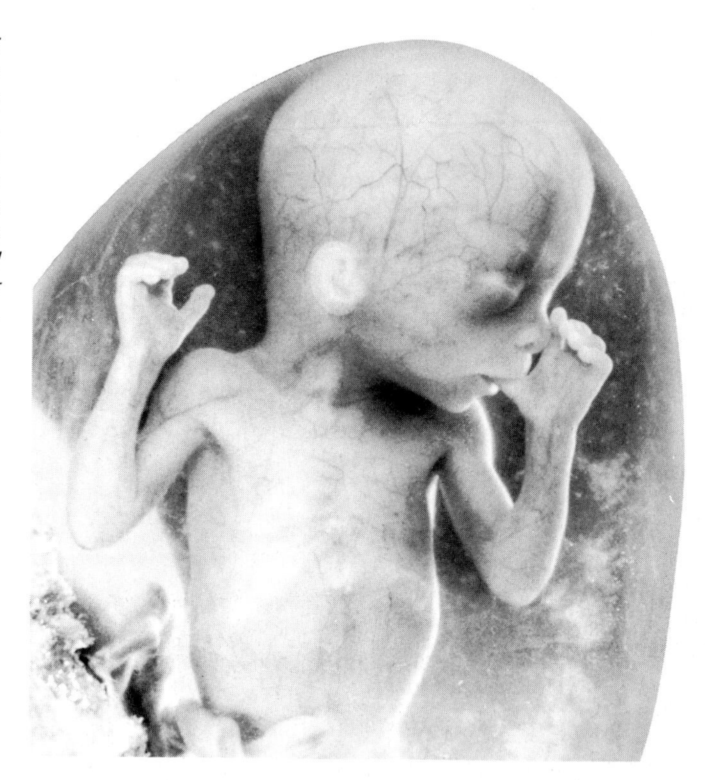

11-5 *During the Nazi era, countless German schoolchildren memorized this poem. But thumb-sucking is quite normal. Within the uterus, the unborn child sucks his thumb; often the newborn will do so moments after birth.*

humiliation of the searching child, will augment the child's sense of a worthy self. Embarrassing the child will interfere with his ability to conquer future crises.

the school-age child

By the time the child enters school he is in what Freud called the "latency period." His sexual interests have abated. This is the fourth stage of Erikson's schema of personality development, *industry versus inferiority.*

"Personality at the first stage crystallizes around the conviction 'I am what I am given,' and that of the second, 'I am what I will.' The third can be characterized by 'I am what I can imagine I will be . . .' The fourth: 'I am what I learn.' "[16]

No other creature has as long a period of dependency as the human, for no other creature has as much to learn before he can become self-sufficient. The child must learn skills, use tools, and do something he considers useful. Returning from school to his parents, he will hold out the result of his labor. "Look," he will say hopefully. If he is met with appreciation, he will attempt to do still better. If parental indifference is his lot, a deep sense of inadequacy and inferiority will overwhelm him. But praise must be merited. Should he receive commendation for an effort he knows is inferior, he will lose respect for the person praising him.[17]

puberty: the teen-ager

"I felt myself isolated, helpless and always shut up in myself: I do not complain of it, for I believe that my early meditations developed and strengthened my thinking powers."[18] So did that celebrated political magician Talleyrand describe his twelfth year. His was a lonely adolescence. Adolescence generally is. Erikson terms this fifth stage *identity versus self-diffusion.*

[16] Erik H. Erikson, "Growth and Crises of the Healthy Personality," p. 211.

[17] Increasingly sick, Joey spent five years in two schools before coming to be treated by Bettelheim. Three months before, he had attempted suicide. It required almost three years of treatment for the boy to accept his humanness. Bettelheim concludes his description of the case of the "mechanical boy" this way: "When Joey was 12, he made a float for our Memorial Day parade. It carried the slogan: 'Feelings are more important than anything under the sun.' Feelings, Joey had learned, are what make for humanity; their absence, for a mechanical existence. With this knowledge Joey entered the human condition." (Bruno Bettelheim, "Joey: A 'Mechanical Boy,'" p. 127.)

[18] From *Memoirs of the Prince of Talleyrand,* quoted in Saul K. Padover, ed., *Confessions and Self-Portraits* (New York, 1957), p. 152.

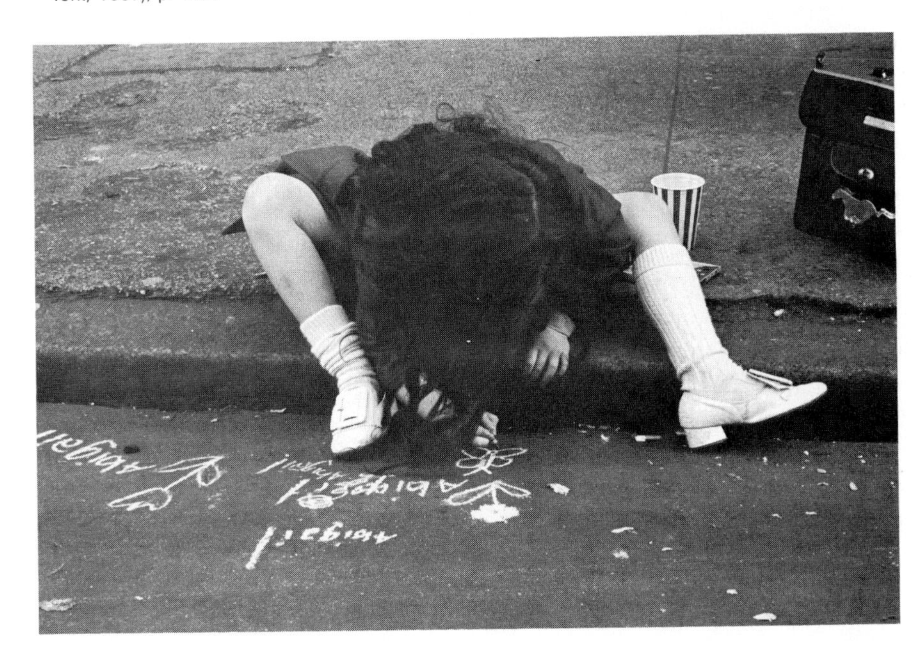

11-6 *"Learning is not child's play" (Aristotle).*

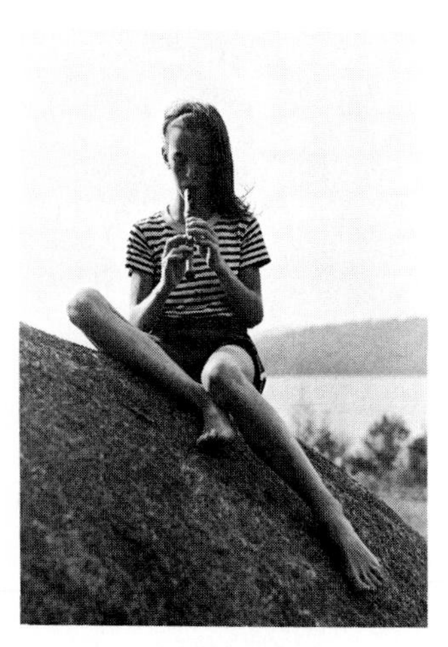

11-7 *Adolescence. "Heard melodies are sweet, but those unheard/Are sweeter"* (*John Keats*).

So many changes happen to the adolescent that he needs to become reacquainted with himself. Powerful new sexual urges send him soaring into confused dream worlds. These frighten him and make him feel vaguely guilty. Added to these disturbances are the "inability to settle on an occupational identity" and "the inexorable standardization of American adolescence."[19] Erikson has further described this stage:

> There is a "natural" period of uprootedness in human life: adolescence. Like a trapeze artist, the young person in the middle of vigorous emotion must let go of his safe hold on childhood and reach out for a firm grasp on adulthood, dependent for a breathless interval on his training, his luck, and the reliability of the "receiving and confirming" adults.[20]

Without reasonably satisfactory resolutions in the previous four stages—without basic trust, for example—adolescence can be a tribulation. Not identity but identity diffusion may result. In this culture this diffusion is common. Temporary identity may be found by some in a gang. With others, self-identity is interminably slow in coming. From his elders, the adolescent hears apprehensive criticism. Parents have been known to say, "Grow up. Stop hanging around the public square and wandering up and down the street. Go to school. Night and day you torture me. Night and day you waste your time having fun."[21] These words are translated from a Sumerian clay tablet four thousand years old. But the confusion of adolescence is no easier to endure today than it ever was before. Emotional illness still may result.

adulthood

> Henceforth I ask not good-fortune, I myself am good-fortune,
> Henceforth I whimper no more, postpone no more, need nothing . . .
> Strong and content I travel the open road.[22]

THE FIRST STAGE Adulthood comprises the next three stages of the Erikson schema of personality development. The first adult stage is *intimacy and distantiation versus self-absorption.* Childhood is over, as is youth. Ostensibly, self-identity is established. Now mature mutual relationships in love, friendship, and work are sought and are possible. The young adult also exhibits what Erikson refers to as "the counterpart of intimacy . . . *distantiation:* the readiness to repudiate, to isolate, and, if necessary, to destroy those forces and people whose essence seems dangerous to one's own." This necessary defensive reaction is not always understood or appreciated by older adults.

THE SECOND STAGE In this stage, *generativity versus stagnation,* the mature person is prepared to share creatively. He understands that taking can be a way

[19] Erik H. Erikson, "Growth and Crises of the Healthy Personality," p. 218.
[20] Erik H. Erikson, "Identity and Uprootedness in Our Time," in H. M. Ruitenbeek, ed., *Varieties of Modern Social Theory* (New York, 1963), pp. 55–68.
[21] From Samuel Noah Kramer, *Everyday Life in Bible Times,* quoted in Jerome Beatty, Jr., "Trade Winds," *Saturday Review* (March 16, 1968), p. 18.
[22] Walt Whitman, "Song of the Open Road," lines 4–7.

of giving, but that there is a difference between taking and exploiting. Generativity includes a mutual desire for parenthood, for creating the next generation. But it is more than mere reproduction. It is the ability to help another person gain those constructive strengths necessary for effective living.

THE THIRD STAGE: TOWARD THE GREAT EXPERIENCE This stage is called *integrity versus despair and disgust.* The first Earl of Balfour (1840–1930) was a gentle man and a gentleman. His had been a good and exciting life in the service of his country. His last words were, "This is going to be a great experience."

An originator and leader, he had met life with courage and verve. The last stages of his life were a continuum of doing. He even died with anticipation. The final stages of his life had given him integrity. His life was a full circle. It excluded despair and disgust.

Thus Erikson unfolds the processes of the development of the human personality. Most people pass through them without too much trouble, gaining the emotional strength to function more effectively. But, at various times during their personality development, some people need help. How much? This may vary from a few quiet conversations with a wise friend to long-term psychotherapy. But help must be available.

Albert Einstein once said that "Every kind of peaceful cooperation among men is primarily based on mutual trust and only secondarily on institutions such as courts of justice and police." Without the basic trust of infancy there cannot be the mutual trust of adulthood.

personality disorders and emotional problems

definitions but not human formulae

The emotionally healthy person is able to meet the stresses of life and to choose appropriate methods of solving problems. He has a realistic sense of his own worth and interacts constructively with others. He is able to find satisfaction in efficiently performing his work. Since he adapts well in his environment, and perceives it with minimal distortion, he functions effectively on the health scale.

Emotionally healthy people behave normally; that is, their behavior is, for the most part, culturally acceptable. Behavior is appraised as normal according to degree and in the context of time and place. For an example of degree, consider two women in this culture. One wears a dress that tastefully shows off her feminine attributes; she is normal. The other sheds all her clothes in the street; her exhibitionism is possibly a sign of illness. Time is another factor in determining normality. The shrieking adolescent girls of seventeenth-century Salem were thought to be possessed by the Devil. Today, comparable behavior at a rock concert draws little attention. Locale is another context for normality. In Java, it is acceptable for two people who are arguing in public to punctuate their epithets with the added insult of shedding their clothes. If this were done on a street in the United States, however, psychiatric investigation might well be suggested. If the concept of normal behavior varies according to degree, time, and place, can normality be defined? Today, many specialists who diagnose and treat emotional problems accept Freud's concept that the ability to work and to love without undue emotional impedimenta is measure enough of normality.

extent of the problem in the United States

During the Second World War, one of every eight U.S. men examined for the draft was rejected because of emotional problems. On any given day, an estimated 2 million people are disabled by emotional illness in this country. From 7 to 12 percent of school-age children and youth need professional help for severe emotional problems. It is estimated that about 10 percent of the population will, at some point in their lives, suffer serious emotional illness necessitating hospitalization.

the limits of labels

It is with reservations that the following limited classification of disorders is introduced. There are many such classifications, and they are convenient for discussing disorders. However, they should not be used to pigeonhole either people or their problems. Indeed, many specialists concerned with emotional health tend to dispense with the labels or classifications altogether, preferring instead to discuss adjustive and maladjustive behavior in broad, uncategorized terms. As Menninger has said:

> We label mental diseases the way little girls label their dolls. And one little girl's *Helen* is not like another little girl's *Helen.* In the same way, Dr. A's "schizophrenia" is different from Dr. B's "schizophrenia." And as long as we think of mental illness as a horrible monster with a name like schizophrenia—we won't be able to prevent it.[23]

"he who can simulate sanity will be sane."
Ovid (43 B.C.–A.D. 18)

Menninger's concept is surely supported by an experiment designed by a Stanford psychiatrist. Eight volunteers (three women and five men), without significant psychiatric histories, presented themselves for admission to psychiatric hospitals. Among the volunteers were three psychologists, a pediatrician, a psychiatrist, a painter, and a housewife. All complained of a single phony symptom: they said they heard hollow voices. In eleven out of twelve tries, the ostensibly emotionally healthy volunteers were admitted with a diagnosis of schizophrenia. They were discharged between one and seven weeks later; the discharge diagnosis: schizophrenia in remission. The twelfth volunteer was both admitted and discharged as having a manic-depressive psychosis.[24] In the hospital, the pseudopatients behaved normally and cooperated fully. The other patients were much more perceptive than the staff. During the first three fake

[23] "A Conversation with Karl Menninger and Mary Harrington Hall on the Psychology of Vengeance," *Psychology Today,* Vol. 2, No. 9 (February 1969), p. 63.

[24] "12 Admissions of Mental Error," *Medical World News,* Vol 14, No. 6 (February 9, 1973), pp. 17–19.

hospitalizations, 35 of a total of 118 patients expressed their suspicions, saying, for example, ''You're not crazy. You're a journalist or professor. You're checking up on the hospital.''[25]

The experiment was then reversed. Staffs at various teaching hospitals were advised of the above results. They were similarly advised that a pseudopatient would soon come seeking admission to their hospitals. Of 193 patients, 41 were alleged to be pseudopatients by at least one staff member. Twenty-three were considered suspect by one psychiatrist, and 19 were thought to be possible pseudopatients by one psychiatrist and one staff member. During all this time, no pseudopatient had presented himself to any of the hospitals.[26]

These experiments raise questions about the definition of schizophrenia, the acumen of some of those who diagnose it, the lack of reassessment of patients in an institutional milieu, the shortages of personnel properly equipped to handle the condition, and the conditioning of those who make diagnoses of individuals in the context in which they are seen.

A Classification of Personality Disorders

A. *Psychotic disorders*
   1. *Organic causes:* Characterized by lesions[27] in the brain.
   2. *Functional:* There is no demonstrable lesion in the brain.
      a. Schizophrenia
      b. Manic-depressive psychoses
      c. Paranoia

B. *Neurotic disorders*
   1. *Psychoneuroses* (neuroses)
      a. Anxiety states
      b. Phobias
      c. Obsessive-compulsive reactions
      d. Hysterias
      e. Traumatic neuroses
   2. *Psychosomatic disorders:* Peptic ulcer and asthma, for example, may be exacerbated by psychosomatic influences.

C. *Character disorders:* Examples include drug dependence, alcoholism, criminal behavior, and the psychopathic personality. Some psychologists include sexual divergences, such as homosexual behavior, in this group. Many psychologists disagree. (In December 1973, the Board of Trustees of the American Psychiatric Association announced its unanimous decision no longer to consider homosexual behavior per se a disease.)

Psychotic behavior disorders are more severe than neurotic disorders. The individual displaying psychotic behavior has lost much contact with reality. However, the psychoneurotic person is still able to view his emotional problems with some degree of objectivity and he attempts to cope with them. Social

[25] ''Being Sane in Unsane Places,'' *Science News,* Vol. 103, No. 3 (January 20, 1973), p. 38.
[26] *Science,* Vol. 179 (January 19, 1973), pp. 250–58.
[27] A lesion is any abnormal or harmful change in the structure of a tissue.

deviance, rather than emotional symptoms, is the main characteristic of a person with a character disorder. For this reason, character disorders are categorized separately.

notes on the various disorders

the psychotic disorders

ORGANIC LESIONS Brain tumors, severe head injuries, and infections such as far-advanced untreated syphilis not uncommonly result in psychoses. The psychotic behavior of *senile dementia* is seen more frequently as greater numbers of people live to be very old. This form of psychosis is due to deterioration of aged brain cells; arterial arteriosclerosis (page 270) resulting in prolonged lessening of blood-carrying oxygen to the brain may be partly causative.

FUNCTIONAL DISORDERS Psychotic behavior is not so easily recognizable as is generally thought. Some people are obviously deranged. Among these are people suffering from the extreme forms of *mania* and the more dramatic types of *schizophrenia.* However, many people whose behavior is occasionally psychotic ordinarily appear quite normal. Suddenly, without warning or cause, they may go berserk. And just as suddenly, they may return for a time to normal behavior. People suffering manic-depressive states, for example, usually experience a temporary period of lucidity between a ''high'' jubilant mood and a ''low'' dejected mood. In this last instance, it is as if the sick individual's moods swing like a pendulum from one extreme to the other, with lucid intervals.

In the United States, schizophrenia[28] (Greek *schizein,* to divide + *phren,* mind) is the most common of all the psychoses, accounting for about 25 to 30 percent of all first admissions to the nation's hospitals for the emotionally ill. Today, about half the beds in those hospitals are occupied by schizophrenic patients. It has been estimated that 2 percent of the U.S. population will have an episode of schizophrenia at some time in their lives. In disadvantaged areas, such as urban slums, the prediction rises to 6 percent. But it is not poverty as such that is the direct cause of the disorder. Poor nutrition, inadequate medical care, the stress of growing up in a disordered family—these can combine to contribute to schizophrenia.

A great deal of recent research has focused on schizophrenia. The electrical brain waves of the schizophrenic may differ from those of nonschizophrenic people. Some investigators consider schizophrenia related to an imbalance of body chemistry and function. Proof of this is as yet lacking. Some studies suggest a genetic aspect to schizophrenia, pointing to a tendency of the condition to occur in families. However, the relative importance of the influence of environment on the incidence of schizophrenia needs study. ''The importance of genetic factors . . . has . . . been established . . . although . . . environment too plays its etiologic role.''[29]

[28] Highly recommended as a source of information on this subject is Department of Health, Education, and Welfare Publication No. (HSM)73-9086, reprinted in 1973, called: ''Schizophrenia, Is There an Answer?'' It can be obtained from the Superintendent of Documents, U.S. Government Printing Office, Washington, D.C. 20402.

[29] Leonard L. Heston, ''The Genetics of Schizophrenic and Schizoid Disease,'' *Science,* Vol. 167, No. 3916 (January 16, 1970), p. 255.

Because of their predominance in the sixteen to thirty age group, schizophrenias have been called the "psychoses of youth." The very young (six to seven years), the middle-aged, and the elderly are not, however, exempt.

People diagnosed as schizophrenic do not usually (as is popularly supposed) split totally from reality into a world of their own. Nor do they generally have sudden character changes of the Dr. Jekyll and Mr. Hyde variety. Unless the person whose behavior is schizophrenic is in a totally disorganized state, he does have some sense of common reality. What is happening to such an individual is that certain aspects of his world, some of his experiences, have no basis in reality. Schizophrenia is a good example of the limitation of labels mentioned earlier in this section. It is not a single disease, with a determined set of symptoms, a known cause, and a single treatment. Indeed, two people diagnosed as schizophrenic may demonstrate entirely different symptoms. Nor does any known single pattern of interaction between an individual and his environment inevitably lead to schizophrenic behavior. People react to different stresses individually. The time in a person's life at which the stress occurs may be as important as the nature of the stress. An emotional experience with which one individual could cope at six years of age might be overwhelming to him at three.

A wide variety of symptom combinations are observed in schizophrenia. Such an individual may suffer from *unusual perceptions of reality. Illusions* may thus torment the schizophrenic person; he falsely interprets a real sensory image: a gentle smile may seem to alter into a threatening scowl. *Hallucinations* may also fill his world. They may be visual, tactile, auditory, or all three. One woman told of evening visits by her long-dead father, who patted her shoulder as he advised her about her marriage plans. Another woman accused her dentist of installing a tiny transmitter in the cavity of a molar. By means of this she received constant threatening coded messages, not only from foreign powers but also from other planets. Perhaps the most pathetic characteristic of many people whose behavior is schizophrenic is their deep sense of utter loneliness. Confused by misperceptions, bedeviled by hallucinations and illusions, the schizophrenic is alone in a sea of fear, and it is this very loneliness that compounds his inner terror. At times, he may remain motionless for hours, totally withdrawn (see Figure 11-8). Paying no attention whatsoever to his environment, he tries to block out his overwhelming fear. It may even be necessary to feed and dress him. Another person, similarly afflicted (or the same one at a different time), moves about constantly, incoherent, wide-awake, watchful, sometimes giggling or babbling senselessly.

11-8 *Assuming the position of a fetus, this catatonic patient has retreated into the womb. Now it is a lonely shelter.*

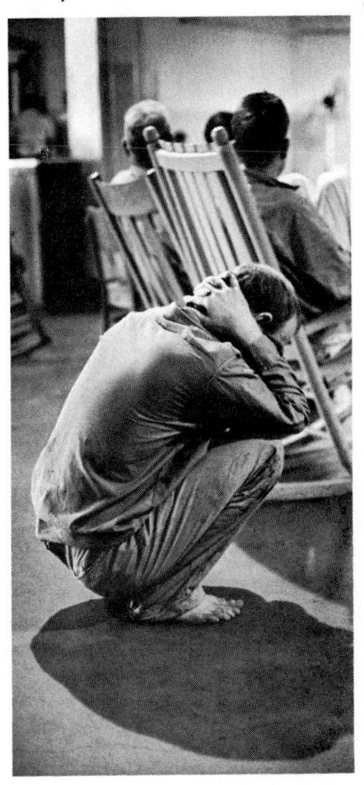

When, in his essay on *Solitude* (in *Walden*) Thoreau asked, "Why should I feel lonely? is not our planet in the Milky Way?" he was writing of an inner peace based on his firm sense of serene reality. But centuries ago, Ecclesiastes (4:10), writing of other matters, described the despair of the schizophrenic: "Woe to him that is alone when he falleth; for he hath not another to help him up."

To communicate to the schizophrenic that there are others to help him up is the basic job of the therapist. Tranquilizing drugs are important because they calm the patient. His behavior becomes socially acceptable. This has a therapeutic effect on the relationship between the patient and the professional staff. Now they can communicate. These beginning social contacts can eventually be enlarged to include family, friends, and the whole community. Sometimes, psychotherapy is helpful; by sharing his experiences with a trained person, the schizophrenic may gradually sort out the real from the unreal. He will not be plunged deeper into fear and isolation. Group therapy is frequently useful. Occasionally, electroshock therapy can be helpful, especially if severe depression is part of the picture. Although a nourishing diet is important, the value of massive doses of vitamins is doubtful. (Such megavitamin therapy has been guaranteed by some ''experts'' as a ''sure cure'' for drug abuse.) From some therapists have come glowing reports that enormous doses of various vitamins, supplemented by other drugs, psychotherapy, sometimes electroshock treatments, hormone injections, special diets—''tailored'' to individual patients—have resulted in remarkable success in the treatment of various emotional disorders.[30] Schizophrenia, severe depressions, drug dependencies, senility, and various emotional disturbances in children have all reported to have been benefited by an individual combination of such treatments. Such claims have not met the tests of scientific appraisal.

That vitamin lack is related to emotional illness is indisputable. For example, patients with pellagra, due to a shortage of the vitamin niacin (see page 654), display psychotic behavior. But then, many people without pellagra display psychotic behavior. Thus, it is difficult to prove that niacin, for instance, can be a cure for a wide variety of psychotic behaviors. It becomes impossible when each individual patient is also provided with a wide range of other therapeutic procedures. Added to these difficulties are questions about the validity of the diagnoses. Both the National Institute of Mental Health and the American Psychiatric Association point to the lack of confirmation of the value of megavitamin therapy, stating that the bulk of research evidence indicates that it adds nothing to usual psychiatric treatments.[31]

It is considered unwise to hospitalize a schizophrenic patient for prolonged periods in a large, distant, impersonal institution. This merely isolates him further. Family therapy, involving the patient, his parents or spouse, and a therapist, is gaining increasing favor.[32] The family can learn much about helping a patient. An interesting California experiment is the Camarillo State Hospital program, in which schizophrenic children aged six to fifteen are placed in the homes of couples who are specially trained to respond to the child's destructive behavior in such a way as to help with the rebuilding of his personality. Early

[30] ''Back to Reality the Megavitamin Way,'' *Medical World News,* Vol. 12, No. 35 (September 24, 1971), pp. 15–18.

[31] Robert J. Trotter, ''Will Vitamins Replace the Psychiatrist's Couch?'' Vol. 104, No. 4 (July 28, 1973), pp. 59–60.

[32] Some recent limited research suggests that the families of patients with schizophrenic behavior seem to have a greater resistance to some viral infections (such as influenza and measles) and a higher rate of fertility than the families of people whose behavior is not schizophrenic. (''Latent Schizophrenics Have a Biological Advantage,'' *New Scientist and Science Journal,* Vol. 51, No. 762 [July 29, 1971], p. 242, citing Michael Carter and C. A. H. Watts, *British Journal of Psychiatry,* Vol. 118 [1971], p. 453.)

results are encouraging.[33] Once recovered, the former patient need not try to forget his schizophrenic experiences. He can learn to accept them as part of his growth, of his humanness.

Next to schizophrenia, the *manic-depressive psychoses* are the most common psychoses (afflicting 10 to 15 percent of psychotics). There is, of course, an enormous difference between the occasional "blue mood" to which all normal people are susceptible and this condition. Its onset usually occurs between the ages of thirty and fifty, and women are more commonly afflicted than men. Classically, the manic-depressive reaction is seen as an elation (*manic phase*) or a deep despondency (*depressive phase*). An attack may consist of elation alone or of depression alone, or of alternating elation and depression. A *manic reaction* may be set off by a chance remark or even a mild witticism. There then follows an excessive response with a tendency to irrationality. The *depressive reaction* is marked by retardation of both thought and activity. The patient maintains an air of general hopelessness. Except in exceedingly severe cases, the manic-depressive suffers no lasting intellectual impairment. Even without treatment, recovery is common. The manic phase ordinarily lasts about three months; the depressive phase lasts about three times as long. There is a tendency for the symptoms to recur; about three-fourths of these patients have one or more recurrences. Today, the classic picture is rare because of the use of drugs.

"The black dog" was Winston Churchill's description of the depression that hounded him throughout his long life. Abraham Lincoln's deep depressions, accentuated by dreams in which he viewed his own coffin, added much to the despair of his marital life (although some suggest that Mary Todd Lincoln was the cause). The most famous recent case of an apparently successfully treated depression was that of Senator Thomas Eagleton. But depression is not limited to the celebrated. Every year in this country, about 8 million people visit their physicians because of depression; about 250,000 require hospitalization for its treatment.[34] A sense of loss is considered to be one of the major precipitants of depression. This is particularly true of an adult who had also lost a parent during childhood or adolescence. Depressions of various degrees can be induced by real or imagined loss of love, public image, career, the security of a familiar job (which explains why job promotion is often accompanied by depression), and a host of other happenings. There is some evidence that certain depressions involve disorders of brain chemistry. Some drugs, for example, have an effect on the chemicals that help carry nerve impulses from one brain cell to another. Some of these chemicals (called *neurotransmitters*) are thought to be involved in depressions, and certain drugs prevent their breakdown. The chemistry of brain function is a whole new field of research in all areas of emotional distress. The social isolation that leads to anxiety, depression, and even psychotic behavior is being investigated biochemically. It is believed that brain

[33] "Foster Parents Trained for Psychotics," *Journal of the American Medical Association,* Vol. 219, No. 11 (March 13, 1972), p. 1411.

[34] An excellent article about this subject has been prepared by psychiatrists David Elkind and J. Herbert Hamsher, "The Anatomy of Melancholy," *Saturday Review of Science,* Vol. 55, No. 40 (October 1972), pp. 54–59.

chemistry may be altered, and this, in turn, may alter responses to various drugs. Thus, there may be a "brain chemistry" involved in extremes of loneliness.[35]

Most mild depressions require no treatment. Severe depressions may require drug therapy or *electroconvulsive* (*ECT*) *therapy*—also known as *electroshock* (*EST*) or *electrocoma* (*ECT*). ECT is quite harmless. Through electrodes held at the temples by a headband, a charge of 100 volts (sometimes 150 to 170) is delivered deep into the brain of the previously anesthetized patient. Within half an hour the patient awakes, somewhat groggy. There is some temporary confusion and forgetfulness; this usually occurs more often after several treatments. Insofar as is known, there are no lasting harmful after effects, unless the patient has had a great number of treatments—perhaps fifty or more. Nobody knows why ECT works. Drugs are also used in the treatment of depression, but their effect is slower than that of ECT; this is singularly important with suicidal patients. Drug therapy of depression needs more research. Psychotherapy to discover the emotional roots of the disorder, and then to learn to handle them adequately, is also a valid treatment. Treatment may involve a combination of procedures.

Paranoia may be manifested by delusions of grandeur or persecution. A paranoid patient might believe himself to be Christ or Mohammed. Persecutions that such individuals feel are generally accompanied by a tendency to seek ulterior motives in the behavior of others. Such was the case of a woman who received the annual prize in law school as the student who had shown the greatest scholastic improvement. Upon graduation, she sued the school for damages. She alleged that the real motive of the faculty, in giving her the prize, was to show the world that in her work was the greatest room for improvement. In this way the faculty was demonstrating that she was not as fit as her associates to be a lawyer.[36]

the neurotic disorders

Every normal individual has his share of neurotic symptoms. These symptoms, resulting from the ordinary stresses and inner conflicts that he has been able to handle, do not interfere with his effective functioning in society. Thus, a person who has neurotic symptoms does not necessarily have a neurotic *disorder,* or *neurosis.* Whether a neurotic disorder actually exists depends on the degree of involvement of the personality. Neurotic symptoms, arising from an unresolved inner conflict of needs, may take command of the personality for a prolonged time. Effective functioning becomes difficult, even impossible. It is then that a neurotic disorder exists and professional help is indicated. (Those who wonder whether their symptoms are severe enough to merit help should seek such help, if only to remove their doubt.) Unlike most people with psychotic behavior, neurotic individuals do not lose contact with the reality of their

[35] Robert J. Trotter, "The Biological Depths of Loneliness," *Science News,* Vol. 103, No. 9 (March 3, 1973), pp. 140–41.

[36] Arthur P. Noyes and Lawrence C. Kolb, *Modern Clinical Psychiatry,* 6th ed. (Philadelphia, 1963), p. 370.

environment. Although limited, sometimes severely, the neurotic person is generally able to carry on his usual functions.

PSYCHONEUROSES Here, briefly described, are the major psychoneuroses.

Anxiety states are one of the most common of psychoneuroses. Everyone shows symptoms of anxiety sometimes, but the neurotic's anxiety is chronic and severe, and he is helpless in handling it. His tension is constant; he feels under severe stress almost all the time. Unbearably acute attacks of anxiety, such as an overwhelming sense of approaching doom, may punctuate his chronic condition. He may suffer a variety of disagreeable physical symptoms such as excessive sweating and heart palpitations. Anxiety states are the most common form of neurosis in young people. Anxiety is so basic to the human experience and so common an emotional problem that it is the subject of the whole of the next chapter.

A *phobia* is a persistent fear of an object or situation that is not really dangerous or that has been blown out of all proportion to the actual danger. Examples are *agoraphobia,* a fear of open spaces; *claustrophobia,* a fear of enclosed places; *acrophobia,* a fear of high places; and *pavor nocturnus,* a fear of the dark, a phobia common to children and some adults.

Obsessive-compulsive reactions are manifested in people who are compelled to think about something that they do not want to think about (obsessive thoughts) or who are compelled to do some act that they do not want to do (compulsive acts). Among the most common compulsive reactions is compulsive hand-washing. For example, an individual who has masturbated may respond to his action with abnormal disgust or a sense of uncleanliness. His excessive thoughts about cleanliness may become obsessive, and he may compulsively wash his hands repeatedly. Such individuals are aware of the absurdity of their thought processes or actions but seem helpless to control them.

There are two types of *hysteria. Conversion hysterias* exhibit the same symptoms as many diseases. They are characterized by body symptoms such as paralysis of the legs, tics, or loss of sensitivity to pain. In *dissociative states,* there is a virtual temporary takeover of the individual to the extent that he no longer dictates his own behavior. An example of this is the *multiple personality.* In this instance, two or more different personalities are found in the same person. *Amnesia,* which is "sleepwalking while awake," is another type of dissociative state. This is a hysterical *fugue,* or flight, in which the individual escapes an intolerable situation by totally disassociating himself from it. Thus, he may suddenly appear far from home one day, able neither to identify himself nor to be identified. He may begin an entirely new life. Amnesia of his past is complete. Upon recovering, he will remember absolutely nothing of his fugue.

Traumatic neuroses occur as a result of the distress of extreme stress. A severe automobile crash may, for example, precipitate a severe neurosis. By no means does stress always result in a traumatic neurosis. Some feel that constant activity was responsible for the low incidence of reported neuroses among Eng-

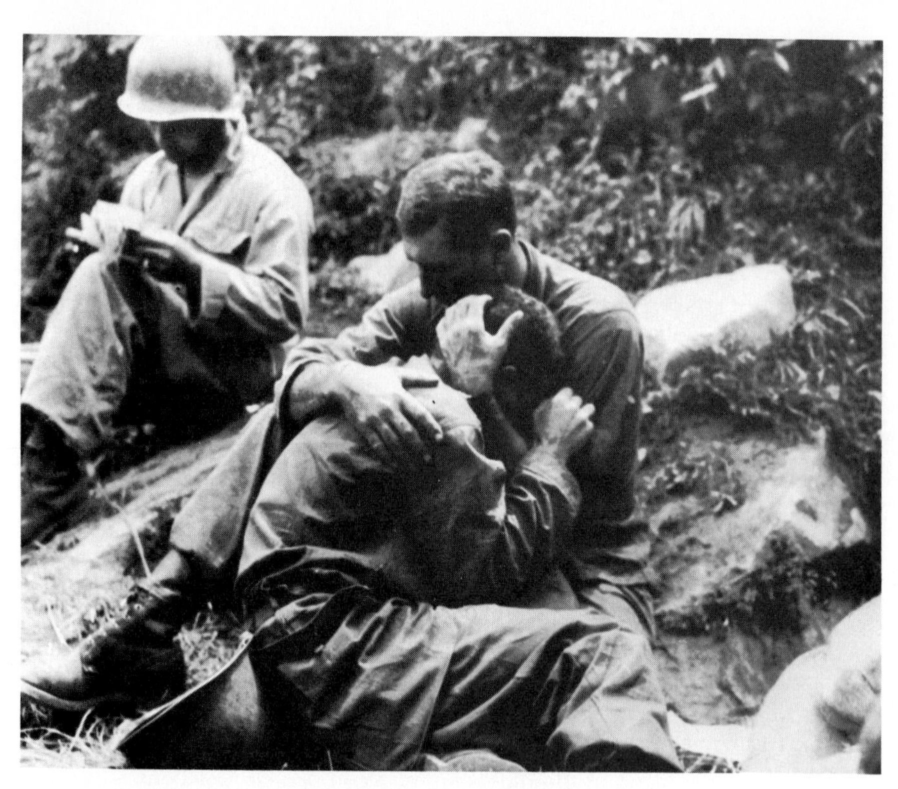

11-9 *Combat stress in Korea. "O brother man! fold to thy heart thy brother" (John Greenleaf Whittier).*

lish, German, and Japanese civilians exposed to bombings during the Second World War. They were too busy to have emotional problems.

Those who study war neuroses usually distinguish between *combat exhaustion* and *combat neuroses.* The neurotic combatant is frequently described as a jumpy, chain-smoking, trembling man. The soldier suffering from combat exhaustion may fall asleep in the middle of a roaring battle. Some soldiers may be more likely to develop chronic war neuroses than others. A soldier who has been raised in a rigid environment, for example, is more inclined to suffer from combat neuroses. The most common feature of the combat neuroses of soldiers of U.S. armies during the Second World War was a deep sense of guilt. (This was not true of soldiers of the First World War.) During the Second World War, these sick men accused themselves of having failed their wounded or dead buddies.

Those with traumatic neuroses may be grievously misjudged. A case in point is the authentic Second World War story of two heroic pilots. After a long history of bravery in the Pacific, both were transferred to England. One would walk to his plane but, once there, was unable to board it. His feet turned him around. He would curse himself, swearing to fly on the morrow. But always, just before boarding, his feet would turn him around. His buddy, on the other hand, boarded his plane easily. But as soon as he passed the English side of the Channel, he would begin to vomit. Since he had to wear an oxygen mask, he was medically disabled. "The man who could not control his feet was defrocked, demoted, dewinged, and sent to Iceland. The man who could not control his stomach was considered a hero whose stomach just could not take it."[37]

The incidence of psychiatric casualties—12 per 1,000—among U.S. soldiers serving in Vietnam was lower than in previous wars. In Korea that incidence was 37 per 1,000; in the Second World War, 101 per 1,000.[38] However, this is only part of the picture. "The single most important factor influencing psychiatric attrition in Vietnam [was] the one year tour."[39] Knowing just when one's personal risk would end was a potent safeguard against collapsing emotionally under the stress of combat. However, this rapid rotation prevented continuity of relationships with those with whom one shared the risks. And, upon the veteran's return, there were no cheering crowds. Many remained emotionally in Vietnam, experiencing "reentry shock" lasting for weeks or months. So unpopular was the war that many returning servicemen felt they had betrayed their own generation. So withdrawn were so many from civilian life that the Vietnam veteran was often called "the invisible veteran." It is of interest that the U.S. soldiers in Vietnam were the youngest and the best educated group of servicemen.[40] These factors, plus rigid Selective Service procedures, doubtless added to their ability to cope.

PSYCHOSOMATIC DISORDERS When the seventeenth-century Englishman John Donne observed that "the body makes the minde," he was not reversing the ancient Roman Ovid. "Diseases of the mind impair the powers of the body," wrote the latter. Both poets understood that reciprocal negotiations between mind and body profoundly affect health. "As white as a sheet" or "hot under the collar" takes due note of the skin as a mirror of man's emotions. Whether he blushes or has gooseflesh, his anxiety is being expressed in a physical way. Why? Because the temporary release of tension via a physical reaction is easier to bear than containing the tension.

The term "psychosomatic" originates from the Greek *psyche,* mind, and *soma,* body. Psychosomatic disorders originate in the mind and are manifested in bodily symptoms. Emotional stimuli are referred by the brain to body organs, resulting in effects ranging from gooseflesh to migraine headaches. Though these symptoms have no actual physical cause, they are nevertheless very real. For example, no condition is seen more frequently by the physician than tension headache. It is caused by sustained muscle contraction about the head and neck. In enduring stress such as cramming for an examination or driving in heavy traffic, the neck muscles contract in positions of maximum alertness. In several patients a physician was able to produce another type of headache, migraine, by discussing with them some of their guilt-producing life situations.

[37] Douglas D. Bond, "Management of the Mentally Disabled," in Oliver Schroeder, ed., *The Mind* (Cincinnati, 1962), p. 280.

[38] Marc J. Musser and Charles A. Stenger, "A Medical and Social Perception of the Vietnam Veteran," *Bulletin of the New York Academy of Medicine,* Vol. 48, No. 6 (July 1972), p. 863, citing P. G. Bourne, *Men, Stress and Vietnam* (Boston, 1970).

[39] Peter G. Bourne, "The Viet Nam Veteran," in *The Vietnam Veteran in Contemporary Society;* Department of Medicine and Surgery, Veterans Administration, Washington, D.C. (May 1972), p. iv-83. (The Veterans Administration publication is available for $2.75 from the Superintendent of Documents, U.S. Government Printing Office, Washington, D.C., 20402. It is highly recommended.)

[40] Marc J. Musser and Charles A. Stenger, "A Medical and Social Perception of the Vietnam Veteran," p. 861.

Helping these patients understand the reasons for their reactions reduced the number and severity of their headaches.[41] *Asthma* can be precipitated by some substances, such as dust or feathers, to which the individual is sensitive (allergic). But emotional tension may also start an attack. Or both an allergic reaction and emotional tension may be involved and overlap to affect the respiratory system in this manner. The eye is also often involved in anxiety reactions. A case related by Menninger concerns a twenty-four-year-old woman with prolonged disabling eye problems. These had started shortly after the death of her brother in the war. Jealous of him, she had wished him dead. Also, to see if he was really different from her, she had once peeped at him. "The guilt, therefore, was associated not only with the envy of the brother but with the peeping."[42] In such cases psychotherapy can be remarkably helpful.

The effects of the emotions on the body's organs are both numerous and common, and patients with psychosomatic illnesses fill doctors' offices.

character disorders

The identification of a person as someone who has a character disorder is not a moral judgment. This is a scientific term used to classify some emotionally sick people. The variation in degree of these problems is considerable. One individual may merely be a neurotic nuisance. Another constantly breaks the law. In this latter group are the *psychopathic personalities.* These individuals are utterly irresponsible. Their sickness is in their lack of conscience. Psychopaths know the difference between right and wrong. However, they are psychologically unable to care about the difference. Preoccupied with the immediate gratification of their own needs, they are oblivious to the needs of others. They lack a sense of guilt and suffer little or no anxiety. Not necessarily lacking intelligence, they are frequently charming. But they feel no love for anyone. Friends, family, minister, and psychiatrist are unable to reach them. Their disorder may result from the lack of an affectionate relationship with an adult during childhood. The antisocial psychopath may reveal bitterness over this deprivation of love.

A habitual criminal of a generation ago, Johnny Rocco, was not a foundling, but, perhaps worse, he felt like one. These lines from the Anglo-Saxon folk epic poem *Beowulf* can aptly be applied to him:

> From a friendless foundling, feeble and wretched,
> He grew to a terror as time brought change.

He suffered his way into crime because of a hostile mother. About his mother's reaction to his brother Davie's death he wrote, "When Davie died, she said she wished it was me instead." He added, pitifully, "Money I stole I would never

[41] R. M. Marcussen and H. G. Wolff, "A Formulation of the Dynamics of the Migraine Attack," cited in *Harold G. Wolff's Stress and Disease,* rev. and ed. by Stewart Wolf and Helen Goodell, 2nd ed. (Springfield, Ill., 1968), p. 47.

[42] Karl Menninger, *Man Against Himself* (New York, 1938), p. 368.

give to my mother.''[43] As a boy, he would only give her money he honestly earned selling the magazine *True Confessions.*

homosexual behavior: character disorder, or just a minority's sexual expression?

In discussing male homosexual behavior, Kinsey and his coworkers wrote: ''Males do not represent two discrete populations, heterosexual and homosexual. The world is not to be divided into sheep and goats . . . nature rarely deals with discrete categories. Only the human mind invents categories and tries to force facts into separated pigeon-holes.''[44] Homosexual behavior is not an all-or-none condition, and in evaluating it considerations of time, place, and degree are especially important. In some of the summary graphs of the Kinsey report the term *heterosexual* is used to denote individuals who had experienced few or no episodes of homosexual behavior throughout their lives. By the Kinsey criterion, however, anyone who has had even one childhood experience of homosexual behavior may be termed a homosexual.[45] However, fantasies, dreams, and the transient homosexual behavior of adolescents can hardly be a basis on which to label people homosexuals. Nor are infrequent, isolated, or situational episodes of homosexual behavior indicative of a true homosexual orientation. The Kinsey data fail to distinguish between homosexual behavior that is a preferential or generally exclusive pattern, in which the individual actively seeks sexual gratification with a member of the same sex, and the vast number of relatively insignificant episodes of homosexual behavior that occur among a large proportion of the population. Such labeling of human behavior can be both misleading and harmful. And it should be reiterated that a number of students of the subject consider homosexual behavior to be divergent behavior—different, rather than deviant.

misconceptions about homosexual behavior

Heredity has not been proved to be directly related to homosexual behavior. Furthermore, it is a mistake to associate body type or mannerisms or occupation with homosexual behavior. A brawny football player may actively and exclusively prefer a homosexual behavior pattern; a graceful male ballet dancer may prefer a heterosexual pattern. Only a small percentage of people whose behavior is homosexual (fewer than one in twenty men and probably the same number of women) can be identified by such attributes as mannerisms or dress.[46]

the extent of homosexual behavior

How many people in this country participate in homosexual behavior? Surely, many millions. Kinsey estimated about 4 percent of the adult white male population in the United States to be exclusively homosexual after the onset of ado-

[43] From Jean Evans, *Three Men,* quoted in Edward A. Strecker and Vincent T. Lathbury, *Their Mothers' Daughters* (Philadelphia, 1956), pp. 179–80.
[44] Alfred C. Kinsey, Wardell B. Pomeroy, and Clyde E. Martin, *Sexual Behavior in the Human Male* (Philadelphia, 1948), p. 369.
[45] *Ibid.,* pp. 474, 658.
[46] Warren A. Ketterer, ''Homosexuality and Venereal Disease,'' *Medical Aspects of Human Sexuality,* Vol. 5, No. 3 (March 1971), p. 119.

lescence. Thirty-seven percent were estimated to have had at least some overt homosexual experience to the point of orgasm between adolescence and old age.[47] However, this last figure must be considered in a new light. The present director of the Institute for Sex Research, founded by Kinsey, recently revealed that this estimate may now be considered high. Since he had ready access to prisoners, Kinsey used them for many of his interviews. He thought that their experience was typical of lower socioeconomic groups. Such is not the case.[48] Indeed, recent revelations of rape of new prisoners by long-term prisoners have shocked the nation.

Available information on the incidence of homosexual behavior among females is, at best, open to question. Female homosexual behavior seems to be treated with studied indifference. Unlike the male, who is often hounded by the police, the female whose behavior is homosexual is rarely arrested. In this culture, deep emotional involvements between women are more acceptable than those between men. Kinsey's data revealed that female homosexual responses had occurred in about one-half as many females as males. Homosexual contacts to orgasm had occurred in about one-third as many females as males. At any age period, about one-half to one-third as many females as males were primarily or exclusively homosexual.[49] Some researchers suggest that the number of females participating in homosexual behavior may approximate the number of males. In addition, there is some reason to believe that more women than men are inclined to engage in both homosexual and heterosexual relationships during the same period.

the roots of homosexual behavior

VARYING INFLUENCES AT VARYING TIMES Basically, human sexuality depends on three factors—*genetic, endocrine,* and *psychological.* All are involved in human sexuality, but the degree of their influence on human development varies at different stages of growth. Genetic combinations are established as a result of fertilization and subsequent cellular division. The cells contain the fundamental arrangement of chemical materials (DNA) necessary for the development of genital, nervous, and muscular structural patterns. Endocrine tissue has an early influence on the direction that the developing embryo will take. The critical role of endocrine hormones in determining nervous and genital system structure is discussed on pages 254–59. But this intrauterine activity is not the only instance in which these glands assume primary importance. Puberty is marked by a second surge of endocrine activity. Androgens in the male and estrogen in the female, along with other hormones, stimulate further growth and development of the sexual organs. Hormones also increase the sensitivity of the sexual structures to stimulation. Still other hormones, such as those from the thyroid gland that affect vitality and strength, have an indirect influence on sexual development.

[47] Alfred C. Kinsey *et al., Sexual Behavior in the Human Male,* pp. 650–51.
[48] "In the News," *Medical Aspects of Human Sexuality,* Vol. 3, No. 7 (July 1969), p. 104.
[49] Alfred C. Kinsey, Wardell B. Pomeroy, Clyde E. Martin, and Paul H. Gebhard, *Sexual Behavior in the Human Female* (Philadelphia, 1953), p. 475.

But neither the genes nor the hormones completely determine the human choice of the sex object. It is culture that most profoundly influences heterosexual behavior. The instruction may be as subtle as a boy's haircut or as blunt as a child with short hair jeering at a smaller boy's shoulder-length curls. So, starting at birth, environmental influences begin to supersede and augment the now visible genetic-endocrine influences on the child. Not until puberty do the endocrine glands temporarily take over again and partly supersede the psychological influence of the environment. In the late teens or early twenties, when endocrine maturity is complete, the psychological factors engendered by the environment again become paramount. To summarize: Within the uterus, the genetic and endocrine factors are decisive. In early childhood, the environment molds most of the sexual response. During adolescence, the endocrine glands again assume primary importance. By the late teens or early twenties, psychological influences again become supreme. Although different influences are dominant at different times, they all operate to a certain extent all of the time. The seesaw effect resulting from the varying influences of genetic, endocrine, and psychological factors at different stages of human development, can hardly be expected to guarantee one single form of sexual behavior. Considering the complexity of these relationships, it is not surprising that there is so much homosexual behavior. It is surprising that there is so little.

PREADOLESCENT SEXUAL BEHAVIOR Before the onset of puberty, when surges of hormonal activity intensify the sexual drive, there is much curiosity and, indeed, sexual play among both boys and girls. Occasionally small groups of children, usually of the same sex, participate in prepubescent sexual play. Unless they are treated with senseless harshness by adults, they experience no particular anxiety as a result of this passing behavior.

EARLY ADOLESCENT NEEDS The increased sexual drive that occurs at puberty can be an overwhelming experience. The anxious young person is usually quite unsure of his relationship to the opposite sex. Understandably, he or she may retreat to more familiar ground—to members of the same sex. Most young people pass through a period of intense interest in the same sex before proceeding to a heterosexual adjustment. They share tremendous secrets and derive needed comfort in the knowledge that they all have problems. The variety of sexual expression during this ordinarily transient period may be considerable. "At this age homosexual behavior should be viewed as a temporary defense against the fear associated with the move towards full heterosexual relationships."[50]

POSSIBLE PARENTAL FACTORS One recent study of New York adolescent girls whose behavior pattern was homosexual identified a disruptive and unstable family background (and not only an unresolved Electra complex; see page 289) as a major contributing factor in their homosexual behavior.[51] A

[50] Group for the Advancement of Psychiatry, Committee on Adolescence, *Normal Adolescence* (New York, 1968), p. 77, cited in Warren J. Gadpaille, "Homosexual Experience in Adolescence," *Medical Aspects of Human Sexuality,* Vol. 2, No. 10 (October 1968), p. 33.

[51] "Research with Adolescents Sheds New Light on Early Lesbianism," *Science News,* Vol. 96, No. 3 (July 19, 1969), p. 45.

British study supports this view: "Children reared in families which are incomplete, disturbed by distortions in personal relationships, or whose sexual attitudes are markedly clouded by repression or ignorance appear to be particularly vulnerable . . . It is particularly important to stress that these homosexual feelings do not inevitably imply homosexuality."[52]

It should be emphasized that parental attitudes are by no means the only (and often not the major) factor in the development of a homosexual behavior pattern. Some investigations reveal that men whose behavior is homosexual may have had reasonably good relationships with their parents. The sons of close-binding, intimate mothers and dominated, detached fathers often develop a homosexual behavior pattern, but just as often develop a heterosexual pattern. This is not to deny the profound effect of parental attitudes on children. However, a simple cause-and-effect relationship between parental behavior and a homosexual orientation in their children has not been established. Nevertheless, parents will do well to understand that homosexual feelings are commonly a part of growing up. They can also show appreciation and encouragement of the child's budding heterosexual interests.

A BIOCHEMICAL BASIS? That the male hormone androgen has a profound effect on the developing embryonic brain is discussed on pages 489–90. The period of this hormonal activity is so critical that any deviation from it may help to explain some divergent male sexual behavior. Research has produced preliminary evidence that some instances of male homosexual behavior may be associated with an imbalance between two chemicals that are related to the male sex hormone *testosterone.* When testosterone is broken down in the male body, two chemicals, *androsterone* and *etiocholanolone,* are produced in the urine. Studies have shown that in men whose behavior is heterosexual the amount of androsterone in the urine is greater than the amount of etiocholanolone. Preliminary research suggests that in men whose behavior is homosexual the ratio is reversed.[53] The researchers emphasize that there is no cause-and-effect relationship between the urine's chemical content and homosexual behavior. Moreover, some British research revealed a low level of urinary testosterone in two men whose behavior was exclusively homosexual.[54] In 1971, a group of U.S. workers reported a significant reduction of blood serum testosterone levels and spermatozoa counts in thirty young males whose behavior was homosexual. In addition, there was a significant correlation between the degree of the biochemical defect and low spermatozoa count and the rated degree of homosexual behavior.[55]

Still other studies of relatively few individuals reveal that "urinary testosterone readings in female homosexuals are higher than in heterosexual con-

[52] "Female Homosexuality," *British Medical Journal,* Vol. 1, No. 5640 (February 8, 1969), p. 331.

[53] M. Sydney Margolese, "Homosexuality: A New Endocrine Correlate," *Hormones and Behavior,* Vol. 1 (1970), pp. 151–55, and "The Homosexual: Is It Chemistry?" *Medical World News,* Vol. 12, No. 16 (April 23, 1971), pp. 4–5.

[54] John A. Loraine, A. A. A. Ismail, D. A. Adamopoulos, and G. A. Dove, "Endocrine Function in Male and Female Homosexuals," *British Medical Journal,* Vol. 4, No. 5732 (November 14, 1970), pp. 381–442.

[55] Robert C. Kolodny, William H. Masters, Julie Hendryx, and Gelson Toro, "Plasma Testosterone and Semen Analysis in Male Homosexuals," *New England Journal of Medicine,* Vol. 285, No. 21 (November 18, 1971), pp. 1170–74.

trols."[56] In addition, levels of the female hormone estrone tend to be lower in women whose behavior is homosexual than in women who are heterosexually oriented.[57]

These findings raise more questions than they answer. Is the hormonal imbalance found in the majority of individuals whose behavior is homosexual? Is it the result or the cause of a homosexual orientation? Does this hormonal imbalance occur at those periods of life during which the direction of future sexual behavior is determined? Today, the answers to these and other questions are being actively sought. It does seem possible that endocrine factors are among the many that are involved in homosexual behavior.

homosexual behavior: dilemma and hope

IS HOMOSEXUAL BEHAVIOR A DISEASE? Many professionals consider homosexual behavior a disease that requires prolonged psychiatric therapy. However, the scientifically based opposition to their view is formidable and merits serious consideration. One group claims that the sickness and misbehavior that can be associated with homosexual behavior is due to society's cruel appraisal. "Educate society," they say, "and the sickness and maladjustment will be lessened." Members of the opposing group declare that this approach is unrealistic and that a practical adjustment to existing cultural mores is essential for emotional health. In this country, they continue, it is impractical to expect society to soon accept homosexual behavior. Moreover, they point out that since heterosexual orientation is begun at an early age, homosexual behavior unavoidably generates conflict, depression, self-denigration, and guilt.

The opposition answers that psychotherapists treat only those homosexually oriented individuals who seek therapy. Millions of individuals whose behavior is homosexual do not wish to change their sexual orientation. They point to ample data showing that people whose behavior is homosexual are no more emotionally maladjusted than are people whose behavior is heterosexual. The work of Evelyn Hooker is often cited to support this view. She expresses the view that "apart from the specific difference in sexual orientation, many of the homosexuals she had studied reveal, on psychological testing, no 'demonstrable pathology' that would differentiate them in any way from a group of relatively normal heterosexuals."[58] Another study group reported that "there was little difference demonstrated in the prevalence of psychopathology[59] between a group of 89 male homosexuals and a control group of 35 unmarried men . . . Despite the slight increase in disability and the changes in their lives, the homosexual men functioned well."[60] Moreover, a study involving almost 1,700

[56] John A. Loraine, D. A. Adamopoulos, K. E. Kirkham, A. A. A. Ismail, and G. A. Dove, "Patterns of Hormone Excretion in Male and Female Homosexuals," *Nature*, Vol. 234, No. 5331 (December 31, 1971), p. 553.
[57] *Ibid.*
[58] Judd Marnor, ed., *Sexual Inversion: The Multiple Roots of Homosexuality* (New York, 1965), pp. 15, 16.
[59] The word *psychopathology* is from the Greek *psyche*, mind + *pathos*, disease + *logos*, word, reason (the science or study of). *Psychopathology*, then, means the study of emotional disorders or disease.
[60] Marcel T. Saghir, Eli Robins, Bonnie Walbran, and Kathye A. Gentry, "Homosexuality: III. Psychiatric Disorders and Disability in the Male Homosexual," *The American Journal of Psychiatry*, Vol. 126, No. 8 (February 1970), p. 63.

males whose behavior was homosexual revealed that those men older than forty-five years were no more lonely, depressed, or unhappy than those who were younger.

However, the professionals who consider homosexual behavior a disease to be treated emphasize the need for integration of sexuality into the total life style. A dynamic adjustment to living today, they state, is hardly compatible with a deep-seated terror of women, fleeting and meaningless sexual involvements, depression, inadequacy, and pathetic passivity. "Sexual relations with a person of the same sex," one psychiatrist recently stated, "represent a deviation or a short-circuiting of a very definite biological intention."[61]

THE HOPE: TREATMENT FOR THOSE WHO WANT IT Several studies have been designed to investigate whether homosexual behavior can be changed through psychiatric treatment. Moreover, it is claimed that many (although not all) of those who seek treatment want to develop a heterosexual behavior pattern. Both men and women have successfully changed their homosexual orientation. In some cases, group therapy has helped to bring a change. One study, extending over eighteen years, included 710 patients drawn from both clinics and private practice. Including partially and fully heterosexual adjustments, the reported "change rate" was about 45 percent.[62]

A recent survey suggested that among many women who are homosexually oriented there is a basic attraction for members of the opposite sex. In this study twenty-four women whose behavior was homosexual were compared to twenty-four nonhomosexually oriented women. Both groups of women were in psychoanalysis. Heterosexual dreams were not significantly fewer in the homosexually oriented group, nor was the desire for pregnancy less prevalent. Even before any psychoanalytic therapy, a majority of these women (53 percent) had experienced heterosexual activity. Indeed, 75 percent overtly sought social contact with men whose behavior was primarily heterosexual. With adequate treatment, the probability of a change to heterosexuality among the homosexually oriented women was considered to be about 50 percent.[63]

wanted: professional help

who is trained to help?

The treatment of emotional disorders by psychological means is called *psychotherapy.* When other methods, such as drugs, shock treatment, or surgery, are used, the procedure is considered *somatotherapy.* Some physicians use both.

[61] Lawrence J. Hatterer, "Debate: Can Homosexuals Change with Psychotherapy?" *Sexual Behavior,* Vol. 1, No. 4 (July 1971), p. 45. Expert but differing opinions as to whether homosexual behavior is a disease are presented in "Viewpoints: Is Homosexuality Pathologic or a Normal Variant of Sexuality?" *Medical Aspects of Human Sexuality,* Vol. 7, No. 12 (December 1973), pp. 10, 15–16, 18, 23–26. The discussants are Judd Marmor, Harold M. Voth, Norman L. Thompson, Jr., Tony Bieber, Evelyn Hooker, John W. Drakeford, and Charles W. Socarides.

[62] Lawrence J. Hatterer, *Changing Homosexuality in the Male. Treatment for Men Troubled with Homosexuality* (New York, 1970), p. 492.

[63] H. E. Kaye *et al.,* "Homosexuality in Women," *Archives of General Psychiatry,* Vol. 17, No. 5 (November 1967), pp. 626–34.

Although somatotherapy is generally limited to physicians, psychotherapy is not. The four professional groups involved with psychotherapy are the psychiatrists, psychologists, psychiatric social workers, and psychiatric nurses. Within their various competencies they all contribute to the total treatment available to the patient.

The *psychiatrist* is a doctor of medicine with extensive training in the diagnosis and treatment of emotional problems. All *clinical psychologists,* although they are not M.D.s, have graduate training in their specialty. In addition to diagnosing and treating the emotionally disturbed, psychologists also administer and interpret psychological tests. After earning a master's degree in social work, the *specialized social worker* obtains special training in interviewing techniques and psychotherapy. Such training is invaluable in gaining insightful information about a patient's home, work, and community. *Psychiatric nurse specialists* do some therapy, supervise medical regimens, and need a master's degree.

Psychoanalysis is a special technique of psychotherapy that uses the basic techniques of Freud. Although clinical psychologists and psychiatric social workers may engage in psychoanalysis, the majority of psychoanalysts are psychiatrists.

In a large *mental hospital,* all four specialists may work together in handling emotional problems. In community mental health centers, the psychiatrist, clinical psychologist, social worker, and nurse specialist are members of a team, each contributing to the patient's recovery. All may also be engaged in private practice in the community. Recent years have seen marked changes in the roles of these professionals. Future years will see even more.[64]

There is a gross shortage of adequately trained personnel to treat psychological problems. Practicing in the United States are only about twenty-three thousand psychiatrists, sixteen thousand psychologists who work with emotional problems, and thirty-three thousand psychiatric nurses.[65]

some psychological methods used to help emotional problems

It is understandable that no single technique is used in dealing with complex emotional problems. The *client-centered* technique of psychotherapy directs the patient neither to his problems nor to his early childhood. The therapist makes no effort to suggest either goals or a new way of life. As the patient talks out his problems, the therapist may help to clarify them, but it is assumed that the patient is able to solve his problem. In this atmosphere of patient esteem, the emotionally distressed person comes to realize his worth and his ability to live fruitfully.

Behavior therapy tries to eliminate the behavior pattern that is distressing the patient. Learning techniques are used. One behavior therapist tells of a patient who was unable to have sexual intercourse with his wife—

[64] Departments of health and mental health (both state and local), local councils of social agencies, and mental health associations are all sources of information regarding local facilities for the treatment of emotional problems. Two national agencies that are especially helpful in providing information about the qualifications of agencies are the National Association for Mental Health, 10 Columbus Circle, New York, New York 10019, and the Family Service Association of America, 44 East 23rd Street, New York, New York 10010.

[65] *Building a National Health Care System;* A Statement on National Policy by the Research and Policy Committee of the Committee for Economic Development (April 1973), p. 51.

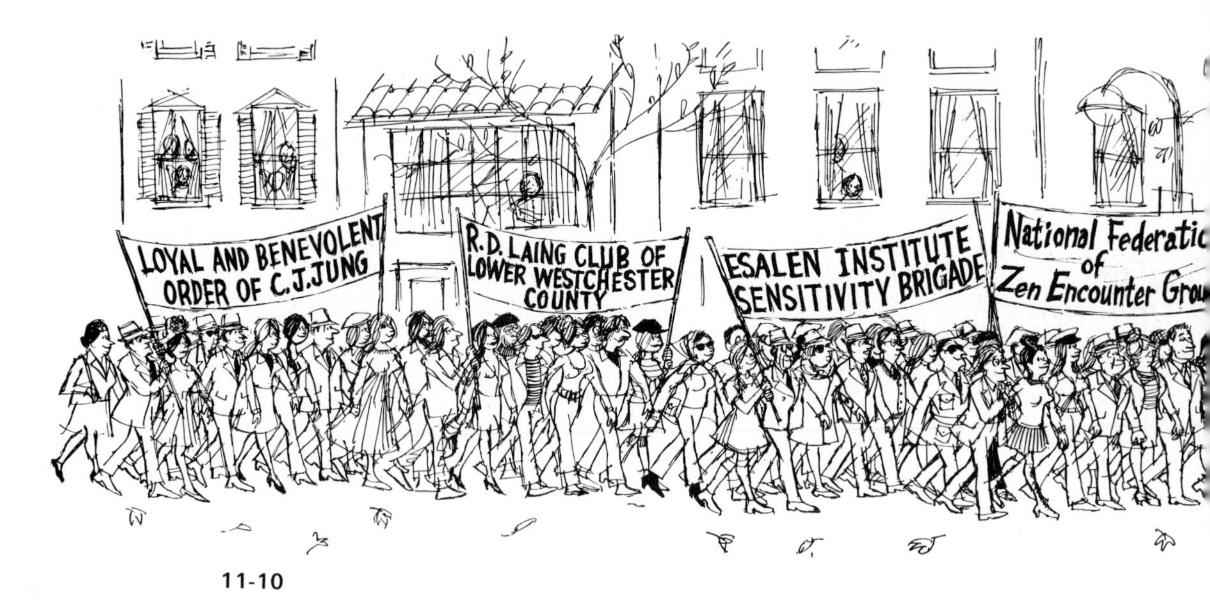

11-10

> unless he first dressed up as a woman, and he frequently went out on the streets at night dressed in this fashion and wearing a wig. This symptom had become especially uncomfortable to the patient because he feared that his young son, as he grew up, would learn about it. The treatment prescribed was extremely simple. Electrodes were fastened into the woman's clothing that the patient habitually wore; he was encouraged to dress up but warned that at some point he would receive a painful shock or hear a buzzer and that the shock or buzzer would then be repeated at irregular intervals until he had removed the clothing. Each session of therapy included five starts at dressing followed by the shock or buzzer, with a one-minute rest period between each trial. After 400 trials, the treatment was considered ended.[66]

The patient apparently recovered. The aversive conditioning by pain and punishment, rather than by pleasure and reward, has also been used in treating homosexual behavior and alcoholism.

Toward the end of the last century, Freud and Breuer originated *psychoanalysis*. Severe emotional distress in a hysterical girl had been manifested in deafness and paralysis of an arm. While under hypnosis, she told of many experiences related to her symptoms. Seemingly as a consequence of this, her symptoms disappeared. Psychoanalysis, as a treatment procedure, had begun. Freud discovered that if a patient was merely asked to relate anything that came to his mind (*free association*), past experiences that had been long repressed in the unconscious and had been causing symptoms eventually came to light. As these unconscious conflicts were revealed to the patient, his symptoms often abated or disappeared. As a result of his earned revelation, the patient developed personality strengths that enabled him to better adjust to his environment. Over the years numerous variations of this procedure have been introduced, but

[66]C. B. Blakemore *et al.*, "The Application of Faradic Aversion Conditioning in a Case of Transvestism," cited in Jerome Kagan and Ernest Havemann, *Psychology: An Introduction* (New York, 1968), pp. 443–44.

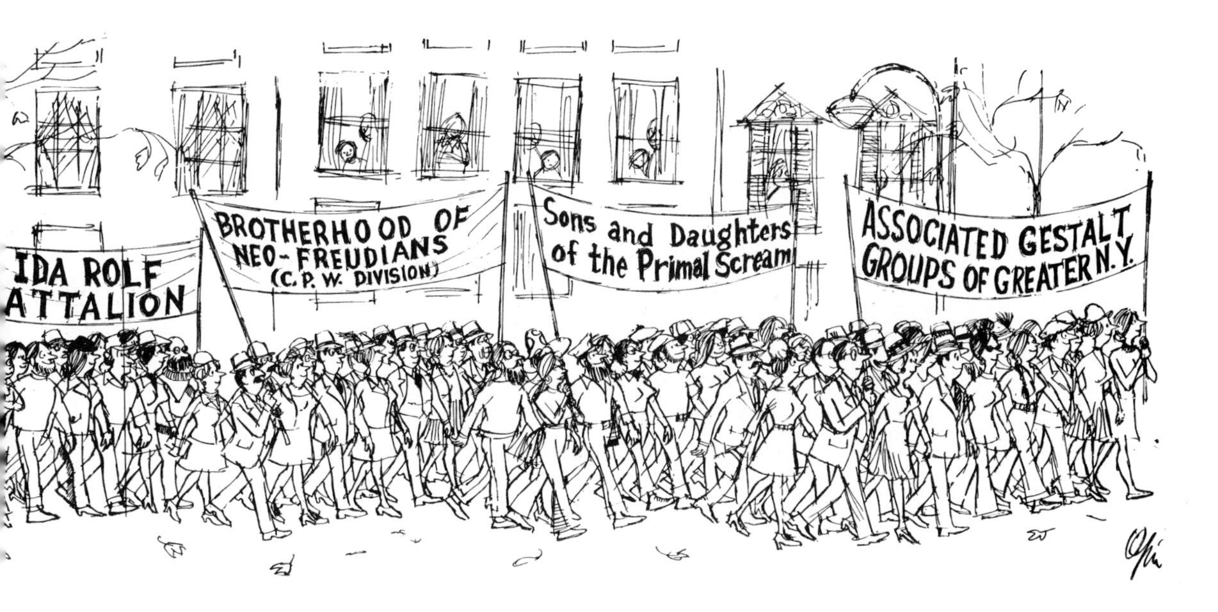

the fundamental approach of psychoanalysis remains unchanged. Dorsey has quoted a little-known poem illustrating what he has called this "growth of self-insight":

> As I walk'd by myself, I talk'd to myself
> And myself replied to me;
> And the questions myself then put to myself
> With their answers I give to thee.[67]

Months or years of from two to five hourly sessions a week may be required for this procedure. Lately, psychotherapy has been abbreviated and, for some, is intermittent. Psychotherapy is work for both therapist and patient. In the very first hours, the therapist tries to comprehend the patient's problem. He then attempts to help the patient understand and then deal with the problem. Again, the techniques used depend on the patient. Insight is required of the patient. He must be able to arrive at it, endure it, and use it. Comprehending and confronting his human problems, he will seek ways of resolving them. Not all patients are suitable for psychotherapy, including those with severely limited intelligence, those who do not come voluntarily, and those who somehow profit financially from their sickness and so remain sick. Persons with severe physical lesions, such as brain tumors, can hardly profit from psychotherapy. By no means, however, does this exclude all people who are physically ill. Many individuals with physical ailments, such as tuberculosis, may do better under psychotherapy. A wide variety of emotional problems are amenable to psychotherapy. Among them are anxieties, psychosomatic problems, and obsessive-compulsive neuroses.

[67] Barnard Barton, "Colloquy with Myself," quoted in John M. Dorsey, Preface, in *Illness or Allness* (Detroit, 1965), p. 13.

psychoactive drugs help bring about change

The use of psychoactive drugs has resulted in a marked drop in the total population of state mental hospitals. Not all of these drugs are new. *Reserpine,* the active principle of the root *Rauwolfia serpentina,* has been used for centuries to treat anxieties and dementias in India, Southeast Asia, and Europe. *Chlorpromazine,* a synthetic drug, is, like reserpine, quite effective in inducing relaxation. Both are particularly useful in treating schizophrenia.

Why are tranquilizers so often superior to barbiturates? The latter are useful in inducing sleep. With them excitement is reduced, but patients are not able to move about. However, tranquilizers reduce the intensity of the excitement itself. Delusions and hallucinations are reduced without a profound soporific (sleep-inducing) effect. Gross symptoms may be abated so that the patient can be reached. Since tranquilizers do cause some drowsiness, patients so medicated should not drive.

Tranquilizers were introduced in the mid-1950s, the first in a series of new therapeutic methods. Between 1950 and 1970 the number of patients in U.S. institutions for the emotionally ill dropped from 560,000 to 340,000. This was a 40 percent decrease; a 40 percent increase might otherwise have been expected. Short-term treatment took a firm hold. During the 1960s, in the nation's hospitals for the emotionally ill, admissions rose from 360,000 to 600,000, yet the number of beds fell from 722,000 to 527,000. And since short-term treatment could be given in outpatient clinics, psychiatric outpatient clinic visits increased from 892,000 in 1962 to 2.7 million in 1970. No longer was the care of the emotionally ill limited to custodial isolation in large institutions. New medications, group therapy, therapeutic community treatment, and mental health centers near patients' homes that were staffed by professionals with a team approach, were among the factors that wrought these massive changes.[68]

Lithium salts have been used by Europeans for many years. During the nineteenth century the spas were particularly popular among Europeans and U.S. tourists who thought themselves revitalized by the lithium-containing water. Recently lithium salts have been approved by the Food and Drug Administration for calming the manic stage of manic-depressive psychosis. It is used with caution, because it may be accompanied by a variety of disagreeable and even dangerous side effects. A preliminary study in Texas revealed that (with a few exceptions) the higher the level of lithium in drinking water, the lower the rate of admissions to hospitals for the emotionally ill.[69] Other research suggests that, in maintenance doses, lithium carbonate may have a preventive effect in both manic and depressive illness. Another compound, *imipramine,* may provide similar benefits.[70]

Nevertheless, grave reservations have been expressed about some aspects of the use of certain psychoactive drugs. Few experts would recommend their

[68] *Building a National Health Care System,* p. 52.

[69] "In Texas: The More Lithium in Tap Water, the Fewer Mental Cases," *Medical World News,* Vol. 12, No. 38 (October 15, 1971), pp. 18–19.

[70] "Prophylaxis for the Mentally Ill?" *Medical World News,* Vol. 14, No. 22 (June 1, 1973), p. 35.

abandonment. Antipsychotic drugs are the single most effective way of managing certain acute or active psychoses, particularly schizophrenia and mania. But concern is growing that antipsychotic drugs are often used indiscriminately and excessively. Decisions that should be made on a strictly individual and medical basis are being influenced by social pressures to reduce taxes by diminishing the number of hospital beds and personnel. At first glance such pressures appear justified. Without medication, 60 to 80 percent of schizophrenic patients are readmitted to the hospital in a year; with medication, that percentage drops to only 20 to 30 percent. However, the difference diminishes with time; over several years it may be only 10 to 15 percent. Moreover, studies show that the majority of hospital-discharged patients remain burdens to their families and society. Mental health centers, outpatient facilities, and private practitioners are also heavy users of these drugs. Within institutions, they have been adjuncts to the solution of management problems. In addition, when one drug dose fails, it may be increased or another drug added.[71]

But perhaps the most serious criticism of the way the drugs are used is the evidence that they become seriously toxic. The accusation has been made that, only too often, a mechanical straightjacket has been replaced by a chemical one; among other side effects, prolonged use often results in a severe reduction of activity. Moreover, "A particular cause for alarm is that certain neurologic complications can occur gradually, can be masked by the drugs themselves and may be irreversible and incurable, and no class of antipsychotic drugs appears to be free of the risk."[72] In addition, these drug-caused diseases of the nervous system are by no means rarities. Careful evaluation of the effect of these drugs on an individual basis, the restriction of dosage to the lowest effective levels, and regular reevaluation of the individual's continued need for them are necessary.

shock therapy and psychosurgery

Shock therapy is more commonly used than insulin therapy; the former is widely employed in therapy regimens by some psychiatrists. This is most effective with depressive states (see page 299), although its use for other emotional disturbances has met with some success. The trend, however, is away from shock treatment toward the use of tranquilizers. Some years ago, there was much publicity about a procedure called *prefrontal lobotomy*. In this operation the lobes of the cerebral cortex that are in front of the motor areas of the brain were separated from the rest of the brain. Results were poor. The procedure has now generally fallen from favor. By no means, however, has psychosurgery (cerebral surgery designed to relieve emotional problems) been abandoned. The removal of the temporal lobe (the cerebral lobe in the

[71] George E. Crane, "Clinical Psychopharmacology in Its 20th Year," *Science,* Vol. 181, No. 4095 (July 13, 1973), pp. 124–28. As of midsummer 1973, this article was among the most comprehensive available on this subject. It is also recommended for its references.

[72] Ross J. Baldessarini and Joseph F. Lipinski, "Risks vs. Benefits of Antipsychotic Drugs," editorial in *New England Journal of Medicine,* Vol. 289, No. 8, p. 428.

area of the temple) resulted in improved behavior in two patients. Both had developed violent behavior patterns following significant accidental brain damage. One of the patients stopped his repeated attempts to strangle his parents; the second patient also relaxed considerably.[73] However, it is in cases of epilepsy related to the temporal lobe that brain surgery seems to have brought an added bonus. One English surgeon reported the surgical removal of a temporal lobe in more than 250 patients with temporal-lobe epilepsy. Not only did he obtain complete relief for some patients who had been victims of uncontrollable seizures, but he also produced improved behavior in a large fraction of the patients.[74] In all cases of psychosurgery, careful selection of patients and sophisticated methods of diagnosis are essential.

In the past twenty years, the drastic prefrontal lobotomies of the past have been replaced by psychosurgery of greater precision and smaller lesions. These have almost eliminated the poor results of earlier extensive lobotomies. Moreover, for many patients they have brought improvement of emotional problems long resistant to other known forms of treatment.[75] Nevertheless, psychosurgery is much less common in this country than in Britain. What little psychosurgery is performed in this country is in university hospitals for some otherwise hopeless emotional disorders, for temporal-lobe convulsive discharges, and to relieve the constant, demoralizing pain of certain advanced cancers.

A major concern of public, political, and some professional groups has been the fear that psychosurgery will deprive potential patients of their free will. (A counterargument is that human beings may, for example, be imprisoned for violent behavior caused by brain disease, and that psychosurgery can free them.) Other objections to psychosurgery are that many patients for whom it is contemplated are incapable of making decisions or that the procedures will rob them of their intellectual capacities. Such fears have resulted in actions like a 1973 bill introduced into Congress to fine any surgeon performing psychosurgery in a federal institution, and the withholding of all research grants relating to psychosurgery by the National Institutes of Health until a special committee reports on ways of protecting the civil rights of potential psychosurgical patients.[76]

Thus, a controversy rages. It cannot be resolved by hysteria but by rational contemplation and calm discussion. One distinguished U.S. specialist has written that "On the one hand all patients for whom behavior-changing surgery is contemplated should be reviewed by independent committees consisting of both professionals and laymen, including women and minority members. On the other hand the time is clearly appropriate for a careful, scientifically

[73] "Lobectomy Ends Violent Episodes in Two Patients," *Journal of the American Medical Association,* Vol. 226, No. 1 (October 1, 1973), p. 19.

[74] Murray A. Falconer, "Reversibility by Temporal-Lobe Resection of the Behavioral Abnormalities of Temporal-Lobe Epilepsy," *New England Journal of Medicine,* Vol. 289, No. 9 (August 10, 1973), pp. 451–55.

[75] William H. Sweet, "Treatment of Medically Intractable Mental Disease by Limited Frontal Leucotomy," *New England Journal of Medicine,* Vol. 289, No. 21 (November 22, 1973), pp. 1117–25.

[76] Lawrence C. Kolb, "Psychosurgery—Justifiable?" *New England Journal of Medicine,* Vol. 289, No. 21 (November 22, 1973), pp. 1141–42.

controlled study of behavior-modifying surgery."[77] Two neurosurgeons have added that

> There is already enough knowledge of environmental and psychopharmacological drugs to control a vast segment of our population, without invoking brain surgery or electrical brain stimulation. The great hope of emotional brain research is that it will free us from our present tyrannies and future dangers of control. To this end, brain scientists need the help of philosophers, ethicists, theologians, social scientists, lawmakers, and jurists working in concert.[78]

self-help by environmental manipulation

Just as environment may induce stress and anxiety, so may it be manipulated to induce relief. Nobody should try to solve severe emotional problems alone. It is worth reemphasizing that early help can prevent progression of an emotional aberration. Moreover, professional advice is valuable in determining the need for help. However, many people with a mild emotional disturbance can help themselves considerably. Often, the mere presence of an understanding listener helps. Thus, marriage, although no substitute for therapy, may help an anxious individual find relief. For the same reason, friendships may also be effective in relieving anxiety. Unfortunately, some individuals attempt to relieve anxiety by repeated extramarital or premarital affairs. Such affairs may heighten conflict, increase guilt, and leave the sensitive individual more disturbed than before.

Interest in games can be decidedly therapeutic. Anxiety brought on by frustration is often relieved by appropriate competitive games. Aggressions from frustrations, which otherwise produce anxiety, are thus harmlessly diverted to sports. Spectators at sporting events also achieve this relief. Athletic contests are planned with great cunning. Why are tension-producing favorite teams so avidly supported? People normally enjoy the pleasure that comes with relief of the deliberately created tensions.

Sublimation of aggressive drives into creative work does not ordinarily resolve conflict. However, sexual and other drives may be sublimated into successful humanitarian efforts.

Noble lives are often led by those who assuage loneliness with humanitarian service. Before he was forty, Albert Schweitzer was world renowned as an outstanding Protestant theologian and as an organ interpreter of Bach. In his middle years, he forsook all the appurtenances of success. He went to medical school, graduated, and became a medical missionary. At lonely Lambaréné, in the African jungle, he built a hospital. "Here at whatever hour you come, you will find light and help and human kindness"[79] is inscribed on a lamp leading

[77] Norman Geschwind, "Effects of Temporal-Lobe Surgery on Behavior," *New England Journal of Medicine*, Vol. 289, No. 9 (August 10, 1973), p. 481.

[78] Vernon H. Mark and Robert Neville, "Brain Surgery in Aggressive Epileptics: Social and Ethical Implications," *Journal of the American Medical Association*, Vol. 226, No. 7 (November 12, 1973), pp. 765–72.

[79] Robert Coope, *The Quiet One* (London, 1952), p. 219.

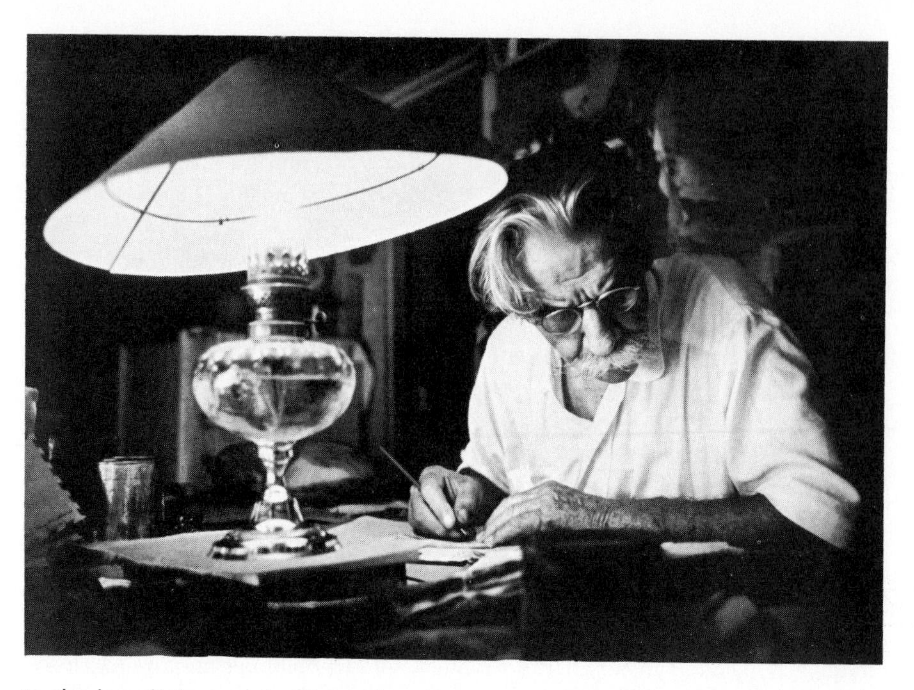

11-11 *Albert Schweitzer in Africa.*

to the hospital quay. In the profoundest sense, Schweitzer used his tensions to good purpose. If the great man's inner world was loneliness, in his work he surely found balm.

what is the best treatment for emotional disorders?

Modern treatment of mental illness has brought emotional strength to countless people who might otherwise have led wasted lives. Today, early diagnosis and treatment offer hope to those who half a century ago would have been forgotten. Nevertheless, therapy for many emotional disorders is still based on empirical methods.

> Recent studies have indicated that results with different treatments are markedly similar. Most statistical studies show that 65 to 70 percent of neurotic patients and 35 percent of schizophrenic patients improve after treatment regardless of the type of treatment received. Long-term follow-up studies of treated patients have also demonstrated no differences among the various treatments.[80]

This statement does little to resolve this question: which type of psychotherapy is best suited for the average emotional problem? Because there is no average emotional problem, the answer to that question will probably never be found. Differences in reactions to different stimuli by different people at different times—such variables do not readily lend themselves to measures of psychotherapeutic success. By relatively simple manipulation of his environment, one individual may relieve considerable anxiety-producing stress. At the other extreme, an individual may fail to overcome his emotional hurdles despite intensive appropriate psychotherapeutic treatment. More important than the kind

[80] Ari Kiev, ed., *Magic, Faith and Healing* (London, 1964), pp. 4, 5.

of help received is receiving it from a competent source when it is needed. It is hardly surprising that treatments vary. Considering the complexity of emotions, it is more surprising that they vary so little. That citadel of the mind, the brain, occupies but a third of a cubic foot of space. Under ordinary conditions it uses only ten watts of energy. A single refrigerator light bulb consumes four times that much energy. And yet, assuming that nothing is ever completely forgotten, the average brain is capable of storing some 280 sextillion (280,000,000,000,000,000,000,000) ''bits'' of information. As to the brain's complexity, consider only that part of its structure controlling behavior that is distinctively human—the cerebral cortex (page 266).

> Charles Herrick,[81] the distinguished American neuroanatomist, attempted to get some conception of the number of possible connections among the millions of cortical cells in a single human brain. Based on a series of computations, he inferred that there were $10^{2,783,000}$ such connections. To print this number written out in figures would take about two thousand ordinary book pages.[82]

In the accepting and sorting of numberless human experiences, in its endless relaying of responses, is it to be wondered that the mind falls sick and needs treatment? And that the treatments are so varied?

> Erikson relates the case of a little boy who ate paper. Nobody, however, paid any attention to him. He ate more and more paper. Still nobody cared. So finally he ate the theatre tickets, and then he received treatment.
>
> One of the ways of looking at symptomatology at any period in any society is: Where is the point where you eat the theatre tickets? We had quite an interesting case brought to the Menninger Clinic of a girl who really didn't need treatment herself, although her parents did. They lived in a house with one bathroom. She used to lock the door and take a three-hour bath. In time, the parents brought her to a psychiatrist, and then she was able to get them treated.[83]

Where is the point where one eats the theatre tickets? Where is the point at which emotional problems must be referred to others for professional diagnosis and treatment? It should be early. A problem that will at first be handled with ease may, if neglected, worsen. To work professionally with emotional problems is difficult. The trained professional understands both his limitations and his potential. He knows how to recognize the need for help in whatever form it appears; he knows when and how to step in and when to leave the disturbed person alone. But most of all, he knows that there are no simple definitions, no easy cures. The mind of man is the most complex and the most autonomous of all created systems. As John Milton wrote in *Paradise Lost* (I.254–55),

> The mind is its own place, and in itself
> Can make a Heaven of Hell, a Hell of Heaven.

[81] Charles J. Herrick, *The Evolution of Human Nature* (Austin, Tex., 1956).
[82] J. Z. Young, *A Model of the Brain,* cited in *Harold G. Wolff's Stress and Disease,* rev. and ed. by Stewart Wolf and Helen Goodell, 2nd ed., p. 172.
[83] Margaret Mead, ''The Changing World of Living,'' *Diseases of the Nervous System,* Vol. 28, No. 7 (July 1967), p. 7.

summary

According to the noted psychologist Erik Erikson, the human personality develops in eight stages, each of which takes place at a particular period of life and each of which is characterized by a particular task that must be satisfactorily accomplished before the individual can healthily enter the next stage (page 285).

1. For the infant, the stage is *basic trust versus basic mistrust* (pages 286–87).

2. The toddler stage is *autonomy versus shame and doubt* (page 288).

3. The preschooler must deal with *initiative versus guilt* (pages 289–90).

4. For the school-age child, the task is *industry;* the alternative is *inferiority* (pages 290–91).

5. In puberty, the teen-ager confronts *identity versus self-diffusion* (pages 291–92).

6. The first adult stage involves *intimacy and self-distantiation versus self-absorption* (page 292).

7. The second adult stage has to do with *generativity versus stagnation* (pages 292–93).

8. The third adult stage concerns *integrity versus despair and disgust* (page 293).

For convenience of discussion, personality disorders may be broadly categorized as:

1. *psychotic disorders,* in which the individual often loses contact with reality. They may be caused by *organic brain lesions* (page 296), or they may be *functional.* Functional psychotic disorders include *schizophrenia* (pages 296–99), the *manic-depressive psychoses* (pages 299–300), and *paranoia* (page 300).

2. *neurotic disorders,* in which the individual remains able to recognize and attempt to deal with his emotional problems. These disorders include the *psychoneuroses* (pages 301–02)—*anxiety states; phobias; obsessive-compulsive reactions; hysterias* (*conversion hysterias* and *dissociative states*); and *traumatic neuroses*—and *psychosomatic disorders* (pages 303–04).

3. *character disorders* are manifested by social divergence rather than by emotional symptoms. Examples of individuals with character disorders are the alcoholic, the drug addict, and the *psychopathic personality* (page 304). Some psychologists consider sexually divergent behavior, notably homosexual behavior (pages 305–10), to be a manifestation of character disorder, though many disagree.

Psychotherapy refers to the treatment of emotional disorders by psychological means (page 310). The treatment is called *somatotherapy* when other methods, such as drugs (pages 314–15), shock therapy (pages 315–16), or psychosurgery (pages 315–16), are used. Four groups of professionals are involved with psychotherapy: psychiatrists, psychologists, specialized social workers, and psychiatric nurse specialists (page 311). Among the approaches to treatment are *client-centered therapy* (page 311), *behavior therapy* (pages 311–12), and *psychoanalysis* (pages 312–13). In addition, many individuals may achieve considerable relief from mild emotional disturbances by altering their anxiety-producing environment (pages 317–18).

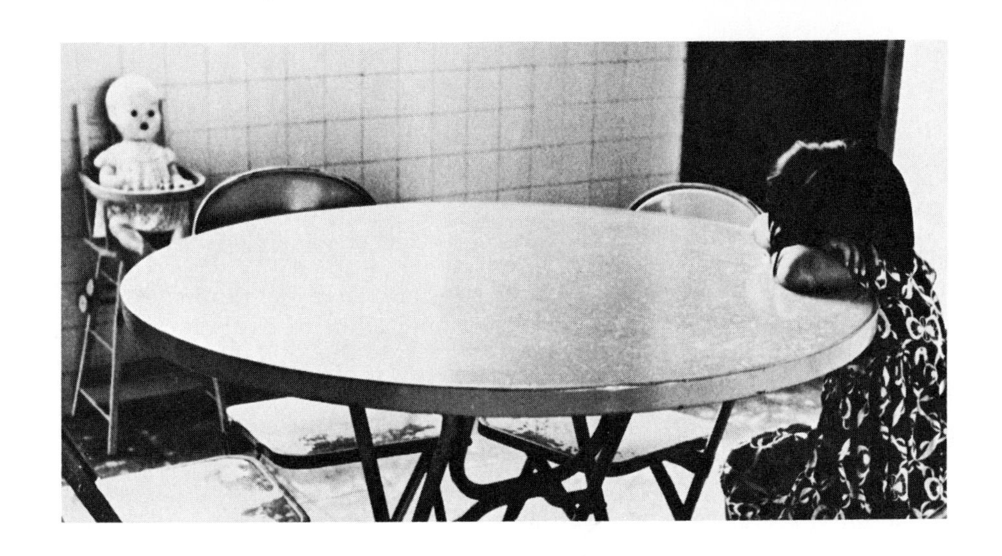

anxieties in the 1970s

12

the nature of anxiety

"The problem of anxiety" wrote Freud more than forty years ago, "is a nodal point, linking up all kinds of important questions; a riddle, of which the solution must cast a floodlight upon our whole mental life."[1] What, then, is anxiety? Anxiety is a feeling of foreboding. It is a premonition that something evil is about to happen. As a descriptive term it may be used synonymously with "worry." What is the difference between fear and anxiety? Fear is caused by an immediate experience. One is fearful of something or somebody specific and one is afraid now. However, one is anxious about something that may be quite vague. Also, anxiety is always a feeling about the future.

People have a reservoir of anxieties. Most of these anxieties are conquered; others are half-remembered or are deeply buried in the subconscious. The first strange face, the initial separation from the mother, the first day at school—these childhood anxieties are added to the countless anxiety-associated strivings, defeats, and victories that are inevitable in normal living.

the power of anxiety

Even savage animals, if you keep them confined, forget their natural courage.[2]

Of the 6,654 U.S. Army men captured in the Korean war, over 90 percent were taken prisoner during the first twelve months. In those days, enemy treatment of prisoners was atrocious. A ninety-mile death march killed 10 percent of 500 men. Indeed, in the three years of war, 38 percent of the 6,654 U.S. prisoners perished. Of these, more than a thousand were victims of atrocities. Even during the beginning weeks of the conflict, the word spread through the U.S. ranks harshly and clearly: capture meant suffering and death. Within him, each man carried this tight knot of anxiety.

12-1 *Fear—an immediate, specific emotion, quite different from anxiety.*

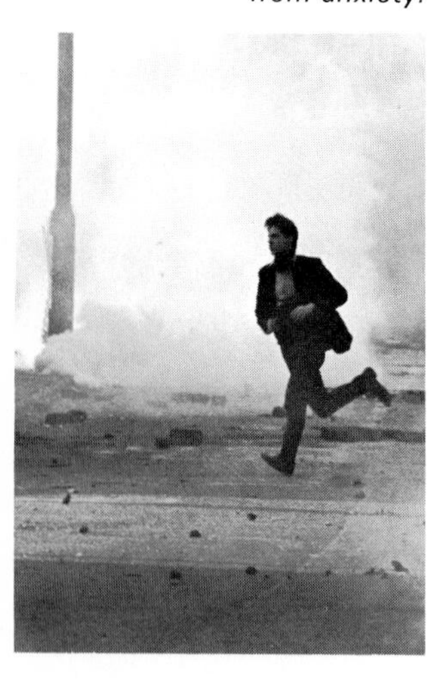

For those who were captured, the stresses of war were intensified. Each man had an ancient and crying need to be relieved of his anxieties. Knowing this, their captors did not immediately fulfill the worst expectations of the prisoners. Instead, they fed them and offered them friendship. To agonizingly anxious men, they held out the lure of tranquility. But there was a price: cooperation with the Korean movement for "world peace." Less than 2 percent of the men collaborated. Doubtless the commitments of most of the men to their own culture induced them to endure. For some, the offer may have even created more tension and anxiety, arising from the conflict between wanting to accept the offer and not wanting to seem cowardly before fellow captives.

So, part of this method of handling prisoners was to offer relief from intolerable anxiety. The plan was intensified by removal of all leaders from their midst. A feeling of abandonment and rejection was cultivated among the prisoners. In a score of ways the men reexperienced a long-forgotten threat of childhood. "If you don't come along, I'll leave you here by yourself!" The unmeant rejections of parents and teachers, the scorn of playmates, the indifference of

[1] Sigmund Freud, *General Introduction to Psychoanalysis,* American ed. (New York, 1920), p. 341.
[2] Tacitus, *History,* Bk. IV, sec. 64.

girls—all these childhood anxieties were consciously or unconsciously renewed, and with their renewal all the old anxious tensions had to be handled again. The newer anxieties were also intensified. Even physical activity of the prisoners was seriously limited—a common source of childhood anxiety. The acute uncertainty of the future, the constant threat of physical and mental harm, the tragic sense of abandonment and rejection, the conflicts and guilts, and the frustration and inactivity of the prison situation—for the prisoners, the cup of anxiety was filled to overflowing.

some variables of anxiety

The prisoners were in an extreme situation. But few life situations are untouched by anxiety. Anxiety moves the whole of the emotional life. Its more severe manifestations are only too recognizable: the dry throat, the quavering whisper, and, in extremes of anxious terror, the stifled scream. Less dramatic (but just as distressing and more common) manifestations of anxiety are restlessness, cold sweat, palpitating heart, muscular tension in the back of the neck, chest pain, and a hopeless, helpless, sinking sense of impending disaster. However, people differ in their reactions to similar situations. One man's financial ruin does not demoralize him. Expending the energies of his anxiety profitably, he works to recover. Another is paralyzed by the mere possibility of a relatively minor loss. Still another man is precipitated into mild anxiety by a spot on his clothes. Yet when someone asked Albert Einstein why he was so indifferent to his clothes, the great physicist merely answered, "It would be a pity if the wrapping proved better than the meat."

anxiety: contagion and conscience

Observe a line of small children waiting to be immunized. As one approaches the needle, he begins to tremble, then to cry. One by one, most of the others will lose control and also cry. So it was with the U.S. Army men captured by the Communists, except that most of them thought themselves too old to cry before their buddies. It was no different with the guilt-ridden flagellants of the fourteenth century (Chapter 5), and it is anxiety that dictators have learned to stir in their screaming hordes. Yet, although anxiety can be contagious, to feel it one must have a conscience. A psychopathic criminal does not possess an adequately developed conscience. He suffers no conflict from his actions. He can know no anxiety. In contrast, the anxiety of irreconcilable conflict destroyed the devout minister of W. Somerset Maugham's indestructible story, "Rain." His lust for the prostitute collided with his conscience. From his powerfully conflicting tensions rose guilt and anxiety. He could bear neither and committed suicide.

anxiety as a motivation

Clearly anxiety is society's tool for maintaining obedience to law and order. But it is more. Because it stimulates man to seek appropriate and constructive solutions to the problems causing it, anxiety may yet save humanity. In this regard, Toynbee[3] drew an illustrative parallel. Fishermen, bringing in herring from the North Sea, noticed that the fish in the tanks became sluggish. Because the fish

[3]Arnold Toynbee, "How to Turn the Tables on Russia," cited in Rollo May, *The Meaning of Anxiety* (New York, 1950), p. 12.

consequently lost some of their freshness, their market value was reduced. By placing catfish into the herring tanks, the fishermen menaced the herring. In the face of this threat, the herring became active, flourished, remained fresh, and retained their market value. Of course, in the end the herrings' "anxiety reaction" did not save them; they were eaten by people. Nonetheless, the threat set in motion constructive defenses against the predatory catfish in their ecosystem. Will human beings turn the tables on anxiety? Will they constructively deal with predators, not only within themselves, but also in their outer ecosystems? A good beginning is to recognize societal threats. Halleck wrote:

> The most idealistic, psychologically sound, and committed students have considerable ability to identify themselves with those who are especially oppressed, the persecuted and the poor. In a commonality of brotherhood they feel the oppression of others as if it were their own. This truly Christian, socially responsible attitude is admittedly only a part of the motivation of activists. Yet at some time or other, for however brief a period, it becomes a powerful factor towards commitment to dissent. Where the attitude of selflessness is persistent, it fosters deep involvement in civil rights work, poverty programs and the Peace Corps.[4]

It is well to remember that the possibility of a destructive reaction to anxiety is in itself cause for anxiety. Fearful, indeed, is "aimless anxiety, which drives us into irrational *action,* irrational *flight*—or, indeed, irrational *denial* of danger."[5]

escape from anxiety

All human reactions to anxiety are designed to relieve or escape it. Sometimes anxiety may be relieved by a simple expedient, such as changing to a less demanding job. It is more difficult to change a boy friend or girl friend. "I can't afford you anymore," one young woman told a man who had caused her nothing but pain. The normal reaction to anxiety is the realistic appraisal of stress, followed by the taking of appropriate action. Sometimes the reaction to anxiety can be costly. A chronically high anxiety level in college students is related to both lower grades and a higher rate of dropout. Unfortunate as these consequences are, they are certainly remediable. A study of 1,454 Harvard dropouts showed that psychiatric disorders were four times as high among the dropouts as among the general undergraduate population. A highly encouraging sign of the ability of these young men to handle anxiety was the finding that the "psychiatric dropouts have the same rate of return, attainment of honors and graduation as those who drop out for other reasons."[6]

Anxiety is a paradoxical human experience. An insistent threat to human welfare, it may nonetheless contain the seeds of human salvation. The ability to tolerate and constructively use anxiety may decide more than human health. It may well determine human existence. For this reason, this chapter is wholly

[4] Seymour L. Halleck, "Why Students Protest: A Psychiatrist's View," *Think,* Vol. 33, No. 6 (November–December 1967), p. 6.
[5] Erik H. Erikson, *Childhood and Society* (New York, 1950), p. 363.
[6] Armand M. Nicholi, Jr., "Harvard Dropouts: Some Psychiatric Findings," *American Journal of Psychiatry,* Vol. 124, No. 5 (November 1967), p. 657.

concerned with several anxiety-provoking problems that are central to modern living.

one deep root of modern anxiety: "I am frightened"

The seventeenth-century French mathematician and philosopher Blaise Pascal wrote:

> When I consider the short duration of my life, swallowed up in the eternity before and after, the little space which I fill, and even can see, engulfed in the infinite immensity of spaces of which I am ignorant, and which know me not, I am frightened, and am astonished at being here rather than there; for there is no reason why here rather than there, why now rather than then. . . The eternal silence of these infinite spaces frightens me.[7]

Three centuries later, men ventured out of the world and tentatively explored the moon's ecosystem. But did these majestic technological triumphs nullify some of the anxiety so long ago expressed by Pascal? Not for most men. The same anxieties—Who am I? What is my relation to other men and to the world outside myself?—remain.

Indeed, modern man's anxieties have increased, partly because of the same technological changes that might have been expected to reassure him. One must forsake the womb. But is it necessary to get out of the very world? With this added degree of separation, this generation will yet have its anxious rendezvous. Moreover, today the very speed of change troubles people. Impermanence and rootlessness are built into their lives—into their jobs, their automobiles, even into the family unit. If change and rootlessness have grown to be the mark of modern times, anxiety is their common symptom. But it is not quite the same symptom of Pascal nor of those who preceded him. It is compounded. Men now fear that they will be unable to control not only what they know, but also what they are about to know. Destruction by nuclear weapons, dehumanization by computers, devastation by pollution, depersonalization by industry—these threats have not given modern man reason to feel secure with his own technology.

It is not technology itself man fears, nor its creators. Man fears man. Why? Because he does not know him. Man's knowledge of himself and his ability to communicate with others has not kept pace with his other discoveries. He has communicated with men on the moon, but not always with men across the table. Man's inner space has not been conquered. Today, the failure to establish human contact disturbs man's relationship with himself, and the group's relationships with other groups. War—the old expression of group conflict—has always been a source of anxiety. Modern war has created the added anxiety of a sense of helplessness. Being able to act positively to reduce one's anxieties is essential for emotional health. But in the face of Armageddon most people feel powerless. Human knowledge has outstripped wisdom.

Global anxieties, then, are assuredly a part of our time. But nearer home, one finds a world of anxieties well worth exploring. What are some of them?

[7] Quoted in Theodosius Dobzhansky, *Mankind Evolving* (New Haven, Conn., 1962), p. 346.

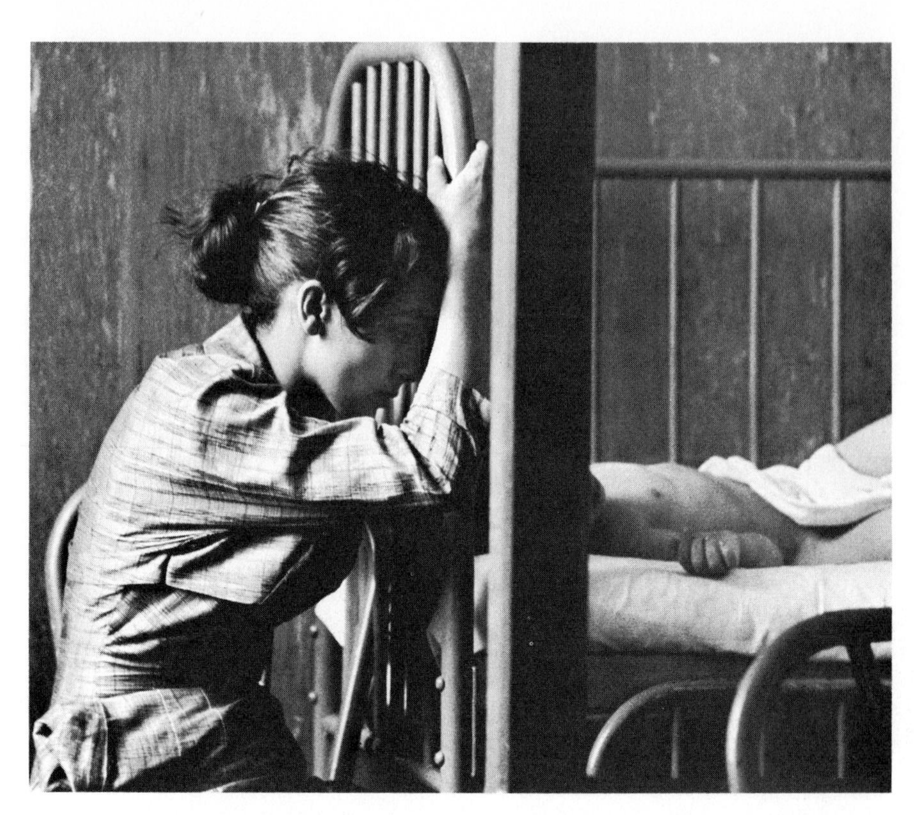

12-2 *Parental anxiety.*

parental anxiety

A distraught young mother presented her dilemma to her family physician this way: "It's my fault," she said, her voice trembling. "I should have breast-fed my baby." Suddenly she was angry. "But I hated it. I couldn't stand it. I never liked it, and I can't hide not having liked it any more. Last month I read an article in this magazine." She held a popular woman's journal. "Is it really that unnatural not to breast-feed the baby? You told me to forget about it. But a friend of mine read that unless you breast-feed your baby, you have lesbian tendencies or something. Is that somebody's idea of a joke?" She wiped her eyes. "I'm beginning to hate this whole thing." She was crying. "I hate it. I hate having a baby. Everybody says something different."

Some women want to breast-feed their babies. They enjoy it, and do it easily. Others, just as normal, do not enjoy breast-feeding. They should not do so. A guilt-ridden mother, resentfully holding her child to her breast, will do that child no good. It is the total experience of dining, of human comfort and tenderness, that is essential to the baby in this, the stage that Erikson calls basic trust versus mistrust.

The young woman described above is still another victim of an endless barrage of conflicting advice. Don't pick up Billie when he screams. Pick up Billie when he screams. Exclude Susie from the bedroom; what if she does feel left out? Don't exclude Susie from the bedroom; she'll feel left out. Never take Willie's hands away from his penis; if you do, he'll masturbate in public. Always divert Willie when he's doing his exploring; if you don't, he'll masturbate in public. And so on, ad infinitum. The result is a confused parent, doubtful of every action, suspicious of his own love, convinced of his inadequacy, and suffering parental guilt.

parent development

Parents develop too. As Friedman has noted,[8] they pass through stages related to the stages of their child's development (see Table 12-1). Parents and child develop together, experiencing singular, yet interwoven, problems. And, like the child, a parent in the throes of one stage may still be occupied with unsolved problems of a past stage.

In the first stage, it takes time for parents to learn how to interpret such cues as the howl of the child. What is the baby trying to tell them? He is dry, fed, fondled. No diaper pin pierces his bottom. Why, then, does he weep? Is it still another gas bubble? Or is it because his bed was accidentally moved six inches from the window and he misses the usual shaft of bright light?

When the recliner becomes a sitter and suddenly a toddler, he is into everything. Again the parents need time. It is not always easy to wholeheartedly accept a child who seems to be winning an all-day footrace with his mother. No sooner may this acceptance come about than Friedman's third stage of parental development—separation—is reached.

The pain of separation is not limited to children. The child's first day at school, punctuated by the peremptory command, ''Mommie, g'wan home,'' is a trauma that mothers (and grandmothers) are not prone to forget. Nor is the fourth stage, manifested by a child's independence, any easier for the parents. Their child's ''declaration of independence'' hurts some parents and angers others. It is almost as difficult for the rejected parents to remember that they are still desperately needed as it is for them to understand the rejection. The fifth stage of parental personality development is marked by an opportunity for the parents to rebuild their lives, not around the child, but with themselves more in mind.

Parental development begins with the parents' own childhood. Parents need help. Many parents come to realize that the child is trying to give that help. This effort, in turn, helps the child to identify with his parents and to grow with them. Their effort can be mutually beneficial.

the child's development: whose responsibility?

The parent has become the scapegoat of modern times. ''Look at how badly you raised me,'' is the accusation and excuse of many an emotionally distressed young person. The parents' sense of guilt is deep. But it is well to remember that someone who points the finger of blame at another person will find three fingers of his hand pointing at himself. ''The fact is that children, too, possess freedom of choice. It appears at an early age and develops with the intelligence

[8] David Belais Friedman, ''Parent Development,'' *California Medicine,* Vol. 86, No. 1 (January 1957), pp. 25–28.

TABLE 12-1 Parent and Child Development	
STAGE ONE: INFANT	**STAGE TWO: TODDLER**
Parent Development: Learning the *cues.* **Erikson:** Trust. **Spock:** Physically helpless; emotionally agreeable. **Ogden Nash:** *Many an infant that screams like a calliope* *Could be soothed by a little attention to his diope.*	**Parent Development:** Learning to *accept growth and development.* **Erikson:** Autonomy. **Spock:** A sense of his own individuality and will power; vacillates between dependence and independence. **Ogden Nash:** *The trouble with a kitten is that* *Eventually it becomes a cat.*
STAGE THREE: PRESCHOOLER	**STAGE FOUR: SCHOOL-AGER**
Parent Development: Learning to *separate.* **Erikson:** Initiative. **Spock:** Imitation through admiration; learns about friends; preliminary interest in sexuality. **Ogden Nash:** *But joy in heaping measure comes* *To children whose parents are under their thumbs.*	**Parent Development:** Learning to *accept rejection*—without deserting. **Erikson:** Industry. **Spock:** Fitting into outside group; independence of parents and standards; developing conscience; need to control and make moral judgments. **Ogden Nash:** *Children aren't happy with nothing to ignore* *And that's what parents were created for.*
STAGE FIVE: TEEN-AGER	
Parent Development: Learning to *build a new life,* in the context of changing family relationships. **Erikson:** Identity. **Redl:** Conflict to be confined to specific and major issues at hand; peer orientation and fair play. **Ogden Nash:** *O adolescence!* *I'd like to be present I must confess* *When thine own adolescents adolesce!*	Source: David Belais Friedman, "Parent Development," *California Medicine,* Vol. 86, No. 1 (January 1957), pp. 25–28.

and other capacities of the youthful personality. Children, then, share the responsibility for their behavior and emerging characters with their parents, relatives, teachers and friends."[9]

And freedom of choice is a durable freedom that may remain when all other freedoms are gone. Frankl writes,

[9] Corliss Lamont, *Freedom of Choice Affirmed* (New York, 1967), p. 32.

> We who lived in concentration camps can remember the men who walked through the huts comforting others, giving away their last piece of bread. They may have been few in number, but they offer sufficient proof *that everything can be taken from a man but one thing: the last of the human freedoms—to choose one's attitude in any given circumstances, to choose one's own way.*[10]

Undeniably, parents need improving, but the child must share in the responsibility for his own development. It is an opportunity. Again, he can help not only himself but also his parents.

the working mother

The life of the average mother today is not like her grandmother's used to be. Her grandmother was not isolated with a runabout child. Her grandmother was not locked up in a carefully measured, stingily allotted, two-room space, a three-dollar telephone call away from her nearest relative. Her grandmother lived among a retinue of relatives and neighbors, all interfering but caring. Her grandmother's time was a time of *kirche, kinder, kochen* (church, children, cooking). Bread was baked at home, not bought practically tasteless and neatly sliced. It was a time of the "superhome" not the supermarket. Her grandmother had a single gadget—a music box given her as a wedding present. And when her grandmother bade farewell to her son, who was leaving to be on his own, she had another child at her breast. When her grandmother died that summer at forty-three, and the child died too, it was very sad. Sad, but not unusual. Most grown people died of some infection before they reached the age of fifty; and, in those days, countless babies died of summer diarrhea.

Today's average mother will live well past seventy. She will have borne three children or fewer by twenty-seven. She will have raised them before she is fifty. Production of basic services outside the home (education, recreation, food), combined with labor-saving automation, add perhaps as much as ten more years during which child-raising can be a reasonably part-time job. Even a woman who manages to keep busy at home throughout all the childbearing years can count on only about twenty years of complete occupation. These are interim years. They come out of the middle of her life. What is more, some 80 percent of married women become widows—many at a young age. If they hope to remarry, they must become involved in activities outside the home. And they must compete with the growing number of divorcees and other unmarried women.

These potential problems do not contribute to the modern woman's desire to consider domesticity a full-time lifetime occupation. Child-rearing is now a temporary full-time job. Since 1950 the number of married working women in the United States has exceeded the number of single working women. Moreover, the acceptance of women by industry testifies to their success in the business world. More than 42 percent of all U.S. mothers now have jobs outside the home. Since the Second World War, the number of U.S. working women has doubled, but the number of working mothers has increased eightfold. More than one-third of these working mothers have children under six years of age;

[10] Victor E. Frankl, *Man's Search for Meaning* (New York, 1959), p. 112.

half of these have children under three. The mothers of more than 25 million U.S. children are working outside the home; about 5.6 million of these children are under six years of age. Most of the children of working mothers under twelve are cared for in their own homes.[11] Millions of mothers work outside the home because of financial necessity. In the past ten years, however, an increasing number of working mothers have been working because they are unhappy at home. For them, the horizons of home are too limited. They make poor full-time mothers and dull, nagging wives. At work they are happier. But many working mothers are anxious that they are failing their children. They feel guilty. Need they?

The mother who is content at home need not be defensive about it. A happy full-time mother always will be best for children. But an unhappy mother, resentfully brooding over her missed life outside the home, is best outside that home. An outside job may well improve her performance with her children. And a smaller amount of high-quality mothering is better than a massive amount of poor mothering.

A job, then, may relieve the guilt she feels about being a dissatisfied mother. But what can she do about her new guilt—her feeling that she has deserted the home? She must remember that, like it or not, the home and children remain primarily her responsibility, not her husband's. And, indeed, recent studies have indicated that the majority of today's young women choose careers that will not lead them into later serious conflicts with their desire to be successful wives and mothers.[12] The greatest problem for the working mother is the care of the infant and preschooler. The care of older children is more easily arranged. People who care for other people's children must have enormous sensitivity, patience, and tenderness. Such people are very hard to find. The degree of the average working mother's guilt will depend in part on her success in meeting the critical problem of substitute care. Also, she must honestly ask herself if she is physically and emotionally able to handle both complex, demanding aspects of her life. A woman who is exhausted and tense from a high-pressure business or professional life may find it difficult to be the warm, relaxed mother of a child waiting at home. Children thrive on love, not ticker tape.[13] Despite "heavy investment in preparing their chosen careers, [women] must impose self-limitations after marriage and children."[14] The working mother who feels guilty and tries to "make it up" to her child for being absent will not mother, but overprotect the child. In the end, the child will fight her off.

What about the father? Without his support, the working mother will fail. If she is prone to constantly remind him of her contribution to the family income, she will receive not support but hate. Work will become for each of them an

[11] "Working Mothers," *Saturday Review of Education,* Vol. 1, No. 2 (February 10, 1973), p. 60.

[12] Harold L. Wilensky, cited in "Woman's Work Is Never Done: Roundup of Current Research," *Transaction,* Vol. 6, No. 7 (June 1969), p. 8.

[13] "Where I come from," Fiorella La Guardia used to shrewdly say, "we knew the difference between ticker tape and spaghetti." The Little Flower was reflecting even deeper feelings than a social conscience. He was saying: "Society should care like a mother."

[14] Louise Sandler, "Career Wife and Mother," *Archives of Environmental Health,* Vol. 18, No. 2 (February 1969), pp. 154–55.

escape from the other. And the child at home will live on a deserted island threatened by the stormy seas of dissension.

Finally, do not the studies of mother-deprived children provide abundant evidence that a mother's absence deprives and sickens a child? (See the following section.) One must guard against glib conclusions. To begin with, the absent mothers in the studies were usually completely absent. Moreover, maternal deprivation was not the only misfortune of many of these children. Other factors—such as bitter family dissension, poverty, and racial discrimination—also contributed to the emotional sickness of children without mothers. Recent evaluations point to little or no direct correlation between working mothers and childhood instability. Children raised in kibbutzim (the cooperative agricultural communities of Israel) are kept in nurseries. The nursery workers are carefully selected to provide affection and warmth for the children. Every day the children are visited by their own parents. A degree of family life is thus part of each child's day. Some investigators claim that the absence of continual parental attention plus the kibbutz emphasis on the community welfare may even enhance the child's development in some ways.[15]

In summary, many working mothers succeed in raising emotionally healthy children. But they must work at it.

childhood anxiety

the need for mothering

The relation between infant and mother is a ballet, in which each partner responds to the steps of the other.[16]

Observe a newborn calf. Shakily it struggles to its trembling legs. Still wet, listing, it totters to its mother's teat. Such is its early independence. The dependence of the human newborn, however, is complete. Even the purpose of the breast must be shown him. To completely deprive the human newborn or infant of mothering is catastrophic.

At birth, threats promptly beset the utterly vulnerable human infant. The respiratory center of the brain, the respiratory muscle (diaphragm) separating the chest from the abdomen, the respiratory muscles between the ribs in the newborn—all these need further development. To meet his consequent threat of inadequate respiration, the newborn human must breathe two or three times as fast as the adult. To the respiratory threat is added a gastrointestinal threat. The gut lining is incomplete. For a time, it will function poorly. A third threat is that of an inadequate relationship between the infant and his mother or mother-substitute. And still a fourth threat is that the infant might not be able to satisfy his needs for pleasure, for example, the oral pleasure of enough sucking. For all people, to a varying degree, these threats become realities.

[15] Earl Siegel, "Child Care and Child Development in Thailand, Sweden, and Israel—Their Relevance for the United States," *American Journal of Public Health,* Vol. 63, No. 5 (May 1973), pp. 396–400.

[16] Jerome Kagan, "The Child: His Struggle for Identity," *Saturday Review* (December 7, 1968), p. 80.

The infant feels hunger. Hunger hurts. He is threatened, anxious. He cries and he is fed. His tension is relieved. But sometimes he cries and the breast (or bottle) does not come. All he can do is cry more. He hurts more. His stress grows. He suffers more anxiety. About six months of a small amount of frustration will teach him how to deal with frustration. Too much frustration, however, will teach him that his most important person cannot be counted upon. He loses his basic trust. At the breast the infant learns, for the first time, love and hate (see pages 286–87).

The effects of prolonged maternal deprivation have long been studied. In 1801, the "wild boy" of Aveyron was found in a French forest. Attempts to help him laid the foundation for present treatment of the mentally retarded. For more than thirty years, reports of children completely deprived of mothering have described their sad expression, pitiable dejection, rigidity, mental and social deterioration, stupor, and even unduly high sickness and death rates.

Animal infants also develop severe emotional problems from maternal deprivation. Laboratory monkeys raised without mothers grieve piteously. At times they clasp their heads in their arms and rock. Some pinch the same patch of skin hundreds of times daily or develop other compulsive mannerisms. Others fail to mate successfully.

One experiment separated young monkeys from their mothers and raised them with mother substitutes constructed of wire. One wire substitute incorporated a bottle containing warm milk from a mother monkey. The other substitute was covered with terry cloth. The young monkeys turned to the bare wire effigy only to feed. Otherwise they clung to the soft terry cloth mother substitute (Figure 12-3). This study indicated "that contact comfort is a variable of overwhelming importance in the development of affectional response, whereas lactation is a variable of negligible importance."[17] Monkeys reared with the never scolding, always warm terry cloth "mother" nevertheless did not mature normally.

Observations such as these, combined with highly defensible, if theoretical, schema of normal personality development (see pages 285–93), correctly emphasize the critical importance of mothering to the normal growth of the child. The fact that most psychiatrists vigorously emphasize this has not helped to diminish the widespread sense of guilt and anxiety among many working mothers of young children. And an anxious mother means an anxious child.

the disciplined, dependent struggle for independence

Months before birth the first human heartbeat pumps not mother's but fetal blood independently produced. Intrauterine life is not mere unremembered slumber. Unborn, the child sucks (often his thumb; see Figure 11-5, page 290), preparing for later oral gratifications of feeding and sex. Within the uterus, jerky movements prelude the initial tottering independence from the mother. Sometime after birth—in body exploration and use, in later creative curiosities at school—the child seeks freedom from dependency. He is dependent, and

[17] Harry F. Harlow, "The Nature of Love," *American Psychologist,* Vol. 13, No. 12 (December 1958), p. 676. Lactation refers to the period of milk secretion.

seeks independence, longer than any other creature. His prolonged dependency gives him the time he needs to learn the behavior expected of him by his culture. But this dependency can also produce frustration, insecurity, hate, guilt, anxiety.

The childhood struggle for freedom takes place in a milieu of love and hate. He loves the breast that gratifies him; he hates it when it frustrates him. He loves his parents when they comfort him; he hates them when they control him. This love-hate ambivalence is carried into later years. It is a major cause of anxiety. The frustrations of dependency continue, as hostility, into adulthood. The adult loves his child. He hates his child. He loves his mate. He hates his mate. This emotional paradox is not peculiar to modern man. Twenty centuries ago the Roman lyric poet Catullus wrote these perplexed lines:

> At once I love and hate
> You ask why this should be,
> I know not, 'tis my fate
> A fate of Agony![18]

When the normality of this ambivalence is recognized, man will not be so governed by the anxiety it creates. The paths to independence are obstructed by parent–child conflict. But the child will travel those paths nevertheless. The loving parent can help. Should help not come, the child will struggle on alone, unaided. Should the parent impede the child in the normal quest for independence, the child will retaliate with hate, and suffer guilt and anxiety because of it. All normal people have dependent needs. Yet a degree of independence is essential for maturity.

During each stage of personality development, the normal child will collect problems. Usually he learns from them. They do not necessarily become serious impedimenta. Problems vary. Should the heart form imperfectly and leak, it will, nonetheless, beat as long as possible. Should a child's oral needs in the first year be thwarted too often, those needs may well be manifested in later life by constant emotional overeating. But the child will, to repeat, develop nonetheless. Well equipped or not, he will seek competence and independence. This, then, the wise parent will accept.

As he strives for independence, the developing child needs to understand discipline, not continuously suffer from it. The more the child clearly comprehends what his parents expect of him, and why, the less will he need discipline and the less will he suffer when disciplined. The mother who literally screams her emotional responses to a child's behavior is more successful, at least in this respect, than the parent who is sanctimoniously silent and ends by being mysterious. Mysterious parents frighten their children. There may be room for mystery in love of God or love between the sexes. There is no room for it in parent-child love. A child who never really knows how a parent feels has problems with discipline.

One day, the little girl pulls the pots and pans from the cupboard. She is

[18] "Ode LXXXV," quoted from *Catullus,* tr. into English verse by T. Hart-Davies (London, 1879), p. 122.

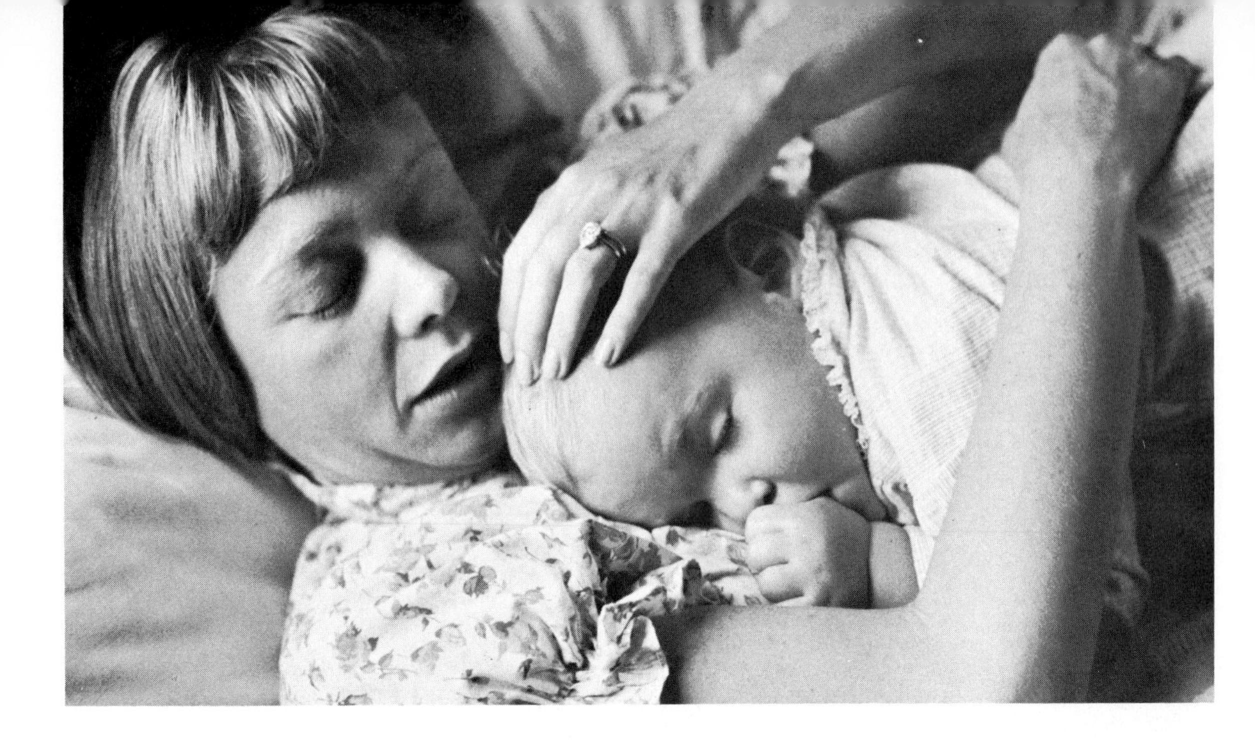

12-3 mother love and maternal deprivation

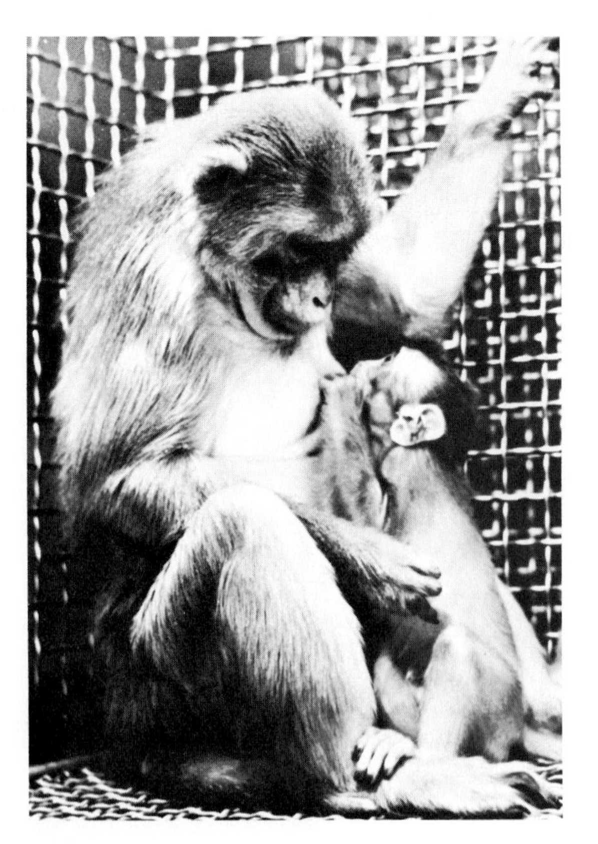

The monkey infant–mother intimacy is a mutual fulfillment (left). *The mother monkey in the photograph below was herself raised with a cloth substitute ''mother.'' She developed abnormally and rejects her infant. Not only food but also cuddling and warmth are the infant's first needs. The normal mother reciprocates by cradling, grooming, caressing, and protecting her baby.*

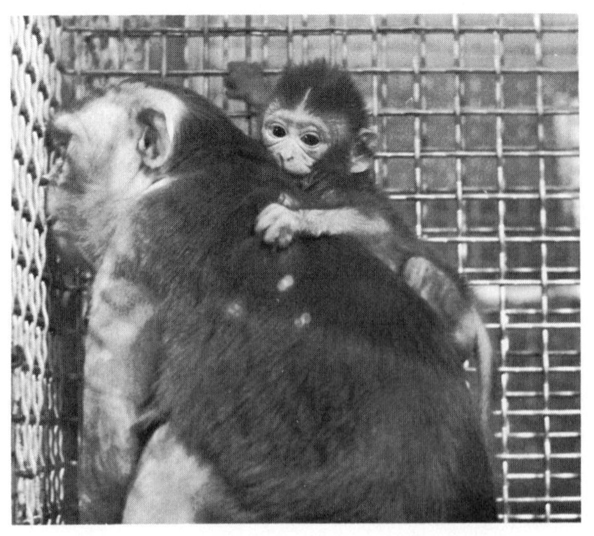

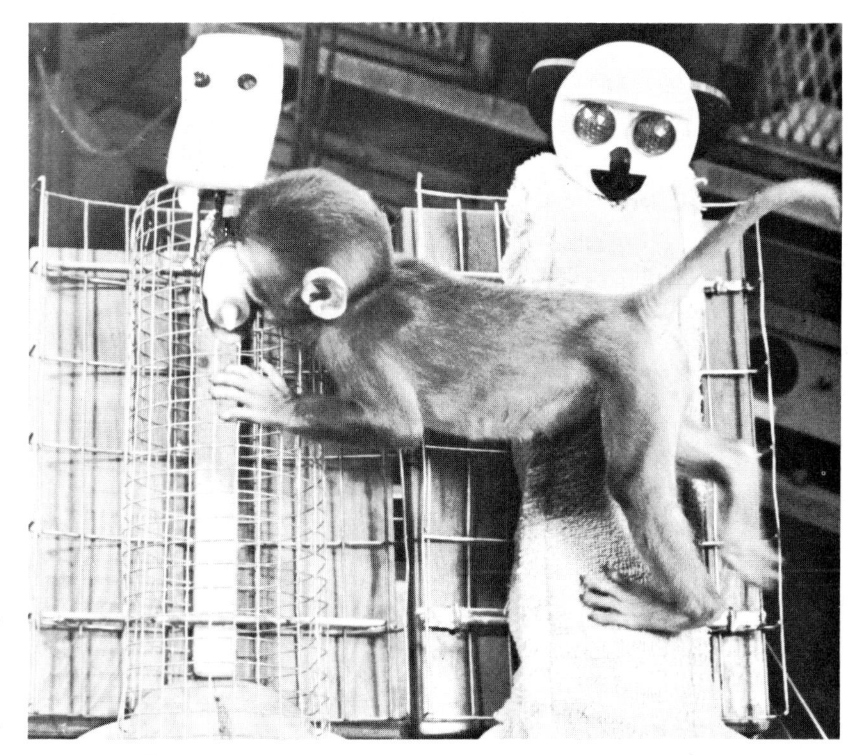

Like the human baby, the infant monkey needs to dine, not just eat. Here, a young monkey clings to the soft, terry-cloth-covered "mother," holding on to it even when feeding from a milk bottle affixed to a plain wire "mother."

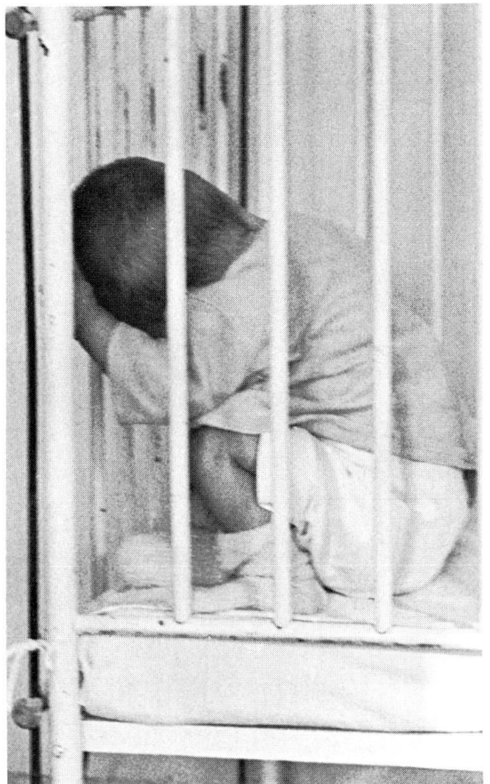

Abandoned and placed in an institution, the Greek child shown at left turned his back on the world. Rejected, he rejects. The depression, immobility, and withdrawal of many children suffering maternal and other deprivations may be worsened by insomnia, loss of appetite, loss of weight, and other grave manifestations.

Like the Greek child, the baby monkey shown below was denied normal contact with mother and peers. Overwhelmed by his sense of abandonment, the monkey infant, no less than the human, shuts out the world.

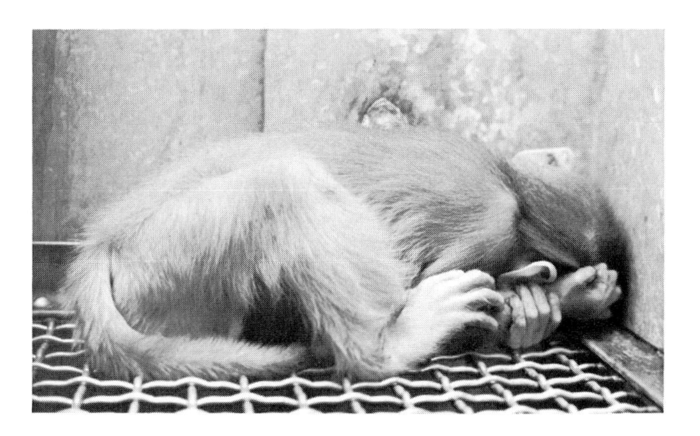

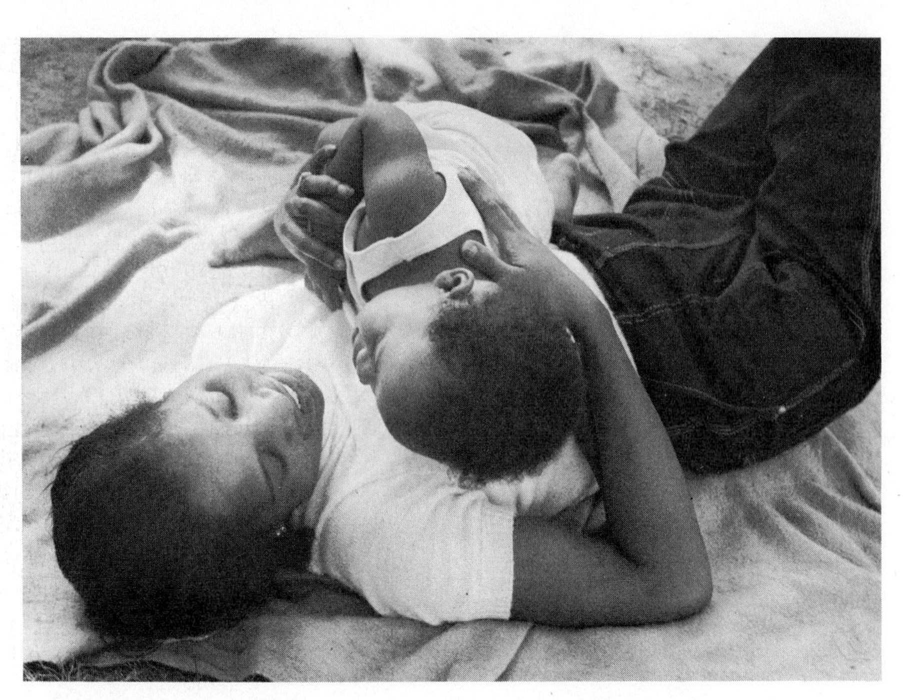

12-4 *The nonmysterious parent.*

kissed and told she is cute. The next day, repeating the same performance, she turns happily to her mother. But a previous marital tiff has angered the mother. The child is scolded and spanked. The child is hurt, not corrected. One day the father answers his little girl's proposal of marriage with "Sure, honey, aren't you my best girl?" (a lying answer to an honest question). The next week, the little girl repeats her proposal. It is met with cold indifference or even harsh hostility (adding injury to error). Or a little girl, living with her divorced mother, must listen to a constant rehearsal of her father's faults. From her father there is nothing but tenderness. She is confused, then angry. The mother retaliates with discipline. The child retaliates with sullen obedience. Children are not miniature adults. They do not spring into adulthood. They do not develop suddenly after a long quiescence. Neither do their anxieties. They need constancy, not confusion. That is why children love peek-a-boo games. That is why they never tire of hearing the same bedtime story. They know what will happen. They can count on it. Discipline of children works best when it arises from constant love, not intermittent hate.

The Oedipal phase in early childhood development demands the utmost of parental sensitivity. To its subtleties attention is now directed.

of Oedipal complexity

Recently, a young man of twenty-two visited a psychiatrist. His chief complaint was that he feared to be alone. Whenever he was by himself, he would become aware of a "creeping" uneasiness. Then slowly terror welled up in him and spread through him "like a stain." He quickly volunteered that he had, for two years, been engaged in homosexual behavior.[19] At present, he was unable to

[19] For a further discussion of homosexual behavior, see Chapter 11, pages 305–10.

relate well to women. But it was not the sexual orientation that disturbed him. It was the loneliness.

Months of psychoanalysis passed. Finally the following story was pieced together. At five, he had worshipped his mother. Now he described her dispassionately. She had been a graceful, beautiful woman, almost childlike. She was fond of picking him up and stroking his hair until he fell asleep. His father was stern and gruff. Sometimes he would grumble, ''Be a big boy. Get off your mother's lap.'' His mother would blush and kiss the child or smooth his hair.

Early one morning his father was ill. The young man remembered every stark detail—the ashen face, the rasping breath, the ambulance, the small clot of onlookers, his own fleeting fright. His mother was inconsolable. All that day she wept. That night he crawled into her bed. ''Don't worry, mommie,'' he said. ''I'll be here and keep care of you. He will die. He'll never come back.'' She slapped him so hard he became confused. She hit him again and again. Then she sent him to his room. In his room he heard her raging at him. Four days later, at his father's funeral, his mother barely spoke to him.

From a five-year-old's normal emotion, an abnormal situation had resulted. The child's guilt about wanting to rid himself of his father (a normal desire at that stage) was heightened by both his mother's immature coquetry and his father's disapproval. He was later unable to identify with a father he had never learned to admire. The father's illness intensified the boy's anxiety. But it was the mother's violent renunciation of him that tore him loose from his most urgently needed moorings.

She might have told him the simple truth: she needed both him and his father. Instead, she lost them both. Instead, she sent the boy to a lonely room from which he never emerged.[20]

masturbation

At about two or three, a normal child explores and stimulates his genitalia. He thereby initiates pleasure in himself and perhaps anxiety in his parents. The parental anxiety originates in conditioning and culture.

The stigma attached to masturbation has ancient beginnings. Early Hebrews and Christians believed children should be seen and sexless. In that period of constant external threat to both groups, it was thought necessary to forbid any practice that might become an internal threat. To strengthen the authority of the family and community, practical controls by adults, including strict sexual repression of the young, were thus deemed essential. During the Dark Ages, fear of disease was added to sin as a deterrent to masturbation. This medieval attitude died slowly. On August 10, 1897, Michael McCormick of San Francisco was granted patent number 587,994 for a male chastity belt. Fathers were to fit them on their adolescent sons to keep them from masturbating. This at least was some improvement over a device used in Victorian times, a padlocked metal cage that was fitted over a boy's genitals at bedtime. To make certain that he did not disturb himself while resting, the cage was outfitted with sharp spikes. In those days the young were led to believe that masturbation

[20] Problems with parents are by no means the only cause of homosexuality. However, in this authentic case there was a definite relationship.

would visit upon them every malady from sterility to stuttering. Even today, there are unfortunates who believe this. Others, who are fully aware that masturbation does not cause disease, still feel ashamed of masturbating. Thus, an aura of anxiety envelops practically all the males and more than half the females in this culture.

''Don't do that!'' This admonition, punctuated with a sharp slap, too often is the two-year-old's introduction to his parent's lack of normal sexual development. The child is taught a crippling lesson: part of him is bad. What is worse, it is a part that feels good. He may never unlearn this. Faced with the catastrophe of losing parental love, he learns early that masturbation is one pleasure that he must enjoy in guilty loneliness. At age two, that is a harsh discovery, especially since he loves his parent with all his dependent heart.

Perhaps he forgets a previous warning. Then he may hear: ''If you don't stop playing with it, I'll cut it off!'' All along the male toddler had fearfully suspected this possibility. Repressed into the unconscious is the child's fear of castration. Years later it will rise, cloaked in anxiety.

The little girl wonders about her absent penis. With a mournful feeling of guilt she remembers her self-manipulation. Did she do something to herself that caused her to lose her penis? Perhaps her parents are punishing her? Unable to dwell on her castration anxiety, she represses it. (It is well to clearly understand that the castration complex can occur without any parental statement or action.) Nevertheless, in the adult woman, this repressed guilt is a common cause of an anxiety neurosis.

The parents who are aware of these possibilities may become overly conscious of them. They are excruciatingly careful not to disturb their child during genital manipulations. There is no reason for this extreme response. A child should be interrupted if his diaper needs changing or for any other sensible reason. Some three- or four-year-olds masturbate publicly. They should be firmly but gently told not to do this. A parent's instruction is better than a stranger's taunt. Ginott writes that parents can help by

> so involving the infant with . . . love, and the child with . . . affection and interest in the outside world, that self-gratification will not remain his only means of satisfaction. The child's main satisfactions should come from personal relationships and achievements. When this is so, occasional self-gratification is not a problem. It is just an additional solution.[21]

Secrecy about sexuality is not conducive to emotional serenity. Many an adolescent girl wants to know about menstruation and pregnancy and delivery, and she wants to know if sexual intercourse hurts. If she sees a magazine double-page spread of children with fins instead of arms, she wants to know all about that, too. She wants to know what kind of sexual activity boys have. And she should know that at least half of all girls masturbate.

Before ''wet dreams'' happen, the boy should know about these entirely normal nocturnal emissions; he will then realize that they are not dirty. Many

[21] Haim G. Ginott, *Between Parent and Child* (New York, 1965), pp. 161–62.

authorities suggest that, for the boy, sex and love are quite unrelated. Unlike the girl, he usually does not romanticize his sexual tensions. Almost all normal adolescent boys (over 95 percent) masturbate. The frequency varies from once or twice to several dozen times a month. This the boy needs to know, and he should be told. The realization that virtually all boys masturbate at his age dilutes his sense of guilt.

The senseless guilt and anxiety to which adolescents have been subjected because of masturbation has abated somewhat. There is considerable agreement among psychiatrists that masturbation is a normal and even valuable transition to mature sexual relations. One thing is certain. In this culture, no other activity indulged in by over 95 percent of all males and 50 percent of females is considered abnormal.

The best answer lies in the Greek ideal of moderation. Boys or girls who masturbate privately and without guilt or a sense of moral unworthiness will be able to give the best of themselves to a mate. Since they look upon themselves as people of worth, and they give something valuable and good.

Those who find in masturbation their only source of gratification and consolation need help. But so does any disturbed person obsessed with one activity to the virtual exclusion of all else in a rich and varied world. From the point of view of body function, however, there is no scientific evidence whatsoever that masturbation can be excessively frequent.

teen-age anxiety

> Each youth sustains within his breast
> a vague and infinite unrest.
> He goes about in still alarm,
> With shrouded future at his arm,
> With longings that can find no tongue.
> I see him thus, for I am young.[22]

Today's teen-age culture is a phenomenon of the wealthy society. True, a lot of teen-agers do not have much money. For many, the only source is an impoverished parent. Other teen-agers marry early. A large number must shoulder other responsibilities, possibly prematurely. In the sodden swamps of Asia there are no pampered teen-agers. Nonetheless, a significant share of this nation's economy depends on this powerfully monied leisure class. Without the money the teen-ager spends on movies, records, cosmetics, clothes, cigarettes, and second-hand cars, business would be sorely shaken. Madison Avenue flatters, cajoles, and caters to the teen-ager. Adults criticize him. Along all the remnant Main Streets of the nation, grown-ups at home, school, and church collectively wag a reproving finger at him. This is not a new phenomenon. Consider, for example, this impatient view written some sixteen hundred years ago:

[22] An Oklahoma high school boy, quoted in Evelyn Millis Duvall, *Family Development,* 2nd ed. (Philadelphia, 1962), p. 297.

> A youth approached me. He was bearded; his clothes were dirty; he wore a student's cloak and he looked a typical New Cynic of the sort I deplore. I have recently written at considerable length about these vagabonds. In the last few years the philosophy of Crates and Zeno has been taken over by idlers who, though they have no interest in philosophy, deliberately imitate the Cynics in such externals as not cutting their hair or beards, carrying sticks and wallets, and begging. But where the original Cynics despised wealth, sought virtue, questioned all things in order to find what was true, these imitators mock all things, including the true, using the mask of philosophy to disguise license and irresponsibility. Nowadays, any young man who does not choose to study or to work grows a beard, insults the gods, and calls himself Cynic.[23]

How long will it take today's teen-ager to straighten out? the modern elders wonder worriedly. By straighten out, they mean, of course, be more like themselves.

The adult desire for self-perpetuation is natural. The Indian poet-philosopher Tagore wrote that "we must not forget that life is here to express the eternal in us."[24] But if the child is truly to meet the parental need for the eternal, if he is to develop the deepest purpose of their lives, his life must have purpose. In the past, the teen-ager made a definite financial contribution to the family. This is generally no longer expected of him. It is not completely true that the teen-ager today has a different set of values than adults. His values are just less complex. (Sometimes his elders are tinged with envy at what he can "get away with.") Like his elders he simply buys the pleasures he can afford. And many a teen-ager mimics the adults he knows. He is out for the bigger, the better, and that ultimate measure of having made it—the most.

But the same things trouble the teen-ager that used to nag his parents. Who am I? What am I? What will become of me? "Be yourself, Debbie," one kindly parent advised his adolescent. "How can I," came her answer, "until I find out who I am?" And hers is not the best age for waiting. Only too keenly does the teen-ager understand the penetrating cowboy laconism: "I ain't what I ought to be, I ain't what I'm going to be, but I ain't what I was."[25]

12-5 *A fortunate adolescent.*

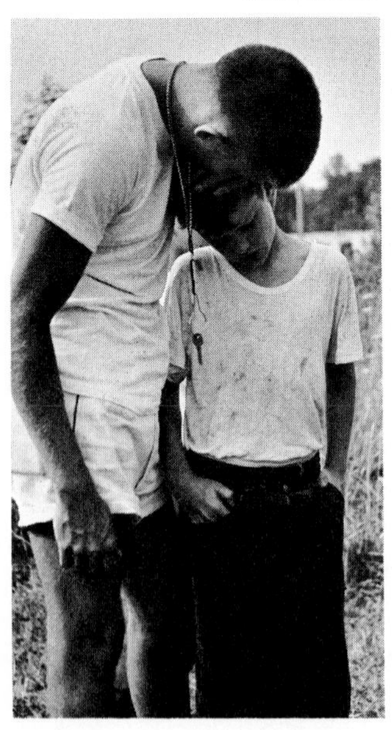

Not often does the adolescent of this culture gain confidence from his elders. In France, for example, a young girl is expected to come to her wedding breakfast transformed overnight from innocent ignorance to mature womanhood. In this country, the girl may hear on one day, "Stay away from those boys," and on the next day, "Why don't you get married?" Too often there is no apprenticeship to adulthood.

In some cultures, the adolescent is given careful preparation for whatever is expected of him as an adult in the community. The ritualistic puberty rites of many African tribal children marks their initiation into the responsibilities of adulthood.[26] "In view of the sudden switch-over, there is, in practice, no defin-

[23] From the memoirs of the Emperor Julian, Vidal's version, cited in "History Repeats," an editorial in *Perspectives in Biology and Medicine,* Vol. 12, No. 3 (Spring 1969), p. 331.

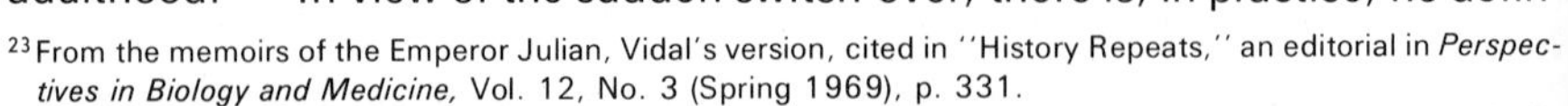

[24] Rabindranath Tagore, "The World of Personality," in Clark E. Moustakas, ed., *The Self* (New York, 1956), p. 82.

[25] Erik H. Erikson, *Childhood and Society,* p. 219.

[26] After circumcision certain African boys understand they are expected to behave like men. The discontinuance of this rite with some African adolescents is thought, by many natives, to be associated with an increase in antisocial behavior. (Laura Longmore, *The Dispossessed* [London, 1959], p. 182.)

able period of 'adolescence' in the traditional African culture.''[27]

Often, however, the adolescent of this culture is on his own. How can he find himself? How can he prevent what Erikson has termed ''self-diffusion''?

In the startling changes of his body, there is no remembered and reassuring sameness—only ungovernable, even unsightly change. In his newly overwhelming feelings he finds fatigue and worry. With the sharp and cruel insight of his age, he perceives the frailties of his elders. Must he seek a place in a society in which he has no growing faith? All is anxiety.

The fortunate adolescent will meet an adult who can listen and who faces both adolescent and adult problems squarely. Such an adult will have learned that love means knowing and being known by another person. Such an adult will help prepare the young person for the dignity of adult intimacy. But finding such an adult is not easy.

where can a person find a person?

''Young men mend not their sight by using old men's spectacles; and yet we look upon Nature but with Aristotle's spectacles, and upon the body of man but with Galen's and upon the frame of the world with Ptolemie's spectacles.''[28] Thus did John Donne, almost 350 years ago, criticize his contemporaries for over-reliance upon those who preceded them. His was an ancient concern and it is a modern one too. However, today's youth has a communication problem. He needs to talk to an older person who sees the past, but not through outworn spectacles.

As ever before, an overwhelming welter of rapid changes besets the modern student. And, as John Donne so clearly saw, yesterday's answers do not always fit today's questions. What is right? What is wrong? Tomorrow is unpredictable, uncontrollable, undependable. Why plan? All this and more must be talked over with somebody. Every place is a crowd. Where can a person find a person to talk to? At home? For some, home is too far away. For others, there is nobody home. Still others have no home. In the church? Too often one goes to church out of habit, not because one really wants to go. Teachers? Some teachers look like listeners. But there is a long line there too. The search for a willing adult ear often ends in forlorn failure.

Adults today must hear and heed these words of Socrates: ''Citizens of Athens, why is it that you turn and scrape every stone to gather wealth and neglect your children to whom, one day, you must relinquish it all?'' If the citizens of Athens heard Socrates, they paid him no mind. Their institutions crumbled. Today's institutions are also shaken. Will they, too, be destroyed in the fires of dispute? Perhaps this next section will suggest some answers. It begins with an extraordinary staff meeting at a famous eastern hospital.[29]

[27] T. A. Lambo, ''Adolescents Transplanted from Their Traditional Environment: Problems and Lessons Out of Africa,'' *Clinical Pediatrics,* Vol. 6, No. 7 (July 1967), p. 439. When the adolescent is transplanted from his rural to an urban environment, however, drug addiction, prostitution, and other delinquency may result.

[28] John Donne, ''Sermon LXXX,'' in John Hayward, ed., *Complete Poetry and Selected Prose* (London, 1930), p. 672.

[29] The incident at the Adolescent and Latency In-Patient Service of Jacobi Hospital, Bronx, Municipal Hospital Center, New York City, is described in a paper by Donald J. Marcuse, ''The 'Army' Incident: The Psychology of Uniforms and Their Abolition on an Adolescent Ward,'' *Psychiatry: A Journal for the Study of Interpersonal Processes,* Vol. 30, No. 4 (November 1967), pp. 350–75.

they found a home in the army

That particular meeting would be long remembered. And looking back, even those with the deepest misgivings realized that they could not have foretold all that would happen. Present this time had been almost all the staff of the adolescent ward of Jacobi Hospital in the Bronx. At best their job was never easy: to help some two dozen eight- to eighteen-year-olds with serious emotional problems. Some routine was often a welcome ally. Change was scrutinized. So the decision to abandon nurses' and aides' uniforms in favor of street clothes could not have been made casually. Almost the whole meeting had been given over to the new proposal. A host of insecurities had surfaced: anxiety about losing status, job identification, lines of authority, controls over patients and one another. At last it had been agreed to try the no-uniform policy for three months.

At a second meeting the young patients were told of the plan. Like the staff, the children were anxious. But their reasons were different. Impostors would come to care for them. Or nobody would. If the uniforms left, so would the nurses. One small boy, a possible runaway, cried worriedly, "The nurses will escape!" Carefully, gently, the basic reason for the change was explained. The atmosphere would be more relaxed. New patients would perhaps feel more comfortable. Nobody made the mistake of saying that the change would make the hospital more like home. Finally, one adolescent wanted to know why. If street clothes were so much better than uniforms, if they made for such better feelings between everybody, why had the change been so long delayed? Nothing can terminate a conversation between an adult and a child so abruptly as a child's penetrating question. This was no exception. The meeting quickly ended.

As with most carefully planned insurrections, there followed a seemingly uneventful period. It lasted six days. Then the adolescent army appeared. It was complete with insignia of rank proclaimed in Magic Marker on pajamas. All was military. An eleven-year-old girl was corps bugler. Around her neck was a carved wooden instrument. Four of the older boys were officers. As allies, they were no longer afraid of one another. There were privates, corporals, and WACs. The disturbed daughter of an army colonel, a pretty and flirtatious girl of sixteen, was the general of the children's army. Accustomed to command, she merely transferred her powers to the military. Armaments (wooden guns) had been manufactured in the occupational therapy shop. The army

> appeared to meet every patient's most acutely felt needs and to solve each one's currently most distressing problems. Depressions lifted. Rivalries waned. Aggression became so bound up in the organization that no one appeared frightened of his own or his fellows' impulses. Individual sexual conflicts were so ingeniously . . . incorporated into the matrix of military roles . . . that they went unnoticed . . . Never were the lines of authority clearer. Never had the dependent and infantile felt better cared for, or the fearful more protected, or the rejected more valued. No one was lonely. Everyone had a vital role and an unmistakable identity. No invading impostors were to be feared. Anyone who craved structure found all he could use. Ambiguities ceased. The vanished uniforms had been restored, as if

to demonstrate their value and function to anyone who had not yet gotten the message . . . The only hitch was that this marvel of a device left out the staff.[30]

And the staff did not accept this lightly.

> Despite its formidable accomplishments the insurgent army was greeted by the now ununiformed staff . . . with distinct displeasure, with dismay and consternation. It was a revolution. The tables were turned . . . Considering how little the army did that was actually disruptive, the near pandemonium that ensued among the staff bears testimony to the extent of their own emotional involvement.[31]

What had actually happened? To both the sick children and some of the staff members responsible for their care, a change in clothing that was emblematic of their institution, authority, codes, or values was threatening. To some extent, their anxiety depended on whether they saw themselves as the sort of people who control others or who accept controls. In varying degrees, all did both. Both staff and patients needed both. Impressed by reported successes of similar clothing changes elsewhere, the staff had agreed to try to adjust to the change. Too, they, unlike the children, clearly understood that loss of uniforms entailed no real loss of those stable elements in their lives that gave them security. Finally, the staff members were free to leave the ward. Their anxieties could be relieved. The sick children had had no such advantages. Poignantly, they too had sought to adjust. They had met the threat to themselves with a threat to others. A usual reaction. A not unusual result.

The children's army reflected in miniature a well-known human reaction. For whole nations do no less than did these emotionally sick youngsters. Whether the threat is real or imagined matters little. Temporarily, at least, martial law establishes authority, security, purpose, direction. But the formation of the children's army excluded the possibility of treatment and cure. It was the order of the desert, not of hope. This the sick children could not see. And it is this that today's mature young student sees only too well. He needs hope within order. Clearly, he understands that "the art of progress is to preserve order amid change and to preserve change amid order."[32]

But he also sees that, too often, nations are like sick children. Why? Why are nations armed camps? In a biology class he learns that even animals that are instinctively hostile to one another can learn to live peacefully together. In an English class he is told of Stephen Crane, the great war novelist who wrote that "the essence of life is war." Bewildered, searching, he turns to the writings of his father's time. In the lyric prose of Thomas Wolfe, one of the celebrated spokesmen of his parents' generation, he reads this:

> War is not death to young men; war is life. The earth had never worn raiment of such color as it did that year. The war seemed to unearth pockets of ore that had never been known in the nation: there was a vast unfolding and exposure

[30] *Ibid.*, p. 362.
[31] *Ibid.*, p. 364.
[32] Alfred North Whitehead, quoted in *Saturday Review* (March 2, 1968), p. 19.

of wealth and power. And somehow—this imperial wealth, this display of power in men and money, was blended into a lyrical music. In Eugene's mind, wealth and love and glory melted into a symphonic noise; the age of myth and miracle had come upon the world again. All things were possible.[33]

And later Wolfe continued:

> With a tender smile of love for his dear self, he saw himself wearing the eagles of a colonel on his gallant young shoulders . . . For the first time he saw the romantic charm of mutilation . . . He longed for that subtle distinction, that air of having lived and suffered that could only be attained by a wooden leg, a rebuilt nose, or the seared scar of a bullet across his temple.[34]

The modern student, reading this, begins to reject the past. He feels a part of a "new race" well described by Emerson a century ago: "There is a universal resistance to ties and ligaments once supposed essential to civilized society. The new race is stiff, heady, and rebellious; they are fanatics in freedom; they hate tolls, taxes, turnpikes, banks, hierarchies, governors, yea, almost laws."

So some students reject the past. All of it. To them, no past values fit the present scene. And since the past is gone, there is no future. What matters is the present. "The most striking change in student value systems is in the direction of values which lead to immediate gratification."[35]

To treat the severely alienated student, the psychiatrist often must start by interviewing the parents in the student's presence. One reason for this is that "the family interview . . . reminds the student that he does have a past and that the past continues to exert an important influence upon his present life."[36] Such a patient is often required to "commit himself to a six-month period of therapy. This emphasizes the existence of a future."[37]

Man need not be retarded by the past nor be worshipful of it. But he does need to understand it. Then he might see, for example, the need for both peace and national defense. The past helps to teach what is solid earth and what is shifting sand. As Eiseley has written,

> Man's story, in brief, is essentially that of a creature who has abandoned instinct and replaced it with cultural tradition and the hardwon increments of contemplative thought. The lessons of the past have been found to be a reasonably secure instruction for proceeding against the unknown future. To hurl oneself recklessly, without method, upon a future that we ourselves have complicated is a sheer nihilistic rejection of all that history, including the classical world, can teach us.[38]

[33] Thomas Wolfe, *Look Homeward, Angel* (New York, 1929), pp. 508–09.
[34] *Ibid.*, p. 533.
[35] Seymour L. Halleck, "Why They'd Rather Do Their Own Thing," *Think*, Vol. 34, No. 5 (September–October 1968), p. 3. How strikingly similar are the emotional states of such college students to those of some small ghetto children beginning school. One school superintendent writes: "A victim of his environment, the ghetto child begins his school career psychologically, socially, and physically disadvantaged. He is oriented to the present rather than the future, to immediate needs rather than delayed gratification, to the concrete rather than the abstract." (Carl J. Dolce, "The Inner City—A Superintendent's View," *Saturday Review* [January 11, 1969], p. 36.)
[36] Seymour L. Halleck, "Psychiatric Treatment of the Alienated College Student," *American Journal of Psychiatry*, Vol. 125, No. 5 (November 1967), p. 103.
[37] *Ibid.*, p. 102.
[38] Loren Eiseley, *The Unexpected Universe*, quoted in *Science*, Vol. 165, No. 3889 (July 11, 1969), p. 129.

So one cannot disregard past institutions, codes, and values. It does not matter whether their symbol is a nurse's uniform, a wedding ring, or a sergeant's stripes. It does matter how a human need for order is met. Institutions, codes, and values need constant, careful reappraisal. Some need changing. Others need to be discarded and, to avoid chaos, replaced by other institutions, codes, and values. In itself, mere rejection of a value is not a value. And mankind cannot do without values.

This much, at least, the emotionally sick children in the Jacobi adolescent ward understood.

Turmoil in a community can arise only from the inner, emotional disorders of its members. The agony of an utter inner chaos, the seemingly total rejection of one's personal worth, provides the subject for the next discussion.

a cry for attention

> Tom sulked in a corner and exalted his woes . . . he pictured himself brought home from the river, dead, with his curls all wet and his sore heart at rest. How she would throw herself upon him, and how her tears would fall like rain, and her lips pray God to give her back her boy, and she would never, never abuse him anymore! But he would lie there cold and white and make no sign—a poor little sufferer whose griefs were at an end.[39]

It is interesting to note that Tom Sawyer (Mark Twain's typical American boy) often envisions his own death.[40] The above passage reflects Tom's response to his Aunt Polly's misunderstanding of him. A short while later Tom reflects in this way about the girl he loves: "She would be sorry someday, maybe when it was too late. Ah, if he could only die *temporarily!*"[41] Later still, Tom, hidden under the bed, watches his aunt weep over his supposed death. In a spasm of self-pity, he even weeps with her. And, as this great story of American boyhood reaches its climax, Tom sees his own funeral services: "at last the whole company broke down . . . in a chorus of anguished sobs, the preacher himself giving way to his feelings and crying in the pulpit."[42]

All this in the gentle, happy summer of boyhood. Yet the novel is among the most beloved of all literature. Why? Because Tom Sawyer's emotions are universally understood. By dreaming of dying, perhaps even by his own hand, the child wreaks the sufferings of guilt on the more powerful. Thus, he avenges his helplessness. A Japanese used to accomplish this by committing hari-kari on the doorstep of his tormentor for all the neighbors to see. He differed in method (though not in basic reasons) from many a Western suicide today.

There are no simple reasons for suicide. Sociological, cultural, physical, psychological—these are among the factors involved. More than 24,000

[39] Mark Twain, *The Adventures of Tom Sawyer* (New York, 1950), pp. 23–24.
[40] It may be similarly significant that, as a boy, Mark Twain deliberately exposed himself to smallpox "to get it over with." He almost perished from the disease.
[41] Mark Twain, *The Adventures of Tom Sawyer,* p. 69.
[42] *Ibid.,* p. 143.

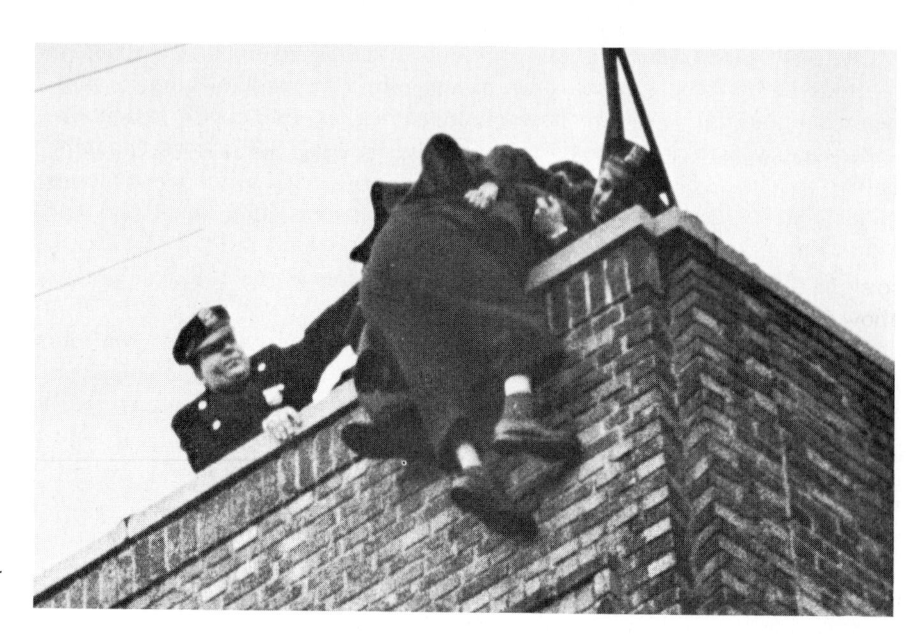

12-6 *A cry for attention—answered.*

people in this country killed themselves in 1972, and an estimated 100,000 to 150,000 tried unsuccessfully to commit suicide. Why "estimated"? Because in this culture suicide is still somewhat taboo and thus is underreported as a cause of death. Rarely is suicide sanctioned. One exception: U.S. U-2 pilots carried with them the means to kill themselves should they be captured. Another example of sanctioned suicide: "In the battle for Khe Sahn, South Vietnam, a young [American] lieutenant fell wounded. As his comrades rushed forward through enemy fire, he waved them back and killed himself with a shot through the head to avoid capture. Preserving the welfare of his unit, he died a hero and it is of note that the newspaper account nowhere referred to his death as a suicide."[43]

Much has been made of the statistic that suicides are the second or third leading cause of death on college campuses. Without underestimating the problem, it should be understood that suicide and other violent deaths (as well as chronic diseases) have become relatively more important because of successes in the control of communicable disease. Nevertheless, suicide is a significant campus problem. It has been estimated that, nationwide, 1,000 students make serious attempts at suicide every year. About 250 succeed.[44] The most important difference between students who kill themselves (or try to) and those who do not, is that the suicidal student is socially isolated. In one tragic case, a student was dead for eighteen days in his room before he was found. Nobody had seemed to know or care that he was missing. Although married people commit suicide less often than single people, there is a paradoxical exception—the married teen-ager. Suspected reasons for this are the stresses

[43] Russel Noyes, Jr., "Shall We Prevent Suicide?" *Comprehensive Psychiatry,* Vol. 11, No. 4 (July 1970), p. 237.

[44] William A. Sievert, "Campus Suicides," *Saturday Review of Education,* Vol. 1, No. 3 (March 10, 1973), p. 55.

inherent in too-early marriage; perhaps many teen-aged people marry to escape an unhappy home. Suicidal students, moreover, usually have a history of emotional disorders; they have a much greater involvement with psychotherapy and have been more often hospitalized for emotional illness. It should be emphasized that suicidal individuals almost always give frequent warnings of their intentions. They should never be ignored.[45]

Do poor grades play a role in student suicides? If they do, it is not nearly so significant as the role played by good grades. Suicidal students perform well above the average, but they often consider themselves frauds. Judging their academic achievements to be phony, they underrate themselves. And U.S. student suicides occur most often not during final exam week, but during the early weeks of the semester. In Japan, however, where suicide leads all other causes of death among those under thirty, academic competition and failure are believed to be a major cause. A major factor associated with student suicides in both the United States and Japan is the early death or absence of a parent.

Suicide among blacks is increasing. Indeed, in some areas, the nonwhite suicide rate has been greater than that of the white for many years. Black suicide is made more tragic by the fact that it occurs most frequently among the young. The main reasons for the increased rate are the stresses of urbanization, enforced unemployment, the absence of fathers, the continued denial of true integration into the larger society, and constant trouble with the police and the courts.[46] One student of suicide, noting the increase of suicide among women in California (from 10 per 100,000 in 1960 to 14.2 in 1970—a 42 percent increase), suggests that women's "drive for success and recognition has increased pressures and opened more possibilities for failure. In precisely those areas where liberated women are making the most progress, the male–female suicide ratio moves towards 'equality.'"[47]

It has been written that suicides among teen-aged U.S. Indians have "shocked investigators." However, the shock could hardly have been one of surprise. In the small Indian community at Fort Hall, Idaho, for example, one study revealed that in a seven-year period (1960–67) the suicide rate was about ten times the national average. Almost half of the suicides were twenty years old or younger. Fort Hall has no high school, no recreation centers, and no jail, and is far from urban areas. Housing is abysmal. Technically, the Indians own the land; but in 1970 the Bureau of Indian Affairs was renting it to white farmers for almost nothing. The unemployment rate among the Indians was ten times the national rate; many families subsisted on incomes as low as $500 a

[45] Richard H. Seiden, "The Problem of Suicide on College Campuses," *The Journal of School Health,* Vol. 41, No. 5 (May 1971), p. 245. Much of the material in this discussion of student suicide is from this source; it is highly recommended for further study and examination of its excellent bibliography.

[46] Richard H. Seiden, "Why Are Suicides of Young Blacks Increasing?" *HSMHA Reports,* Vol. 87, No. 1 (January 1972), pp. 3–8. This article is also recommended for its content and bibliography.

[47] "Drugs and Suicide—A Problem on Both Sides of the Atlantic," *Psychology Today,* Vol. 7, No. 4 (September 1973), p. 20, citing Nancy Allen, "Suicide in California: 1960–1970," California State Department of Health, 1973. It is of interest to note in this regard that "Chinese men [in San Francisco] committed suicide in the past with four to five times the frequency of Chinese women, but this ratio has gradually changed in the last four years with an increasing incidence of Chinese women committing suicide." (Peter G. Bourne, "Suicide Among Chinese in San Francisco," *American Journal of Public Health,* Vol. 63, No. 8 [August 1973], p. 749.) However, whether this is due to the extra stresses associated with women's liberation is surely open to question.

year. Alcoholism and tuberculosis were rampant. Before one twenty-year-old hanged himself, his mother got her third divorce, his grandmother died, and his sister wrecked his car.[48] Six months later his sister also hanged herself.

In the general U.S. population, the most common suicide takes place on a Monday in the spring when a single or divorced elderly white male Protestant kills himself. In this country, the annual suicide rate among physicians is triple that of the whole population. Suicide is more frequent in urban than in rural areas, and suicide rates vary too from city to city; in San Francisco, for example, the rate is five times that of New York City. Today, of all cities, West Berlin has the worst suicide rates. Political tensions are not necessarily the cause. Suicide rates in that city were high long before the Second World War. Among the twentieth century's highest overall suicide rates are in Austria and Switzerland.

An attempt at suicide is a cry for help. In his play *Death of a Salesman,* Arthur Miller put meaningful words into the dialogue of Linda, the wife of the suicidal salesman. To her self-centered sons she speaks of their father:

> Willy Loman never made a lot of money. His name was never in the paper. He's not the finest character that ever lived. But he's a human being, and a terrible thing is happening to him. So attention must be paid. He's not to be allowed to fall into his grave like an old dog. Attention, attention must be finally paid to such a person . . . A small man can be just as exhausted as a great man.[49]

But, later, Willy commits suicide.

In the great gulf, in the long years, between the normal vengeful dreamings of Tom Sawyer, the boy, and the despairing agony of Willy Loman, the salesman, much happens. But again and again do people like these, who are as one in their loneliness, cry out for the attentions of help and love. If attention is not paid, an American childhood may become an American tragedy. In recognition of this, the American Association of Suicidology was organized on a nonprofit basis. Its purpose: to provide a forum about suicide and its prevention. Also, numerous crises centers have been established; at the University of Colorado, for example, students conduct a twenty-four-hour telephone Rap Line. Using it, distressed students can talk with other students of their own age. Professionally, research is bringing about new techniques to deal with the sense of hopelessness and helplessness felt by the potential suicide.[50] And vigorous efforts are being made to make physicians more aware of the problem.[51]

Human loneliness has many costs. In the next section still another of those costs is considered.

[48] Most of this discussion is from "Indian Teen-Age Suicides Shock Investigators," *Roche Medical Image & Commentary,* Vol. 12, No. 6 (June 1970), pp. 11–13.

[49] Arthur Miller, *Death of a Salesman* (New York, 1949), Act 1.

[50] Frederick T. Melges and Alfred E. Weisz, "The Personal Future and Suicidal Ideation," *Journal of Nervous and Mental Disease,* Vol. 153, No. 4 (1971), pp. 244–50. That suicide prevention centers have reduced the suicide rate in the major cities of the United States has been seriously questioned by one recent study. A comparison was made between the suicide rates in cities with such centers (for the years 1960 and 1968) and those in cities without such centers. The data failed to support the notion that suicide prevention centers significantly reduce the suicide rate. ("Suicide Prevention Centers Don't Reduce Suicide Rate," *AMA Health Education Service,* Vol. 13, No. 8 [October 1973], p. 3.)

[51] "Suicide—A Tragic Toll, but Still a Taboo Topic," *American Medical News,* Vol. 16, No. 49 (December 17, 1973), p. 12.

Sitting up straight in her chair, almost primly, a little defiant, tightly clasping ringless fingers, she tells the social worker her name. She is nineteen and came to town eight months ago. It has been five months since she has menstruated. She is not sure who the father is. And then, suddenly, she begins to cry.

''I don't care,'' she says, ''I hate him anyway.''

Scenes like this are twice as common in this country today as they were twenty years ago. More than 300,000 out-of-wedlock babies were born in the United States in 1970; more than 9 percent of the total number of births.

What do we know about the unwed mother? Who is she? What are some of her problems?

One anxiety of many an unwed mother is in her sense of being unloved. Yet often she cannot love. She may come from an overcoercive home. Perhaps her parents do not respect the person in the girl. Her individual speed and pattern of doing things are faults to be constantly corrected. She is directed and overdirected. Her parents do not realize the significance of this poetic advice:

> You may give them your love but not your thoughts,
> For they have their own thoughts.
> You may house their bodies but not their souls,
> For their souls dwell in the house of tomorrow, which
> you cannot visit, not even in your dreams.
> You may strive to be like them,
> but seek not to make them like you.[52]

Constant coercion causes anxiety in the child. It is met in various ways. The child may dilly-dally, daydream, and develop a fine ''forgettory.'' Or the anxiety may be manifested by rebelliousness. Any parental advice then becomes a tyranny to be ignored. Moreover, the child feels unworthy. She may think everything she does is wrong. She feels rejected. She is thrown back on herself.[53] She loses the ability to give love to others. How can she again risk giving love when the people who mean the most to her, her parents, think her very existence a wrong? Out of rebellion, out of desire to retaliate, or in a desperate search for appreciation, she has sexual intercourse. But this arises from a feeling of rejection, not love.

Other girls are the victims of the opposite extreme. The parents are oversubmissive and overindulgent. No whim of the child is denied. The child is showered with unneeded gifts in such profusion that their meaning is lost. Such a girl is bored. She need consider nobody but herself. A severe anxiety about her health (hypochondriasis) may develop. As an attention-getting mechanism, it is useful. She may, moreover, fix all her expectations on the all-powerful, always sacrificing parents. Her ability to love anyone else is diminished. Even the very thought of loving someone else may be threatening. She is without

[52] Kahlil Gibran, *The Prophet* (New York, 1923), p. 18.
[53] Percival M. Symonds, *The Dynamics of Human Adjustment* (New York, 1946), p. 552.

discipline, without the ability to love, for to love requires discipline. Passion requires compassion. Her doting parents have impoverished her with indulgence.

The disadvantages of the unwed mother are considerably more than emotional. Some are socioeconomic. Others are manifested by an increased risk to health, even to life.

Relatively few unwed mothers give birth in private hospitals. More than 50 percent of unmarried mothers get late or no prenatal care. Eighty percent of married women, on the other hand, receive prenatal care in the first six months of pregnancy. In the first three months of pregnancy, less than 10 percent of unmarried mothers get prenatal care. But almost 50 percent of married mothers get this crucial early care in the first three months.

The poorer care of the unwed mother is apparent in the greater threat to the life of both herself and her child. Eclampsia (a toxic condition of pregnancy, once common) and syphilis are both more frequent in unmarried mothers than in married mothers. Unmarried-mother maternal death rates are over three times higher than those of married mothers. The life of the unmarried white mother is at tragic risk. Her pregnancy ends in her death eight times more often than the married white mother's. Both black and Puerto Rican unmarried mothers have a better chance of surviving pregnancy than the white unmarried mother.[54]

The reasons for this are cultural. Black and Puerto Rican unmarried mothers are generally more accepted by their families. The white unmarried pregnant girl is cruelly cast out of her milieu. Often she cannot share her great burden with those who brought her into the world. She must skulk on the perimeter of society. Former friends shun her. By delaying prenatal care as long as possible, she risks her life.

Compared to the baby of the married mother, the baby of the unmarried mother is twice as likely to be premature, is twice as likely to die in the first month, and is twice as likely to be stillborn.

Maimed by emotional maldevelopment, more than 300,000 young girls of this wealthy country every year experience hazards that alienate them still further. They need help. Their help must start with the education of parents.

Moreover, too often only the plight of the unmarried mother has been considered. Whenever possible, the unmarried father should be helped.[55] The popular idea of the older, uneducated, totally maladjusted seducer is not accurate. In one study, most unmarried fathers were found to have at least a high school education, were but a few years older than the mother, and functioned quite adequately in school or work. Delinquency patterns were not usual. Nor is the relationship between unmarried parents so casual as has often been assumed. On the other hand, both young people may be suffering emotional inadequacies established in childhood. Deferment of personal gratification for the more last-

[54] National Council on Illegitimacy, *Illegitimacy: Data and Findings for Prevention, Treatment and Policy Formulation* (October 1965), pp. 34–36.

[55] Not uncommonly, a man may question or vigorously deny that he is the father of a child. If wrongfully named, paternity blood tests may prove him right. They are not always conclusive. Only about 60 percent of men who are improperly accused may be cleared by paternity tests.

ing satisfactions of societal approval is difficult enough for the mature, let alone the immature. Thus "when neither sexual partner possesses any strong identity, and when neither one is strong in the area of responsibility and maturity, each reinforces the other to satisfy personal needs, with little regard for the consequences of the act."[56]

love versus anxiety

> There is a land of the living and a land of the dead and the bridge is love, the only survival, the only meaning.[57]

Life begins and ends with separation. Both are inevitable. Each has its own poignancy.

There is separation at birth. Filling the gulf is love. Without mothering, without embracing love, the infant suffers. Yet, mothering is not smothering. True mother love teaches further separation. The constancy of the mother's love, even after her child's departure, is mirrored by the child's ability to learn to love others in later life.

As the normally learning child explores his body, he learns the glories of self-love. This self-love is not necessarily selfish. The child was born selfish. He will remain selfish only if he learns to hate himself. But if he learns self-worth, he will love this worthy self. And, by giving of a worthy self, he will be able wholeheartedly to enter into the long learning process of loving others. He must, for example, learn to love his neighbor. Were he born with the ability, he would not have had to be commanded.

But how may the child learn to hate himself? He can be taught that he is evil. He can be told a thousand times that he is naughty, that he is bad, that he should be ashamed of himself. A devaluated child devaluates himself still further. And such a child has been cruelly robbed of life's paramount need—the need to give a worthy love. When it is necessary, the child should be corrected, even punished, briefly and to the point, but never heartlessly. He must never feel unloved.

Love is not lust. Love gives. Lust takes. True, both find expression through coitus. Yet, coitus satiates lust, but continues love. With neither animals nor man is love a prerequisite for coitus. However, the profound need of love is characteristic only of man. Sexual desire may result from loneliness, vanity, a desire to conquer or be conquered, a need for social status, a desire to hurt or destroy someone. Any strong emotion (of which love is but one) can stimulate sexual desire.[58] After that desire is satiated, the individual may experience physiological relief. But the deeply significant mutuality, the need to do for another without direct reward, so characteristic of human love, has evaded him.

[56] Reuben Pannor, Fred Massarik, and Byron W. Evans, *The Unmarried Father,* Final Report, Children's Bureau, Welfare Administration, U.S. Department of Health, Education, and Welfare (February 1967), pp. 230–31.
[57] Thornton Wilder, *The Bridge of San Luis Rey* (New York, 1927), p. 235.
[58] Erich Fromm, *The Art of Loving* (New York 1951), p. 54.

He has given the least of himself. He has not given tenderness nor given up greed. He remains separate, alone.

In Chapter 17 there is some discussion of the techniques of sexual intercourse. These are important. However, the techniques of sexual intercourse do not replace the art of loving. Both may be learned. But, as food without love leaves the infant emotionally starved, so does sexual intercourse without love leave the adult still hungering. Only love can solve the anxiety of separation.

Entering adolescence with self-esteem unshaken, convinced of a wholesome personal value, the young person can further develop the vital enrichments of his humanness. Since he has self-respect, he respects. For a few years, a "best friend" occupies the interest, then members of the opposite sex. In these years, slowly, now clearly, then beclouded, but ever recurring, there comes to the youth a new perception. Love is the art of giving. And part of the art of giving love lies in taking it without exploitation. When he has learned to give and to take love, the young person is ready for adulthood. Prepared to exchange separation for union, he seeks a mate. For, as Plato wrote, "Love is the child of need."

summary

Anxiety may be defined as a feeling of foreboding, a premonition that something evil is about to happen (page 322). Anxiety touches almost every life situation and moves the entire emotional life (page 323). The normal human reaction to anxiety is to realistically appraise the stressful situation and then to take appropriate action to relieve or escape the stress (page 324).

The rapid development of technology has given rise to anxiety in humans about their very ability to survive in the modern world (page 325). But the roles humans play in their private lives are often also sources of anxiety. Many adults, for example, feel anxiety in their role as parents. Women may feel anxious and guilty over the question of breast-feeding (page 326) or working outside the home (pages 329–31). Children can become anxious as a result of maternal deprivation (pages 331–32), the struggle for independence from the parents (pages 332–36), his or her feelings toward the parent of the opposite sex (pages 336–37), and guilt feelings about masturbation (pages 337–39). Teen-agers experience anxiety in their search for identity and self-knowledge (pages 339–41). Two costly manifestations of the hopeless loneliness of severe anxiety are suicide (pages 345–48) and unwed motherhood (pages 349–51). Love is the basic need that, when satisfied, leads to the feeling of self-worth that can ward off the stress of anxiety (pages 351–52).

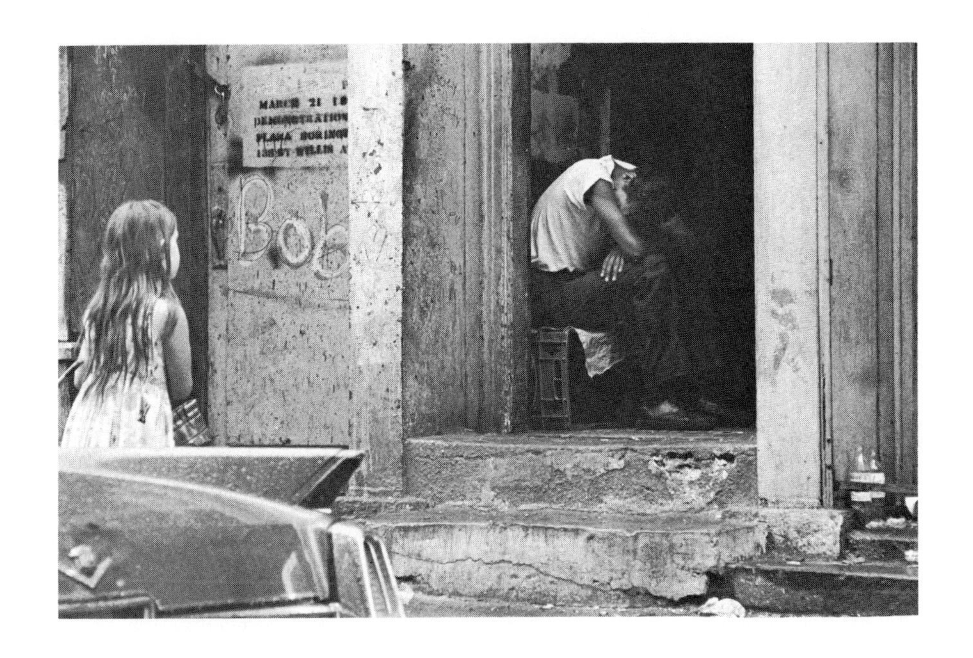

escape into captivity, part 1: older drugs of abuse in the U.S.

13

CLEOPATRA. . . . *Give me to drink mandragora.*
CHARMIAN. *Why, madam?*
CLEOPATRA. *That I might sleep out this great gap of time*
My Antony is away.[1]

Mandragora, or mandrake, may have lent rest to the Egyptian queen; the plant contains sedative properties. Another plant, the deadly nightshade, produces altogether different effects. A few years ago a Riverside, California, professor brewed some and took a large dose of it. His wife became so alarmed by his droll behavior that she called the family physician. In a nearby hospital, a barred-window cell was found for the befuddled pundit. There he was tied hand and foot, spread-eagle, to the bedposts. From this vantage point he could clearly watch the goings-on in his tiny cell. Part of his published report reads as follows:

> Most rooms usually have shuttered air vents situated either near the ceiling or floor. The vent in my cell was located just above the door. To my amazement it began to fill up like a small football stadium with tiered rows of my former students. They were wearing brightly colored berets and horn rimmed colored glasses. Each had a bottle of coke and a bag of popcorn. They single filed into the bleachers, finally filling it to capacity. Now they sat very rigid without appearing to notice my presence. However, when I turned my head as if to look at some other area of the room the scene suddenly became highly animated. As they guzzled their cokes and stuffed popcorn into their mouths they pointed their fingers at me and laughed sardonically. Whenever I focused my eyes on their antics, they suddenly froze and took no notice of me. It is of interest to note that I recognized every face in the group and that I had given each and every one of them the D or F grade in beginning Biology.[2]

"My beloved sweet darling," Sigmund Freud wrote to Martha Bernays almost ninety years ago,

> my tiredness is a sort of minor illness; neurasthenia it is called . . . the bit of cocaine I have just taken is making me talkative . . . Here I am making silly confessions to you, my sweet darling, and really without reason unless it is the cocaine.[3]

Mrs. Margaret Thompson took snuff, as did other London ladies of her day. She died on April 2, 1776, leaving a will that has caused her to be long remembered:

> I, Margaret Thompson, . . . being in sane mind . . . desire that all my handkerchiefs that I may have unwashed at the time of my decease . . . be put . . . at the bottom of my coffin, which I desire may be large enough for that purpose,

[1] William Shakespeare, *Antony and Cleopatra,* I.v.4–6.

[2] Cecil E. Johnson, "Mystical Force of Nightshade," *International Journal of Neuropsychiatry,* Vol. 3, No. 3 (May–June 1967), p. 274.

[3] Ernest L. Freud, ed., *Letters of Sigmund Freud,* Letter No. 94 (New York, 1960), pp. 201–02. This letter was written from Paris on February 2, 1886. Freud had married Martha Bernays in 1884. He died in 1939 at eighty-three. Martha Freud died in 1951 in her ninetieth year.

together with a quantity of the best Scotch snuff . . . as will cover my deceased body.

According to the will, her bearers were to be the six greatest snuff-takers of the parish of St. James, Westminster. Snuff-colored, not black, hats were to be worn. As they went along, six maidens bearing her pall were to take snuff for refreshment. Her servant was "to walk before the corpse, to distribute . . . snuff to the ground and upon the crowd."[4]

She was not the only one to desire interment with her vice. Some years ago in Camembert, France, a man obeyed his wife. He preserved her in the town's best Calvados brandy cider and so buried her. In her memory, he composed this touching rhyme:

Here lies my wife. Her dying wish:
"I think it would be dandy
To be preserved, when comes the end,
Like a ripe plum in brandy."[5]

What is buried in some graves is surprising. What is inscribed on some of the stones marking them is no less startling. Consider this memorial found in a churchyard at Burlington, Massachusetts:

Here lies the body of Susan Lowder
Who burst while drinking a
Sedlitz Powder.
Called from this world
to her heavenly rest,
She should have waited till it
effervesced. 1798[6]

Cleopatra took her drug to ease the pain of separation. The California professor perhaps took his to publish (though he almost perished instead). Freud took cocaine because it stimulated him—maybe to write better love letters. Mrs. Thompson snuffed for sheer pleasure. The French lady willingly left these earthly premises stewing in brandy cider. And poor Susan Lowder probably never revealed why she took a powder.

People have found a variety of purposes for a variety of drugs and have developed profound attachments to some of them. As these attachments are considered in this chapter and the next, the substances that produce depend-

[4] H. V. Morton, *Ghosts of London* (New York, 1940), pp. 33–34.
[5] Lucia Masson, *La Belle France* (New York, 1964), p. 23.
[6] Ann Parker and Aaron Neal, "What a Way To Go!" *Ciba Journal,* No. 39 (1966), pp. 20–29. It may be that this eighteenth-century diagnosis was not incorrect. Seidlitz powder is a laxative that is sold in two separate packets: one contains sodium potassium tartarate with sodium bicarbonate; the second contains tartaric acid. They should be mixed together in cold water. Much of the gas is then given off and the fluid is then drunk while effervescing. One young man swallowed the acid first and followed it with the bicarbonate. All the CO_2 gas was liberated in his stomach. "He afterwards declared that his stomach exploded and that he was thrown against a wall . . ." Emergency surgery revealed "a long tear in the stomach, unassociated with any ulcer." The patient survived. ("Below the Belt," editorial in *The Lancet,* Vol. 11, No. 7718 [July 31, 1971], p. 253, citing "Acute Gastric Distension in Man and Animals," *Proceedings of the Royal Society of Medicine,* Vol. 52 [1959], p. 379.)

ence will be discussed; however, as much attention will be given to those who abuse drugs. Recent years have seen a remarkable increase in the abuse of some drugs in this country. The welter of opinion evaluating this phenomenon has not always been scientifically based. Considerable reliable effort is now being made to rectify this. In appraising the available information, it is well to remember that the effects of a drug may vary from individual to individual, and from time to time with the same individual. (This is particularly true when there is a change in dosage or social setting.)

why drugs?

To this question there is no single answer. Poverty, increased mobility, loosened family ties, the nuclear threat, permissiveness, the information explosion, city tensions, youthful disillusionment, a frustrating war—all have been variously indicted.

Often it is during toddlerhood that the subtle education to use drugs begins. Many an exhausted mother finds that the television set is an ideal babysitter for her tiring runabout. Long before the child can read or reason he has been given a single message again and again: for every hurt there is a drug. By the time adolescence is reached, the child has spent thousands of hours riveted in front of the television set. Only a very slow child could fail to get the drug-balm message.

At times it hurts to be an adolescent. It hurts to be angry at one's parents. It hurts not to know what to do. The adolescent wants to grow up. But he doesn't want to hurt. How can he stop the pain of adolescence? He has been carefully indoctrinated with the answer. He need not confront and decide how to solve his problems. He need only decide which drug to take. The solution is not within him. It is outside of him. The search is not for the good life. It is for the right drug.[7]

13-1 *Education to use drugs often begins in early childhood, as the child spends hours watching television.*

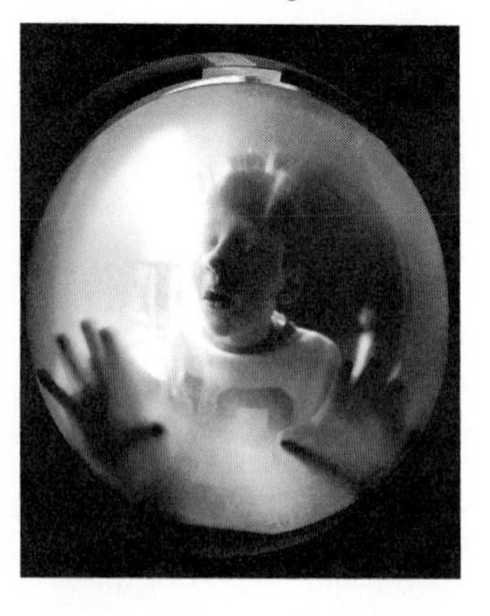

In his search, the adolescent need not go far. Drugs of all kinds fill the family medicine cabinet. When he was a small child, plenty of pills had been popped into his mouth. Some had made him feel better. Rarely had he received any explanation about them. Also, do not his mother and his father constantly use drugs to calm down, to wake up, to get to sleep? And the radio, the television, the newspapers, keep hammering away. For every problem there is a drug. The education against using drugs has been comparatively feeble. Besides, it is just confusing. A television "doctor" tells a teacher which drug to take so as to relax after a hard day. But at school, the teacher lectures about the dangers of drugs. It's no different with parents. And then there is the matter of adolescent rebellion.

[7] John A. Ewing, "Students, Sex, and Marihuana," *Medical Aspects of Human Sexuality,* Vol. 6, No. 2 (February 1972), pp. 102–03.

Kids say that the "pot, acid and speed" drugs are a marvelous way "to blow their parents' minds." In Utah, the kids are not using these drugs to express rebellion. That's because Mormons don't smoke or drink. All the kids have to do to drive *their* parents wild is to leave a cigarette wrapper or a beer can around.[8]

Some rebelliousness combined with a need to imitate makes drug-taking very hard for the adolescent to resist. Surveys suggest that about one in four U.S. adults uses one or more kinds of psychotropic drugs. *Psychotropic drugs* are the mind-benders (the word is derived from the Greek *psyche,* "mind," and *tropē,* "a turning"). They include the sedatives and tranquilizers ("downers") and the stimulants ("uppers"). Nearly half the adult U.S. population reports having used a psychotropic drug at some time.[9] How does this widespread drug use affect the learning young? One recent survey of seventeen thousand Toronto students revealed these comparative data:

Compared to the children of a mother who does not use tranquilizers, the children of a mother who does will be twice as likely to use marihuana or LSD, three times as likely to inhale glue or solvents, four times as likely to use opiates, speed, stimulants, and other hallucinogens, five times as likely to use tranquilizers . . .[10]

Such results have led to the opinion that drug use seems to run in the family. To reduce adolescent drug abuse, it would thus appear that it will be necessary to reach both the parent and child.[11]

However, there is some research to indicate that this concept is too simplistic. The survey conclusions were based not on parental reports, but on the perception of parental drug use by the young. Using also parental reports, one New York study[12] found the relationship between parental drug use and adolescent marihuana use to be grossly overestimated. By far a greater influence was the behavior of friends. Together, peer and parental influence had the strongest effect: "Marihuana use occurs most frequently [when] both friend and parents are drug users."[13] Only further research, over a longer period of time, can answer the question: Which comes first, drug use or drug-using friends?[14]

[8] J. Thomas Ungerleider, "Pot, Acid, Speed," a transcript of a taped review at the Western Regional Conference, sponsored by the U.C.L.A. Alumni Association, *The UCLA Monthly,* Vol. 1, No. 2 (November 1970), p. 9.

[9] Hugh J. Parry, "The Use of Psychotropic Drugs by U.S. Adults," *Public Health Reports,* Vol. 33, No. 10 (October 1968), p. 809.

[10] "Child Addiction Likelier if Mother Is Pill Taker," *Internal Medicine and Diagnostic News,* Vol. 3, No. 23 (December 1, 1970), pp. 1, 14. Other references in which it is assumed that the young begin to use drugs as a result of parental consumption of psychoactive compounds are: R. H. Blum *et al., Horatio Alger's Children: The Role of the Family in the Origin and Prevention of Drug Risk* (San Francisco, 1972); H. S. Lennard, L. J. Epstein, and D. B. Ransom, *Mystification and Drug Misuse* (San Francisco, 1971); G. H. Mellinger, *Journal of Drug Issues,* Vol. 1 (1971), p. 274.

[11] "Research Indicates—Drug Use Runs in Families," *Canada's Mental Health,* Vol. 19, No. 2 (March–April 1971), pp. 28–29, citing *The Medical Post* (October 20, 1970). Surveys that lend support to the concept that parental abuse of psychoactive drugs leads young people to use illegal drugs are considered by M. Lavenhar, E. A. Wolfson, A. Sheffet, S. Einstein, and D. B. Louria, in *Student Drug Surveys,* S. Einstein and S. Allen, eds. (Farmingdale, N.Y., 1972), pp. 33–54; R. G. Smart and D. Fejer, in *Journal of Abnormal Psychology,* Vol. 79 (1972), p. 153.

[12] Denise Kandel, "Adolescent Marihuana Use: Role of Parents and Peers," *Science,* Vol. 181, No. 4104 (September 14, 1973), pp. 1067–70.

[13] *Ibid.,* p. 1067.

[14] *Ibid.,* p. 1069.

How can the family physician help? In 1970, the pharmacists of this nation filled 225 million prescriptions for stimulants, sedatives, and tranquilizers.[15] "Prone to drug dependence ourselves," the prestigious *New England Journal of Medicine* editorialized, "We have turned on our client, white, middle-class America—and the kids came tripping after . . . We do control our prescription pads and should control our professional organizations and the advertising policies of their journals."[16]

for the gullible: a new credibility gap

Those who purchase drugs from street sellers invite deception. For example, in 1971, analyses of Philadelphia street drugs, as well as drugs peddled at rock concerts in the area, revealed that an animal anesthetic, phenylcyclidine (PCP) was commonly substituted for THC, which is the active ingredient of marihuana.[17] PCP is used with caution by veterinarians. In large doses the drug can cause an animal to convulse. Human beings deceived into using the PCP did not have the advantages accorded to animals.

In 1972 were published the results of four studies that had analyzed various illicit drugs. Table 13-1 summarizes these investigations.[18]

terms and classification

"The terms 'habituation' and 'addiction' plagued scientists for years and ultimately came to have a distorted sociological rather than scientific import . . . Fortunately, better perspective has been brought to this complex field by the abandonment of the terms habituation and addiction as having meaningful scientific value."[19] In 1964, the World Health Organization Expert Committee on Addiction-Producing Drugs recommended substitution of the term *drug dependence* for both drug addiction and drug habituation. Agreement in this country was promptly obtained from the Committee on Drug Addiction and Narcotics of the National Academy of Sciences–National Research Council. "Drug dependence is a state of psychic or physical dependence, or both, on

[15] Bruce R. Ditzion, "Psychotropic Drug Advertisements," in "Letters, Comments and Corrections," *Annals of Internal Medicine,* Vol. 75, No. 3 (September 1971), p. 473, citing *The New York Times* (March 4, 1971), p. 36.

[16] Robert Seidenberg, "Advertising and Abuse of Drugs," *New England Journal of Medicine,* Vol. 284, No. 14 (April 8, 1971), p. 789.

[17] S. H. Schnoll and W. H. Vogel, "Analysis of Street Drugs," *New England Journal of Medicine,* Vol. 284, No. 14 (April 8, 1971), p. 791.

[18] A 1973 study showed that "of 572 consecutive street drugs obtained by anonymous donors . . . 54.8% contained none of the substance that they were represented to be. In 4.4% the samples contained not only what they were sold as, but also other drugs." (George C. Lundberg, "Adulteration of 'Street Drugs,'" *Journal of the American Medical Association,* Vol. 235, No. 7 [August 13, 1973], p. 758.)

[19] Nathan B. Eddy *et al.,* "Drug Dependence: Its Significance and Characteristics," *Bulletin of the World Health Organization,* Vol. 32, No. 5 (May 1965), pp. 721–33.

<table>
<caption>TABLE 13–1
Some Common Deceptions in the Illicit Drug Market</caption>
<tr><th>SOLD AS</th><th>MOST OFTEN IS</th><th>ADULTERANTS OR ADMIXTURES</th><th>MAY CONTAIN INSTEAD</th></tr>
<tr><td>Marihuana</td><td>Marihuana</td><td rowspan="2">DMT (dimethyltryptamine)
PCP
LSD
Scopolamine
Opium</td><td>Oregano
Parsley</td></tr>
<tr><td>Tetrahydrocannabinol (THC)</td><td>Not THC but one of many other things</td><td>PCP or inactive substances</td></tr>
<tr><td>LSD</td><td>LSD</td><td>STP
PCP
Strychnine
Amphetamine
Atropine</td><td>STP
PCP</td></tr>
<tr><td>Mescaline</td><td>PCP
STP
LSD</td><td></td><td></td></tr>
<tr><td>Heroin</td><td>Heroin</td><td>Quinine*
Barbiturates</td><td>Inactive material</td></tr>
</table>

*Quinine as an adulterant, and not overdose, is believed to be the major cause of heroin-related deaths.
Source: Edward A. Wolfson and Donald B. Louria, "Prevention of Drug Abuse," *Postgraduate Medicine,* Vol. 51, No. 1 (January 1972), p. 164, citing the following: A. Reed, Jr., and A. W. Kane, "STASH Notes: Phenylcyclidine (PCP)," *Student Association Study Hallucinogens,* Vol. 2 (December 1970); F. E. Cheek, S. Newell, and M. Jaffe, "Deceptions in the Illicit Drug Market," *Science,* Vol. 167, No. 3922 (February 27, 1970), p. 1276; S. A. Marshman and R. J. Gibbons, "The Credibility Gap in the Illicit Drug Market," *Addictions,* Vol. 16 (1969), p. 22; S. H. Schnoll and W. H. Vogel, "Analysis of Street Drugs," *New England Journal of Medicine,* Vol. 284, No. 14 (April 8, 1971), p. 791.

a drug, arising in a person following administration of that drug on a periodic or continuous basis."[20] Considerable confusion had also arisen as to the definition of *drug abuse.* In 1969 the WHO Expert Committee on Drug Dependence defined *drug abuse* as "persistent or sporadic excessive drug use inconsistent with or unrelated to acceptable medical practice."[21] A variety of chemical substances affect man's central nervous system to cause only a psychological (psy-

[20] *Ibid.,* p. 722.
[21] *WHO Expert Committee on Drug Dependence, Sixteenth Report,* World Health Organization Technical Report Series, No. 407 (Geneva, 1969), p. 6.

TABLE 13-2

Some Characteristics of Certain Types of Drugs That Induce Dependence

TYPE OF DRUG DEPENDENCE*	BASIC ACTION	PSYCHOLOGICAL (PSYCHIC) DEPENDENCE	PHYSICAL DEPENDENCE	WITHDRAWAL SYMPTOMS (ABSTINENCE SYNDROME)	DEVELOPMENT OF TOLERANCE
Morphine and morphinelike drugs	Depressant	Yes, strong	Yes, develops early	Severe, but rarely life-threatening	Yes
Barbiturate-alcohol	Depressant	Yes	Yes	Severe, even life-threatening	Yes, but only partial for alcohol
Cocaine†	Stimulant	Yes, strong	No	Possibly	Yes
Cannabis (marihuana)	Stimulant or depressant‡	Yes, moderate to strong	No	None	Yes, slight
Amphetamine	Stimulant	Yes	No	Possibly	Yes
Hallucinogen (LSD)	Stimulant	Yes	No	None	Yes, rapid
Nicotine	Depressant	Yes, strong	No	Yes, variable	Yes
Caffeine	Stimulant	Yes, mild	No	No	Yes, slight

*Khat is not included here because the chewing of its leaves (producing an amphetaminelike drug effect) is not yet a problem in this country.
† Cocaine use in this country is increasing; see pages 413–14.
‡ Since the WHO Expert Committee on Addiction-Producing Drugs classified cannabis as a stimulant in 1965, further research has suggested that it can act either as a stimulant or as a depressant (see pages 418–19).

chic) dependence. However, other drugs also provoke a physical dependence. This latter type of dependence becomes manifested by withdrawal symptoms (the *abstinence syndrome*) when the effects of the drug are interrupted. A physically dependent drug abuser undergoes withdrawal symptoms when he can no longer obtain the drug, or when he is given another drug that nullifies the effects of the one on which he is dependent. If he has had experience with the more severe evidences of the abstinence syndrome, the drug abuser has reason to fear it. A delirium may occur, which is often characterized by hearing strange voices and seeing alarming things that are nonexistent (*hallucinations*) as well as by unreasoning, false beliefs (*delusions*). These, combined with body-shaking tremors and other discomforts, cause the individual to suffer intensely. Some investigators suggest that drugs that produce the abstinence syndrome, such as alcohol, the barbiturates, and the opium derivatives, interfere with the "dream sleep" that is characteristic of the last third of the night and that is associated with rapid eye movements (REMs). Abrupt withdrawal of such drugs, they theorize, results in a sudden, overwhelmingly chaotic resurgence of the dream sleep, which precipitates the delirium of the abstinence syndrome. Many drugs that produce dependence, both psychic and physical, also produce *tolerance;* that is, the drug abuser finds that he must use increasingly larger doses of the drug to achieve the effect obtained with the initial dose. As will be seen below, tolerance to a drug may become so great that doses that would ordinarily be lethal are used without killing the drug abuser. Tolerance to one drug can result in tolerance to a similar one, as in the case of heroin and morphine. This is called *cross-tolerance.*

The World Health Organization Expert Committee has described seven different types of drug dependence according to the patterns of their action and the responses they bring about.[22] These are:

1. morphine type
2. barbiturate-alcohol type
3. cocaine type
4. cannabis (marihuana) type
5. amphetamine type
6. khat type
7. hallucinogen (LSD) type

Table 13-2 indicates some of the basic criteria by which part of this classification was made. Added to this table, moreover, are nicotine (see pages 394 and 395) and caffeine (see page 245, footnote 59).

depressants

THE JUNKIES

When they are
in the street
they pass it
along to each
other but when
they see the
police they would
just stand still
and be beat
so pity ful
that they want
to cry.

Marie Ford, 12 years old[23]

the morphine type of drug dependence: the opiates

some historical notes

Ancient Egyptian mothers used poppy juice to bring slumber to their fretful children. Much later the Chinese used opium dependingly. Not until Ch'ung Ch'en outlawed tobacco smoking in 1641 did they savor the poppy. Two cen-

[22] *Ibid.,* pp. 721–33.
[23] From Herbert Kohl, *36 Children* (New York, 1967), p. 147.

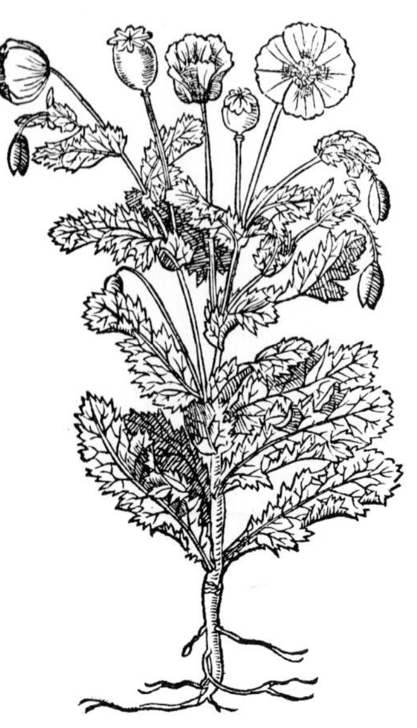
13-2 *The delicate opium poppy.*

turies before, Chaucer had mentioned ''nercotikes[24] and opie'' (''The Knight's Tale,'' line 1472), and Shakespeare's Othello refers to the poppy and ''all the drowsy syrups of the world'' (III.iii.331–32). In *Samson Agonistes* (lines 629–30) John Milton, too, wrote of ''death's benumbing Opium.'' Throughout the ages, writers have woven the poppy into their plots. It is a good device. For mankind, the flower has powerful and exotic meanings.

The sleep-producing poppy, *Papaver somniferum* (see Figure 13–2), flowers in beguiling white, red, and purple. A century ago, John Ruskin eulogized its beauty. The poppy is painted glass . . . always, it is a flame, and warms the wind like a blown ruby.''[25]

The poppy's milky juice oozes not from its delicate petals, however, but from the cut pods. For centuries, its use has released man. Its abuse has imprisoned him. Most of the world's opium used to be grown in Turkey, Burma, India, Persia, China, Laos, Thailand, and Mexico. Legal opium was auctioned ''in such ports as Istanbul and Calcutta by quotas submitted via the Commission on Narcotic Drugs in Geneva and filed with the United Nations Economic and Social Council (handled in the U.S.A. under the Internal Revenue Code).''[26] By the summer of 1973, the U.S. government was reconsidering its policy of trying to prevent the cultivation of the poppy worldwide (see page 366, footnote 48).

the drugs

The risk of dependence on *morphine,* the principal active component of opium, is great, as are its pain-killing properties. Heating morphine with acetic acid (acetylation) synthetically produces the more potent *heroin.* Other synthetic opium derivatives are *dilaudid* and *methadone.* Because of its singular properties, which are described below, methadone is used in the treatment of chronic heroin users. *Codeine,* a derivative of morphine, is commonly used in cough medicines. Many drug abusers start with this substance. *Nalline* (nalorphine hydrochloride; see page 372), an antagonist of opium, does not produce a euphoria. Injection of nalline will dilate the constricted pupils of the chronic heroin user and will also start withdrawal symptoms within half an hour. The careful use of nalline is helpful in diagnosing heroin dependence. However, its more frequent use is in the treatment of overdoses of heroin. *Opioids* is a word designating those synthetic compounds which are not obtained from opium but which have effects like those of opium. Thus, dilaudid and methadone are opioids.

the action

Opiates are depressants. ''The depressant actions include analgesia (relief of pain), sedation (freedom from anxiety, muscular relaxation, decreased motor

[24] In the broadest meaning, however, any agent producing insensibility or stupor is a narcotic. Medically, in the U.S., the term narcotic is today usually limited to opium derivatives such as morphine and heroin. Since morphine is derived from opium, and heroin from morphine, these three terms will be used interchangeably in this section.

[25] John Ruskin, ''Love's Meinie'' and ''Proserpina,'' in E. T. Cook and Alexander Wedderburn, eds., *The Works of John Ruskin,* Vol. XXV (London, 1906), p. 258.

[26] W. Z. Guggenheim, ''Heroin: History and Pharmacology,'' *International Journal of the Addictions,* Vol. 2, No. 2 (Fall 1967), p. 329.

activity), hypnosis (drowsiness and lethargy), and euphoria (a sense of well-being and contentment).''[27] The chronic opiate user, moreover, loses interest in sexuality. Research indicates that in mammals, opiates hit the brain most in that area which plays a role in integrating motor activities and perceptual information. The cerebral cortex, which regulates higher intellectual functions, and the brain stem, which controls sleep and wakefulness, do not seem to have as many specific sites at which opiates can produce their effects.

As was said above, opiates chain man in two ways. The first way is by the development of a physical dependence. This can be initiated by repeated small doses of the drug. If he is without the drug for about twelve hours, the dependent opiate user gets sick (the withdrawal or abstinence syndrome). The second chain is forged by the body's ability to adapt to the drug (tolerance). Because of tolerance, increasing quantities of the drug are required to produce the same effects and to avoid the intense discomforts of withdrawal. Eventually, to experience the original euphoria, the abuser may take doses that would previously have been lethal. And, with this increased dosage, the degree of both the dependence on and the tolerance to the drug also increases. This distinguishing characteristic of morphine and morphinelike drugs is the trap of the abuser.

It is not only a fear of withdrawal that enslaves the opiate abuser. It is also a fear of life. The word ''narcotic'' is derived from the Greek *narkotikos,* meaning ''a benumbing.'' Emotional numbness is what this drug abuser seeks. Uninvolvement is his goal. Life's problems are not encountered. The drug answers all. Hovering on the border of withdrawn sleep, he is easily awakened. This he calls ''being on the nod.'' For the abuser of opiates, however, there is one reality. Somehow, more drug must be gotten. The irony of his situation is complete. He takes the drug to escape. Yet he lives in a constant pressure cooker.

The opiate abuser is haunted by sickness and death. Nor is the newborn spared. Irritability, trembling, vomiting, and a peculiarly high-pitched cry—these are among the warnings to the physician that the mother of a newborn infant is opiate-dependent. So, now, is the baby.[28] For the baby, it may mean the agony of withdrawal. For some babies the symptoms are mild; for others they are so severe that, unless the dependence is diagnosed and treated promptly, the child may perish.[29] Among adult dependents, a dreaded complication is overdose. The opiate abuser has no way of being certain how much drug is contained in the substance he is shooting into his veins. An opiate abuser thought by a pusher to be a police informant may be deliberately sold a lethal overdose. Infections, among them serum hepatitis, caused by infected

[27] David P. Ausubel, *Drug Addiction* (New York, 1958), p. 18.

[28] For a consideration of the extent of this condition, see page 368.

[29] Carl Zelson, Estrellita Rubio, and Edward Wasserman, ''Neonatal Narcotic Addiction: 10-Year Observation,'' *Pediatrics,* Vol. 48, No. 2 (August 1971), pp. 178–89. One study has revealed that the newborns whose mothers were methadone-dependent (see page 368) suffered more severe symptoms of withdrawal than those whose mothers were heroin-dependent. Moreover, compulsive seizures occurred more frequently among the methadone infants. (Carl Zelson, Sook Ja Lee, and Mary Casalino, ''Neonatal Narcotic Addiction: Comparative Effects of Maternal Intake of Heroin and Methadone,'' *New England Journal of Medicine,* Vol. 289, No. 23 [December 6, 1973], pp. 1216–20.)

needles and syringes and careless injection techniques, plague and often kill the opiate abuser.[30] Indeed, there is growing evidence that overdose deaths from heroin are not as likely as fatalities caused by hypersensitive reactions to impurities. A large proportion of street heroin contains quinine. Intravenous injection of quinine can precipitate a marked dilation of blood vessels, a drop in blood pressure, and lethal heart-muscle and respiratory depression. Also responsible for many so-called heroin deaths is the interaction between the injected heroin and other drugs in the body.[31] The practice of sharing needles and syringes is common among opiate abusers. In this way returning soldiers have transmitted to their buddies the malaria they contracted in Vietnam. In this country, cases and deaths from malaria are increasing sharply.[32] The wide variety of microbes and other contaminants that dirty needles, syringes, and drugs are responsible for a particularly dangerous infection of the heart lining, lung abscesses and clots, lung fungus infections, various other pneumonias, and lung lesions caused by injected cornstarch,[33] cotton fiber, and talc.[34] Tetanus has also been commonly reported, as have skin abscesses and vein infections.[35] In a misguided attempt to counteract an overdose, some heroin abusers have had milk injected into their veins. This is potentially catastrophic.[36] The "crush syndrome" has also been recently reported. After injecting heroin the abuser may lose consciousness and lie for hours with the weight of part of his body pressing on a limb, crushing it. Kidney and muscle damage, even paralysis, may result.[37] The use of contaminated needles by heroin dependents may also be responsible for infection in the disc spaces between the spinal vertebrae. Treatment is prolonged and includes immobilization in a plaster cast.[38]

Does heroin have a deleterious effect on menstrual function? Yes. Absence of menstruation (amenorrhea; see page 480) and irregularity may be due to heroin. This also occurs with methadone. With methadone, however, the menstrual difficulties often disappear or improve in about a year. This does not happen with heroin. Ninety percent of women on methadone maintenance therapy (see pages 370–72) return to normal within three years. Both heroin and metha-

[30] Donald B. Louria, Terry Hensle, and John Rose, "The Major Medical Complications of Heroin Addiction," *Annals of Internal Medicine,* Vol. 67, No. 1 (June 1967), pp. 1–22; Charles E. Cherubin, "Infectious Disease Problems of Narcotic Addicts," *Archives of Internal Medicine,* Vol. 128, No. 2 (August 1971), pp. 309–13; Richard B. Jaffe and Edgar B. Koschmann, "Intravenous Drug Abuse," *American Journal of Roentgenology,* Vol. 109 (1970), pp. 107–20.

[31] Mark Weisman, Nathan Lerner, Wolfgang Vogel, Sidney H. Schnoll, and Thomas Banford, "Quality of Street Heroin," *New England Journal of Medicine,* Vol. 229, No. 13 (September 27, 1973), pp. 698–99.

[32] "GI Drug Users May Spread Malaria," *American Medical News,* Vol. 14, No. 3 (January 25, 1971), p. 8; "Malaria Associated with Self-Injection of Drugs," *California Morbidity* (March 5, 1971), p. 1.

[33] William H. Johnson and Jerry Waisman, "Pulmonary Corn Starch Granulomas in a Drug User," *Archives of Pathology,* Vol. 92 (September 1971), pp. 196–202.

[34] "Junkies Have Funny Lungs," *Medical World News,* Vol. 14, No. 30 (August 10, 1973), p. 51.

[35] Donald B. Louria, Terry Hensle, and John Rose, "The Major Medical Complications of Heroin Addiction," pp. 1–22.

[36] Ernst J. Drenick and Kenneth M. Younger, "Heroin Overdose Complicated by Intravenous Injection of Milk," *Journal of the American Medical Association,* Vol. 213, No. 10 (September 7, 1970), p. 1687.

[37] Sara N. Schreiber, Martin R. Leibowitz, Leslie H. Bernstein, and K. Scrinivasan, "Limb Compression and Renal Impairment (Crush Syndrome) Complicating Narcotic Overdose," *New England Journal of Medicine,* Vol. 284, No. 7 (February 18, 1971), pp. 368–69.

[38] "Heroin Addiction Can Lead to Disc Space Infection," *Journal of the American Medical Association,* Vol. 225, No. 10 (September 3, 1973), p. 1167.

done alter menstruation by affecting the hypothalamus of the brain, which controls the cyclic release of hormones affecting ovulation, menstruation, and other functions (see pages 255–58).[39]

the extent of heroin abuse

In the early months of 1972, it was believed that there were from 350,000 to 400,000 heroin abusers in New York City and at least 650,000 in the nation. The estimate for New York City was based on data from previous years and from two sources: the number of heroin dependents listed in the city's Narcotics Register and the number of narcotics-related deaths reported by the medical examiners. In 1971, the New York City medical examiner reported 1,259 such deaths.[40] In 1961, there had been 311 drug-abuse (largely heroin-related) deaths.[41] From 1961 to 1971, the number of narcotics-related deaths in New York City alone had about quadrupled. Heroin had become the greatest killer of teen-agers in the city of New York.[42]

Added to this was disturbing news from Vietnam. There, U.S. servicemen were paying $2.50 for a quarter gram of pure heroin; in the U.S. that amount cost $500. U.S. soldiers had not used narcotics very much in 1969; it was not until 1970 that they started to use both heroin and raw opium. Later, it was shown that narcotics-related deaths among U.S. soldiers were highest in December 1970; during the peak of the epidemic, one in five of the U.S. Army's enlisted men in Vietnam considered himself dependent on some form of narcotic; about one-third had tried one of them once.[43] The prospect of thousands of heroin-dependent veterans returning home filled public and health officials with apprehension. The existing problem at home, combined with the picture in Vietnam, gave ample reason for gloomy predictions.

By midsummer of 1973, however, the outlook had turned from one of apprehension to one of hope. In every region of the United States except the West, deaths due to narcotic overdose were diminishing. Such deaths were lower in 1972 than in 1971; mid-1973 data revealed that narcotics-related deaths had dropped to the 1970 level and were still declining. Moreover, in 1972, fewer people in the United States developed the liver infections associated with the use of dirty needles than did in 1971. From local areas came examples of an improving outlook. In Washington, D.C., the number of people arrested who had a positive urine for heroin dropped from 39 percent in 1972 to 9 percent by mid-1973. The percentages of military inductees rejected for drug abuse

[39] "Methadone: Menstrual Defects?" *Medical World News,* Vol. 14, No. 28 (July 20, 1973), p. 6.
[40] "Heroin-Addict Estimates Soar," *Medical World News,* Vol. 13, No. 7 (February 18, 1972), p. 20.
[41] Louise G. Richards and Eleanor E. Carroll, "Illicit Drug Use and Addiction in the United States," *Public Health Reports,* Vol. 85, No. 12 (December 1970), p. 1040.
[42] "Heroin Leading Death Cause Among Teen-Agers in NYC," *Medical Tribune,* Vol. 11, No. 48, pp. 1, 24.
[43] T. George Harris, "'As Far as Heroin Is Concerned, the Worst Is Over,' A Conversation About the Drug Epidemic with Jerome Jaffee," *Psychology Today,* Vol. 7, No. 3 (August 1973), p. 71. For two years, ending in 1973, Dr. Jerome H. Jaffee was Director of the Special Action Office for Drug Abuse Prevention. Except where indicated, most of the material in this section is from Mr. Harris' interview with Dr. Jaffee.

also declined. And in 1972, property crimes, many of which are attributed to heroin dependents as a source of income for drugs, also declined from the previous year.[44] "In early 1973 the heroin epidemic appeared to be waning in the District of Columbia."[45] Good news also came from New Haven and the rest of Connecticut. Heroin-related deaths had diminished sharply; so had the number of persons seeking detoxification.[46]

WHY THE SEEMINGLY SUDDEN CHANGE? It is now known that, for much of this country, the peak of the heroin epidemic came as early as 1968 and 1969. Peaks of such epidemics are measured by the largest known number of people who used the drug for the first time. But this is followed by a time lag. For many a heroin dependent, it was a year or two before he began to truly realize the cruel trap he was in and to seek escape from it through treatment. Or a few years elapsed before he had to steal to obtain money for heroin. Only then did his growing police record gain attention. For these reasons, heroin abuse seemed to increase in the years following the peaks. It is believed that the downward trend began in about 1970, and continued into 1971 and 1972; mid-1973 also saw reduced abuse of heroin throughout the nation (except in the West, where in some areas, such as San Diego, the peak had not yet been reached). Will the national decline continue and take hold in the West? Only time can tell. One must not be lulled into inactivity by an unwary optimism. There is much to be done. It must be clearly understood that it is not the total number of opium dependents that is decreasing, but rather the number of dependents who are using the drug for the first time. The total number of U.S. opium dependents will diminish only when "the number of new addicts each year becomes smaller than the number of addicts who die, go to jail, or leave the active pool through spontaneous recovery or active treatment."[47]

However, another encouraging sign is the behavior toward heroin of the returned Vietnam veteran. In Vietnam, most of the U.S. soldiers who used heroin or other opiates, did not inject it. They either smoked it or "snorted" (inhaled) it. Also, in June 1971, a testing program was begun to detect heroin in the urine of returning soldiers. This prevented actively dependent heroin abusers from going home without treatment. Eight- to twelve-month follow-up of these veterans showed that a remarkably small number had returned to heroin abuse. Given the short period of follow-up, one must nevertheless be impressed by the impact of environmental change, relative unavailability of opiates, reduced peer pressure, and the noninjecting method of drug self-administration. Each played a significant role in reducing the perpetuation

[44] *Ibid.,* p. 70.

[45] Robert L. DuPont and Mark H. Greene, "The Dynamics of a Heroin Addiction Epidemic," *Science,* Vol. 181, No. 4101 (August 24, 1973), p. 716.

[46] Hans H. Neumann, "Progress in the Other War: The Heroin De-escalation," *Hospital Tribune,* Vol. 7, No. 22 (June 11, 1973), p. 7.

[47] T. George Harris, "As Far as Heroin Is Concerned, the Worst Is Over," p. 71.

of the dependency.[48] Indeed, it was estimated that "of the more than 300,000 Army enlisted men who served in Vietnam in the years 1970 and 1972, only perhaps 2000 to 3000" were opiate-dependent by May 1973, "and most of these were narcotics users before their military service."[49]

An important word of caution is needed here. To carelessly extrapolate the data concerning experience with heroin from U.S. soldiers in Vietnam to civilians is both misleading and dangerous. Some have gone so far as to suggest that "mere experimentation" with heroin presents no dangers. This is not true. Consider the facts. First, about 28 percent of those U.S. servicemen in Vietnam who abused heroin had already begun to use narcotics before they were sent there. Second, the stresses of soldiers in war zones cannot be compared to those of people in civilian life. Third, peer pressure is of a different quality in a war zone; peer pressure was one cause of the spread of dependency from one person to another. Fourth, opiates were cheaper and far more readily available in Vietnam. Fifth, smoking and "snorting," the major methods of self-administration in Vietnam, are not as conducive to quick enslavement by opiates as the injection method. It is true that situations can be created in which early heroin abusers can change their behavior. Preliminary data indicated this to be the case with U.S. Vietnam veterans. However, even in Vietnam, "in the group studied the chances of getting addicted while experimenting were almost 50–50."[50] To experiment with heroin, then, is treacherous; no data exist to contradict this.

Whether heroin dependency will continue to be a problem in this country remains to be seen. But two new federal information-gathering techniques will certainly help. One, the Client-Oriented Data Acquisition Process (CODAP), permits surveys of federally supported treatment programs across the United States; an undue increase in new users will merit further investigation. The other, the Drug Abuse Warning Network (DAWN), provides rapid information on drug-related deaths as well as the drug-associated problems seen in emergency hospital admissions. Such centrally located information systems can help local areas pinpoint their drug problems. Today, more federal funds, when needed and available, and perhaps teams of advisory personnel, may be sent into a problem area to help the frequently bewildered, and often panicked, citizenry with their local drug abuse problems.

[48] *Ibid.*, p. 76. The relative unavailability in the United States of street heroin may be traced largely to the efforts of the Nixon administration to prevent growth of the poppy worldwide. Turkey, in an agreement with the United States, now forbids cultivation of the poppy. India cannot supply enough legitimate opium. U.S. physicians face a shortage of opiate drugs. Among these are paregoric, morphine, nalorphine, nalotene, and codeine. In a June 1971 message to Congress, President Nixon noted that supplying morphine and codeine was the only legitimate reason for cultivation of the opium poppy. For morphine, he also noted, there were already adequate substitutes; research could provide the necessary alternatives for codeine. Many physicians feel that morphine remains the best of the painkillers in certain clinical conditions. And although nobody questions the need for research, there is considerable question that patient pain can await its practical results. ("Opiate Squeeze Is Getting Painful," *Medical World News*, Vol. 14, No. 23 [June 8, 1973], pp. 29, 31; "Halt in Turkish Poppy Output Backfires in Opiates Pinch," *Hospital Tribune*, Vol. 8, No. 1 [January 7, 1974], p. 1.)

[49] "GI Drug Study Belies a Vietnam Connection," *Medical World News*, Vol. 14, No. 19 (May 11, 1973), p. 20.

[50] T. George Harris, "As Far as Heroin Is Concerned, the Worst Is Over," p. 78.

HEROIN DEPENDENTS ARE GETTING YOUNGER Nowadays, the average New Yorker who abuses heroin is about seventeen years old. Four years ago, he was twenty-one; ten years ago, twenty-five. It has been estimated that today, as many as 30 percent of New York's estimated 350,000 heroin abusers have yet to reach their fifteenth birthday. The youngest opiate-drug dependents, however, are newborn babies whose mothers abuse heroin or methadone, or receive methadone from clinic physicians. In 1970, New York City municipal hospitals reported 489 such births. In 1971 the number was 706. In 1960, at the New York Medical College–Metropolitan Hospital Center one in every 164 deliveries was of a drug-dependent mother. In 1972, in the same hospital, one in every 27 babies was born to such a mother—an increase of over six times. All the mothers took heroin; many used other opiates, as well as barbiturates, amphetamines, and a host of other drugs. About 85 percent of women drug abusers are of child-bearing age.[51] "Many of the babies will grow up to be addicts—although they are detoxified before they leave the hospital—because they are brought up in 'addict' households."[52]

Though 85 percent of heroin abusers live and die in the major cities of New York, New Jersey, Maryland, Illinois, and California,[53] heroin abuse is no longer limited to the urban poor. In 1970, it was considered "a plague that is spreading to the suburbs"[54]—and to the white middle class. "Of those under 25 years of age dying from heroin use in Philadelphia [in that year], 50 percent are white."[55] In 1970, "jumping death rates [were] found from New England to Miami, Florida, from New Orleans to Seattle."[56]

Most people who are dependent on opiates need to commit crimes. It is only through stealing, prostitution, and "pushing" narcotics that they obtain sufficient funds for their drug. Many drug abusers, beset by increasing tolerance, develop a prohibitively expensive problem. Their drug may cost as much as $125 or more daily. Often, to control this expense, they voluntarily commit themselves, undergo withdrawal, and then promptly return to lesser doses.

the treatments

Various methods of treatment for opiate dependency have been used. The choice must be tempered by the nature of the patient and "there is no 'typical' drug-dependent person."[57] "The withdrawal method of treatment of the patient with drug-dependence of the morphine-like type should have the combined goal of abstinence, resolution of general medical and psychiatric prob-

[51] Carl Zelson, "Infant of the Addicted Mother," *New England Journal of Medicine,* Vol. 288, No. 26 (June 28, 1973), p. 1393.

[52] "Heroin-Addict Estimates Soar," *Medical World News,* p. 20.

[53] Carl Zelson, "Infant of the Addicted Mother," p. 1393, citing J. S. Lin-Fu, *Neonatal Narcotic Addiction* (U.S. Children's Bureau Publication), Washington, D.C., Government Printing Office, 1967.

[54] Philip H. Abelson, "Death from Heroin," *Science,* Vol. 168, No. 3937 (June 1970), p. 1289.

[55] "Heroin Leading Death Cause Among Teen-Agers in NYC," *Medical Tribune,* pp. 1, 24.

[56] Joseph W. Spelman, "Heroin Addiction: The Epidemic of the 70's," *Archives of Environmental Health,* Vol. 21, No. 5 (November 1970), p. 589.

[57] Herbert A. Raskin, "Treating Today's Heroin User," *American Family Physician,* Vol. 8, No. 2 (August 1973), p. 80.

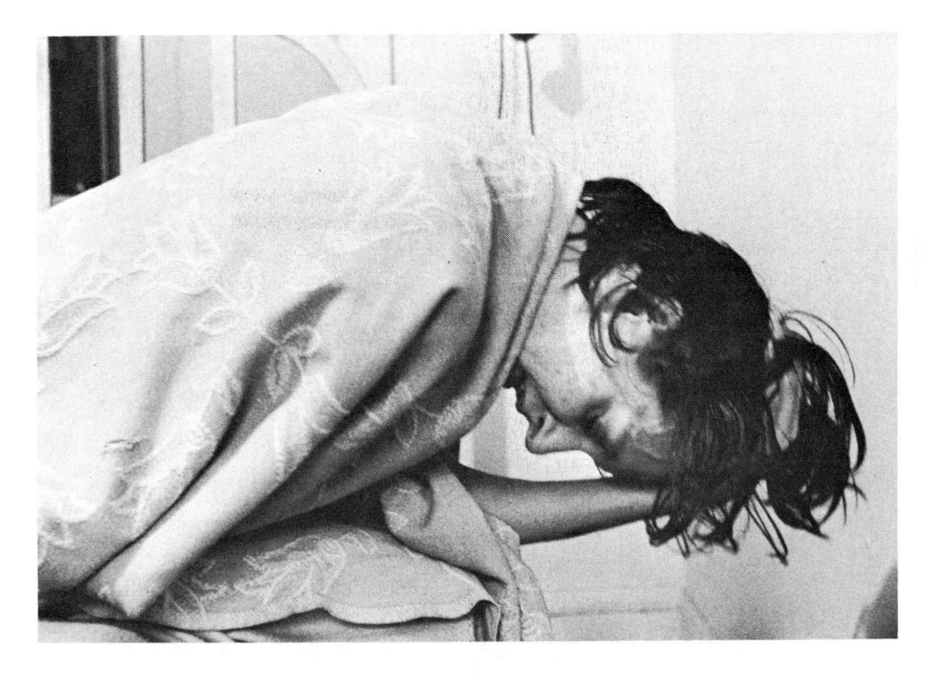

13-3 *Withdrawal.*

lems, and social rehabilitation. The initial step in this treatment procedure is withdrawal from the dependence producing drug . . ."[58] This withdrawal is called *detoxification.*

"COLD TURKEY" "Cold turkey" refers to detoxification without treatment. Because "cold turkey" is a cruel experience, no physician approves of it.

After six to eight hours without the drug or treatment, the heroin dependent begins to suffer the agonies of withdrawal. "I've got superflu, man," he will say. His nose runs and his eyes water. He sweats profusely. Twelve to fourteen hours after his last dose, he may fall into a fitful sleep. This he calls "yen." When he awakens, his "superflu" is worse. He can neither sleep nor eat. His muscles twitch. He yawns and sneezes uncontrollably. Vomiting and diarrhea may also be uncontrollable. One moment he is shaken by a violent chill, the next moment he feels that he is burning with fever. Sometimes he will have an orgasm. His skin, crawling with gooseflesh, resembles that of a plucked turkey; that is why withdrawal without treatment is called "cold turkey." His bones ache and his muscles hurt cruelly. He may make jerky kicking movements; this may be the basis for the expression "kicking the habit." Worst of all, he has a consuming craving for the drug. No plea, no manipulation of others, no mimicking of symptoms, is beyond him. Between thirty-six and forty-eight hours after his last dose of the drug, the symptoms peak. For about seventy-two hours their severity persists, but unless he is very old, or very ill from other some disease, the person undergoing withdrawal will not die. Over

[58] AMA Council on Mental Health and Committee on Alcoholism and Drug Dependence, "Treatment of Morphine-Type Dependence by Withdrawal Methods," *Journal of the American Medical Association,* Vol. 219, No. 12 (March 20, 1972), p. 1612.

a period of five to ten days the symptoms gradually abate. Slowly the physical dependence on the drug diminishes. But the psychic dependence lingers on. It may well persist for the rest of his life.

WITHDRAWAL PLUS SUPPORTIVE THERAPY Another method of treatment involves abrupt withdrawal accompanied by supportive therapy. The supportive therapy may include daily group ''rap'' sessions and a variety of nonnarcotic drugs to alleviate the withdrawal symptoms. When carried out in a nonhospital environment, it usually fails.

WITHDRAWAL PLUS METHADONE Still a third method, approved by most physicians in this country, is gradual withdrawal plus the substitution for heroin of daily diminishing doses of *methadone.* Symptoms, such as muscle cramps, vomiting, and diarrhea, are treated as they occur. When the patient is opiate-free and feeling better, rehabilitation is attempted.

This methadone treatment is now recommended for prisoners. In October 1970, riots broke out in the Manhattan House of Detention for Men (''the Tombs''). Among the major causes were overcrowding and the lack of medical care for heroin-dependent prisoners. Half of the thirty-four thousand annual admissions to the Tombs are opiate dependents, but before the riots prisoners' withdrawal symptoms had not been treated. During the first week of their incarceration, prisoners had endured all the discomforts of withdrawal without treatment. Today the overcrowding has been somewhat relieved. Every day between thirty and fifty prisoners are being gradually withdrawn from heroin. Carefully measured doses of methadone replace the heroin. Other palliative drugs are used when indicated. About ten days are allowed for detoxification before drugs are discontinued.[59] Authorities in other prisons are beginning similarly humane programs.

METHADONE MAINTENANCE Methadone detoxification should not be confused with *methadone maintenance.* With methadone detoxification the heroin is replaced by methadone, which in turn is gradually withdrawn over a number of days. With methadone maintenance, heroin is also replaced by methadone, but the methadone may be continued indefinitely. In hundreds of clinics throughout the country, more than seventy-five thousand former heroin dependents are maintained on methadone. That number is steadily increasing. *Methadone* is a synthetic narcotic (an opioid) that is taken orally. In treatment clinics it is usually dissolved in orange juice. Like heroin, it causes severe dependency. Why, then, is its professional use so widespread? Because it is believed to have a number of advantages over heroin. To understand those advantages it is necessary to first discuss the basic theories explaining its effectiveness.

There are two major theories about the way methadone works. The first and original one is that a chronic heroin (or other narcotics) abuser has altered his

[59] Vincent P. Dole, ''Detoxification of Sick Addicts in Prison,'' *Fourth National Conference on Methadone Treatment: Proceedings* (San Francisco, January 8–10, 1972), pp. 65–67.

body metabolism at the cellular level. (Metabolism refers to the chemical changes that take place in the body). This metabolic alteration is such that narcotics produce a ''high''—an exaggerated sense of well-being. Without heroin, the dependent person experiences a feeling called ''narcotics hunger.'' It can be relieved only by opioids. Based on these concepts, methadone maintenance consists of the daily administration of a specified dose of methadone in fruit juice. Meanwhile, attempts at rehabilitation are made. In six to eight weeks a state of stabilization is reached. At this time, the patient has achieved a high degree of cross-tolerance (see page 419). This means that his level of body methadone prevents him from experiencing a high from other narcotics, even when they are injected. This is called ''narcotics blockade.''[60] This theory presumes that the patient will need to take methadone as long as he lives. The second theory of methadone maintenance holds that the reason for heroin dependency is not entirely metabolic, nor does methadone correct a metabolic defect. Environment, peer-group pressure, predrug social and environmental problems are among the factors that are involved. This theory suggests that eventually the methadone-maintained patient can be successfully withdrawn from the drug. With psychosocial support he can be a functioning, drug-free member of society.[61]

In any case, there is little doubt that methadone maintenance has succeeded in getting a great number of people to discontinue heroin. The effects of methadone last from twenty-four to forty-eight hours, whereas the heroin-dependent person must seek another dose every four to five hours. Moreover, the patient taking oral methadone every day in a clinic setting is no longer subject to the threats of a ruthless pusher; nor is he a victim of impure drugs, infected needles, and dirty syringes. No longer must he prey on society, leading a life of crime to obtain his drug. Nor does he continue to entice others into heroin abuse. With his heroin hunger controlled, and his intellectual and physical capacities essentially unimpaired, the methadone patient can seek employment. And the economic cost to society is greatly diminished. But for these patients, methadone is not enough. Intensive rehabilitation, tailored to the individual patient, is essential.

There is considerable controversy about methadone maintenance. Because methadone maintenance involves switching patients from one narcotic to another, the treatment has been decried as immoral. However, nobody questions

> the legitimacy of providing insulin for diabetics, antipsychotic agents for schizophrenics, antiseizure medication for epileptics and a variety of other medicaments to other chronically ill people . . . Even that ancient and useful device, the crutch,

[60] Jerome H. Jaffee, ''Drug Addiction and Drug Abuse,'' Chapter 16 in *The Pharmacological Basis of Therapeutics* (New York, 1970), pp. 305–06.

[61] T. George Harris, ''As Far as Heroin Is Concerned, the Worst Is Over,'' p. 79; Paul Cushman and Vincent P. Dole, ''Detoxification of Rehabilitated Methadone-Maintained Patients,'' *Journal of the American Medical Association,* Vol. 226, No. 7 (November 12, 1973), pp. 747, 752; and Vincent P. Dole, ''Detoxification of Methadone Patients and Public Policy,'' pp. 780–81 of the same issue.

is not debased by calling it "*merely* a crutch" when it permits a person to ambulate who otherwise could not do so.[62]

Methadone maintenance is by no means a panacea for the treatment of all heroin abusers. For example, with most adolescent patients, it is recommended that a program of detoxification, psychotherapy, and intensive vocational rehabilitation be tried first. Although this approach has had some success, it has resulted in dishearteningly few permanent cures. The risks of sickness and death to the adolescent are great, as is the economic cost of the treatment. For these reasons methadone maintenance of adolescents is being attempted in several clinics.[63]

ALTERNATIVES TO METHADONE A possible improvement on methadone, L-methadyl acetate, is now being studied.[64] It suppresses narcotic hunger twice as long as does methadone. With its use the patient's visits to the clinic are reduced to two or three a week.

There is also hope of a preventive "chemical vaccination" against heroin use. Unlike methadone, several drugs, such as cyclazocine, naloxone, and nalorphine, are opioid antagonists. They can also block the high from heroin. Such compounds are being researched by the Federation Against Drug Addiction.[65]

TREATMENT CENTERS Programs that offer a variety of treatments are also being tried. Among these are methadone plus weekly group therapy and multimethod residential treatment centers.[66]

Federal narcotic treatment centers in this country include the Public Health Service hospitals at Lexington, Kentucky, and Fort Worth, Texas. Despite active therapy designed to help the patient deal with conflicts between his ego and environment, the follow-up studies of released patients show a disappointingly high rate of return to drug dependence. California also maintains an advanced treatment program. The California State Rehabilitation Center program involves compulsory civil commitment, detoxification, diagnostic study, and transfer to a rehabilitation center for mandatory treatment periods lasting from six to fourteen months. Halfway houses, for those not quite ready for societal onslaughts, are provided.[67] In both the federal and California institutions the patients are

[62] John C. Kramer, "Methadone Maintenance for Opiate Dependence," *California Medicine,* Vol. 113, No. 12 (December 1970), pp. 7, 10. Excellent discussions of the pros and cons of methadone maintenance are Amitai Etzioni, "Methadone Best Hope for Now," *Smithsonian,* Vol. 4, No. 1 (April 1973), pp. 50, 52, 53, and Henry L. Lennard, Leon J. Epstein, and Mitchell S. Rosenthal, "The Cure Becomes a New Problem," in the same issue, pp. 51, 54–57.

[63] Stuart L. Nightingale, "Adolescent Addiction: Does Methadone Have a Role?" *Fourth National Conference on Methadone Treatment: Proceedings,* pp. 41–43.

[64] Jerome H. Jaffee and Edward C. Senay, "Methadone and L-Methadyl Acetate Use in Management of Narcotic Addicts," *Journal of the American Medical Association,* Vol. 216, No. 8 (May 24, 1971), pp. 1303–05.

[65] "Immunization Against Drug Addiction," *Newsletter of the World Medical Association,* Vol. 4, No. 3 (May–June 1971), p. 1.

[66] "Out of One Program, Many Treatments," *The University of Chicago Reports (Division of Biological Sciences and Pritzker School of Medicine)*, Vol. 21, No. 1 (Fall 1971), pp. 3–7.

[67] It was in Santa Monica, California, that Synanon, a private foundation, was founded. Today, for some abusers, it offers a haven and a hope. Not all applicants are admitted. Not every resident can obey its rigid rules. It affords harsh reality for a harsh sickness. Synanon has survived because other methods have not. It deserves careful professional evaluation. The two facilities of Daytop Lodge and Daytop Village are in Staten Island, New York, and in Sullivan County, New York. Here again, the rules are strict and the program rigid. Narcotics Anonymous and Teen Challenge also work voluntarily to help the individual with a drug problem, as does Exodus House.

detoxified and must remain until there is hope that they are cured.

Unfortunately, it is easier to get a willing patient off drugs than to keep him off. Except for physician-patients, relapse rates are as high as 90 percent. That less than 10 percent of physicians return to drugs indicates the importance of having some life interest apart from drugs—of having "something to go back to."[68]

A PILOT HEROIN–MAINTENANCE PROGRAM FOR THE U.S.? It is certainly true that methadone maintenance does not prevent many patients from using other drugs with which it has no cross-tolerance, such as alcohol, barbiturates, and stimulants. Too, there have been some methadone overdose deaths; many of these occur because of the illegal sale of methadone on the streets. Others complain that, in this drug-attuned culture, it is unfortunate but predictable that a cure for the abuse of a drug would be—another drug. Still others are critical about the lack of attention being paid to such excellent heroin treatment centers as Phoenix House, Daytop, and Synanon. Here the dependency is upon the human environment rather than methadone. However, these are limited institutions; to provide them for the hundreds of thousands of heroin dependents would seem an impossible job. Lack of funds is not the only problem; a lack of competent personnel would preclude a massive effort in this direction. They should, nevertheless, be expanded as much as possible. There has been some discussion about heroin maintenance for heroin dependents. An American Bar Association committee "has recommended starting pilot heroin-maintenance programs to explore their feasibility."[69] There is something to be said for a well-researched, carefully controlled pilot program of this nature.

THE BRITISH APPROACH Some experts laud the British approach to morphine or morphinelike-drug dependence. Although methadone maintenance is used extensively in Britain, specialist physicians may legally prescribe heroin. Prescribing is now limited to approved doctors operating from specified clinics. Registration of narcotic dependents is mandatory. By 1968, these were among the requirements that were added to the British system.[70] Previously, in the early 1960s, the British system had been failing. One reason: lack of controls

[68] The rate of drug dependency among physicians is thought to be considerably greater than among other groups of U.S. adults. Increased availability, the stress of overwork, and the personality of the individual are of critical importance in such instances. One physician became so dependent on his phenylephrine nose drops that when, during military service, he was assigned to a ship, he brought four gallons aboard, because he did not know when he would return to a port for a new supply. He thought he was treating a sinusitis and that the drug prevented him from smothering. Psychotherapy helped this man. (Ralph B. Little, "Hazard of Drug Dependency Among Physicians," *Journal of the American Medical Association,* Vol. 218, No. 10 [December 6, 1971], pp. 1533–34.)

[69] Lorrin M. Korran, "Heroin Maintenance for Heroin Addicts: Issues and Evidence," *New England Journal of Medicine,* Vol. 288, No. 13 (March 29, 1973), pp. 654–60. This article is particularly recommended for both its thorough presentation and its excellent bibliography. An article opposing a heroin maintenance program in the United States is Edward Lewis, Jr., "A Heroin Maintenance Program in the United States?" *Journal of the American Medical Association,* Vol. 223, No. 5 (January 29, 1973), pp. 539–46. This article is recommended for its well-reasoned point of view; it is particularly valuable in differentiating between the problems of heroin dependency in the United States and in Great Britain.

[70] "Transatlantic Debate on Addiction," editorial in *British Medical Journal,* Vol. 3, No. 5770 (August 7, 1971), pp. 321–22.

over prescribing physicians. How well the new system works remains to be seen. It is believed that the severity of the heroin problem in Britain has not equaled that in this country since the First World War.[71]

the barbiturate-alcohol type of drug dependence

Unlike the abstinence syndrome induced by withdrawal of morphine and morphinelike drugs, the abstinence syndrome following discontinuance of both barbiturates and alcohol depends on a prior prolonged and continuous ingestion of relatively high doses. In addition, the signs and symptoms resulting from the prolonged excessive use of alcohol and barbiturates are similar. So are the signs and symptoms ensuing from the withdrawal of either drug. Also, barbiturates will suppress the withdrawal symptoms of the alcoholic and, to some extent, alcohol will suppress withdrawal symptoms for the chronic barbiturate abuser. These are among the reasons for the grouping of these drug dependencies into one type. However, for the sake of convenience, they will be discussed separately in this section.

sedatives: barbiturates and barbituratelike drugs

Since they allay excitement, barbiturates are sedatives. Among these are the short-acting *Seconal* and *Nembutal* and the longer-acting *Phenobarbital*. Recently, a host of nonbarbiturate sedatives have been developed including *Doriden, Dormison,* and *Quaalude.* (Because of its increasing abuse, Quaalude is discussed separately on pages 375–76.) Tranquilizers, such as *Equanil* and *Miltown* (trade names for the same drug) and *Librium,* also have a barbituratelike action. There is no question that these drugs, and the many others like them, have great medical value. They are generally used to control signs and symptoms resulting from psychic, circulatory, respiratory, and gastrointestinal distress. However, all barbiturates and barbituratelike drugs can be abused. They should never be used without the advice of a physician. As with all other drugs, new information constantly comes to the physician about both their uses and dangers. He is particularly concerned with the patient who will attempt to conceal a dependence because of shame or the desire to obtain still another prescription. Some patients in large cities go from physician to physician seeking a prescription for the drug on which they have become dependent. Of all the sedatives, the barbiturates are the most abused.

Every year barbiturates kill more people (more than 3,500) in this country than any other drug; many die as suicides. As with the opium derivatives, prolonged and excessive use causes not only profound psychological and physical dependence but also rapid tolerance. The true barbiturate abuser may pop between ten and twenty pills or capsules into his mouth every day. They are not hard to get. Counting refills, millions of prescriptions for sedatives are filled every year in the nation's drug stores. The U.S. consumption of barbiturates is close to a million pounds per year, or about 4.5 billion average doses.[72]

[71] *Ibid.*, p. 322, citing F. B. Glaser and J. C. Ball, *"The British Narcotic 'Register' in 1970,* A Factual Review," *Journal of the American Medical Association,* Vol. 216, No. 7 (May 17, 1971), pp. 1177–82.
[72] Henry B. Murphree, "The Continuing Problem of Barbiturate Poisoning," *American Family Physician,* Vol. 8, No. 2 (August 1973), p. 108.

Acute barbiturate poisoning may, at first, make an individual seem sociable. This is because of the alcohol-like effect on inhibitions. As has been pointed out, barbiturate and alcohol intoxication are similar. Soon moodiness and depression replace the cheerfulness. The barbiturate abuser slurs his speech, staggers. He seems to suffer an inner agony. Finally, he may sink into a coma. Without attention, he may not waken.

This is not the only way to die of barbiturate poisoning. To avoid a sleepless night, a barbiturate abuser may take one or two pills at bedtime. An hour or two later he awakens, his mind a cloud of cotton. Two more pills. Again he sleeps. A deeply disturbed person may awaken repeatedly, each time more confused, each time gulping down more barbiturates. "The average lethal dose [of barbiturates] is only about 15 times the average hypnotic dose."[73] With the respiratory and cardiovascular systems depressed, this individual, too, eventually may not awaken. Should he ingest alcohol before bedtime, he runs an even greater risk. Both alcohol and barbiturates are depressants. One adds to the action of the other. Worse, between the two drugs there is a cross-tolerance. Tolerance to alcohol produces increased tolerance to barbiturates, and vice versa. For this reason alcoholics tend to take higher than usual doses of barbiturates. The combined effects of barbiturates and alcohol are disastrous. Often people are found dead with amounts of barbiturates and alcohol in the blood that, if either had been taken without the other, would not have been fatal. And, tragically, "among the drugs that alcoholics combine most frequently with alcohol, the barbiturates are the most common."[74] Indeed, alcoholics soon find that barbiturates not only provide an intoxicating effect similar to that of alcohol, but also boost the effect of alcohol.

Without adequate treatment withdrawal from barbiturates may be hazardous. During the first six to eight hours, the patient may seem improved. Then he begins to experience trembling, anxiety, headache, and vomiting, which in turn give way to grave threats to life. Toxic delirium and psychoses occur and the patient may die during a convulsion. The danger of convulsions may persist for the first week of withdrawal or even longer. Thus, withdrawal from barbiturates should take place in a hospital; it is usually much more dangerous than withdrawal from heroin. A patient undergoing withdrawal from barbiturates may require as long as six weeks of scrupulous care. The temporary substitution of long-acting for short-acting barbiturates has been found to make the withdrawal period far less dangerous.[75] Psychotherapy to examine and treat the cause of the dependence is essential.

"LUDE" ABUSE[76] "Luding out" is a street term referring to the sedative-hypnotic effects of a depressant drug called methaqualone. Introduced to the

[73] *Ibid.*

[74] Paul Devenyi and Mary Wilson, "Barbiturate Abuse and Addiction and Their Relationship to Alcohol and Alcoholism," *The Canadian Medical Association Journal,* Vol. 104, No. 3 (February 6, 1971), p. 215.

[75] David E. Smith and Donald R. Wesson, "A New Method for Treatment of Barbiturate Dependence," *Journal of the American Medical Association,* Vol. 213, No. 2 (July 13, 1970), pp. 294–95.

[76] This section is based on an article by Darryl S. Inaba, George R. Gay, John A. Newmeyer, and Craig Whitehead, "Methaqualone Abuse," *Journal of the American Medical Association,* Vol. 224, No. 11 (June 11, 1973), pp. 1505–09.

U.S. medical profession by a single drug company in 1965 (under the trade name *Quaalude*), by 1972 its sales had increased 360 percent.[77] Thus motivated, by 1972 several other drug companies had joined in the manufacture of the drug, marketing it under different trade names. The drug was first synthesized in India in 1955; during the next five years it was available in Japan. In this country, methaqualone has been alleged to cause little or no dependency, minimal suppression of REM sleep, and no initial excitement phase—all of which are common dangers with barbiturate use. But almost twenty years ago the Japanese knew better. Japanese physicians had observed both physical and psychological dependency on methaqualone, and withdrawal symptoms as severe as delirium and life-threatening convulsions.[78] ''Luding out'' can be permanent. Of the 275 U.S. cases of acute methaqualone intoxication reported in 1972, sixteen died.[79] Combined with another depressant, such as alcohol, methaqualone can be particularly hazardous. Methaqualone is mistakenly believed by some to stimulate sexual desire. Like alcohol and other drugs, it may appear to do this by lowering the sexual inhibitions of some people. But, also like alcohol, increasing doses diminish the sexual function. In June 1973, the *Journal of the American Medical Association* editorialized: ''Methaqualone, in addition to being widely abused, . . . may produce serious toxic reactions, and has a potential for both physical and psychological dependence. It cannot be considered, therefore, to be a drug essential to medical practice.''[80]

alcohol

''How sweet is everything that is moderate . . . For Mnesitheos says that one should always avoid excesses in everything.''[81]

CULTURAL CONCEPTS The primitive Cocomas Indians of the Amazon Valley grind the bones of their dead to a fine powder that they then gulp down with their beer.[82] Sometimes Jivaro Indians dip enemy shrunken heads in beer before tasting the brew.[83] And so devoted are the primitive Dusun to potent drink that writers have reported entire village populations, including children, quite drunk.[84] Among primitive peoples, every important event, from birth to marriage to death, was and is celebrated with alcohol.

[77] *Ibid.*, p. 1505, citing D. Zwerdling, ''Methaqualone: The Safe Drug That Isn't Very,'' *The Washington Post* (November 12, 1972), p. B-3; D. Zwerdling, ''Methaqualone, Hottest Drug on the Streets,'' *The San Francisco Chronicle* (November 13, 1972), p. 15; ''Methaqualone—A Dr. Jekyll and Mr. Hyde?'' *The Pharm-Chem Newsletter,* Vol. 2, No. 1 (1973), pp. 1–4.

[78] *Ibid.*, citing M. Kato, ''An Epidemiological Analysis of the Fluctuation of Drug Dependence in Japan,'' *International Journal of Addictions,* Vol. 4 (1969), pp. 591–621.

[79] *Ibid.*, p. 1508, citing ''Warning on 'Sopors,''' *Newsweek* (February 28, 1973), p. 65.

[80] ''Methaqualone,'' Editorial in the *Journal of the American Medical Association,* Vol. 224, No. 11 (June 11, 1973), p. 1521.

[81] Athenaeus (419 B.C.), quoted in Sterling Dow, ''Two Families of Athenian Physicians,'' *Bulletin of the History of Medicine,* Vol. 7, No. 1 (June 1942), p. 18.

[82] Ernest Crawley, *Dress, Drinks, and Drums* (London, 1931), p. 219.

[83] William Curtis Farabee, *Indian Tribes of Eastern Peru, Papers of the Peabody Museum of American Archaeology and Ethnology,* cited in Chandler Washburne, *Primitive Drinking* (New York, 1961), p. 105.

[84] Owen Rutter, *British North Borneo,* cited in Chandler Washburne, *Primitive Drinking,* p. 250.

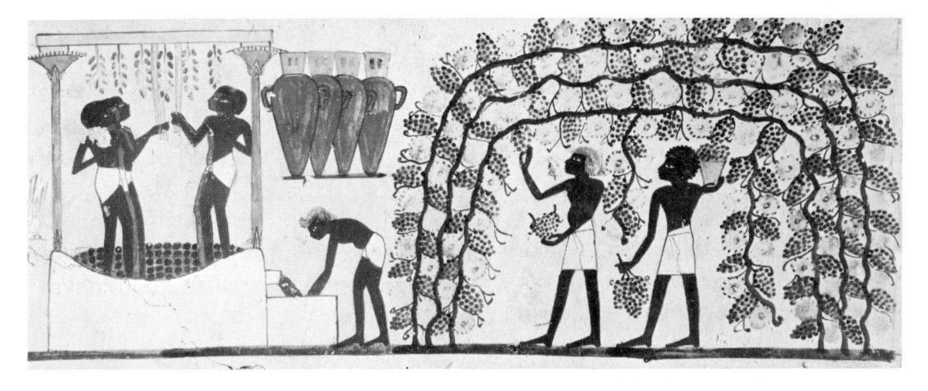

13-4 *Grape-harvesting and wine-making in ancient Egypt.*

Where did the word "alcohol" begin? The Arabic *al kohl* originally referred to a fine antimony powder used for staining the eyes. From it was derived the word *alcohol.* Whether this is the origin of the toast "here's mud in your eye" is unknown.

Nor is it known when alcohol was first made. Stone age beer jugs, ten to fifteen thousand years old, have been discovered. Forty centuries ago, the Babylonian Code of Hammurabi provided careful regulations for the sale of beer. In about 1500 B.C., an ancient Egyptian book of etiquette warned: "Make not thyself helpless in drinking in the beer shop . . . Falling down thy limbs will be broken, and no one will give thee a hand to help thee up, as for thy companions . . . they will say, 'Outside with this drunkard.' "[85] Alcohol seems to have been a problem even at ancient Greek athletic events. The Greek stadium at Delphi still has a sign, *circa* 5 B.C., forbidding wine in the stadium. Violators were to be fined five drachmas. Today, the Southern Methodist University stadium boasts a comparable prohibiting sign.[86] One of Harvard College's first projects was a brewery.[87] Nevertheless, a similar regulation now forbids drinking in the Harvard University stadium.[88]

Nor is the Bible short of references to alcohol. As soon as he left the ark, Noah built an altar (Genesis 8:20). But then he planted a vineyard and got drunk (Genesis 9:20, 21). That his inebriety led to poor behavior and a bad example for his sons is, however, made abundantly clear. Use of alcohol was permitted among the Jews—wine "cheereth God and man" (Judges 9:13)—and was even part of religious life. But to be intoxicated was considered an abomination; self-control was the rigid rule.

The early Romans were also abstemious. Nevertheless, the later progressive societal decay, during and following the years of the Punic Wars, saw drunkenness rampantly accompany promiscuity. Both Roman debauchery and Hebrew restraint profoundly influenced the early Christians (see page 439). Those desiring to be known as followers of Christ were instructed, "Be not drunk with

[85] Sir E. A. Wallis Budge, "The Dwellers on the Nile," cited in "Alcoholism as a Disease," *World Health* (January 1966), p. 21.
[86] Arthur P. McKinlay, "Non-Attic Greek States," in Raymond G. McCarthy, ed., *Drinking and Intoxication* (Glencoe, Ill., 1959), p. 51.
[87] J. C. Furnas, *The Life and Times of the Late Demon Rum* (New York, 1965), p. 20.
[88] Arthur P. McKinlay, "Non-Attic Greek States," p. 51.

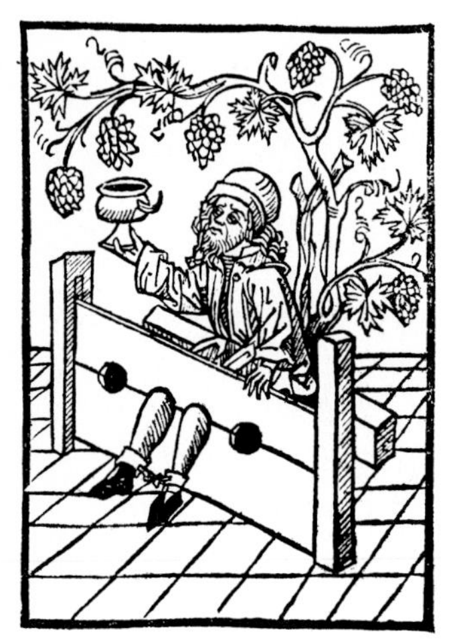

13-5 *A 15th-century alcoholic in the stocks.*

wine'' (Ephesians 5:18). However, the use of wine was not completely forbidden, as Paul's advice to Timothy makes clear: ''But use a little wine for thy stomach's sake and thine often infirmities'' (I Timothy 5:23). Today, to the Catholic, temperance is an important virtue. Although neither Luther nor Calvin was an absolute teetotaler, modern Protestant churches tend strongly to support abstinence.

Primitive peoples drank partly to relieve anxiety. Added to relief from tension were pleasures of the senses, such as taste and smell. Enveloping the pleasant package were companionship and religious meanings. The ancient civilized peoples doubtless had some reasons for drinking that were similar to those of the primitives. But a remark of Sholem Asch might be considered to have a universal application to drinking: ''Not the power to remember, but its very opposite, the power to forget, is a necessary condition of our existence.''[89] A Guatemalan Indian expressed this even more succinctly: ''A man must sometimes take a rest from his memory.''[90]

THE FATE OF ALCOHOL IN THE BODY According to a Japanese proverb,

> First the man takes a drink,
> Then the drink takes a drink,
> Then the drink takes the man!

Swallowed, alcohol stops first at the stomach. This often mistreated organ promptly helps its owner. Its walls allow only about 20 percent of the alcohol to be absorbed into the circulation. Absorption is delayed by foods rich in protein and fats (milk, eggs, meat) and by dilution (water, milk, juices). It has been said that for this reason Russian diplomats consume large quantities of milk before trying to impress their foreign guests with their ability to ''hold their vodka'' at a state banquet. Alcohol not absorbed by the stomach mucosa must await entrance into the small intestine, where complete absorption is quick regardless of the presence of food. But this entrance is slowed or even temporarily halted (depending on the amount of alcohol taken) by the spastic closure of the pyloric valve at the juncture of the stomach and small intestine. The delay prevents a sudden absorption (and a walloping dose) of all the ingested alcohol into the circulation. Whether absorbed into the circulation from the stomach or small intestine, alcohol in the blood means rapid access to the next stop, the liver. It is in the liver that most (90 percent) of the ingested alcohol is processed.

[89] Sholem Asch, *The Nazarene,* tr. by Maurice Samuels (New York, 1939), p. 3.

[90] Louis Lewin, *Phantastica: Narcotic and Stimulating Drugs,* cited in Norman Taylor, *Flight from Reality* (New York, 1949), p. 17. Apparently, many of the early developers of the U.S. West sought frequent respites from their memories. The Western saloon was a unique institution and it often doubled as a courthouse, jail, political campaign headquarters, or gambling parlor. (Richard Erodes, ''How the West Was Wan—The Morning After,'' *Signature,* Vol. 8, No. 6 [June 1973], p. 29.) And, to go back to earlier times, the U.S. national anthem, ''The Star-Spangled Banner,'' is based on an English drinking song. (Kenneth Keating, ''Mine Enemy—The Folk Singer,'' in *A Treasury of American Political Humor,* ed. by Leonard C. Lewin [New York, 1964], p. 301.) Nor was it a disgrace to brew beer in Colonial times. William Penn brewed and sold beer; taverns were the hotbeds of the Revolution, and on December 4, 1783, George Washington delivered his farewell address to his officers in a tavern. (Ernst and Johanna Lehner, *Folklore and Odysseys of Food and Medicinal Plants* [New York, 1962], pp. 34–35.

Relatively little passes out through the lungs as expired air or via the kidney as urine.

Alcohol is a toxin, or poison. *Detoxication,* the destruction of its poisonous properties, is accomplished by *oxidation*—a chemical process involving body oxygen. During the body detoxication of alcohol, three oxidation processes occur.

1. The first occurs in the liver. The liver receives much more alcohol than it can handle at one time. It oxidizes a tiny amount of its received alcohol into acetaldehyde. (The fate of this irritating substance is detailed in 2 below.) The rest of the alcohol leaves the liver utterly unchanged. It is then carried by the blood to the right side of the heart and then continues on to the lungs. As the blood in the lungs goes through its usual process of exchanging carbon dioxide waste for fresh oxygen, it also rids itself of a very little of its freeloader, alcohol. Thus, a tiny amount of alcohol is evaporated with breathing. This is not the alcohol that can be smelled, though it can be accurately measured. The alcohol that can be smelled is that in the mouth.

From the lungs, the alcohol that has not evaporated on the breath (and this is, by far, the greatest part of it) returns, with the newly oxygenated blood, to the left side of the heart. Then, not yet detoxicated, still not oxidized, the alcohol is pumped throughout the body.

So, the hitch is in the liver. It cannot oxidize all the alcohol it gets in one fell swoop. The liver works slowly, oxidizing alcohol a little at a time. The rest gets into the circulation via the heart and lungs. The alcohol distributed throughout the body must wait its turn for bit-by-bit detoxication by the liver. It is during that waiting period that the famed reactions to alcohol occur. Thus, alcohol acts with relative rapidity, but it leaves the body slowly.

2. While alcohol travels unchanged over the circulatory route, the liver busily, but slowly, oxidizes a few drops at a time to acetaldehyde. The acetaldehyde is very toxic. Fortunately, it quickly undergoes a second oxidation. This occurs not only in the liver but throughout the body. Acetic acid is formed.

3. A third, and final, oxidation also takes place throughout the body. Acetic acid is oxidized to water, carbon dioxide, and caloric energy.

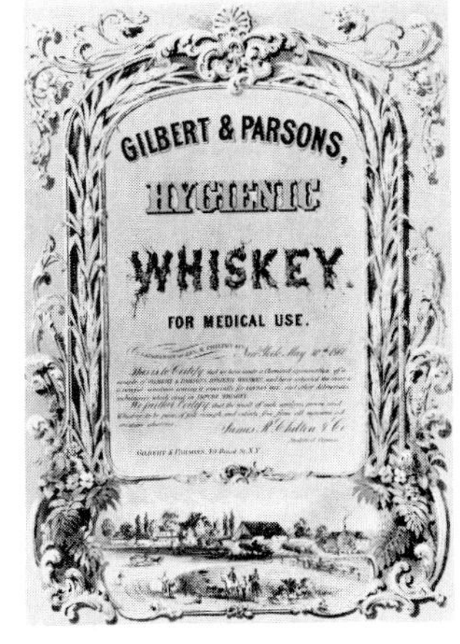

13-6 *Before the discovery of anesthetics, whiskey was used to relieve pain. Some 19th-century doctors in frontier America found an additional use for it. To keep their adult patients from scratching their smallpox vaccinations, for several days they kept them too drunk to raise their arms.*

THE EFFECT OF ALCOHOL Alcohol is not a stimulant. It is a depressant. But most people who drink spirits moderately do not seem depressed. On the contrary, they are relaxed, even gay. Those drinking too much were described by Benjamin Rush, a Quaker doctor and signer of the Declaration of Independence, as "singing, hallooing, roaring . . . tearing off clothes . . . dancing naked."[91]

Depression only comes later. Why the delay? Alcohol does indeed depress and anesthetize the nervous system. But it also releases inhibitions. Carried by the blood through the brain, it courses through the cerebral cortex. It is in the cortex that the numberless nerve connections of learning are laid. Alcohol

[91] Benjamin Rush, "Inquiry into the Effects of Ardent Spirits upon the Human Body and Mind," reprinted in *Quarterly Journal of Studies in Alcohol,* Vol. 4, No. 2 (September 1943), p. 325.

numbs them. If one has learned to hold his tongue, for example, alcohol loosens it. If it slips enough, he may halloo.

How do hangovers happen? How does too much drink take the man? The body cells lose fluid. There is thirst. Circulatory changes cause headaches. Decreased inhibitions promote overactivity. There is fatigue. The alcohol irritates the stomach. There is nausea. The alcohol assaults the nervous system, causing dizziness.

ALCOHOL, SEXUALITY, AND MARRIAGE Alcohol releases sexual inhibitions. In moderate amounts before sexual intercourse, it is certainly not contraindicated. Routine use of alcohol to diminish anxiety about coitus may signal a need for psychiatric help. Confirmed alcoholics lose interest in sexual intercourse. Male alcoholics often become impotent. The Porter in Shakespeare's *Macbeth* says of alcohol, that "it provokes and unprovokes. It provokes the desire, but it takes away the performance" (II.iii.33–35). Marriages complicated by excessive drinking are four times as likely as other marriages to end in divorce.

ALCOHOL AND DRIVING There is little question of the relationship between driving, drinking, and death. In more than half the fatal traffic accidents in this country, a driver is involved who has been drinking.[92] In Wisconsin, it was found that the fatality rate from this cause among young people aged sixteen to twenty was more than twice that of the general population. Most fatalities of sober drivers were the result of two-car accidents; the drinking driver usually was killed in a single-car crash.[93]

Some recommend a reevaluation of the "don't mix drinking and driving" rule.[94] Others, however, point out that "the variable effects of food taken with drink, tiredness, minor illness and remedies taken for it, and other factors including habituation to alcohol, make it impossible to advise any 'safe' upper limit for alcohol consumption before driving."[95] Several chemical tests are available for measuring the alcohol content in the system. The spinal fluid, saliva, blood, urine, and breath all have been accurately tested. Such evidence can, of course, be used in court (as was noted in Chapter 3).

Before driving, a drunken person may be walked around the block a couple of times to "sober him up." But this is to no avail. Muscle tissue cannot utilize alcohol. Exercise will not materially reduce the level of alcohol in the blood.

THE INCIDENCE OF DRINKING Two out of three adults in this country drink some kind of alcoholic beverage. Half of these use distilled spirits. One-fourth of them drink at least three times weekly. Among occasional drinkers, men outnumber women three to two. Three times as many men as women drink regularly. Among the better educated and the more affluent, drinking is more

[92] W. Haddon, Jr., and V. A. Bradess, "Alcohol in the Single Vehicle Fatal Accident: Experience of Westchester County, N.Y.," *Journal of the American Medical Association,* Vol. 169, No. 14 (April 4, 1959), p. 1587.
[93] Ronald H. Laessig and Kathy J. Waterworth, "Involvement of Alcohol in Fatalities of Wisconsin Drivers," *Public Health Reports,* Vol. 85, No. 6 (June 1970), p. 548.
[94] Robert F. Borkenstein, "A Realistic Approach to Drinking and Driving," *Traffic Safety,* Vol. 67, No. 10 (October 1967), p. 11.
[95] "Drinking Drivers," an editorial in *British Medical Journal,* Vol. 2, No. 5544 (April 8, 1967), p. 67.

common. City people drink more than rural dwellers. Protestant abstainers outnumber the Jewish three to one, and the Catholic two to one. Blacks drink as commonly as do whites.[96]

Until a few years ago, it was believed, with some validity, that—with a few overpublicized exceptions—teen-agers rarely got drunk. But there is increasing evidence that many teen-agers do drink to intoxication and, indeed, become dependent on alcohol.[97] Too many high school students no longer drink merely to taste adulthood.[98]

ALCOHOLISM Of the estimated 100 million people in the United States who drink some alcohol, about 9½ million are alcoholics.[99] Thus, for one in eleven alcohol is a poison. That person is an alcoholic. Without treatment he may become human backwash, gutted, guttered.

Why can one person drink alcohol convivially, while another becomes a confirmed alcoholic? There are no simple answers. The causes of alcoholism are many and complex. In some cases the reasons reach into childhood. For example, as a child, an alcoholic may have been grossly overprotected. He comes to need this excess protection. He learns to fear its loss. To keep it, he remains dependent. Then, one day, he is an adult. Suddenly he must compete. He must be independent. He is bereft. He may reach for alcohol, which, he may have learned, will embolden him.

There are women who begin to drink heavily in their middle years. Their menopause may have begun. Their children are gone, their husbands are at work all day. They feel alone, unneeded. Unprepared for these events, they suffer what has been called the "empty nest syndrome."[100] Instead of expanding their horizons, they try to drown their grief in a bottle. Of course, there are other reasons for alcoholism among women, but the condition is more serious than in men for at least one reason: women tend to hide the affliction more, and this deception is more readily abetted by their families.[101]

Some researchers suggest that alcoholism tends to run in families,[102] or to have a genetic basis. Some recent studies do suggest that different susceptibilities to alcohol may be due to differences in rates of metabolism between racial groups.[103] Moreover, family-history studies have shown high rates of

[96] Harrison M. Trice, *Alcoholism in America* (New York, 1966), p. 22.

[97] Jules Salzman, *The New Alcoholics: Teenagers,* Public Affairs Pamphlet No. 499 (October 1973).

[98] Donald L. Hinder, "Drug Use by Students of Drug Abuse," *Journal of Drug Education,* Vol. 3, No. 3 (Fall 1973); Margaret R. Porter *et al.,* "Drug Use in Anchorage, Alaska: A Survey of 15,634 Students in Grades 6 Through 12, 1971," *Journal of the American Medical Association,* Vol. 223, No. 6 (February 5, 1973).

[99] "Alcoholism: America's Most Destructive Drug Problem," *Medical World News,* Vol. 12, No. 8 (February 26, 1971), p. 43.

[100] Joan Curlee, "Alcoholism and the Empty Nest," *Bulletin of the Menninger Clinic,* Vol. 33, No. 3 (May 1969), pp. 165–71.

[101] "Alcoholism in Women," *Journal of the American Medical Association,* Vol. 225, No. 8 (August 20, 1973), p. 988.

[102] George Winokur, Theodore Reich, John Rimmer, and Ferris N. Pitts, Jr., "Alcoholism: III. Diagnosis and Familial Psychiatric Illness in 259 Alcoholic Probands," *Archives of General Psychiatry,* Vol. 23 (1970), pp. 104–11.

[103] D. Fenner, L. Mix, O. Schefer, and J. L. Gilbert, "Ethanol Metabolism in Various Racial Groups," *Canadian Medical Association Journal,* Vol. 104, No. 472 (1971).

familial incidence of alcoholism.[104] A young person's peers also have a profound influence on his drinking patterns.

Alcoholism generally develops in three phases, each of which is characterized by certain symptoms. Even before the potential alcoholic reaches the first phase, he has warnings. His very first drink may be an unexpected delight. He can hardly wait for another. His course begins.

The symptoms of alcoholism need not follow in sequence. Some come together. Others may not occur. Throughout the first blank period or amnesia that marks the first phase, the potential alcoholic will act normally. He may be cheering at a football game with friends. On the following day, he remembers nothing. Deep within him is a gnawing uneasiness. Later, this will be a wild fear. What did he do and say? He cannot recall. He drinks more. For many alcoholics the tolerance for the liquid drug increases. For others it seems to decrease. The first phase may last five years—sometimes less.

The second phase, which begins with loss of control of drinking, is the milestone in the alcoholic's journey. Without adequate treatment, it marks the beginning of a downhill course. In this stage the moral argument over alcohol does the alcoholic the greatest disservice. That quarrel helped create the concept of the average alcoholic as a skid-row bum. Less than 10 percent of the nation's alcoholics inhabit skid row. The rest live with their families, desperately hanging on to their jobs. It is the skid-row caricature of the alcoholic that his important people—his wife, children, friends, boss, and even minister—cannot accept of him. He is not really that, they say. He will straighten out. The alcoholic helps with the delusion. Tomorrow will be sober. Pale, trembling, furtive, he pulls himself together. To those worrying about him, he gives false hope. They vacillate. He is not treated. He rejects such help as Alcoholics Anonymous. Then he is drunk again. His remorse is their despair.

The last phase is a haunting torment that he will run out of alcohol. Hours are spent in searching for and then hiding it. Often he cannot keep the alcohol down. Days are spent on his knees, like an animal, crawling, vomiting, perhaps resting his throbbing head on a toilet bowl.

His body, long resentful, is now in angry protest. He may have already become hoarse from his swollen throat (''brandy voice''). His bloodshot eyes, pasty skin, red ''brandy nose'' have become part of him. Poor nutrition wastes him. Vitamin-deficiency diseases plague him. Without alcohol he may develop *delirium tremens* (the abstinence syndrome). Numberless ''worms'' or ''ants'' torture him. ''Snakes'' bite into him. Delirium tremens is a true psychosis. Five percent of alcoholics develop delirium tremens. Without attention, perhaps 25 percent of those with delirium tremens die. With care, less than 5 percent die.

Other signs of vitamin deficiency may occur. Prickly burning of the hands and feet heralds the pain and paralysis of *polyneuritis*. Prompt treatment with

[104] Marc Alan Schuckit, ''Family History and Half-Sibling Research in Alcoholism,'' *Annals of the New York Academy of Sciences,* Vol. 197 (May 25, 1972), pp. 121–25; Donald W. Goodwin, ''Is Alcoholism Hereditary? A Review and a Critique,'' *Archives of General Psychiatry,* Vol. 25 (December 1971), pp. 545–49; and Donald W. Goodwin, Fini Schulsinger, Leif Hermansen, Samuel B. Guze, and George Winokur, ''Alcohol Problems in Adoptees Raised Apart from Alcoholic Biologic Parents,'' *Archives of General Psychiatry,* Vol. 28 (February 1973), pp. 238–43.

vitamin B can prevent permanent disability. *Korsakoff's psychosis* (also seen with diseases other than alcoholism) is characterized by periods of amnesia filled in by the patient with all sorts of preposterous tales. Full recovery has not been reported. *Wernicke's syndrome* is the result of impeded brain tissue metabolism. With vitamin B therapy, improvement is likely.

In addition, recent research suggests that "the long-term ingestion of alcohol plays a probable causative role in the commonly observed heart disease of alcoholic patients."[105] It is now believed that alcohol is toxic directly to the heart.[106]

There is no evidence that moderate consumption of alcohol causes brain damage; this does occur with long-term excessive intake of alcohol. Studies with rats support the conclusion that, with prolonged use, "it is the alcohol itself and not malnutrition [as was previously thought] that inflicts brain damage."[107] Recent work suggests that problems of blood circulation caused by alcoholism also contribute to brain disease.

ALCOHOL, CALORIES, AND MALNUTRITION Alcohol, in itself, does not cause one to be fat. Its calories are not directly stored as fat. They do, however, replace food calories, which are then stored. Unless the drinker cuts down on his food calories to the extent of his alcohol caloric intake, he will fatten.

As a rule alcoholics, no matter what their body weight is, are malnourished. This is true despite the high caloric content of alcohol (a pint of bourbon—not an unusual daily intake for an alcoholic—contains 1350 calories). Alcoholic beverages have little food value. Also, during drinking bouts the alcoholic diminishes his food intake. He is not hungry. Years of excessive drinking have irritated and inflamed his stomach lining. His small intestine has lost some of its ability to absorb fats, fat-soluble vitamins, proteins, and other essential nutrients. His euphoria—his exaggerated sense of well-being—is not conducive to hunger. Even if he were hungry, the alcoholic is frequently so penniless that he could not afford food.

The malnutrition of acute alcoholism contributes to increased fat deposition in the liver. The cells of a fatty liver are only mildly injured. However, with the more serious liver inflammation called *hepatitis,* numerous liver cells are killed. Sometimes the hepatitis is fatal. When it is not, a healing process occurs as fibrous tissue infiltrates the liver. *Cirrhosis of the liver* results. This healing process does not help liver function. Why? The fibrous tissue cannot function as liver tissue. Cirrhosis of the liver is primarily the result of malnutrition, although the alcohol may play a direct role.

THE TREATMENT OF ALCOHOLISM The treatment of alcoholism must begin with evaluation of the physical, emotional, social, and cultural factors influ-

[105] Dean T. Mason, James F. Spann, James L. Hughes, Robert Zelis, and Ezra A. Amsterdam, "Alcohol and the Heart," *The Heart Bulletin,* Vol. 20, No. 1 (January–February 1971), p. 3.

[106] "Alcoholism: America's Most Destructive Drug Problem," p. 46.

[107] "Alcohol Isn't Really Dangerous, Is It?" *New Scientist,* Vol. 60, No. 872 (November 15, 1973), p. 460, citing Don W. Walker and Gerhard Freund, "Impairment of Timing Behavior After Prolonged Alcohol Consumption in Rats," *Science,* Vol. 182, No. 4112 (November 9, 1973), pp. 597–98.

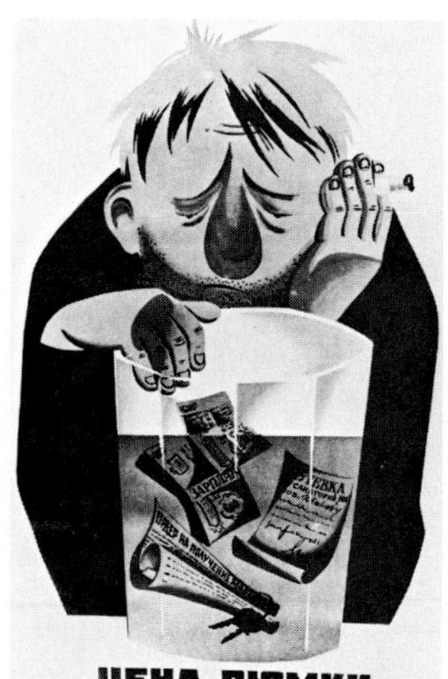

13-7 *"The Price of a Drink" is the title of this Russian anti-alcoholism poster. Sinking into the glass of vodka are rubles, tickets for a vacation, and a certificate for an apartment.*

encing both the alcoholic and his or her family. According to the patient's needs, either inpatient or outpatient services may be used. Various carefully supervised methods may be used in the treatment of the alcoholic, including *aversion therapy, antabuse, adjustment,* and *Alcoholics Anonymous.* In *aversion therapy* the patient is first given injections of a nauseant drug. He then drinks various kinds of liquor. He may come to associate his resultant nausea with the ingested alcohol. For many, this treatment has been successful. *Antabuse* makes even a small amount of ingested alcohol a dangerous experience—the patient becomes seriously ill. Various tranquilizers may also be used. Psychological *adjustment* may be achieved with the aid of group therapy. *Alcoholics Anonymous* is a splendid supportive organization offering much psychological and spiritual aid, which may, however, need *professional supplementation.* The best approach is multidisciplinary.[108] Some health departments have embarked on alcoholism prevention and treatment programs.

In 1970 the Comprehensive Alcohol Abuse and Alcoholism Prevention, Treatment, and Rehabilitation Act was passed. One result was the establishment of the National Clearinghouse for Alcohol Information of the National Institute of Alcohol Abuse and Alcoholism. This federal agency has done much to educate the public as to the need to treat alcoholism as an illness.[109]

It used to be thought that once an alcoholic starts drinking, he cannot stop. For some alcoholics, this may not be the case. Studies at the University of Oklahoma suggest that "for the phenomenon of 'craving' to occur . . . the drinking must be done in a social setting."[110] In an open hospital setting the alcoholic's drinking patterns seemed considerably easier for him to control. Possibly, then, alcohol might be incorporated into the treatment program of the alcoholic. In this way he may learn that he can, indeed, control his alcohol intake.[111] It has been demonstrated that alcoholics can "give up excessive drinking and stabilize on a normal drinking pattern."[112] But this accomplishment requires carefully supervised treatment.

some minor depressants: sniffing for dreams

Greek mythology refers to the priestess Pythia, seated on the side of the mountain Parnassus. From the earth she inhaled cold vapors that already had convulsed goats and a goatherd. Her vapor-inspired thoughts were carefully interpreted by the priests. Thousands of years later, stylish English gentry of the early nineteenth century used laughing gas to sniff themselves silly at dinner parties. Soon college students in this country were sniffing and laughing too. Ether sniffing became popular both in this country and abroad; one nineteenth-century report states that "the students at Harvard used to inhale sulfu-

[108] Ruth Fox, "A Multidisciplinary Approach to the Treatment of Alcoholism," *International Journal of Psychiatry,* Vol. 5, No. 1 (January 1968), pp. 34–46.
[109] "Chafetz Cites Rising Momentum," *Alcohol & Health Notes,* Experimental Issue (June 1973), pp. 1, 7.
[110] "Alcoholics Who Can Handle Their Liquor," *Medical World News,* Vol. 12, No. 46 (December 10, 1971), p. 16.
[111] *Ibid.,* p. 17.
[112] Oliver Gillie, "Drug Addiction—Facts and Folklore," *Science Journal* (December 1969), pp. 75–80.

ric ether from their handkerchiefs, and it intoxicated them and made them reel and stagger.''[113] Nowadays, chloroform seems to have replaced ether in some circles. A recent report of ''chloroform parties'' in central Wisconsin has been cause for concern. A bottle of chloroform is passed around the room and each participant inhales the vapors from a saturated cloth. Some drink some of the chloroform. As an anaesthetic chloroform is little used today. Among the reasons for its limited use are the high incidence of liver damage and the undesirable side effects such as heart stoppage and drop in blood pressure.[114] At one chloroform party a nineteen-year-old boy ingested enough chloroform to hospitalize him in a coma. He had suffered severe liver damage.[115]

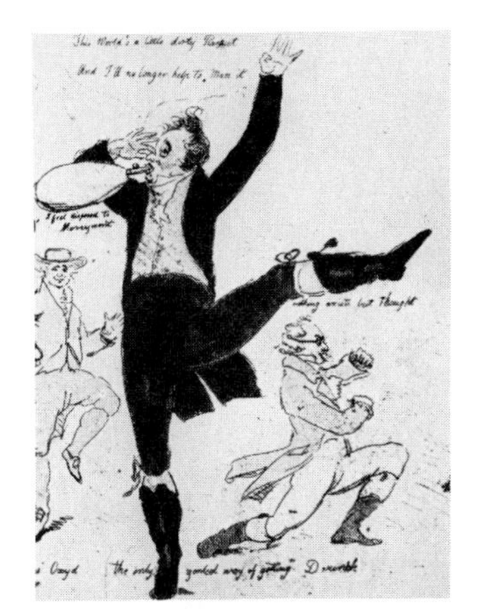

13-8 *Nitrous oxide (laughing gas) was discovered in 1806 by the great chemist Sir Humphrey Davy. It caught on as a party fad, as evidenced in this cartoon.*

A tube of glue and a paper bag provide some children and adolescents with their dreams. Model-airplane glue is most popular. However, plastic cement, antifreeze, paint thinner, cleaning and lighter fluids, gasoline and kerosene—all have their followers. The vapors are central nervous system depressants. With chronic abuse, tolerance has been reported. With discontinuance of the drug, withdrawal symptoms can be severe but are usually mild. Nausea, vomiting, dizziness, and ringing of the ears have all been reported. At first, the sniffer is exhilarated. As he sniffs, euphoria and hallucinations may occur. Occasionally hallucinations persist for several hours. Homicides have been associated with the abuse of the vapors of glue, lacquer thinner, and plastic cement. With the beginnings of the sniffing experience, there is no established evidence that irreversible physical damage results.[116] However, there is considerable clinical opinion that physical damage to both kidney and central nervous system is likely.[117] Persistent glue sniffing can result in severe anemia and bone marrow and liver damage.[118] Chronic gasoline sniffers can develop lead poisoning.

By decreasing the supply of oxygen to the lungs the Freon aerosol spray sniffer risks his life. By the beginning of 1971, aerosol sniffing had caused at least 110 deaths.[119] Particularly popular as inhalants are underarm deodorants, hair sprays, insecticide sprays, and the propellant gases used for all of these.[120] It is the propellant gas that is believed to cause the fatal heart attacks,[121] although other mechanisms may be involved.[122]

[113] W. T. G. Morton, ''A Memoir to the Academy of Sciences at Paris on a New Use of Sulfuric Ether,'' cited in Sidney Cohen, *The Drug Dilemma* (New York, 1969), p. 99.

[114] Louis S. Goodman and Alfred Gilman, *The Pharmacological Basis of Therapeutics* (New York, 1970), p. 84.

[115] William W. Storms, ''Chloroform Parties,'' *Journal of the American Medical Association,* Vol. 225, No. 2 (July 9, 1973), p. 160.

[116] Edward Preble and Gabriel V. Laury, ''Plastic Cement, The Ten-Cent Hallucinogen,'' *International Journal of Addictions,* Vol. 2, No. 2 (Fall 1967), p. 275.

[117] John C. Pollard, ''Teen-Agers and the Use of Drugs: Reflections on the Emotional Setting,'' *Clinical Pediatrics,* Vol. 6, No. 11 (November 1967), pp. 618–19.

[118] E. T. O'Brien, W. B. Yeoman, and J. E. A. Hobby, ''Hepatorenal Damage from Toluene in a 'Glue Sniffer,''' *British Medical Journal,* Vol. 2, No. 5752 (April 3, 1971), pp. 29–30.

[119] ''Cardiac Toxicity of Aerosol Propellants,'' editorial in *Journal of the American Medical Association,* Vol. 214, No. 1 (October 5, 1970), p. 136, citing M. Bass, ''Sudden Sniffing Deaths,'' *Journal of the American Medical Association,* Vol. 212 (1970), pp. 2075–79.

[120] Charles F. Reinhardt, Alex Azar, Mary E. Maxfield, Paul E. Smith, and Linda S. Mullin, ''Cardiac Arrhythmias and Aerosol 'Sniffing,''' *Archives of Environmental Health,* Vol. 22, No. 2 (February 1971), p. 265.

[121] George J. Taylor IV and Willard S. Harris, ''Cardiac Toxicity of Aerosol Propellants,'' *Journal of the American Medical Association,* Vol. 214, No. 1 (October 5, 1970), pp. 81–85.

[122] ''Sniffing Death in Aerosols,'' *Medical World News,* Vol. 12, No. 1 (January 8, 1971), pp. 24–25.

tobacco

> A filthie noveltie . . . A custome lothsome to the eye, hatefull to the nose, harmefull to the braine, dangerous to the Lungs, and in the black stinking fume thereof, neerest resembling the horrible Stigian smoke of the pit that's bottomlesse.[123]

some historical notes

There is no evidence of ancient Greek, Roman, or German smoking. In West Indian, Central American, and Mexican antiquity, Mayan Indian relics testify to the use of tobacco. In a report dated 1497, a priest, Romano Pane, first described the habit. The Indians inhaled smoke through a Y-shaped pipe called a ''tabaco.'' The two forks of the Y fitted into their nostrils.

Tobacco was the first commercial export from the New World to the Old. Without it, the colonization of Virginia might have been long delayed. First explored by Sir Walter Raleigh (who enjoyed a pipe of tobacco before going to the scaffold in 1618), the colony was constantly threatened by disease, hunger, and Indian attack. Nevertheless, it prevailed. How? The gallant Captain John Smith made friends with the Indians. And food came from England. Most important, however, John Rolfe, the settler who married the Indian princess Pocahontas, discovered a method of curing tobacco. In England, despite the bitter antagonism of James I, demand for the leaf grew. Still the lonely Virginians were unhappy. Then a major problem was solved. Ninety marriageable girls were sent to them from London. The settlers, mostly young men, paid only traveling expenses. Since tobacco took the place of money, from 120 to 150 pounds of good Virginia leaf were traded for each girl.[124]

James and his supporters persisted in their opposition to tobacco. Darkly, they suggested that it caused impotence:

> It dulls the sprite, it dims the sight,
> It robs a woman of her right.[125]

In those days, the Russians whipped tobacco smokers or slit their noses. In 1642, a Papal Bull exorcised ''infecting the churches with . . . noxious fumes.''[126] Excommunication was threatened.

But nothing stopped smoking. Today, even the threat of possible death fails to accomplish this.

why do people smoke?

Curiosity probably prompts the average adolescent to start smoking. To prove his adult status, he continues despite his initial distaste. The young mimic becomes a rebel. Smoking demonstrates resistance to parental authority. But no single theory can account for the eventual profound hold of tobacco on the young person. Nor will any single theory of cure help break the habit.

[123] James I of England, in *A Counterblaste to Tobacco* (1604), cited in E. Corti, *A History of Smoking,* tr. by Paul England (London, 1931), p. 83.
[124] *Ibid.,* p. 92.
[125] C. M. Fletcher *et al., Common Sense About Smoking* (Baltimore, 1963), p. 81.
[126] E. Corti, *A History of Smoking,* p. 129.

Some aspects of the origins of tobacco dependency merit particular mention.

emotional roots

Even in the security of the womb, an unborn baby will suck his thumb (see Figure 11-5). At birth, and before the cord is cut, the newborn may pop a thumb into his mouth. To eat, healthy babies must suck. Many babies normally continue to suck after their hunger is satiated. Sucking, then, is a basic instinctive need of the infant, a drive associated with the mother's warmth, with food, with security. Some babies are more avid suckers than others, rejecting cup and spoon, weaning late. A child to whom sucking is not so important may be weaned earlier. Others wait three years or longer. A content child, satisfied with his early sucking experience, will usually venture easily into the next phase. An insecure child, not satiated by his sucking experience, perhaps because of a constantly agitated mother, will only reluctantly part with early comforts. Sucking can become excessive (see page 289). This is seen with older children who continuously suck their thumbs or with chain-smokers.

The infant relieves the pain of hunger by sucking the nipple. The child finds succor with a blanket or thumb. The adult drags on a cigarette or pipe. This can be a continuous behavior pattern, a prolonged emotional shelter.

"Sucking or smoking, therefore, is innately capable of reducing the negative effect of distress and of evoking the positive aspect of enjoyment . . . Many adults experience distress frequently enough every day to seek to reduce this distress by smoking."[127]

economic aspects of smoking

It has been claimed that the $3.7 billion collected in tobacco taxes (federal, $2.0 billion; state, $1.6 billion; local, $0.1 billion) makes the tobacco industry an indispensable contributor to the U.S. economy. A recent Canadian study[128] singled out only four cigarette-induced diseases—lung cancer, coronary heart disease, chronic bronchitis, and emphysema—and fires caused by cigarette smoking. For these were estimated the annual costs of medical care, income lost because of illness, loss of future income because of death, and the value of property lost in cigarette fires. The results, applied to the United States: in hard cash, the people of this nation pay far more for cigarettes every year than the $3.7 billion in presumed benefits they receive from their cigarette taxes.[129]

[127] Silvan S. Tomkins, "Psychological Model for Smoking Behavior," *American Journal of Public Health,* Vol. 56, No. 12 (December 1966, supplement), p. 18.

[128] James L. Hedrick, "The Economic Costs of Cigarette Smoking," *ASMHA Health Reports,* Vol. 86, No. 2 (February 1971), citing "Canadian Department of National Health and Welfare: The Estimated Costs of Certain Identifiable Consequences of Cigarette Smoking on Health, Longevity, and Property in Canada in 1966," *Research and Statistics Memo* (Ottawa, 1967), Appendix 1(a).

[129] James L. Hedrick, *ibid.,* pp. 179–82.

social aspects of smoking

Smoking is a socially contagious disease . . .[130]

Some people smoke to feel more intimately a part of a convivial group, to share a relaxing group activity. For others, a cigarette provides a protective smoke-screen in an uncomfortable social situation, such as a party at which the smoker feels ill at ease. For still others, smoking provides an outlet for the tensions of a busy world. These are but a few of the social aspects of smoking.

What specific human harm comes of tobacco smoking? Before examining the evidence, one must visualize the airway system.

the normal respiratory tree

Inhaled air traverses the nasal and (if the mouth is open) oral cavities, passes the *pharynx* to the *larynx,* and reaches the hollow, stiff *respiratory tree* (see Figure 13–9 and body charts 11 and 12 in the color section). This is indeed a tree, but upside down, with its branches spreading out on each side of the chest cavity.

The main trunk, the four-inch-long *trachea* (windpipe) divides into two main branches, the *bronchi* (singular, *bronchus*). Division and subdivision continue until tiny twigs are reached called the *bronchioles.* These end in thin-walled air sacs, the *alveoli* (see Figures 13–9 and 13–10). There, through the capillary network embedded in the alveolar walls, oxygen is absorbed into the blood and carbon dioxide is eliminated. The oxygen from the inhaled air is carried in the blood from the lungs to the heart through the pulmonary veins, and it reaches the rest of the body via the aorta, the great artery from the heart. The carbon dioxide has been delivered to the alveolar capillary network through the pulmonary arteries, which feed blood to the lungs from the heart. The carbon dioxide is expelled from the alveolar capillaries when breath is exhaled.

The trachea and bronchi are kept rigid and open by regularly spaced, *C*-shaped rings of hard fibrous tissue called *cartilage.* The bronchioles, however, are not held open by cartilage but by *elastic fibers.* Thus, they get larger with inhalation and smaller with exhalation.

Covering the whole respiratory tract, from nose to bronchioles, is a thin, moving film of mucus. Every day about three ounces of mucus are produced by glands in the lining of the air passages. The mucus is kept moving toward the throat by countless sweeping, hairlike *cilia.* Like millions of tiny brooms, the cilia project from the lining of the bronchial tubes (see Figure 13-9). The moving mucus blanket keeps the air passages moist and protects them. Inhaled dust, germs, and other foreign particles stick to the mucus blanket and are swept away by the ciliary brooms. Anything that interferes with ciliary action interferes with the normal housekeeping of the respiratory system.

cigarette smoking: harbinger of sickness and death

On January 11, 1964, *Smoking and Health,* the report of the Advisory Committee to the Surgeon General of the Public Health Service, was released. In 1967, a second report, *The Health Consequences of Smoking,* was made available by

[130] "Cowardice About Smoking," editorial in *British Medical Journal,* Vol. 1, No. 5751 (March 27, 1971), p. 683.

the Surgeon General, and supplements to it were issued in 1968, 1969, 1971, and 1973. The later reports reinforce the first one. What are some of the accumulated findings?

1. Because of illness, cigarette smokers spend over a third again as much time away from their jobs as persons who never smoke. Women who smoke are sick in bed 17 percent more than women who never smoke.[131]

2. Total death rates for cigarette smokers are nearly 70 percent higher than for nonsmokers. Heavier smoking means higher death rates. For example, with those smoking forty or more cigarettes daily, the death rate rises to 120 percent more than that of nonsmokers.[132] The ratio of smoker to nonsmoker death rates is greatest in the precious peak years, forty to fifty.[133] Furthermore, "life expectancy among young men is reduced by an average of 8 years in 'heavy' cigarette smokers, those who smoke over two packs a day, and an average of 4 years in 'light' cigarette smokers, those who smoke less than one-half pack per day."[134]

3. The death rates from cancers of the lung, larynx, oral cavity, esophagus, kidney, urinary bladder, and pancreas are all markedly higher with cigarette smokers than nonsmokers.[135]

Other studies reveal that some nations in which people smoke the most have enjoyed the least advance in the length of life of its men. Among these are the United States and Scotland. Poor countries such as Portugal, Albania, and Costa Rica today record higher life expectancies for its men at age thirty-five than does Scotland or the United States.[136]

The earlier smoking is started, the sooner death occurs. Children are mimics. The impact of advertising, the example of parents and others important to the child, the child's search for symbols of maturity—all combine to impress the pre–teen-ager with a favorable picture of the smoker.[137] The rapid increase of smoking among high school students has led to recommendations that education against smoking begin no later than the third grade.[138]

emphysema and chronic bronchitis: chronically obstructed lungs

The smoke from cigarette combustion produces gases that paralyze cilia. Mucus cannot move. In the bronchioles, a traffic jam is created. How? With inhaling, the bronchioles expand. Air can squeeze in past the unmoving mucus. But as

[131] *Smoking and Illness* (1967), prepared by the National Clearinghouse for Smoking and Health, Public Health Service, and based on a report issued by the National Center for Health Statistics, *Cigarette Smoking and Health Characteristics.*

[132] "Summary of Research," *Smoking and Health, Report of the Advisory Committee to the Surgeon General of the Public Health Service* (1964).

[133] *Ibid.*, "Summary and Conclusions."

[134] "Summary of the Report," *The Health Consequences of Smoking,* 1969 Supplement to *The Health Consequences of Smoking, A Public Health Service Review,* Public Health Service Publication No. 1696 (1967) p. 3.

[135] "Smoking and Cancer," *The Health Consequences of Smoking,* 1968 Supplement, pp. 94–106.

[136] "Aged Mortality and Cigarette Smoking Linked," *Geriatric Times,* Vol. 4, No. 11 (November 1970), p. 14.

[137] Charles L. Leedham, "Pre-Teen Smokers," *Clinical Pediatrics,* Vol. 6, No. 3 (March 1967), p. 135.

[138] Eva J. Salber and Theodor Abelin, "Smoking Behavior of Newton School Children," *Pediatrics,* Vol. 30, No. 3 (September 1967), p. 371.

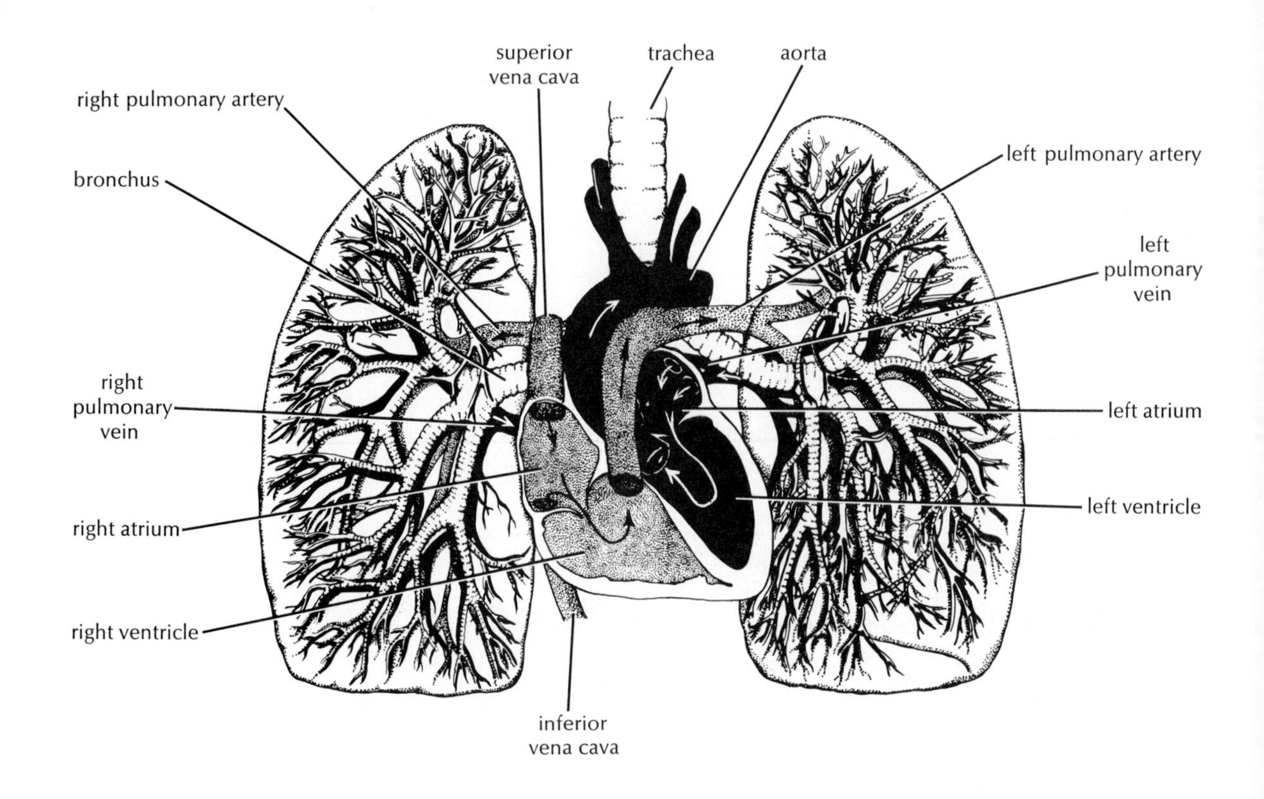

13-9 the respiratory system

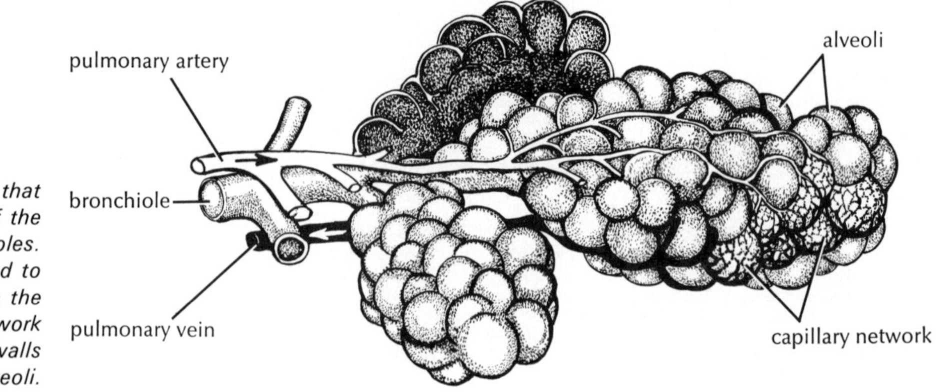

Alveoli: air sacs that are terminals of the lung's bronchioles. Oxygen is supplied to the blood through the capillary network embedded in the walls of the alveoli.

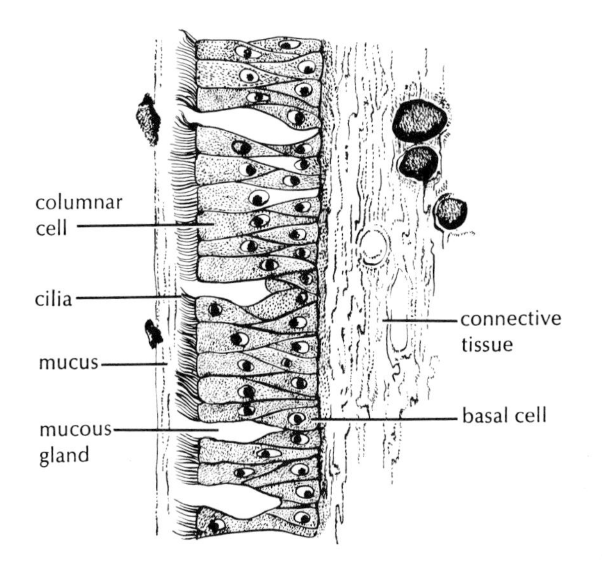

Respiratory epithelium resting on connective tissue. When the surface layer of epithelial cells is damaged, the damaged cells are cast off and replaced by upgrowing deeper cells, which grow cilia when they reach the surface. Although the epithelial cells lie at different levels, they all reach the underlying connective tissue and are in contact with the nerves in connective tissue, which control the beat of the cilia. The columnar cells reach the connective tissue by narrowing. The cells of this type of respiratory epithelium are found throughout the entire respiratory tract except in the alveoli and in the smallest air passages leading directly to the alveoli. The extremely thin epithelium in the alveoli is unlike the rest of the respiratory epithelium to permit an efficient exchange of oxygen and carbon dioxide gases. In addition, cilia are absent in the passage of the vocal cords. Were they present there, voice production would be hampered. Therefore, this passage is cleared by clearing the throat or by a slight cough.

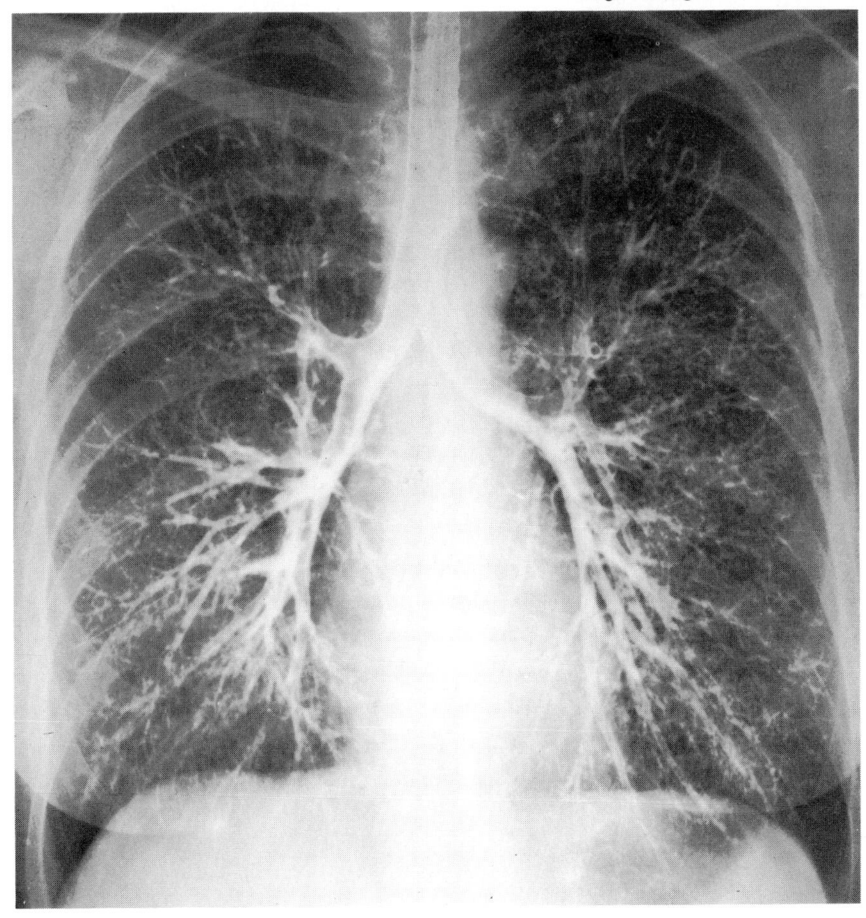

A bronchogram, an X-ray of the lungs taken after instilling an opaque medium in the bronchus.

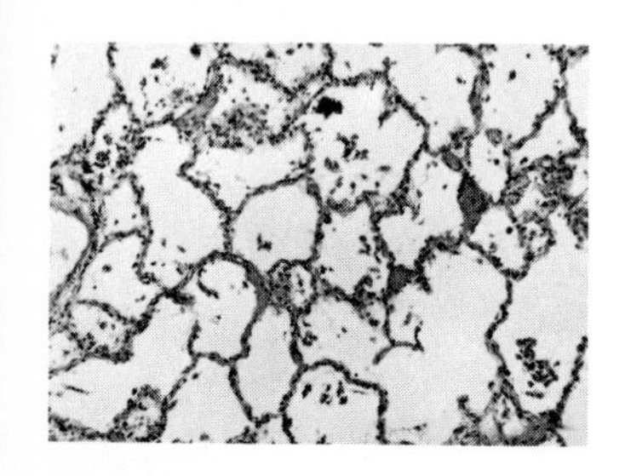

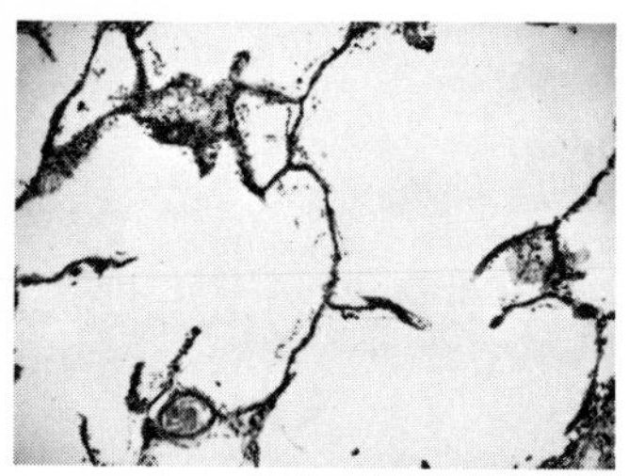

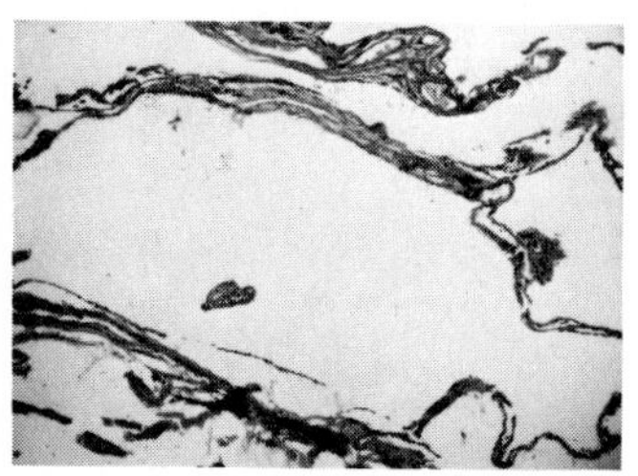

13-10 *Normal lung alveoli* (top), *alveoli partly destroyed* (center), *and extensively destroyed alveoli* (bottom).

air is exhaled, the bronchioles diminish in size. They clamp down on the trapped, accumulated mucus. Air cannot get out. It stretches the air sacs (alveoli). These balloon. They form large air blisters. Some rupture. Lung tissue is destroyed (see Figure 13-10). Breathing efficiency is diminished. To accommodate the damaged, overstretched lung, the entire bony chest cage enlarges. Then the diaphragm, the breathing muscle separating the chest and abdomen, loses efficiency. All this is *emphysema.*

Emphysema is generally seen in conjunction with *chronic bronchitis.* The accumulation of mucus and the paralysis of cilia combine to prevent the elimination of germs. These, in turn, infect the bronchial tubes.

''Cigarette smoking is the most important cause of chronic bronchitis . . . [and] evidence indicates that cigarette smoking is the most important agent in the development of pulmonary emphysema in man.''[139] Moreover, ''for chronic bronchitis and emphysema . . . the death rate for cigarette smokers is 500 percent higher than for nonsmokers.''[140] This deadly duo comprise the major elements of chronic obstructive disease of the bronchi and lungs. The past twenty years have seen a more than sixfold increase in the number of deaths from these conditions. Smoking is a much more significant cause of these diseases than is atmospheric pollution or occupational exposure.[141]

smoking and cancer

''Carcinoma of the lips occurs most frequently where men indulge in pipe smoking: the lower lip is particularly affected by cancer, when it is compressed between the tobacco pipe and the teeth.''[142] This was written 175 years ago. In our own time, the study of cancer and smoking has taken on new urgency. The following statement was issued by the Public Health Service in July 1969:

> Additional evidence substantiates the previous findings that cigarette smoking is the main cause of lung cancer in men. Cigarette smoking is causally related to lung cancer in women but accounts for a smaller proportion of cases than in men. Smoking is a significant factor in the causation of cancer of the larynx and in the development of cancer of the oral cavity. Further epidemiological data strengthen the association of cigarette smoking with cancer of the bladder and cancer of the pancreas.[143]

The relationship between cigarette smoking and lung cancer has been intensively studied. These are some of the findings: (1) The average male cigarette smoker has nine to ten times the chance of the nonsmoker of developing lung cancer. For heavy smokers this risk doubles.[144] (2) If smoking is discon-

[139] ''Smoking and Chronic Obstructive Bronchopulmonary Disease,'' *The Health Consequences of Smoking,* 1969 Supplement, pp. 37, 38.

[140] ''Summary and Conclusions,'' *Smoking and Health* (1964), p. 29.

[141] ''Chronic Obstructive Bronchopulmonary Disease,'' *The Health Consequences of Smoking, A Report to the Surgeon General,* U.S. Department of Health, Education, and Welfare Publication No. (HSM)71-7513 (1971), p. 153.

[142] S. Th. Sömmering, ''De Moribus Vasorum Absorbentium Corporis Humani'' (1795), p. 109, tr. in Ernest L. Wynder and Dietrich Hoffman, *Tobacco and Tobacco Smoke* (New York, 1967), p. 1.

[143] ''Summary of the Report,'' *The Health Consequences of Smoking,* 1969 Supplement, p. 4.

[144] ''Summary and Conclusions,'' *Smoking and Health* (1964), p. 31.

tinued, the risk of dying from lung cancer sharply decreases.[145] (3) Since 1930, the lung cancer death rate in women has increased more than 400 percent. Compared to the increase in the male lung cancer rate, after 1960, there was noted a "greater relative rise in mortality from lung cancer in the female population."[146] This increase continues. (4) Only one of twenty diagnosed lung cancers is now cured.[147] Of all the common malignancies, lung cancer offers by far the least hope of cure (see page 205). (5) The microscopic appearance of about 100,000 specimens of lung tissue (taken from people who had either died or were undergoing lung surgery) was correlated with smoking history. The results:[148]

Those who had never smoked had normal lung tissue.

"Pre-cancerous lesions" were found in proportion to the amount of cigarette smoking.

The tissue of those who had smoked and stopped showed less lung disease changes. Reversibility is possible when smoking is stopped.

If smoking continues, precancerous cells go on to malignancy. Deeper tissue is invaded. The changes then do not reverse. Man suffers few illnesses so presently incurable as cancer of the lung.

Other research indicates that heavy smokers are more likely to have a more highly malignant form of lung cancer than are light smokers.[149]

Those interested in promoting tobacco sales have long claimed that cigarette smoking has never been proved to cause lung cancer. Why? Because it never produced lung cancer in the experimental animal that smoked. In a definitive study, cancer of the lung has been induced in dogs by the actual inhalation of tobacco smoke.[150] The dogs learned to enjoy the tobacco, "begging and wagging their tails for a cigarette."[151]

cigarette smoking: the heart and blood vessels[152]

Increasing evidence suggests that "cigarette smoking can contribute to the development of cardiovascular disease and particularly to death from coronary heart disease . . . Some of the harmful cardiovascular effects appear to be reversible after cessation of cigarette smoking."[153] Depending on other risk factors (such as high blood pressure and high serum cholesterol), the death rate of cigarette-smoking males is from 70 to 200 percent higher than that of non-

[145] "Smoking and Cancer," *The Health Consequences of Smoking,* 1969 Supplement, p. 55.
[146] "Smoking and Cancer," *The Health Consequences of Smoking,* 1968 Supplement, p. 97.
[147] Alton Blakeslee, *It's Not Too Late to Stop Smoking Cigarettes,* Public Affairs Pamphlet No. 386 (New York, 1966), pp. 10–12.
[148] *Ibid.,* p. 10.
[149] "More Smoking: Worse Malignancy," *Medical News, Journal of the American Medical Association,* Vol. 211, No. 13 (March 30, 1970), pp. 2081–82.
[150] E. Cuyler Hammond, Oscar Auerbach, David Kirman, and Lawrence Garfinkel, "Effects of Cigarette Smoking on Dogs," and Oscar Auerbach, E. Cuyler Hammond, David Kirman, and Lawrence Garfinkel, "Pulmonary Neoplasms," *Archives of Environmental Health,* Vol. 21, No. 6 (December 1970), pp. 740–53 and 754–68, respectively.
[151] *Newsweek,* February 16, 1970, p. 86.
[152] The material in this section is drawn from "Smoking and Cardiovascular Disease," *The Health Consequences of Smoking* (1967), pp. 25–28, and its 1968 and 1969 Supplements.
[153] "Summary of the Report," *The Health Consequences of Smoking,* 1969 Supplement, pp. 3–4.

smoking males. And the tragedy of these figures is deepened by the fact that it is young smokers who die more often. "Additional evidence . . . indicates that young smokers between the ages of forty-five and fifty-four have the highest mortality ratios—three times as great for men, and twice as great for women, if they smoke ten or more cigarettes per day, as compared to nonsmokers."[154]

How does cigarette smoking affect the heart? Experimental evidence suggests that cigarette smoking contributes to the release of chemicals that mimic the effect of the impulses from certain fibers of the sympathetic nervous system.[155] The result: the tension of the heart wall is increased, as is the heart rate. The heart muscle must work harder. It needs more blood, for only by an increased blood supply can more oxygen and other nutrients be brought to the more active heart. Ironically, having created the need for more blood, cigarette smoking decreases the body's ability to meet it. How? In several ways.

It is nicotine that increases the work of the heart by causing a rise in both the heart rate and the blood pressure. And it is the blood hemoglobin that carries oxygen to all the tissues. But cigarette smoking means the inhaling of carbon monoxide (cigarette smoke is 3 to 4 percent carbon monoxide). "Smokers generally have 3 percent to 7 percent of their hemoglobin saturated with carbon monoxide."[156] This decreases the amount of oxygen available for the needy heart muscle. "Carbon monoxide interferes with the ability of the heart to extract oxygen from the . . . blood. The combination of increased oxygen requirements and decreased oxygen availability may well lead" to a lack of blood to the heart muscle, "particularly in patients with coronary artery disease."[157] In addition, cigarette smoking impairs lung function. No longer can the breathing process deliver enough oxygen to the tissues. Again the heart is short-changed. If the coronary arteries are partially occluded with atherosclerosis, the danger is multiplied. Atherosclerotic arteries have lost some elasticity and cannot dilate enough to bring more blood and other nutrients to the heart. What is worse, the absorbed nicotine and carbon monoxide from cigarette smoking is believed to contribute to the development of atherosclerosis. The harmful effects of cigarette smoking are not limited to the heart, the lung, the hemoglobin, and the blood vessels. It is now thought that cigarette smoking makes platelets, a type of blood cell involved in clotting, more adhesive. As a result, clots may be formed more readily within the coronary arteries that bring blood to the heart. And since such clots obstruct the blood flow, a heart attack is hastened.

Cigarette smoking delivers blow after blow to the heart. It is not surprising that those more susceptible to coronary disease have heart attacks more often if they smoke—and recover less often.[158] Recent evidence suggests that im-

[154] E. C. Hammond, "Smoking in Relation to the Death Rates of One Million Men and Women," quoted in *The Health Consequences of Smoking* (1967), p. 25.

[155] For discussions of the sympathetic nervous system and of blood circulation, see pages 267–69 and 215–23.

[156] Stephen M. Ayers, "Role of Carbon Monoxide and Nicotine in Circulatory Effects of Cigarette Smoke," *Journal of the American Medical Association,* Vol. 219, No. 4 (January 24, 1972), p. 520.

[157] *Ibid.*

[158] "General Considerations" and "Cardiovascular Diseases," *The Health Consequences of Smoking* (1971), pp. 8–9, 21–134.

pending fatal heart attacks may be precipitated by cigarette smoking. In such a situation, "the patient can be told not merely that he is killing himself slowly but that the next cigarette could be his last."[159]

cigarette smoking and peptic ulcers

Peptic ulcers (see page 686) afflict the mucous membrane of the esophagus, stomach, or duodenum. Such ulcers are more prevalent among cigarette smokers than nonsmokers. Cigarette smoking has a stronger association with stomach ulcers than with duodenal ulcers.[160] Cigarette smoking reduces the effectiveness of medical and surgical treatment of both. Complications following surgery for peptic disease are more frequent among cigarette smokers. So is recurrence of peptic disease.

One reason for the serious incidence of duodenal ulcers in cigarette smokers may be chemical. Recent studies suggest that nicotine "may be lifting protection from the duodenum by inhibiting pancreatic and biliary buffering secretions while gastric output of hydrochloric acid continues at its usual rate."[161] It has moreover been found that when a person starts inhaling cigarette smoke, some of his intestinal contents squirt back into the stomach. The bile juice from the duodenum has an emulsifying effect (an effect in which one liquid is distributed throughout another liquid in small globules). This effect combines with the acidity of the stomach to damage the stomach wall.[162]

cigarette smoking and tooth loss

Periodontal disease (particularly gum inflammation, bony-tissue destruction, and loss of teeth) is much more common among smokers than nonsmokers. For example, women smokers between twenty and thirty-nine years of age have twice the chance of losing their teeth, even all their teeth, than nonsmoking women in that age group. Among men smokers, the chance of becoming toothless between thirty and fifty-nine years of age is double that of nonsmokers.[163]

smoking and the woman

> You've come a long way, baby,
> To get where you've got to today.
> You've got your own cigarette now, baby.
> You've come a long, long way.

So ran the happy jingle in a recent television advertising campaign. "Baby" had indeed come a long way. So had the cigarette advertiser. However, his

[159] "Sudden Death by Cigarette," *New Scientist,* Vol. 53, No. 785 (March 2, 1972), p. 462.
[160] "General Considerations" and "Peptic Ulcers," *The Health Consequences of Smoking* (1971), pp. 13, 423.
[161] "Ulcer 'Smoke Ring' Clarified," *Medical World News,* Vol. 12, No. 22 (June 4, 1971), p. 23.
[162] "Smoking Irritates the Stomach Wall as Well as Other People," *New Scientist,* Vol. 59, No. 859 (August 16, 1973), p. 373, citing N. W. Reed and P. Grech in the *British Medical Journal,* Vol. 3 (1973), p. 313.
[163] Harold A. Solomon *et al.,* "Cigarette Smoking and Periodontal Disease," quoted in *Medical Bulletin on Tobacco,* Vol. 6, No. 4 (December 1968).

journey had been more profitable than hers. That particular message had helped to sell $4\frac{1}{2}$ billion of the new brand of cigarettes in 1970.[164] But what had woman's journey brought her?

First, she was beginning to smoke at an earlier age. In 1969, 8.4 percent of girls between twelve and eighteen years of age were regular smokers. By 1972, the percentage had risen to almost 12 percent. (And younger smokers become heavier smokers.) Moreover, compared to a nonsmoking woman, she was spending more time sick in bed, had more chronic disease, and was losing more time from work. Her risk of dying? In a short time it had gone up 20 percent. In 1972, her chance of dying of lung cancer was twice that of a non-smoker, and so was her chance of developing a host of other smoking-related diseases. Among the most serious of these are chronic bronchitis, emphysema, and heart disease.[165] She was becoming equal to man, not in her necessary human fulfillment, but in her unnecessary sickness and death.

SMOKING AND PREGNANCY Yes, woman has come a long way down Tobacco Road. And if she is pregnant, she is taking her baby with her. Smoking during pregnancy apparently increases the risk of spontaneous abortion[166] and stillbirth.[167] The child born of the mother who smokes during pregnancy is more likely to die during the early weeks of life.[168] (Should the woman give up smoking by the fourth month of her pregnancy, the risk to the baby seems to diminish sharply.)[169] His chances of having congenital heart disease may be greater.[170] He is more likely to be underweight.[171] Even at the age of seven, the child whose mother smoked during her pregnancy may be smaller and slightly (four months) retarded in reading ability.[172] His chances of being rated "significantly less well adjusted" at that age are greater.[173] Fortunately, reassessment at age eleven is more encouraging. Around that age the child born of the smoking

[164] As of January 1, 1971, radio and television advertising of cigarettes was outlawed in this country. One reason: the influence of the ads on potential smokers—particularly children.

[165] "Women and Smoking, Latest Brief," National Clearinghouse for Smoking and Health, U.S. Department of Health, Education, and Welfare Publication No. (HSM)72-7512 (December 1971); Public Health Service, U.S. Department of Health, Education, and Welfare, *The Health Consequences of Smoking* (January 1974), pp. 99–149.

[166] J. Fredrick, E. D. Alberman, and H. Goldstein, "Possible Teratogenic Effect of Cigarette Smoking," *Nature,* Vol. 231, No. 5304 (June 25, 1971), citing C. S. Russell, R. Taylor, and C. E. Law in the *British Journal of Social Medicine,* Vol. 22, No. 119 (1968), and Alton Ochsner, "The Health Menace of Smoking," *American Scientist,* Vol. 59, No. 2 (March–April 1971), p. 250, citing E. Athayde, "Incidencia de abôrtos e mortinatalidade nos operarias da industria de fumo," *Brasil-Medico,* Vol. 62 (1948), pp. 237–39; P. Berhard, "Sichere Schaden des Zigarettenrauches bei der Frau," *Medicinische Wochenschrift,* Vol. 104 (1962), pp. 1826–31; C. S. Russell, R. Taylor, and R. N. Madison, "Some Effects of Smoking in Pregnancy," *Journal of Obstetrics and Gynaecology of the British Commonwealth,* Vol. 73 (1966), pp. 742–46; and G. S. Hudson and M. P. Rucker, "Spontaneous Abortion," *Journal of the American Medical Association,* Vol. 129 (1945), pp. 542–44.

[167] *Ibid.,* p. 529, citing N. R. Butler and E. D. Alberman, *Perinatal Problems* (Edinburgh, 1969), and Alton Ochsner, "The Health Menace of Smoking," p. 250.

[168] *Ibid.*

[169] John Bardin, *Today's Health News,* Vol. 51, No. 4 (April 1973), p. 9.

[170] J. Fredrick, E. D. Alberman, and H. Goldstein, "Possible Teratogenic Effect of Cigarette Smoking," pp. 529–30.

[171] *Ibid.,* p. 529, citing N. R. Butler and E. D. Alberman, *Perinatal Problems.*

[172] *Ibid.,* citing R. Davie, N. R. Butler, and H. Goldstein, *From Birth to Seven* (New York, 1972) and "More on Smoking in Pregnancy," *Footnotes on Maternity Care,* Vol. 34, No. 8 (October 1970), pp. 120–21, citing "Gravida's Smoking Seen Handicap to Offspring," *Ob-Gyn News,* Vol. 5, No. 12 (June 15, 1970), p. 16.

[173] *Ibid.,* p. 121.

mother usually catches up to his contemporaries. But the cost to both mother and child has been high, and it may prove to be higher than was originally suspected. Incomplete studies suggest that seven-year-olds born of mothers who smoked during pregnancy are 40 percent more prone to epileptiform convulsions. Does this tendency persist with eleven-year-olds? That is now being studied.[174]

Why is the unborn child so adversely affected? Smoking causes the flow of blood through the placenta to decrease. It increases the poisonous carbon monoxide content of the placental blood. It decreases the supply of oxygen and other nutrients to the baby. The nicotine in cigarette smoke has a directly toxic effect on the fetus.

mouldy tobacco: a possible danger

Healthy tobacco leaf is host to a large population of fungi. But some fungi can make the tobacco leaf sick. Can they do the same to man? Workers at the North Carolina State University and the U.S. Department of Agriculture are seeking the answer. Fungal cultures were isolated from both freshly harvested and cured tobacco and injected into mice. More than 75 percent of the fungal cultures from fresh tobacco and 49 percent of those from cured tobacco killed the mice. The most lethal fungi were among the most common. Other tests compared tobacco that was diseased because of fungi with tobacco that was not. The diseased tobacco caused severe illness and death.[175]

are pipes and cigars safer than cigarettes?

More research is needed, but in some respects pipes and cigars do seem to be safer than cigarettes. One recent study[176] compared urinary excretions of nicotine by cigarette, pipe, and cigar smokers. Cigarette smokers excreted three times as much nicotine as the others. This was thought to be due to the lesser inhalation by pipe and cigar smokers. Moreover, "evidence indicates that there is little risk of coronary heart disease associated with cigars and/or pipe smoking."[177]

In addition, "there is a much smaller increase of the lung cancer death rate associated with pipe and/or cigar smoking than with cigarette smoking."[178] Why? Alkaline pipe and cigar smoke gives up its nicotine readily. It is quickly absorbed into the blood stream through the mucous membranes of the mouth, pharynx, and larynx. But the acid smoke of cigarette tobacco parts with its nicotine more reluctantly.[179] Only the deep lung tissue provides a vast enough area for the exchange of such a chemical between inhaled air and the blood. So in

[174] "Smoking During Pregnancy Is Linked to Convulsions and Fits in Offspring," *Medical Tribune,* Vol. 11, No. 40 (July 20, 1970), reporting the work of E. M. Ross (1970) as described at the Third European Symposium on Epilepsy. The work of Ross is also cited by Alton Ochsner, "The Health Menace of Smoking," p. 250.

[175] "Watch Out for Mouldy Tobacco!" *New Scientist,* Vol. 45, No. 682 (January 1, 1970), p. 7, citing the work of P. B. Hamilton *et al.,* published in *Applied Microbiology,* Vol. 18, p. 570.

[176] Alfred Kershbaum *et al.,* "Effect of Cigarette, Cigar and Pipe Smoking on Nicotine Excretion," *Archives of Internal Medicine,* Vol. 120, No. 3 (September 1967), p. 314.

[177] *The Health Consequences of Smoking* (1967), p. 25.

[178] *Ibid.,* p. 34.

[179] A. K. Armitage and D. M. Turner, "Absorption of Nicotine in Cigarette and Cigar Smoke Through the Oral Mucosa," *Nature,* Vol. 226, No. 5252 (June 27, 1970), pp. 1231–32.

order to absorb enough nicotine to achieve the desired tobacco effect, the cigarette smoker must inhale. Since the inhaled smoke contains cancer-causing substances, the cigarette smoker's lungs are put at greater risk of developing cancer than are the lungs of the pipe or cigar smoker.[180]

However, cigar and pipe smokers still run the risk of developing cancers of the mouth, pharynx, and larynx. Their chances of developing such cancers are higher than those of nonsmokers and about the same as or slightly lower than those of cigarette smokers. Pipe smokers are particularly prone to oral cancer, especially of the lip.[181] There is also an unduly high incidence of cancers of the bladder and kidney among pipe and cigar smokers.[182] Some smokers are trying to escape smoking by the use of snuff and chewing tobacco. Fortunately, snuff is no longer used to quiet babies. Like chewing tobacco, it is a distinct cause of cancer of the oral cavity.[183] Not surprisingly, one study concludes that "heavy cigar and pipe smoking may be more hazardous than previously thought and should not be considered a safe alternative to cigarette smoking."[184]

As for the recently introduced "little cigars," preliminary data indicate that the concentrations in them of such harmful substances as carbon monoxide, hydrogen cyanide, and certain hydrocarbons are comparable to those found in cigarettes. Also, cigarette smokers who switch to little cigars tend to use them as they used cigarettes. Thus, according to the 1973 Public Health Service report on *The Health Consequences of Smoking,* little cigars must be considered hazardous at this time.

the best tip?

Do filters strain out the cigarette sickness? Research workers report "no." In studying the effects of nine popular filter tip cigarettes in reducing tar and nicotine, they concluded that "cigarette filters did not offer protection against the health hazards of smoking."[185] The best tip, then, is to quit smoking.

even for most nonsmokers, there's no escape—as yet

In this country, state legislators are making efforts to pass laws limiting cigarette smoking in public places. Adverse reactions to tobacco smoke are the bane of many allergic people.[186] And the carbon monoxide in cigarette smoke may be hazardous to nearby nonsmokers. The carbon monoxide content of polluted city air rarely contains more than thirty parts of carbon monoxide per million parts of air, while cigarette smoke streams have been found to contain from 400 to 40,000 parts per million (p.p.m.) of carbon monoxide.[187] Among relatively

[180] "The World Is an Addict," *The Lancet,* Vol. 2, No. 7681 (November 14, 1970), pp. 1019–20.

[181] *The Health Consequences of Smoking* (1971), A Report to the Surgeon General, pp. 12, 277–78, 281, 284–89.

[182] "Smoking and Cancers of the Bladder and Kidney," *The Lancet,* Vol. 1, No. 7700 (March 27, 1971), p. 635, citing K. Lockwood, *Acta Path. Microbiol. Scand.,* 1961, Supplement 145, p. 1.

[183] George E. Moore, "Hazard of Snuff," *Journal of the American Medical Association,* Vol. 223, No. 3 (January 15, 1973), p. 336.

[184] Theodor Abelin and Otto R. Gsell, "Relative Risk of Pulmonary Cancer in Cigar and Pipe Smokers," *Cancer,* Vol. 20, No. 8 (August 1967), pp. 1295–96.

[185] Alfred Kershbaum *et al.,* "Regular, Filter Tip and Modified Cigarettes," *Journal of the American Medical Association,* Vol. 201, No. 7 (August 14, 1967), pp. 545–46.

[186] Herbert Savel, "Clinical Hypersensitivity to Cigarette Smoke," *Archives of Environmental Health,* Vol. 21 (1970), pp. 146–48; Bernard M. Zussman, "Tobacco Sensitivity in the Allergic Patient," *Annals of Allergy,* Vol. 28 (1970), pp. 371–77.

[187] Bertram D. Dinman, "Carbon Monoxide and Cigarette Smoking," *Journal of the American Medical Association,* Vol. 212, No. 11 (June 15, 1970), p. 1785.

healthy people, a ninety-minute exposure to only 50 p.p.m. of carbon monoxide can result in diminished hearing discrimination; visual acuity, particularly at low levels of light intensity, is also lessened. These hazards must be added to those already suffered by individuals with diseases of the heart, bronchi, and lungs, to whom an increased concentration of carbon monoxide may present a genuine threat.[188] "Adult non-smokers . . . spending several hours in smoke-filled rooms are inhaling the equivalent of one or two cigarettes a day. This may be enough to double their chances of dying from lung cancer."[189] There is, moreover, mounting evidence that exposing children to cigarette smoke is harmful.[190]

worldwide antismoking activity

In countries from Israel to Iceland, antismoking recommendations are part of public policy. Recently, a Japanese government agency questioned the need for health warnings on cigarette packs. Japanese health experts denounced this as "putting the national treasury before the national health."[191] In the United States, research projects include studies of tobacco genetics, tobaccoless cigarettes, and filtered cigarettes. The search is on for a safer cigarette.[192] The World Health Organization has sought and received recommendations from its 131 member nations for diminishing the problem on an international scale.

helping the smoker to quit

In numerous antismoking clinics ways are being sought to help the individual smoker to stop smoking. The most difficult phase is the first period of withdrawal. This stage is basically a learning task. Previously, the former smoker had used cigarettes to help him through periods of stress. Now he must learn new ways of handling old stresses. It is difficult to give up a meaningful and comforting object during a period of unusual stress. After the initial withdrawal phase, the former smoker enters on a more prolonged, but less difficult, period of withdrawal. Like the first, it requires learning.[193]

Some people gain weight as they stop smoking. Many smokers find it better to defer a concentrated effort to lose weight until a less difficult time. Antismoking tablets may help, but frequently they are stomach irritants.

Stimulus satiation has helped many smokers to quit. The subject is instructed to double his smoking amount for four days and then to treble it for two days. For the next few days, at least, not smoking is more a relief than a trial.[194] An intensification of this technique requires the smoker to smoke almost continuously—at least four packs a day—for several days. Eventually, smok-

[188] "Cigarette Smoke Pollutes Non-smokers' Environment," *Medical News, Journal of the American Medical Association,* Vol. 219, No. 7 (February 14, 1972), p. 821.

[189] Jon Tinker, "Should Public Smoking Be Banned?" *New Scientist,* Vol. 59, No. 858 (August 9, 1973), pp. 313–15.

[190] Donald A. Dukelow, "'Cigarette Smoke-Filled Room': A Hazard to Nonsmokers and Children," *Journal of the American Medical Association,* Vol. 223, No. 3 (January 15, 1973), p. 336.

[191] Emil Corwin, "Smoking—A World Problem," p. 504.

[192] "The Search for Safer Tobacco," *Health News,* Vol. 48, No. 2 (February 1971), pp. 12–13.

[193] M. A. H. Russell, "Cigarette Dependence: II—Doctor's Role in Management," *British Medical Journal,* Vol. 2, No. 5758 (May 15, 1971), p. 394.

[194] *Ibid.,* pp. 394–95.

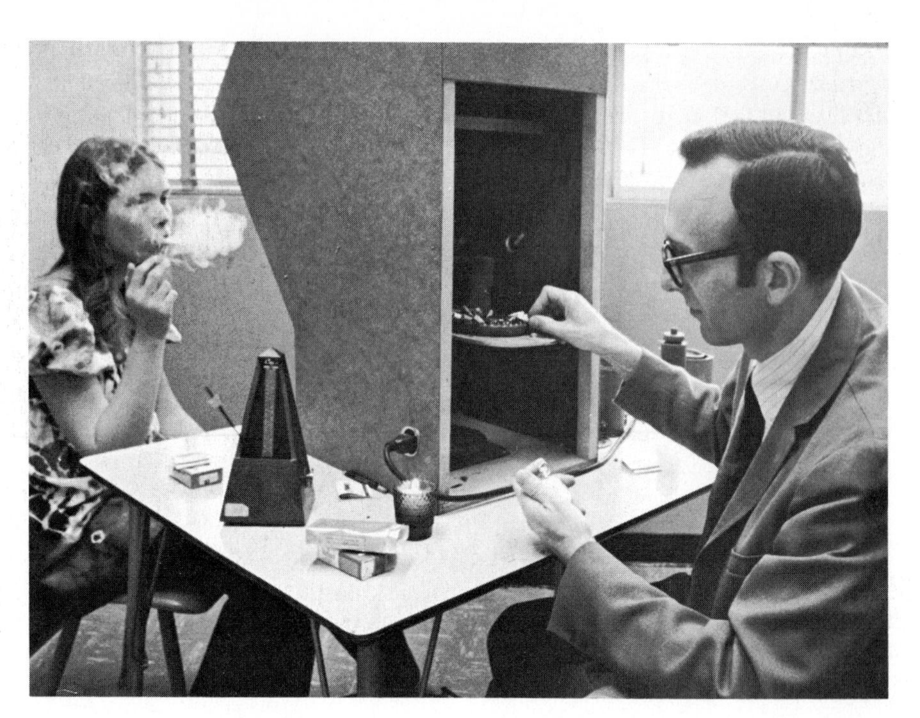

13-11 *Aversion treatment to quit smoking. A student smokes while smoke is blown into her face.*

ing even one more cigarette becomes almost overwhelmingly distasteful.

Other aversion techniques have been used with some success. In one, the smoker takes a puff on a cigarette every six seconds. At the same time a smoke machine blows hot puffs of smoke into his face (Figure 13-11). His nose and throat burn, his eyes water, he coughs miserably, he wants to vomit. After a brief rest, the process is repeated. For this course of treatment the smoker pays a deposit. If he quits the course instead of the smoking, he loses the deposit.

Electric shock has also been tried. In a laboratory setting, the smoker occasionally and unpredictably receives an electric shock as he brings the cigarette to his mouth and inhales. Pain and anxiety, rather than comfort and peace, become associated with smoking. What if the smoker persists with his cigarettes away from the laboratory? He is instructed to use a special cigarette case. It is electrically wired and so is he. Every time he reaches for a cigarette, he receives a painful shock.[195]

The English writer Charles Lamb once rhymed: "For thy sake, tobacco, I/ Would do anything but die."[196] Every year thousands of smokers go him one better.

[195] Edward Lichtenstein, "How to Quit Smoking," *Psychology Today,* Vol. 4, No. 8 (January 1971), pp. 42, 44, 45.

[196] Charles Lamb, "A Farewell to Tobacco," in *Bookman's Pleasure,* comp. by Holbrook Jackson (New York, 1947), p. 164.

summary

One manifestation of the anxieties of the 1970s is the increasingly widespread use—and abuse—of drugs. This chapter considers the types of drug dependence resulting from the abuse in the United States of older types of drugs, namely

1. *depressants*. These drugs reduce psychic and motor stimuli. The *morphine type of drug dependence* is produced by such depressants as *opium* and its derivatives, especially *morphine* and *heroin* (page 362). The opiate abuser develops a *physical dependence* on the drug, which means that deprivation results in the *withdrawal* or *abstinence syndrome;* his body also develops a *tolerance* to the drug, which means that greater quantities are needed to produce the same effects and to avoid withdrawal (page 363). Among the treatments for opiate dependence are "cold turkey" (pages 369–70), withdrawal plus supportive therapy (page 370), withdrawal plus methadone (page 370), methadone maintenance (pages 370–72), treatment centers offering a variety of approaches (pages 372–73), and heroin maintenance (pages 373–74).

The *barbiturate-alcohol type of drug dependence* is produced by *sedatives* (page 374)—*barbiturates* (Seconal, Nembutal, Phenobarbital), *nonbarbiturate sedatives* (Doriden, Dormison, Quaalude), and *tranquilizers* (Equanil or Miltown, Librium)—and by *alcohol*. Alcohol can affect sexuality (page 380), driving ability (page 380), and the process of nourishment (page 383). *Alcoholism* is a major drug problem in this country (pages 381–83). Treatment of alcoholism involves one or a combination of methods, including aversion therapy, antabuse, adjustment, and Alcoholics Anonymous (pages 383–84).

A less common form of drug abuse involves the inhalation of depressant vapors from such substances as chloroform, glue, and aerosol sprays (pages 384–85).

2. *tobacco.* An important *emotional aspect* of the origins of tobacco dependence is the relief from stress provided by the sucking reflex (page 387). As for the *economic aspects* of smoking, though the U.S. tobacco industry is big business, the revenue derived from tobacco taxes is more than offset by the costs of smoking-induced disease and fire damage (page 387). Smoking also has various *social aspects* (page 388).

The 1964 Surgeon General's report on *Smoking and Health* indicated a link between smoking and increased illness rates, higher death rates, and shorter life expectancy (pages 388–89). Subsequent reports have supported these findings. Cigarette smoking is the main cause of *emphysema* and *chronic bronchitis* (pages 389–92). It is also associated with lip and lung cancer (pages 392–93), cardiovascular disease (pages 393–95), peptic ulcers (page 395), and tooth loss (page 395). Increased smoking among women has led to increased incidence of associated diseases (pages 395–96). Smoking by a pregnant woman has adverse effects on the child (pages 396–97). Another smoking hazard may be the fungi that cause tobacco-leaf mould (page 397). Pipes and cigars—but not "little cigars"—may be safer than cigarettes (pages 397–98). Filters do not eliminate the dangers of smoking (page 398). Health warnings on cigarette packs, research for safer cigarettes, and programs to help individual smokers quit are part of worldwide antismoking activity (pages 399–400).

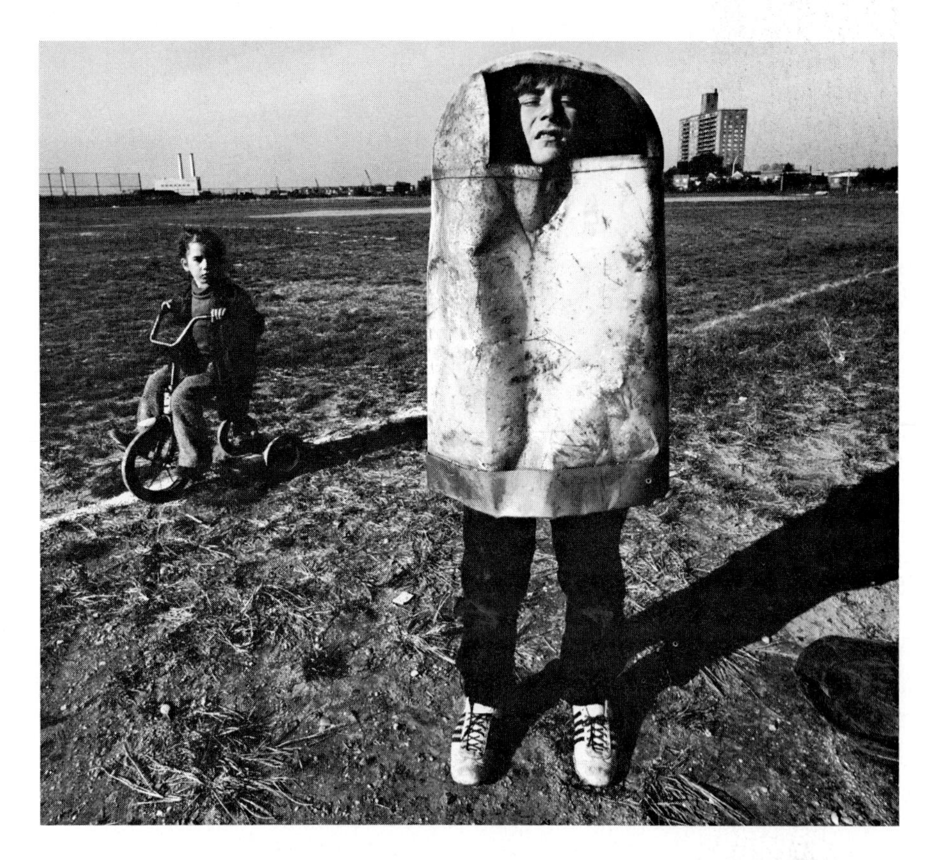

escape into captivity, part 2: newer drugs of abuse in the U.S.

14

stimulants

differences among the stimulants: speed freaks vs. acid heads

the amphetamine type of drug dependence

Basically, depressants such as morphine, the barbiturates, and alcohol reduce psychic and motor stimuli. The depressive drug abuser is often psychically and physically incapacitated. His senses are deadened, and he exists on the foggy border between consciousness and unconsciousness. He drifts into a troubled sleep. This loss of consciousness limits the amount of drug he takes. His antisocial behavior, such as stealing, is rooted in the need to secure more drug. Stimulants, on the other hand, excite psychic and motor activity. Thus, hallucinogens such as LSD and marihuana are discussed with the stimulant group, along with the amphetamines. Nevertheless, although the amphetamine-type abusers (''speed freaks'') and the LSD abusers (''acid heads'') both take stimulants, their choice of stimulant is largely determined by their needs and their personalities. And each of these stimulants produces bizarre but different behavior. Moreover, as will be seen, marihuana is unique in that it can act as either a stimulant or a depressant.

The speed freak seeks one result; the acid head, another. The amphetamine-type drug abuser takes the drug primarily to experience a ''flash'' or ''rush.'' This he describes as a ''full body orgasm.'' The acute anxiety and the hallucinations and paranoia associated with amphetamine abuse are secondary. This psychic storm may combine with an undiminished, even a temporarily increased, physical strength. This mixture of irrationality and strength can suddenly explode with the murderous violence of a hand grenade. The LSD abuser wants a different drug reaction and his secondary behavior is different from the speed freak's. ''Rather than seeking a *flash* or a thrill as do the speed freaks, the chronic LSD user develops a complex set of motivations for his drug use, involving self-psychoanalytic, pseudoreligious and creative aspirations.'' The speed freak is often violent; this the acid head rejects. Thus ''speed always drives out acid.''[1]

amphetamine misuse?

''Despite 30 years of extensive use . . . the place of amphetamines in clinical practice is far from established. . . . The effectiveness of amphetamines in treating obesity and depressive reactions is minimal and controversial.''[2] Amphetamines are, however, useful in the treatment of *hyperkinetic* (abnormally overactive) children with learning disorders (see below). But this and the few other conditions for which amphetamines are helpful hardly justify their massive production.

[1] David E. Smith, ''Speed Freaks vs. Acid Heads,'' *Clinical Pediatrics,* Vol. 8, No. 4 (April 1969), pp. 187–88.

[2] George R. Edison, ''Amphetamines: A Dangerous Illusion,'' *Annals of Internal Medicine,* Vol. 74, No. 4 (April 4, 1971), p. 608. Amphetamines and barbiturates are now being combined in a single capsule. Thus, the downers reduce the effect of the uppers while the sleeping individual ostensibly loses weight. Now sold in the illicit market, these present a singular hazard. (Richard Kunner, ''Double Dealing in Dope,'' *Human Behavior,* Vol. 2, No. 10 [October 1973], p. 22.)

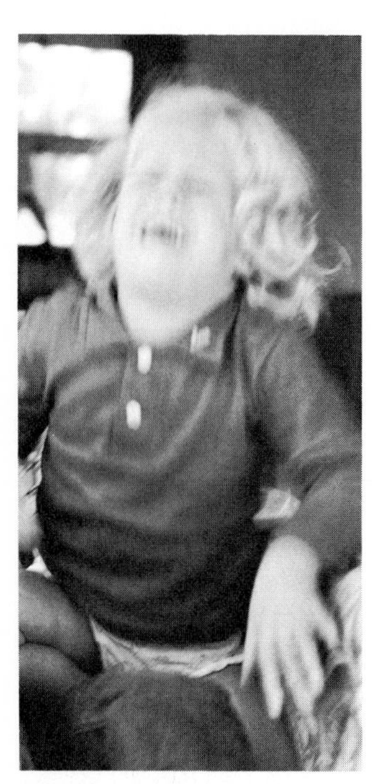

14-1 *A hyperkinetic child.*

In 1967, the governments of Britain and Sweden restricted the prescribing of amphetamines by physicians. In October 1970, the U.S. Food and Drug Administration prohibited physicians from prescribing amphetamines, except for *narcolepsy* (uncontrollable sleepiness), hyperkinetic behavior disorders in children, and the short-term treatment of obesity.[3]

a note about the hyperkinetic child

The child behaves ''as if there were an inner tornado.''[4] The hyperactivity, hyperexcitability, short attention span, frequent impulsiveness, learning and reading disabilities, low tolerance to frustration—all these become the bane of the teacher's life. One such child can destroy order in any classroom. The child's condition is called a ''hyperkinetic disorder'' or ''minimal brain dysfunction.'' Although both diagnoses are commonly used interchangeably, most of these children have no signs of structural damage to the central nervous system.[5] A hyperkinetic disturbance may have many causes. It is believed by some that the basic condition is a disorder of the mechanisms in the central nervous system that inhibit behavior. Irrelevant stimuli are not filtered out; the child is literally at the mercy of all of his environmental stimuli.[6] It is important to differentiate such children from those who are merely responding to stresses at home, poor teaching, overcrowded classrooms, and frustrated, rigid, punishing adults who respond with disfavor to an active, normally ebullient, questioning child of high intelligence.[7] Of the estimated 3 percent of all U.S. children who are said to be hyperkinetic, most are believed to have normal or superior intelligence.[8]

Many hyperkinetic children are dramatically improved by treatment with amphetamine-type drugs. Amphetamines may act as tranquilizers with these children. For them, stimulant drugs seem to activate or strengthen the inhibitory mechanisms in the central nervous system. In this country, more than 150,000 children are now being treated with these drugs. Massive screening for the condition is being proposed.[9] Some physicians believe that such drugs are too often used without real justification or adequate supervision. Others

[3] ''FDA Commissioner Restricts Use of Amphetamines,'' *California Medical Association News,* Vol. 15, No. 15 (August 31, 1970), p. 1.

[4] ''Amphetamine-Type Drugs for Hyperactive Children,'' *The Medical Letter,* Vol. 14, No. 7 (March 31, 1972), p. 21.

[5] *Ibid.*

[6] Taranath Shetty, ''Alpha Rhythms in the Hyperkinetic Child,'' *Nature,* Vol. 234, No. 5330 (December 24, 1971), p. 476.

[7] ''Classroom Drugs: Treatments or Pacifiers?'' *Medical World News,* Vol. 12, No. 15 (April 16, 1971), p. 4. (This is a brief news review of a fifteen-page report of a conference on the hyperkinetic child organized by the U.S. Department of Health, Education, and Welfare. The essence of the majority opinion was published by D. X. Freedman *et al.* in *Psychopharmacology Abstract* Vol. 7 [1971].)

[8] *Ibid.*

[9] L. Alan Sproufe and Mark A. Stewart, ''Treating Problem Children with Stimulant Drugs,'' *New England Journal of Medicine,* Vol. 289, No. 8 (August 23, 1973), p. 407, citing R. Richard, ''Drugs for Children—Miracle or Nightmare?'' *Providence Sun-Journal,* February 6, 1972; D. J. Safer, ''Drugs for Problem School Children,'' *Journal of School Health,* Vol. 41 (1971), pp. 491–95; L. A. Sproufe, ''Drug Treatment of Children with Behavior Problems,'' *Review of Child Development Research,* Vol. 4, ed. by Frank Horowitz (in press); G. G. Steinberg, C. Troshinsky, and H. R. Steinberg, ''Dextroamphetamine-Responsive Behavior Disorder in School Children,'' *American Journal of Psychiatry,* Vol. 128 (1971), pp. 174–79; P. H. Wender, *Minimal Brain Dysfunction in Children* (New York, 1971).

point out that limited studies indicate that children treated between the ages of eight and eleven years still have severe behavioral problems in their teens.[10] Others suggest that "the basic flaw of drug treatment is that it cannot teach a child anything, and it is not yet established that drug treatment makes the child more accessible to other intervention techniques."[11] Although most workers in this area would not discontinue the treatments in properly selected and supervised cases, all are agreed that more caution and research are indicated. Amphetamine dependence from this treatment has not been proved.

amphetamine: the bitter pill

The proprietary names for methamphetamine central nervous system stimulators are *Methedrine* and *Desoxyn.* For dextroamphetamine, they are *Dexedrine* or *Benzedrine.* In street terminology, "speed," "crystal," or "meth" usually refers to an amphetamine.

Amphetamine abusers develop no physical dependence. Withdrawal is, therefore, neither dangerous nor painful. However, psychological dependence is marked. So is tolerance. An abuser may gobble as many as 150 "pep pills" a day to attain the effect first experienced with just one. The ability of the amphetamines to induce tolerance is almost unique among stimulants of the central nervous system. So great can the clearly developed tolerance become that an abuser of this group of stimulants is eventually able to withstand a dose several hundred times greater than that ordinarily prescribed by physicians.

When swallowed, amphetamines are tasteless, but they can become a bitter pill. With abuse, the drugs cause sleeplessness, extreme hyperactivity, profound behavior changes, and hallucinations. Even relatively moderate doses may cause such marked psychic changes as to make college attendance, for example, impossible.[12] Chronic amphetamine abuse has led to brain damage.[13] In addition, methamphetamine may be the common denominator in a condition that recently killed four of fourteen afflicted drug abusers. Inflammation of the blood vessels resulted in bulging, blocked arteries that could not supply blood to affected organs. Kidney failures are believed to have caused the deaths. Also affected were the liver, pancreas, stomach, small and large bowels, and heart.[14]

Most people who abuse amphetamines begin by taking these drugs orally, but many individuals go on to "shoot" the drug by vein. After many injections, scars develop along the veins; these the abuser calls "tracks." A strong tolerance

14-2 *The spider, perhaps the greatest architect among living creatures, loses its cunning when fed "speed."* Top: *A normal web.* Bottom: *A web spun twelve hours after the spider was given a dose of dextroamphetamine.*

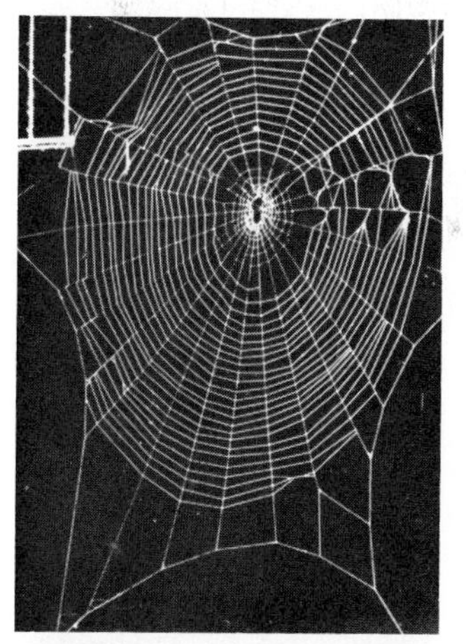

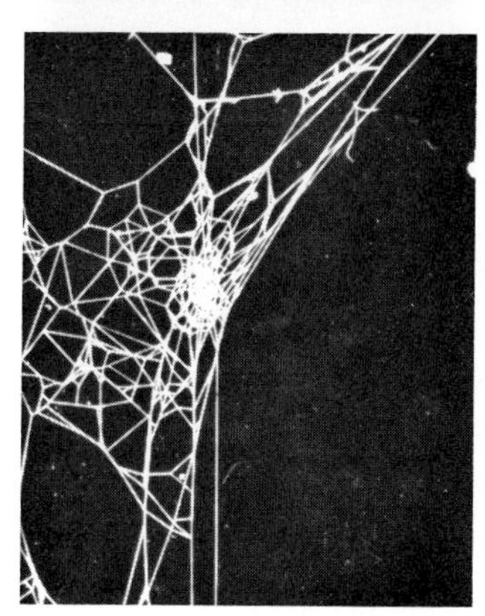

[10] *Ibid.,* p. 409, citing G. Weiss *et al.,* "Studies on the Hyperactive Child, VII: Five Year Follow Up," *Archives of General Psychiatry,* Vol. 24 (1971), pp. 409–14; and W. Mendelson, N. Johnson, and M. A. Stewart, "Hyperactive Children as Teen-Agers: A Follow-up Study," *Journal of Nervous and Mental Diseases,* Vol. 153 (1971), pp. 273–79.

[11] Arthur R. DeLong, "What Have We Learned from Psychoactive Drug Research on Hyperactives?" *American Journal of Diseases of Children,* Vol. 123, No. 2 (February 1972), pp. 177–80.

[12] Richard M. Steinhilber and Albert B. Hagedorn, "Drug Induced Behavioral Disorders," *GP,* Vol. 35, No. 5 (May 1967), pp. 115–16.

[13] "Drug Dependency," the UCLA Interdepartmental Conference, Anthony Kales, moderator, *Annals of Internal Medicine,* Vol. 70, No. 3 (March 1969), p. 591.

[14] B. Philip Citron, Mordechai Halpern, Margaret McCarron, George D. Lundberg, Ruth McCormick, Irwin J. Pincus, Dorothy Tatter, and Bernard J. Haverback, "Necrotizing Angiitis Associated with Drug Abuse," *New England Journal of Medicine,* Vol. 283, No. 19 (November 5, 1970), pp. 1003–11.

is developed. Soon the amphetamine abuser gives himself astronomic amounts. With each fresh injection he experiences the "rush." He is then known as a "speed freak." How much does he take? It is impossible to be certain. His drug source is the black-market laboratory. Dosage and content vary widely (see Table 13-1, page 359).

A perilous pattern develops. The drug is injected about every two hours around the clock for three to six days (rarely more). During this period the abuser remains continuously awake. This is called a "run" or "speed binge." The abuser then "falls out." Exhausted, tremulous, disorganized, enduring terrifying visual and auditory hallucinations, and paranoid, he goes to sleep. Once asleep, he cannot be awakened. Following a three- or four-day run, the drug abuser sleeps twelve to eighteen hours. He awakens hungry. His paranoia is largely gone. But now he is plagued by a depression of extraordinary intensity. One seventeen-year-old girl put it this way: "Without speed I feel so lousy that I'd rather shoot speed and live for one week than live for forty years without it."[15] To escape the terrible depression, the abuser must start another run. If the drug is available, he does. If not, the desperate search for it begins.

During a run, appetite disappears. The experienced abuser may force himself to eat. To control the growing anxiety, hallucinations, and paranoia, barbiturates or opiates may be added to the regimen. It is with the first injection that the severe paranoia may appear, though usually it is delayed several days. Everyone is suspect. Friends "bug" the phone. Every car is a police cruiser. Trees are detectives. To track down his enemies one abuser set out with his pet Doberman. Excited, the abuser is likely to become violent. He may hurt or kill somebody. "If the patient is large or violent, the physician may be in some immediate jeopardy."[16] But often the sick and suspicious person will not go to the doctor.

During a run, the "meth head" has purposeless compulsions. One abuser may shine his shoes, again and again, all day long. Another will take a radio or an automobile motor apart. Completely absorbed, he seems untroubled by his lack of coordination and failure to "repair" it.[17] For extended periods a male abuser may engage in nonejaculatory intercourse. Eventually this will lead "to the inability to get or maintain an erection at all, and a chemically produced total impotence."[18] With discontinuance of the drug, this impotence disappears. But the psychotic symptoms often persist.

During a period of chronic use, twenty to thirty pounds may be lost. Commonly seen, and in part because of malnutrition, are abscesses, nonhealing ulcerations, and brittle fingernails. Among amphetamine abusers, serum hepatitis is common. It is caused by a virus transmitted by dirty needles and syringes. The mortality from this liver disease is much higher than that seen with infectious hepatitis (see pages 166–67).

[15] Quoted in David E. Smith, "Speed Freaks vs. Acid Heads," p. 185.
[16] *Ibid.*, p. 186.
[17] John C. Kramer, V. S. Fischman, and Don C. Littlefield, "Amphetamine Abuse," *Journal of the American Medical Association*, Vol. 201, No. 5 (July 31, 1967), pp. 89–93.
[18] Jordan Scherer, "Patterns and Profiles of Addiction and Drug Abuse," *International Journal of Addictions*, Vol. 2, No. 2 (Fall 1967), p. 75.

It is estimated that, in the major cities of this nation, thousands of young people take intravenous amphetamines. Those amphetamine abusers who want to stop taking it find that difficult. Why? ''Meth'' abusers generally live together, communally. They cannot bring themselves to leave their friends.[19] Yet even in this human need for companionship, there is an added and ironic danger. Amphetamine toxicity is augmented in a crowded ecosystem. Aggregation of animals increases the toxicity of amphetamine fourfold. ''It has become obvious that taking the drug in a high-density population situation increases its toxicity.''[20]

A particularly dangerous complication has developed. LSD is now often contaminated with methamphetamine crystal. ''The tachycardia [excessively rapid heart rate], muscle tremor and anxiety produced by 'speed' is often magnified by the LSD-sensitized mind into a panic reaction.''[21]

the hallucinogen (LSD) type of drug dependence

The drugs causing dependence of the hallucinogen (LSD) type include *LSD, psilocybin* (a drug found in a mushroom), and *mescaline* (found in the buttons of a small cactus—''mescal'' or ''peyote''—and in the seeds of varieties of the morning glory). In this country, some Indian tribes use the mushrooms, cactus buttons, and morning-glory seeds during their religious rites. Their medicine men and women also use them for treatment. Like the amphetamines, the LSD type of hallucinogens have the capacity to induce tolerance. This, however, is not characteristic of drug dependence of the cannabis, or marihuana, type (see pages 418–19).

LSD

Elephants interest some psychiatrists. The adult male elephant periodically goes berserk and, for two weeks, is a menace. To study this cyclically recurring emotional distress, investigators gave Tusko, a 7,000-pound resident of Oklahoma City's Lincoln Park Zoo, a dose of LSD to simulate the behavior. Why? Because of LSD's ''well-known personality-disrupting effect upon humans and other animals.''[22] An elephantine dose killed Tusko in one hour and forty minutes.

Tusko had received 297 milligrams (297,000 micrograms) of LSD. The human dose is only 0.1 to 0.2 milligrams (100 to 200 micrograms). No human death directly attributable to LSD has been reported. The effective dose of LSD is tiny. One ounce would provide 300,000 adult doses. Two pounds, equally distributed, ''would mentally dissociate every man, woman, and child in greater New York for an eight-hour period . . . 'an average dose' . . . 100 micrograms . . . can barely be seen with the naked eye.''[23] Taken by mouth, LSD does not

[19] David E. Smith and Alan J. Rose, ''Observations in the Haight-Ashbury Medical Clinic of San Francisco,'' *Clinical Pediatrics,* Vol. 7, No. 6 (June 1968), p. 316.
[20] David E. Smith, ''Speed Freaks vs. Acid Heads,'' p. 187.
[21] David E. Smith and Alan J. Rose, ''Observations in the Haight-Ashbury Medical Clinic of San Francisco,'' p. 319.
[22] Louis Jolyon West, Chester M. Pierce, and Warren D. Thomas, ''Lysergic Acid Diethylamide: Its Effect on a Male Asiatic Elephant,'' *Science,* Vol. 138, No. 3545 (December 7, 1962), p. 1101.
[23] Sidney Cohen, *Drugs of Hallucination* (London, 1964), pp. 34–35.

act for about forty-five minutes. About four hours after consumption, the effects begin to decrease. In six to twelve hours, they are gone. Tolerance to LSD is rapidly developed. Unlike opium tolerance, LSD tolerance may be developed in a few days and is usually lost in two or three days. Over a period of days, therefore, some users build up an LSD tolerance of 1,000 or 2,000 micrograms (sometimes even more). Since the average dose is but a tenth this size, massive doses must be taken to build up a tolerance. There is no evidence of physical dependence on LSD.

Two major types of reactions are attributed to LSD, one psychic and the other nonpsychic. Each will now be examined.

PSYCHIC EFFECTS For thirty to forty-five minutes after ingestion of LSD, usually nothing happens. Then, for a brief period, there is a sense of well-being. This is followed by a feeling of unreality, of depersonalization and loss of body image. In new users this may be terrifying. The following case was reported from Bellevue Hospital in New York:

> A 21-year-old woman was admitted to the hospital along with her lover. He had had a number of LSD experiences and had convinced her to take it to make her less constrained sexually. About half an hour after ingestion of approximately 200 microgm., she noticed that the bricks in the wall began to go in and out and that light affected her strangely. She became frightened when she realized that she was unable to distinguish her body from the chair she was sitting on or from her lover's body. Her fear became more marked after she thought that she would not get back into herself. At the time of admission she was hyperactive and laughed inappropriately. Stream of talk was illogical . . . Two days later, this reaction had ceased. However, she was still afraid of the drug and convinced that she would not take it again because of her frightening experience.[24]

The illusions following LSD ingestion may include an orgy of vividly colored shapes and patterns, some beautiful, others bizarre. These are called "pseudo-hallucinations." While knowing that the perception of bizarre designs has no basis in external reality, the individual sees them anyway. True hallucination, in which one perceives something that is not actually there, is not common with LSD abusers. What does occur is a perceptual change. The LSD abuser sees what is in the environment, but for him it has changed markedly in shape or color and in meaning. These are illusions not strictly hallucinations. *Synesthesia,* the translation of one type of sensory experience into another, may also occur. Music may be felt as body vibrations. Colors may beat in rhythm with music.[25] (The song "Good Vibrations" refers to synesthesia.) Some individuals seem to recall long-forgotten events. Others claim feelings of transcendence. Smith has described a *psychedelic*[26] *syndrome.* A belief in nonviolence, a desire

[24] William A. Frosch, Edwin S. Robbins, and Marvin Stern, "Untoward Reactions to Lysergic Acid Diethylamide (LSD) Resulting in Hospitalization," *New England Journal of Medicine,* Vol. 273, No. 23 (December 2, 1965), p. 1236.

[25] David E. Smith and Alan J. Rose, "The Use and Abuse of LSD in Haight-Ashbury," *Clinical Pediatrics,* Vol. 7, No. 6 (June 1968), p. 318.

[26] The word *psychedelic* is derived from the Greek *psychē,* "the organ of thought and judgment," and *delos,* meaning "manifest or evident." The psychedelic drugs are differentiated from other drugs by their capacity "to induce or compel states of altered perception, thought, and feeling that are not (or cannot be) experienced except in dreams or at times of religious exaltation." (Louis S. Goodman and Alfred Gilman, *The Pharmacological Basis of Therapeutics* [New York, 1970], p. 296.)

to return to nature, a belief in magic, signs, and mental telepathy, and a tendency to live in groups are often among its characteristics.[27]

Today, legal use of LSD is limited to research. Its official distribution is by the National Institute of Mental Health. As it is a colorless and tasteless substance, its illegal handling is difficult to detect. A reasonably sophisticated chemist can make it. The chemical search for "soul" has become a spreading cult. What objective data are available regarding the psychic effects of LSD?

> . . . 21 reports . . . contained the details of . . . adverse reactions to LSD . . . there were 142 cases of prolonged psychotic reactions, 63 nonpsychotic reactions, 11 spontaneous recurrences, 19 attempted suicides, 4 attempted homicides, 11 successful suicides, and 1 successful homicide . . . An additional 9 cases shared possible suicidal intent . . . There were 6 cases of convulsions which may be seen as tic reactions.[28]

Many more adverse reactions to LSD occur than are reported. Ungerleider and others surveyed 2,700 psychiatrists, psychiatric residents, general practitioners, and psychologists in the Los Angeles County area. They found that more than twenty-three hundred adverse reactions had been noted in just one and a half years. They consider this figure conservative. What percent of LSD users have adverse reactions? This is unknown because a reasonably accurate estimate of LSD-dependent abusers is not available.[29]

Some individuals who experienced prolonged psychoses after taking LSD had had no previous psychiatric disturbance.[30] A single dose of LSD has, in many cases, produced a psychosis (the duration of the psychoses varies).

There is no explanation for the "flashback" phenomenon of an LSD experience weeks or months after the last ingestion of the drug. Despite discontinuance of LSD, one woman had spontaneous recurrences of hallucinations for months. "She . . . had terrifying involuntary illusions of people decomposing in the street in front of her and had nightmares in vivid color. She continued to have these experiences five months after her last drug experience."[31]

So it was with Stevenson's Dr. Jekyll. Without his drug, and while sitting in the park, he "was once more Mr. Hyde."[32] The "reappearance of LSD symptoms a month to over a year after the original use, without reingestion,"[33] is ominous indeed.

Some nonpsychotic reactions have been prolonged. Acute panics, confusions, and psychopathic behavior have been reported. Of these, panic reactions are most frequent. Some of these have required long-term psychotherapy.

[27] David E. Smith. "Speed Freaks vs. Acid Heads." p. 318.

[28] Reginald G. Smart and Karen Bateman, "Unfavorable Reactions to LSD," *Canadian Medical Association Journal,* Vol. 97, No. 20 (November 11, 1967), p. 1214.

[29] J. Thomas Ungerleider *et al.,* "A Statistical Survey of Adverse Reactions to LSD in Los Angeles County," *American Journal of Psychiatry,* Vol. 125, No. 3 (September 1968), pp. 352–56.

[30] Medical Society of the County of New York, Public Health Committee, Subcommittee on Narcotics Addiction, cited in Reginald G. Smart and Karen Bateman, "Unfavorable Reactions to LSD," p. 1216.

[31] Saul H. Rosenthal, "Persistent Hallucinosis Following Repeated Administration of Hallucinogenic Drugs," *American Journal of Psychiatry,* Vol. 121, No. 3 (September 1964), pp. 240–41.

[32] Robert Louis Stevenson, "The Strange Case of Dr. Jekyll and Mr. Hyde," in Damon Knight, ed., *A Century of Great Short Science-Fiction Novels* (New York, 1964), p. 59.

[33] "LSD—A Dangerous Drug," editorial in *New England Journal of Medicine,* Vol. 273, No. 23 (December 2, 1965), p. 1280.

LSD-associated suicide has occurred. One successful suicide (of the eleven reported) was of a twenty-year-old college student. "A few days prior to his death he discussed plans for the immediate and distant future with friends . . . He took LSD in the company of others . . . and without explanation, while by himself, disrobed and took his life."[34]

There has been some research on the psychic effects of LSD. It may enhance, though not replace, skilled psychotherapy. Its successful use with a woman dying of cancer has been reported. Four LSD treatments combined with psychotherapy spread over two years had a beneficial effect on the patient's attitude toward her illness. Previously, she had been markedly depressed. With treatment she

> left the hospital in good spirits and was able to participate actively in her daughter's wedding. She fulfilled her desire to walk down the aisle without the aid of even a cane, and during the reception she amazed all the guests by dancing with her husband. Her sister said she had been the life of the party.[35]

The patient died soon afterward, but her last days had been made immeasurably happier.

LSD is also being tried in the treatment of alcoholism and narcotic dependence. As yet it is too early to evaluate the effect.

DOES LSD HAVE NONPSYCHIC EFFECTS? In determining whether LSD has lasting physical effects, scientists have sought the answers to four questions:

1. Does LSD damage chromosomes?
2. Does LSD cause cancer?
3. Does LSD cause genetic mutations? Does it induce modifications or new combinations of genes or chromosomes that are transmissible from one generation to another?
4. Does LSD have a *teratogenic* effect? That is, does it produce physical defects in offspring while in the uterus?

In 1971, much of the pertinent scientific literature relating to these questions was reviewed by several California workers. They examined sixty-eight studies and case reports that had been published over a period of four years. Their conclusions: "From our work, and from a review of the literature, we believe that pure LSD ingested in moderate doses does not damage chromosomes in vivo [within the living body], does not cause detectable genetic damage, and is not a teratogen or a carcinogen in man."[36]

It was noted that "in a study of human pregnancies, those exposed to illicit [probably impure] LSD had an elevated rate of spontaneous abortions."[37]

[34] Martin H. Keeler and Clifford B. Reifler, "Suicide During an LSD Reaction," *American Journal of Psychiatry,* Vol. 123, No. 7 (January 1967), p. 885.

[35] Walter N. Pahnke, Albert A. Kurland, Sanford Unger, Charles Savage, and Stanislav Grof, "The Experimental Use of Psychedelic (LSD) Psychotherapy," *Journal of the American Medical Association,* Vol. 212, No. 11 (June 15, 1970), p. 1860.

[36] Normal J. Dishotsky, William D. Loughman, Robert E. Mogar, and Wendell R. Lipscomb, "LSD and Genetic Damage," *Science,* Vol. 172, No. 3982 (April 30, 1971), p. 439. A *teratogen* is an agent or factor that causes physical defects in the developing embryo, A *carcinogen* is an agent that causes cancer.

[37] *Ibid.*

These investigators, therefore, suggested ". . . that, other than during pregnancy, there is no present contraindication to the continued controlled experimental use of pure LSD."[38] They noted in addition that a further review of fifteen studies resulted in conclusions similar to their own.[39]

the seeds of psychoses

As has been pointed out above, other hallucinogens, producing reactions similar to that of LSD, include *mescaline, psilocybin,* and *morning-glory seeds.* A suicide following the use of morning-glory seeds has been reported.[40] Another disturbed twenty-four-year-old man "first learned of the hallucinogenic effects of morning-glory seed ingestion through a newspaper article cautioning against the use of the seeds."[41] Before going into shock, he experienced a variety of hallucinations. Four months later hallucinations were occurring both at will and against his will.

Recent years have seen a revival of interest in the use by North American Indians of peyote, the hallucinogenic plant containing mescaline (see page 407). Considered Mexico's original "peyote tribe," about ten thousand Huichols have lived for centuries (separated from European culture) in the remote regions of the high Sierra Madre. Their *nearikas*—wool paintings based on visions resulting from ingesting peyote—are collector's items. "Unlike other North American Indians who have adapted peyote rituals as a symptom of withdrawal and despair, and have often abused its use, the Huichols are abstemious and disciplined."[42] The use of peyote and whiskey by the Indians of the Plains has a different history, in which the white man played an evil role. There is an old Indian legend that, when Henry Hudson landed at the southern tip of Manhattan Island, he opened a keg of whiskey and fed it to the Indians. The Indian name "Manhattannick" means "the place where we all got drunk."[43] It is of interest to note that until the coming of the white man, the Plains tribes did not use hallucinogenic plants such as mushrooms and Jimson weed. Tobacco was used only in a few ritual puffs. However, the Plains tribes greatly respected visions. To achieve them they would inflict excruciating self-torture, imploring the spirits to pity their suffering. Peyote was native to northern Mexico. It spread from one tribe to another as far north as the Canadian plains. At first, it provided a new way to seek visions. Later, it provided escape from the humiliations of defeat by the white man.[44]

Today, the Native American Church of North America is comprised of reli-

14-3 *An Indian eating mind-affecting mushrooms before the god Mictlanteccuhtli, from a 16th-century manuscript.*

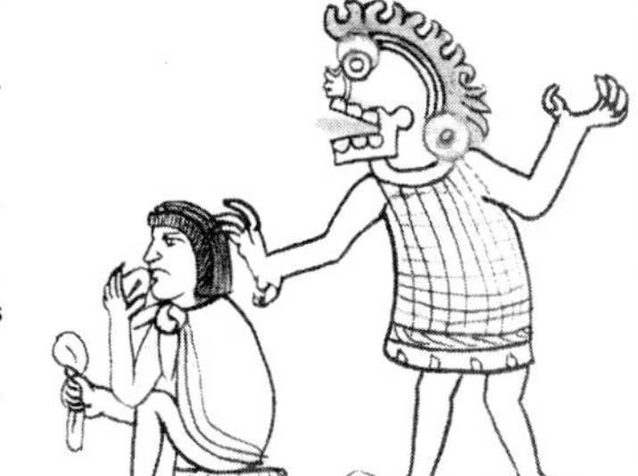

[38] *Ibid.,* citing William H. McGlothlin, Robert S. Sparkes, and David O. Arnold, "Effects of LSD on Human Pregnancy," *Journal of the American Medical Association,* Vol. 212, No. 9 (June 1, 1970), pp. 1483–91.

[39] *Ibid.,* citing B. K. Houston, *American Journal of Psychiatry,* Vol. 126, No. 2 (1969), p. 251.

[40] Sidney Cohen, "Suicide Following Morning-Glory Seed Ingestion," *American Journal of Psychiatry,* Vol. 120, No. 10 (April 1964), pp. 1024–25.

[41] P. J. Fink, M. J. Goldman, and I. Lyons, "Morning-Glory Seed Psychoses," *Archives of General Psychiatry,* Vol. 15, No. 2 (August 1966), p. 210. Many experts hold that the wide publicity concerning dangerous drugs has piqued the curiosity of the vulnerable and promoted drug use.

[42] Raymond Friday Locke, "The Huichol Indians of the Mexican Sierra Madre: Introduction," *Mankind,* Vol. 3, No. 9 (October 1972), p. 29.

[43] Alexander B. Klots, "Indigens and Immigrants," *Natural History,* Vol. 78, No. 4 (April 1969), p. 41.

[44] Peter Farb, "Rise and Fall of the Indian of the Wild West," *Natural History,* Vol. 77, No. 8 (October 1968), p. 41.

TABLE 14-1

Comparative Strengths of LSD and Other Hallucinogens (Approximate)

HALLUCINOGEN	COMPARATIVE STRENGTH*
Marihuana (leaves and tops of *Cannabis sativa,* swallowed)	30,000 mg.
Peyote buttons (*Lophophora williamsii*)	30,000 mg.
Nutmeg (*Myristica fragrans*)	20,000 mg.
Hashish (resin of *Cannabis sativa*)	4,000 mg.
Mescaline (3,4,5-trimethoxyphenylethylamine)	400 mg.
Psilocybin (4-phosphoryltryptamine)	12 mg.
STP (2,5-dimethoxy-4-methyl-amphetamine)	5 mg.
LSD (d-lysergic acid diethylamide tartarate)	0.1 mg.

*That is, each of these dosages has an equivalent effect.
Source: Sidney Cohen, "Pot, Acid and Speed," *Medical Science,* Vol. 19, No. 2 (February 1968), p. 31.

gious Indian groups of almost all tribes. They believe that the cactus plant peyote is a God-given sacrament. During their religious ceremonies they eat considerable amounts of it. One population of Navajo Indians was studied for rates of emotional illness that might be traced to their ceremonial ingestion of peyote. The rate was found to be very low, "probably because the feelings evoked by the drug experience are channeled by church belief and practice into ego-strengthening directions and there are built-in safeguards against bad reactions."[45]

"the pink wedge"

On November 11, 1967, a tablet called "the pink wedge" was sold to some young people in San Francisco. It was not much larger than a saccharine tablet. Users thought they were buying LSD. They were. But it was contaminated with STP (named for a motor fuel additive, Scientifically Treated Petroleum). On analysis, STP was found to be DOM,[46] an experimental compound developed by the Dow Chemical Company. Somehow, the formula had fallen into illicit hands. It was not long before the Haight-Ashbury Medical Clinic was deluged by young people in a toxic panic. After treatment, many could remember nothing of their experience.[47]

"STP" has other meanings. A Canadian psychiatrist writes:

> The letters stand for Serenity, Tranquility and Peace—and any associations with a tombstone may not be inappropriate in view of the occasional fatal outcome

[45] Robert L. Bergman, "Navajo Peyote Use: Its Apparent Safety," *American Journal of Psychiatry,* Vol. 128, No. 6 (December 1971), pp. 51–55.
[46] DOM is 2,5-dimethoxy-4-methyl-amphetamine, which is the chemical present in STP. (Solomon H. Snyder, Louis Faillace, and Leo Hollister, "2,5-Dimethoxy-4-Methyl-Amphetamine [STP]: A New Hallucinogenic Drug," *Science,* Vol. 158, No. 3801 [November 3, 1967], pp. 669–70.)
[47] David E. Smith and Alan J. Rose, "The Use and Abuse of LSD in Haight-Ashbury," p. 321.

> of STP ingestion . . . The actual psychedelic experience lasts for four to five days, with effects similar to though much more intense than those of LSD. The subject is unable to sleep for the first 20 hours or so, then sleeps for 4 to 10 hours; on awakening he finds himself in an even more intense psychedelic experience than before sleep, and the effects are highest at this time, gradually wearing off in the next few days and leaving the subject exhausted.[48]

over-the-counter hallucinogens

Not all hallucinogens are illegally sold. A number of intoxications have been reported recently from a considerable diversity of over-the-counter products. Many, such as cold tablets, cough suppressants, and sleep inducers, are intensely advertised. They should be kept ''under the counter'' and sold only by prescription.

cocaine

The street name for cocaine is still ''snow'' (or ''coke'' or ''girl''); at about the turn of the century, in this country, its abusers were called ''snowbirds.'' Derived from the leaves of certain coca plants growing on the eastern slopes of the Andes in Peru and Bolivia, cocaine's most important modern medicinal action is as a local anesthetic. In the mid-sixteenth century, the Spaniards invaded Peru. They bought millions of pounds of cocaine to feed to the Indians. Since cocaine is a central nervous system stimulant, causing very profound psychic dependency and possibly tolerance, the Indians were hardly able to resist working long hours in unspeakable conditions, mining gold and silver for their oppressors. The Indians chewed the leaves. In this country the white powder is snorted or sniffed from the back of the wrist, or from a small spatula. Tiny ''coke spoons'' have been sold as fashionable jewelry. In early 1973, about $50 would buy an evening's dose.

The effects of cocaine are similar to those of the amphetamines. As with the amphetamines, acute cocaine intoxication is marked by excitability, confusion, anxiety, restlessness, and headache. There may be a sudden rise in temperature preceded by a chill. The individual may become nauseous or vomit. Cocaine can be highly toxic. Why? It is absorbed from all sites of application, including the mucous membrane. The rate of absorption may exceed the rate of excretion and detoxification, and it thus may build up in the body. This does not occur when cocaine is swallowed, because in the gastrointestinal tract the drug undergoes chemical changes.

As with the amphetamines, chronic cocaine poisoning can lead to exhaustion, hallucinations, delirium, and paranoia. Cocaine sniffers report that the drug is a sexual stimulant, but the depression that follows its abuse may be accompanied by the temporary inability to have an orgasm. Also reported among chronic cocaine sniffers is an inflammation of the mucous membrane of the nasal septum. Complicating this may be a reduced resistance to infection, a perforation of the nasal septum, and eventual facial disfigurement. Cocaine has also been used by abusers as an injection, with results similar to the am-

[48] J. Robertson Unwin, ''Illicit Drug Use Among Canadian Youth: Part I,'' *Canadian Medical Association Journal,* Vol. 98, No. 8 (February 24, 1968), p. 405.

phetamines when administered in the same fashion (see pages 405–07). Some males have taken advantage of cocaine's anesthetic properties, rubbing it on the head of the penis to achieve prolonged erection without orgasm—a desired sexual "ego trip." Occasionally a woman who abuses cocaine, or whose male sexual partner does so, must be treated for spasms and a painfully raw vaginal mucous lining. A similar condition is seen resulting from coitus under the influence of amphetamines. The amphetamines have a drying effect on the vaginal secretions; this plus the unusually prolonged coitus produces the symptoms.

marihuana

historical notes

Forty-seven centuries ago the Chinese emperor Shen Nung knew of the seductive powers of a plant that was known throughout his empire as "the Liberator of Sin." In India, however, it was named "the Heavenly Guide." Today that plant is called *Cannabis sativa.* In this country its most widely known product is *marihuana.* Marihuana is a Mexican term that originally denoted an inferior tobacco. It is Spanish for Mary Jane.[49]

In some places all cannabis products are called *hashish,* after a Moslem fanatic of the eleventh century named Hasan ibn-al-Sabbah. To embolden his men to assassinate Christian Crusaders, he is reputed to have fed them cannabis. It has been claimed that the word "assassin" is derived from Hasan's full name, Hashishin. Many scholars believe that the drug Hashishin used was opium, not cannabis. Tongue in cheek, some students of words have pointed to 2 Kings 4:40, which says, "There is death in the pot." But this passage merely refers to a "pot of pottage" made of wild herbs.

The male cannabis plant is used to make rope fiber or hemp.[50] The Greek word for "hemp" is *kannabis;* cannabis plants are thus sometimes called "hemp." The value of the plant as a source of rope may account for its cultivation in so many parts of the world. The early settlers of the American colonies planted *Cannabis sativa* and made rope from it. During the Second World War, the U.S. government cultivated the plant in six Midwestern states because it was feared that the Philippine source of hemp would be lost to the Japanese. Early in 1944, the War Production Board issued a directive forbidding the nonmilitary use of hemp to make rope, even for hangings.[51]

the plant source of cannabis

The annual plant *Cannabis sativa* grows wild in most temperate and tropical areas, and almost everywhere in the United States. Maturing in about four to five months, it often reaches a height of six feet or more. Although some varieties of *Cannabis sativa* have both male and female characteristics in a single plant, the plant usually occurs in separate male and female forms. All parts of both the male and female plants contain *psychoactive* (mind-affecting) chemi-

[49] *The Use of Cannabis, Report of a World Health Organization Scientific Group* (Geneva, 1971), p. 6.
[50] "What They're Saying," *Medical World News,* Vol. 12, No. 41 (November 5, 1971), p. 6.
[51] Negley K. Teeters, *"Hang by the Neck . . ."* (Springfield, Ill., 1967), p. 172, citing Louis Blake Duff, *The Country Kerchief* (Toronto, 1929).

cals. It is in the young, small leaves surrounding the seeds of the plant, and in its flowering tops, that most of the psychoactive ingredients are found. Decreasing percentages of the psychoactive chemical are found in the leaves, smaller stems, larger stems, roots, and seeds.[52] The flowering tops of the female plant secrete a clear, varnishlike resin. This substance is *hashish*.

In the freshly reaped cannabis plant, heredity is the most important single factor in determining the amount of psychoactive chemicals. Climate, soil, and weather also influence the intoxicating properties of the plant. In addition, time of harvest and duration and temperature of storage affect potency.

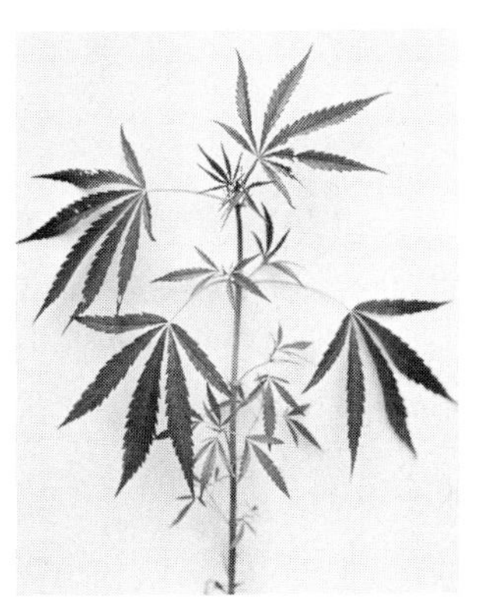

14-4 *A cannabis plant.*

cannabis chemistry

The chemical constituents of the cannabis plant are divided into two major groups: the *cannabinoids* and the *noncannabinoids.* Among the constituents of the noncannabinoids are waxes, oils, starches, and a variety of other substances, some of which are as yet unidentified. Their effect on human health is unknown.

Numerous cannabinoids have been isolated from cannabis. Most are not known to affect human beings. A few are lethal to bacteria. Several are known to have psychoactive as well as other effects. Of these last, chemists have named the two most important. These are Delta-9-tetrahydrocannabinol (Delta-9-THC) and Delta-8-tetrahydrocannabinol (Delta-8-THC).[53] Both are now available in synthetic form. Delta-9-THC is thought to produce most of the effects of cannabis in animals and humans.

cannabis preparations

In the United States, the two most common cannabis preparations are marihuana leaf and hashish. The leaf is most often cut and crushed and rolled into a thin cigarette, usually called a ''joint.'' It may also be smoked in a pipe, baked in brownies, or boiled in water to make a tea. Hashish (or ''hash'') is a hard brown cake of the pure cannabis resin. It is five to ten times more potent than marihuana. It is most often smoked in a pipe, but it too may be eaten or drunk. Today, the great majority of cannabis users in this country use marihuana rather than hashish, and smoke it rather than swallow it. In India, cannabis is widely eaten or drunk.

Experienced marihuana and hashish smokers are able to control the dose and, therefore, the effect of the drug. Those who ingest it orally have no control over the dose. Marihuana smokers experience some effect within a few minutes. The ''high'' usually begins in about fifteen minutes and lasts about three hours. The effects of oral intake of cannabis do not begin for one-half hour to

[52] *Marihuana and Health, Second Annual Report to Congress from the Secretary of Health, Education, and Welfare* (1972), p. 135, citing P. S. Fetterman, E. S. Smith, C. W. Waller, O. Guerrero, N. J. Doorenbos, and M. W. Quimby, ''Mississippi-Grown *Cannabis sativa* L: Preliminary Observation on Chemical Definition of Phenotype and Variations in Tetrahydrocannabinol Content Versus Age, Sex, and Plant Part,'' *Journal of Pharmaceutical Sciences,* Vol. 60, No. 8 (1971), pp. 1246–49.

[53] Not all chemists use this nomenclature. For example, Delta-9-THC is sometimes called Delta-1-THC. Agreement on a universal nomenclature is expected shortly.

two hours, reach a peak in about three to four hours, and continue in a diminishing fashion for about eight hours. Those few who have injected suspensions of marihuana or hashish into a vein have not produced the result they desired. They have, however, produced grave physical symptoms.

the fate of marihuana in the body

The effect of THC, the active principle of cannabis, on the human being is not easy to determine. In part, this is because of the difficulty in determining the dose taken. When marihuana is smoked as a cigarette or in a pipe, a certain amount of the active material is lost when the smoke escapes into the air. It is estimated that only between 20 and 50 percent (perhaps even less) of the THC in a marihuana cigarette is absorbed by the lungs.[54] Thus the dose of THC that is actually delivered to the smoker varies greatly.

Animal research has shown that, once they get into the circulation, some of the active cannabinoids (the forms of THC) rapidly begin to disappear from the blood.[55] What happens to them? It is believed that they are quickly converted into other chemicals, or *metabolites.* (A metabolite is a product of *metabolism,* which, as has been said, refers to the chemical changes that take place in the body.) THC metabolites are rapidly taken up by nervous and other body tissues.[56] It may be (though this has not been proved) that it is the metabolites, rather than the original cannabis constituents, that are responsible for the drug's effects.

An unusual chemical event is believed to occur with the metabolism of THC. THC metabolites pass from the liver via the bile duct and gallbladder to the gastrointestinal tract. In the gastrointestinal tract these metabolites are reabsorbed and then secreted again into the liver-gastrointestinal circulation.[57] The significance of this is not yet understood. But it has been suggested (although, again, not proved) that there is an enzyme (see page 531, footnote 22) in the liver involved in the metabolism of THC.

Moreover, it has been noted that, in man, if Delta-9-THC is administered intravenously, it will persist in the blood plasma for several days.[58] In rats, after a single injection of the drug beneath the skin, the concentration of Delta-9-THC in fat "was ten times greater than in any other tissue examined, and persisted in this tissue for two weeks. With repeated injection [it] and its metabolites accumulated in fat and brain."[59]

Special notation should here be made about the distribution of the drug in pregnant animals. THC does cross the placenta. It may concentrate in the fetus in sizable amounts.[60] The effect on the fetus is not yet known.

[54] *Marihuana and Health, Second Annual Report to Congress from the Secretary of Health, Education, and Welfare* (1972), pp. 170–72.
[55] *Ibid.,* p. 159.
[56] *Ibid.,* p. 173.
[57] *Ibid.,* citing H. A. Klausner and J. V. Dingell, "The Metabolism and Excretion of Delta-9-Tetrahydrocannabinol in the Rat," *Life Sciences,* Vol. 10 (1971), p. 49.
[58] David S. Kreuz and Julius Axelrod, "Delta-9-Tetrahydrocannabinol Localization in Body Fat," *Science,* Vol. 179, No. 4071, p. 391.
[59] *Ibid.,* pp. 391–92.
[60] *Marihuana and Health, Second Annual Report to Congress from the Secretary of Health, Education, and Welfare,* (1972), p. 173, citing the following: R. I. Freudenthal, J. Martin, and M. E. Wall, "The Distribution of Delta-9-Tetrahydrocannabinol in the Mouse," *Journal of Pharmacy and Pharmacology* (1972, in preparation);

Most cannabis metabolites are excreted from the body via the feces and urine. In man a large proportion is excreted in the feces. This may be a result of the increased activity associated with the liver-gastrointestinal recirculation.

the extent of marihuana use and abuse

According to a survey by the National Commission on Marihuana and Drug Abuse,[61] made available on January 21, 1972, about 24.6 million people in this country had used marihuana at least once. But only about 8.34 million were still using it. Why had so many people forsaken marihuana? Boredom. Sheer loss of interest had caused 81 percent of the reporting adults to quit the drug. The second most common cause for discontinuing the use of marihuana was its illegality.

How often were people using marihuana by mid-1971? Another study has shown that, of an estimated 9 percent of the population aged eleven and older who had used marihuana at least once, 3 percent smoked marihuana daily (about three cigarettes per occasion); 11 percent, three to six times a week; 40 percent, one to eight times a month; 46 percent had used marihuana fewer than ten times or had stopped using it.[62]

marihuana and the U.S. soldier

Much was written about the abuse of marihuana among U.S. army personnel in Vietnam. Two studies indicated that from 25 to 31 percent of the troops went beyond the experimentation stage.[63] Among officers and senior noncommissioned officers, marihuana use was uncommon.

It is known that a majority of treated U.S. Army personnel were able to forsake heroin upon their return to the U.S. (see pages 365–67). Whether there is any relationship between this and their present consumption of cannabis products or other drugs is unknown.

In summary, then, many millions of young people of all classes in this nation have experimented with, or are chronically using, marihuana. After the age of twenty-five, most people discontinue the drug. Millions, however, continue to use it. It is estimated that, by 1975, some 44.4 million people in the country will be between fourteen and twenty-four years old.[64] That will amount to almost 20 percent of the entire population. So pervasive a practice among such a large segment of the population merits close study. Consider both the knowns and the unknowns. Both are important in making a personal or national decision about the drug.

R. D. Harbison, "Maternal Distribution and Placental Transfer of C^{14} Delta-9-Tetrahydrocannabinol in Pregnant Mice," *Journal of Pharmacology and Experimental Therapeutics* (1972); J. Idanpaan-Heikkila, G. D. Fritchie, L. F. Englert, B. T. Ho, and W. M. McIsaac, "Placental Transfer of Tritriated (1) Delta-9-Tetrahydrocannabinol," *New England Journal of Medicine,* Vol. 281 (1969), p. 330.

[61] "Marihuana Commission Finds Usage High," *Science News,* Vol. 101, No. 5 (January 29, 1972), p. 72.

[62] *Marihuana and Health, Second Annual Report to Congress from the Secretary of Health, Education, and Welfare* (1972), p. 38a, citing William H. McGlothlin, "Marihuana: An Analysis of Use, Distribution and Control," U.S. Bureau of Narcotics and Dangerous Drugs, SCID-TR-2 (1971).

[63] Edward Colback, "Marihuana Use by GI's in Viet Nam," *American Journal of Psychiatry,* Vol. 128, No. 2 (August 1971), p. 205.

[64] *Population Estimates,* Bureau of the Census, U.S. Department of Commerce, Series P-25, No. 381 (December 18, 1967), p. 6.

marihuana: a drug in a class by itself

Marihuana can be classified with no other drugs. It can act as either a stimulant or a depressant.[65] Give a mouse a barbiturate depressant. It sleeps. Give a mouse both a barbiturate and marihuana. Together the drugs have a greater depressant effect than the barbiturate alone. The marihuana has increased the depressant effect of the barbiturate. Give a mouse a stimulant amphetamine. It becomes excited. Give a mouse both an amphetamine and marihuana. Together the drugs have a greater stimulant effect than the amphetamine alone. The marihuana has increased the stimulant effect of the amphetamine. When the combined effect of two drugs is greater than the effect of either drug used alone, a phenomenon called *potentiation* has occurred. Thus it may be said that, paradoxically and remarkably, ''marihuana potentiates both barbiturate sleeping time and amphetamine excitement in mice.''[66]

In the matter of tolerance, there is even more to suggest that marihuana is unique.

tolerance to marihuana

Tolerance is a fundamental characteristic of such drugs as the opiates, the barbiturates, and alcohol (see page 361). Thus, repeated administration of given doses of these drugs produces a decreasing effect. With narcotics, for example, tolerance is manifested by a shortened duration of the drug's action and a marked elevation of the killing dose. Unlike many lower animals, man develops only a slight degree of tolerance to marihuana. By no means is it as profound as his tolerance to opiates, barbiturates, and alcohol. Like lower animals, man may develop tolerance to some of the effects of marihuana and not to others.[67] What is more, numerous longtime marihuana smokers report that they need less—not more—of the drug to achieve the same effect. This phenomenon is called *reverse tolerance.* Various explanations have been suggested for it.

WHY REVERSE TOLERANCE? SOME CONJECTURES The metabolites of THC (see page 416) continue to be excreted in the urine and feces of a chronic marihuana smoker for several days. This indicates that repeated intake of marihuana results in an accumulation of the drug's active chemicals in the body tissues.[68] Therefore, residues of the drug remain in the body of the chronic user for considerable periods. For this reason it is possible that reverse tolerance would develop—that the drug would have increasing effects with repeated smaller doses. Moreover, some researchers theorize that repeated doses of the drug may increase the ability of the liver to produce an enzyme that might be necessary to convert THC into the truly psychoactive chemicals.[69] Increasing

[65] Some researchers consider it neither a stimulant nor a depressant for this reason.

[66] Richard Colestock Pillard, ''Marihuana,'' *New England Journal of Medicine,* Vol. 283, No. 6 (August 6, 1970), p. 295.

[67] *Marihuana and Health, Second Annual Report to Congress from the Secretary of Health, Education, and Welfare* (1972), p. 17.

[68] Louis Lemberger, Stephen D. Silberstein, Julius Axelrod, and Irwin J. Kopin, ''Marihuana: Studies on the Disposition and Metabolism of Delta-9-Tetrahydrocannabinol in Man,'' *Science,* Vol. 170, No. 3964 (December 18, 1970), pp. 1320–22.

[69] ''Marijuana,'' a report prepared with the technical assistance of Richard Lance Christie and Joel Simon Hochman, *Human Behavior,* Vol. 1, No. 1, p. 61.

effects with repeated smaller doses could also occur in this manner. Still a third reason for reverse tolerance may be found in the fact that people must learn how to smoke marihuana efficiently and what effects to expect from it. Suggestibility, or the user's anticipation of the effect of the drug, plays a major role in this learning process. This "anticipation factor" has been demonstrated in the laboratory. Longtime users frequently report a marihuana high after they have smoked placebos, "marihuana" cigarettes from which, unbeknownst to them, all the active principle has been removed. They are thus deceived into anticipating an effect. It may be that this "learned sensitization" to marihuana, based on prolonged past experience, minimizes the mild tolerance to the drug that actually may occur.[70]

CROSS-TOLERANCE In large doses, marihuana can cause hallucinations in man. So can the stimulant hallucinogens LSD, mescaline, peyote, and DMT. But LSD, mescaline, peyote, and DMT show a *cross-tolerance* for one another. This means that a person who takes increasing doses of any one of these four will develop tolerance not only to the drug he is taking, but also to the other three. For example, increasing doses of LSD cause tolerance not only to LSD but to mescaline, peyote, and DMT as well. But marihuana shows no cross-tolerance with any of these four hallucinogens.[71] In addition, the chemical structure of THC does not suggest that marihuana is primarily a hallucinogen.

PHYSICAL DEPENDENCE AND DEATHS UNPROVED Unlike opiates, the barbiturates, and alcohol, marihuana does not seem to cause physical dependence. There is little evidence that withdrawal or abstinence symptoms of consequence occur with abrupt discontinuance of marihuana. In addition, as the drug is now ordinarily used in this country, the margin of safety is very wide between the dose of cannabis required to produce an effect and the dose necessary to kill. "Death from an overdose of cannabis is apparently extremely rare and difficult to confirm."[72]

dose, set, and setting affect individual signs and symptoms

A *sign* of a condition is objective; it is observed. A *symptom* is subjective; it is felt. The signs and symptoms of marihuana intoxication in humans vary with *dose, set,* and *setting.*

"*Set* refers to the attitudes, moods, expectations, and beliefs which the individual brings to the drug-using experience. *Setting* represents the external circumstances surrounding the experience."[73] The set depends on the personality. The setting is the environment, whether a laboratory or a lonely living room. How may dose, set, and setting affect even scientific reporting about marihuana? Consider a mechanical task such as a driving test, the results of which are particularly affected by dose, set, and setting.

[70] Leo F. Hollister, "Marihuana in Man: Three Years Later," *Science,* Vol. 172, No. 3978 (April 2, 1971), p. 27.
[71] It is worth noting, however, that Delta-9-THC shows a cross-tolerance for Delta-8-THC.
[72] *Marihuana and Health, Second Annual Report to Congress from the Secretary of Health, Education, and Welfare* (1972), p. 21.
[73] *Marihuana and Health, Summarized Version: A Report to the Congress from the Secretary, Department of Health, Education, and Welfare* (January 31, 1971).

marihuana and driving

Three students volunteer to serve as experimental subjects in a university laboratory. Their job: to take a laboratory-simulated driving test under the influence of a measured dose of THC in a marihuana cigarette. It should be promptly noted that one particular method of administration of the drug is used. If the drug were swallowed instead of smoked, for example, the test results would be different. Note too that street marihuana would produce different results because the amount of THC varies in street-sold marihuana. Also, for all three subjects the setting is artificial. The laboratory is neutral, impersonal; it can hardly be compared to the crawling, choking, exasperating, demanding, smoggy freeway traffic at the end of a working day.

Consider, too, the personality of each of the three students participating in the experiment. The first is an avowed believer in the benefits of marihuana. He proclaims it his salvation from stress. Would he not be inclined to try to do as well as possible on the driving test? Indeed, were he so inclined, he should also be able to regulate his high, even experience reverse tolerance, and thus regulate to some extent the results of his driving test.

The second student professes utter indifference to marihuana. ''It's not my bag,'' he says. If this is true, he has nothing to prove. The results of his driving test will reflect that fact. The third student expresses a distaste for drugs. He quotes Ogden Nash: ''For me, 'pot is not.' The whole idea gets me uptight.'' In the analysis of the results of his test, this feeling cannot be ignored.

So each student is set to respond to the experimental marihuana in his individual way. And each student's simulated driving performance will be profoundly affected by his personal response to the drug. Moreover, individual attitudes toward drugs are not clear-cut and easy to measure. The confirmed smoker's approach to marihuana may be an expression more of rebellion against society than of conviction about the drug. The indifferent student may not be so indifferent as he seems or even as he believes himself to be. The student who proclaims his hatred of marihuana may really be masking his fearful desire to try it. Add to these variables still another. The three students may not have the same ability to metabolize drugs. Their bodies may respond differently. All these factors make it very hazardous indeed to draw general conclusions about the effect of marihuana on driving.

Now complicate the experiment. Attempt to measure the comparative effects of marihuana and alcohol on simulated driving. In the case of alcohol, one at least has a beginning. There are known relationships between the amount of alcohol in the blood and dangerous driving. As yet no such fixed relationships are available for marihuana. And it was not until midsummer of 1973 that the first reliable test for detecting low levels of marihuana in human blood was announced by scientists at Sweden's Karolinska Institute.[74] Noting these and other problems, one investigator wrote: ''Since our first experiments

[74] ''The First Blood Test for Marihuana in Humans,'' *New Scientist,* Vol. 59, No. 856 (July 26, 1973), p. 181. The application of this technique to legal medicine will be hampered by the drug's rapid disappearance from the blood soon after ingestion and by the extreme complexity of the testing equipment.

we have simply asked subjects when they were 'high,' 'Do you think you could drive a car now?' Without exception the answer from those who had really gotten high has been 'No!' or 'You must be kidding!' "[75]

SOME STUDIES OF MARIHUANA AND DRIVING One study[76] that compared the effects of marihuana and alcohol on driving performance found that speedometer errors increased with marihuana, but alcohol produced even more errors. Although the investigators were careful to state their results precisely, the study has been widely misinterpreted. Moreover, it had many of the shortcomings mentioned above. Other and more recent studies indicate that marihuana smoking does make driving an automobile dangerous.

Numerous investigators have found that marihuana impairs memory of recent events. "Persons high on marihuana have subtle difficulties in speech, primarily in remembering from moment to moment the logical thread of what is being said. Marihuana may interfere with retrieval of material from immediate storage in the brain."[77] One young student described this phenomenon in this way:

> I often drive my automobile when I'm high on marihuana . . . I'll come to a stop light and have a moment of panic because I can't remember whether or not I've just put my foot on the brake. Of course, when I look down, it's there, but in a second or two afterward, I can't remember having done it. In a similar way I can't recall whether I've passed a turn I want to take or whether I've made the turn.[78]

Another hazard of driving while under the influence of marihuana is a marked and persistent increase in the time required to recover from glare.[79] Thus, marihuana smokers who drive at night may risk serious consequences, to themselves and to others. Also, a significant dose-related increase in braking time has been reported.[80] Added to these marihuana-induced hazards are those related to "flashbacks," a phenomenon discussed on page 426.

marihuana use: early symptoms

This old Persian tale is still told today in southwestern Asia:

> Three men arrived at Ispahan at night. The gates of the town were closed. One of the men was an alcoholic, another an opium-addict, and the third took hashish. The alcoholic said: "Let us break down the gate"; the opium smoker

[75] Leo F. Hollister, "Marihuana in Man: Three Years Later," p. 24.

[76] A. Crancer, Jr., J. M. Dille, J. C. Delay, J. E. Wallace, and M. D. Haykin, "Comparison of the Effects of Marihuana and Alcohol on Simulated Driving Performance," *Science*, Vol. 164, No. 3881 (May 16, 1969), pp. 851–54.

[77] Andrew T. Weil and Norman E. Zinberg, "Acute Effects of Marihuana on Speech," *Nature*, Vol. 222, No. 5192 (May 3, 1969), p. 434.

[78] *Ibid.*, p. 437.

[79] *Marihuana and Health, Second Annual Report to Congress from the Secretary of Health, Education, and Welfare* (1972), p. 219, citing I. M. Frank, R. S. Hepler, S. Stier and W. Rickles, "Marihuana, Tobacco, and Functions Affecting Driving," paper presented at the American Psychiatric Association, Annual Meeting, Washington, D.C. (May 1971).

[80] *Ibid.*, citing P. Bech, J. Christiansen, H. Christrup, B. Kofod, J. Nyboe, I. Rafaelson, and O. J. Rafaelson, "Cannabis and Alcohol: Effect on Simulated Driving," paper presented at the Meeting on Biochemical and Pharmacological Aspects of Dependence and Reports on Marihuana Research, Amsterdam (September 30–October 1, 1971).

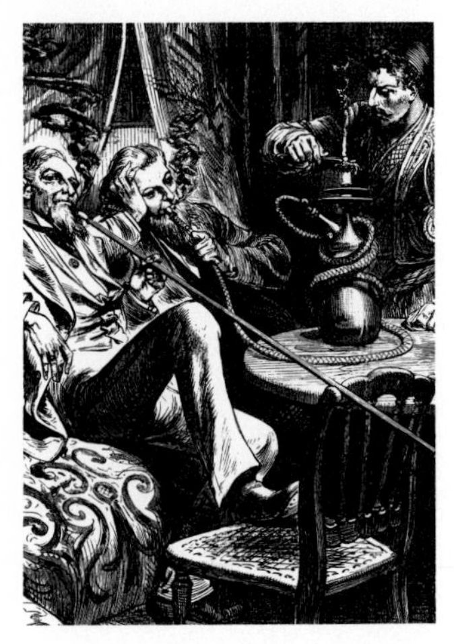

14-5 *Nineteenth-century U.S. visitors to the Middle East smoking opium and hashish.*

suggested: "Let us lie down and sleep until tomorrow"; but the hashish-addict said: "Let us pass through the keyhole."[81]

Keeping in mind the variable effects of dose, set, and setting, consider the early symptoms—subjective effects—of cannabis use as experienced by marihuana smokers.

At doses ordinarily used in this country at the present time, smokers report varying degrees of a variety of symptoms. Within seconds to minutes many people feel a series of jittery *"rushes."*[82] Then comes *euphoria*—a pleasant, relaxed tranquility. Time passes slowly. Space may seem diminished. So are inhibitions. Attention is dulled. Thought processes fragment. The user may be either hilarious and friendly or silent and distant. "There is an awareness of being intoxicated not unlike that produced by alcohol. The user becomes acutely conscious of certain stimuli to the extent that his whole attention is focused, immersed and at times lost with the sensory experience."[83] Less commonly, *dizziness* and a sense of *lightness* are reported. *Nausea* and *increased hunger* have also been experienced. The increased hunger, like some other symptoms, may be due in part to the increased suggestibility caused by the drug. Marihuana smoking is often a "lonely group" affair: "The group pressure of a majority experiencing a particular effect would be strong for the others."[84]

What symptoms occur with *higher than ordinary doses? Depersonalization*—loss of the sense of personal ownership of one's body—has been reported. One user described the loss of his sense of body reality in this way: "I float up and up and up until I'm miles above the earth. Then, Baby, I begin to come apart. My fingers leave my hands, my hands leave my wrists, my arms and legs leave my body."[85] Visual distortions and imagery are also not uncommon. For example, colors may appear to shimmer. (This effect is not nearly so intense as with LSD.) The higher the dose of marihuana, the more likely it is that such symptoms as depersonalization and hallucinations will occur. (A few marihuana smokers experience these effects with small doses.)

Panic, depression, and *toxic psychoses,* although very rare, sometimes do occur, especially among inexperienced marihuana users. *Panic* is the most common of these unusual adverse reactions. The floating feeling of unreality, the eerie sense that the body has lost its place in space, frightens some people. Terrified, they panic. The best treatment: quiet, nonjudgmental, nonthreatening reassurance. A temporary *depression* has also been infrequently observed with marihuana smoking. Whether the drug itself produces the depression is unknown, but doubtful. Recovery is the rule. Usually it needs little or no treatment.[86] Both depression and panic occur more frequently among those who are

[81] *World Health: The Magazine of the World Health Organization,* Vol. 13, No. 1 (January–February 1960), p. 24.
[82] Richard Colestock Pillard, "Marihuana," p. 296.
[83] *Ibid.,* p. 296.
[84] Leo F. Hollister, "Hunger and Appetite After Single Doses of Marihuana, Alcohol and Dextroamphetamine," *Clinical Pharmacology and Therapeutics,* Vol. 12, No. 1 (January–February 1971), p. 49.
[85] Quoted in Edward R. Bloomquist, "Marihuana: Social Benefit or Social Derangement?" *California Medicine,* Vol. 106, No. 5 (May 1967), p. 348.
[86] Andrew T. Weil, "Adverse Reactions to Marihuana," *New England Journal of Medicine,* Vol. 282, No. 18 (April 30, 1970), pp. 997–98.

new to the drug or who attach much emotional meaning to their use of it. It may well be that the drug precipitates these adverse reactions in individuals already predisposed to emotional disorders. The extremely rare *toxic psychoses,* which are poison-induced reactions to marihuana, are discussed on pages 425–26.

marihuana use: early signs

The immediate signs—objective, physical indications—of marihuana smoking are few. Most researchers report a reddening of the delicate membrane that lines the eyelids and covers the exposed surface of the eyeball (the conjunctiva; see pages 277–78) and an increased pulse rate. These signs may last as long as the psychic effects of the drug. (It is not the smoke that causes the red conjunctiva. Oral ingestion of cannabis has the same effect.) Some investigators have also noted a slight contraction of the pupils, accompanied by a drooping of the eyelids. It is not true, as was formerly claimed, that marihuana causes the pupils to dilate. Some impairment of muscle strength has also been reported among marihuana users. However, blood pressure, body temperature, and knee-jerk reflexes usually remain unaffected. Both smoked marihuana and oral Delta-9-THC cause dilation of airways lasting as long as sixty minutes and six hours, respectively. This is in contrast to the airway constriction that follows cigarette smoking.[87] (It would be of interest to research the effect of cannabis on asthmatic people; see page 428 for a discussion of cannabis as a possible source of medications.) Unlike opiates, marihuana smoke does not cause depression of the center in the brain that controls respiration.[88] Brain waves, measured by the encephalogram, may show minimal changes.[89] It used to be thought that the hunger evidenced by some marihuana smokers was a result of a drop in the blood sugar. This has been shown to be not true, but the cause of the professed hunger is unclear (see page 422). Despite some hand and body unsteadiness, there seems to be no gross impairment of ability to coordinate and to control muscle action.

With people who are new to the drug, moderate doses of marihuana significantly impair reading comprehension and impede performance on learning tests. Even with experienced users the drug interferes with logical thinking. Thus "cannabis significantly impairs cognitive [understanding, reasoning] functions, the impairment increasing in magnitude as the dose increases or the task is more complex or both."[90]

marihuana use: delayed effects

Research is being conducted both in the United States and abroad on the delayed effects of the prolonged use of cannabis.

From India have come reports associating chronic cannabis use with loss of

[87] Donald P. Tashkin, Bertrand J. Shapiro, and Ira M. Frank, "Acute Pulmonary Physiologic Effects of Smoked Marijuana and Oral Delta-9-Tetrahydrocannabinol in Healthy Young Men," *New England Journal of Medicine,* Vol. 289, No. 7 (August 16, 1973), pp. 336–40.

[88] Louis Vachon, Muiris X. FitzGerald, Norman H. Solliday, Ira A. Gould, and Edward Gaensler, "Single-Dose Effect of Marihuana Smoke," *New England Journal of Medicine,* Vol. 288, No. 19 (May 10, 1973), pp. 985–89.

[89] Robert G. Heath, "Marihuana: Effect on Deep and Surface Electroencephalograms of Man," *Archives of General Psychiatry,* Vol. 26 (June 1972), pp. 577–84.

[90] *The Use of Cannabis, Report of a World Health Organization Scientific Group* (Geneva, 1971), p. 25.

appetite and weight, anemia, and constipation.[91] But are these due to the drug or to the pervasive poverty and malnutrition in that country? Nobody can be certain.

A recent report from England[92] may have great significance. Evidence of *cerebral atrophy* (a permanent wasting away of part of the main portion of the brain) has been reported in ten young male patients who had smoked cannabis for three to eleven years. These patients had also used amphetamines and LSD, but in much smaller amounts. Among the symptoms noted were behavior changes, inability to recall recent events, hallucinations, depression, and headaches. By no means does this research present adequate proof that brain changes are caused by the use of cannabis.[93] True, in young people this type of permanent brain damage is rare. It may be caused by other afflictions, such as head injuries and certain infections, but none of the ten patients had a history of such illness. There are some deficiencies in the study. The technical methods used in making the diagnoses are not acceptable to all workers.[94] In addition, if cerebral atrophy was indeed present, the relatively small amount of other drug use reported by the patients could have had some role in causing the disease. Moreover, the investigators compared the brains of the heavy marihuana smokers with the brains of other patients without nervous system damage. It would have been better to have made a comparison with the brains of people with the same deterioration who did not smoke marihuana. Also, if the amphetamines the patients had abused were intravenously self-administered, the brain changes might conceivably have been due to blood-vessel inflammation. Nevertheless, to ignore this study would be foolhardy. More research in this direction is surely indicated.

Some will find comfort in the fact that whereas it has been proved that prolonged alcoholism often results in cerebral atrophy, it has not been proved that chronic use of marihuana does. However, answers regarding alcoholic brain disease came only after many years of study. For example, careful examination of actual human brain tissue obtained after death was necessary. "The full impact of the massive drug exposure of youth during the '60's may not be adequately assessed for another decade."[95]

Another possible delayed effect of chronic use of cannabis is damage to chromosomes, but some recent studies have failed to prove any cannabis-related chromosomal damage in man or rats.[96] The results of one study suggest

[91] *Ibid.*, pp. 26–27, citing the following: I. C. Chopra and R. N. Chopra, "The Use of Cannabis in India," *Bulletin of Narcotic Drugs,* Vol. 9, No. 1 (1957), pp. 4–29; J. E. Dhunjibhoy, "A Brief Résumé of the Types of Insanity Commonly Met With in India with a Full Description of 'Indian Hemp Insanity' Peculiar to the Country," *Journal of Mental Science,* Vol. 76 (1928), pp. 254–64; J. Sterne and C. Ducastaing, "Les Artérites du Cannabis Indica," *Archives des Maladies du Coeur et des Vaisseaux,* Vol. 53 (1960), pp. 143–47.

[92] A. M. G. Campbell, M. Evans, J. L. G. Thompson, and M. J. Williams, "Cerebral Atrophy in Young Cannabis Smokers," *The Lancet,* Vol. 2, No. 7736 (December 4, 1971), pp. 1219–24.

[93] "Cannabis Encephalopathy?" editorial in *The Lancet,* Vol. 2, No. 7736 (December 4, 1971), p. 1240.

[94] For example, J. Bull, "Cerebral Atrophy in Young Cannabis Smokers," *The Lancet,* Vol. 2, No. 7739 (December 25, 1971), p. 1420, and Colin Brewer, "Cerebral Atrophy in Young Cannabis Smokers," *The Lancet,* Vol. 1, No. 7742 (January 15, 1972), p. 143.

[95] Lincoln D. Clark, "Marihuana and Human Behavior," p. 45.

[96] *Ibid.*, p. 27, citing the following: P. A. Martin, "Cannabis and Chromosomes," *The Lancet,* Vol. 1 (1969), p. 370; R. L. Neu, H. O. Powers, S. King, and L. J. Gardner, "Cannabis and Chromosomes," *The Lancet,* Vol. 1 (1969), p. 675.

an increase of chromosomal breakage among marihuana users as compared to nonmarihuana users. However, the investigators do not consider their results conclusive, urging that further similar studies be conducted.[97] High doses of cannabis extracts given to rats, hamsters, and rabbits do cause the birth of abnormal offspring. However, these doses are much higher than those ordinarily obtained from marihuana smoking in this country at this time. In addition, the birth of abnormal children has not yet been attributable to marihuana use.[98]

A significant study of U.S. soldiers in West Germany[99] concerns thirty-one daily hashish smokers. "Every patient described the development of his tremendous hashish tolerance as one that simply occurred by consuming increasing amounts over a few weeks' period . . . most claimed that chronic smoking was done more out of habit, similar to tobacco smoking."[100] In these cases the severity of the signs described below were apparently not associated with previous smoking of either marihuana or tobacco. Nor were they prevented by the filtering action of a small piece of window screen placed in the bottom of the bowl of the hashish pipe. Among the conditions reported among the soldiers were inflammation of the mucous membranes of the nose, throat, bronchi, and sinuses. Particularly common was swelling of the uvula, the fleshy tissue that hangs from the soft palate.

does marihuana cause toxic psychoses?

It is well to emphasize the difference between *true psychoses* (see pages 296–300), which are usually deep-seated and prolonged, or *chronic,* and *toxic psychoses,* which are of brief duration, or *acute.* Toxic psychoses also differ from true psychoses in that they are the result of the presence of toxins (poisons) in the body, which cause a temporary malfunction of the brain's cerebral cortex. This may be due to many intoxicants (and medications), including marihuana.[101]

A novice in marihuana use may experience an immediate marihuana-associated toxic psychosis, and a long-term user may experience a delayed toxic psychosis. But the occurrence of toxic psychosis among both new and long-term users is very rare.

Sometimes a person with a history of true psychosis (such as schizophrenia), or an individual whose personality structure borders on the abnormal, will be precipitated into psychotic behavior by marihuana. However, it is the person-

[97] "Marihuana Users Show Breaks in Chromosomes," *Hospital Tribune,* Vol. 7, No. 15 (April 16, 1973), p. 3.

[98] Lincoln D. Clark, "Marihuana and Human Behavior," citing the following: W. F. Gerber and L. C. Schramm, "Effect of Marihuana Extract on Fetal Hamsters and Rabbits," *Toxicology and Applied Pharmacology,* Vol. 14 (1969), pp. 276–82; W. F. Gerber and L. C. Schramm, "Teratogenicity of Marihuana Extract as Influenced by Plant Origin and Seasonal Variation," *Archives of International Pharmacodynamics,* Vol. 177 (1969), pp. 224–30; T. V. N. Persaud and A. C. Ellington, "The Effect of *Cannabis sativa* L. (Ganja) on Developing Rat Embryos—Preliminary Observations," *West Indian Medical Journal,* Vol. 17 (1968), pp. 232–34.

[99] Forrest S. Tennant, Jr., Merle Preble, Thomas J. Prendergast, and Paul Ventry, "Medical Manifestations Associated with Hashish," *Journal of the American Medical Association,* Vol. 216, No. 12 (June 21, 1971), pp. 1965–69.

[100] *Ibid.,* p. 1966.

[101] Some writers object to the application of the word "psychedelic" to LSD or marihuana. The term has the connotation that these drugs induce highly creative thought patterns. There is little reason to believe this. A better term would indeed seem to be "toxic psychosis."

ality structure of the individual, and not the chemical structure of the drug, that is instrumental. ''The intoxication merely triggers the psychosis, as is seen with a variety of other drugs including alcohol, amphetamine and LSD.''[102]

marihuana: delusion of early adolescence

As a child approaches adolescence, he must begin to

> relinquish his dependence on his parents for emotional support and learn to base his self-esteem on his own achievements. These achievements not only involve success in the path towards his profession, but also social and sexual success . . . Before the adolescent reaches maturity he has to deal with many disappointments, frustrations, feelings of helplessness and wishes to escape . . . The question now is how are these inevitable conflicts of adolescence going to be settled? Is the adolescent going to tackle them by asking himself after a disappointment, ''What did I do wrong?'' ''How can I do it differently?'' Is he going to be able to base his self-esteem on his own achievements? Or is he going to fall back on external ''magic'' [such as marihuana] that can elevate his self-esteem at command just as the traditional objects [such as a teddy bear or a blanket] that he used when he was a toddler did?[103]

It may be argued that many adults also use alcohol, tobacco, and marihuana for some emotional support. True. The difference lies in this: usually the adult has already established the realistic patterns of his life, whereas the adolescent has yet to do so. Adult and adolescent marihuana abuse cannot be compared. Not only has the adolescent far more to lose, but his temptation to rely on the magic of marihuana is much greater. For these reasons, it is doubtful ''that Margaret Mead and some others are justified when they criticize parents and ask, 'What do parents expect if they tell their teen-age children not to smoke marijuana when they themselves have a martini in one hand and a cigarette in the other?' ''[104]

''flashbacks''

''Flashbacks'' are another possible, albeit infrequent, delayed effect of marihuana use. For example, under the influence of marihuana, a person may see a flower ''breathe.'' Later, without the drug influence, that person may have the same experience. There are reports of marihuana-induced flashbacks of visions that had previously occurred under the influence of a hallucinogen such as LSD.[105] Some people enjoy flashbacks. Others are so terrified by them that they have to go to the hospital. Usually flashbacks disappear after the drug is discontinued.

[102] Andrew T. Weil, ''Adverse Reactions to Marihuana,'' p. 1000, citing D. E. Smith and C. Mehl, ''An Analysis of Marihuana Toxicity,'' *Journal of Clinical Toxicology* (in preparation).

[103] Klaus Angel, ''No Marijuana for Adolescents,'' *The New York Times Magazine* (November 30, 1969), pp. 170–78.

[104] *Ibid.*

[105] Andrew T. Weil, ''Adverse Reactions to Marihuana,'' p. 999.

the amotivational syndrome

Some chronic marihuana smokers exhibit a constellation of characteristics manifested by a disinterest in self and in social improvement. It has been termed the *amotivational syndrome.*[106] Is there something in marihuana, as a drug, that causes this lack of motivation, this lack of interest in the purposeful pursuit of goals? Is chronic marihuana abuse a part of the amotivational syndrome or a cause of it? There is much disagreement over the answers to these questions. Some people point to the numerous individuals in this country who regularly smoke mild preparations of marihuana without such discernible personality changes.[107] Others, stressing the individuality of reactions to marihuana, state that the drug has not been used long enough in this culture to permit such an evaluation of its effect. There are many chronic users of marihuana who exhibit the amotivational syndrome, but there are also many who do not. In addition, many nonusers of marihuana demonstrate the amotivational syndrome. In one controlled study of Jamaican farmers, the work records of thirty chronic marihuana smokers did not differ significantly from those of thirty nonsmokers. In fact, the smokers often worked harder after smoking, but more movements were required to complete a particular task, such as hoeing or weeding, apparently because of a need for repetition to correct inaccuracies. It is important to note that the work demands on Jamaican farmers are different from those on U.S. truck drivers or students, for example.[108] More controlled studies in this country are indicated. But they must never lose sight of the individual's response. No matter what the results turn out to be, if they are not clearly applicable to considerable numbers of people, they will be the kind of ''proof'' upon which to concentrate doubts.

marihuana and increased awareness

Many marihuana users report increased sensitivity to and appreciation of music. Some tests (such as for pitch discrimination) of nonmusicians do not support this. In one interview study, 357 jazz musicians listened to music before and after taking cannabis. After taking the drug, 31 percent reported their appreciation of the music impaired, and 19 percent reported it bettered; the rest could not decide or could not perceive any difference.[109]

Nor do some available tests support the commonly described marihuana-

[106] W. H. McGlothlin and L. J. West, ''The Marihuana Problem: An Overview,'' *American Journal of Psychiatry,* Vol. 125, No. 3 (September 1968), pp. 370–78.

[107] Paul A. Walters, George W. Goethals, and Harrison G. Pope, ''Drug Use and Life-Style Among 500 College Undergraduates,'' *Archives of General Psychiatry,* Vol. 26, No. 1 (January 1972), pp. 92–96.

[108] Study commissioned by the U.S. Department of Health, Education, and Welfare and conducted by the Research Institute for the Study of Man, New York, in collaboration with the Faculty of Medicine, University of West Indies, Kingston. Findings as reported in ''No Harm Found in Chronic Use of Marijuana,'' *Hospital Tribune,* Vol. 7, No. 35 (October 15, 1973), pp. 1, 21. In addition to concluding that chronic marihuana use by these subjects ''did not produce demonstrable intellectual or ability deficits,'' the study found ''no evidence to suggest schizophrenic effects or brain damage.''

[109] Paul A. Walters, George W. Goethals, and Harrison G. Pope, ''Drug Use and Life-Style Among 500 College Undergraduates,'' citing C. Winick, ''The Use of Drugs by Jazz Musicians,'' *Social Problems,* Vol. 7 (1959), pp. 240–53.

increased awareness of touch, taste, and smell.[110] But it may be that the tests are inadequate to measure such subtle responses. It may also be that increased suggestibility and the environment (set and setting) account for some of the reports by users. What is the explanation for the remainder of the great number of reports of such increased awareness? Normally, a person ignores a stimulus that is not needed for what he wants to do. In some way, marihuana causes a loss of this habituation to irrelevant stimuli. This loss, plus the user's frequently changed perception of time and space, accounts for some of the sensory novelty caused by marihuana.[111]

marihuana and sexual behavior

An individual who strongly opposes drug abuse will probably find that marihuana interferes with sexual desire and pleasure. On the other hand, a man and woman who are attracted to each other may find that marihuana stimulates their sexual desire. For some people, the conspiratorial aspect of using an illegal drug is exciting enough to seem to enhance sexual expression.

Marihuana apparently causes varying degrees of distortion and heightening of sound, taste, touch, and vision, all of which are involved in sexual expression. Since marihuana makes time seem to pass more slowly, the sexual act, including orgasm, may appear to be prolonged. Moreover, like a small amount of alcohol, a low dose of marihuana reduces sexual inhibitions.

As a drug, does marihuana itself stimulate physical sexual expression? As one researcher has noted, ''Neither our random samplings nor my psychiatric interviews with marihuana users have led us to conclude that marihuana use is a significant precipitant of sexual behavior.''[112]

marihuana: stepping stone to other drugs?

Does marihuana abuse lead to the abuse of other drugs, including heroin? Those who answer negatively base their reply on two points:

1. There is nothing in the pharmacological action of cannabis per se that disposes a user to resort to other drugs. (Pharmacology refers to the study of drugs.)

2. Millions of people in this and other countries use marihuana and other cannabis products regularly without regularly using other drugs.

Although not proved, the first of these statements is probably correct. The degree of its truth depends largely on the chemical formulae of the cannabinoids (see page 415).

It is the second statement that needs examination. It cannot stand alone. Its accuracy depends, not on the nature of the cannabinoids, but on the nature

[110] *Ibid.,* citing the following: D. F. Caldwell, S. A. Myers, E. F. Domino, and P. C. Mirriam, ''Auditory and Visual Threshold Effects of Marihuana in Man,'' *Perceptual and Motor Skills,* Vol. 29 (1969), pp. 755–59; E. G. Williams, C. K. Himmelsbach, A. Wikler, and D. C. Ruble, ''Studies on Marihuana and Pyrahexyl Compound,'' *Public Health Report,* Vol. 61 (1946), pp. 1059–83.

[111] Lincoln D. Clark, ''Marihuana and Human Behavior,'' *Rocky Mountain Medical Journal,* Vol. 69, No. 1 (January 1972), p. 43.

[112] John A. Ewing, ''Students, Sex, and Marihuana,'' *Medical Aspects of Human Sexuality,* Vol. 6, No. 2 (February 1972), p. 113.

of the highest of the hominoids—man. And man, unlike drugs, has no formulas. Numerous studies[113] support the following two statements:

1. ''No one has failed to find a statistical relation between marihuana and the use of other drugs—legal and illegal.''[114]

2. ''Use of other drugs is clearly related to frequency of marihuana use.''[115]

In the study that led to the second statement the statistical test for the reliability of the data was termed ''fantastic.'' Studied were young, functioning college students.

> One hundred percent of the daily marijuana users and 84% of the weekly marijuana users had tried other drugs, in contrast to 22% of the monthly marijuana users, 18% of the less frequent users, 20% of the ones who had experimented, and zero percent of the subjects who had never tried marijuana. Five percent of the students in this sample had tried opium derivates (heroin, opium, cocaine). In the order of frequency of mention were the hallucinogens, ''downers,'' ''uppers,'' and the stronger cannabis preparations [such as hashish].[116]

In summary: there is no evidence at present that the pharmacological properties of cannabis per se lead to the abuse of other drugs. Such secondary drug abuse would appear to be due to the personality and environment of the individual. That there are many such personalities is no longer open to dispute. Many people in this country who use marihuana do not abuse other drugs. Many do.

can cannabis be a medicine?

There is a growing interest in the medical possibilities of cannabis preparations. Preliminary evidence suggests that a synthetic cannabis product called synhexyl may be useful in controlling severe epilepsy.[117] Favorable results have also been reported with the use of cannabis to treat chronic middle-ear infections, sinusitis, and a variety of skin conditions.[118] Because marihuana de-

[113] *The Use of Cannabis, Report of a World Health Organization Scientific Group,* p. 12, citing the following: R. H. Blum and associates, *Drugs, II, Students and Drugs* (San Francisco, 1969); E. Goode, ''Multiple Drug Use Among Marihuana Smokers,'' *Social Problems,* Vol. 17 (1969), pp. 48–64; M. I. Soueif, unpublished data.

''In many parts of the United States, especially the northern urban centers, opiate addiction is related to prior use of marihuana. Yet it is also apparent that only a small number of all marihuana users follow such a progression. If anything is clear, it is that the availability of a drug is directly related to its nonmedical use and that such use of any drug increases the likelihood of any multiple drug use. As the phenomenon of widespread use of marihuana by youth in our country is still comparatively recent, it remains to be seen whether the number of persons in their early 20's who are dependent upon narcotics will increase during the early 1970's, when such a phenomenon might be expected to occur if there is progression from marihuana to more potent agents. During the past two years, it appears that multiple drug use among our youth has led many to become heroin addicts. The present pattern of heroin use by white middleclass, native-born, suburban youth contrasts sharply with the pattern of use by poor, culturally unassimilated, central city residents which had been stable for the past 25 years.'' (Leo F. Hollister, ''Marihuana in Man: Three Years Later,'' p. 26, citing J. C. Ball, C. D. Chambers, M. J. Ball, *Journal of Criminal Law, Criminology and Police Science,* Vol. 59 [1968], p. 171.)

[114] Richard Colestock Pillard, ''Marihuana,'' p. 30.

[115] ''The Marijuana Problem,'' an edited transcription of the Clinical Case Conference arranged by the Department of Psychiatry at the UCLA School of Medicine, moderator, Norman Q. Brill. This excerpt is from the discussion by Evelyn Crumpton. Reprinted in *Annals of Internal Medicine,* Vol. 73, No. 3 (September 1970), p. 43.

[116] *Ibid.*

[117] *Marihuana and Health, Second Annual Report to Congress from the Secretary of Health, Education, and Welfare* (1972), p. 265, citing J. A. Davis and H. H. Ramsey, ''Antiepileptic Action of Marihuana—Active Substance,'' *Federation Proceedings,* Vol. 8 (1949), pp. 284–85.

[118] *Ibid.,* citing J. Kabelik, Z. Krejci, and F. Santawy, ''Cannabis as a Medicament,'' *United Nations Bulletin of Narcotics,* Vol. 12, No. 3 (July–September 1960), pp. 5–23.

creases pressure within the eye, it may be helpful in treating glaucoma (see page 275).[119] The tetrahydrocannabinols show some limited promise in the treatment of high blood pressure.

Not long ago, physicians at a major medical center noticed that some teen-aged leukemia patients were unexplainably suffering less than formerly from nausea and extreme lassitude, the side effects of their antileukemia medication. The teen-agers had found that smoking marihuana seemed to diminish their symptoms. Their personal investigations are being investigated by their physicians.[120]

In laboratories throughout the country, much more carefully controlled initial research than that of the teen-agers on the medical properties of marihuana is today being carried out. The standardized marihuana used in these studies is a ''U.S.-government–grown leaf produced at Uncle Sam's own pot plantation in Mississippi.''[121]

marihuana and the law

> A year ago, if I had $100 in gold in my pocket, I was a law-abiding citizen; if I perchance had a pint of whiskey, I was a criminal. Today, if I have the whiskey, I am a law-abiding citizen; but if I have the gold I am a criminal violating the law.[122]

This statement was made in 1934. The year before, the Banking Act had prohibited gold transactions and the prohibition of alcohol had been repealed. Not infrequently the citizen is left bewildered by rapidly changing laws. So it is with the laws regulating marihuana. The U.S. Pure Food and Drug Act of 1906 merely required that the amount of cannabis in any drug or food sold to the public be clearly indicated. Today, cannabis is governed in this country by narcotics laws.[123] But it is not a narcotic. Testifying before a Senate subcommittee studying juvenile delinquency, the former director of the National Institute of Mental Health stated that marihuana ''should not be associated with narcotics—either medically or legally,''[124] Recent years have seen widespread public opinion favoring the legalization of marihuana. What are some of the arguments on which this view is based? How do they stand up under scrutiny?

1. *Enforcement of marihuana laws is costly.* True. In arresting and imprisoning thousands of adult and juvenile marihuana offenders, California alone has been spending millions of dollars a year. On the other hand, outright legalization of marihuana would hardly be cost-free. Licensing, production, processing,

[119] R. S. Hepler and I. R. Frank, ''Marihuana Smoking and Intraocular Pressure,'' *Journal of the American Medical Association,* Vol. 217, No. 10 (September 6, 1971), p. 1392; ''Marijuana Works in a Legal Study, Too,'' *Medical World News,* Vol. 14, No. 33 (September 14, 1973), pp. 20–21.

[120] ''Marijuana Works in a Legal Study, Too,'' p. 43.

[121] *Ibid.,* p. 37.

[122] L. J. Dickinson in René A. Wormser, *The Story of the Law* (New York, 1962), p. 443.

[123] The 1937 Federal Marihuana Regulations required every person who deals in or prescribes marihuana to pay an annual tax. It also levied a tax on each transfer of the drug. A subsequent ruling by the Commissioner of Narcotics designated marihuana as a narcotic. However, the Narcotics Manufacturing Act of 1960 did not authorize the manufacture of marihuana preparations. Thus, marihuana has been practically eliminated from regular medical practice. A special Marihuana Act licensed certain physicians to prescribe the drug. Also, specific amounts of it are available for research upon special authorization of the Director of the Bureau of Narcotics and Dangerous Drugs. (Louis S. Goodman and Alfred Gilman, *The Pharmacological Basis of Therapeutics,* p. 1718.)

[124] ''Pinning Down the Weed,'' *Science News,* Vol. 96, No. 13 (September 27, 1969), p. 263.

distribution, and sale of marihuana—all would need to be government-controlled so as to prevent overpricing, adulteration, and other abuses. Huge bureaucracies, similar to those needed for alcohol, would be required. "Then tax marihuana to pay for government control," say the proponents of legalization. But, as with alcohol, the cost does not stop there. Should chronic marihuana abuse, like alcoholism, be responsible for an amotivational syndrome, it (combined with the proved association with other drug abuse) would inevitably increase welfare costs. All taxpayers would also have to pay the costs of treatment and rehabilitation of those whose dependence on various other drugs would be associated with freer availability of marihuana (see pages 428–29). True, millions of people who use no drug but marihuana today would never need treatment, rehabilitation, or welfare after legalization—but many people would. This much is clear: those who do not want marihuana legalized would have to pay as much for it as those who do and perhaps more.

2. *Use of marihuana is nobody else's business.* Those who put forth this argument should remember that there is no such thing as a purely private vice. "He who overindulges . . . with respect to drugs . . . alters the lives of others . . . he is unavailable for civic obligations."[125] Society must pay heavily for individual drug abuse. Tax-supported drug abuse programs are already costing millions of dollars every year. And one might speculate about an added danger. Should chronic drug abuse become a pervasive way of life for enough people in the nation, it would not be the first time that a drugged population might be governed by a smaller group that is not, while both call it freedom. To this, China's history is a bitter testament; the opiate dependency of millions of its people was hardly of help in providing the strength needed to resist cruel domestic rulers and foreign interventions.

3. *Marihuana is no more harmful than alcohol.* Mounting evidence, though incomplete, tends to support this statement. However, neither the human mind nor the answers to social problems are found in the laboratory. Alcohol is deeply rooted in Western culture. Indeed, for many it is part of a religious sacrament. Nevertheless, the cost of alcohol to society includes at least $9\frac{1}{2}$ million emotional and physical cripples. The cost in money? Every year alcoholism drains the U.S. economy of an estimated $15 billion. Marihuana is not ingrained in this culture. Why risk adding to the already massive problems of society?

4. *Tobacco is more harmful than marihuana.* No responsible observer can ignore the dangers of tobacco (see pages 388–97). However, in some respects tobacco is safer than marihuana. For example, while smoking tobacco one can drive a car, but driving under the influence of marihuana must be considered distinctly hazardous[126] (see pages 420–21). Moreover, tobacco does not lower inhibitions, as does marihuana.

Does marihuana smoking cause cancer? Marihuana smoke contains about 40 percent as much tar as tobacco smoke. When applied to the skin of mice it does cause cancerlike cellular changes. At present, it is believed not to pose

[125] Charles E. Wyzanski, Jr., "Marijuana: It's Up to the Young to Solve the Problem," *New Republic,* Vol. 157, No. 17 (October 21, 1967), p. 16.
[126] Lincoln D. Clark, "Marijuana and Human Behavior," p. 45.

a major lung cancer threat. In any case, marihuana now seems less likely than tobacco to cause cancer because the number of marihuana cigarettes consumed by the average marihuana smoker is small compared to the number of tobacco cigarettes consumed by the average tobacco smoker. It is not known at this time whether the combination of marihuana and tobacco increases the risk of cancer.

5. *Since marihuana can be made more cheaply and acts more quickly than alcohol, legalization would drive the alcohol industry out of business.* This argument is invalid. When cannabis was legally bought in India, that country still had serious alcohol problems. In addition, people who use alcohol do so for reasons different from the motivations of those who use cannabis. Moderate alcohol users do not take the drug for the express purpose of getting ''stoned.'' Marihuana users do. (The term ''stoned'' used to be reserved for people who got drunk.) In this culture, moderate use of alcohol is involved with its palatability and the social amenities of which it is a part. Oral marihuana has an unpleasant taste that is difficult to disguise, and ''in considering the social use of marihuana one must justify drug-taking in its own right without the various social conventions surrounding the use of alcohol, nicotine, or caffeine, as these drugs are presently used socially.'' Interestingly, to increase the effect of marihuana, many users drink sweet, fortified wines. Also, marihuana smokers use alcohol more frequently and in larger amounts than do those who abstain from marihuana.[127]

6. *People of other countries use marihuana without problems.* This is not true. The use of marihuana is now legally restricted in almost every country in the world. African nations are searching for better methods of control. Indeed, in some parts of Africa the penalty for growing and distributing marihuana may be death. After twenty-five centuries of use, during which cannabis became part of its religious life, India has undertaken a program aimed at the elimination of its ''pot skid rows.'' (It is worth noting that the United States is a cosigner of the United Nations treaty controlling marihuana. To legalize the drug, this nation would have to abrogate the treaty.)[128]

7. *In the doses ordinarily taken in this country, marihuana is usually harmless.* It is true that no physical harm has been demonstrated under these circumstances. The psychological harm that prolonged marihuana use does to some people has yet to be evaluated. As with alcohol, many people may begin moderate marihuana use only to find themselves trapped in chronic abuse. The use of cannabis in this country may not long be limited primarily to marihuana, any more than alcohol consumption is limited to 3.2 percent beer. As yet, relatively little is known about chronic abuse of stronger cannabis preparations such as hashish.

8. *Present marihuana laws are unenforceable and unfair.* That some government regulation of drugs is necessary is beyond dispute. Legal restrictions apply to alcohol and, to a lesser extent, tobacco. Protection of the public de-

[127] Leo F. Hollister, ''Marihuana in Man: Three Years Later,'' p. 26.
[128] Sidney Cohen, ''Pot, Acid and Speed,'' *Medical Science,* Vol. 19, No. 2 (February 1968), p. 33.

mands no less. The controversy surrounding the laws against marihuana is rooted in the criminal sanctions that are presently directed against the user. It is argued that punishment of the marihuana user is self-defeating; if anyone should be prosecuted, it is the grower and seller. Another objection to present marihuana laws is that, in their enforcement, constitutional guarantees of privacy are violated. Many have suffered the stigma of arrest who are not otherwise deviant. Penalty structures are said to be unfair because they are unduly harsh and because they vary from state to state. Moreover, the ease with which marihuana can be grown makes uniform enforcement impossible. "Bootlegging of beer and wine is possible, but not especially easy. Anyone with a window box can bootleg marihuana."[129]

"Laws and institutions are constantly tending to gravitate. Like clocks, they must be occasionally cleansed and wound up, and set to true time."[130] Marihuana exploded on the national scene so suddenly that there was no time to adjust existing laws. New laws cannot be enacted precipitately. But a considerable body of responsible opinion has recently urged that existing marihuana laws be reviewed so that they do "not routinely make felons out of students seeking a thrill."[131] Such recommendations have already borne fruit. In July 1973, for example, Oregon's governor signed a bill making possession of up to one ounce of marihuana a violation, rather than a criminal act. Thus, the penalty for the possession of that amount is more like a traffic violation; the smoker may be fined up to $100. A month before, Texas had markedly eased what had been the nation's most punitive marihuana laws. Indeed, as of autumn of that year, Rhode Island was the only state in which marihuana possession was an automatic felony, although in four states (Arizona, California, Nevada, and Mississippi), it was left to the judge's discretion as to whether possession was a felony or a misdemeanor. Moreover, as of early 1974, bills to ease marihuana laws had been introduced into the U.S. Congress and nine other states besides Oregon and Texas.[132]

As times change, marihuana legislation will change even more. And as with all social change, young people will need to participate. "Constructive idealism is the badge of youth. Society renews itself from the oncoming generation. Liberty and order rest more upon the harnessing of adventurous insights than on a mere repetition of ancient patterns."[133] If this society is to solve its drug problem, it will have to enlist the aid of its young people in seeking that solution.

[129] Leo F. Hollister, "Marihuana in Man: Three Years Later," p. 26.

[130] Henry Ward Beecher, *Life Thoughts.*

[131] Neil L. Chayet, "Law, Medicine and LSD," *New England Journal of Medicine,* Vol. 227, No. 5 (August 3, 1967), p. 254. See also Richard Colestock Pillard, "Marihuana," p. 301, citing the following: R. H. Blum, "Mind-Altering Drugs and Dangerous Behavior: Dangerous Drugs," *President's Commission on Law Enforcement and Administration of Justice, Task Force Report, Narcotics and Drug Abuse, Annotations and Consultant's Papers* (1967), pp. 21–39; J. Lister, "Cannabis Controversy and Other Sundry Troubles," *New England Journal of Medicine,* Vol. 280, No. 13 (March 27, 1969), pp. 712–14; Council on Mental Health, "Marihuana and Society," *Journal of the American Medical Association,* Vol. 204, No. 13 (June 24, 1968), pp. 1181–82.

[132] "Marijuana Laws Today: The Move Toward Decriminalization," *Psychology Today,* Vol. 7, No. 5 (October 1973), pp. 20, 22, 123.

[133] Charles E. Wyzanski, Jr., "Marijuana: It's Up to the Young to Solve the Problem," p. 16.

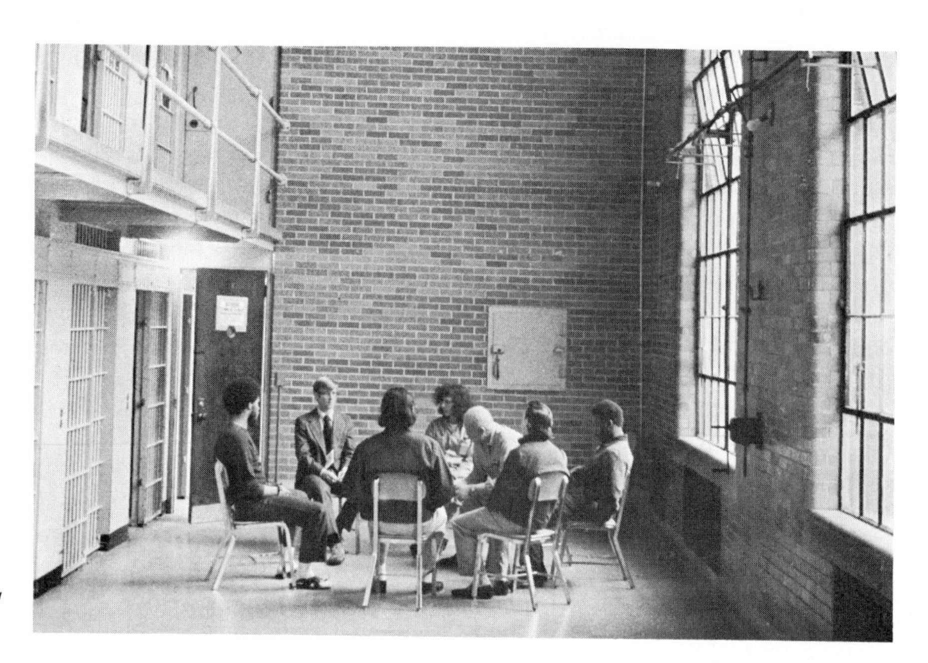

14-6 *Transcendental meditation in a prison.*

transcendental meditation: new hope?[134]

Drug abuse has long been discouraged by leading mystics. The great Indian mystic Meher Baba wrote: "The [drug] experience is as far removed from Reality as is a mirage from water. No matter how much one pursues the mirage, one will never reach water and the search . . . through drugs must end in disillusionment."[135] Now it appears that the system of transcendental meditation developed by another Indian mystic, Maharishi Mahesh Yogi, may offer hope to some drug abusers.

The Maharishi drew his method from the ancient traditions of Hinduism. In the United States, an estimated 76,000 people have learned its techniques. It is not to be confused with either hypnosis or sleep. No change of religion or life-style is required. Students are taught a systematic method of transcending, or "going beyond," their bodies by repeating a particular sound while concentrating on a "suitable" thought. The sounds, which are called *mantras,* have no special meaning. A commonly used mantra is the syllable *om*.

A research team at Harvard Medical School has discovered some startling effects of transcendental meditation on the human body.[136] The subjects were thirty-six student volunteers. During their meditation, the volunteers' oxygen consumption fell by a remarkable average of 17 percent. A lower breathing rate can be faked, but lowered use of oxygen cannot because of the body's need for it. Breathing rates were in fact diminished, as were rates of carbon dioxide elimination and heart rates. Electroencephalographic brain patterns were markedly altered.

[134] An excellent discussion of the effect of meditation on body function is: Robert Keith Wallace and Herbert Benson, "The Physiology of Meditation," *Scientific American,* Vol. 226, No. 2 (February 1972), pp. 84–90.
[135] *God in a Pill? Mehar Baba on L.S.D. and the High Roads* (San Francisco, 1966), p. 2.
[136] Robert Keith Wallace, Herbert Benson, and Archie F. Wilson, "A Wakeful Hypometabolic Physiologic State," *American Journal of Physiology,* Vol. 221, No. 8 (September 1971), pp. 795–99.

Transcendental meditation also had an astonishing effect on the level in the blood of a chemical called lactate. People suffering from anxiety neuroses (characterized by severe apprehension, psychic tension, uncertainty, and fear) experience a rise in lactate level while under stress. In normal people, injection of lactate causes symptoms of anxiety neuroses. During and after transcendental meditation, lactate levels dropped markedly. These results "suggest an intriguing biochemical tie-up with the feelings of restful tranquility subjects describe during and after meditation."[137]

Interestingly, many people who begin to practice transcendental meditation begin to cut down on their abuse of drugs. Before learning transcendental meditation, twenty of the volunteers in the Harvard study had abused drugs, including marihuana, amphetamines, LSD, and heroin. Of the twenty, nineteen stopped their abuse of drugs completely. They found that compared to the feelings induced by meditation, the sensations resulting from drug abuse were extremely distasteful.[138] Intrigued, the same group of Harvard scientists in 1970 sent questionnaires to 1,950 people on some thirty U.S. college campuses who had been practicing transcendental meditation for three months or more. Replies came from 1,862 people, 1,081 men and 781 women. The results:[139]

1. The vast majority had progressively decreased their abuse of all drugs, including cigarettes. By the time they had been practicing transcendental meditation for twenty-one months, most of the respondents had completely stopped using drugs.
2. Drug sellers reported similar results. Of 384 subjects who had been selling drugs, 71.9 percent had stopped during the first three months of transcendental meditation and 95.9 percent had stopped after twenty-one months.
3. Transcendental meditation had altered the respondents' attitude toward drugs. Instead of encouraging or tolerating drug abuse among their friends, they now actively discouraged it.

All these results need further study, but they do tend to confirm a line spoken by Iago in Shakespeare's *Othello* (I.iii.324–25): "Our bodies are our gardens, to the which our wills are gardeners."

summary

Recent years have seen increasing abuse of newer types of drugs in the United States, including

1. *stimulants.* These drugs act on the central nervous system to excite psychic and motor activity (page 403). The *amphetamine type of drug dependence* is not characterized by physical dependence; it does, however, result in psychological dependence and tolerance (page 405). Am-

[137] "The Physiology of Meditation; Or How to Give Up Drugs," *New Scientist and Science Journal,* Vol. 51, No. 771 (September 30, 1971), p. 724.
[138] *Ibid.*
[139] "Meditation May Find Use in Medical Practice," *Journal of the American Medical Association,* Vol. 219, No. 3 (January 17, 1972), pp. 295, 298–99.

phetamine abuse causes sleeplessness, hyperactivity, profound behavior changes, and hallucinations (page 405).

The *hallucinogen (LSD) type of drug dependence* (page 407) also induces tolerance (page 407), but not physical dependence (page 408). Among the hallucinogens are *LSD* (pages 407–11); *mescaline, psilocybin,* and *morning-glory seeds* (pages 411–12); "the pink wedge" (LSD contaminated with STP; page 412); and numerous preparations sold over the counter, such as cold tablets (page 412). These drugs induce hallucinatory perceptual changes (pages 408–10).

Cocaine is a stimulant that causes physical and psychological dependence as well as tolerance (page 413). Its effects are like those of the amphetamines (pages 413–14).

2. *marihuana.* The plant *Cannabis sativa* has two major groups of chemical constituents: *cannabinoids* and *non-cannabinoids.* Of the cannabinoids that have psychoactive effects, the two most important are Delta-8-THC and Delta-9-THC (page 415). The two cannabis preparations most often used in the United States are *marihuana leaf* and *hashish* (page 415). Marihuana can act as either a stimulant or a depressant (page 418). Only a slight degree of tolerance results in humans from marihuana use (page 418). Many long-time smokers report that they need less rather than more of the drug to obtain the same effect—a phenomenon called *reverse tolerance* (pages 418–19). Marihuana is unlike LSD and other stimulant hallucinogens in that it has no *cross-tolerance* for other drugs (page 419). It does not seem to cause physical dependence, withdrawal symptoms, or death from overdose (page 419).

The individual signs and symptoms of marihuana use are affected by *dose, set,* and *setting* (page 419). Thus conclusive findings about its effects are difficult to obtain, though it has been established that marihuana use impairs driving ability (pages 420–21). Among the *early symptoms* (subjective effects) of marihuana use are (with ordinary doses) "rushes," euphoria, dizziness and lightness, nausea, and increased hunger (page 422); and (with higher than ordinary doses) depersonalization, panic, depression, and toxic psychoses (pages 422–23). The *early signs* (objective, physical indications) may include reddening of the conjunctiva of the eyes, increased pulse rate, slight contraction of the pupils, impairment of muscle strength, or dilation of the air passages (page 423). The *delayed effects* of prolonged marihuana use are being investigated. They may include cerebral atrophy (page 424) and chromosomal damage (pages 424–25), though neither has been proved. In one study habitual hashish smoking was shown to cause inflammation of the mucous membranes of the nose, throat, bronchi, sinuses, and uvula (page 425). Other possible delayed effects include toxic psychoses (pages 425–26); psychic dependence in the immature (page 426); "flashbacks" (page 426); the amotivational syndrome (page 427); increased sensory awareness (pages 427–28); and varying effects on sexual behavior (page 428).

Present evidence indicates that marihuana use does not lead to the abuse of other drugs. Secondary drug abuse seems to depend on individual personality and environment (pages 428–29). A number of arguments—of varying degrees of validity—have been advanced in favor of the legalization of marihuana (pages 430–33). The mystic technique of transcendental meditation has helped a number of people stop their abuse of drugs (pages 434–35).

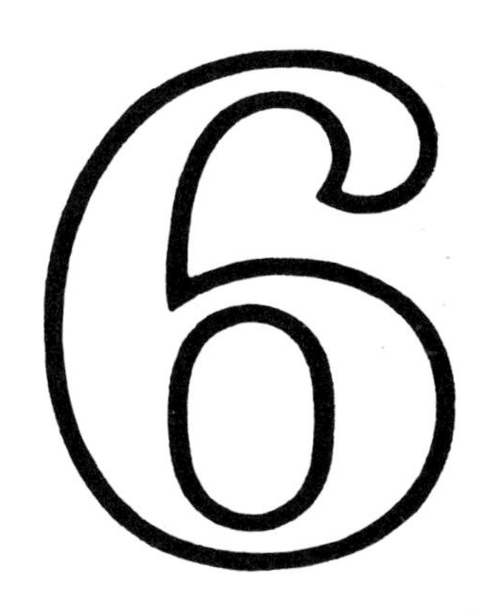

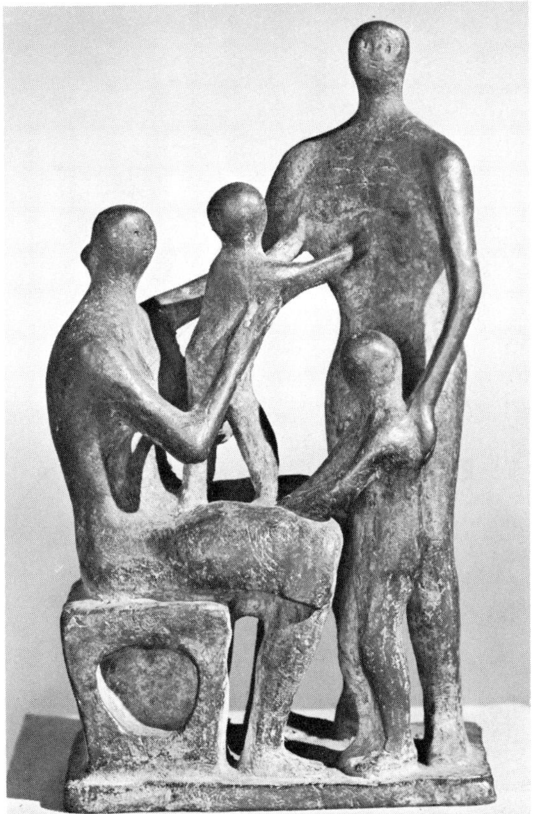

marriage: preparation and realities

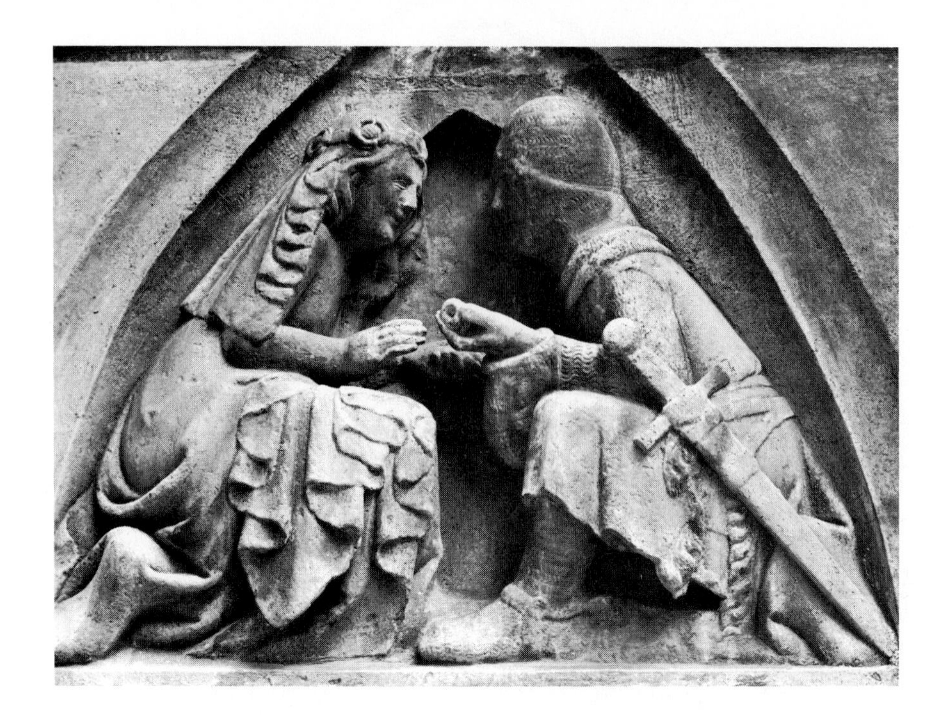

some premarital and marital considerations

15

courtship and conquest: animal instinct, human learning

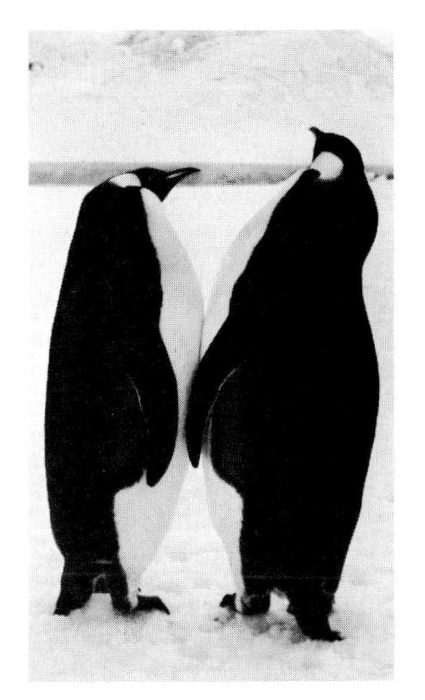

15-1 *Penguins courting.*

"The snail is a hermaphrodite: male and female are incorporated into one; there is no he and no she. Perhaps that is why snails are so sluggish; they have nothing to stir them, nothing to fight for, nothing to pursue, nothing to win."[1] Almost all other creatures, however, actively differentiate between the sexes, and engage in elaborate mating rituals too. For elegance and variety, nonhuman love-planning is both instructive and humbling. The fighting fish of Siam do an underwater courtship ballet, of which the color, grace, and timing would delight the most exacting choreographer. And the female cricket knows true devotion. Responding to a phonograph record playing the ardent chirp of a long-dead male cricket, she will desert locally available swains. Hurrying a considerable distance, she will lovingly seek an approach into the record player.[2] Gift-giving, too, is not unknown to creatures that go courting. Indeed, with some species of spider, an empty-handed male may become a snack. So, instinctively, he often arrives with a fly, carefully gift-wrapped in silk. Dancing a specific pattern and displaying his markings, he can only trust to luck. As for higher animals, the complex courtship that goes on among penguins, for example, or among monkeys and apes, has long fascinated zoologists.

And so, all in season, the nonhuman world is a rhythmic maneuvering of love, a pervasive, instinctive planning for new life. Instinctive, not learned. But people need to be taught the art of love. Among earth's creatures, man is almost alone in becoming confused by such matters. His confusion is created by his culture, for in no other aspect of his life are his self-imposed regulations more rigid.

on the establishment of marital codes

Family life of this culture is based on Judeo-Christian traditions. These can be traced to the age of the biblical Hebrew patriarchs. The family was established as an institution to provide stability and protection for the group. In the home of the ancient Hebrews, the father was the head and the mother the heart.

From the Hebrews, the early Christians got a model for building a stable family structure. From the Romans, they learned the price of excessive societal laxity and disruption of normal family life. Three Punic Wars against Carthage (in the second and third centuries B.C.) occupied Rome for over a century. These had made many Roman families enormously rich. Roman sons were constantly off at war. Fathers consequently placed their daughters in positions of wealth and indirect power. Roman women of leading families began to vie with one another and with men for power. The Elder Cato complained bitterly: "All men rule over women, we Romans rule over all men, and our wives rule over us." The new preoccupations of women led them to neglect their families. Con-

[1] James Kemble, *Hero Dust* (London, 1936), p. xiii. "Hermaphrodite" derives from the names Hermes (the Greek god who served as messenger to the gods) and Aphrodite (the Greek goddess of love and beauty).
[2] H. Smythe, *The Female of the Species* (London, 1960), p. 58.

temptuously, Roman men rejected marriage. "Why do I not marry a rich wife?" asked a Roman writer. "Because I do not wish to be my wife's maid."[3] Laws penalizing celibacy were to no avail. The upper classes, remaining childless, customarily adopted children for purposes of inheritance. Divorce, previously rare, became widespread. Marriage became a cynicism. Slaves cared for children. Children were spoiled. "Expressions which would not be tolerated even from the effeminate youths of Alexandria," wrote Quintilian, "we hear from them with a smile and a kiss."[4] With the family structure crumbling, morals declined. Rome underwent a sexual revolution. Luxury and sloth replaced the formerly strict family life. The public amorality of the highborn also became a way of life for the middle classes. Other factors, such as widespread malaria and an overextended economy, certainly helped to enfeeble the once mighty empire. But a basic flaw marred Rome. The vitality of the family had been wasted. Rome collapsed. Upon its ruin, Christianity began to build.

why the rigidity? why the guilt?

The year 312 saw Christianity legally recognized by the decaying Roman Empire. Observing the social disarray about them, the early Christians were determined not to repeat the errors of their predecessors. Polygamy, practiced by the Hebrews, was rejected. Roman sexual laxity was anathema. The abortion and infanticide, the divorce and adultery of the Greeks and Romans were condemned. In this atmosphere, sexual permissiveness was out of the question. Sexuality was sinful. Centuries passed before even marital sexual intercourse became more than a base need, to be tolerated only because it provided children.

This is not to say that rigid sexual regulations immediately took hold in the Christian world. Controls developed gradually. It was not until 786 that the Anglo-Saxon Synod passed a decree ensuring permanence to marriage. Indeed, up to the Reformation, one year's trial marriage was practiced in Scotland. The Church, however, held fast. Gradually its precepts took hold. Yet, even as sexual intercourse became a sanctified part of marriage, restrictive rules were retained. Those who took short cuts found society harsh indeed. Why? Because their actions threatened the family as the basic unit of society and, therefore, threatened society itself. If humanity were to survive, it was essential that sexuality and mating be controlled.

The Judeo-Christian culture, then, established basic marriage codes that have endured for the Western world. Often, these codes have been supported by threat and guilt, two powerful tools of Western society. "In the last analysis, guilt feelings, for most people, are simply a realization that they have failed to follow societal convictions of right and wrong."[5]

But guilt promotes anxiety. Many people who ignore marital codes may reject their own sense of guilt, but it does not go away. Prolonged, unresolved guilt may become disease. That is why the origins of marital codes merit some exploration in a health book.

[3] Quoted in Willystine Goodsell, *A History of Marriage and the Family* (New York, 1934), p. 136.
[4] *Ibid.*, p. 152.
[5] William M. Kephart, *The Family, Society, and the Individual* (Boston, 1961), p. 117.

the lover, whom all the world does not love

primitive courtships

The tribulations of love and courtship vary from culture to culture. Among the Macusis of British Guiana, a young swain may not choose a wife until he has proved his courage. One way to demonstrate it is by allowing himself "to be sewn up in a hammock full of fire ants."[6] The hopeful Arab bridegroom of Upper Egypt displays his valor by undergoing a severe whipping by the bride's relatives.[7] The romantic maneuvering among the young of one Bolivian Indian tribe is no less hazardous:

> Ordinarily young people of nubile age are supposed to be shy of one another, and while tending herds pass one another by many times without apparently seeing each other. Around Camata, if a boy . . . wishes to take notice of a girl, he picks up a handful of fine earth or dust and throws it at her. This is a first step of courtship . . . The next time they meet, the boy picks up some fine gravel, and the girl may do likewise. If they continue to be interested this goes on until finally they throw rocks at each other. Informants told me that there were two cases of deaths in Camata during the last four years from such a cause; one woman received a fractured skull and the other a broken back.[8]

yesterday's courtships

In 1700, the British Parliament enacted the following:

> That all women of whatever age, rank, profession or degree, whether virgin maid or widow, that shall from and after such Act impose upon, seduce and betray into matrimony any of His Majesty's subjects by means of scent, paints, cosmetic washes, artificial teeth, false hair, Spanish wool, iron stays, hoops, high-heeled shoes or bolstered hips, shall incur the penalty of the law now in force against witchcraft and like misdemeanors, and that the marriage upon conviction shall stand null and void.[9]

It was perhaps such legislation that prompted the degree of cautious honesty, if not outright optimism, so often proclaimed as proper in eighteenth-century English books on model letter-writing. One such volume, the *New London Letter Writer,* includes a model letter entitled, "From a Young Lady After Having Smallpox to her Lover." Apparently, the young man had led her to believe that "the beauties of my person were only exceeded by the perfection of my mind." She was, therefore, not regretting too much the loss of her good looks, for "it gives you a happy opportunity to prove yourself to be a man of truth and veracity."[10]

Many years later, in the nineteenth century, English lovers, for reasons of their own, were wont to go skating. Since chaperones rarely skated, they were benched on the sidelines. In 1876, *Punch* published a cartoon of these scandalous goings-on (Figure 15–2).[11] Not all was raucous humor, however. A Mrs.

[6] Edward Westermarck, *The History of Human Marriage,* 5th ed., Vol. I (New York, 1921), p. 49.
[7] *Ibid.,* p. 51.
[8] Weston La Barre, "The Aymara Indians of the Lake Titicaca Plateau, Bolivia," *American Anthropologist,* Vol. 50, No. 1, Part 2 (January 1948), p. 129.
[9] Quoted in Henry A. Bowman, *Marriage for Moderns* (New York, 1960), p. 129.
[10] E. S. Turner, *A History of Courting* (London, 1954), p. 121.
[11] *Ibid.,* p. 178.

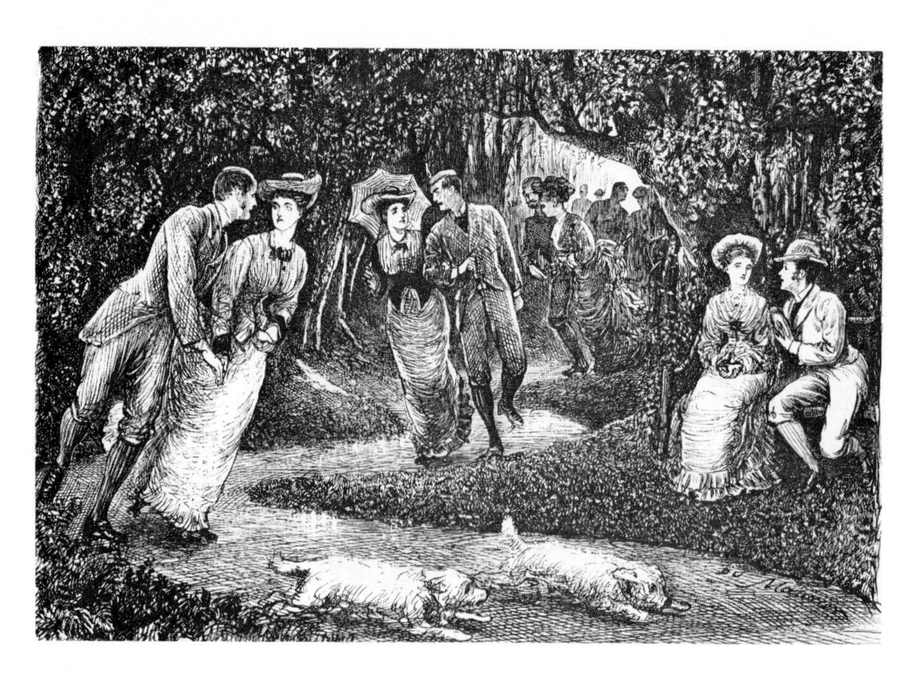

15-2 *"Rink to me only with thine eyes"* (*from* Punch, *1876*).

Burton Kingsland, composing for the *Ladies Home Journal* (*circa* 1900), prepared this brief, but presumably effective, speech to be made by a young lady whose debauched swain had slipped his arm about her waist: "Don't you think it rather cowardly for a man to act toward a girl as you are doing when she has trusted him and is in a measure powerless to resist such familiarity?"[12]

Things have changed.

modern courtship

In this culture, basic training for marriage begins early, with group dating. This is followed by random dating. Perhaps it is during a shopping tour with their mothers that modern children gain the first unconscious tips for random dating. Random dating is just shopping around. One does not have to buy. There is time for window-shopping. If one chooses, one may come in and browse. Sometimes, a small investment is made. By telephone, one learns a lot and overcomes much. Everybody gets stung a little, some more than others. But one gets to know the game. And, in the end (hopefully), one sees enough and adds up enough experience to get some idea of what one needs, what to look for, and what commitment may be safely made. People of some other countries view random dating with astonishment. For them, the sheer number of dates per teen-ager is fickleness amounting to immorality. And the absence of a chaperone—an open invitation to family dishonor.

Admittedly superficial and often hurtfully competitive, random dating is instructive as a prelude to the next stage of mating, "going steady" (a status often anxiously sought both by high school and by many college students). Since the random dater is but a recent graduate of the shy group-dating system, his sexual behavior is usually not a problem. It is not until the going-steady stage that

[12] *Ibid.*, p. 195.

the problems associated with sexual relationships arise. Fearful that their children will drift or be forced into a poor marriage, many parents who regarded random dating with tolerance are suspicious of the going-steady stage of courtship. Nevertheless, going steady does relieve the competitive pressures of random dating. Moreover, it gives priceless training in such virtues as tolerance, patience, and gentleness that will be useful in the married state.

It is in the turbulent, searching years of adolescence that a person must begin learning the mating game. In this anxious time of searching for a self-acceptable self, of trying to settle on a life's work, of attempting to cope with overwhelming bodily changes, and of beginning a separation from one's parents—it is in these years that the dating dilemma occurs. The dilemma is this: without being clearly told what is expected of him, the teen-ager is nevertheless given to understand that much is expected of him. "Grow up," he is told, yet he is forbidden to do what he sees grownups do. Driven by urges he has not yet learned to understand or control, he attempts to answer them as grownups do. With the paraphernalia of sexual activity, such as cars and condoms, readily available, what is missing? A chaperone? In this society, she is all but extinct.

premarital sexual activity

In this age of laboratory-observed sexual intercourse and a welter of sexual statistics, it should not be forgotten that people, not numbers, do the loving. No matter how informative the numbers seem to be about people, each person has a secret heart. Discussions of premarital sexual activity are incomplete without an exploration of individual answers to a variety of questions. In what context does the premarital sexual intercourse occur? What does premarital sexual intercourse do to the relationship of the participants? How much love is involved? The uses and abuses of sex are numerous. Valid uses of sexual expression vary from reproduction and pleasure to deep desires to share and cooperate with and to give and belong to someone. Its abuses range from destructive domination to sheer revenge. How much premarital sexual activity is based on emotional problems having little to do with love needs? How much results from genuine mutual caring and how much from attempts to rebel or to escape anxiety or other problems, such as loneliness or a sense of personal worthlessness? How often does a young person engage in a premarital sexual experience because of the conviction that any pain or humiliation must be endured to get love? When is premarital sexual intercourse an exploitation of one person by another? Do premarital sexual experiences relieve these nonsexual problems or merely accentuate them? Is the young person who has just terminated a first premarital sexual experience more vulnerable to becoming promiscuous? Is the decision to engage in a premarital sexual experience based on a realistic appraisal of the self, or is it part of a glamorized view of a constantly shifting "scene"? Statistics of coital rates among the unmarried hardly reveal adequate information about the actual causes or significance of these rates. Moreover, although this discussion will be primarily concerned with premarital coitus, premarital sexual experiences of course include varying degrees of petting which stop short of coitus. Not enough is known about the incidence or significance of these. More research is needed in all these areas. And that research must be tempered with the understanding that premarital sexual experiences, like all experiences, affect different people differently.

One study[13] of college students and their parents indicates that a majority of the college females (66 percent) and males (52 percent) considered sexual intercourse between engaged couples acceptable. This compared with only 20 percent of their fathers and 17 percent of their mothers approving. That so many of the males—48 percent of them—considered premarital intercourse unacceptable is not surprising. Some men expect to marry a virgin yet attempt to seduce every woman they date. In *Hamlet,* Ophelia notes this male paradox in a little song that relates a lovers' conversation:

> "Young men will do't, if they come to't.
>
> . . .
>
> Quoth she, before you tumbled me,
> You promised me to wed."

He answers:

> "So would I ha' done, by yonder sun,
> An thou hadst not come to my bed."[14]

Another college study[15] emphasizes the difference in opinion between the generations. Only 55 percent of the coeds questioned considered virginity at marriage very important. Eighty-eight percent of the coeds' mothers considered it very important. Why the disparity? Why are mothers generally less tolerant of premarital sexual intercourse than their daughters? There are many reasons. However, this is certain. Although mother and daughter share the same basic cultural values, their positions within that culture are quite different. So are the pressures to which they are exposed. It is much easier for an anthropologist to explain the benefits of premarital coitus among South Sea Islanders than it is for a mother to explain them in Dubuque, Iowa.

premarital sexual activity: the data

It should be emphasized that most studies made to determine the extent of premarital sexual intercourse are out of date. They relate not to today's college students but to their parents and grandparents. Within limitations the sexual activities of young people today can be compared with data gathered decades ago by varying sampling techniques. They cannot, however, be logically measured by these data.

In a questionnaire study reported in 1968 by Vance Packard, an attempt

[13] Seymour L. Halleck, "Sex and Mental Health on the Campus," *Journal of the American Medical Association,* Vol. 200, No. 8 (May 22, 1967), pp. 684–90.
[14] William Shakespeare, *Hamlet,* IV.v.61–66.
[15] Seymour L. Halleck, "Sex and Mental Health on the Campus" pp. 684–90.

was made to ascertain premarital coitus rates among juniors and seniors from all regions of the United States.[16] Great care was exercised to respect privacy and ensure accuracy of reporting. The work lacks much in method and as interpretative social science. Moreover, the report is more than six years old. Some results, to be viewed within these limitations, are:

1. The coital experience of the college males had increased little since earlier studies.

2. Among the junior and senior female respondents, 43 percent reported coital experience. Bearing in mind the hazards of comparing results of Packard's and earlier studies, one can suggest that this represents a 60 percent increase over any data gathered before 1960. Despite this, it should be noted that most junior and senior women in the group remained virgins, as did 43 percent of the men. Unless there has been a radical change in just a few years, the Packard report hardly supports the concept that promiscuity is a general practice among U.S. college students. Moreover, as will be pointed out in the following paragraphs, the Packard data may be illusory.

3. Coital rates by regions, as reported by this study, were as follows:

	MEN	WOMEN
South	69%	32%
East	64%	47%
West	62%	48%
Midwest	46%	25%
National totals	57%	43%

Several previous studies, wrongly applied by some to the entire U.S. college population, were based on merely regional results. The unreliability of such a procedure can be illustrated by comparing the regional percentages with the national percentages in the Packard report.

the "myth of an abstinent past" and of a promiscuous present[17]

Compared to previous generations, the prevalence of unwed teen-age mothers has risen markedly. This fact has often been used to support the idea that today's teen-agers experience more sexual intercourse than formerly. But this is disputed by an analysis of the changing nature of menstruation during the adolescent years. In both this country and Europe, the onset of menstruation (*menarche*) occurs at a younger age than in previous generations. "The present mean age at menarche in the United States (12.54 years) implies that 94 percent of girls aged 17.5 years are fully fecund [fertile]. When the mean age of menarche was 16.5 years, around 1870 in Europe, only 13 percent of girls were fully fecund at age 17.5"[18] In the United States, the average age at menarche declined one year in the period from the 1930s to the 1960s. Thus, today's teen-ager has an increased risk of pregnancy. One reason for the earlier menarche and longer fertile period of the modern teen-ager is her improved

[16] Summarized from Vance Packard, *The Sexual Wilderness* (New York, 1967), Chapters 9–11 and Appendixes.
[17] Phillips Cutright, "The Teen-Age Sexual Revolution and the Myth of an Abstinent Past," *Family Planning Perspectives,* Vol. 4, No. 1 (January 1972), pp. 24–31.
[18] *Ibid.,* p. 24.

preadolescent health and nutrition.[19] These factors also reduce the number of spontaneous abortions and, therefore, increase the number of illegitimate births.

> In the past, relatively poor health conditions may have moderated the consequences of nonmarital teenage sex. Improved health conditions appear to have increased the chances that an out-of-wedlock conception will be carried to term (hence, become visible, and a problem), and have also increased the capacity of sexually active young girls to conceive . . . Aside from substantial increases in premarital sex among young whites with their future husbands, we find no evidence that a change in nonmarital sex of 'revolutionary' proportions has occurred since 1940 among the white or nonwhite teenagers.[20]

These conclusions are based on statistical analyses that also include the effects of such variables as fetal loss and contraceptive use.

an analysis by Gagnon and Simon

Does the increased proportion of nonvirginal college girls indicate a sexual revolution? A superficial glance at the statistics might bring a quick affirmative reply. Unfortunately this is the kind of affirmation that is all too characteristic of many anxious observers of sexual mores today. A careful analysis of the Packard data fails to support the prevalent notion that premarital coitus has materially increased in the past forty-odd years. As Gagnon and Simon have written about the prevalence of premarital coitus:

> It does not appear that there is any body of research evidence leading to a belief that the figures generated by Kinsey et al. for the period 1925–45 from an admittedly limited sample have radically changed. Data recently gathered for Mr. Vance Packard indicate there may be an increase in proportion of college-going females who are not virgins. The ultimate meaning of these figures, however, is still in doubt. The proportion of a population having coitus before marriage can only be calculated from a population that has completed the premarital period, that is, from interviews with those married. What Packard's data do indicate is that for the college-educated the arena for premarital coitus has moved from the post-college to the college level.[21]

Among girls who do engage in premarital sexual intercourse is the actual frequency of coitus increasing, and is it occurring with a greater number of different men? It would seem not. In this country the average age at which girls first have coitus has not declined. The average age at which girls first marry has declined, although it has recently stabilized. Thus young people have, on the average, fewer years in which to engage in premarital sexual activity. Gagnon and Simon conclude that "the evidence that girls now have intercourse with a larger number of males than in the past must also rest upon very weak grounds."[22]

[19] Research with mice has indicated that although dietary protein has an accelerating effect on the ovulation of prepubescent mice, the presence of mature male mice (or their odors) seems to have a much greater influence. The researchers observe, "[The fact that] social stimulation was more effective than protein intake may have relevance to the phenomenon of accelerated sexual maturation in human females." ("The Male Presence," *Scientific American,* Vol. 226, No. 6 [June 1972], p. 53.)

[20] *Ibid,* pp. 30–31.

[21] John H. Gagnon and William Simon, "Prospects for Changes in American Sexual Patterns," *Medical Aspects of Human Sexuality,* Vol. 4, No. 1 (January 1970), p. 103.

[22] *Ibid.*

The very insignificance of the increase in the percentage of coitally experienced college men (as revealed by the Packard data) may well have a special significance. Kinsey found that young men in the lower socioeducational levels engaged in premarital coitus with a much greater number of girls and to a considerably greater extent than did young men in the upper socioeducational groups. That was more than twenty-five years ago. In the past two decades, the number of men from the lower socioeconomic levels that go on to college has increased. In an educational milieu that their fathers did not have, they are meeting middle-class men (and women) with middle-class values. It is reasonable to believe that the long-established middle-class patterns, such as deferment of gratification, so characteristic of a striving group, are being assimilated by a new population. "It is therefore possible," wrote Gagnon and Simon, "that previously discovered high rates of coitus on the part of lower class men may be declining towards the lower middle class patterns . . . If middle and lower class patterns converge, it will be far closer to the style of the former than the latter."[23]

And so there is considerable reason to question seriously the highly advertised notion that premarital sexual intercourse without commitment is more prevalent than formerly, that it is occurring with greater frequency among those who do practice it, and that promiscuous sexual behavior without rules is the way of life among young people today. "What is observed is a continued development of a process which has continued for some forty years in American society. . . . the mating process has become more and more one of exchanging increasing levels of sexual intimacy on the part of the female for increasing emotional commitments on the part of the male."[24] If a major change in the pattern of premarital coitus had occurred in the past forty years, two factors would have been recognized as contributing much to that change. First, unmarried women would be having sexual intercourse with a large number of men without marriage plans with any of them; second, it would be the woman's responsibility to prevent pregnancy. However, the reverse is true. When premarital coitus occurs, it is usually in the context of a marital commitment. And contraception has generally remained the responsibility of the male. The unmarried woman in this country who does engage in premarital coitus does not usually use contraceptives in order to have sexual intercourse with a variety of uncommitted men.[25]

Why, then, have so many people been led to think otherwise? First, there has been a delay in the recognition of the sexual revolution that began almost

[23] *Ibid.*

[24] *Ibid.*

[25] Sociologist Ira L. Reiss considers "the causal connection between birth control pills and participation in premarital sexual intercourse on the part of the young . . . quite difficult to establish." Pointing out that "starting in the late 1960's a rise in premarital sexual intercourse did seem to occur particularly among college girls," he nevertheless cautions that "this is not by any means fully substantiated." Nevertheless, "most of the small studies done since 1965 do seem to find that the proportion of 20-year-old college girls who are nonvirginal reaches about 40% . . . I would think," he continues, "that the basic attitudes would have to change before a woman would participate in premarital intercourse and use the pill . . . The paths leading to these attitudes do not depend as much on the availability of the pill as they do on such factors as love experiences with men, exploration of one's own sexuality, and the general acceptant sexual attitude that prevails in close friends and elsewhere in the social context." (Ira L. Reiss, "The Pill and Adolescent Sexuality," *Medical Aspects of Human Sexuality,* Vol. 6, No. 6 [June 1972] p. 178.)

fifty years ago. Second, the open mind of the citizen is a great receptacle for gossip and exceptions. As was the case with their parents and grandparents, this generation of college students has not escaped the accusatory press. Some newspapers, conveniently ignoring the behavior of most students, publish the flamboyant opinions or actions of the smaller percentage. There is a relatively small group of unmarried young people whose sexual behavior has become strikingly less than ordinary. But as one student counselor of long experience recently noted:

> The much-publicized growing sexual promiscuity is not general practice on the campus. Shyness, introversion, vestigial guilt, self-doubt, and the fear of rejection keep students from the practice of their preaching, even with pills and intrauterine devices to reduce their fear of pregnancy. Actually, premarital pregnancies are on the wane, "sleeping around" is not admired and premarital sex is practiced most often in a semiresponsible and monogamous relationship.[26]

There are people in every culture who see a sexual revolution as mankind's salvation. Others see it as mankind's destruction. It is neither.

> As one looks around, most young people, even those who protest, are busily going about the business of mate selection that will eventuate in marriage and children. Among the vast silent, but not necessarily happy, middle class that still dominates the landscape of American youth, getting married and getting a job and a house are still their central concerns. What else was really expected to happen? What was expected was that young people, when the constraints on freedom of all sorts were released, would do what adults thought they might do (but also would not have): go out and have a sexual ball.[27]

It did not happen, of course. And it is to the credit of young people that they are so patient with those elders who thought it would. Whether in Samoa or Dubuque, sexual behavior in a culture changes rather slowly.

promiscuity: sexual behavior without rules

In the present context, promiscuity refers to indiscriminate sexual behavior. Promiscuous men and women have sexual intercourse without rules. As a chronic behavior pattern promiscuous sexual behavior is often seen among those who fear love. They are afraid to be committed, to be vulnerable. To them, love is not a fulfillment but a threat. Promiscuity may be a symptom of deep-seated unmet needs. The promiscuous woman may have had an unresponsive mother. Hungry for affection, she turned to her father. As an adult she seeks other sources of affection. Her constant search involves her in numerous short-lived sexual experiences. Sometimes promiscuity is the unhappy result of severe childhood denigration. The man who has numerous liaisons with women whom he considers inferior to himself may be seeking revenge on an overly critical mother. Some college students, separated from their parents for the first time, attempt to relieve their anxiety through promiscuous behavior.

[26] Robert E. Kavanaugh, "The Grim Generation," *Psychology Today,* Vol. 2, No. 5 (October 1968), p. 55.
[27] John H. Gagnon and William Simon, "Prospects for Changes in American Sexual Patterns," p. 110.

Some people are sexually promiscuous because they fear that abstinence is harmful to health. There is no doubt that, for some, prolonged sexual repression may give rise to emotional problems. However, an extremely high percentage of patients undergoing psychiatric care can hardly be considered to be sexually repressed. A recent survey of twenty-four psychiatrists treating 107 unmarried female students at a Midwestern university revealed that "86 percent had had sexual relations with at least one person, and almost three-fourths (72 percent) had had relations with more than one person . . . Patients may be promiscuous but the population is not."[28] In this respect, however, further study of some of the nonvirginal college women of the Packard report[29] might have been helpful. As was stated above, a considerable percentage had reported coitus with "several" or "many" males. Whether any of these young women were receiving psychiatric therapy is not known.

It is by no means here inferred that promiscuous sexual behavior inevitably leads to severe emotional distress for everyone. But neither does abstinence inevitably result in emotional illness. The former president of the American Academy of Psychoanalysis recently wrote: "There is no reason to believe that one will develop a mental or physical illness unless one's sex needs are satisfied, or that an individual patient's sex life must be paramount in his emotional adjustment."[30] Seymour Halleck, another psychiatrist, supported this statement in these words: "The proposition that gratification of sexual needs is highly correlated with mental health seems to be at least questionable."[31]

In examining the causes of student despair, Halleck discussed the campus "elite" group. They are so named because of their considerable influence on other students. Devoted to the present, apprehensive of the future, the members of this group work actively, if intermittently, for political causes. Their attitude toward sex is certainly more casual than that of the average student. Halleck wrote of them:

> Rollo May, professor of graduate psychology at New York University, has described the new sexuality as sex without passion . . . There is reason to doubt the capacity of such students to make successful marriages . . . The student psychiatrist sees more and more recently married couples who find themselves unable to tolerate the possibility of loving one person intimately or remaining faithful to that person . . . The new era of promiscuity seems to have done little to enhance the female student's image of herself as a productive and responsible person. The elite female student shows little inclination to seek a career but seems to be trapped in a new feminine mystique which deprives her of meaningful goals and self-respect. Her status as a whole person is subtly degraded.[32]

Almost five hundred years ago, the Dutch theologian Erasmus may have best described the true pain of the promiscuous: "I ask you: will he who hates

[28] Seymour L. Halleck, "Sex and Mental Health on the Campus," pp. 684–90.
[29] Vance Packard, *The Sexual Wilderness,* p. 163.
[30] Leon Salzman, "Recently Exploded Sexual Myths," *Medical Aspects of Human Sexuality,* Vol. 1, No. 1 (September 1967), p. 9.
[31] Seymour L. Halleck, "Sex and Mental Health on the Campus," pp. 684–90.
[32] Seymour L. Halleck, "The Roots of Student Despair," *Think,* Vol. 33, No. 2 (March–April 1967), pp. 22–23.

himself love anyone? Will he who does not get along with himself agree with another? Or will he who is disagreeable and irksome to himself bring pleasure to any? No one would say so, unless he were himself more foolish than Folly."[33]

searching for someone to marry

why marry?

> We who dwell in the heart of solitude are always the victims of self-doubt. Forever and forever in our loneliness, shameful feelings of inferiority will rise up suddenly to overwhelm us in a poisonous flood of horror, disbelief, and desolation, to sicken and corrupt our health and confidence.[34]

Thomas Wolfe could make an episode of solitude seem stimulating. It may be. But as a way of life solitude is nothing to be desired. As the Creator observed: "It is not good that the man should be alone" (Genesis 2:18).

Basically, men who are alone seek wives, and single women husbands, so that they will not be alone. True, there are other reasons, such as societal pressure. But by far the greatest majority of ordinary people seek a meaningful, sharing relationship with another person.

There have been studies in which respondents rated "the relief of loneliness" last as a need they wanted satisfied. But to be loved, to have someone to confide in, to show affection—these were mentioned most often. Without these, one is indeed lonely. But marriage is not merely an escape from a self-centered downbeat emotion. It is a positive and creative way to work for self-realization. Successfully married people can take and give affection. They can confide in each other without fear of harsh judgment. They can cry together and not be ashamed. They can disagree, even quarrel violently, and know it is not the end. They are busy, not only with each other, but with a variety of life's challenges. In no other human relationship can this kind of mutuality be developed. But the skills involved in building and sustaining such a relationship are not inherent, nor are they easily acquired. They require effort. So to conquer loneliness through marriage is to gain many things. One should seek not a person with whom to share loneliness but one to help dispel it.

courtship: reflexive? reflective? or both?

The right person means contentment. The wrong one can indeed entwine two lives in grief. "Though thou canst not forbear to love," wrote Sir Walter Raleigh to his son, "yet forbear to link."[35] The brilliant Elizabethan knight was not advising against marriage. He was advising caution. Of the three most elemental events in human life—birth, death, and marriage—marriage is most open to intelligent personal decision. Love has been too simply defined as a conflict between reflex and reflection.[36] Reflection can enrich the expression of love that molds a good marriage.

[33] Erasmus, "The Praise of Folly," in Louis Kronenberger, ed., *The Pleasure of Their Company* (New York, 1946), p. 564.
[34] Thomas Wolfe, "God's Lonely Man," in *The Hills Beyond* (Garden City, N.Y., 1941), p. 187.
[35] Quoted in Alan C. Valentine, ed., *Fathers to Sons; Advice Without Consent* (Oklahoma City, 1963), p. 16.
[36] *Szpilki* (Warsaw, Poland), cited in *Atlas,* Vol. 16, No. 3 (September 1968), p. 58.

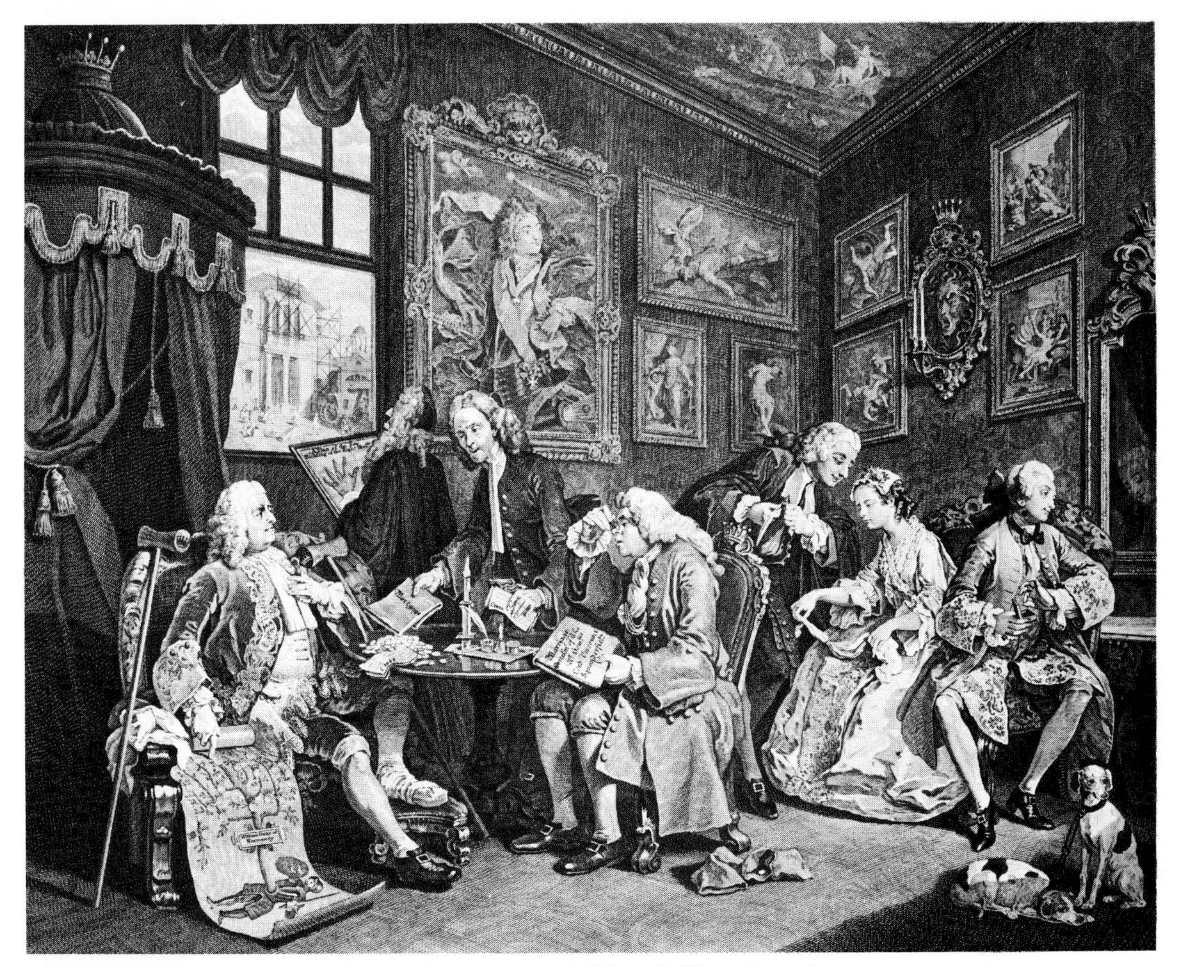

15-3 *"The Contract" from "Marriage à la Mode"* (*1745*) *by William Hogarth* (*1697–1764*). *The wealthy, socially ambitious merchant and his lawyer offer gold, bonds, and mortgages, while the impoverished earl points to his impeccable family tree and favors his aristocratically gouty foot. As for the bartered couple, the merchant's daughter seems less than ecstatic at the match; the future groom admires himself in the mirror.*

At twenty, one can hardly contemplate fifty years of living. A marriage choice is thus all the more difficult. It is not easy to make one decision do for half a century. The wonder is not that such a high percentage of U.S. marriages end in divorce. The wonder is that there are not more failures.

There are those, like H. G. Wells, who consider it foolhardy to leave so vital a decision "to flushed and blundering youth . . . with nothing to guide it but shocked looks and sentimental twaddle and base whisperings and cant-smeared examples."[37] Samuel Johnson grumbled that all marriages should be arranged by the Lord Chancellor "without the parties having any choice in the

[37] H. G. Wells, *Tono-Bungay,* quoted in E. S. Turner, *A History of Courting* (London, 1954), p. 15.

matter.''[38] Some sixteen centuries ago, Father Tertullian (160?–230?) gloomily regarded the corrupt Roman society and its tottering empire. ''Divorce,'' he said, ''was now looked upon as one fruit of marriage.''[39]

To avoid tasting of that bitter fruit, what thoughts and questions should occur to the person who is considering someone as a potential mate?

some general pointers

1. How confident are both members of the couple that their marriage will be successful? Studies show that lack of confidence in this respect is a good indicator of future failure.[40]

2. Does the relationship survive loss of glamor? In the moonlight most girls look lovely. In a similar light most young men get by pretty well. However, how do matters seem when one of the parties is miserable with a bad cold?

3. How is conflict handled? Do the inevitable problems that erupt during a disagreement always get buried only by mutual physical attraction? Or do conflicts teach insight and better understanding of each other? It is as important to learn from a quarrel as it is to make up. But the courting couple whose quarreling is constant and unresolved will find little happiness in marriage.

4. Is conversation easy? Perhaps the pair have never really talked to each other. Can one endure the occasional long silence of the other when necessary?

5. What happens when the pair is with a group? Does either of them embarrass or persistently criticize the other? Is one ashamed of the other? Do they avoid groups altogether? Why? Courting is a private affair, but most married people have get-togethers with friends.

6. How are decisions made? Does one member of the pair expect the other to ''like it or lump it''? Some couples say that ''we have been married for forty years and have never had a word of disagreement.'' When two people agree on everything, only one is thinking.

7. Is that knitting or stamp collecting or watching pro football or interminable chattering on the telephone going to be bearable for fifty years?

8. What is the home life of the possible life partner like? Studies have repeatedly shown that people from relatively happy homes are the best marriage risks. (There is the exception, of course, of the child of divorced parents who works all the harder to make a marriage succeed. Too, there is the occasional case of the marital partner who sacrifices an entire life to the wounding memory of a parental divorce. Fearful of marriage failure, he or she may scrupulously avoid all disagreement and never express his or her individuality.) Moreover, although it need not be decisive, the attitude of the family toward the prospective mate is important.

9. What are his or her best friends like? Off-beat? If so, it is well for the marriage partner to be a trifle off-beat too. Of course, there may be limits. Not

[38] Boswell's *Life of Johnson,* quoted in Holbrook Jackson, *Bookman's Pleasure* (New York, 1947), p. 77.

[39] Willystine Goodsell, *A History of Marriage and the Family,* p. 145.

[40] Judson T. Landis, ''Danger Signals in Courtship,'' *Medical Aspects of Human Sexuality,* Vol. 4, No. 11 (November 1970), p. 40.

long ago, a Boston woman "sued for final separation because her husband insisted on coming to bed with his pet monkey wrapped around his neck," and a Seattle woman complained that her husband "maintained a spring-fed trout pool in their marital bedroom, together with pipelines providing wine and beer on tap."[41]

10. What is the physical health of the potential marital partner? A slight anemia may add a bewitching pallor to the complexion, but it may become wearing after a few years of marriage.

11. How self-sufficient is the proposed mate? How dependent? How much dependency does one need of the other? Overdependency can become an illness. That it is an illness only when carried beyond a certain point is not well understood. It is degree that often determines mental aberration. To some extent almost all people are dependent. Marriage provides the individual with one way of satisfying this need. However, dependency may be extreme and unresolved. Manifesting itself in marriage, overdependency may cause one partner to unconsciously expect the other to be a substitute parent. This role the second partner may summarily reject. Frustrated, the dependent partner may seek attention by becoming a hypochondriac or an alcoholic. When this happens, the marriage is endangered.

12. What role does each potential marital partner expect the other to play? There is the man who wants to marry a pretty girl who is a good housekeeper. He understands and wants the responsibility of making money to support his family. Other men have a less traditional approach. They emphasize companionship and education. Those who contemplate marriage need, then, to examine the role they expect to play and the role they want their intended partner to perform in the marriage situation.

13. Has the relationship been frequently broken off and renewed? Such a relationship is predictive of trouble if the couple marries.

some special premarital considerations

A paradox in this nation's culture is this: the attributes of which the nation is proudest endanger an institution on which it depends—marriage. Individualism is revered; yet marriage is hardly an individual enterprise. The people of this country draw strength from the cultural melting pot; yet from this same pot come mixed marriages, and mixed marriages are risky.

There are, in this nation, at least a dozen Protestant denominations with membership totaling more than 69 million people. The Roman Catholic church includes in its membership 46 million people with an almost bewildering variety of tongues and customs. Other Christians belong to such groups as the Eastern Orthodox church and the Polish National Catholic church. The Jews—Orthodox, Conservative, and Reform—number 5½ million. There are also quite a few Buddhists and Mohammedans in this country. Then, there are those who do not believe in God or in any divine personality or meaning.

Today, the great majority of the U.S. population is white. There are more than 22 million blacks, hundreds of thousands of American Indians, Chinese,

[41] Patrick Ryan, "And the Last Word . . . On Divorce," *New Scientist and Science Journal,* Vol. 49, No. 743 (March 18, 1971), p. 595.

and Japanese. Filipinos, Hindus, Koreans, Hawaiians, and Malayans all add spice to the melting pot. Most countries of the world have added some stock to the mixture. But total racial amalgamation is unlikely to occur during the lifetime of anyone alive today.[42]

This wonderful conglomeration of people marry and reproduce in a society dominated by one belief—the sanctity of the individual. A clash of interests is inevitable. The demand for the satisfaction of individual needs is opposed by the demands imposed on each individual by his cultural background. Too often the resulting conflicts lead to divorce.

interfaith marriages

People of different religious faiths often fall in love. Rebellion or status-seeking by no means accounts for all interfaith marriages. But those who contemplate marrying someone outside their own faith should comprehend their chances of happiness. Unfortunately, there have been methodological problems in the study of this matter. Still, the following data do provide food for thought.

Interfaith couples are less likely to adjust well to marriage. One study [43] showed that only 50 percent of Protestant–Catholic marriages scored *high* adjustments in this study, while 61 percent of Catholic–Catholic marriages, 71 percent of nonchurch marriages, and 80 percent of Protestant–Protestant marriages scored high.

Another study indicates that, by marrying a non-Catholic, a Catholic woman increases her chances of divorce or separation by about 50 percent. A Protestant woman, by marrying outside her religion, increases her risks of divorce or separation by more than 300 percent.[44]

Other research gives similar results. Some 5 percent of unmixed Jewish and Catholic marriages end in divorce or separation. This increases to about 6 percent in unmixed Protestant marriages. However, some 15 percent of mixed Catholic–Protestant marriages end in divorce. The most hazardous of all is the marriage of a Catholic man to a Protestant woman. More than 20 percent end in divorce. The same study indicates too that the marriage of a Catholic woman to a man without a religion is only half as risky as the marriage of a Protestant woman to a man who does not profess a religion.[45]

There are growing signs of permissiveness among some members of the major religious bodies. However, the general reaction of the religious leadership in the United States to interfaith marriage is negative.

Although the Jewish intermarriage rate is the lowest of the three major faiths in this country, it is certainly increasing. In 1963, Rosenthal[46] reported the

[42] David M. Heer, "Intermarriage and Racial Amalgamation in the United States," *Eugenics Quarterly,* Vol. 14, No. 2 (April 1967), p. 120.

[43] James A. Peterson, *Education for Marriage,* 2nd ed. (New York, 1964), p. 223.

[44] *4,108 Marriages of Parents of Michigan State University Students,* cited in Robert O. Blood, *Marriage* (New York, 1964), p. 83.

[45] Judson T. Landis, "Marriages of Mixed and Non-Mixed Religious Faith," *American Sociological Review,* Vol. 14, No. 3 (June 1949), pp. 401–07.

[46] Erich Rosenthal, "Studies of Jewish Intermarriage in the United States," *American Jewish Year Book* (New York, 1963), pp. 3–53.

Jewish intermarriage rate in the nation's capital to have risen from 1 percent with first-generation Jewish marriages to 10.2 percent for those of the second to 17.9 percent by the third generation. It is of interest that the number of children of these marriages raised in the Jewish religion fell spectacularly when compared to earlier generations. In 1964, Sklare[47] accepted the 17.9 percent figure as "probably very close to the current rate." Reform Jewish congregations are more tolerant of Jewish intermarriage than those of the Orthodox or Conservative tradition. Although a large number of such marriages are known to be successful, more adequate studies are indicated.

What are some major sources of disharmony in interfaith marriages? Despite ardent premarital agreements, conflicts often occur over the religious training of children. (This may account for the very high divorce rates of Protestant mothers from Catholic fathers.) Artificial birth control, a practice opposed by the Catholic religion, is another source of deep disagreement. Then, there are the multitudinous cultural differences. Religion is a way of life. Even those whose relationship to their own faith has been casual may find the rituals of another church an imposition.

Many interfaith marriages succeed. Nevertheless, it is well to remember that love alone does not necessarily conquer all.

interracial marriages

In 1967, the U.S. Supreme Court invalidated a Virginia law forbidding marriages between whites and blacks. That Virginia and sixteen other states had passed such laws testifies to the considerable hostility against such marriages. Nevertheless, they are increasing. In one study[48] of data from Hawaii, Michigan, Nebraska, and California, it was found that the rate of white–black marriages rose during the period studied. Hawaii had the highest reported incidence of black–white marriages, with California, Michigan, and Nebraska following. Interestingly enough, 1959 data, the latest available from California and Michigan, showed that the black–white marriage rate in Michigan was half that of California. Both are industrial states with similar proportions of black populations. An exploratory study in Indiana[49] indicated that such marriages generally occur between people who are, by and large, equals in education, economics, and culture. Kelley[50] suggests that those contemplating an interracial marriage would do well to carefully consider all the issues, varying from personal motivations to the possibilities of varying values, whether they be social, ethical, educational, or religious. Of course, these considerations, among others, are important in all marriages. As to the potential for marital success

[47] Marshall Sklare, "Intermarriage and the Jewish Future," *Commentary,* Vol. 37, No. 4 (April 1964), pp. 46–52.
[48] David M. Heer, "Negro–White Marriage in the United States," *Journal of Marriage and the Family,* Vol. 28, No. 3 (August 1966), pp. 262–73.
[49] Todd H. Pavela, "An Exploratory Study of Negro–White Intermarriage in Indiana," *Journal of Marriage and the Family,* Vol. 26, No. 5 (May 1964), pp. 209–11.
[50] Robert K. Kelley, *Courtship, Marriage, and the Family,* 2nd ed. (New York, 1974), Chapter 11.

of these and other interracial marriages, adequate appraisal awaits more intensive study.

Not enough research attention has been given to the children born of interracial marriages. One group of investigators found that "interracial offspring of white mothers obtained significantly higher IQ scores at four years of age than interracial offspring of Negro mothers, suggesting that environmental factors play an important role in the lower intellectual performance of Negro children."[51] Preliminary results of a Los Angeles study suggest that the quest for identity of the child of a black–white marriage is even more difficult than that of the black child in this country. The child often resents both parents, is unable to identify with either, and also resents his siblings with characteristics that are racially different. These are among the problems of the small number of children who have been studied.[52]

interclass marriages

Numerous studies show that adjustment rates are poor in marriages in which the partners come from widely separated social classes. The wider the class difference between husband and wife, the lower is the percentage of good adjustment.[53]

Men are more likely than women to have a successful marriage with a partner slightly below their own class. The college English professor may marry the colorful truck driver and get away with it. She is more likely to end by criticizing his fingernails, and he will puzzle why she never noticed them before. Each will be right about the other and wrong for the other.

money

> "My other piece of advice, Copperfield," said Mr. Micawber, "you know. Annual income twenty pounds, annual expenditure nineteen nineteen six, result happiness. Annual income twenty pounds, annual expenditure twenty pounds ought and six, result misery. The blossom is blighted, the leaf is withered, the god of day goes down upon the dreary scene, and—and, in short, you are for ever floored. As I am!"[54]

In this, the most affluent of nations, countless couples attribute their marriage failures to "money problems." One major study[55] pointed out that it is not the amount but the manner of expenditures that is the major cause of marital friction. One young wife told this story:

> It's twenty years ago, but it's like yesterday. I was seven. I knew my father had just lost his job, but I pretended I didn't. He came out of the bedroom and told my mother, "I don't know. I just don't know where our next piece of bread

[51] Lee Willerman, Alfred F. Naylor, and Ntinos C. Myrianthopoulos, "Intellectual Development of Children from Interracial Matings," *Science,* Vol. 170, No. 146 (December 18, 1970), p. 1329.

[52] Joseph D. Teicher, "Some Observations on Identity Problems in Children of Negro–White Marriages," *Journal of Nervous and Mental Disease,* Vol. 146, No. 3 (March 1968), pp. 249–56.

[53] Ruth Shonle Cavan, *The American Family,* 2nd ed. (New York, 1953), p. 232.

[54] Charles Dickens, *David Copperfield* (London, 1849–50), Chapter 12.

[55] Lewis M. Terman, *Psychological Factors in Marital Happiness* (New York, 1938), pp. 167–71.

is coming from." Sometimes, I can still hear him. His voice was quiet. In two years he was dead.

What's this got to do with my husband? He doesn't understand. He'll go out and spend two hundred dollars on a suit. Or he'll buy white-wall tires. He just doesn't know that being poor can kill a person like it killed my father. He doesn't know what it's like not to know where your next piece of bread is coming from.

It is true; he does not know. And the danger to their marriage is that he does not want to know. He has never known a day of financial want. His side of the story is typical:

We've been married eleven years. I've never made less than twenty thousand a year. We've got money in the bank. Even if we didn't, my folks could help. They have always had more than they need. What's she so scared about?

The problems of this couple spring from their widely disparate economic pasts. Spending patterns are learned in childhood from family experience. She will forever tighten the purse strings that he will forever loosen.

Similar tensions overtake the rich girl–poor boy marriage. The woman who once drove her own expensive car may well find a crowded bus irksome. The early fun of making a budget work often becomes a weary trial. Sadly, she may soon see the sum of her expenditures as the dreary sum of her marriage.

How can these pitfalls be avoided? One should know not only the financial behavior pattern of the proposed mate, but also his or her ability to plan expenditures. How one fits finances into married life is often critical.

age

In no other Western country do people marry so young as in the United States. Prosperity, the income of the working woman, the changing role of the teen-ager from a family financial asset to a costly burden—all these promote marriage at an early age (see pages 459–62).

Teen-age marriages are particularly prone to failure. Numerous studies repeatedly emphasize the high divorce and poor adjustment rates of teen-age unions. One investigator found "that the proportion of remarried women among those who first married below the age of 18 years was about three times as high as that for women who first married between the ages of 22 to 24 years."[56] Particularly hazardous are marriages between the very young. The divorce rates of marriages between people sixteen or younger is 400 percent higher than for marriages in which husbands were from twenty to twenty-six years old and wives twenty-two to twenty-four.[57] In addition, "teen-age marriages forced by pregnancy are the most unstable of all."[58]

How old should one be before getting married? Some students of marriage

[56] Paul C. Glick, "Stability of Marriage in Relation to Age at Marriage," in Robert F. Winch *et al.*, eds., *Selected Studies in Marriage and the Family,* rev. ed. (New York, 1962), p. 624.
[57] Thomas P. Monahan, "Does Age of Marriage Matter in Divorce?" *Social Forces,* Vol. 32, No. 10 (October 1953), p. 86.
[58] Judson T. Landis, "Danger Signals in Courtship," p. 43.

recommend twenty-nine for the man and twenty-four for the woman. Others suggest twenty-five and twenty-two. Setting the same age for everyone is pointless. Emotional stability and maturity are better indices of marital success than chronological age. One good way of deferring a possibly premature marriage while at the same time learning more about a potential partner is a reasonably long engagement. How long should the engagement period be? A year should tell the couple enough. "The best insurance policy against divorce in our society is a thorough engagement."[59] As Chaucer wrote, more than five hundred years ago:

> It is no childes pley
> To take a wyf with-oute avysement.[60]

Seek, then, advisement for marriage.

marriage: "the craft so long to lerne"

prologue

> Next, when they had got them huts and skins and fire and woman was appropriately mated to one man, and the laws of wedlock became known and they saw offspring born of them, then first mankind begun to soften. For the fire saw to it that their shivering bodies were less able to endure cold under the canopy of heaven and Venus sapped their strength and children easily broke their parents' proud spirit by coaxing. Then also neighbors began eagerly to join in a league of friendship amongst themselves to do no hurt and suffer no violence, and asked protection for their children and womankind, signifying by voice and gesture, with stammering tongue, that it was right for all to pity the weak. Nevertheless concord could not altogether be established, but a good part, nay the most part, kept the covenant in good faith or else the race of mankind would even then have been completely destroyed, nor would birth and begetting have availed to prolong their posterity.[61]

So did the Roman poet Lucretius (96?–55 B.C.) tell about the beginnings of the family of man. Families banded together and established protective societal rules. Those breaking the rules imperiled the group and were punished. Sexuality and love, and marriage too, were truly controlled by the group. In that sense, man's deepest intimacy was public business. So it is today. Although marriage has ancient origins, it remains as rich and complex an adventure as life itself. And just as six centuries ago the poet Chaucer described life as "the craft so long to lerne," so is marriage a craft no more quickly learned.

No known human society allows promiscuity to be its governing way of life. In every society, marriage and the family exist. All societies, moreover, have chosen marriage as the arrangement for having children. And "in every known

[59] Ersel Earl LeMasters, *Modern Courtship and Marriage* (New York, 1957), p. 168.
[60] Geoffrey Chaucer, *The Merchant's Tale,* lines 1530–31.
[61] Lucretius, *On the Nature of Things,* quoted in Felding H. Garrison, *Contributions to the History of Medicine* (New York, 1966), p. 25.

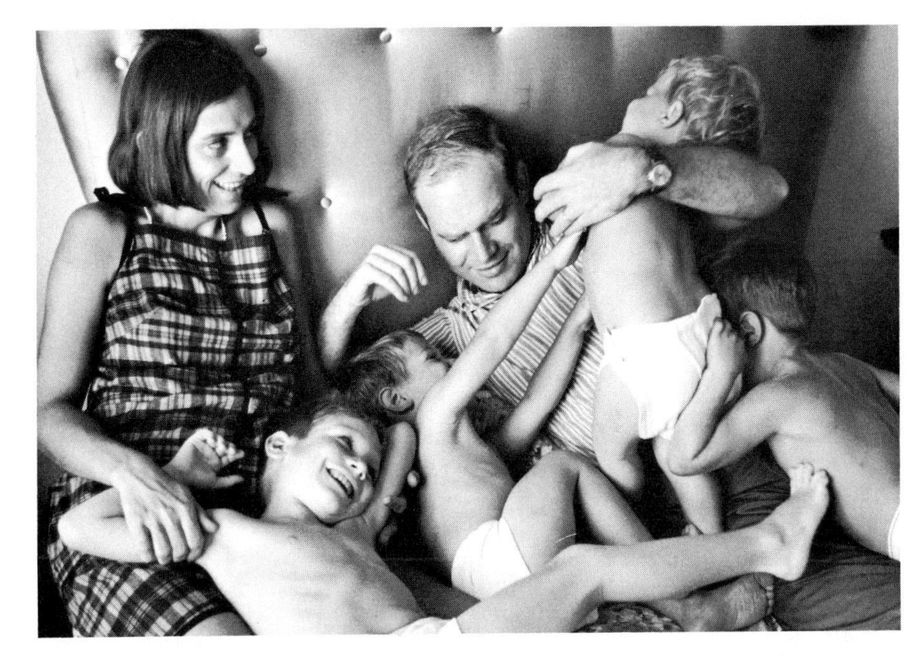

15-4

human society, there is a prohibition against incest.''[62] These pervasive behavior patterns prevent social convulsions that would be inimical to child-rearing. Without such restrictions, the group would die, the victim of its own rulelessness. ''It is marriage which is the basic social instrument of man's survival . . . for survival there must be an accommodation between the sexes . . . enduring enough to provide protection, care, and reasonable security for the offspring.''[63]

Marriage serves man's needs to resolve loneliness and to perpetuate his kind. And society pressures him to resolve these needs through marriage. In relatively recent years, however, new dimensions of marriage have developed. Have they weakened the married state?

Although there have been great societal changes, the family based on monogamous marriage stubbornly prevails in this country. It has been repeatedly said that it is losing its popularity among the young, but in 1970 both the number and rate of marriages in the United States had increased for the twelfth consecutive year. In addition, approximately three-quarters of all marriages occurred in the eighteen- to twenty-four-year age group.[64] However, in 1970 the rate of divorce had also increased from approximately one in four marriages in 1960 to approximately one in three, although it did not reach the peak rate

[62] Bernard Berelson and Gary A. Steiner, *Human Behavior* (New York, 1964), pp. 313–16. Let it not be assumed, however, that the avoidance of mating with relatives (the ''incest taboo'' in humans) is limited to the culturally learned and determined influences of human beings. Behavioral mechanisms for the avoidance of inbreeding seem to have evolved in many creatures lower in the evolutionary scale, such as the white-throated sparrow and a species of moth.

[63] William M. Kephart, *The Family, Society, and the Individual,* p. 64.

[64] *Monthly Vital Statistics Report, Provisional Statistics, Annual Summary for the United States, 1970,* U.S. Department of Health, Education, and Welfare, Public Health Service, Health Services and Mental Health Administration, Vol. 19, No. 13 (September 21, 1971), pp. 8, 9.

recorded after the Second World War between 1945 and 1947.[65] Despite the divorces, marriages in this country are far more prevalent today than they were at the turn of the century. In 1900 only 52.8 percent of men over fourteen years of age were married; in 1970 76 percent of men over eighteen years were married. In 1900 only 55 percent of women were married; in 1970 some 68 percent were married.[66] (The reason that the 1970 percentage for married women was lower than that for men is due to the greater number of women than men in this country.)

Today, the date of the marriage does not await the completion of education. Never before have so many students married. And they share with all recently married people a new awareness of sexual relationships. No longer, for example, are woman's sexual needs regarded as incidental. Rapid social change, moreover, has added threats to the stability of marriage. The mobility of the family and the emancipation of the woman are but two of the factors contributing to fresh perspectives of marriage. Consider two major aspects of marriage so characteristic of these times.

the campus marriage

It was not until the Second World War was over that married students were first seen in appreciable numbers on the nation's college campuses. Thousands of veterans used their benefits to obtain an education. Today's graying professors remember them well. They were not college boys. They were older, tougher men. Some were filled with a speechless anger. Most were intensely purposeful. They had no time to fool around. They had been through a war and knew something about time. Many were married. Their wives worked. There was always pregnancy to think about. It was, for most vets, a difficult time. It was, for their wives, a time for marking time. Veterans were used to waiting. Their wives quickly learned.

One of the chief concerns of married students is money. A recent nationwide survey showed that parents pay for 61 percent of students' expenses.[67] Marriage changes that picture. Some married students want to make it on their own. Often parents are reluctant to help because of a sincere belief that such a prolonged dependency might harm the marriage. Others are more abrupt: "If you're old enough to get married, you're old enough to support yourself." Many parents do help. Nevertheless, married students receive much less parental cash than do single students. Some married students are aided by the GI Bill. Most work. Not uncommonly the wife supports her student husband. Whatever the plan, it is beset with risks. That the vast majority of campus marriages succeed speaks well for the maturity of those who venture into them.

It is the campus wife's education that is at greatest risk. Marriage may dilute her motivation; the purchase of an economics text cannot compare with her first investment in a Picasso reproduction for the bedroom wall. No philosophy professor will gain her attention as a whimpering baby will. Yet, occasionally, an

[65] *Monthly Vital Statistics Report, Final Statistics,* Center for Health Statistics, U.S. Department of Health, Education, and Welfare, Public Health Service, Health Services and Mental Health Administration, Vol. 19, No. 19, Supplement (2) (January 26, 1971), p. 1.

[66] *U.S. Bureau of the Census, Statistical Abstract of the United States: 1971* (92nd edition), p. 33.

[67] Robert O. Blood, *Marriage,* p. 163.

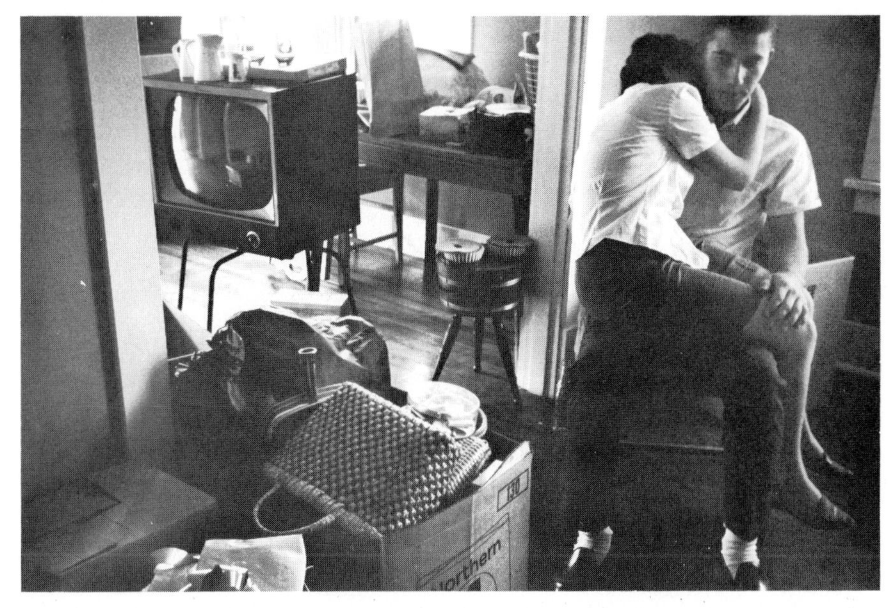

15-5 *Move-in day.*

educationally mixed marriage may result, and her sacrifice multiplies. Her husband becomes involved in the world of the slide rule or the stethoscope or Byzantine art. Her world may become a matter of warming a typewriter or yesterday's stew. Or she may seek contentment in recipes and afternoon TV shows. (There is no evening TV. He has to study.) A conversation gap occurs and widens. In a class in Russian literature, the student husband hears a quote: "If you are afraid of loneliness, do not marry."[68] But he is already married. He studies guiltily. She is lonely too. "If it hadn't been for you . . ." they both think. The bubble of love bursts, and mutual blame takes over.

Moreover, the married student is pressed for time. He may need to devote every evening of the week to study. Restlessly, his wife remembers the ruthless exclusion of the married from campus activity. She seeks to be busy. She may read or do mechanical things or perhaps go to the movies alone. Conflicts over leisure time are a major cause of marriage failure among college students. The wife also worries about their inadequate sexual relationship, a surprisingly common problem among married college students.[69] Her youth does not help the situation. Campus marriages now occur at earlier ages than they used to. The college student must bring security into a student marriage. To count on finding security within marriage is a mistake.

Pregnancy may also complicate the student marriage. It ends the wife's immediate plan for a college education. Often it concludes her husband's schooling. Some college fathers successfully lead a tripartite life. Their time is divided among job, school, and family. In one study it was found that "only 52 percent of the graduate-student fathers were going to school full-time compared to 79 percent of the childless graduate students."[70]

[68] *The Personal Papers of Anton Chekhov,* intro. by Matthew Josephson (New York, 1948), p. 75.
[69] James A. Peterson, *Education for Marriage,* p. 216.
[70] Robert O. Blood, *Marriage,* p. 166.

Grades may be a problem. Some studies do indicate that married students' grades are equal to, or even better than, single students'. However, marriage can hardly be recommended as a means of improving grades. There is a significant lack of data regarding the number of married students who drop out of school because of poor grades. The relationship between the married student's age and grades needs further study. Sometimes grades, as such, create dissension. The wife who consistently does better than her husband may find herself in the same position as the unmarried coed who feels it necessary to "play dumb" with her dates. The young, nonbreadwinning husband, his masculine role further diminished, may add resentment to regret.

The problems of campus marriage must be dealt with early. Indeed, they are best discussed and planned for before the marriage takes place. Another aspect of marriage is rarely considered, even expected. So insidiously does it develop that neither partner clearly sees it as a threat to their future. Too, for some it hardly exists. Others accept it. Still others resent it. It is the problem of monotony in marriage.

marriage, monotony, and the appreciation of both

> And may her bride-groom bring her to a house
> Where all's accustomed, ceremonious;
> For arrogance and hatred are the wares
> Peddled in the thoroughfares.
> How but in custom and in ceremony
> Are innocence and beauty born?[71]

In the pattern of everyday married life, there is much that is honored by time. Custom and ceremony, no matter how subtle, add to the richness of the marital fabric. But mere repetition makes for a drab cloth. Individuality and custom can, however, be compatible. Indeed, customs provide an opportunity for sharing individuality. Her custom may be as simple as a best tablecloth for dinner. But unless he occasionally brings a bunch of flowers to decorate the table too, the time will come when neither sees the tablecloth. What is left? Monotony.

Many people find some marriage monotony a comfort, not a problem. They see it as a mark of their certainty about each other. Whether one can count on the other is a valid test of courtship. In marriage it is part of the loving. Life cannot be perpetual excitement. There is surely some truth in this reasoning.

Others refuse to even recognize tedium as a possible part of marriage. They hark back to the "good old days," when people (meaning women) had no time for nonsense like boredom. "In the past," they say, "women knew their place; they never thought about being bored, and they never got a divorce either." Just how far back the good old days go for such philosophers is never clear. That Grandpa was a kindly soul, in whose beneficent light Grandma was ever content, may be true. Maybe.

In the early nineteenth century, *The Ladies' Book* quoted the following advice of a minister to a bride: "Your duty is submission . . . Your husband is, by the Laws of God and of man, your superior; do not ever give him cause to re-

[71] William Butler Yeats, "A Prayer for My Daughter."

mind you of it.''[72] So wifely self-expression continued to be discouraged and total obedience to be expected. But the role of woman changed. The shackling notion of feminine obedience was discarded. Millions of women in this country found work outside the home. (Some of the problems of working mothers are discussed on pages 329–31.) But a great number of those who remain at home are bored. This is not to say that the working woman is never oppressed by monotony. Nor is homemaking a tedious occupation for many women. But many a stay-at-home woman certainly finds little opportunity to relieve the monotony of housekeeping. Sheer boredom then erodes her marriage. And her husband, tired and perhaps also bored with his work, joins her in an unrelieved tedium.

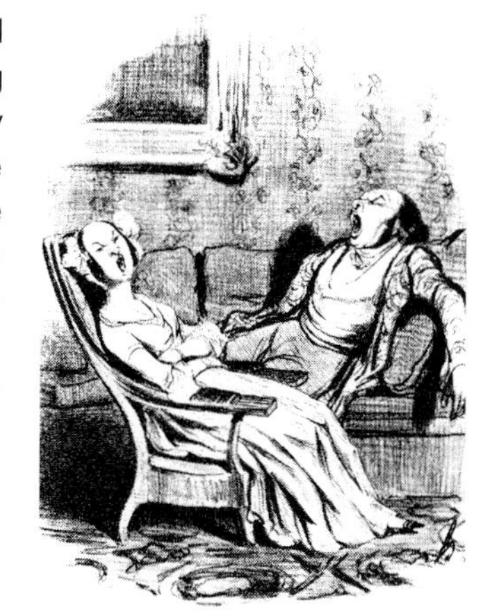

15-6 *''Marital Harmony: Six Months After the Honeymoon,'' a cartoon by Honoré Daumier (1809–1879).*

Many marriages, then, die on the vine. Husband and wife simply stop noticing each other. True, the arithmetic of living—the baby's allergy, the leaking roof, the clogged sink—does not add up to romance. But to keep a marriage alive takes work and planning. The couple must make time to do things together both at home and away from the home and office. Daily opportunities to share thoughts and feelings must be created. Privacy is not always easy to achieve. But no home needs to be the private preserve of a small child. Often a good babysitter will help. Timing is also crucial. A woman, exhausted by a toddler, may find it hard to end the day by concentrating on her husband's office difficulties. In turn, he may be too weary, at the moment, to be concerned about the TV repairman. And so, at times, silence is the wisest and most appreciated course.

In a marriage marred by boredom, a word of appreciation is usually long overdue. Sincere praise for accomplishment is a need of both marital partners. There is the story of the unhappy man who ran around with other women, not because his wife did not understand him, but because she understood him only too well. To her, knowing him meant undermining him. The woman who cannot regard her husband without foil in hand, ready to pierce his ego, will destroy her marriage. Marriage is not a competition. One does not gain by the other's loss. Between the married, ''one-upmanship'' is a dangerous game. There is no victim in a good marriage. Moreover, the husband who does not accentuate his marriage with expressed appreciation may reap (and deserve) a bitter harvest.

''It was a lot of little things,'' then, explains many a happy marriage as well as many a divorce. The difference is that the happily married couple, having worked at it, will know what happened to them. They will know why the customs and ceremonies of their marriage never lost freshness and meaning.

Campus marriage, monotonous marriage—all marriage is profoundly influenced by the topic of Chapter 17, sexuality. As has been pointed out, human beings are unique in needing instruction in the art of love. Complex products of this demanding culture, modern people usually bring to marriage an accumulation of information and misinformation about sexuality. Everywhere, the cultural influence on sexual behavior is profound. Some primitive cultures (the

[72] Cited in Vance Packard, *The Sexual Wilderness,* p. 244.

Muria of India, for example) expect women to be as sexually aggressive as men. In other cultures, the women are frigid and find coitus humiliating. In this country, only recently have a growing number of males felt the need to sexually gratify their partners. In Samoa this attitude has long existed.[73] Sexual mores are not often directly changed as a result of biological discovery, but such changes may yet come about in Western culture. Consider first the male and female reproductive systems in the next chapter, and then in Chapter 17 consider mutuality in the sexual life.

summary

In the nonhuman world, mating behavior is governed by simple instinct. Among humans, the unique element of culture, of learned behavior, has given rise to confusion over the rituals of courtship and marriage (page 439). In the Western world, the marital codes established by the Judeo-Christian culture endure, often reinforced by threat and guilt—which give rise to anxiety (page 440).

The accepted rituals of courtship vary from culture to culture and from time to time. In the United States today, the usual pattern progresses from group dating to random dating to "going steady" (page 442). The extent of and motivations for premarital sexual activity vary widely with the individual (pages 443–44). Studies of the extent of premarital sexual activity, such as those made by Vance Packard (pages 444–45) and by Gagnon and Simon (pages 446–48), provide generalizations that are useful for comparison with previous generations but that cannot be considered definitive.

Promiscuity may be defined as indiscriminate sexual behavior—sexual intercourse without rules (page 448). Among the emotional motivations for it are the fear of commitment, an unmet need for affection, revenge on an overly critical parent, relief from anxiety, or the belief that sexual abstinence causes emotional problems (pages 448–49).

Most people seek an enduring, meaningful, sharing relationship with one other person, almost always in the context of marriage (page 450). Marriage should be an intelligent personal decision based on a number of considerations, including those listed on pages 452–53. Couples contemplating marriage should give special consideration to differences between them that may affect the success of their marriage—such as differences in religious faith (pages 454–55), in race (pages 455–56), in social class (page 456), in attitudes toward money (pages 456–57), and in age (pages 457–58).

Marriage has come under renewed scrutiny in recent years as a result of such rapid social changes as higher divorce rates, increased mobility, and the emancipation of women (pages 459–60). Two kinds of marriage that merit particular attention by today's young people are the campus marriage (pages 460–62) and the marriage that succumbs to monotony and boredom (pages 462–64).

[73] Harvey D. Strassman, "Sex and the Work of Masters and Johnson," *GP,* Vol. 38, No. 4 (October 1968), p. 111.

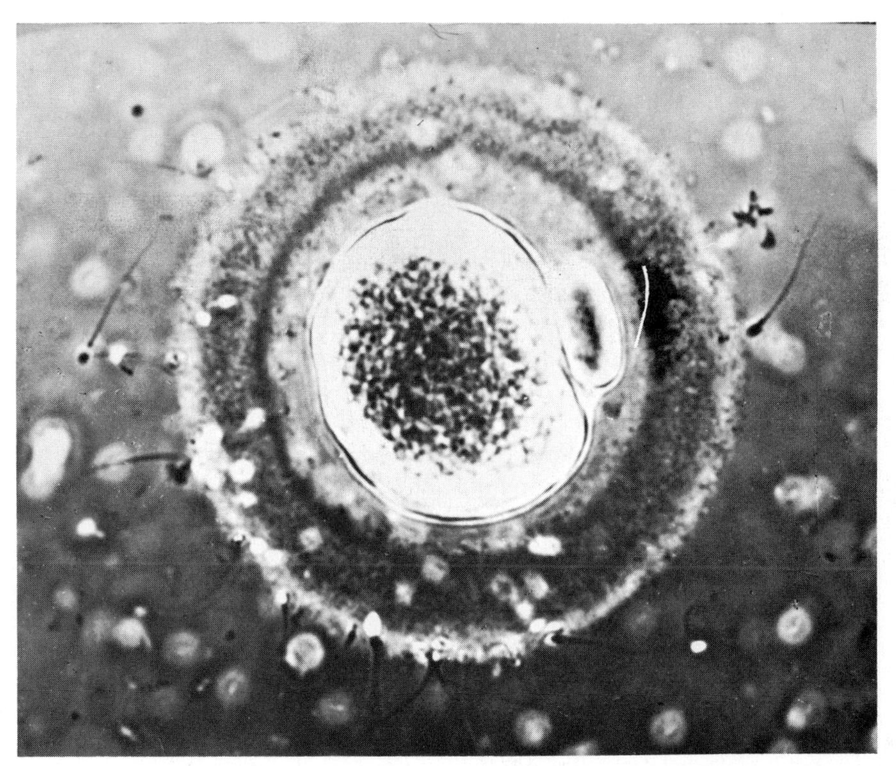

Human spermatozoa enter an ovum. Only one will fertilize it.

human reproductive structure and function

16

the brain's chemical "fertility switch"[1]

In the discussion of the pituitary gland (Chapter 10, pages 254–58), it was pointed out that its posterior lobe stores and releases several hormones; one stimulates contraction of the uterus at the beginning of childbirth. The anterior lobe both produces and releases hormones. They activate and control other glands—the thyroid, adrenals, and ovaries and testes. But it is upon the function of certain cells in the brain's hypothalamus that both lobes of the pituitary gland depend. As was discussed, the products of the posterior lobe of the pituitary gland are manufactured in the hypothalamus. And both the manufacture and release of the hormonal products of the anterior lobe are controlled by chemicals from the hypothalamus called *releasing hormones* or *factors.* The releasing hormones from the hypothalamus that are of present major concern are those stimulating the anterior lobe of the pituitary to, in turn, produce and release the hormones that control the sex glands—the ovaries and testes. Before these are discussed, however, it would be well to consider the pineal gland (or pineal body). Increasing knowledge suggests that this structure may play an important role in the activities controlling sexual function and reproduction.

the pineal gland

Buried near the center of the brain, and attached to its cerebellar portion by a slender stalk, the pineal gland was once thought to be the seat of the soul. Today, this single, pea-sized body is usually regarded as a sort of relay station, sending messages to the nervous system that influence the body's "biological clock." This still mysterious timing system within the body synchronizes with the external cosmic clock that determines day and night (see pages 6–8). (Body temperature, for example, is lower in the morning than in the late afternoon.)

The pineal gland is rich in chemicals, some of which are secreted in synchronization with the ebb and flow of daylight. *Melatonin,* a chemical that acts as a hormone, is found in the pineal gland. In lower animals it appears that melatonin has an inhibiting effect on the sexual function. Moreover, it has been found, by animal experimentation, that light can affect the sexual cycle by controlling the synthesis of melatonin in the pineal gland. This may account for the seasonal mating periods of many animals. Human beings are almost unique in that they do not mate according to season. If and how light generates nervous activity into pineal gland function in human beings is being investigated. Also being considered is the possible relationship of the pineal gland to the hypothalamus.

[1] Graham Chedd, "The Switch of Fertility," *New Scientist and Science Journal,* Vol. 51, No. 758 (July 1, 1971), pp. 11–13.

the reproductive systems

the male reproductive system

The male reproductive system consists of a pair of male gonads (testes) and excretory ducts (the epididymis, vas deferens, and ejaculatory ducts). The accessory structures are the seminal vesicles, prostate gland, Cowper's glands (also called the bulbo-urethral glands), and penis.

the male reproductive organs

About two months before birth, the *testes* usually descend from the abdomen into the external sac, the *scrotum.* It is crucial that this occur before adolescence. Only at a temperature cooler than that of the abdominal cavity can the development of spermatozoa in the testes occur. Should both testes fail to descend, sterility results. Should only one testicle reach the scrotum, there would probably be enough normal spermatozoa to ensure fertility. In some males only one testicle descends and years may elapse before the other descends. In many cases, surgery and hormones have been successful in the treatment of undescended testicles.

A basic purpose of the testes is to produce *spermatozoa* (Greek *sperma,* seed). This first function is carried on by germinal cells of the *seminiferous tubules.* These coiled little tubules (straightened out in both testes they would be a mile long) are supported by connective tissue in which special cells carry out the second basic function of the testes—the production of the hormone *testosterone.* The same hormone of the anterior pituitary that maintains the corpus luteum (see page 478) in the female is responsible for the production of testosterone in the male. It is the testosterone that causes the male genitalia to develop, the voice to deepen, the bones to increase in size, the beard to appear, and the psyche to change. The growth of the external genitalia is the first sign of puberty in the boy.[2]

Eventually, the seminiferous tubules unite into a single convoluted tube at the back of each testis called the *epididymis.* Mature spermatozoa leave the

[2] *Androgens* are substances capable of producing masculine body characteristics. Thus *testosterone* and *androsterone* are among the androgens. Testosterone is the predominant androgen produced by the testes; it is, therefore, the major hormone of male sexual development. Its functions are both numerous and profound. It is essential in the fetus for male internal and external genital differentiation (see pages 488–89). After puberty, it contributes to spermatogenesis. In addition, testosterone stimulates the development of the seminal vesicle and prostate, is necessary for the contribution of the seminal vesicle and prostate to semen and ejaculation, and matures the secondary sex characteristics of the adult male, such as the deepening voice, penile enlargement, muscularity, and facial hair. (Daniel D. Federman, "The Assessment of Organ Function—The Testis," *New England Journal of Medicine,* Vol. 285, No. 16 [October 14, 1971], p. 901.)

By their action on the *sebaceous glands* of the skin, androgens predispose teen-agers to acne. The intense self-concern characteristic of the pubescent person does not make acne easy to bear. This disease of the sebaceous glands in the skin occurs in some 75 percent of children at puberty. Usually it is mild. The normal sebaceous glands produce an oily substance called *sebum.* In acne an abnormal amount of sebum blocks the outlet of the gland. It enlarges. The outer part of the lesion turns black, not from dirt, but because of chemical changes. These are the "blackheads." Infection may occur and spread deep into the skin. Washing several times daily with a disinfectant soap is wise. However, there is no evidence whatsoever that the initial lesion of acne begins because of uncleanliness. Moreover, the prevalent belief that acne is caused by masturbation is utterly untrue. Even mild cases of acne are often best seen by the family physician. He may refer severe cases to a skin specialist (dermatologist). Many physicians forbid their acne patients to partake of chocolates, nuts (peanut butter), and soft drinks. The understandable emotional distress caused by severe acne makes professional counsel desirable.

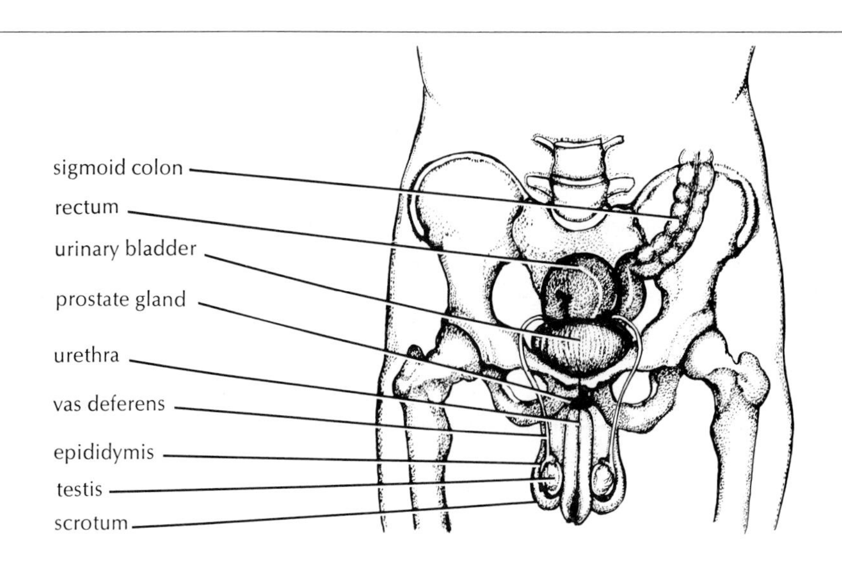

16-1 The male reproductive system

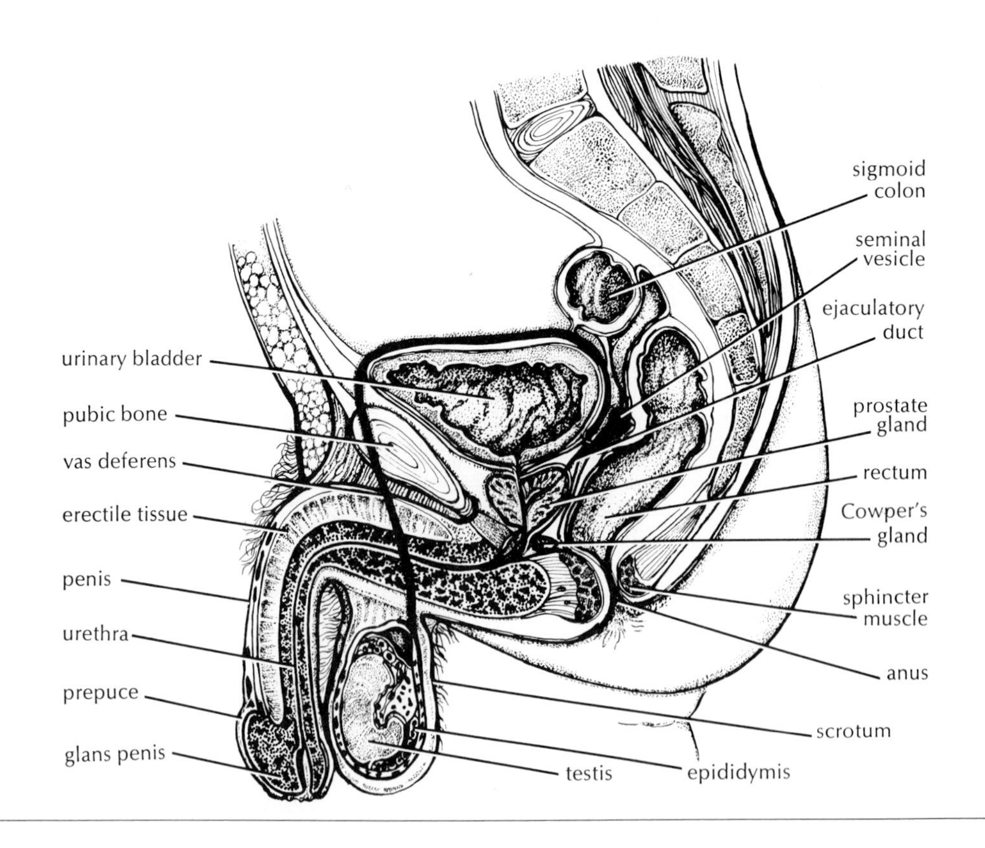

seminiferous tubules and are temporarily stored in the epididymis. At maturity, enough spermatozoa have accumulated in the epididymis for ejaculation.

The *vas deferens* (or spermatic cord) is a continuation of the epididymis. It goes upward along the back of the testes and, by way of a canal in the groin, into the abdomen. Eventually the vas deferens joins the duct of the *seminal vesicle* of its side of the body. The two seminal vesicles are located between the bladder and rectum and produce a secretion that adds to the volume of the seminal fluid. The seminal vesicles empty their secretions into the *ejaculatory ducts* which, in turn, empty into the *urethra.* The urethra is the canal of the male organ for sexual intercourse, the *penis.* Through the penis, the semen is discharged and urine is passed from the bladder. Through a remarkable engineering mechanism (see page 471), urine and semen never pass at the same time.

The first one-and-one-half inches of the urethra, as it leaves the bladder, is surrounded by the chestnut-sized *prostate gland,* which also contains many muscle fibers. The gland part secretes a thin fluid that helps carry the semen and provides it with a necessary alkaline medium. The muscle part of the pros-

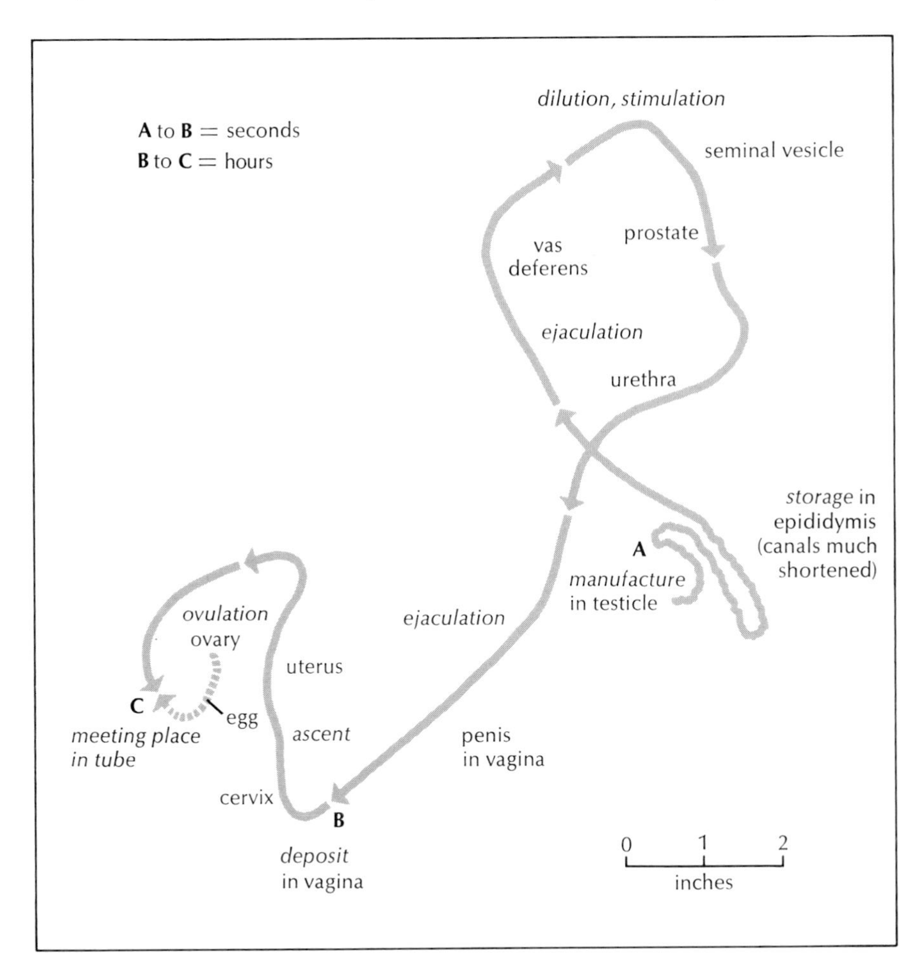

16-2 *The route of a spermatozoon from its origin to its fertilization of an ovum.*

tate helps eject the semen out of the penis. On each side of the prostate glands is one of the two *Cowper's glands.* They look like peas and secrete the thick material characteristic of seminal fluid.

The penis hangs in front of the scrotum. At the tip of its head (*glans*) is the slitlike opening of the urethra. The thin skin of its body is loose. At the neck of the penis, the skin folds upon itself to form the *prepuce* (foreskin). This is the portion of the skin of which part is removed at circumcision. Circumcision is associated with a decrease in the incidence of cancer of the penis. There is, moreover, some evidence that cancer of the cervix is more common among wives of uncircumcised men. However, there is considerable opinion that both cervical and penile cancers are more closely associated with poor personal hygiene than with the presence of the prepuce. Not all physicians agree that routine circumcision is essential.

The belief, moreover, that the uncircumcised male has more control over his ejaculations than the man who is circumcised is a fallacy. It doubtless arose from the mistaken notion that since the glans of the uncircumcised male is largely covered by the prepuce it would be less exposed to friction during coitus. The fact is that the prepuce of the uncircumcised male is significantly retracted during sexual intercourse (it may not be when he masturbates). He is, therefore, no more likely to be able to control his ejaculations than is a circumcised male.[3]

Another fallacy is the belief that a larger penis is more effective during coitus than a smaller one. This misconception is discussed on pages 508–09.

mechanism of erection of the penis and ejaculation

Not every penile erection is due to increased sexual stimulation. For example, partial erection may result from lifting heavy loads or from straining while having a bowel movement. This is due to stress on the muscles of the perineum. Newborn males may have a penile erection; this is probably related to the infant's increased muscle and nerve irritability, such as may be caused by crying. When a penile erection is due to sexual excitement, its stimuli begin in the higher brain centers; the erection itself is the result of a spinal reflex. Cerebral influence is apparently not always necessary for an erection; indeed, it may inhibit penile erection. Man does not have voluntary control of an erection; he cannot will it. To understand how the spinal nerve reflex causes erection, consider first some of the internal structure of the penis.

The penis contains three cylindrical bodies of erectile tissue (see Figure 16-1). They run the length of the penis to its head. These cylindrical bodies contain many small vascular spaces; they are thus a spongy erectile tissue. For an erection to occur, nerve stimuli cause dilatation of the little penile arteries (arterioles). At the places where the arterioles and the vascular spaces join are valvelike structures. When the penis is flaccid these structures (called *polsters*) cause blood to be shunted away from the vascular spaces and directly into the

[3]William H. Masters and Virginia E. Johnson, *Human Sexual Response* (Boston, 1966), pp. 189–91.

veins. With adequate nerve stimuli these polsters relax. This permits rapid inflow of blood into the spaces of the cylindrical erectile tissue of the penis. The rate of the inflow of blood from the arterioles is then temporarily greater than the rate of the outflow from the veins. This causes an increase of blood volume in the penis. When a steady state is reached, in which blood inflow equals outflow, penile enlargement ceases, and the penis is stiff. The veins of the penis are also equipped with valvelike structures, which some investigators think slow down the return of blood from that organ. Others disagree with this.

Before ejaculating, the male frequently has an emission of a few drops (or more) of fluid that may contain active spermatozoa. (This accounts for pregnancies that may result despite the practice of coitus interruptus [see page 616].) The ejaculatory process begins with contractions of the ducts leading away from the seminiferous tubules in the testes. These contractions continue along the epididymis to the vas deferens. The vas deferens then contracts along with the seminal vesicles. The contents of the vas deferens, as well as those of the seminal vesicles, are expelled into the part of the urethra that passes through the prostate. The prostate has also been contracting rhythmically to add fluid to the ejaculatory content. At the onset of the ejaculatory process, the ringlike band of muscle fibers (the sphincter) surrounding the exit from the urinary bladder contracts. Semen is thus prevented from entering the urinary bladder; semen and urine are not ordinarily expelled together. After ejaculation, nerve stimuli cause constriction of the penile arterioles, and the erection is gradually lost.

16-3 *A spermatozoon in diagram* (top) *and as seen through a scanning electron microscope* (bottom), *showing the head, neck, middle piece, and part of the tail.*

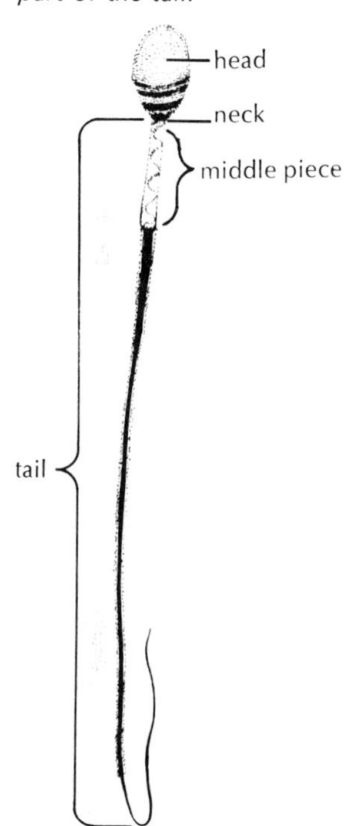

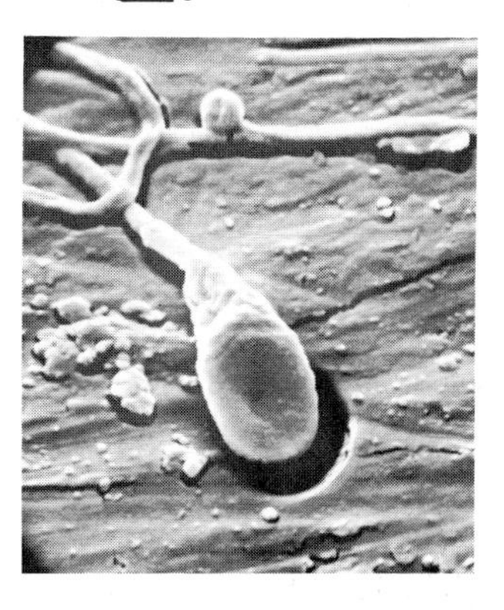

semen

The ejaculated fluid containing the sperm is a thick, whitish material. It is about a teaspoonful in amount. However, the consistency and amount of the seminal fluid may vary, for example with the age of the male. In healthy men, the ejaculatory amount is reestablished in about twenty-four hours or less. During ejaculation, the entire transit from testes to vagina occupies but a few seconds. Although sperm can remain motile in the vagina for as long as two hours, some can reach the cervix in seconds. Indeed, ejaculation may well take place directly on the cervix. However, hours may be required for ascent of the sperm through the uterus and part of the Fallopian tube in order to fertilize an ovum (a distance of about six inches). On an average, the journey probably requires about an hour (see Figure 16-2). Each spermatozoon has a bulbous head. Its long mobile tail propels it to its destination (see Figure 16-3). When one compares the size of a spermatozoon with the relatively enormous distance it must travel to fertilize an ovum, one cannot help but be struck by its vigor. Yet, of the millions of spermatozoa emitted in each ejaculum, usually only one manages the task of fertilization. Why? It may be that the destiny of a spermatozoon is determined by differences in the structure of the membrane surrounding it.[4]

[4] Garth L. Nicolson and Ryuzo Yanagimachi, "Terminal Saccharides on Sperm Plasma Membranes: Identification by Specific Agglutinins," *Science,* Vol. 177, No. 4045 (July 21, 1972), pp. 276–78.

the female reproductive system

The essential glands of the female reproductive system are the pair of female gonads (ovaries). The female reproductive *duct* system is composed of the Fallopian tubes (named after the Italian anatomist Gabriello Fallopio [1523–62], the structures are also called the oviducts or uterine tubes), the uterus (womb), and the vagina, and the associated structures—the external genitalia. The mammary glands (breasts) may also be considered as part of the female reproductive duct system (see Figure 16-8).

the ovaries and ova

The two *ovaries* (egg containers) are the fundamental organs of femininity. About the size and shape of a shelled almond, each ovary is situated on one side of the *uterus* and is attached to it by ligaments. Just as the organs of masculinity (the testes) produce male sperm, so do the ovaries produce mature *ova* in the female. When the female child is born, each of her ovaries contains about 200,000 tiny sacs or follicles.[5] In each follicle lies a microscopically small primordial sex cell (or *oögonium*). Each female is born with all the primordial sex cells she will ever have. At this primitive, unripened stage, no sex cell is capable of fertilization. The ripening process whereby a primordial sex cell becomes an ovum must await puberty. This usually occurs between the ninth and seventeenth years (twelve and a half years is the average). During a woman's lifetime, only about 400 (perhaps 1 in 1,000) ova leave either of the ovaries.

Every month the mature human female experiences a series of changes basically involving the hypothalamus in the brain, the anterior lobe of the pituitary gland, the ovaries, and the *endometrium* (the lining of the uterus). The purpose of these changes is to prepare for possible pregnancy. For pregnancy to occur, an egg must leave the ovary, be fertilized, and then be firmly implanted in the endometrium of the prepared uterus.[6]

What happens to the ovary (ovarian cycle) is related to what happens to the uterus (menstrual cycle). *Ovulation* and *menstruation* are different events, happening at different times, to different organs. But each intimately affects the other.

OVULATION To follow the events leading to the release of a mature egg from the ovary (days 1–8 in Figure 16-5), start with a landmark—day 1, the beginning of the menstrual period. Why day 1? Because the woman can observe the first day of her period more easily than her last. She can thus count from that day more reliably. Also assume that every twenty-eight days the average female menstruates five days. With different people these time periods vary normally. They are used here only as examples. Note, however, that the ovarian and menstrual cycles are correlated here.

1. Menstruation begins on day 1 and continues through day 5 (see Figures 16-5 and 16-6). Chemicals from the hypothalamus stimulate the anterior lobe

[5] Estimates of the number vary enormously. Some scientists believe that, at birth, there are as many as half a million follicles in each ovary.

[6] The Roman Catholic church teaches that conception occurs with fertilization. Other bodies, such as the American College of Obstetrics and Gynecology, consider biological life to begin with implantation.

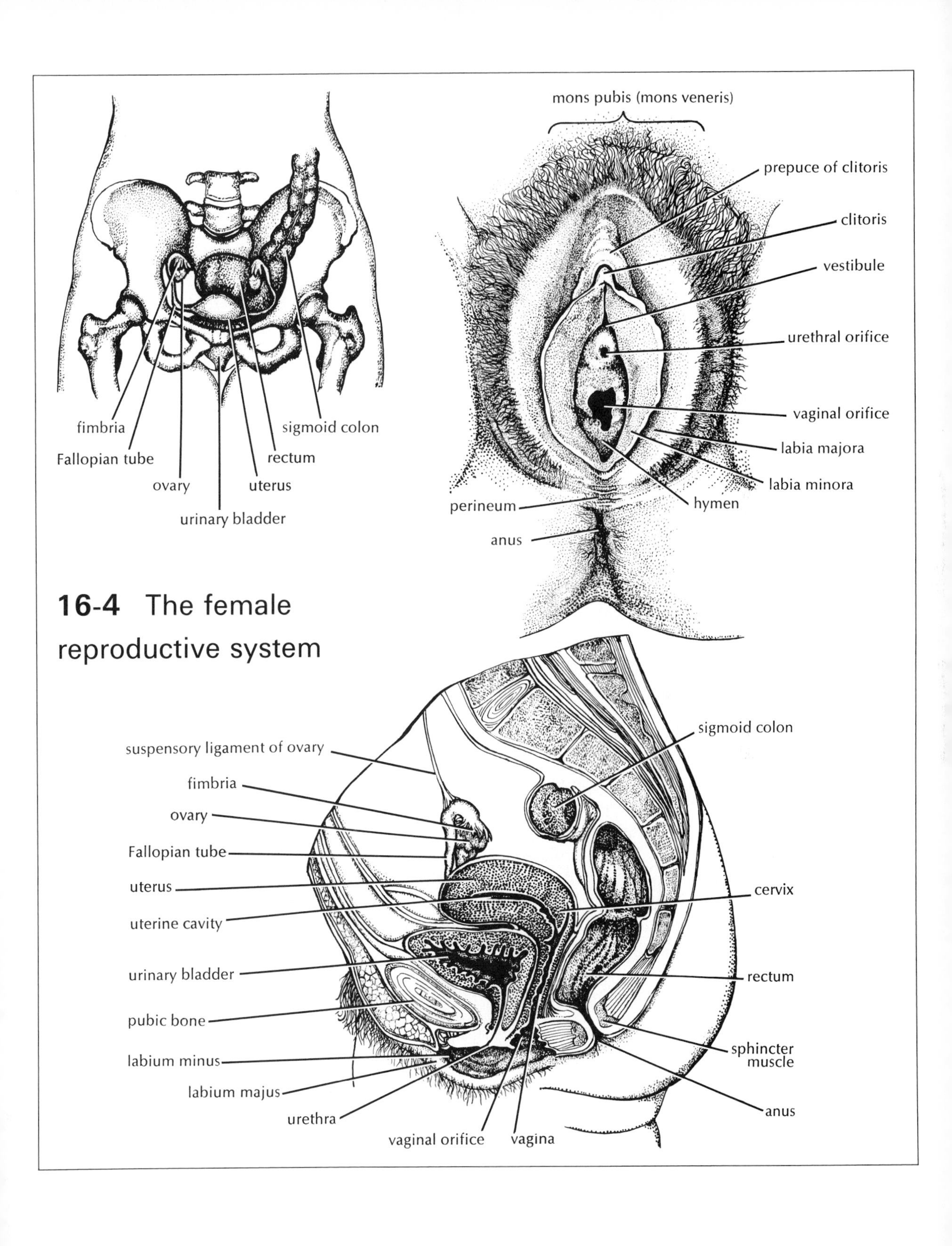

16-4 The female reproductive system

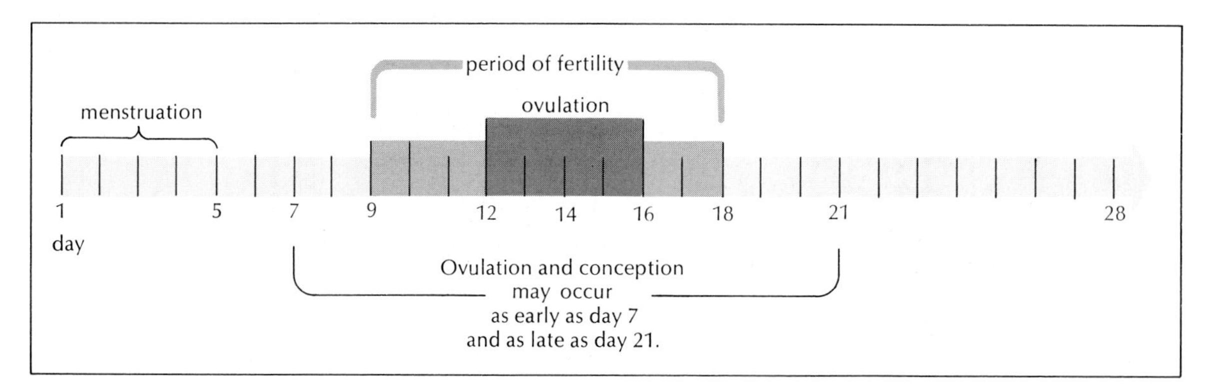

16-5 *The menstrual cycle.*

of the pituitary gland to produce and release the follicle-stimulating hormone (FSH) directly into the venous blood stream.

2. The FSH reaches and activates the ovaries. Not one but several (of the many thousands) of immature ovarian follicles in one or both ovaries respond to the FSH and begin to ripen. Which ovary is more affected is unpredictable. Estimates of the number of immature follicles that respond to the FSH usually vary from two to thirty-two.

3. The cells of those ovarian follicles that are ripening multiply greatly and the single maturing ovum within each follicle increases in size. The increased layers of follicular cells secrete a *follicular fluid.* This fluid forms tiny pools, which first separate groups of cells but which then run together to form a little lake within each follicle (see Figure 16-6). The follicles mature at different rates of speed, so some are at earlier stages of development than others. By about day 10, a few of the most mature follicles look like fluid-filled rounded sacks. The developing ovum is in the wall of the sack and is surrounded by follicular cells, which separate it from the lake. The follicle is now called a *Graafian follicle,* after a seventeenth-century Dutch anatomist, Regner de Graaf, who first described it.

4. As they ripen, the cells of maturing follicles also produce a hormone of their own called *estrogen.* Its function at this stage is to begin the preparation of the uterus for implantation of a fertilized ovum.

5. On about day 10, one (or, very rarely, two) of the follicles undergoes a sudden spurt of growth. In three or four days it is completely mature. As a rule only one follicle and ovum matures and only one ovum leaves the ovary. (If a woman has a tendency for multiple births, there may be more than one.) No one knows what determines which follicle (and ovum) will be selected. The other follicles, and their contained ova that are not destined to leave the ovary, develop to varying extents, only to regress, die, and be replaced by small scars. No other trace of them remains.

6. A few hours before the ovum is ready to leave, the follicle that contains it migrates to the surface of the ovary. By day 13 or 14 the ovum is ready to go. It has been seen at surgery as a tiny protrusion from the ovarian surface.

7. A few days before, the anterior lobe of the pituitary gland had begun the release of a second hormone, the luteinizing hormone (LH), directly into the

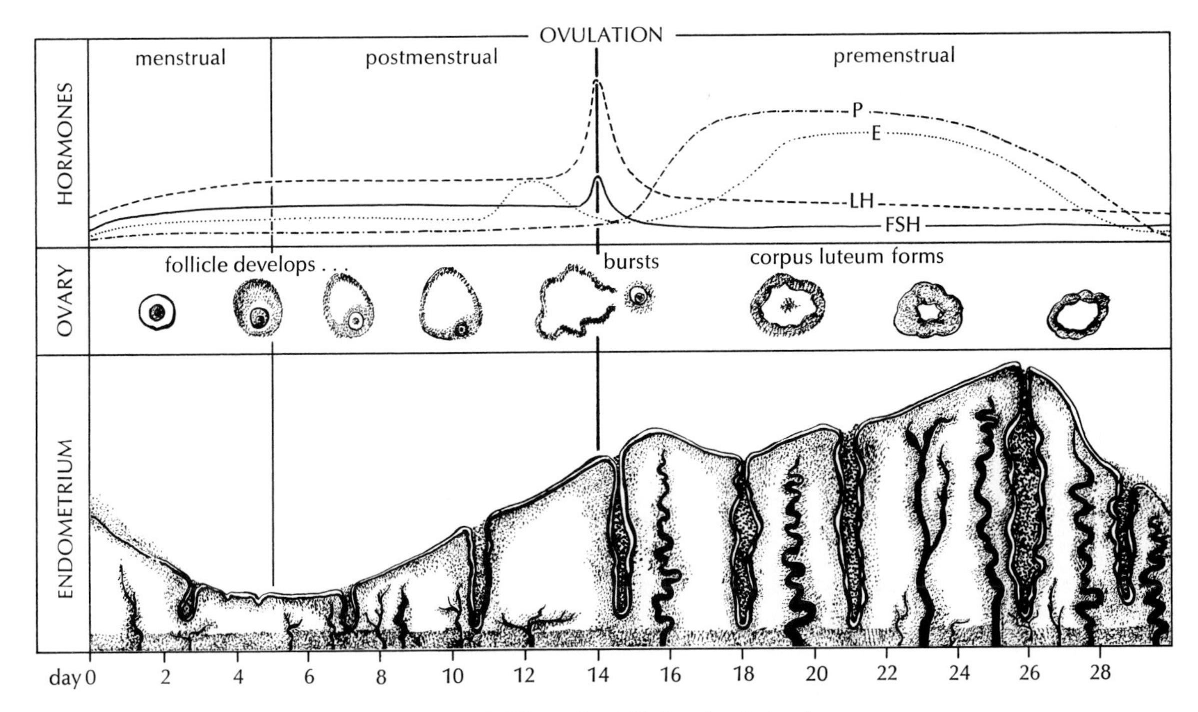

16-6 *The menstrual and ovulatory cycles. (FSH = the follicle-stimulating hormone; E = estrogen; LH = the luteinizing hormone; P = progesterone.) Note that the progesterone level is detectably higher within twenty-four hours after ovulation occurs.*

venous blood. Like the FSH, the release of LH is governed by hypothalamic chemicals from the brain. Moreover, it is believed that the same hypothalamic chemical governs the manufacture and release of both FSH and LH.

8. The LH causes the follicle to rupture, and the ovum is released. This is *ovulation.* On the average, ovulation occurs on day 14. Ovulation, then, occurs at about the middle of the menstrual cycle. In 1972, it was reported that the ovary contracts slightly to gently squeeze the ovum loose and send it on its way.[7] Apparently, just a few ennervated muscle cells are responsible for one of the most significant squeezes in biology.

To this point it has been seen that, influenced by releasing chemicals from the brain's hypothalamus, the anterior lobe of the pituitary gland has produced and released two hormones. One, FSH, stimulated the growth of follicles that, as they developed, produced estrogen. The second pituitary hormone, LH, caused rupture of the follicle, releasing the egg.

Three parenthetical observations will be made here. First, *conception,* the fertilization of an ovum by a sperm, cannot occur unless both mature sex cells are viable. Upon being released from the ovary, the ovum usually survives for twenty-four to thirty-six hours. For the ovum, assume a maximum survival time

[7] "The Gentle Squeeze That Sent You on Your Way," *New Scientist,* Vol. 53, No. 783 (February 17, 1972), p. 366.

of two days. Upon being deposited in the vagina, sperm usually survive for one to three days. (This would include the several hours of survival in the vagina and the two or three days in the cervix and above.) For sperm, assume a maximum survival time of three days. Usually ovulation occurs, in the average woman, about fourteen days before the onset of the next menstrual period, give or take two days. Keeping in mind the average maximum survival times of the ovum and of sperm, as well as the average day of occurrence of ovulation (with its two-day leeway), refer to Figure 16-5 for an illustration of the average period of fertility of the woman who menstruates every twenty-eight days. Counting from day 1 of the menstrual period, she will ovulate between day 12 and day 16. However, her ovum will survive for about two days. A viable ovum may thus be available for fertilization until approximately day 18 of the menstrual cycle. The woman may have ovulated as early as day 12. For about three days a sperm can survive to fertilize an ovum. It then follows that conception can occur if a sperm is deposited in the vagina as early as three days before ovulation. If the woman menstruates regularly every twenty-eight days (and many normal women do not), she will, on the average, be most likely to become pregnant if sperm are deposited in the vagina between day 9 and day 18 of her menstrual cycle. Throughout this book human individuality is stressed. Menstruation and ovulation are hardly exceptions. Some women menstruate every twenty-one days, others, every thirty-five days. They should calculate their periods of maximum fertility accordingly. For example, the woman who menstruates every twenty-one days can set an ovulation date on day 7 of the menstrual cycle. The woman who menstruates every thirty-fifth day will usually ovulate on day 21. In either case her calculations of maximum fertility must make allowances for a two-day leeway for ovulation and the viability of both ovum and sperm. There are many women whose menstrual cycles from month to month are irregular. Without obtaining a reliable average over a year, they cannot calculate a reasonably reliable period of maximum fertility.

Second, when ovulation occurs, the rupture is accompanied by a small amount of ovarian bleeding. This blood may be irritating and may cause brief abdominal discomfort. With right-side middle-of-the-month pain, the woman may worry that she has appendicitis. Only the physician is equipped to differentiate between the two.

Third, as the follicle develops, its estrogen (step 4 above) affects the uterus. In preparation for implantation of the developing product of the fertilized egg (the embryo), the lining (endometrium) of this organ thickens, as does the muscle layer. Estrogen also affects the cervical secretions, making them more receptive for the sperm if it is there. It also causes the Fallopian tubes to contract more rapidly. (Estrogen, the basic female sex hormone, is responsible for many of the female sex characteristics, such as growth of breast tissue (page 483).

THE DESTINY OF THE RELEASED OVUM   Where does the ovum go? It enters the *Fallopian tube* (see Figure 16-7)[8] nearest the ovary from which the egg

[8] Obstruction of these tubes by inflammation is one of the most common causes of sterility, for the egg cannot reach the uterus. Sometimes, with a partially blocked tube, the sperm does reach the egg to fertilize it. But then the larger fertilized egg cannot get through the tubes to the uterus. A tubal pregnancy results, which can be terminated surgically (see page 179 and footnote 10 on page 478).

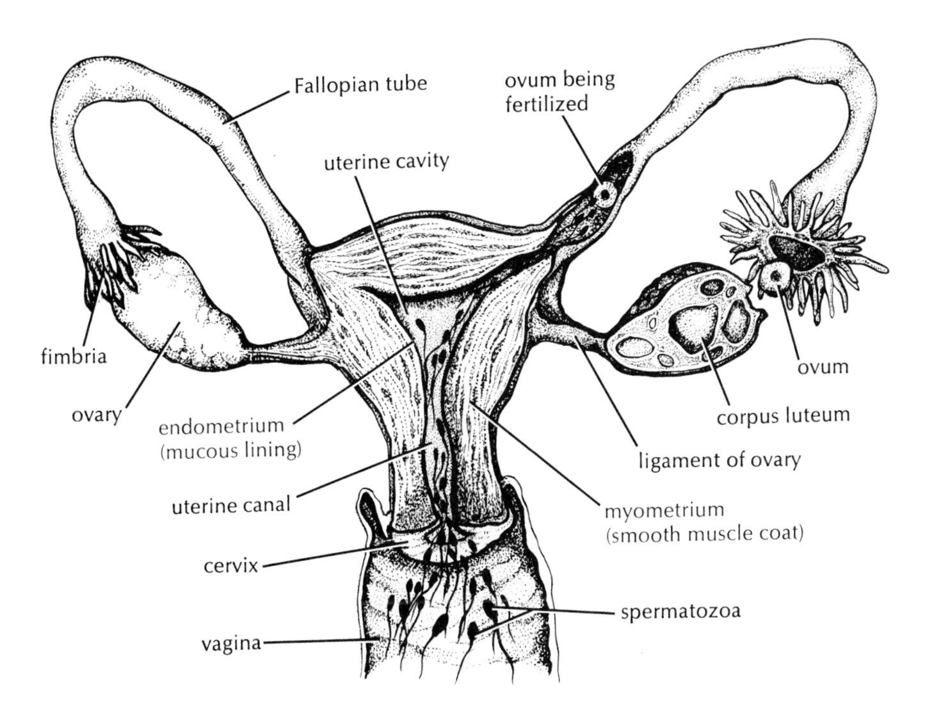

16-7 *An ovum is shown leaving the ovary. The same ovum is shown later being fertilized in the upper Fallopian tube. The fertilized ovum (zygote) will cleave daily (becoming a blastocyst) as it continues down the Fallopian tube to the uterus. After floating in the uterus for several days, it will be implanted in the uterine wall. It should be noted that this is a highly schematic representation.*

came. At its lower end, each of these three- to five-inch tubes opens into the upper uterine cavity. At its upper end, each Fallopian tube lies close but not directly attached to its corresponding ovary. This free end of the Fallopian tube ends in fingerlike projections called *fimbria.* And it is the fimbria that draw the escaped ovum into the Fallopian tube. Now the ovum is ready to be fertilized, to make the journey to the uterus. Unlike spermatozoa, however, it cannot move alone. By the gentle sweeping motions of hairlike cilia lining the Fallopian tube, and by waves of contractions passing along the tube itself, the ovum is helped along its way.

As the ovum begins its journey down the Fallopian tube, what goes on in the emptied follicle that remains behind in the ovary? Under the influence of LH it closes, grows to the size of a lima bean, and takes on a yellowish tint. Now it is called the *corpus luteum* (Latin *corporis,* body + *leuteum,* yellow). Its future function depends on whether or not the ovum is fertilized.

If the ovum is not fertilized within forty-eight hours, it continues down the Fallopian tube to the uterus. There it disintegrates. Any remnant of it is eliminated through the vagina with the menstrual flow. (As was stated on page 476, the time period of ovum viability (its ability to be fertilized) is somewhere between twenty-four hours and about two days.) In the ovary, triggered by LH, the corpus luteum produces the hormone *progesterone,* which means "to promote pregnancy." Indeed, this is its function. Acting upon the uterine endometrium, progesterone causes it to mature in preparation for a fertilized ovum. In the absence of fertilization, the corpus luteum continues to produce progesterone until late in the menstrual cycle. Not until about day 25 does the corpus luteum begin to degenerate to become a small depressed scar in the ovarian tissue. Progesterone is then diminished. Fragments of the uterine endometrium and mucus from the uterine glands slough off with an average of one to three ounces of menstrual blood. A new ovarian cycle is ready to begin.

If the ovum is fertilized (usually in the upper part of a Fallopian tube), the sequence is entirely different. The fertilized ovum (*zygote*) divides, becoming a tiny mass of cells (*blastocyst*), during its two- to four-day trip down the tube to the uterus. Once there, it is not immediately implanted in the uterine wall. Several days may go by before the uterine endometrium is entirely ready. So it is about five to seven days following ovulation that implantation occurs. The elaborately prepared uterine endometrium receives the new life. The zygote is now an embryo. Implantation usually happens between day 18 and day 22. It may, however, occur as late as day 23 of the menstrual cycle.[9] After implantation, the membranes of the embryo produce a *gonadotropic hormone.* This hormone, like LH, stimulates the corpus luteum to produce progesterone.[10]

Indeed, with pregnancy the corpus luteum in the ovary continues its activity for twelve weeks before some of its functions are taken over by the *placenta* (afterbirth). By its timely continued production of estrogen and progesterone, it promotes persistent endometrial growth, so essential in sustaining the intrauterine being. It also prevents the maturation of new follicles. And this last fact makes possible one type of contraceptive pill—a synthetic chemical combination of progesterone and estrogen. Properly taken, the pill prevents ovulation (see Table 21-1, pages 618–21).

the uterus and menstruation

The hollow uterus, about the size and shape of a pear, is a muscular pelvic organ. Nourished and sheltered in this abode, the developing child is an *embryo*

[9] This assumes ovulation occurs on about day 14. Add approximately two to four days in the Fallopian tube, and about another two to four days in the uterus. The subsequent history of the embryo is described in Chapter 19.

[10] Rarely, in about 1 in 350 pregnancies, implantation occurs outside the uterus. These are ectopic pregnancies (Greek *ektopos,* displaced). The extrauterine implantation most commonly occurs within a Fallopian tube, but it can take place in an ovary or even within the abdomen. Within the abdomen the developing embryo may be attached to the large intestine. Severe pain is usually the pregnant woman's first warning that her pregnancy is ectopic. With a pregnancy in the Fallopian tube, this pain usually occurs at about the sixth week. The cure is surgical. Almost all ectopic pregnancies fail to survive. Very rarely, an ectopic pregnancy results in a healthy baby. Perhaps the most unusual of all instances of misplaced pregnancies was reported from Hong Kong. "A three-month-old boy . . . had three fetuses removed from his abdominal cavity after his mother became suspicious of his swelling condition. Of the three fetuses one was 2 inches long and well formed." (Anthony Smith, *The Body* [New York, 1968], p. 109.)

for two months, then a *fetus,* and, upon birth, an *infant.* The upper part of the uterus, its *body,* is mostly muscle. During pregnancy, the uterus enlarges to about sixteen times its normal size. Its muscle enlarges enough to produce contractions adequate to help expel the baby. The smaller lower end of the uterus, the *cervix,* points downward and tilts slightly toward the back into the vagina. It can be felt by the woman and has the consistency of the tip of the nose. Its identification is important to the woman who uses a diaphragm for birth control. The physician can both see and feel the cervix with ease. This is fortunate, for it affords early diagnosis of cancer of the womb, which most commonly begins at this site. There are small mucous glands in the cervix that may become infected. Sometimes they become clogged, causing a mucoid discharge.

The uterus is loosely moored to the bony pelvis by tough fibrous bands called *ligaments.* It is thus suspended in the pelvic cavity between the bladder, in front, and the rectum, behind. The stretching of these ligaments during pregnancy may cause a pulling sensation in the groin. The enlarging pregnant uterus diminishes space for the bladder and rectum (see Figure 16-4). This explains the frequent urinary dribbling that occurs during late pregnancy and the importance of emptying both bladder and rectum to facilitate delivery of the child.

As has been mentioned, the endometrium (the lining of the uterine cavity) is elaborately prepared in anticipation of a viable fertilized egg. Hospitality for the fertilized egg is the basic function of the uterus. Under the influence of estrogen from the maturing ovarian follicle, the endometrium thickens. Fluid accumulates. Blood engorges the tissue. When, however, these preparations are met with naught but an unfertilized and, therefore, degenerating egg, the uterus bleeds. With *menstruation,* the excess endometrium loosens and is discharged, with the mucus from the uterine glands, as blood-filled tissue through the cervical opening and vagina.

SOME UNTRUTHS ABOUT MENSTRUATION The Greeks, wrongly considering menstruation to be a cleansing process, called it *katharsis.* In the first century, Pliny the Elder wrote that menstrual blood dulled razors, and Aristotle thought menstruating women ruined mirrors. The early Hebrews punished those who had intercourse during menstruation (Leviticus 20:18). During medieval times, menstruating women were excluded from churches and wine cellars alike. In the latter case it was believed they would spoil the wine. Menstruating women are still segregated in ''blood huts'' by some African tribes. Child marriage developed among the Hindus because they incorrectly believed that the menstrual blood is essential for the embryo. To lose menstrual blood before pregnancy is still considered irreligious by many Hindus. Not long ago, in rural Russia, menstrual blood was collected in flasks by unmarried girls from as many village women as possible. It was then used by the village witch to determine fertility. Elsewhere in Europe a drop of menstrual blood used to be placed in a swain's wine to help him win the love of its owner.

SOME TRUTHS ABOUT MENSTRUATION During menstruation an absorbent pad is used to absorb the *menses,* or menstrual flow. It may be worn externally, although many women prefer an internal tampon. Tampons may be worn by girls who have just begun to menstruate. That they cannot or should not be used by virgins is a myth. To lessen chances of infection, tampons should be changed at least twice daily. There is no reason whatsoever to limit activity during menstruation. The menstruating woman may engage in any normal activity that she enjoys when she is not menstruating. Bathing, swimming, horseback riding, hairwashing, bicycling, dancing, gym classes—all these are perfectly permissible. Some couples enjoy sexual intercourse during menstruation and there is usually no contraindication to this. The mild abdominal cramping that sometimes occurs during menstruation may require an aspirin or two, but usually even this is not necessary. Douching at the end of menstruation is neither necessary nor recommended. The action of normal vaginal bacteria maintains vaginal cleanliness and health. Because of fluid retention some women may gain a pound or two during the week before the onset of menstruation. This does not call for a change in diet; with the onset the weight is lost, as is an occasional heavy feeling in the pelvis and legs. *Premenstrual tension,* manifested by increased moodiness and irritability, even mild depression, is not uncommonly experienced during the few days prior to the onset of menstruation. These are not usually significant symptoms. In a very few cases, the mild physical discomfort and increased emotional sensitivity combine to make a woman a trial both to herself and to others. Occasionally a woman will even use this situation to gain sympathy. The very rare personality change associated with menstruation usually indicates other deeply rooted problems. The vast majority of women handle their monthly menstrual periods as what they are—an entirely normal indication of femininity during the reproductive years.

Dysmenorrhea, or painful menstruation, does not refer to the ordinary discomfort mentioned above; it is more severe. It may have a wide variety of causes, either physical, psychological, or both. *Menorrhagia* refers to excessive and usually prolonged uterine bleeding occurring at regular intervals. *Metrorrhagia* is uterine bleeding at completely irregular intervals. The amount may be normal; the flow may be prolonged. *Amenorrhea* refers to the cessation of menstruation before the menopause. Sudden changes in climate or emotional distress are among the variables that may cause a change in the amount of menstrual flow; a period may be delayed or may even be skipped because of such factors. Amenorrhea of longer duration is, of course, most commonly due to pregnancy. However, endocrine disorders or severe malnutrition and anemia may cause amenorrhea. Dysmenorrhea, menorrhagia, metrorrhagia, and prolonged amenorrhea all indicate prompt consultation with the family physician.

NORMAL DIFFERENCES AMONG WOMEN Women who desire to be different from other women surely accomplish this with their menstrual histories. The onset of menstruation (*menarche*) varies. On the average, as noted above, it occurs at about twelve and a half years. First menstruations are usually irregular. They may not be associated with ovulation. Some girls menstruate for months or even years without ovulating; so the onset of menstruation does not always mean fertility has begun (see page 498). Abnormally early onsets of menstruation and ovulation are rare. Lena Medina, a classic case in medical history, was delivered of a healthy child when she was only five years and nine months old. An ovarian tumor had accelerated her sexual maturity. Her pregnancy had been caused by rape.

Women normally differ as to the duration (one to six days, with an average of four or five days) and the amount (one to eight ounces, with an average of about two or three ounces) of menstrual bleeding. Individual women also vary from month to month in their onsets of bleeding. For women who calculate "safe periods" for sexual intercourse based on the first day of menstruation, it is essential to keep an accurate record of monthly onsets for at least a year.

An important note: *it is vital for a particular individual to know what is ordinary for her. Any marked departure is the signal for an immediate visit to a physician.* A gross change in menstruation, such as excessive bleeding or spotting between periods, may be of minor significance. It may, however, signify disease such as cancer that, treated early, is easily curable. The diagnosis of such cancers by means of the Papanicolaou test is a painless procedure.

THE MENOPAUSE The age of the cessation of menstruation (*menopause*) varies widely. Today, the U.S. average is about forty-nine. Some women may cease menstruating even before forty, though this is rare. Many modern women menstruate in their fifties. It is possible that the better general health of the woman of today is responsible for the later occurrence of menopause. Although both ovulation and menstruation may stop abruptly, the menopause is usually not a sudden event. With most women, ovulation and menstruation taper off gradually; failure to realize this may result in pregnancy. Because of the irregularity of ovulation at this time, the "change of life" baby is not a common event. Nevertheless, many physicians advise that family planning be continued until no menses have occurred for six months. Just as puberty is accompanied by body changes and the beginning of menstruation, so is the menopause accompanied by body changes and the cessation of the function. The *climacteric* refers to those phenomena, both physical and psychological, which are associated with the end of menstruation in women and, in both sexes, with a diminution in the production of certain chemical compounds, including sex hormones. In the woman, it is the period that is begun by the menopause and during which she enters her postreproductive years. In the man, it is generally marked by some lessening of sexual activity.

Several grossly cruel and senseless untruths should be dismissed. First, the menopause heralds neither old age nor obesity. Second, it is not a common cause of insanity. By far the greatest majority of menopausal women need no medical treatment. As a rule, sexual activity continues. Frequently, it improves. For many women, the feeling of warmth and flushing of the face, neck, and upper body ("hot flashes") and the sweating are mere annoyances. For an unknown reason, they seem to occur most often at night. Some women suffer embarrassment because they believe their hot flashes are noticed by others.

This is not so. There are no outward indications of hot flashes. With a considerable number of women they do not occur. For a few, other symptoms include headaches, irritability, insomnia, and depression. In such cases, overeating results in overweight. Results of the treatment of these symptoms are generally excellent. Her children raised, relieved of some of her pressures, the postmenopausal woman can anticipate thirty or more happy, productive years.

An important note: *a heavier menstrual flow, or "flooding," is not a usual characteristic of the menopause. Excessive bleeding and bleeding between periods* (*regardless of the time of life*) *always indicate immediate consultation with a physician. Delay has cost many a woman her life.*

the vagina

The *vagina* is a tube about three and one-half inches long. The vaginal walls are composed of muscle. The inner surface of the vagina is lined with transverse folds. During childbirth both muscle and folds expand tremendously. Cells from vaginal fluid are useful in determining not only the time of ovulation but also cancer of the uterus. In both instances the cells characteristically reflect these changes. In the virgin, the external opening of the vagina may be partially closed by a fold of mucous membrane called the *hymen* (see Figure 16-4). The hymen is frequently absent in females who have never had sexual intercourse. Rarely, the hymen interferes with the passage of menstrual blood. This is easily corrected by the physician. The normal reaction of the vagina is acid. A bacillus is involved in maintaining this normal reaction. If this acid reaction is not maintained, the vagina is prone to infection. Douching may be advised by a physician to encourage the acidity of the vagina. A woman should not douche unless advised to do so by her physician. Some popular douches not only harm delicate tissues but remove beneficial bacteria (see page 514).

the external genitalia

The *mons pubis* is a rounded fatty pad above the labia majora and over the front pubic region (see Figure 16-4). The word *pubes* refers to the hair growing over the pubic region.[11] The *labia majora* are skin folds that pass backward from the mons pubis. Like the mons they are fatty pads covered, in the adult, with hair. The *clitoris,* at the upper end of the labia minora, is extremely sensitive. Its sole purpose is to stimulate sexual desire. The *labia minora* are about as thick as a large rubber band. They arise from the clitoris and then pass backward and enclose an area called the *vestibule.* The *urethra* (leading from the urinary bladder) and vagina open into the vestibule, as do the *Bartholin's glands* (*vulvovaginal glands*). During prolonged sexual excitement, the Bartholin's glands secrete a small amount of lubricating material; it should not be confused with the vaginal lubrication that occurs early (within seconds) in the woman's sexual response (see page 493). On either side of the opening of the female urethra are

[11] *Pubes* is also the plural of *pubis,* which refers to the pubic bone.

the several small *Skene's ducts.* These and the Bartholin's glands may easily become infected, particularly by the gonococcus.

the mammary glands

Before puberty there is little difference between the male and female breasts. In adult males they remain rudimentary. However, with the onset of puberty in the girl and the production of certain hormones by the ovaries, the breasts begin to develop. With each menstrual cycle the breasts enlarge slightly; they feel heavier, and the nipples are more sensitive. Just below the center of the adult female mammary gland is the raised *nipple,* surrounded by the circular pigmented *areola* (see Figure 16-8). Small openings on the surface of the nipple mark the openings of the ducts of the underlying glandular elements. With pregnancy, these are quite visible during the secretion of milk (*lactation*). The numerous small elevations on the areolar area are due to sebaceous glands. The breast structure is composed of about twenty distinct tubular glands or *lobes,* which, in turn, are composed of many *lobules.* The lobes are embedded in loose connective tissue and fat, which give the breast its shape. Each lobe eventually drains into the *lactiferous duct* of the nipple. Just before the duct terminates into the nipple it is dilated as a *lactiferous sinus.*

During pregnancy the nipples and areolae darken. Around the areola a secondary, lighter areola usually develops. The sebaceous glands of the areola enlarge. They are then called *Montgomery's glands.* They secrete an oily material that keeps the nipple supple and prevents the skin from cracking. Early in pregnancy a thin, scanty, yellow-white precursor of milk is secreted. This continues throughout the entire pregnant period. This secretion is called *colostrum.* During the first days of the baby's life, colostrum is a good food. Before the milk is produced, colostrum may be drawn off to stimulate milk flow. The sense of fullness and the tingling of the breasts sometimes felt in the early months of pregnancy soon abate.

LACTATION: MILK SECRETION At times the lactating woman's provision of milk takes on economic overtones. Even today primitive women, such as the Papuans, suckle an infant at one breast as they suckle a wolf cub or a piglet at the other. In more civilized but stricken societies breast milk has been used to feed the starving adult.

In John Steinbeck's *Grapes of Wrath,* Rose of Sharon smiles mysteriously as she feeds a starving migrant. Wet nurses have long profited from the prime value of their product. During two lactating periods, one woman not long ago expressed thirty thousand ounces of surplus milk that brought her $3,717. Another woman earned $2,020 for her twenty thousand ounces of surplus milk produced during only one lactation. Yet another wet nurse maintained seven babies at one time with her daily product.[12] The buyers are mothers who desire

[12] Ronald S. Illingsworth, *The Normal Child* (Boston, 1968), p. 13.

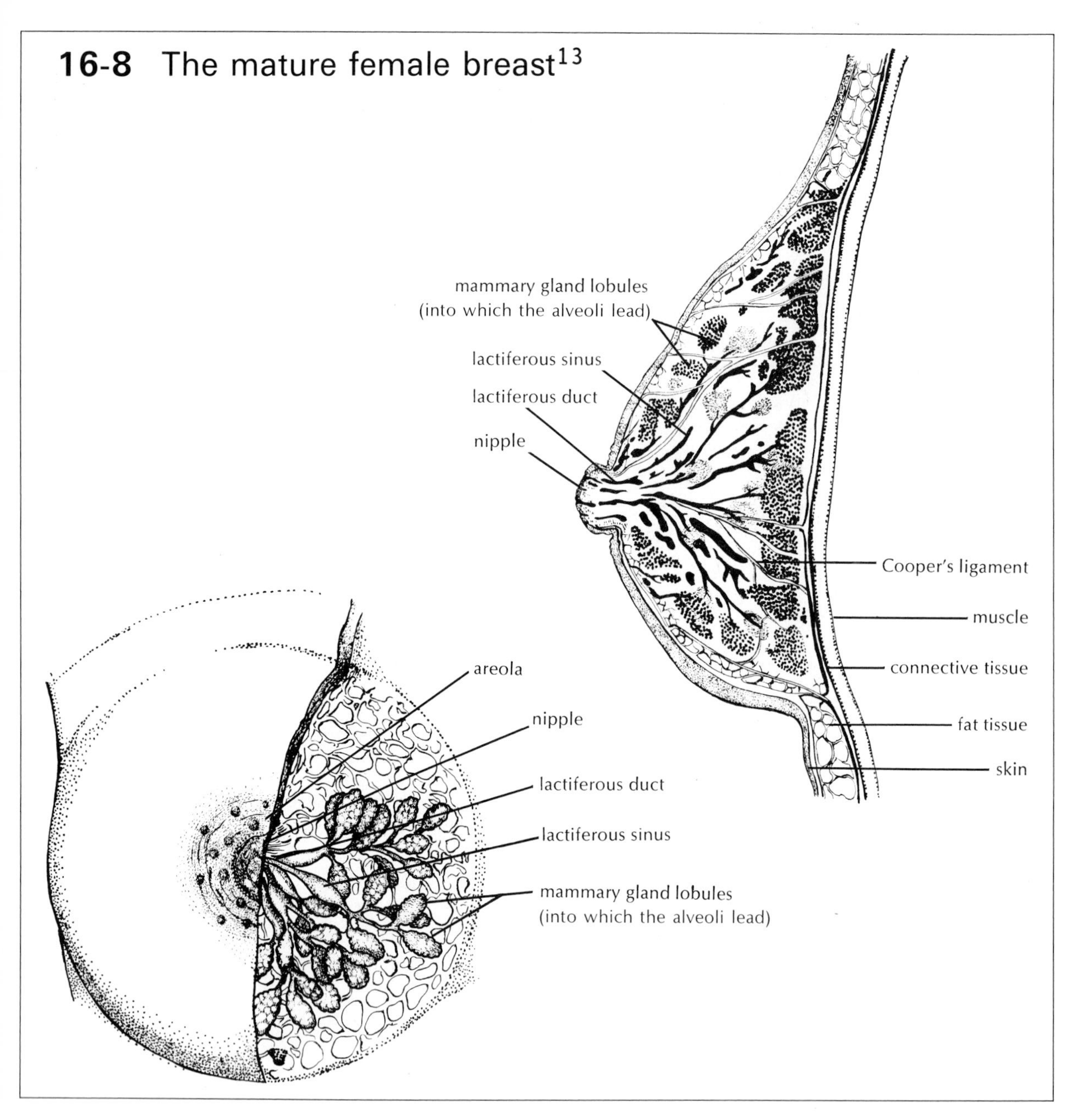

[13] The significance of Cooper's ligaments has recently been reemphasized by two consultant surgeons. These fibrous attachments help to support the breasts. Without adequate brassiere support the ligaments stretch, as does the intrinsic connective tissue. This causes the breasts to droop. No amount of exercise will restore the ligaments. However, exercise may embellish breast contour (sagging or otherwise) by improving posture and increasing the thickness of the underlying pectoral muscle. Modern surgery can restore severely pendulous breasts. Patients who have had such surgery may find that they do not need brassieres as consistently as do other women. (John H. Wulsin and Milton T. Edgerton, "Cooper's Droop: Mystique of the Bra-Less Mamma Maligned," *Journal of the American Medical Association,* Vol. 219, No. 5 [January 31, 1972], p. 625. The term "Cooper's Droop" is credited to Dr. Carl Manion of the University of Kansas Medical Center.)

to feed their babies breast milk, but are unable to produce it in adequate amounts.

However, such mass production and distribution is not ordinarily desired or needed by the average mother who wishes to breast-feed her baby. Breast milk has been called the ideal food. Some of its advantages include its freedom from contamination, its immunity-imparting qualities, its cheapness, and its superior protein balance. In areas where sanitation is poor, such as the tropics, milk that does not come from the mother's breast may be so contaminated as to imperil the baby's life. Moreover, the colostrum of mother's milk contains antibodies that provide the child with immunity to various ailments. Breast-fed babies endure fewer respiratory infections. Among breast-fed babies allergies are less common, as is the likelihood of soreness about the anus. The protein balance of mother's milk is superior for the baby's growth to the protein balance of cow's milk, but there is little evidence that, in the long run, bottle-fed babies suffer as a result of this nutritional difference. Cow's milk contains more protein, thiamin, riboflavin, and calcium, but less iron and vitamin C. In the more affluent countries, the nutritional deficiencies of cow's milk are easily corrected with supplements. Also, although difficult to prove by controlled studies, many psychiatrists feel that, to a varying extent, bottle-feeding deprives both the child and mother of some psychological advantage that is gained by intimacy. But it is doubtless just as true that the mother who unhappily breast-feeds her baby has and gives a more harmful experience than the mother who happily bottle-feeds her baby.

Although the lactating mother must eat more to have an adequate milk supply, breast-feeding is probably cheaper. Breast-feeding may mean less work for the mother. True, the stools of bottle-fed babies are firm, and the looser stools of breast-fed babies make diapers more difficult to clean. But these days this advantage is negated by the use of disposable diapers. And breast-feeding obviates sterilization of bottles as well as measuring and mixing and warming the food.

There are also some disadvantages to breast-feeding that should be considered. Not uncommonly, breast-fed babies are underfed, a fact that may never occur to the willing mother. This may be due to an inadequate milk supply. The drugs and chemicals to which the mother is exposed and which then pass into her milk constitute a serious modern problem. The nursing mother should be extremely careful about drug use, for her milk may become dangerously contaminated. The toxicity of a drug depends, in part, on body weight. A safe dose for the mother may be an unsafe dose for her breast-fed baby. Among those drugs that should be used with caution or not at all are alcohol, tobacco, oral contraceptives, and marihuana. A daily cocktail or two is not a contraindication to breast-feeding. More alcohol may be. The woman who smokes heavily should not breast-feed her baby because of the toxicity of the nicotine. Oral contraceptives interfere with the production of milk and should not be used by nursing mothers. The effects of marihuana on a baby are unknown—reason enough to contraindicate its use by the mother who desires to breast-feed her child. Although in the future contamination of the mother's milk by DDT or radiation may become a problem in some countries, there is not enough evidence to indicate that present levels of DDT or radiation in the environment in the U.S. are high enough to make mother's milk dangerous to the child.

summary

Like other body structures, the sex glands—male *testes* and female *ovaries*—are controlled by hormones from the anterior lobe of the pituitary gland, which in turn is controlled by hormones from the hypothalamus of the brain (page 466). Hormones from another gland in the brain, the *pineal gland,* or *pineal body,* may also affect the sexual function (page 466).

The major structures of the *male reproductive system* are the two *testes,* which are contained in an external sac called the *scrotum* and which produce *spermatozoa* and the hormone *testosterone* (page 467); and the *penis,* which can become erect in response to a spinal nerve reflex (page 470) and through which *semen* containing spermatozoa (page 471) is transmitted and deposited in the female vagina during *ejaculation* (pages 470–71).

The major structures of the *female reproductive system* are the two *ovaries,* in which *follicles* are formed—which, while maturing, produce the hormone *estrogen* (page 474). A mature follicle is called an *ovum* (egg). One of the ovaries ordinarily releases one ovum every month in a process called *ovulation* (pages 472–76). The ovum travels through one of the two *Fallopian tubes* (pages 476–78). If it is not fertilized by a spermatozoon, it continues to the *uterus* (pages 478–79), where it disintegrates and is eliminated through the vagina (page 482) in *menstruation* (pages 479–82). If the ovum is fertilized, it is called a *zygote;* it continues down the tube, dividing (and now called a *blastocyst*) and becoming implanted as an *embryo* in the prepared wall of the uterus (page 478). Other structures of the female reproductive system are the external genitalia—*mons pubis, labia,* and *clitoris* (pages 482–83). The *mammary glands,* or *breasts,* may also be regarded as part of the female reproductive duct system (pages 483–86).

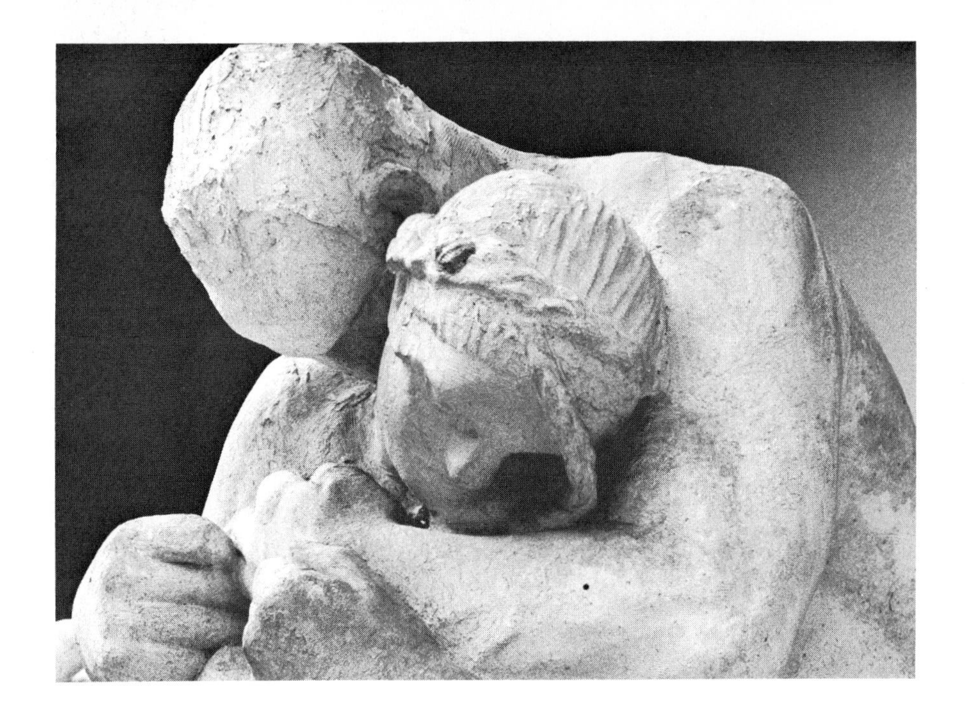

the sexual life

17

the biological logic of mutuality

the primordial female

"In the beginning, we were all created females; and if this were not so, we would not be here at all."[1] This remarkable statement is the culmination of years of biological research. In their first stage of development, the sex organs of the mammalian embryo (including the human) consist of two elevations of tissue. These are the *genital ridges.* Each ridge contains the cells necessary for the development of either an ovary or a testis. Since it can develop in either direction—female ovary or male testis—each genital ridge must be considered an undifferentiated primitive gonad. (A gonad [Greek *gone,* seed] is a gland producing spermatozoa or ova.) The outer rind of each undifferentiated gonad is capable of becoming an ovary; the inner core is capable of becoming a testis. However, although genetic sex is established at conception, the sex genes do not exert their influence until the fifth or sixth week of life. At that time, if the genetic instruction is to produce a male, the inner cores of the embryonic gonadal ridges develop into testes. For this to occur, it appears that some active secretory process is necessary. (Should this process fail to happen, the tendency of the embryo's genital ridges is to develop ovaries.) Once the primitive testes have been formed, they secrete both the male hormone androgen and a second substance. This other substance inhibits the development and causes the regression of those embryonic tissues that could become the organs of the female internal reproductive system (tubes, uterus, and vagina). The androgen causes the development of the male internal and external reproductive system. The male substances thus overcome the female pattern.

However, if the genetic instruction is to produce a female, the processes by which testes, androgen, and female-inhibiting substance are produced do not take place, nor do the subsequent events. The outer rinds of the genital ridges—the female cellular potentials—proliferate into ovaries. In the absence of androgen and the female-inhibiting substance, a female results from the already existing, and thus primordial, tissue.

Scientists have conclusively proved that in the absence of embryonic androgen the female potential develops regardless of the genetic sex. They have removed the undifferentiated gonads of a male rabbit embryo within the uterus by means of exquisitely delicate surgical techniques. In the absence of testes (and, therefore, androgen), the genetic male was born with completely female external genitalia. When the undifferentiated gonads of a female embryo in the uterus were removed, the genetic female rabbit was, of course, born without ovaries, but with completely female genitalia. The ovarian hormone estrogen is not needed for differentiation into a female; however, androgen is essential for differentiation into a male. Clearly, then, the external female sex organs are not rudimentary, imperfect, inadequate versions of the male sex organs. "Na-

[1] Mary Jane Sherfey, "The Evolution and Nature of Female Sexuality in Relation to Psychoanalytic Theory," *Journal of the American Psychoanalytic Association,* Vol. 14, No. 1 (January 1966), p. 43.

ture's prime disposition is to produce females; maleness only results from something added—androgens.''[2] In other words, ''only the male embryo is required to undergo a differentiating transformation of the sexual anatomy; and only one hormone, androgen, is necessary for the masculinization of the originally female genital tract.''[3] The female genital tract develops independently, without cellular transformation by a hormone. Thus, it is the female whose tissue is primordial; and the sex organs of the male are an out-growth of her original tissue. The penis develops from the primordia of the clitoris; the scrotum, from the primordia of the labia; the male, from the female. Embryologically, man comes from woman.[4]

the male brain: an androgenized female brain

Recent research has revealed some startling additional information about androgen. The results of experiments with laboratory animals support the following concept:

> It does appear that one of the principle actions of androgen during development is to organize the immature central nervous system into that of the male . . . we are talking about an active process; that is, the presence of androgen during development acts upon the brain to program, in effect, patterns of maleness. The absence of androgen permits the ongoing process of femaleness to pursue its natural course. The evidence to support this theory is now abundant.[5]

Thus ''the brain makes do with one type of anatomic system . . . The male brain is an androgenized female brain.''[6]

What do some of these findings suggest? As has been pointed out, modern biological knowledge militates against the sexual subordination of woman. In addition, these studies suggest an explanation for the greater prevalence of divergent sexual behavior among males. Most behavioral scientists agree that homosexual behavior, for example (see pages 305–10), is more prevalent among men than women. This difference is even more marked with other forms of divergent sexual behavior.

[2] Warren J. Gadpaille, ''Research Into the Physiology of Maleness and Femaleness,'' *Archives of General Psychiatry,* Vol. 26, No. 3 (March 1972), p. 195.

[3] Mary Jane Sherfey, ''The Evolution and Nature of Female Sexuality in Relation to Psychoanalytic Theory,'' p. 45.

[4] These findings lend themselves to speculation. Is woman ''superior,'' since she was embryologically first? Is man ''superior,'' since he is ''furthest along the evolutionary line''? Doubtless it is most sensible to put aside the notion of ''superiority'' and, instead, to use this new information for a more mature, realistic, and therefore enjoyable appreciation of the opposite sex.

[5] Seymour Levine, ''Sexual Differentiation: The Development of Maleness and Femaleness,'' *California Medicine,* Vol. 114, No. 1 (January 1971), p. 13. Other research has indicated a relationship between a high IQ and an overproduction of fetal androgen or hormones with an androgenlike side effect. Included in the study were fifty-three female hermaphrodites and seventeen males who, it was determined, had also experienced an overproduction of fetal androgen. Sixty percent displayed an IQ of over 110; in the general population the expected percentage of such an IQ is 25 percent. An astonishing 13 percent had an IQ of over 130; this level is reached by only 2.2 percent of the general population. Corrective hormone therapy after birth apparently does not change the disproportionate ratio of high IQ's. The significance of this discovery is being studied. In the general population, there are no marked differences between the sexes in IQ. (John W. Money, ''Pre-natal Hormones and Intelligence: A Possible Relationship,'' *Impact of Science on Society,* Vol. 21, No. 4 [1971], pp. 285–90.)

[6] Robert J. Stoller, ''The 'Bedrock' of Masculinity and Femininity: Bisexuality,'' *Archives of General Psychiatry,* Vol. 26, No. 3 (March 1972), p. 209.

Elsewhere in this book, reference is made to the fragility of the male as compared to the female (see pages 544–46). It has been suggested that his comparative weakness is not limited to the more physical aspects of life. The male's "reproductive function and psychosocial development is much more easily tipped off-balance or derailed than that of the female."[7] It is the male embryo that is subject to the added chances for error caused by formidable androgenic changes. It is the male whose embryonic brain patterns must be radically altered. The female embryo is the original one; it develops autonomously. Furthermore, the changes necessary for the production of a male take place at a critical period in the development of the embryo.

> The power of the critical period is so great that a single pulse of hormone in the laboratory may set for life the gender behavior as masculine or feminine (without there being any anatomic change in the body, for by this time the development of the reproductive anatomy is complete).[8]

the roots of sexual behavior

The presence or absence of androgen does more than determine physical reproductive function. By its organizing effect on the hypothalamus and nearby nervous tissue, it produces a change that predictably affects masculine or feminine sexual behavior. "Only if the fetal brain (hypothalamus) is organized by androgen does masculine behavior result. And, if normally occurring androgens are blocked in the male, then . . . femininity appears."[9] This has now been established beyond question by both clinical observation and laboratory experimentation with animals.

the role of learning in gender identity

There are, however, more pervasive factors influencing the child's gender identity than the hormonal influences. These are the culturally learned patterns of behavior and thought that are inculcated in the child from birth by the parents and by society as a whole. What the child is taught by the culture concerning gender identity transcends the effects of chromosomes, hormones, and other physiological factors.

> It is . . . clear that gender of assignment and rearing predictably take precedence over and override all contradictory determinants: chromosomes, hormones, gonads, internal and external sexual morphology [structure] and secondary pubertal changes . . . the critical period for core formation of gender identity may be between 12 and 18 months . . . after about 2 to $2\frac{1}{2}$ years of age, shift of core identity cannot take place, even when *all* sexual determinants are those

[7] Warren J. Gadpaille, "Research Into the Physiology of Maleness and Femaleness," p. 203.
[8] Robert J. Stoller, "The 'Bedrock' of Masculinity and Femininity: Bisexuality," p. 210.
[9] *Ibid.*, p. 209. See also Warren J. Gadpaille, "Research Into the Physiology of Maleness and Femaleness," p. 194. Significantly, moreover, it is the male hormone testosterone (see page 467) that most strongly influences sexual desire in both sexes. Females secrete most of their male hormones in the adrenal glands. Women who have had their adrenal glands surgically removed lose their sexual desire. Women who have had their ovaries removed, with subsequent loss of estrogens, rarely lose their sexual desire.

of the other sex. Thus far in the literature there are no reported cases of successful shift after that age; there are, on the other hand, numerous case reports of psychological havoc and tragedy brought about by efforts to effect or enforce such a shift after the critical period."[10]

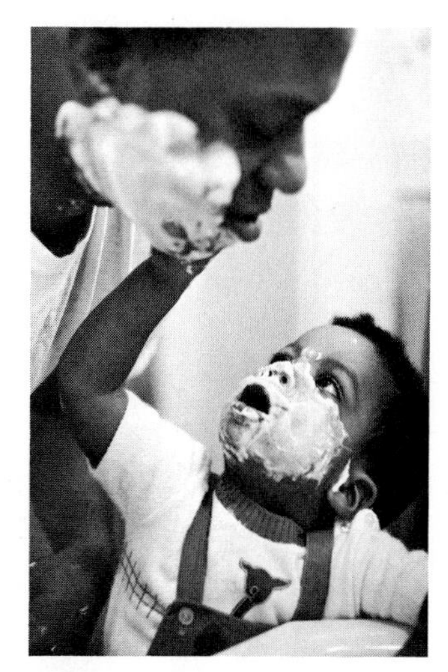

17-1 *Learning gender identity.*

The higher a creature is placed on the evolutionary scale the greater is the importance of learning in sexual behavior. Among all animals, it is most important in man. The learning experience of peer group juvenile sex play seems to be of greater significance for the achievement of competent adult sexual function than even mothering.[11]

The overwhelming influence of learning on the child's sense of gender identity can be most clearly seen in the case of hermaphrodites. There are various kinds of hermaphrodites; a *true* hermaphrodite, however, has both ovarian and testicular tissue either separate or in the same gonad.[12] The individual is physically a member of both sexes and the appearance of the external genitalia is inconclusive. If the parents are continuously uncertain about the sex to which their hermaphroditic child should be assigned, the child will go through life believing that he or she is of neither sex or of both sexes. However, if the parents are certain of the child's gender (whether male or female), the child will also be certain. This is true even when the genitalia are ambiguous. "There is no genetic or innate mechanism to preordain the masculinity or femininity of psychosexual differentiation . . . The analogy is with language. Genetics and innate determinants ordain only that language can develop . . . but not whether the language will be Arabic, English or any other."[13]

Different interpretations of maleness and femaleness have been made not only in various cultures but also during various periods of history. Is it the male who is always sexually aggressive? Not among the Muria in India. As was mentioned in Chapter 15, they expect the woman to be as aggressive as the man. "The Andaman Islanders like to have a man sit on his wife's lap in fond greetings, and friends and relatives, of the same or opposite sex, greet one another in the same manner after absences, crying in the affected manner of the mid-Victorian woman."[14] In many European countries embracing men are unnoticed. In the United States such behavior in everyday encounters would be noticed with amused (and hopefully tolerant) doubts about gender identity, although embracing among women is acceptable. However, men may publicly embrace with impunity in this country under specific circumstances. Upon scoring a touchdown, football players not only embrace vigorously, but have been known to weep and to add an affectionate pat on the bottom to their expressions of affection.

[10] Warren J. Gadpaille, "Research Into the Physiology of Maleness and Femaleness," p. 200.
[11] *Ibid.*, p. 202.
[12] John W. Money, *Sex Errors of the Body* (Baltimore, 1968), pp. 42–43. (This wise and authoritative little book is highly recommended to anyone interested in this field.)
[13] Judd Marmor, "'Normal' and 'Deviant' Sexual Behavior," *Journal of the American Medical Association,* Vol. 217, No. 2, citing John Money, "Developmental Differentiation of Femininity and Masculinity Compared," in S. M. Farber and R. H. L. Wilson, eds., *Man and Civilization* (New York, 1963), pp. 56–57.
[14] Judd Marmor, "'Normal' and 'Deviant' Sexual Behavior," citing M. K. Opler, "Anthropological and Cross-Cultural Aspects of Homosexuality," in Judd Marmor, ed., *Sexual Inversion: The Multiple Roots of Homosexuality* (New York, 1965), pp. 108–23.

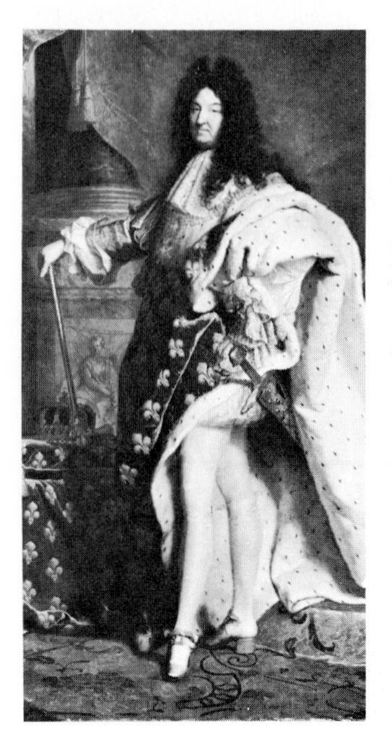

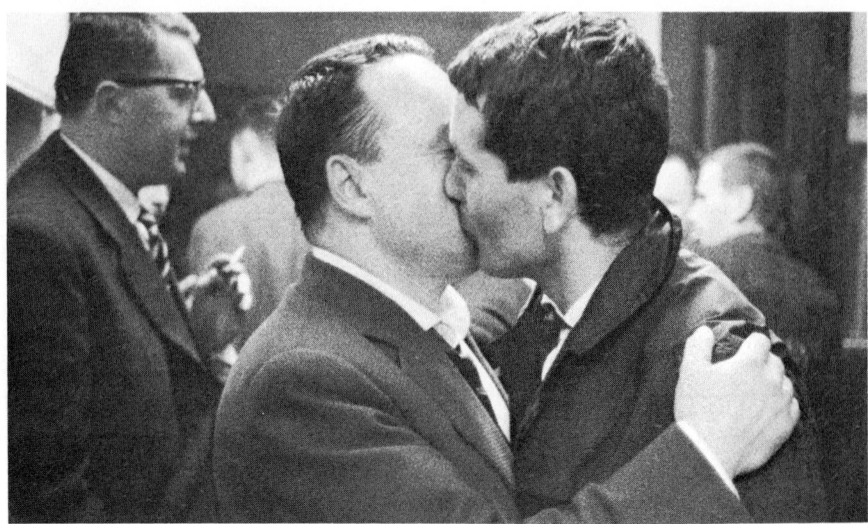

17-2 *Ideas of acceptable male and female behavior and appearance vary with the culture and the time.* Above: *Bar patrons in Czechoslovakia pay no attention as two men embrace and kiss in greeting.* Left: *King Louis XIV of France (1638–1715).*

Nor do clothes make the man—or woman. The colorful beads and shirts worn by many young men in this country today were worn by many young men in this country years before them—the Navajo Indians. Nor were the bejeweled, berouged, perfumed, powdered, curly-wigged, girdled, miniskirted, panty-hosed, high-heeled males of former days particularly noted for their indifference to women. Indeed, it was not until relatively recent times that women's legs replaced men's as objects of sexual admiration, and "unmentionables" were anything else but male garments.[15]

on the physiology of the human sexual response

William H. Masters and Virginia E. Johnson, of the Reproductive Biology Research Foundation at St. Louis, have written the most authoritative recent account of the physiology of the human sexual response.[16] Most of the discussion in this section is based on their work.

In their discussion Masters and Johnson divide the sexual responses of both sexes into four phases: the *excitement phase,* varying from a few minutes to hours; the intense, shorter (thirty seconds to three minutes) *plateau phase;* the three- to ten-second *orgasmic phase* (sometimes longer in women); and the *resolution phase,* lasting ten to fifteen minutes with an orgasm and, without orgasm, lasting as long as twelve to twenty-four hours.

[15] Una Stannard, "Clothing and Sexuality," *Sexual Behavior,* Vol. 1, No. 2 (May 1971), p. 30.
[16] William H. Masters and Virginia E. Johnson, *Human Sexual Response* (Boston, 1966).

It should be emphasized that sex is more than a total body experience. It is an experience of the whole personality. One psychiatrist considers the female orgasm to be "the manifestation of that all-pervading instinct for survival of the child that is the primary organizer of the woman's sexual drive and by this also of her personality."[17] Other people reject this notion; they believe it to be still another outmoded and restrictive idea about woman's sexual expression. Whatever the opinion, it is well to remember that since there is no human equation, some individual variations are common and should be expected.

in the female

Even the early feminine responses to adequate sexual stimulation (during the excitement phase) are not limited to the pelvis. They are widely distributed. From contracting great muscles of the thighs, abdomen, and back, to the tiny muscle fibers often erecting the nipples, the woman's sexual attention is total. The distention of the breast veins as they become engorged with blood and the marked increase in breast size is called *tumescence*—swelling. (Tumescence occurs in all distensible parts of the body and is the major feature of the sexual response in both sexes. It results from the enormous increase of blood in the surface circulation. In these areas blood is forced in through the arteries faster than it can leave via the capillaries and veins. The presence of a special erectile tissue in some areas—the walls of the inner nose, the nipples, vaginal entrance, clitoris, and penis—makes them particularly susceptible to the swelling tensions of tumescence.) During the late excitement phase, or early in the plateau phase, in perhaps three-fourths of women and one-fourth of men, there begins the *sex flush.* Much more noticeable in fair-skinned people, this temporary, measleslike rash first appears on the skin of the abdomen. As sexual excitement intensifies, the rash spreads but it will disappear immediately after coitus. Often it does not occur. The clitoris also undergoes tumescence, and the vagina had begun early to secrete a lubricating fluid by a process not unlike sweating. This fluid aids penetration of the penis, thereby facilitating coitus. As sexual excitement continues, a sudden contraction of muscles encircling the vagina may cause some of this accumulated fluid to spurt out. This has led to the completely mistaken notion that women ejaculate as do men. In this first phase, the inner two-thirds of the vagina increases in size and the uterus contracts rapidly and irregularly. The reaction of the labia depends on whether the woman has given birth. If she has not, the labia majora will thin and flatten, if she has, they will enlarge. In both instances the labia minora increase in size. Bartholin's glands may, in this stage or the next, and during prolonged coital activity, produce a slight secretion to ease the entrance of the penis. The heart rate quickens, and, as is to be expected with sexual excitement, the blood pressure rises.

In the second phase, the plateau phase, tumescence and the sex flush reach their peak. From head to toe, muscle tension reflects the physical and emotional absorption with the impending climax. Evidence of this is in the facial grimace, the flaring nostrils, rigid neck, arched back, and tensed thighs and buttocks.

[17] From "Female Sexuality," a panel meeting of the American Psychoanalytic Association held in Detroit, Michigan, May 6, 1967, and reported by Warren J. Barker, *Journal of the American Psychoanalytic Association,* Vol. 16, No. 1 (January 1968), p. 126.

Now respiration increases and the heart rate and blood pressure remain high. It is in the plateau phase that the clitoris withdraws from its normally overhanging position, pulling back deeply beneath its hood. Contraction of the encircling muscles of the vagina causes it to tighten about the penile shaft. Within these vaginal muscles, the veins become engorged with blood. Added to this venous congestion is that occurring in the veins of the irregularly contracting uterus as well as the other pelvic organs. And it is when the woman reaches the plateau phase of her sexual tension that her labia minora change color in a remarkable way. The color change of the labia minora with the woman who has never borne a child varies from a pink to a bright red. The labia minora of the woman who has borne a child varies from a bright red to a deep wine. So specific are these color changes of the labia minora that they have been termed the "sex skin." In the premenopausal woman, the sex skin is absolutely indicative of impending orgasm. The *pelvic congestion* is relieved by the third level of the woman's sexual cycle, the orgasmic phase.

The orgasm is the pleasurable peak of the sexual experience. This explosive release of body-wide, purposively developed, neuromuscular tension lasts from three to ten seconds. Hearing, vision, taste—all the senses are diminished or lost. It was during the excitement phase that this loss of sensory awareness had begun. It has been said that only a sneeze is as physiologically all-absorbing as an orgasm. But a sneeze is mostly a local experience and an orgasm is not. Although the sensation of orgasm is centered in the pelvis, the whole body responds to it. Of all the widespread muscle responses, the contractions of the muscles in the floor of the pelvis that surround the lower third of the vagina cause the most unique phenomenon. These muscles contract against the engorged veins that surround that part of the vagina and force the blood out of them. This creates the orgasm. These contractions, in turn, cause the lower third of the vagina and the nearby upper labia minora to contract between three and fifteen times. The strength and number of these orgasmic contractions vary greatly and normally, as does the whole sexual experience.

The resolution phase of the woman's sexual response is marked by prompt disappearance of the sex flush, the fading of the sex skin color, the decline of muscle tension and tumescence (detumescence), and her general return to the prestimulated condition.

in the male

Masters and Johnson have emphasized the physiological similarities of the sexes in their sexual responses. All the phases and the general changes, such as muscle contractions and tumescence, also occur in the male. In the excitement phase, blood that is delivered to the penis enters the spaces of its spongy erectile tissue. The structure within the penis efficiently prevents return of most of the blood from that organ into the general venous circulation. Penile enlargement and stiffening result. (There is no relationship whatsoever between the size of the penis and either virility or fertility.) During the male's plateau phase, the tumescent testes are elevated and become so congested with blood that they increase in size from 50 to 100 percent.

Orgasm and *ejaculation* occur simultaneously. The contractions of the epididymis, vas deferens, seminal vesicles, and prostate produce the sensation of imminent ejaculation. The force of perineal muscle contractions causes the seminal fluid to squirt out from the penis. This ejaculation accompanying the male orgasm is the most singular physiological difference in sexual response between the sexes.

General detumescence of the male is rapid (resolution phase). Penile detumescence usually occurs in two stages. After ejaculation the penis quickly returns to be about 50 percent larger than its prestimulated flaccid state. Although complete erection increases the actual size of the penis considerably, it often seems that the initial stage of penile detumescence has not actually caused much diminution of the erection. Depending largely on the kind and duration of the stimuli of the excitement and plateau stages, final detumescence requires a longer time. After orgasm, the male experiences a *refractory period*—a temporary resistance to sexual stimulation. During this period, the sexual stimulation that excited him earlier is no longer effective. It may be distasteful.[18] But restimulation of the woman after her orgasm may result in one or more orgasms. Nothing will help more in understanding this complex human difference than honest communication. The man, for example, may learn to delay his orgasm until his wife has been satisfied. Consistent premature ejaculation with loss of erection is a frequent problem that can be effectively helped (see pages 516–17).

sexual similarities

Some essential similarities between the male and female sexual response may be noted from the preceding sections. The sexual response of each may be divided into four phases. Both sexes respond to touch, and a variety of stimuli may serve to arouse either sex. Nor is it true that the female responds much more slowly to sexual stimuli than does the male. Her history of a tardy response is due to cultural repression. When the female is able to time her own responses, when she herself regulates the rhythm and intensity of her stimuli (as occurs with masturbation), the time she requires to reach an orgasm approximates that of the male. In addition, both the male and female share the phenomenon of tumescence. And, despite the male ejaculation, the physiology of orgasm is similar in both sexes.

[18] Recent research suggests that the male rat has a way of notifying the female of his sexual disinterest during his refractory period. After ejaculation he sings an ultrasonic song. The song corresponds to the period during which he cannot spontaneously initiate copulation. His song signals the female, who then refrains from sexually provocative behavior such as ear-wiggling and darting about. The measured frequency of the ultrasonic sounds of the male rat's "I'm out of action" song is exactly that of males who have been beaten in a fight, or of females who resist overattentive males. Thus "in general they appear to be desist-contact signals." (Ronald J. Barfield and Lynette A. Geyer, "Sexual Behavior: Ultrasonic Postejaculatory Song of the Male Rat," *Science,* Vol. 176, No. 4041 [June 23, 1971], p. 1349.) Demonstrating that the truly scientific mind is never idle, nor ever at a loss to turn pure science into some practical application, one journal published this reflection: "It should now surely be interesting to know what would happen if a rat colony was played continuous recordings of these antisocial signals. Could one devise an ultrasonic rat contraceptive?" ("A Song for the Male Who Has Had Enough," *New Scientist,* Vol. 55, No. 803 [July 6, 1972], p. 7.)

17-3 the embrace of life

The sculptures on these two pages and page 487 are by the Norwegian artist Gustav Vigeland (1869–1943).

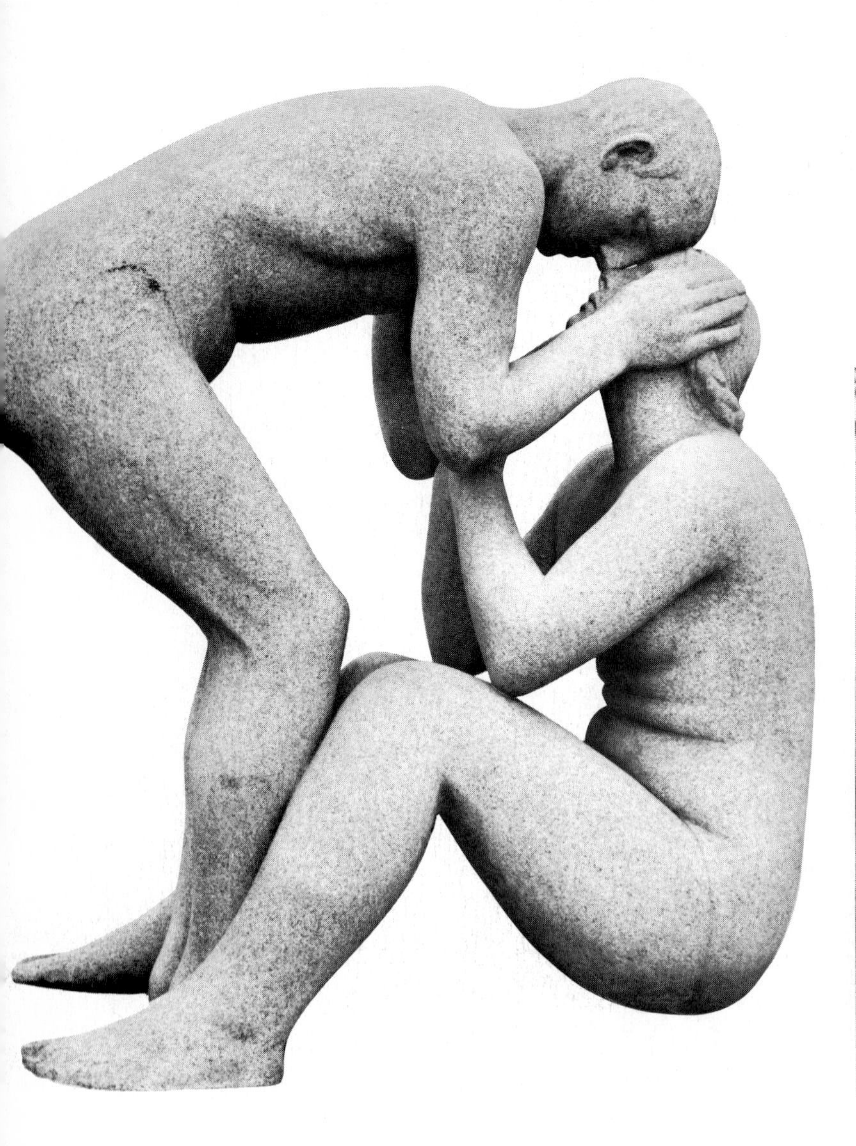

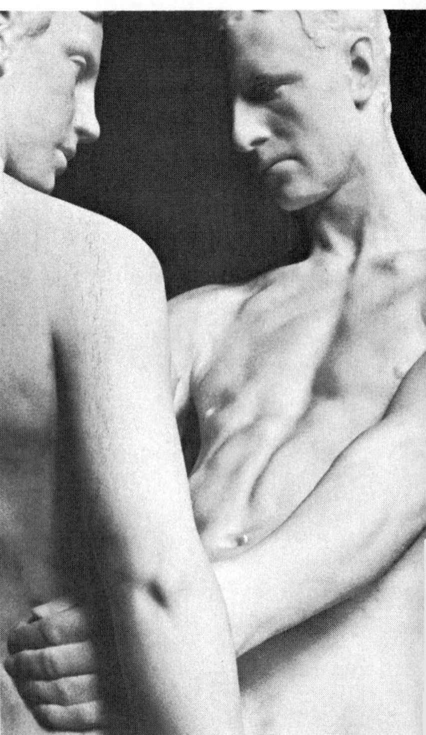

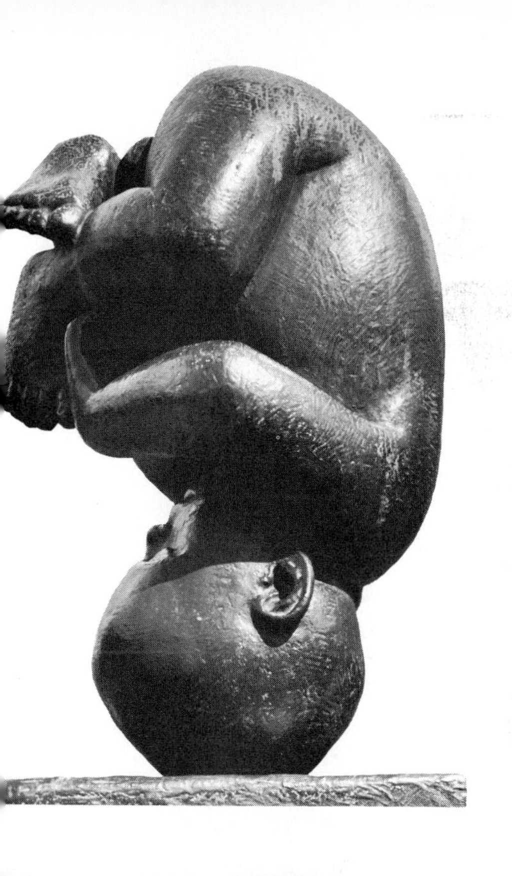

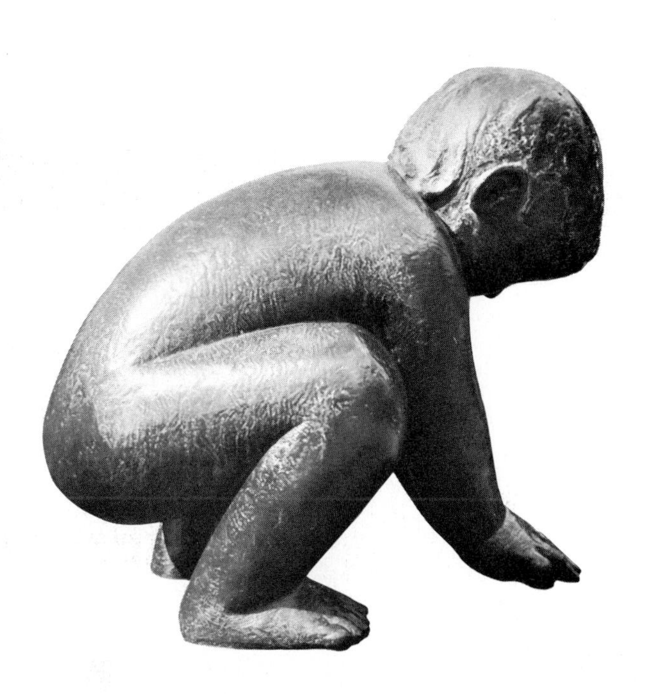

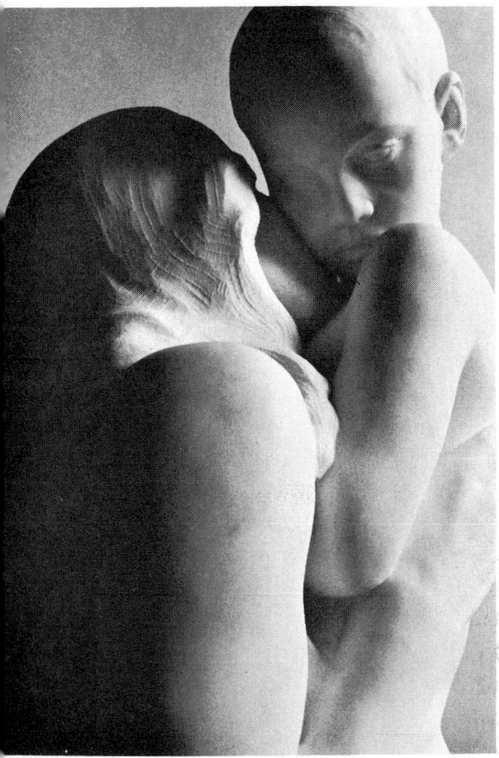

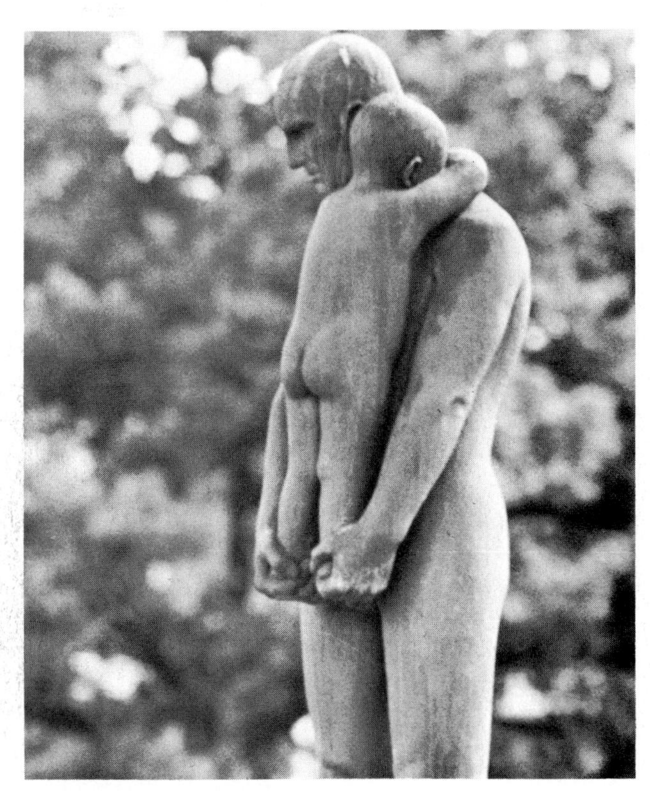

sexual differences

differences in adolescent sexuality

Nevertheless, there are some basic differences in the sexual responses of the male and female. These differences begin to be noticeable at puberty. True puberty is marked by change in the ovaries and testes and changes in their secretions. With the first ejaculation, or soon after, most boys produce viable spermatozoa. In the female, however, puberty does not necessarily include the ability to become pregnant. And if pregnancy should occur, it does not follow that the child can be carried to term. Ancient physicians were aware of this distinction. Puberty (Latin *pubes,* hair) indicated the time that certain body parts became covered with hair. Nubility (Latin *nubis,* veil) meant the time that a girl was able to wear the nuptial veil and be married. A girl may experience a period of *adolescent sterility.* Although this is ordinary, there are exceptions. And the length of time that the adolescent female remains sterile varies greatly. Many adolescent menstrual cycles do not include ovulation. This developmental difference between the adolescent boy and girl may account for the subtle yet profound differences in sexual arousal and response. In addition, the dissimilar development of the sexual cells may explain why a physically mature adolescent girl generally is not strongly impelled to seek physical expressions of her sexuality, while a boy is.

When ova do begin to mature completely, they do so singly and are discharged without accumulating. Unlike the female, the male adolescent is vexed by accumulated and trapped sexual fluids, which must escape by ejaculation. In the young girl, sexual stimulation results in a rather diffuse reaction that is dominated by the cerebral cortex. Her increased adolescent sexuality is socially oriented toward marriage. In the adolescent male, a similar amount of sexual stimulation results in the increased production of spermatozoa and the flow of secretions from the accessory sex glands. With this pressure the ejaculatory reflex is excited. His tensions can be relieved only by ejaculation. In the male this is not a diffuse but a local reaction. It is not as cerebral as it is genital. His increased adolescent sexuality is genitally orientated. Although he is capable of great tenderness at this age, only later does his sexuality become social. "This contrast points to a basic distinction between the developmental processes for males and females: males move from privatized personal sexuality to sociosexuality; females do the reverse and at a later stage in the life cycle."[19] Combine this with the ordinarily greater sexual imagery of the young male, and the reasons for his earlier interest in sexual relief becomes clear. However, despite his sexual urgencies, the young adolescent boy finds that girls his own age are quite indifferent to him. Indeed, they may be contemptuous of his clumsy shyness. The early sociosexual orientation of the young adolescent girl explains her interest in dating older boys. It is not sexual expression that she seeks; it is social expression. The awkward boys of her age lack the social sophistication that is necessary to gratify her needs.

[19] William Simon and John Gagnon, "Psychosexual Development," *Trans-action,* Vol. 6, No. 5 (March 5, 1969), p. 13.

The average man can more frequently achieve sexual gratification independent of love than can the average woman. For many women, sexual expression, particularly coitus, is inseparable from love. Married men rate sexual intercourse with the woman for whom they feel affection as the most important feature of their marriage. Most married women tend to rank sexual intercourse lower than security. For them a home and children are the most important elements of marriage. This difference the husband will do well to heed. For the male to bring casualness to the marital bed is to invite rejection or, worse, resentful submission. The wise husband will "seduce his wife romantically rather than erotically, to put her in the right frame of mind by romantic words and settings that appeal to her."[20] The greater emphasis on security rather than sexuality by most women may well be associated with their greater ability to endure sexual deprivation.

differences in attitude toward sexuality

The sexes are not equally aroused by the same stimuli. It is believed that fewer women than men are sexually stimulated by nudity, erotic movies, or sexual stories. The fact that upper-class men seem to be more susceptible to stimulation by these than men of lower socioeconomic levels indicates that the response may be learned. Women seem to be more easily aroused by such stimuli as romantic movies and stories, although, again, cultural conditioning doubtless plays a part in their response. Moreover, sexual fantasies are much more common among men than women. During both masturbation and sexual intercourse, many more men than women are inclined to make use of sexual fantasies. Frequently the fantasy in which the man engages during these sexual expressions varies considerably from the actual expression. This is not usually the case with women.[21]

psychological differences in sexual arousal

Among women, the variations in the degree of sexual response are much greater than among men. Some women, perhaps 10 percent, never reach an orgasm. Others do not have an orgasm until they are thirty or forty years of age. Among men, this is exceedingly rare. At the other end of the scale, however, women far exceed men in number of orgasms they can achieve in a given time

differences in degree of sexual response

[20] Robert O. Blood, *Marriage* (New York, 1969), p. 360.

[21] A newly developed method of determining human sexual preferences involves the use of the electroencephalogram (EEG). This instrument provides traces of the electrical activity of the brain. It has been useful in the diagnosis of a variety of conditions such as brain tumors and epilepsy. One of the brain waves that can be recorded is related to anticipation. For this reason it is called the *expectancy wave,* or *E-wave.*

Twelve single male and twelve single female students between the ages of eighteen and twenty-two were selected for a study. They were not screened for sexual experience or preference. They were shown a series of photographs of male and female nudes, and their electroencephalographic tracings were recorded. Although the pictures were not erotic, the genitalia were fully visible. Also included among the photographs was the shadowy outline of a fully clothed woman; her gender could not be readily determined. The results: the electroencephalographic tracings of the male students showed a markedly elevated E-wave response to the photographs of female nudes; the E-wave response of the female students clearly showed their preference for the male nudes. As the experiment continued, the male E-waves increased as they viewed the clothed, shadowy figure of the woman; her gender had become revealed to them.

A whole new area of investigation into thought processes is opened by this experiment. What are the expectancy waves of a patient on viewing a mother and father? How is the therapy of a drug-dependent person progressing? What will the expectancy waves reveal when the patient is shown a picture of a needle and syringe or of a liquor bottle? (Ronald M. Costell, Donald T. Lunde, Bert S. Koppel, and William K. Wittner, "Contingent Negative Variation as an Indicator of Sexual Object Preference," *Science,* Vol. 177, No. 4050 [August 25, 1972], pp. 718–20.)

period. Among a group of college students, for example, a few young women reported an average of twenty-five or more orgasms every week throughout their four-year college careers.[22]

The sexes also vary in regard to the age at which they reach their peaks of sexual activity. When all kinds of sexual activity are considered, the average male of this culture reaches his peak before he is twenty years old. The average female starts engaging in sexual activity at an older age and increases her responses and activity more slowly to a peak at about age thirty. Until she is about fifty, and in many cases beyond that age, the average woman's sexual drive and activity remains at a relatively even plateau. There are, of course, individual variations.

the periodic (cyclic) increase in the woman's sexual desire

Still another difference between the sexes may be partly attributable to female physiology. Many women report increased sexual desire before the onset of menstruation. A lesser number experience this heightened sexual interest following menstruation or at the time of ovulation, which occurs at the midpoint of the menstrual cycle. Women whose sexual desire is greatest before the onset of menstrual bleeding may be stimulated by the pelvic congestion that is consequent to the increased amount of blood in that area.

This periodicity (or cyclicity) can be related to the activity of the hypothalamus of the female brain. It will be remembered that in the human embryo androgen acts on the brain to program maleness; the absence of androgen permits the ongoing pattern of femaleness to develop (see pages 488–89). It has also been shown that brain (hypothalamic) chemicals are responsible for the release of luteinizing and follicle-stimulating hormones from the anterior lobe of the pituitary gland (see page 474). On the average, the human female ovulates every twenty-eight days. This phenomenon depends on the periodic (or cyclic) release of (1) follicle-stimulating hormone (FSH) to promote the growth of the Graafian follicle, which produces estrogen and also houses the ova to be released at ovulation (see page 474) and (2) luteinizing hormone (LH), which induces the formation of corpora lutea and triggers ovulation (see pages 475 and 477). Only pregnancy (see pages 571–77) interferes with this normal cycle in the female.

Male reproductive function shows no such cyclicity. Androgen organizes the hypothalamus of the brain of the male embryo to behave differently. Like the female, his hypothalamic brain patterns are organized to also provide chemicals to stimulate the release of both luteinizing hormone (LH) and follicle-stimulating hormone (FSH) from his anterior pituitary. In the male, however, the LH causes the development of those cells in the testes that are largely responsible for testosterone production (see page 467, footnote 2), and the FSH initiates spermatogenesis. But the LH from the anterior pituitary is produced not cyclically, but continuously. And the release of FSH is timed to meet the demands of spermatogenesis, not oögenesis (the development of ova). That the pituitary gland itself is not sexually differentiated has been proven by transplantation

[22] *Sexuality and Man,* compiled and edited by the Sex Information and Education Council of the United States (New York, 1970), p. 28, citing Alfred C. Kinsey *et al., Sexual Behavior in the Human Female,* pp. 537–43.

experiments. A female pituitary transplanted into a male will not interfere with normal male functions; a male pituitary transplanted into a female will not interfere with completely female functions.[23] Thus, the cyclicity of the female's reproductive system and the acyclicity of the male's both appear to originate in the hypothalamus of the brain.

differences in desired frequency of sexual intercourse

How often do married couples have sexual intercourse? The answer depends on a wide variety of factors, such as how old they were when they got married and their individual needs. There are no rules, just differences. There is evidence (some of which is derived from the work of Kinsey[24]) that the average male desires sexual intercourse more frequently than the average female. The word *average* is here stressed. Some women desire sexual intercourse more often than their husbands, although the majority of women report that they want it less often. It is noteworthy that husbands and wives often may give significantly different estimates of the actual number of times they have sexual intercourse. This may be revealing of both their attitudes toward sexuality and their satisfaction with the marriage. For example, a woman who desires less intercourse may overestimate the number of times she has it, or a husband who wants to have sexual intercourse more frequently might estimate the actual frequency to be closer to what he wants it to be, rather than to what it actually is. He may also report a greater frequency to emphasize his masculinity.[25]

The frequency of sexual intercourse is not as significant as is the frequency of rejection—and how the rejection is handled.

differences in sexual potency

One of the most significant differences between the sexes lies in their relative potency. The fate of the comparatively frail male is considered on pages 490 and 544. Compared to woman, man becomes ill much more often, and he dies at a younger age. In addition, his psychosexual structure appears to be comparatively fragile. But there is yet another area in which the male is relatively feeble. Man is not as sexually potent as woman.

> Aside from ejaculation, there are two major areas of physiological difference between male and female orgasmic expression. First, the female is capable of rapid return to orgasm immediately following an orgasmic experience if restimulated before tensions have dropped below plateau-phase response levels. Second, the female is capable of maintaining an orgasmic experience for a relatively long period of time.[26]

Not only, then, are women able to be multiorgasmic, but they are also able to experience longer orgasms than men. Moreover, they need not undergo profound nervous system coordinations to prepare themselves anatomically for

[23] Seymour Levine, "Sexual Differentiation: The Development of Maleness and Femaleness," p. 14, citing A. Jost, "Embryonic Sexual Differentiation," in H. W. Jones and W. W. Scott, eds., *Hermaphroditism, Genital Anomalies and Related Endocrine Disorders* (Baltimore, 1958), pp. 15–45.
[24] Alfred C. Kinsey *et al.*, *Sexual Behavior in the Human Female*, pp. 348–49.
[25] George Levinger, "Husbands' and Wives' Estimates of Coital Frequency," *Medical Aspects of Human Sexuality*, Vol. 4, No. 9 (September 1970), pp. 42–43, 47–48, 53, 57.
[26] William H. Masters and Virginia E. Johnson, *Human Sexual Response*, p. 131.

sexual intercourse as men do. For the man an erection is a prerequisite to intercourse. He cannot submit; he must always perform. For countless people, the stress of constant submission or performance is not conducive to sexual competence. The striking difference between the sexes in their postorgasmic needs has been mentioned (page 495). During his refractory period, the man rejects further sexual stimulation; the woman may desire further stimulation in order to enjoy more orgasms. The man and woman who are experienced with each other are usually able to resolve this. He, for example, can learn to defer his orgasm until she has had one or more. On the other hand, the female ability to be multiorgasmic should not lead one to assume that more than one orgasm is desired by all women. There is as much variability in orgasmic wants as in any other complex human function. Moreover, many young men are able to have several orgasms and ejaculations closely following the first; however, this capacity is generally lost by most males by the age of thirty.

problems arising from differences in sexuality

The differences in sexual expression between the sexes must be appreciated by both husband and wife. Otherwise lack of harmony may result. For example, the husband may misinterpret his wife's lesser interest in sexual intercourse. Convinced that she is indifferent to him, he may look elsewhere for a seemingly more agreeable sexual partner. Better communication may help the husband to find that his wife is more receptive than he had imagined.

The wife may attempt to meet her husband's sexual demands by submitting to intercourse and pretending orgasm. This is essentially insignificant if it happens only occasionally. When it persists, a deep-seated emotional disturbance may be suspected. (This is no less true about the husband who recognizes the pretense and accepts it.) Indeed, in these instances, differences in sexual desire may not be the basic problem. One woman may fear the abandon of orgasm. Another may be concerned that its very abandon makes her appear less attractive. By her pretense, a wife may express her hostility toward her husband. Subconsciously, she dares her husband to notice the fraud. When the husband fails to do so, the wife may then point to his deficiencies. A woman who has gone through a period of pretending orgasm may eventually begin to have and enjoy them. Then she may fear that her husband will notice the difference in her response. He may not. He might merely believe that "things are getting better and better."[27]

Not uncommonly, marital-sexual dissension arises not from the wife's lesser interest in sexual intercourse but from her greater desire. This, coupled with her potential for more and longer orgasms and her later development of peak sexuality, may make her husband feel threatened. Fearing a loss of masculinity, he may begin to reject sexuality. He may even become impotent (see pages 515–16). What he should realize is that "the female's orgasm most plausibly represents nature's gift to femininity and not woman's bonus to masculinity."[28] If he can learn to accept this, he may also come to enjoy it.

[27] Salo Rosenbaum, "Pretended Orgasm," *Medical Aspects of Human Sexuality,* Vol. 4, No. 4 (April 1970), p. 84.
[28] *Ibid.*

on woman's release from sexual slavery

The modern interest in the orgasm should surprise nobody. In this technological age, it is the technique rather than the art of love that sells marriage manuals. Yet, apparently technique alone does not suffice. Some college girls, who consider themselves sophisticated about sex, are often reduced to frustrated failure in achieving an orgasm. One psychiatrist writes:

> An emphasis on orgasm pervades all age groups of our society . . . Among university students the search for the ultimate orgasm has become almost a competitive matter. I have seen girls who admitted cheating, stealing . . . and promiscuity with little shame but who wept violently when they confessed that they could not have orgasms.[29]

It has been repeatedly observed that until recently in this culture the female half of the human species had much less experience with orgasm than the male. Not more than a hundred years ago, the opinion was held in Western cultures that only evil women ever admitted, even to themselves, that they enjoyed the sexual act. Sexual anesthesia was the price most women paid for the protection and support of their home and children. Society supported the male as ruler of the roost, and the double standard entended to the double bed. The male's sexual needs were gratified according to his, not his wife's, wishes. He chose the time. He felt no need to give. Once satisfied, he rarely gave his docile mate a second sexual thought. Moreover, he had deeply founded memories of another woman who, presumably, had also been a wife. She had provided for other hungers. With affection he remembered his mother. For such various reasons, then, did the male accept his monogamous arrangement. (And this one-sided relationship doubtless helped lead to the justified (and remarkably patient) resentment felt by many married women. Women's liberation is for both sexes.

The long overdue liberation of women changed all that. Enfranchised, and finding new employment and enjoyment opportunities open to them, women also, at last, expected equality in the marital bed. Many of their husbands then imposed upon themselves an unaccustomed husbandly duty—the sexual satisfaction of their wives. Many, but not all. College-matriculated men are apparently more concerned with wifely sexual gratification than are those with less education. In one study only 7 out of 51 men without college matriculation "expressed the slightest concern with responsibility for coital-partner satisfaction . . . Out of a total of 261 . . . subjects with college matriculation, 214 men expressed concern with coital-partner satisfaction."[30]

This concern of some men with the sexual satisfaction of their wives is to their credit; perhaps college is a civilizing influence, after all.[31]

[29] Seymour L. Halleck, "Sex and Mental Health on the Campus," *Journal of the American Medical Association,* Vol. 200, No. 8 (May 22, 1967), p. 687.

[30] William H. Masters and Virginia E. Johnson, *Human Sexual Response,* p. 202.

[31] Increased knowledge about female sexuality doubtless plays some part in the college male's interest in his sexual partner's satisfaction. The cultural double standard has progressed from the notion that sexual behavior is something that the man does *to* the woman, to something that he does *for* her. Now men (and women) must act on the premise that it is something he does *with* her. ("MDs Held Lacking in Sex Function Training," *Internal Medicine News,* Vol. 5, No. 14 [July 15, 1972], p. 24, quoting Virginia E. Johnson.

variations in orgasmic quality

"There is good evidence that the capacity for orgasm or sexual climax is a natural birthright of almost every healthy adult human being."[32] The quality of a human orgasm is to a great extent a matter of individual interpretation. Although an orgasm involves the same nervous pathways and the same total body responses in all humans, the degree of involvement varies with individuals and situations. This may be a factor causing subjective differences in the quality of different orgasms. On one occasion, for example, a woman may have sexual intercourse while she is depressed and tired. If her partner is matter-of-fact and pays no heed to her mood, she may have no orgasm or perhaps only a local clitoral sensation. But if her partner is sensitive to her mood, if he expresses his love and waits for her participation, she knows he cares. Then, even if her orgasmic experience is not intense, the totality of her sexual experience will more likely be satisfying.

some myths and misconceptions about human sexuality

"The little rift between the sexes," wrote Robert Louis Stevenson, "is astonishingly widened by simply teaching one set of catchwords to the girls and another to the boys." Only too often is that rift widened even more by teaching them misconceptions about one another's sexuality. This is not usually deliberate. Most of the modern open-minded discussion about sexual matters is of recent origin. Unfortunately, much of today's talk about sexuality is based on yesterday's misinformation. What are some of the more common of these misconceptions?

Misconception No. 1: To have a satisfactory marital experience, the wife and husband must have an orgasm with each intercourse.

This generally unrealized ideal has been a hazard to many a marriage. The difference in the degree of sexual interest between the sexes has already been mentioned. As a marriage matures and intimacy deepens, the frequency of the wife's orgasms may increase. However, the wife will accomplish orgasm, and more often sooner, when she realizes that "the husband's enjoyment of the act has to take precedence over his efforts to please his wife. Otherwise, sooner or later, neither of them will have any pleasure at all."[33]

Both the young husband and the young wife approach their new roles with some guilt and anxiety. They do not suddenly awaken to maturity after a long period of sexual somnolence. Nevertheless, instead of preparing adolescents for their future sexual function, society merely controls them. Many of these controls are necessary. (Today, almost the only adult pleasure usually forbidden the unmarried teen-ager is sexual intercourse.) But this sexual control is matched by a conspiracy of parental silence about the subject. The growing boy is not helped by the slick magazine, nor by the refusal of his parents to talk

[32] *Sexuality and Man,* p. 25.
[33] Milton R. Sapirstein, *Paradoxes of Everyday Life* (New York, 1955), p. 28.

about sexuality, nor by the embarrassment of his teachers. Too often, his education is a compound of the sniggering anxieties of his contemporaries and furtive, short-lived, basically uncomfortable liaisons. He drifts alone on the murky waters of opinionated misinformation. Sexuality is associated with something evil.[34] It may then be loaded with guilt and anxiety.

His young wife may be similarly ill-equipped. Her secret anxiety may be matched by her dreamy determination to equal the seemingly satisfactory creatures her husband sees in some magazine gatefolds. She owes it to him, the man she loves, to be the responsive and adequate wife.

No matter what their previous experience has been, marriage has ceremoniously thrust the couple into a new, often threatening role. They must prove themselves. Right now. Every time.

Thus does marriage pose anxieties that require patience, enormous understanding, and a sense of humor about oneself and one's mate. It will relax the couple to know that orgasm with each intercourse is not necessary to a happy marriage. Terman's research indicates that a wife's capacity for orgasm is not highly related to the couple's happiness.[35] And more recent research by Masters and Johnson suggests that the intensity and duration of a woman's orgasm is not necessarily related to her sense of sexual gratification. An orgasm of relatively low intensity and short duration, during a sexual experience with a husband she loves, may indeed be evaluated by the wife as a complete and fulfilling sexual experience.[36] The consistent sexual competency of the wife is not as important to marital happiness as understanding and patient communication. Feeling safe and feeling a sense of trust are no less profoundly involved with marital happiness than the orgasm.

Misconception No. 2: Simultaneous orgasm is absolutely essential for ultimate and satisfactory sexual expression.

This nonsense, a favorite of some marriage manuals, is another anxiety producer. The woman must, after all, either begin to have, or have, an orgasm before the man. If the former is true, simultaneous orgasms are possible. These are delightful experiences. However, many couples never have them; nor do they miss them. To insist on a simultaneous orgasm is another way of putting oneself on trial. The man who is on constant trial does not relax. He may become unable to have an erection. This failure may, in turn, make him fear that he has lost his sexual prowess. Shame torments him. Sometimes a man may become impotent with a wife with whom he feels on trial. Instead he finds himself potent with "another woman." Or, with his wife, he may have premature ejaculations, with attendant guilt feelings. As will be pointed out later: "Problems of premature ejaculation . . . disturbed the younger members of the study-subject population." This was particularly true of college-matriculated men: "with these men ejaculatory control sufficient to accomplish partner satisfaction was con-

[34] This association may have begun long before adolescence—on the day the small child was punished for examining the genitalia.

[35] L. M. Terman, "Correlates of Orgasm Adequacy in a Group of 556 Wives," in M. F. De Martino, ed., *Sexual Behavior and Personality Characteristics* (New York, 1966).

[36] Warren R. Johnson, *Human Sexual Behavior and Sex Education* (Philadelphia, 1968), pp. 50–51.

sidered a coital technique that must be acquired before the personal security of coital effectiveness could be established."[37]

With premature ejaculation, there is anxiety. Again the male doubts his potency. It is worth repeating that male sexual activity is circumscribed by a basic requirement. He must feel certain of his active role. He cannot, like his mate, submit to sexual intercourse. Although constant submission may relieve her of some of the stress of performance, it will bring her not the fulfillment of a satisfying sexual expression, but the bitterness of sexual repression. For her, too, coitus should neither be a test nor a contest.

Some marriage manuals make effective chaperones.

Misconception No. 3: Direct clitoral stimulation during sexual intercourse is essential.

There are some misguided writers who detail the crucial importance of direct clitoral stimulation to arouse sexual desire. Research disputes this advice. For a great number of women the difference between clitoral excitement and irritation is slight. To their surprise (and in contradiction to many marriage manuals) many husbands discover that their wives find manual clitoral stimulation distinctly disagreeable, if not painful. Many, instead, prefer manual stimulation of the general mons area. There is only one best way to find out. Ask.

Effective manual stimulation of the general mons area results in a clitoral retraction reaction (see page 494). The clitoris normally retracts upward.

> This physiological reaction to high levels of female sexual tension creates a problem for the sexually inexperienced male. The clitoral-body retraction reaction frequently causes even an experienced male to lose manual contact with the organ. Having lost contact, the male partner usually ceases active stimulation of the general mons area and attempts manually to relocate the clitoral body. During this "textbook" approach, marked sexual frustration may develop in a highly excited female partner. . . Once . . . clitoral retraction has been established, manipulation of the general mons area is all that is necessary for effective clitoral-body stimulation.[38]

Misconception No. 4: This is a double mistake: (1) *that there is a vaginal orgasm distinct from the clitoral orgasm, and* (2) *that clitoral orgasm is immature; only vaginal orgasm is mature.*

These false concepts go back to the outmoded idea that female sexual organs are but incomplete male organs, nothing more than a perpetual case of arrested genital development. It was thought impossible, if not indecent, for women, thus hopelessly sexually retarded, to enjoy, much less desire, sexual intercourse. Freud did not fall into this trap, but he did fall for the idea of the female as an incomplete, hence inferior, male. He considered woman biologically dependent on man. He thought that, lacking a penis, she was passively envious. "Freud's theories buttressed all the prevailing prejudices and promoted the notion that the female was a deficient male and a second-class citi-

[37] William H. Masters and Virginia E. Johnson, *Human Sexual Response,* p. 202.
[38] *Ibid.,* pp. 65–66.

zen."[39] Reflecting the patriarchal culture of his time, he attributed to biology what was, in reality, culturally prescribed. To this was added another error. Girls who masturbated usually did so by manual clitoral stimulation. This, it was decreed by many early writers, was immature. Hence, manual clitoral stimulation to orgasm by adults was immature. Although clitoral stimulation during intercourse was acceptable, only vaginal orgasm was the mark of the normal and sexually mature woman.

The trouble with all this is that it is wrong. What are the facts?

1. The sexually sensitive areas of the female genitalia are the clitoris, labia minora, and the lower third of the vagina (see pages 482–83). (As a source of erotic arousal, the mons area ranks with the clitoris and the labia minora; it is, however, not strictly a part of the genitalia. The labia minora are not as sensitive as the clitoral shaft and the mons area.)

2. The upper two-thirds of the vagina has a different embryological origin than the lower third; that is, it arises from a different group of cells. The lower third of the vagina and the labia minora have the same embryological origin; they arise from the same group of cells. Nor are the clitoris and the lower third of the vagina separable structures.

3. The upper two-thirds of the vagina plays no part in the orgasm. Nor does it play a part in the development of erotic feelings.

4. During sexual arousal, the lower third of the vagina and the labia minora function as a unit. They are thought to be about equally sensitive to sexual stimulation. The clitoris is more sensitive than either.

5. With one exception, there are no nerve or muscle or blood vessel connections between the clitoris and the vagina. The exception is a network of veins from the clitoris that merges into a network of veins lying along the walls of the vagina. During sexual excitement, these veins are engorged with blood, causing tumescence. Within ten to thirty seconds after sexual excitement, a lubricating fluid appears on the vaginal walls. This fluid seeps onto the vaginal walls directly from the plexus of veins surrounding the vaginal barrel.

6. Like the penis, the clitoris is generously endowed with nerves and is capable of tumescence, spasmodic contraction, and detumescence.

7. During coitus, the penis rarely comes in direct contact with the clitoris. This is because of the above-mentioned retraction reaction. The traction of the penis on the sensitive labia minora stimulates the shortened, hidden clitoris. The thrusting movements of the penis

> create simultaneous stimulation of the lower third of the vagina, labia minora, and clitoral shaft and glans as an integrated, inseparable functioning unit with the glans being the most important and, in by far the majority of instances, the indispensable initiator of the orgasmic reaction . . . it is a physical impossibility to separate the clitoral from the vaginal orgasm.[40]

[39] Leon Salzman, "Psychology of the Female," *Archives of General Psychiatry,* Vol. 17, No. 2 (August 1967), p. 195.

[40] Mary Jane Sherfey, "The Evolution and Nature of Female Sexuality in Relation to Psychoanalytic Theory," p. 78.

8. During the female orgasm, the male often feels contractions on the shaft of his penis. What are they? Does the vagina produce these contractions of orgasm? No. Then what does contract? It was pointed out above that the orgasmic contractions are of the muscles located in the floor of the pelvis that surround the lower third of the vagina. With female orgasm, these muscles contract, not directly against the vaginal wall, but against the network of engorged chambers of veins and blood channels about that part of the vagina. In this way the venous passages are emptied of blood (detumescence). These muscle contractions about the vaginal veins cause the lower vaginal walls to be passively pushed in and out. Moreover, these muscle contractions cause the upper labia minora to contract. That is what the male feels. "Therefore there is no such thing as an orgasm of the vagina. What exists is an orgasm of the circumvaginal venous chambers."[41]

9. Thus, one cannot distinguish between vaginal orgasm and clitoral orgasm. Regardless of how it was stimulated, the nature of the orgasm is the same.

Present knowledge of the origin, anatomy, and function of the female genitalia should help to dispel many a female fear. Long depressed by the idea of the inferiority of the clitoral orgasm, many women blamed either themselves or their husbands for their failure to achieve "vaginal orgasm." The whole notion, however, of a vaginal orgasm separate from clitoral orgasm is biologically impossible and, therefore, utterly invalid. And to consider clitoral orgasm immature and vaginal orgasm mature is senseless. "The tendency to reduce clitoral eroticism to a level of psychopathology or immaturity because of its supposed masculine origin is a travesty of the facts and a misleading psychologic deduction.[42]

Misconception No. 5: The size of the genital organs (penis or vagina) is related to sexual prowess.

This error is based on myths that have been dispelled by considerable research, most recently by that of Masters and Johnson.[43]

First, the size of the penis is in no way related to the size of the man. In a group of 312 men ranging from twenty-one to eighty-nine years, it was found that the longest penis in the flaccid (soft) state belonged to a man five feet seven inches tall who weighed 152 pounds; the smallest penis was that of a man four inches taller and twenty-six pounds heavier.

Second, upon erection, a larger penis does not necessarily increase to a greater size than does a smaller penis. For example, one man's penile measurement in the flaccid state was 7.5 cm. (2.95 in.); in the erect its length increased to more than double its flaccid state—it lengthened 9 cm. (3.5 in.) to equal 16.5 cm. (6.5 in.). Another man's flaccid penis was 11 cm. (4.3 in.) long; it increased only 5.5 cm. (2.2 in.) as a result of erection; erect, its length also

[41] *Ibid.*, p. 84.
[42] Leon Salzman, "Psychology of the Female," p. 196.
[43] William H. Masters and Virginia E. Johnson, *Human Sexual Response*, pp. 191–95.

totalled 16.5 cm.[44] The extent to which misinformation about penile length can concern some individuals is demonstrated by the young man who reportedly tied weights of increasing size to his penis every day in an attempt to lengthen the organ. He failed.[45]

Third, during the late excitement or early plateau phases, the vagina lengthens and also expands in its upper (deeper) area of the cervix. This creates a receptacle to receive the seminal pool that is about to be deposited. This overdistention of that upper part of the vagina makes some women feel that the penis is "lost in the vagina." This sensation has nothing to do with penile size. It is more apparent in the woman whose vagina has been traumatized during childbirth and then inadequately repaired. However, under ordinary circumstances, it is most unusual for the vagina to be so large as to interfere with coital pleasure. A vagina is rarely so small that accommodation of the penis is difficult unless the woman is highly aroused. The same is occasionally true in the case of the woman who has passed the menopause or who has not had sexual intercourse for a long time. In summary,

> penile size usually is a minor factor in sexual stimulation of the female partner. The normal or large vagina accommodates a penis of any size without difficulty. If the vagina is exceptionally small, or if a long period of continence or of involution [shriveling] intervenes, a penis of any size can distress rather than stimulate, if mounting is attempted before advanced stages of female sexual tension have been experienced.[46]

Misconception No. 6: Permanent or even temporary abstinence from sexual intercourse will invariably result in neurotic or psychotic behavior.

Sexual intercourse is a means of fulfillment for the human personality. It can be a way of providing basic human needs for intimacy, sharing, and commitment. True, as in the animal world, coitus is a biological act of procreation. But it can also be a profound expression of humanness.

However, to equate temporary or permanent abstinence from sexual intercourse with invariable emotional disorder is an error. Coitus is an expression of the whole personality, but it is not the personality per se. Neurotic and psychotic behavior are expressions of a disorder of the whole personality. Sexual disorders may be part of disordered personality expressions, but they are usually the result, not the cause, of neurotic or psychotic behavior. It should, however, be stressed that people may suffer disturbances of sexual function without demonstrating severely neurotic or psychotic behavior.

Coitus is the only physiological function that a person can choose to keep unfulfilled. Some people choose to permanently refrain from sexual intercourse.

[44] Does the penis ever decrease in size from the flaccid (soft) state? Yes. Cold, severe exhaustion resulting from undue and prolonged physical strain, advanced age, surgical castration—these are among the reasons that the size of the penis diminishes from that of its usual flaccid state in an individual. Prolonged impotence (see pages 515–16) of over two years may also have this effect. It may also occur immediately after a man has attempted but failed to have sexual intercourse. This last cause fortifies the belief that lessening of penile size, like erection, is not only the result of a spinal reflex, but is also profoundly influenced by stimuli from the higher brain centers. (William H. Masters and Virginia E. Johnson, *Human Sexual Response,* pp. 180–81.)

[45] Eugene Schoenfeld, *Dear Doctor Hip Pocrates* (New York, 1968), p. 19.

[46] William H. Masters and Virginia E. Johnson, *Human Sexual Response,* p. 195.

In his "On the Good of Marriage," Saint Augustine wrote: "To many, total abstinence is easier than perfect moderation." (In his *Confessions,* however, he wrote: "Give me chastity and continence but not yet.") Many people have led long and purposeful lives without experiencing the meaningful pleasures that can be part of sexual intercourse.

Of course, such individuals are in the minority. However, at various times in their lives, many people defer sexual intercourse for considerable periods of time. There is no evidence whatsoever that this leads to emotional illness.

Misconception No. 7: The treatment of sexual inadequacy is always difficult, costly, and time-consuming.

By no means is this true. Sometimes seemingly severe sexual problems have simple causes and need relatively minor adjustment for their solution. To cite some examples: one man was delighted with the totality of his wife's sexual responses, yet they embarrassed and inhibited him, particularly when her uninhibited screaming and shouting during orgasm occurred while their children or guests were in the house. A second man lost penile sensation and also worried about the adequacy of the size of his penis because his wife was prone to use an excessive amount of spermicidal jelly "just to be on the safe side." Another man was married to a demure little woman whose pelvic movements during coitus were so vigorous that penis and vagina were too soon parted. Instead of an uncontrollable desire to have an orgasm, the husband had an uncontrollable desire to laugh. Fearing to hurt his wife's feelings, he controlled his merriment, but his sexual life was adversely affected. To avoid soiling the bed sheet, still another couple were wont to rush to the bathroom immediately after the husband's ejaculation. Soon they found the price of this tidiness too high; their sexual life suffered. All such problems, if they are candidly discussed, can be corrected with obvious minor adjustments.[47] They require neither prolonged nor expensive attention.

Masters and Johnson's study of human sexual inadequacy

In the development of their various treatments for sexual inadequacies, Masters and Johnson were guided by certain basic concepts. First, they emphasized that sexual activity is a form of communication and personal interaction. Their second concept (a corollary of the first) was the principle that it was the sick marital relationship, and not only the sick individual, that required treatment. Here Masters and Johnson parted company with tradition. Previous failures by some therapists to understand that there is no such person as an uninvolved partner in a marital relationship, or, when that was understood, the lack of practical effort to treat the relationship itself may well explain some of the failures of more traditional approaches.

[47] The cases cited above are from John L. Schimel, "Some Practical Considerations in Treating Male Sexual Inadequacy," *Medical Aspects of Human Sexuality,* Vol. 5, No. 3 (March 1971), pp. 24, 29–31.

A third concept resulted in another treatment innovation. Masters and Johnson believed that no man can fully comprehend a woman's sexual response; no woman can fully comprehend a man's sexual response. This realization has resulted in their development of the *dual-sex treatment team.* Composed of a man and a woman, the treatment team deals with the sexual inadequacies consequent to the ailing marital relationship. This approach now seems obvious and logical. Yet in the past it was not generally taken. Single therapists, usually men, saw patients alone. The patients' marital partners were not included in the therapeutic process. Again the results were often disappointing.

The fourth concept was the necessity of taking careful histories of all patients as well as paying meticulous attention to a complete physical and laboratory examination. A patient's history might reveal, for example, that she was taking an oral contraceptive. Occasionally, this could cause her inadequate sexual response. In such a case, the cure could be the simple discontinuance of the pill. In another case, a physical and laboratory examination might reveal a diabetic husband. This, rather than a psychological problem in the marital relationship, could cause his impotence. Purely physical factors are but a small percentage of the total causes of sexual inadequacy. But if these factors are not first eliminated therapy might be based on mistaken diagnoses and may even magnify problems rather than alleviate them.

critics of Masters and Johnson

The treatment procedures for sexual inadequacy practiced by Masters and Johnson are not without their critics. Nor are all their critics ill-informed traditionalists. The distinguished psychiatrist Rollo May has said that "they put the emphasis on orgasm when it should be on love. They help some couples, and I congratulate them for that, but their total impact on society is to send us further down the road of misunderstanding ourselves and our need to love one another."[48] In a recent review of *Human Sexual Inadequacy* in the *Journal of the American Medical Association,* psychiatrist Natalie Shainess wrote:

> The ideas within this book can be summed up quite briefly: marital units (not couples, please!) are advised to "pleasure" (touch) each other—a leaf taken from sensitivity and encounter groups—but to delay actual coitus until given permission by the therapists; wives are taught to squeeze the penis to prevent ejaculation; husbands are taught to use metal dilators on wives who have vaginismus. In short, each is placed in the power of the other, depending on the condition. This reviewer cannot resist asking: can faulty and inadequate sex truly be corrected in this joyless way, and ignoring the psychological forces at work?[49]

It is doubtless too early to judge the total societal effect of Masters and Johnson's work. However, both May and Shainess do emphasize a valid concern held by other investigators. The sheer objectivity of the approach to sexuality by Masters and Johnson might indeed lead some to unthinkingly consider

[48] Quoted in Paul Wilkes, "Sex and the Married Couple," *The Atlantic Monthly,* Vol. 226 (December 1970), p. 92.
[49] Natalie Shainess, review of *Human Sexual Inadequacy, Journal of the American Medical Association,* Vol. 213, No. 12 (September 21, 1970), p. 2084.

sexual expression as a mechanical event. The danger would certainly seem greatest with those who have not considered sexuality as an expression of the whole personality. However, Masters and Johnson can hardly be said to make this error. Masters has defined sexuality as "a dimension of the personality and sex as a specific physical activity."[50] Recently, the authoritative journal *Medical Aspects of Human Sexuality* devoted a considerable portion of one issue to a careful and generally appreciative description of the Masters and Johnson technique. In an introductory statement the editors emphasized that *"the following descriptions constitute the physical procedures utilized in treatment of sexual dysfunctions. It is to be emphasized that the techniques are of little or no value without supportive psychotherapy for the marital relationship, for the* relationship *and the interaction of the couple are the primary focus of Masters' and Johnson's therapeutic program."*[51]

Masters and Johnson classify and treat sexual inadequacy

After preliminary interviews and medical examinations, the patients meet with therapists at the Reproductive Biology Research Foundation in a series of round-table conferences. At the first meeting, the therapists discuss their initial findings with the couple. So begins an education program about sexuality. It is an integral and continuing part of the therapy. Long-held misapprehensions and myths about sexuality are aired. Problems revealed by the history of each patient are explored. Sometimes one member of the marital pair wishes a secret fact kept from the other. This desire is generally respected, although there are occasions in which the sharing of such information is necessary for the resolution of a sexual problem. Permission to discuss the secret is usually obtained in a private interview between one of the therapists and the patient.

If the first round-table conference is successful the couple is given their homework. This consists of "sensate focus exercises" to be carried out in the privacy of their hotel room. The exercises are simple, but they have profound meaning. Lying naked, the pair stroke and feel each other. The breasts and genitals are not touched. At this stage coitus is not to take place. This pleasing of one another is free from any demand by either member of the pair. Neither is required to perform. People who have been married for many years may, at first, be clumsily self-conscious. Sometimes the exercises seem very funny to them. This is good. Humor and sexual expression are old companions, and they get along well with each other. After a few such sessions, most couples look forward to these experiences. They may come to have a poetic quality. It is as if Robert Browning's lines had truly come to pass:

[50] Mary Harrington Hall, "A Conversation with Masters and Johnson," *Psychology Today,* Vol. 3, No. 2 (July 1969), p. 52 (see also page 84).

[51] "Highlights of Masters and Johnson Therapy Techniques," *Medical Aspects of Human Sexuality,* Vol. 4, No. 7 (July 1970), p. 36.

> Your soft hand is a woman of itself,
> And mine the man's bared breast she curls inside.[52]

Following the fourth day increased sexual expression is permitted. The breasts and genitals are now touched and stroked. The communicating wife or husband guides the hands of the partner. They tell each other what is most pleasurable. They share information about the areas of greater pleasure, the speed of stroking, the degree of pressure desired.

In this manner the marital partners learn to contribute to each other's sexual pleasure via nerve endings called the *end organs of touch.* These nerve endings are distributed throughout the skin and some of the body's deeper organs. Certain of these nerve endings are organized in a unique way. Some parts of the adult body are so richly supplied with these uniquely structured end organs of touch that, under certain circumstances, their stimulation leads to sexual excitement. These are the *erogenous zones.* However, the human being can learn to be sexually excited as a result of the stimulation of a wide variety of end organs of touch that are not strictly within the erogenous zones. The sensitivity of the erogenous zones varies greatly with different people, but touch is part of the language of love. As two lovers seek to discover one another's erogenous zones, they embark on an adventure in intimacy. The explorations and discoveries, the givings and takings of love can bring about a transcendent and mystical enthrallment in which (as the poet John Milton wrote) two people are "Imparadis'd in one another's arms."[53] In the clinic the round-table discussions are continued. The various aspects of the developing sexual experience are discussed. The couple, moreover, receives information on the next procedure.

On the fifth day the therapy is directed to the specific problem affecting the partners.

on inadequate sexual response

in the female

Among the contributions of Masters and Johnson has been their clarification of the definitions of various human sexual problems. For example, because of its vagueness they reject the use of "frigidity" as a diagnostic term. They regard "inadequate sexual response" as a more satisfactory general term to describe such problems in both men and women.

Three aspects of inadequate female sexual response have been studied by Masters and Johnson.

dyspareunia

Dyspareunia (painful coitus) may result from physical causes, such as vaginal infection, an irritating collection of *smegma* (an oily, ill-smelling secretion of the

[52] Robert Browning, "Andrea del Sarto," lines 21–22.
[53] John Milton, *Paradise Lost,* Book IV, line 506.

sebaceous glands; see page 515) around the clitoris, or a chemical irritation (as occurs with some douches or inserted chemical contraceptives). Older women may experience dyspareunia due to thinning of the vaginal mucous membrane; this is easily treated.

Dyspareunia may also be caused by psychological problems that result in insufficient vaginal lubrication. Among these emotional impediments may be the woman's fear of injury or pregnancy, hostility toward her husband, or conflict over her sexual role (as may result from a highly repressive childhood).

orgasmic dysfunction

As recently as the nineteenth century, the famed London physician William Acton wrote that ''most women happily for them [or, in a later edition, ''happily for society''] are not troubled with sexual feeling of any kind.''[54] Today, happily for both society and its men and women, this misconception is being corrected. But it did contribute to the social acceptance of the notion that decent women were not supposed to have orgasms (see page 503). Orgasmic dysfunction, which refers to difficulties encountered by women in reaching orgasm, is even today often rooted in mid-Victorian rejection of woman's sexual humanness and sexual identity. A woman with *primary* orgasmic dysfunction is one who has never attained an orgasm.[55] ''There is good evidence that the capacity for orgasm or sexual climax is a natural birthright of almost every healthy adult human being.''[56]

The treatment of orgasmic dysfunction requires the couple's understanding of each other's past sexual experiences and sexually tinged memories. Those factors that sexually stimulate or depress the woman should be discussed. The married nonorgasmic woman is often one whose husband ejaculates prematurely.[57] Should this be a chronic experience, the husband will need professional help. If successful, that help will increase his sense of shared responsibility. Heedless of his wife's needs, he may have succeeded in having an orgasm, but failed in providing one. And his wife, anxious to please, may have feared that he would not have an orgasm. Distracted by her worry, she may have been unable to achieve the sexual tension necessary for orgasm. Discovering such intimacies about each other, and resolving them together, can be a rich and enduring experience in marital mutuality.

vaginismus

Vaginismus is a spasm of the vagina that results in a constriction of the vaginal outlet. The spasm is involuntary; it is in no way under the control of the woman who experiences it. It is brought about by ''imagined, anticipated, or real attempts at vaginal penetration. Thus, vaginismus is a classic example of a psy-

[54] Quoted in Melva Weber, ''Sexual Inadequacy: How Masters and Johnson Treat It,'' *Medical World News,* Vol. 11, No. 18 (May 1, 1970), p. 47.
[55] William H. Masters and Virginia E. Johnson, *Human Sexual Inadequacy,* p. 227.
[56] *Sexuality and Man,* p. 25.
[57] William H. Masters and Virginia E. Johnson, *Human Sexual Inadequacy,* pp. 228–29.

chosomatic illness."[58] (See pages 303–04.) Since penile penetration is impossible or, at best, extremely difficult, vaginismus is commonly the cause of unconsummated marriages and marriages in which coitus is very infrequent. Understandably, the husband may be severely affected by his wife's disability. Male sexual inadequacies, such as impotence, are not uncommonly associated with vaginismus. This emphasizes the importance of a diagnostic and treatment approach that involves both husband and wife. Among the causes of vaginismus is repressive sex education from which the child learns that sex is dirty and sinful. The psychic trauma of rape or a painful initial coital experience may also result in vaginismus. A previous homosexual orientation may be another cause.

in the male

dyspareunia

The causes of male dyspareunia are generally physical in nature. Poor personal hygiene may lead to an infection beneath the foreskin. The resultant inflammation may be painful even without the stimulation of sexual intercourse. Old scars within the urethra from a subsided gonorrheal infection may cause a stricture of the urethral passage, which not only may result in painful coitus but, indeed, may interfere with the passage of the urine through the penis. Many, but by no means all, strictures are due to untreated gonorrhea. Early and adequate treatment of gonorrheal infection is the best preventative of gonorrheal strictures. A third cause of male dyspareunia is phimosis (Greek *phimosis,* muzzling, closure). Men with phimosis have an unusually long prepuce (foreskin) that is so tight that it cannot be drawn back from over the glans penis. As with many other penile problems, the condition may be painful even when the man is not attempting sexual intercourse. Phimosis can become quite complicated if it is not treated. Fibrous tissue may grow between the prepuce and the glans. These fibrous adhesions make the prepuce even less retractable. Smegma may collect and cause infection, inflammation, and even ulceration, all of which may be very painful. Fortunately, these disagreeable and inhibiting circumstances are easily rectified—usually by circumcision and administration of medication to relieve the infection. Still another cause of male dyspareunia may be found within the environment of the vagina. Not uncommonly contraceptive chemicals and douche preparations may cause allergic manifestations in sensitive penile tissue.

impotence

"It is the heaviest stone that Melancholy can throw at a man, to tell him he is at the end of his nature." So did the seventeenth-century English physician and writer Sir Thomas Browne describe the despair of impotence. Men who suffer

[58] William H. Masters and Virginia E. Johnson, *Human Sexual Inadequacy,* p. 250. The term *psychosomatic* is from the Greek *psychikos,* mind + *soma,* body. Psychosomatic disorders originate in the mind and are manifested as physical symptoms. Emotional stimuli are referred by the brain to body organs, resulting in effects ranging from goose flesh to vaginismus. The ancients were well aware of psychosomatic influences. "Diseases of the mind impair the powers of the body," wrote Ovid. Nor did the seventeenth-century Englishman John Donne contradict Ovid when he wrote that "the body makes the minde."

from *primary impotence* have either never had an erection or have been unable to maintain an erection long enough to have sexual intercourse. Those who suffer from *secondary impotence* were once sexually capable but have lost the ability to have an erection and maintain it long enough to enjoy coitus.

Primary impotence usually is the result of a deep-seated psychological problem. A boy may grow up to be impotent if he is denigrated, or taught that sex is sinful and dirty, or is overwhelmingly impressed by his mother that her sex is preferable to his.

Secondary impotence has a wide range of causes. Biological-physical causes include disease, injury, and impotency-inducing medication. Among the psychosocial factors are rigidity during childhood training, an affiliation with an orthodox religious group with highly restrictive sexual mores, and an orientation toward homosexual behavior. The major cause of secondary impotence in the Masters and Johnson population is premature ejaculation (see the next section). Such impotence may take years to develop. Drinking too much alcohol is the second major cause of secondary impotence. Impotence from this cause may occur suddenly (see page 380). Sometimes excessive alcohol consumption can lead to a single episode of impotence. In most cases this is no cause for undue concern. However, to be convivial or to build up his courage a man may consistently drink a small amount of alcohol before engaging in sexual intercourse. If this becomes habitual, he may increase his intake. Then he experiences an episode of impotence. Anxiety about the next performance may result in another failure. He may try to drown his fear of failure in more alcohol. Soon fear of failure to have an erection haunts the afflicted man. Like an angry bystander he observes himself with anxiety. No longer does an erection occur as naturally to him as does breathing. He watches to see if he will perform, and he cannot. He hopes that by his very frustration he can will his penis erect. But no man can will an erection. If he seeks treatment, this is one of the first facts that he has to learn.

premature ejaculation

With this condition, the male loses much of his erection as soon as he ejaculates. He is thus unable to continue intravaginal intercourse. Should the ejaculation occur before his partner is sexually satisfied, it may be considered premature. A variety of reasons may account for premature ejaculation. By no means are all of them unusual. The time between his sexual contacts may have been too long. Or he may have enjoyed too prolonged a period of foreplay. An occasional premature ejaculation should not concern either partner. When it becomes a chronic part of the sexual pattern, serious problems arise.

Many men in this culture regard the ability to satisfy their sexual partner as one measure of masculinity. Persistent failure to do so causes the man to lose confidence in his masculinity. Even a few failures may make him feel that he is on trial. This makes him anxious, and his mounting anxiety causes him to ejaculate prematurely—often even before his penis enters the vagina. At first his wife may be patient with him. She avoids stimulating him before intromission. If this fails, she may resort to self-pity. "You're just using me," she may tell him bitterly. Now their sexual experience is out of its context of love. It is no longer an expression of understanding mutuality. It is surrounded by embarrassment, anxiety, failure—even hate.

Masters and Johnson consider premature ejaculation a problem if the male cannot control his ejaculation during vaginal containment long enough to satisfy his partner for at least 50 percent of their coital exposures. Of all the male dysfunctions, they find premature ejaculation the easiest to cure.

ejaculatory incompetence

The man with ejaculatory incompetence usually has no difficulty in having an erection. However, he cannot ejaculate in the vagina. This disability is "the clinical opposite of premature ejaculation . . . separate from impotence."[59] Fortunately, it is rare. A severely restrictive upbringing, a fear of causing pregnancy, or a shocking emotional upset may cause ejaculatory incompetence. Sometimes a single traumatic event may cause the problem. It has been noted that wives of husbands with this condition may feel rejected. Despite this, they may frequently experience multiple orgasms.

Today, careful studies have revealed new ways of helping those with many of these sexual inadequacies—not only the young but also the elderly. It is as if scientific investigators, respectful of human significance and dignity, have helped bring to pass these wistful lines from the *Rubáiyát:*

> Ah Love! could you and I with Him conspire
> To grasp this sorry Scheme of Things entire,
> Would not we shatter it to bits—and then
> Remold it nearer to the Heart's desire![60]

summary

The primordial human reproductive tissue is female. The male reproductive system results from production of the hormone *androgen* and of a substance that inhibits the development of embryonic tissue into female reproductive structures (pages 488–89). Moreover, androgen acts upon the brain to produce male patterns of behavior (pages 489–90).

Transcending genetic and hormonal influences, culturally learned patterns of behavior and thought powerfully influence gender identity (pages 490–91). Acceptable modes of male and female behavior and appearance vary from culture to culture and from time to time (pages 491–92).

In their studies of the physiology of human sexual response, William H. Masters and Virginia E. Johnson divided the sexual responses of both men and women into four phases: the *excitement phase* (page 493), the *plateau phase* (pages 493–94), the *orgasmic phase* (page 494),

[59] William H. Masters and Virginia E. Johnson, *Human Sexual Inadequacy,* p. 126.
[60] *Rubáiyát of Omar Khayyám,* tr. by Edward FitzGerald.

and the *resolution phase* (page 494). Male sexual response is also characterized by *ejaculation* and a subsequent *refractory period* (pages 494–95).

There are a number of differences in sexual response between the sexes. These include differences in adolescent sexuality (page 498); differences in attitude toward sexuality (page 499); psychological differences in sexual arousal (page 499); differences in degree of sexual response (pages 499–500); cyclic variation in female sexual desire (pages 500–01); differences in desired frequency of sexual intercourse (page 501); and differences in sexual potency (pages 501–02). Such differences may give rise to dissension between marital partners, which can often be resolved by communication and consideration (pages 502–03). An individual may experience variations in the quality of orgasm at various times (page 504). Many marital-sexual problems are a result of myths and misconceptions about sexuality (pages 504–10).

Masters and Johnson have written about the classification and treatment of inadequate sexual response (pages 510–13). They studied three aspects of inadequate female sexual response: *dyspareunia,* or painful coitus (pages 513–14), *orgasmic dysfunction* (page 514), and *vaginismus,* an involuntary spasm of the vagina that prevents penetration (pages 514–15). Inadequate male sexual response may involve *dyspareunia* (page 515), *impotence* (pages 515–16), *premature ejaculation* (pages 516–17), or *ejaculatory incompetence* (page 517).

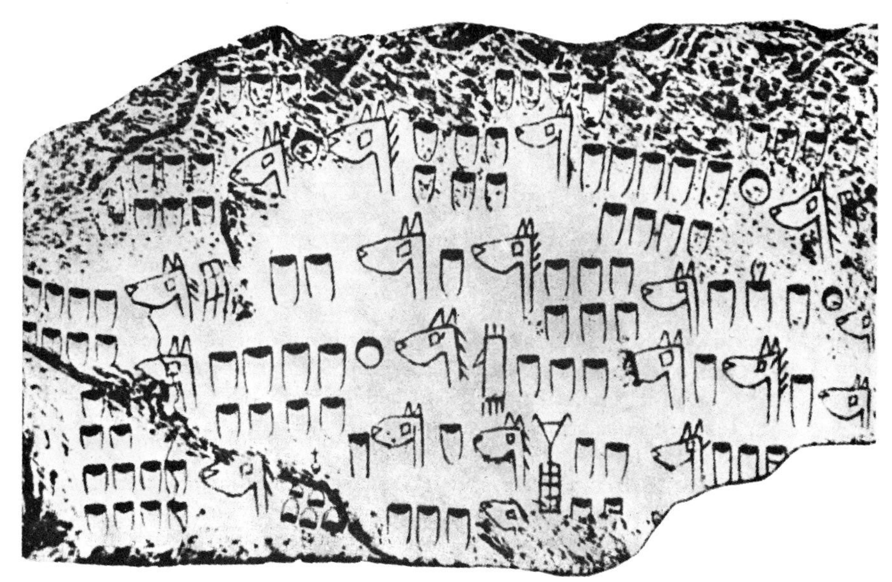

Heredity is an ancient concern. This horse pedigree is 6,000 years old.

the human beginning

18

Before I was born out of my mother generations guided me[1]

''in the beginning . . .''

Many millennia ago there was no life in the world. In a certain right time and environment, however, chemicals combined and were sparked into living fragments. That is, they reproduced themselves exactly. Sometimes they failed to do this and reproduced themselves inexactly. This accident was then duplicated exactly.

In time the living fragments became cells. Cells became tissue. Tissues were formed into creatures. Countless trillions of different individuals were born into a million species, and died. Some, like the dinosaur, perished forever. Others, like man, endured and became more complex. But, although man has found a way to get out of this world and back again, he still has, as an embryo, ''gills'' like a fish's. His genes send ancestral messages, but his needs have modified the message. His ''gills'' become glands and major blood vessels. Genetic instruction and evolution dictate this.

genetics: molding a new person

The reasons for interest in heredity are several. First, the chromosomes within the nucleus of the human cell give directions that help decide the characteristics of man. Change those directions and man can be changed. Many scientists are apprehensive that man will ''tamper with heredity.'' To better understand and control human destiny, every generation must understand some genetics.

A generation ago, the British novelist and critic C. S. Lewis wrote these warning words:

> What we call Man's power over Nature turns out to be a power exercised by some men over other men with Nature as its instrument . . . And all long-term exercises of power, especially in breeding, must mean the power of earlier generations over later ones . . . If any age really attains . . . the power to make its descendants what it pleases, all men who live after it are the patients of that power.[2]

By late 1973, scientists had synthesized the first gene that had the potential for functioning in a living cell. Moreover, its product could also be detected in a living cell.[3] Such work has the ultimate aim of repairing defective human

[1] Walt Whitman, ''Song of Myself,'' line 1162.

[2] Quoted in Paul Ramsey, ''Shall We 'Reproduce'?'' *Journal of the American Medical Association,* Vol. 220, No. 11 (June 12, 1972), p. 1483.

[3] ''A 126-Unit Artificial Gene,'' *Science News,* Vol. 104, No. 9 (September 1, 1973), p. 132, and Thomas H. Maugh II, ''Molecular Biology: A Better Artificial Gene,'' *Science,* Vol. 181, No. 4106 (September 28, 1973), p. 1235.

genes. But knowledge is not wisdom, as human history has amply shown. It is the unwise use of knowledge—knowledge without judgment—that today imperils humankind.

Atomic energy provides a second reason for concern with genetics. The fallout from atomic testing may produce an effect, most likely deleterious, on human genes. But more than bombs are involved. Future generations will see a greatly expanded industrial use of atomic energy. The effect of possible atomic radiation on the progeny of posterity is urgent health business, and only an informed public can influence government policymakers to safeguard health.

The involvement of genetics with illness is yet a third reason the subject requires study. More than 1,600 varieties of birth defects perplex man. Some, like flat feet, are minor. Other, like Mongolism, are more serious. In all such disorders, genes play a varying role. Sometimes it is the gene that is basically at fault. In other cases it is the environment that disturbs genetic processes. And there are conditions for which the primary cause is unclear. But one concept is clear: all genetic processes must be considered within their ecosystems. Every gene interacts with its environment and is inexorably influenced by it.

the cell, unit of life

The *cell* (Figure 18-1) is the basic unit of life. The *protoplasm* is the chemical life of the cell. Protoplasm is made mainly of cellular proteins, fats, carbohydrates, and inorganic salts in a watery medium. It contains thousands of *enzymes* (see footnote 22). Many enzymes contain *vitamins.* Enzymes are eventually used up and must continuously be created anew by the cell from available nutrients. Their vitamin component must be made by the cell or taken in with food. Cells also contain special materials involved with their particular activity, such as the *glycogen* seen as granules in the liver cell.

The ministructures in the cell's protoplasm, the *organelles,* function in concert with their intracellular environment. The membrane-encircled *nucleus,* the largest of the cell's organelles, contains and is surrounded by protoplasm. Protoplasm outside the nucleus is called *cytoplasm.* Thus, the two major parts of most cells are the nucleus and the cytoplasm. The events that occur in the cytoplasm, such as digestion, respiration, secretion, and excretion, depend on the activity within the nucleus. The nucleus is also essential for the reproduction of the cell.

the nucleus

Within the nucleus are the *chromosomes* (Figure 18-2). The chromosomes contain the *genes* (Figure 18-3). A gene is the unit of heredity. But it is even more. Because each gene is composed of *DNA,* it governs the life of the cell. Because DNA can reproduce itself during cell division, its code is transmitted to subsequent cells. The *nucleolus,* or "little nucleus," is an organelle that is not visible in some stages of cell division. It has no membrane. It may be a storehouse of chemicals for the reproduction of DNA.

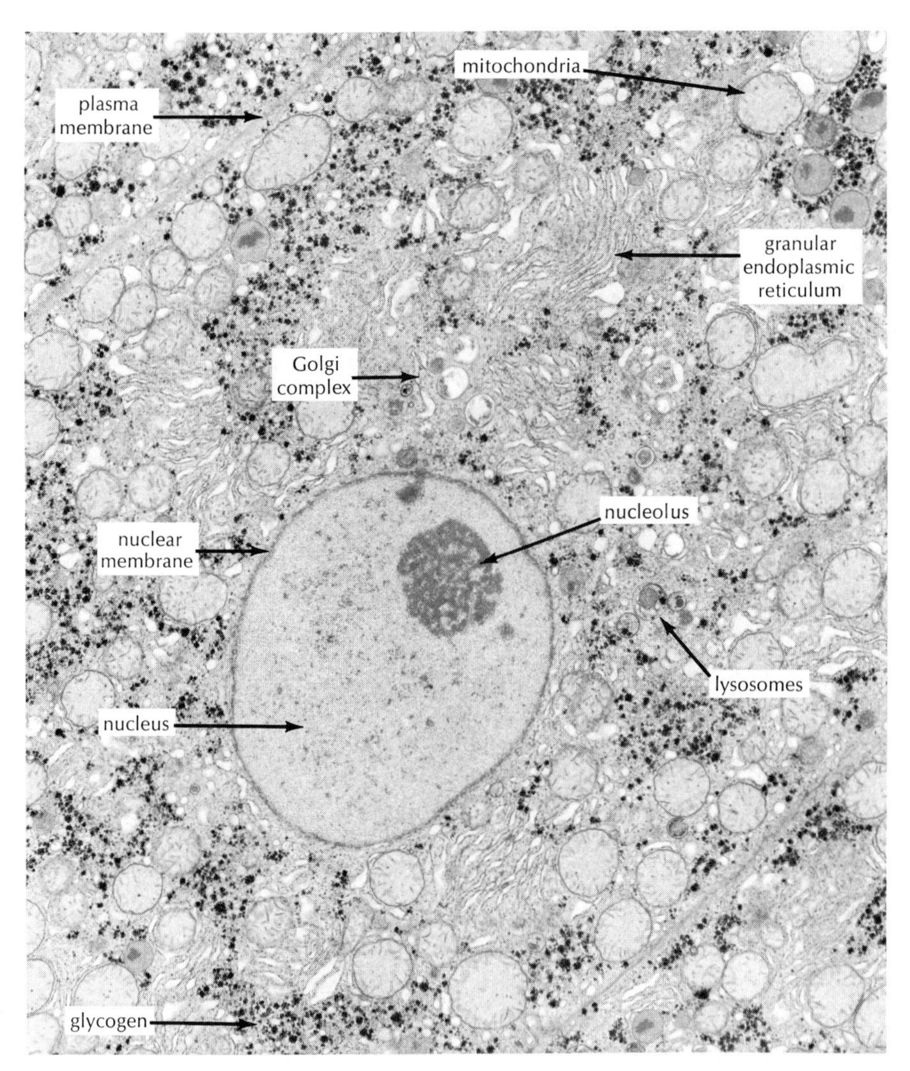

18-1 *A mammalian cell. Visible in this liver cell are granules of glycogen.*

In the cell community, red blood cells are unique. During their maturation in the bone marrow they lose their nuclei. Bereft of DNA, these cells cannot synthesize protein. Red blood cells live only so long as their enzymes last—about 120 days. Every second some 2.5 million red blood cells must be released into the circulation.

the cytoplasm, its membranous wall, and the endoplasmic reticulum

Policing the kind and amount of material entering the cell is its enveloping, porous *plasma membrane.* The plasma membrane, made up of fats, proteins, carbohydrates, and other components, does more than merely delineate cell boundaries. It is a complex structure performing a wide range of tasks that are essential to health and life. It admits some molecules that seek to enter the cell; it rebuffs others. It also permits the escape of waste materials from the cell but fastidiously retains essential substances.

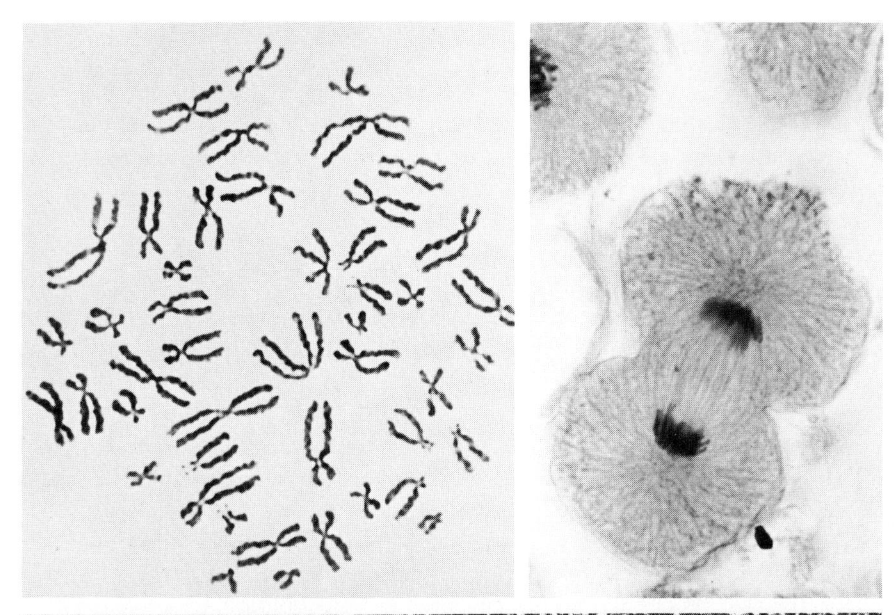

18-2 *Chromosomes of a normal human male* (left) *and of a whitefish* (right). *The chromosomes of this whitefish cell have duplicated themselves, and the cell itself is dividing into two cells* (*see mitosis, page 529*).

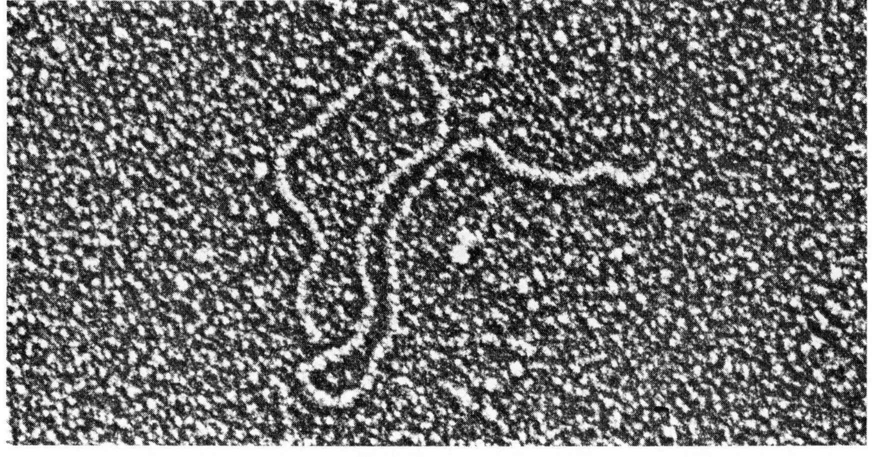

18-3 *A single gene, isolated from a common intestinal bacterium* (*see Chapter 25, page 773*).

> All chemical and electrical information that reaches the cell does so through its membrane. Hormones, insulin [page 260] for example, initiate their effects through interactions with receptor sites on cell surfaces . . . Many drugs act through cell-surface contacts, muscle contractions are triggered by electrical stimuli acting on membranes, and a host of enzymatic activities are carried out on the cell surface.[4]

When cancer occurs, disorders of the cell membrane are common. A better understanding of the cell membrane has a high priority in the science of the seventies.[5]

At various places the plasma cell membrane appears to fold inward to extend

[4] Barbara J. Culliton, "Cell Membranes: A New Look at How They Work," *Science,* Vol. 175, No. 4028 (March 24, 1972), p. 1350.

[5] How the study of cell membranes has been absorbing scientists in numerous laboratories is described in "The Cell Wall," *Medical World News,* Vol. 12, No. 30 (August 13, 1971), pp. 35–39, 43.

into the cytoplasm of the cell as the *endoplasmic reticulum.* Thus is created a membranous transportation system of canals along which needed materials move deep into the cell's cytoplasm. The endoplasmic reticulum communicates with the nuclear membrane. By this route nutrients for the nucleus are delivered. Wastes can be carried out via these canals too. Guiding the transport of materials within the cell and helping the cell to maintain its shape, then, is a system of tiny tubules.[6]

the organelles within the cytoplasm

On part of the endoplasmic reticulum granules are clustered; these are *ribosomes*—the sites of protein synthesis. Seemingly continuous with the nongranular endoplasmic reticulum is the *Golgi complex.* This may be a sort of enzyme storage bin; protein enzymes, completed at the ribosomes, penetrate the membrane of the endoplasmic reticulum and possibly migrate, via its channels, to the Golgi complexes, to be kept and released when needed by the cell. Also in the cytoplasm of most cells are the *mitochondria* and *lysosomes.* Mitochondria are the cell's energy sources. Like tiny fuel furnaces distributed throughout the cellular cytoplasm, mitochondria convert the chemical energy of cellular nutrients into a high-energy compound called *adenosine triphosphate* (*ATP*). ATP is released as needed for the cell's work. Mitochondria are enclosed by a membrane.[7] So are the lysosomes, the cell's digestive organelles. Each lysosome contains enzymes that break down complex nutrients into simpler substances. Another duty of the lysosome is to act as a minute garbage disposal, ridding the cell of bacteria or worn-out materials.

Consider the treasure of past and future generations contained within the cell: the nucleus, the power-packed mitochondria, the digesting lysosomes, the Golgi complex of storage facilities for completed protein enzymes, the membranous network of endoplasmic reticulum that provides a transportation system for cellular nutrients and wastes and a ribosomal site for protein synthesis—all these active islands surrounded by a small sea of protoplasm, which, in turn, is enveloped by the meticulously selective plasma membrane. They speak of the balanced organization within the cellular ecosystem. Two tools

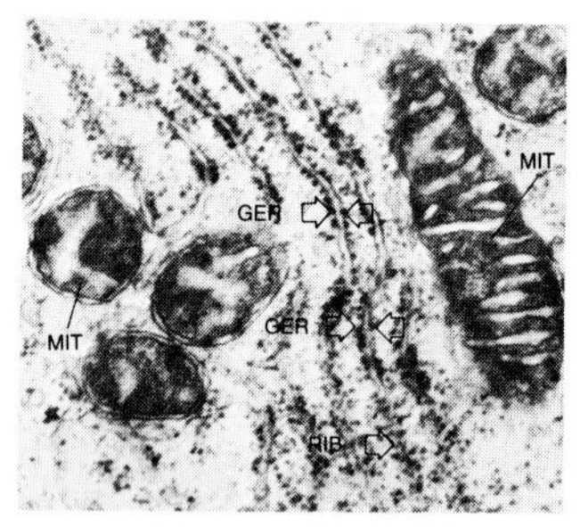

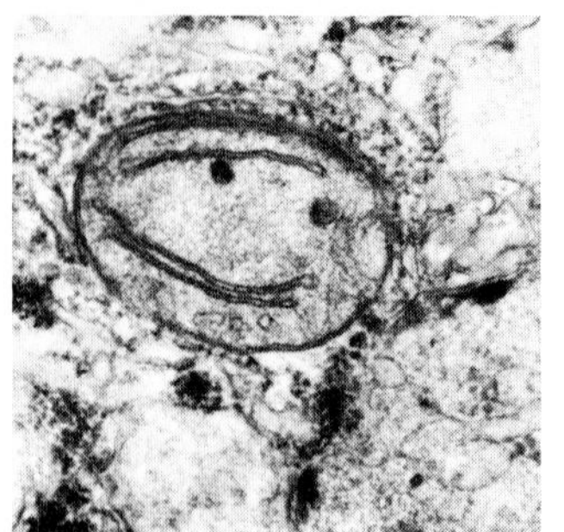

18-4 Top: *Electron photomicrograph showing granular endoplasmic reticulum* (*GER*), *mitochondria* (*MIT*), *and ribosomes* (*RIB*). Bottom: *A mitochondrion that happened to form a smiling face. The "eyes" of the mitochondrion are granules and the "mouth" and "eyebrows" are distorted crests of a diseased human liver cell.*

[6] Keith Roberts, "Signposts of the Cell," *New Scientist,* Vol. 53, No. 777 (January 6, 1972), p. 13.

[7] The origin of mitochondria remains one of the mysteries of the cell. These organelles contain their own DNA and RNA, which, some scientists believe, replicate independently of nuclear DNA and RNA. Thus they may have a system of protein synthesis that is independent of the protein synthesis system of the rest of the cell. Mitochondria resemble bacteria, and one evolutionary theory about their presence postulates that the first primitive cells to be formed did not need oxygen to survive. Threatened with extinction when the environment was enriched by oxygen, the primitive cells ingested oxygen-using bacteria that provided adenosine triphosphate to carry on the cell's respiration. In this view, mitochondria are thus derived from bacteria. Another theory suggests that during early cellular evolution, cells used oxygen but needed a larger surface. This was achieved by a folding inward of the cell membrane with eventual formation of membrane-bound vesicles—now known as mitochondria. The membrane acted as a permeable but selective barrier between the elements of respiration and the cell's cytoplasm. Since the membrane was impermeable to DNA and RNA, the cell implanted a system of protein synthesis within the mitochondria. (Samuel Vaisrub, "The Mystery of the Mitochondria," *Journal of the American Medical Association,* Vol. 222, No. 11 [December 11, 1972], p. 1422, citing F. A. Raff and H. R. Mahler, "The Nonsymbiotic Origin of Mitochondria: The Question of the Origin of the Eukaryotic Cell and Its Organelles Is Reexamined," *Science,* Vol. 177 [1972], pp. 572–82.) This second concept would seem to be partly supported by the discovery that there is DNA not only in the nucleus and mitochondria but also in the cytoplasm. It is theorized that these cytoplasmic molecules of DNA are "being ferried from nucleus to mitochondria." ("Is Cytoplasmic DNA Just Passing Through?" *New Scientist,* Vol. 54, No. 794 [May 4, 1972], p. 250.)

have made the cell more accessible to scientific scrutiny—the *electron microscope* and the *ultracentrifuge.* The first has afforded magnifications of over 100,000. The ultracentrifuge can whirl treated cell suspensions at speeds of sixty thousand revolutions per minute. Trapped in such an intense separating force, the microlayers of the cells separate to provide materials for the study of organelles. A new science, *molecular biology,* reveals both the normal and the abnormal at this level.

some chemical regulators of cellular life

But scientific investigation of the cell is not limited to ultramicroscopic searches for its ministructures. By what mechanisms do these ministructures operate so that health and life occur? In recent years an increasing amount of attention has been drawn to three chemical substances of enormous importance to cell (and body) function and dysfunction.

1. *Cyclic AMP* is the abbreviation for a small molecule with a big name: cyclic nucleotide adenosine 3′, 5′-monophosphate. It was first identified in 1957; the clarification of its function earned a 1971 Nobel Prize for Vanderbilt University's Earl W. Sutherland. Cyclic AMP has been called a "second messenger" within the cell. Why? Because (among other things) it acts as a mediator for many hormones.[8] Consider this example: epinephrine is a hormone secreted by the inner part of the adrenal gland (see page 258); among its functions are increasing the blood pressure and stimulating the heart. When it approaches a cell it does not act directly. Rather, it interacts with a receptor on the cell membrane. In this way an enzyme is stimulated into action. This enzyme, in turn, synthesizes cyclic AMP from ATP (see the preceding section). Thus the level of cyclic AMP within the cell is increased. The cyclic AMP then goes on to do the actual work of the hormone in the cell. The result of elevating the level of cyclic AMP in different tissues varies with the chemical makeup (and biological needs) of that tissue. In fatty tissue cells, for example, increased decomposition of fats occurs. In the liver cell, a rise in the level of cyclic AMP results in the increased splitting up of the body's chief stored carbohydrate—glycogen.[9] It is apparent, then, that this "second messenger," cyclic AMP, is a chemical mediator between "the hormone of the cell surface and the central control of cellular activity in the nucleus."[10]

Clearly, many of the basic regulatory processes that control the growth, differentiation, and hormonal responses of the cell are affected by its concentration of cyclic AMP. Thus, cyclic AMP is believed to regulate the all-important enzymes that, in turn, trigger reactions in body cells resulting in the storage of sugars and fats. It is, moreover, involved in the activities of genes. It may be that cancer is, in part, due to an inadequate supply of cyclic AMP.[11] In the labo-

[8] Earl W. Sutherland, "Studies on the Mechanism of Hormone Action," *Science,* Vol. 177, No. 4047 (August 4, 1972), pp. 401–08. This article is recommended for advanced students in this area.
[9] Alan Boyne, "Is Cyclic AMP a Key Chemical in Memory?" *New Scientist,* Vol. 58, No. 842 (April 19, 1973), p. 145.
[10] "Secluded Cancer Viruses Are Stirred by Cyclic AMP," *New Scientist,* Vol. 59, No. 861 (August 30, 1973), p. 484. Paradoxically, cyclic AMP not only is involved in switching off cell division; it may also switch on the production of certain viral particles. This whole area of research is attracting much attention. Of particular interest is the cell surface, for cyclic AMP is involved in the profound changes on that surface, as is cancer.
[11] Ira Pastan, "Cyclic AMP," *Scientific American,* Vol. 227, No. 2 (August 1972), pp. 97–105.

ratory, for example, cells in a culture can be triggered into dividing in a cancerous fashion by cancer-causing agents; the addition of cyclic AMP to the culture medium can stop the cancerous divisions. There are a number of other diseases in which a possible abnormality of cyclic AMP is involved. Among these are hay fever, asthma, some emotional disorders, eczema, and psoriasis.

Consider this last condition. It has been found that tissue from the lesions of psoriasis patients contains considerably less cyclic AMP than the uninvolved skin of a psoriasis patient or the skin of a normal person. As has been noted, elevation of cyclic AMP levels in the cell inhibits cell division. The cells of psoriasis tissue are characterized by abnormally rapid division. Much research must yet be done, but, theoretically, a treatment for psoriasis might be a compound that would elevate cyclic AMP in the cell. Such compounds have already been identified.[12]

2. For those inclined to chemistry, *cyclic GMP* is cyclic nucleotide, quanosine 3′, 5′-monophosphate. Like cyclic AMP, it is present in all living cells. By 1974, much more was known about cyclic AMP than cyclic GMP. It was theoretically held that many cellular regulations may be influenced by the interaction of cyclic AMP and cyclic GMP. However, it was suggested that their interactions occur only in those body cells in which occur strongly contrasting events, such as contraction–relaxation. Some researchers do not agree that (as was stated above) all the regulatory changes attributed to cyclic AMP are due only to variations in its concentration in the cell. They believe that an antagonist to cyclic AMP, namely cyclic GMP, operates in cell organizations (that is, tissues) that are bidirectionally or oppositely controlled. And, indeed, it has been shown that a number of cellular responses to body hormones and other agents occur with a rapid increase in cyclic GMP, and that these body responses to the same hormones and agents are opposite to those produced by cyclic AMP. These opposing variations between cyclic AMP and cyclic GMP have not yet been shown to *cause* regulatory events, but merely to be *associated* with them.[13]

3. *Chalones* are protein-like substances that are synthesized within the mature cells of various tissues. By late 1973, every kind of tissue that had been examined, including human tissue, had been found to contain its own chalone. Acting as chemical messengers, chalones inhibit, and thus control, cell division (*mitosis;* see the following section). Chalones are not *species-specific.* Thus, for example, chalone from a dog muscle will be effective in limiting cell division of cat muscle cells, or the muscle cells of any other animal. Yet chalones are *tissue-specific*—that is, they inhibit cell division only in the specific tissue from which they arise, without affecting any others; liver-tissue chalone, for example, will inhibit proliferation only of liver cells, skin-cell chalone only of skin cells, and so on. Clearly, then, a chalone maintains the correct number of cells in any given tissue. This fact, combined with the knowledge that its action is reversible

[12] "Evidence Shows 'Second Messenger' (AMP) May Have Role in Psoriasis," *Journal of the American Medical Association,* Vol. 220, No. 7 (May 15, 1972), pp. 907–08.
[13] Gina Bari Kolata, "Cyclic GMP: Cellular Regulatory Agent?" *Science,* Vol. 182, No. 4108 (October 12, 1973), pp. 149–51.

and that it does not poison the cell,[14] endows it with great potential for treatment of human health problems characterized by excessive cell division. Of these, two immediately come to mind: tissue or organ graft rejections and cancer.

Consider the first. To the body, tissue or organ grafts are intruding foreign antigens (see pages 144–45). Faced by them, lymphocytes (see page 141) react by proliferating in large numbers, thus producing cells to attack the invaders. Researchers have already applied lymphocyte chalone to reduce the immune response to tissue grafts in mice.[15] Moreover, in regard to cancer, two Helsinki investigators have successfully used a specific chalone to treat a mouse tumor. Why did raising the level of chalone work? Tumor cells continue to produce the chalone of their tissue of origin. Abnormally high concentrations of it are released in the body. Then why is the tumor not controlled? Because the cell membrane cannot contain the chalone. It is lost so quickly that its concentration within the cell soon becomes less than 10 percent of normal. Thus, raising the chalone level by treatment did heal one type of tumor—in the mouse.[16] What would happen in man is the subject of eager investigation.

meiosis and mitosis

There are two basic kinds of cells in the human body: germ cells (*gametes*) and somatic cells (Greek *soma,* body). A germ cell is a cell of an organism the function of which is to reproduce the kind; these are the ova (eggs) and the spermatozoa.[17] All other body cells are somatic.

When a mature sperm fertilizes a mature ovum, the resultant fusion is a cell called the *zygote.* To achieve the maturity necessary to participate in zygote formation, the germ cells, starting from *primordial sex cells,* must go through a special process of cell division called *meiosis.* Primordial sex cells have forty-six chromosomes, but when meiosis of a primordial sex cell is complete, the mature gamete has only twenty-three chromosomes (see Figure 18-5). Twenty-two of these are single, nonsex chromosomes and are called *autosomes.* The remaining chromosome is either an X or a Y *sex chromosome.* At the end of meiosis, the mature ovum carries a single X-chromosome; the mature sperm either an X-chromosome or a Y-chromosome (see Figure 18-6). It is a basic (although not the only) function of the Y-chromosome to direct the production of the male sex glands (testes).

When fertilization of the mature ovum by the mature sperm occurs, each parent contributes twenty-three chromosomes to the resultant zygote—twenty-two autosomes and one sex chromosome. A normal ovum always con-

[14] Thomas H. Maugh II, "Chalones: Chemical Regulation of Cell Division," *Science,* Vol. 176, No. 4042 (June 30, 1972), pp. 1407–08.

[15] "Chalones Come Out of Obscurity," *New Scientist,* Vol. 59, No. 865 (September 27, 1973), p. 734.

[16] David Moreau and William Bullough, "A Cellular Switch to Stop Cancer," *New Scientist,* Vol. 60, No. 866 (October 4, 1973), pp. 28–29.

[17] Women are born with their total supply of primitive eggs, which nestle immature in the ovary until puberty. Beginning at puberty, men continually replenish their supply of sperm cells.

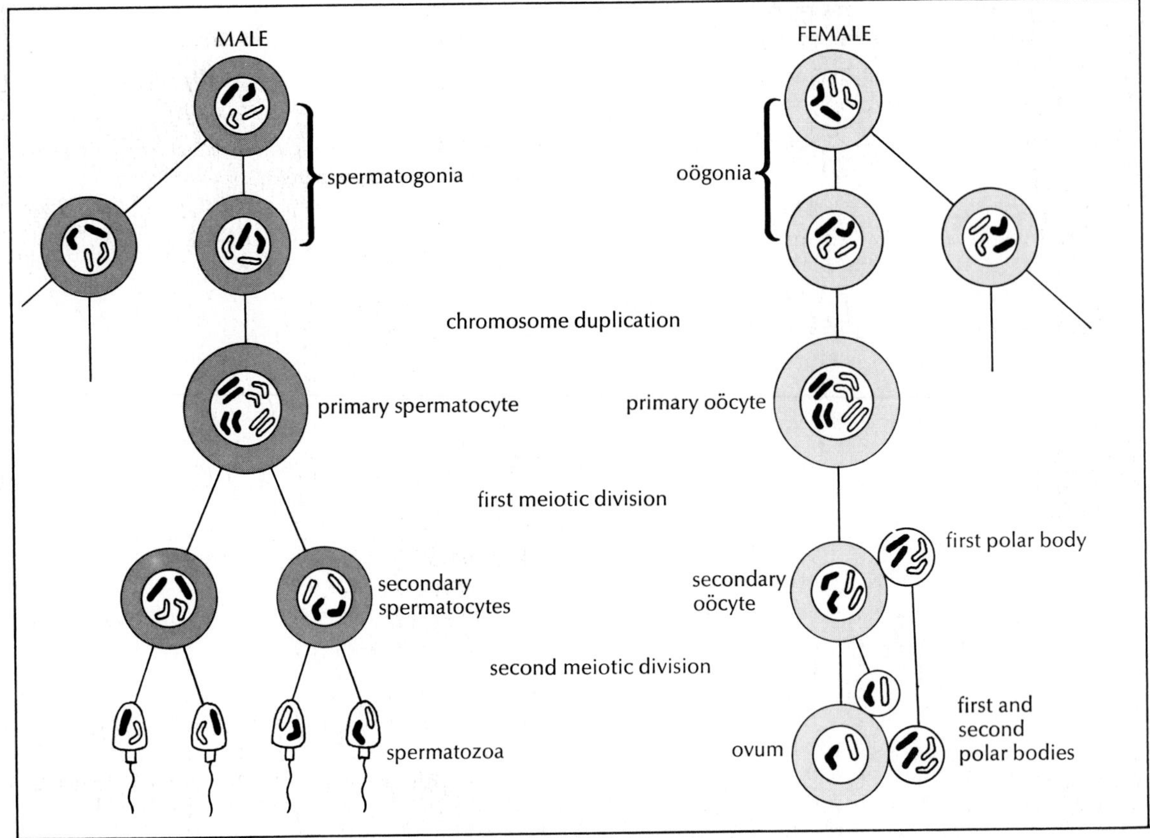

18-5 *Meiosis. The mature gametes (spermatozoa or ova) have half the number of chromosomes that the primordial sex cells (spermatogonia or oogonia) had. During the maturation process, polar bodies simply degenerate. For simplicity, cells shown here have only four chromosomes.*

tains an X-chromosome. If an ovum is fertilized by a normal sperm containing an X-chromosome, the result is XX (female):

$$\text{X (ovum)} + \text{X (sperm)} = \text{XX (female)}$$

If an ovum is fertilized by a sperm containing a Y-chromosome, the result is XY (male):

$$\text{X (ovum)} + \text{Y (sperm)} = \text{XY (male)}$$

So the zygote and all subsequent body (somatic) cells normally contain twenty-three pairs of chromosomes (a total of forty-six chromosomes), of which twenty-two pairs are autosomes and one pair are sex chromosomes. Each autosomal pair is different in genetic content and usually in appearance from all other pairs. Figure 18-7 shows the chromosomes arranged in pairs to form a chromosomal chart called a *karyotype.* Note that each autosomal pair is numbered from 1 to 22 and the sex chromosomes are appropriately labeled X or Y.

As noted above, only the primordial sex cells increase in number by meiosis. The zygote and all subsequent body (somatic) cells multiply by *mitosis.* In the process of mitosis, the threadlike chromosomes in the nucleus of a cell duplicate themselves; the duplicate sets are separated, with one set going to each of the two "daughter" cells produced by the division of the original cell. Thus in *mitosis* each of the two cells produced by the division of a single cell has a full set of chromosomes, whereas in *meiosis* each of the cells has *half* the number of chromosomes the original cell had. By mitosis the body replaces discarded cells and grows. In both meiosis and mitosis there are plenty of chances for errors. Should a cell, be it germ or somatic, fail to receive its proper share or composition of chromosomes, abnormality results.

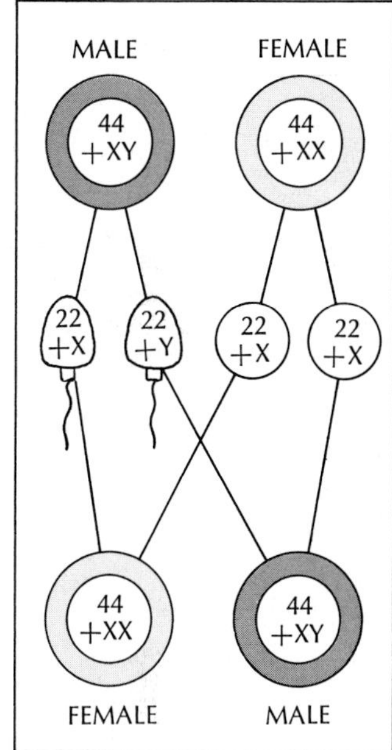

18-6 *If a sperm carrying an X-chromosome fertilizes an ovum, a female (XX) results; if a sperm carrying a Y-chromosome fertilizes an ovum, a male (XY) results.*

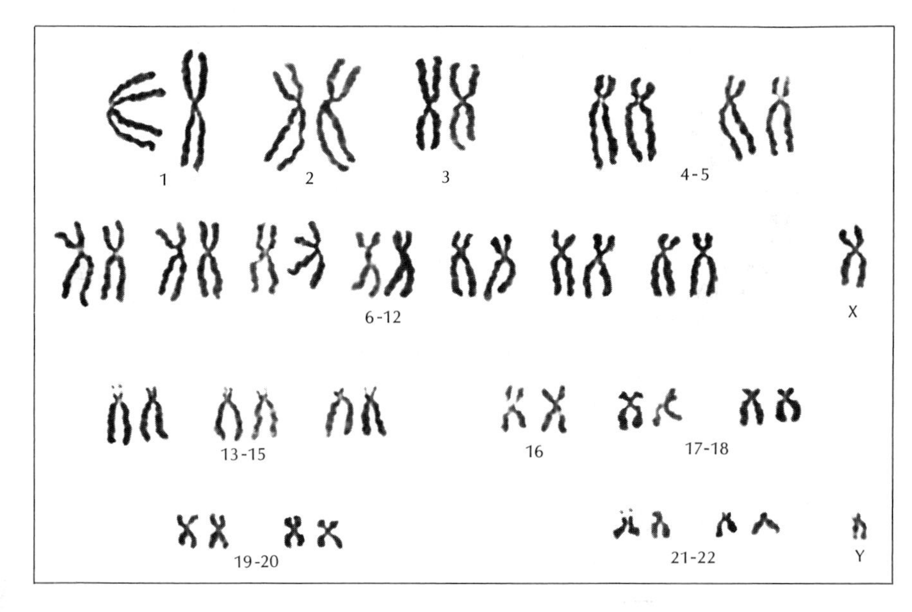

18-7 *Karyotype (chromosomal chart) of a normal human male. The karyotype of a female has two X-chromosomes where the X- and Y-chromosomes appear here.*

genetic order

By their union in the Fallopian tube (pages 477–78) the mature sperm and egg contribute their twenty-three single chromosomes to the fertilized egg to form a zygote with its full normal complement of forty-six. Mitosis begins. The zygote prepares to divide. Each of the forty-six chromosomes splits into two parts, which are exact replicas of each other. The cell divides. Now there are two body cells. Normally, each has its full share of forty-six chromosomes. Several hours later the two somatic or body cells cleave again. There are then four body cells.

Normally, each still contains forty-six chromosomes. And so cell multiplication continues. Every day the somatic cell cluster continues to divide as it travels down the Fallopian tube toward the uterus. With each division these cells double in number. Normally, they never have fewer or more than forty-six chromosomes. At last the tiny, multiplying cellular mass is implanted in the uterine endometrium. Membranes begin to form. Within two or three weeks after fertilization, the embryo is being fed via these membranes. In another week there is a heart. A week later the heart begins to beat. Now cell differentiation continues rapidly, and so does organ development. Differentiation began with the earliest division. For each cell must multiply in the limited space allotted to it and under pressures from every other cell. And, as will be seen, each cell is instructed as to its future function. This is the nature of the cellular ecosystem.[18]

The cells of various organs are specific for those organs. In other words, the cells of the heart are different from those of the gut, which, in turn, are different from those of the nerves, and so on. By birth, roughly fifty successive cell divisions have taken place, resulting in trillions of marvelously organized cells. With normal cell division, every one of those trillions of cells contains the identical number of chromosomes as the original individual single zygote contained. How did this happen? How does one kind of cell end up as a part of a bladder muscle, another kind in the eye, still another in a toenail, and yet a fourth in a mole on the left cheek? How does each cell get the message telling it what to become? The answer lies within the nucleus of the cell, in the chromosomes.

DNA, the master plan; RNA, the obedient worker

Chemically, a chromosome consists mostly of proteins combined with a substance called *deoxyribonucleic acid* (*DNA*). The chromosomal DNA is the material of the gene.[19] Within it is stored the genetic information. Chromosomal DNA may not itself leave the nucleus.[20] It appears imprisoned within it, capable of duplicating itself with each cell division, and serving as a blueprint for the formation of *ribonucleic acid* (*RNA*) molecules. Thus, chromosomes also contain RNA. As will be seen, several kinds of RNA are made, and each plays a specific role in the building of cell proteins.

Outside the nucleus, as part of the cell's cytoplasm, there are still other proteins. Like all body proteins they are originally derived from food. Like all other proteins they are composed of amino acids. It is from this nutrient pool of cytoplasmic proteins that amino acids are taken and brought to the ribosomes.

how the ribosomal factory is made

Peering through the electron microscope at an amphibian oöcyte[21] (Figure 18-8), biologists believe they have discovered how ribosomes originate. A gene is spindle-shaped. Each gene is linked with every other gene like the beads of a necklace. Running from the broad base of the spindle to its tip is a thread.

[18] *Embryology,* the science dealing with the development of the embryo, is discussed in Chapter 19, pages 571–73.

[19] For a discussion of viral DNA, see pages 155–60.

[20] DNA has been demonstrated outside the nucleus, both in mitochondria and in the cytoplasm. Whether these DNA molecules originate from the nuclear chromosomes has yet to be determined (see page 524, footnote 7), nor have scientists as yet clarified the function of DNA outside the nucleus.

[21] An *amphibian* is a vertebrate animal (a frog or a toad, for example) able to live both on land and in water; an *oöcyte* is a female gamete that has not reached full development; mature, it is an ovum.

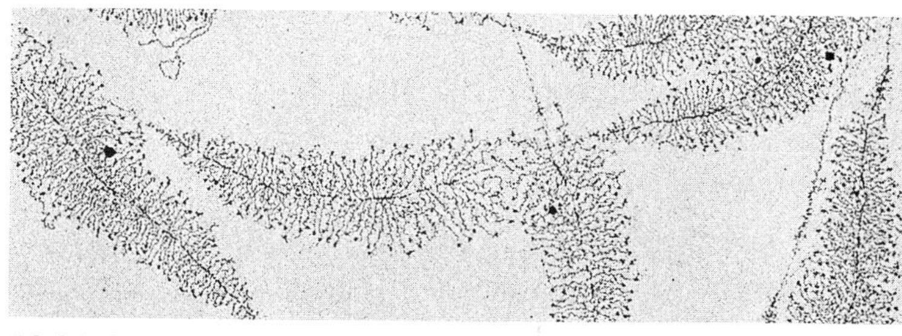
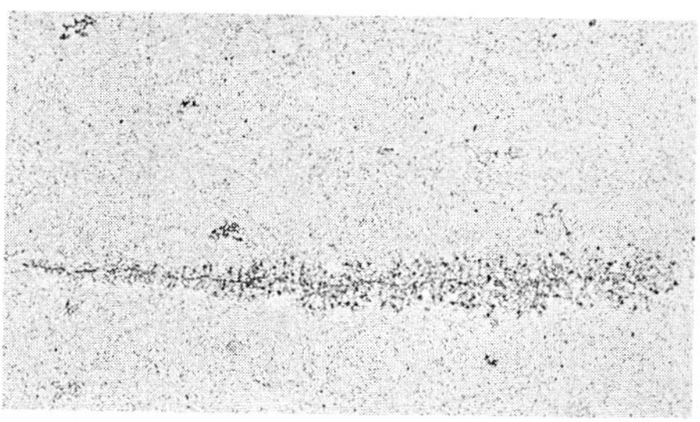

18-8 Left: *This electron photomicrograph of a salamander oöcyte is one of the first to show genes (the spine of the spindle-shaped structure) in the process of producing molecules of ribosomal ribonucleic acid (rRNA), seen as hairlike fibers extending from the genes* (×25,000). Right: *The only electron photomicrograph that shows what are presumed to be ribosomal RNA genes of a human cell* (×36,000).

This thread is DNA—a tiny segment of a chromosome. The DNA of the gene directs the production of molecules of ribonucleic acid (RNA). These hairlike molecules, extending from the gene, spiral about the DNA thread and decrease in size from the base to the tip of the spindle. (The RNA is not an inherent part of DNA; the DNA merely governs the synthesis of RNA according to its present code.) The length of the RNA fiber and its structure are dictated by the DNA, which directs its synthesis from cytoplasmic amino acids. As it is synthesized, the RNA molecules appose themselves to part of the DNA pattern in such a way as to reflect specific chemical configurations. RNA is thus instructed by the DNA. According to DNA instructions, each RNA fiber breaks off and, when free in the nucleus, is broken up into segments, probably by an enzyme.[22] First one, and then a second part of the original RNA fiber leaves the nucleus, deserting the nuclear DNA, which may not leave. Bearing the specific instructions of the DNA, these segments of the RNA fiber meet in the cellular cytoplasm to form a single ribosome. John Lear has described this remarkable process:

> According to the biochemical evidence, the opening event in the sequence of the spindle's operation is the extrusion of the RNA fiber from the main thread of DNA. As the extrusion proceeds, the fiber is strung with a protein coat according to coded instructions from the DNA. This process goes on until each fiber reaches a predetermined length . . . , after which that particular RNA fiber separates from the DNA thread like a quill from a porcupine's back. The fibers depart individually after attaining individual maturity. En route they pass under an unidentified biological knife (presumably an enzyme) that chops each fiber into segments. The first segment to be severed is about one-sixth the length of the whole fiber. This segment moves into the cytoplasm very quickly and at once coils into a tiny sphere. The coiling apparently occurs in response to instructions the DNA thread imprinted on the RNA fiber before setting the fiber loose. That part of the fiber that remains in the nucleus is subsequently chopped several times, until the surviving segment is about one-third as long as the original fiber had been. The final segment then moves out through the nuclear membrane into the cytoplasm, finds a tiny sphere formed by an earlier segment of fiber, and coils into a larger sphere alongside the tiny sphere. The two spheres together make a ribosome.[23]

[22] An enzyme is frequently a protein and has the power to initiate or accelerate certain chemical reactions in plant or animal metabolism.

[23] John Lear, "Spinning the Thread of Life," *Saturday Review* (April 5, 1969), pp. 63–64.

how body protein is made

Consider what happens at a single ribosome.

An amino acid is brought and attached to it. Then a second amino acid is brought to it. With the assistance of an enzyme, the second amino acid is linked to the first. But only in a predetermined way. A third amino acid is brought to the ribosome. It is linked to the second—again in a manner previously decided, and helped by an enzyme. A fourth amino acid then reaches the assembly line at the ribosomal factory. It is linked to its predecessor. Still another follows it. Then another and another. To all the ribosomal depots, in all the body cells, whether in a developing embryo or in an aging man, amino acids, derived from the nutrient pool of cytoplasmic proteins, are brought and linked one to the other. At each ribosome, then, a series of linked amino acids, a chain, is formed. Bonds between these amino acid chains form complex proteins. The manner of arrangement of the amino acids determines protein structure. And protein structure decides body structure and, therefore, function. So the chemical arrangement of the amino acids at the ribosomes results in proteins that will become blue eyes or black eyes, liver or heart, a short or tall person. The variations in the arrangement of amino acids at the ribosomal workbench are no less endless than the variations of hereditary characteristics.

18-9 *Ribosomes: the sites of protein synthesis. The top photo shows granular endoplasmic reticulum (×60,000), on which ribosomes (R) are located (see also Figure 18-1 and page 524). The bottom photo shows ribosomes (R) at a higher magnification (×88,000). Numbers of ribosomes are connected by filaments (M), which are believed to be messenger RNA.*

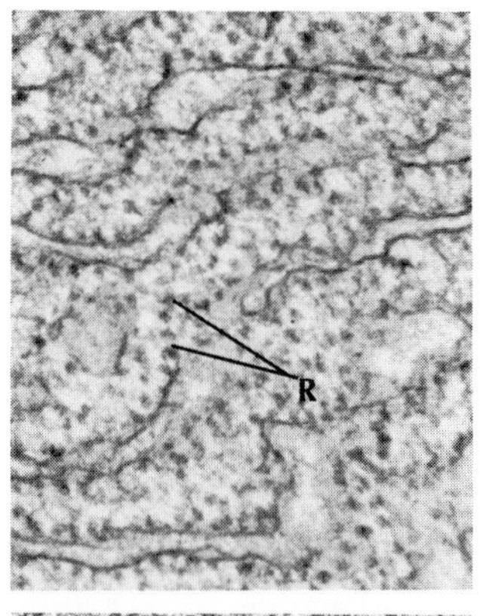

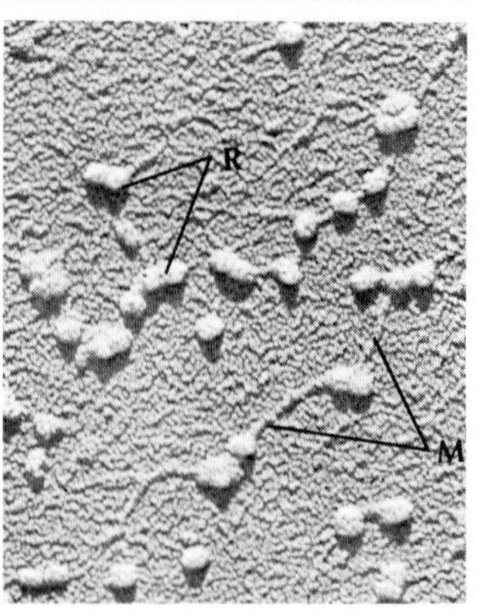

How do the amino acids get selected out of the cytoplasmic protein? How is their sequence determined? How are they brought to the ribosome? And, once at the ribosome, how does it happen that amino acids are so properly arranged? It is the nuclear DNA that governs all this. Only that DNA contains the genetic formula, so only that DNA can impart the genetic code, the hereditary instructions. But how can these DNA instructions reach the ribosome? It has been seen that the DNA may not itself leave the nucleus to direct protein structure at the ribosome. It seems imprisoned within the nucleus, irrevocably locked within the chromosomal pattern. It appears fixed, a template, a mold of chemicals. Since that DNA is unable to carry its own message outside the nucleus, an intermediary is needed—a messenger.

That messenger must somehow obtain the exact complex message, the specific instructions, of the DNA. Like the ribosomal RNA before it, that messenger must, therefore, in turn become a template, a mold of the DNA code. And unlike that DNA, that messenger must be able to leave the nucleus. Obediently that messenger must wend its way to the waiting ribosome, bringing to it the DNA message of instructions. A special kind of RNA is that messenger. Somehow, *messenger RNA* (as it is called) must obtain the patterned message, established by the coded position of certain chemical elements in the DNA. (As will be seen, the message obtained by the messenger RNA is for a different purpose than that obtained by ribosomal RNA.)

Within the cell's nucleus, messenger RNA places itself in apposition to part of the DNA code. It arranges its chemical structure to exactly match that of the DNA. The RNA transcription of the DNA template is thus formed.[24] In this way the messenger RNA has itself become a template, a mold, a momentous master

[24] The rate at which messenger RNA is transcribed from the DNA is determined by the arrangement or sequence of the chemicals of the DNA. In some manner light affects this rate. It sets the biological clock.

copy of the DNA basic chemical structure. Having incorporated within itself the instruction of the DNA, having acquired within its very structure the position of the coded chemical elements of the DNA, the messenger RNA deserts the DNA. It traverses the nuclear membrane. It enters into the midst of the cellular cytoplasm. There the DNA-code-carrying messenger RNA heads for a waiting ribosome. For, as has been stated, it is at the ribosomal workbench that protein is manufactured. And these synthesized proteins contribute to the specific characteristics of the creature-to-be.

Upon finding a ribosome, the messenger RNA is associated with it. Thus is established, at the ribosome, the copy of the DNA code of instructions. Now amino acids, taken from the surrounding cytoplasmic protein, must be brought to the ribosome. And, with the instructions awaiting their arrival, the amino acids must be properly arranged at the ribosome. This can be done only as instructed by the nuclear DNA. For although that DNA seems imprisoned, it remains the master. The traveling messenger RNA, associated with a ribosome, remains but a copy, a slave. And now the readied ribosomal workbench (the synthesis of which was also specifically directed by that DNA) awaits amino acid delivery. To construct specific proteins, to create specific tissue as instructed, amino acid building blocks must be brought to the ribosomal factory from the nutrient cytoplasmic protein pool.

How is this accomplished?

While the ribosome was receiving its instructing messenger RNA, the DNA in the nucleus was not idle. It kept busy directing the production of still another, smaller type of RNA. This third RNA is called *transfer RNA.* Also instructed by the nuclear DNA, in a fixed sequence, transfer RNA leaves the nucleus and enters the cytoplasmic protein pool of amino acids. For each separate amino acid there is a separate transfer RNA. On its way to the ribosome the transfer RNA picks up its selected amino acid from the protein pool. On reaching the ribosome, the amino acid leaves the transfer RNA and, helped by enzymes, attaches itself to the ribosome. One after another, in assembly line fashion, and as instructed by the messenger RNA, the amino acids are linked one to the other.

So transfer RNA keeps leaving the nucleus, picking up selected amino acids from the cytoplasmic protein pool, and delivering them to be linked to the growing amino acid chain at the ribosomal protein factory. But recent work suggests that this factory is not merely an inert organelle—that it is more than a passive building site. It is postulated that the ribosome moves. The message brought to the ribosome from the nuclear DNA by the messenger RNA is in the form of a string of chemicals arranged in a specific sequence. Along this messenger RNA these chemicals are arranged in groups of three, and each group is called a *codon.* Each codon specifies a particular amino acid. So the messenger RNA associated with a ribosome is like a string of beads; each bead is a codon, which is composed of an exact sequence of three chemicals. And each codon waits for transfer RNA to bring to it an allocated amino acid. It is the codon, then, that the transfer RNA must recognize to know at what point at the ribosome to bring its amino acid. Imagine such a string of messenger RNA beads or

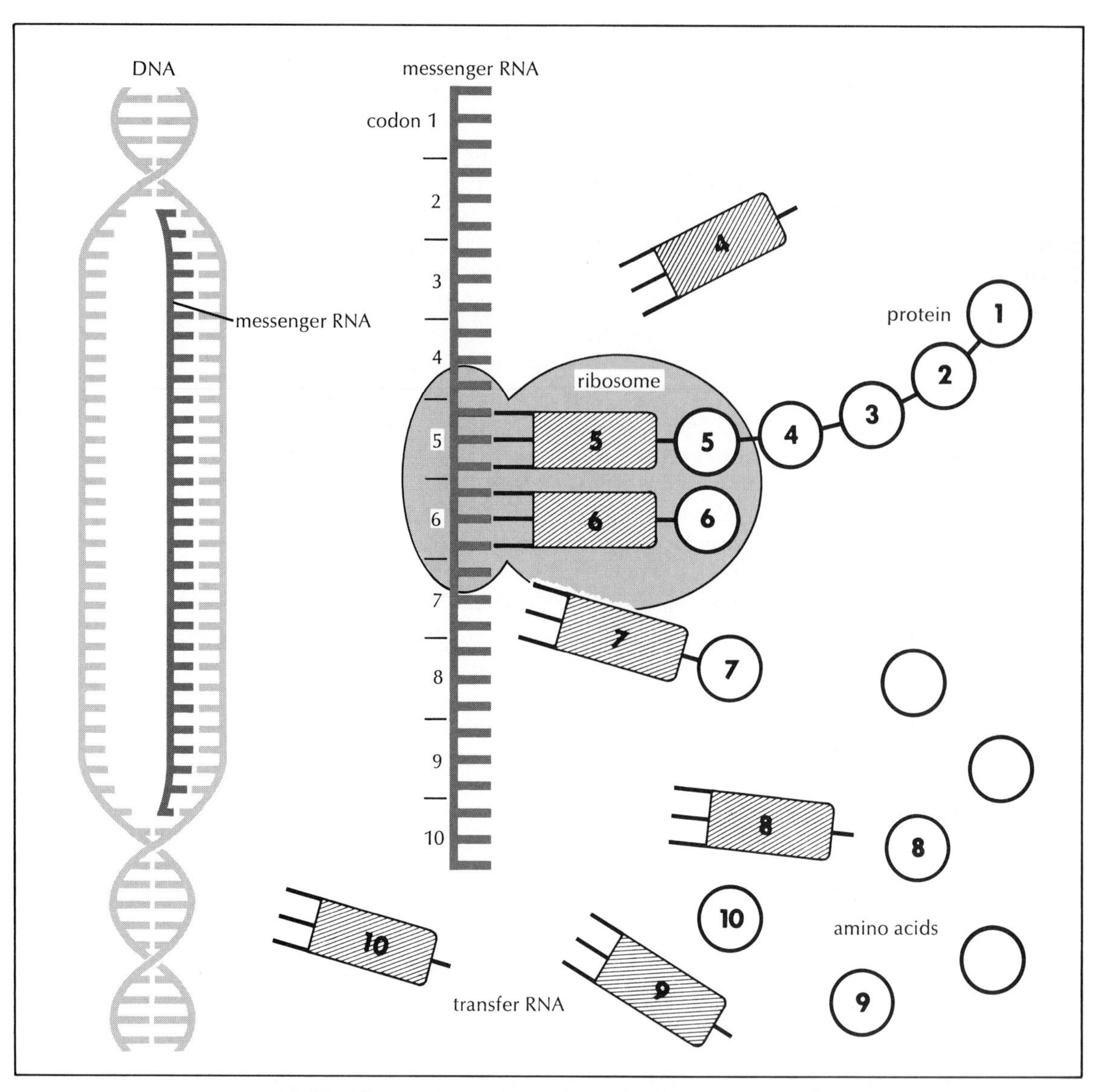

18-10 *The synthesis of proteins. The diagram at the left represents the transcription of genetic information from DNA to messenger RNA. The rest of the illustration schematizes the process by which transfer RNA brings its specified amino acid to the ribosome, which is situated at the codon specifying that particular amino acid. Here amino acid number 6, specified by codon number 6, has just been bound to its site on the ribosome by the corresponding transfer RNA. Amino acid number 6 will bond to amino acid number 5, adding to the growing chain. Then the ribosome will move along the messenger RNA to codon number 7. In this example, the chain will be complete when amino acid number 10 has been bonded to it. (Most proteins, however, consist of two or more chains of amino acids.)*

codons (see Figure 18-10) and, for the sake of explanation, give each codon a number from 1 through 10. (There are many more.) Also for convenience, number each molecule of transfer RNA carrying its particular amino acid. Transfer RNA number 1 brings its specific amino acid, number 1, from the cytoplasmic pool to the ribosome, which is now located at codon number 1 of the messenger RNA. There, amino acid number 1 is attached to the ribosome. Transfer RNA number 1 is then released to seek another of its specific amino acids. Carrying its first amino acid, the ribosome moves on to codon number 2. There another transfer RNA (number 2) waits with its amino acid number 2. Amino acid number 2 is then bound to amino acid number 1. The ribosome moves on to the third bead (or codon) of the string of messenger RNA. The process is repeated and amino acid number 3 is bound to amino acid number 2. In this way one after another specific amino acids are bound to one another, as shown in Figure 18-10. In this sense the ribosome makes its own string of beads, and each bead is an amino acid. The completed amino acid chains are the components of complex proteins. Thus, the ribosome conducts the synthesis of proteins. Finally and, as always, according to DNA instructions, the ribosome has had enough. There are no more codons for it to move along. The ribosome then rids itself of its linked chain of amino acids—of its protein component. What becomes of the complete protein? It contributes to the body structure and function. It will contribute to the eye, or to the heart, or to an enzyme. Multiplied billions of times, this process accounts for the creation of a unique person.[25] The wonder is not that an occasional error or defect occurs. The wonder is that it occurs so rarely.

How extensive is all this activity?

> If it were possible to assemble the DNA in a single human cell into one continuous thread, it would be about a yard long. This three-foot set of instructions for each individual cell is produced by the fusion of egg and sperm at conception and must be precisely replicated billions of times as the embryo develops.[26]

After birth too, and so long as the individual grows, develops, and ages, the genetic process by which cellular proteins are manufactured is repeated still more billions of times. As long as the person lives, it goes on.

the new person: product of genetics? environment? or both?

DNA instructions are many and they are related one to the other. And the whole genetic process takes place in, and is affected by, an all-encompassing environment. Each cell, each nucleus within the cell, each strand of DNA within the nucleus, each chemical component within the DNA, functions within the context of its environment. So there are genetic ecosystems.

If the whole genetic process operates in an environment, it is inexorably influenced by it. An individual is not merely the result of the *genotype.* "The

[25] Here one can best comprehend the individuality of the single being. Within each new zygote formed by the union of sperm and ovum is a completely new organization of DNA, a new master plan, a new set of instructions. Never before had there been a zygote with exactly the same DNA code.

[26] Marshall W. Nirenberg, "The Genetic Code; II," *Scientific American,* Vol. 208, No. 3 (March 1963), p. 82.

genotype is the sum total of the heredity the individual has received, mainly . . . in the form of DNA in the chromosomes of the sex cells. The cytoplasm may also contain some heredity determinants; if so, they are likewise constituents of the genotype.''[27] But with cell division and the resultant increase in the number of cells, with the growth of the organism, the constituents of the genotype must continuously reproduce themselves (replication). The material for this replication is taken from the environment. Consider just the change in size that occurs from man's beginning as a fertilized ovum to full adulthood.

> A human egg cell weighs roughly one twenty-millionth of an ounce; a spermatozoon weighs much less; an adult person weighs, let us say, 160 pounds, or some fifty billion times more than an egg cell . . . The phenotype is, then, a result of interactions between the genotype and the sequence of the environments in which the individual lives . . . The ''environments'' include, of course, everything that can influence man in any way. They include the physical environment—climate, soil, nutrition—and, most important in human development, the cultural environment—all that a person learns, gains, or suffers in his relations with other people in the family, community, and society to which he belongs.[28]

Thus, to say that an individual is genetically predetermined is more than an unjustified limitation on human potential. It is also scientifically invalid. And there is an element of absurdity to the ''heredity versus environment'' argument. For whatever happens in the genetic system is a happening in an environment. Genes are not fateful. By themselves, they decide little.

Nevertheless, practicality does require an answer to the question, ''To what extent can genes predispose an individual to develop certain illnesses?'' Some disorders are dependent on the presence of a particular genetic error (though not all individuals who carry such errors will necessarily manifest the disorders). Then what is the role of the surrounding environment? This varies. In some instances, such as hemophilia, the environmental influence, compared to the genetic, is surely small. With other conditions, the environment plays a more distinct role. Coronary artery disease, as an example, is greatly influenced by both genetic instruction and environment. Short stocky men with a history of heart attacks in their families are more prone to coronary heart disease than tall thin men without such a history. But diet (environment) plays an important role too. How long the condition remains latent and, when revealed, how severely it is manifested—these may be profoundly influenced by the environment. Another example: much has been written of the relationship between an XYY chromosomal pattern and aggressive behavior (see page 542). The association may have some validity. However, most aggressive behavior is unrelated to the XYY chromosome. Moreover, a gentle, well-adjusted person may carry an XYY chromosomal aberration and harm nobody. Another with the same genetic disorder will be a violent, homicidal menace. The difference may be in the environment.

[27] Theodosius Grigorievich Dobzhansky, *Heredity and the Nature of Man* (New York, 1964), pp. 49–50.
[28] *Ibid.*, pp. 50–51. The *phenotype* is the appearance of the trait; the *genotype* is the genetic basis of the trait.

A few years ago, Charles J. Whitman, a twenty-five-year-old architectural engineering major, climbed to the observation deck of the University of Texas tower in Austin. He shot and killed fourteen persons who were on the campus below. Thirty-one others were injured. A few hours before, he had killed his wife and mother. Whitman's chromosomal pattern is unknown. This, however, is known: autopsy revealed a highly malignant brain tumor. Could his brain tumor have contributed to his aggression? Perhaps. (He had presented no known neurological abnormality.) The chromosomal patterns of Lee Harvey Oswald and Jack Ruby are also unknown. But Oswald's terrible childhood certainly helped lay the groundwork for the terrible act of his adulthood.[29] On the other hand, Ruby suffered from psychomotor epilepsy—a seizure disorder singularly resistant to treatment. During a seizure from this type of epilepsy, violence is not uncommon. Twice in his lifetime Ruby had been struck on the head by a pistol butt. Where did genetic influence begin? Where did the environment enter the behavioral picture? It is now impossible to tell. But neither factor can be ignored. What is needed is more alert study.

genetic disorder

Human genetic problems are related either to (1) an error in the physical or chemical *structure* of a chromosome or (2) an error in the *amount* of chromosomal material in the cell. This is generally expressed in terms of the *number* of chromosomes in the cell.

disorders of chromosomal structure

spontaneous mutations

Man was once fishlike, and within the uterus he still lives submerged in water like a fish. Slowly, over millions of years, he left the sea, and over still more millions of years he adapted to a new environment. All his adaptive changes were made possible by infinitely gradual gene changes, or mutations (Latin *mutare,* to change). There are much more rapid changes due to environmental influence, as occurs when the German measles virus attacks the embryo. However, some genetic changes, although occurring in the environment, do not seem to be primarily caused by it. These are called *spontaneous.* A spontaneous change of some part of the chemical structure of the DNA takes place. If the change is not basically molded by the surrounding environment, how, then, may one account for the existence of a mutation in chromosomal structure? What causes a spontaneous change in DNA? The answer to this question remains unknown. Yet even one spontaneously mutant gene can result in profound developmental changes and hereditary health problems. Anatomical and, therefore, functional deviations from the normal ensue. There may be in-

[29] David Abrahamsen, "A Study of Lee Harvey Oswald: Psychological Capability of Murder," *Bulletin of the New York Academy of Medicine,* Second Series, Vol. 43, No. 10 (October 1967), pp. 861–88.

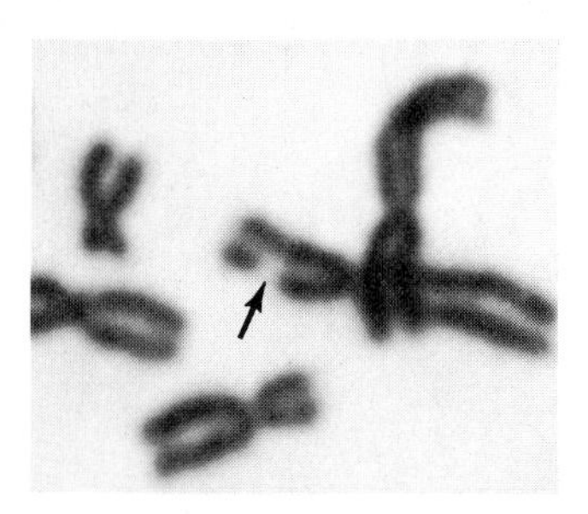

18-11 *A chromosomal break* (arrow) *due to radiation.*

born errors of metabolism. Disorders of carbohydrate metabolism, such as diabetes mellitus, and of amino acid metabolism (phenylketonuria—PKU; see page 558) are examples. Or disease of the blood or blood-forming organs may result. Hemophilia is one of these. By no means are all mutations spontaneous, however. Some are plainly *induced* by an external environmental stimulus. An example is genetic disorder caused by radiation (see page 551).

chromosomal translocation and deletion

This, too, may occur spontaneously, or there may be a direct external cause, such as radiation. Sometimes a chromosome breaks. DNA structure is disrupted. The chromosome may heal into a new and different structure. Or it may remain in fragments. Or it may be just partly repaired, leaving a piece out of its structure. Or two chromosomes may exchange pieces. *Translocation* occurs when a segment or a fragment of one chromosome shifts into another part of a noncorresponding chromosome. Sometimes, one of the products of such an exchange is so small it gets lost. This is called *deletion.* Whatever occurs, the chromosome is adversely altered. Genetic instruction by the DNA of the affected chromosomes is awry. Usually a fertilized egg that contains a broken or wrongly formed chromosome dies. Occasionally, the zygote lives. The individual develops to suffer various deficiencies.

disorders of chromosome number during meiosis or early mitosis

Sometimes it is not a changed chromosomal structure that results in disease. Rather it is an error in the total number of chromosomes that find their way into the cells. Normally, there are forty-six. With genetically related sickness, there may be too many or too few. How can this happen?

errors during meiosis

Study again Figure 18-5 illustrating meiosis. This shows how the chromosomes, having duplicated themselves, separate. Consequently, after the first cell division, when two cells are formed, each cell normally has duplicates of only a single member of each original pair of chromosomes. Sometimes, though, something goes wrong. Nobody really knows why. During meiosis, the chromosomes of a pair do not separate. This is the basic error. One cell receives both chromosomes of the pair, while the other gamete receives none. This is called *meiotic nondisjunction.*

It will be further noted in Figure 18-5 that there are two meiotic divisions. Meiotic nondisjunction can also occur during the second meiotic division after a normal first division. Upon fertilization, should a gamete with a missing chromosome unite with a normal gamete, the zygote and all the cells consequent to its multiplication will have forty-five chromosomes instead of the normal forty-six. This condition is called *monosomy.* Should a gamete with an extra chromosome unite with a normal gamete, the zygote will have forty-seven chromosomes. This is *trisomy.* The trisomy and monosomy of meiotic nondisjunction can affect both the autosomal chromosomes and the sex chromosomes.

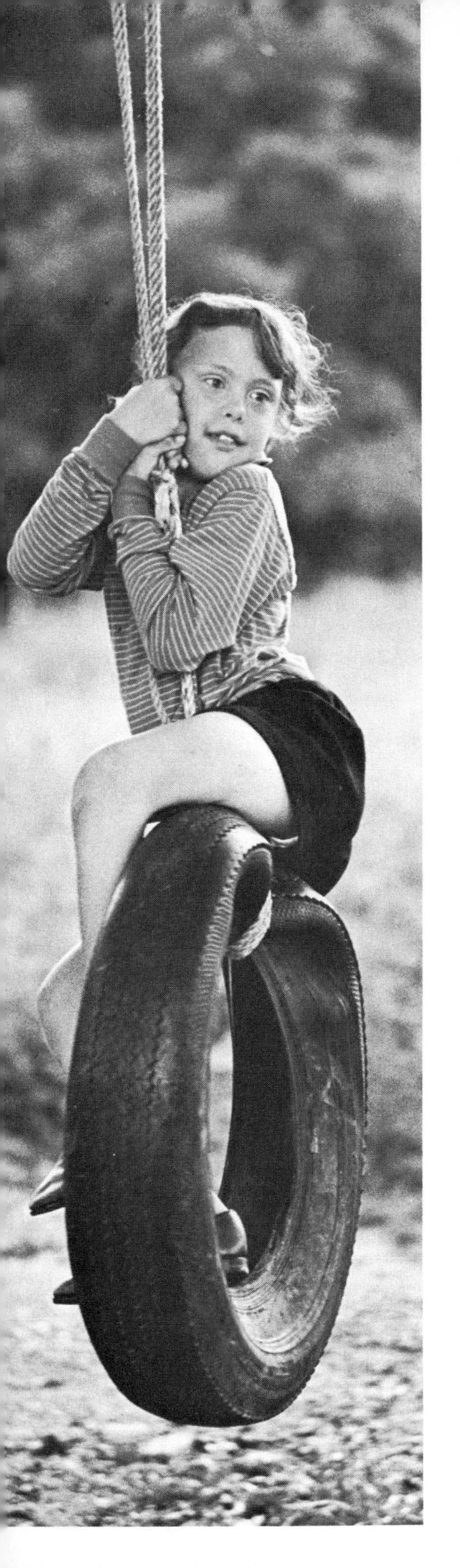

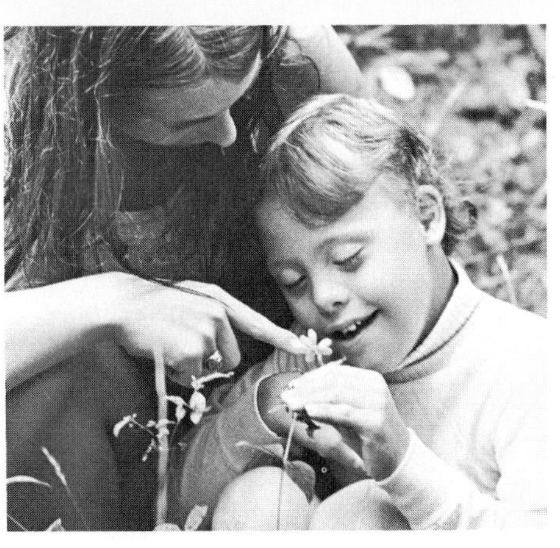

18-12 *These pictures show some moments in a day of ten-year-old David Roberts' life. David has Down's syndrome (Trisomy 21). A loving and generous boy, his I.Q. is only 52, but expressed in terms of emotional development it is a superior 115. David is more fortunate than most children with Mongolism. He has understanding parents. His father, a professional photographer, took these pictures; his mother, a writer, collaborated with her husband on a moving book urging that children like David be kept in a warm family environment if possible. David also has an informed physician, and leads a rich social life. With his special friend in special classes in the Charlotte, North Carolina, school system, David learns at his own pace. For him coordination comes less easily than for most other children, but there is a joy of achievement as he rides a tire-swing. Fortunately, unlike 40 percent of Mongoloid children, David has no heart defects; nor is he unduly susceptible to infection. A host of senseless myths have victimized children like David. Some think they are too stupid to be sensitive; thus the child suffers inadvertently cruel comments. Many believe they are sexually aggressive; the reverse is true: rape by retarded males is almost unknown. Within the past few years the average Mongoloid's life expectancy has risen from twelve years to twenty, and it is increasing. With care, patience, and understanding, the Mongoloid child can lead as full a life as many a person without the condition who lives three times as long.*

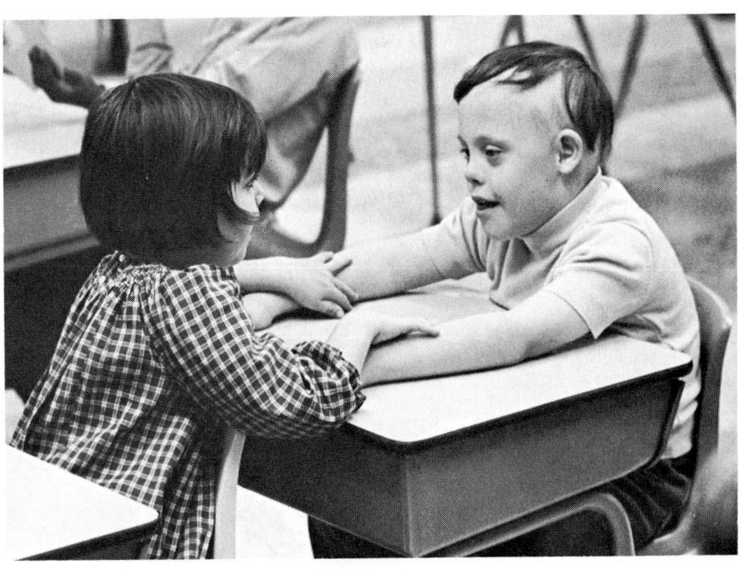

TRISOMY 21 The most common trisomy affects the twenty-first autosome. *Trisomy 21* is one cause of *Mongolism,* or *Down's syndrome* (Figure 18-12), in which nondisjunction occurs with chromosomes other than the X and Y. As a result of this autosomal aberration, the individual has forty-seven instead of forty-six chromosomes. Children with Down's syndrome[30] (named after a nineteenth-century English physician, John Down) are physically and mentally retarded. Muscle tone is poor. The tongue is large. The eyes are slanted, which accounts for the other name of the condition—Mongolism. Palmprints and footprints are abnormal. As the age of the mother increases, so do her chances of giving birth to a child with Mongolism.

Meiotic nondisjunction involving the X and Y sex chromosomes can result in gametes that may unite to produce zygotes that manifest some aberrant sex chromosome arrangements. How do these disorders occur?

TURNER'S SYNDROME (*Figures 18-13 and 18-14*) Illness may result from nondisjunction of sex chromosomes during meiosis. Assume that during an error in meiotic division an ovum receives no X-chromosome. It is fertilized by a normal sperm containing an X-chromosome. The resultant individual acquires a chromosomal pattern as follows:

$$\text{No X (ovum)} + \text{X (sperm)} = \text{0X}$$

(0 refers to the missing X chromosome.)

An 0X zygote develops into an individual with a combination of characteristics called *Turner's syndrome* (*monosomy X*). At birth the baby appears to be a female. But the child has tiny ovaries and does not develop secondary sexual characteristics. She is abnormally short and never menstruates. Turner's syndrome also results if a sperm with no X-chromosome fertilizes a normal ovum.

KLINEFELTER'S SYNDROME (*Figures 18-13 and 18-14*) Sometimes, during meiosis, a single ovum receives both (XX) chromosomes. With fertilization by a sperm carrying a Y-chromosome, what happens? This:

$$\text{XX (ovum)} + \text{Y (sperm)} = \text{XXY}$$

Here there is an excess X (female) chromosome (*intersex*[31]). The result: a *Klinefelter male,* as this individual is called. These people may appear normal, or be quite tall. They may have underdeveloped sexual structures. Ordinarily, they are sterile and are often mentally retarded.

Illness from nondisjunction of sex chromosomes during male meiosis can also result in the Klinefelter male.

[30] A *syndrome* refers to a set of signs and symptoms occurring together, as a group, in a disease state.

[31] Intersexuality should not be confused with homosexual behavior. The former is a genetic disorder. It refers to the abnormal intermingling, in varying degrees, of the characteristics of each sex in one individual. The incidence of homosexual behavior among intersexually abnormal patients is not higher than in the general population.

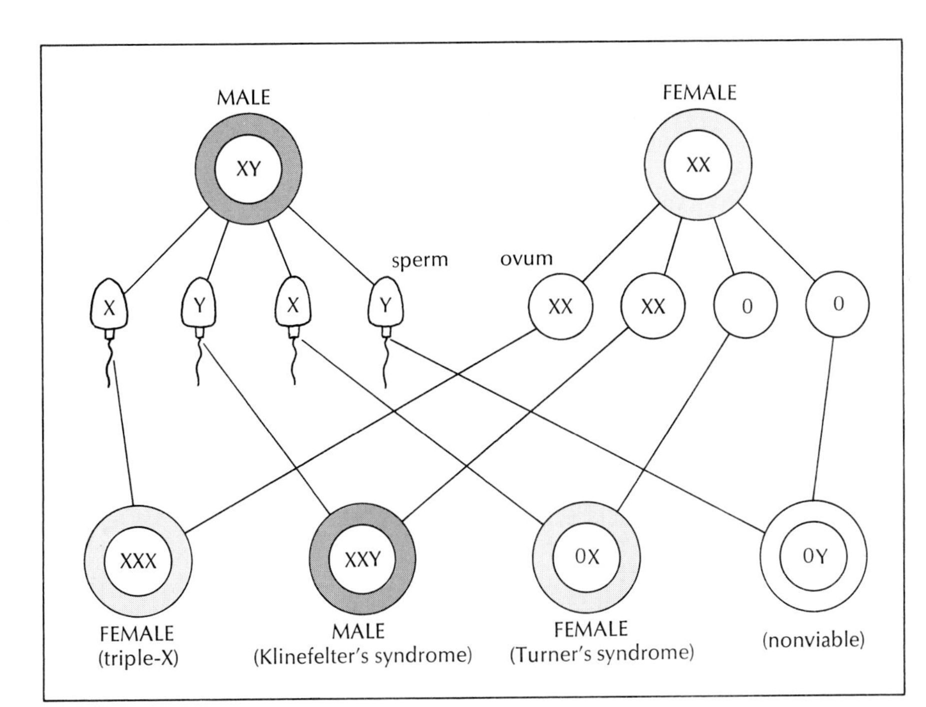

18-13 *Nondisjunction in the mother, resulting in ova with either two X-chromosomes or none. When fertilized, these ova can give rise to the four chromosome combinations shown here. Three of them are abnormal; the fourth is nonviable—the complete absence of an X-chromosome is lethal to a zygote. (This diagram presents an abbreviated view of the development of spermatozoa and ova from the primordial sex cells. The process of meiosis is shown in greater detail in Figure 18-5.)*

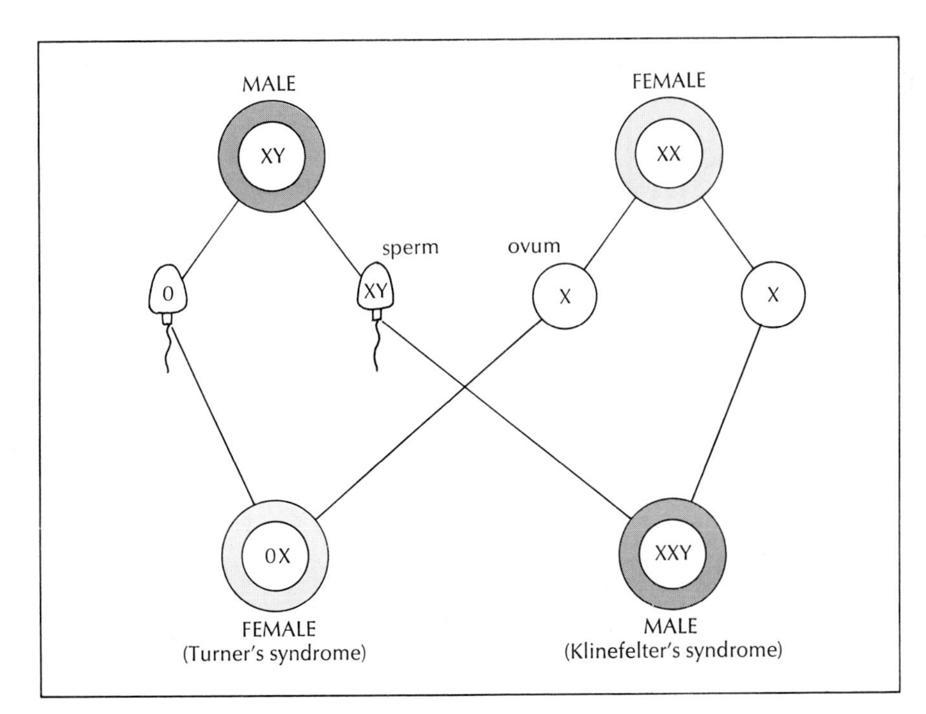

18-14 *Nondisjunction in the father, resulting in spermatozoa with either no sex chromosomes or both an X- and a Y-chromosome. Ova fertilized by such spermatozoa can give rise to the two chromosome combinations shown here. Both of them are abnormal. (As in Figure 18-13, this diagram omits the step-by-step process of meiosis, which is shown in Figure 18-5.)*

18-15 *The XYY syndrome. Nondisjunction in the father may produce spermatozoa with two Y-chromosomes, as shown here. When such a sperm fertilizes a normal ovum (which has an X-chromosome), the result is the XYY male.*

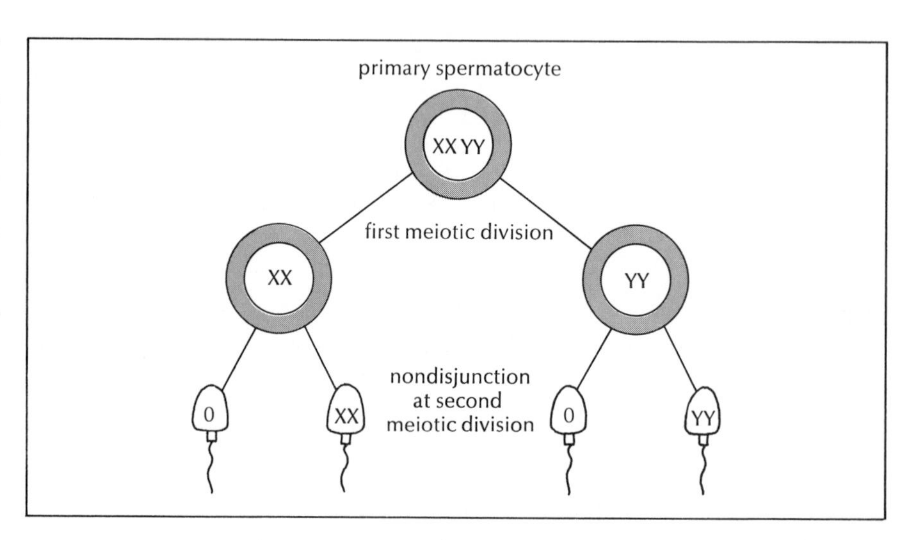

CHROMOSOMES AND CRIME Another abnormal arrangement of chromosomes that can result from nondisjunction of sex chromosomes in male meiosis involves an extra Y-chromosome. When a sperm carrying two Y-chromosomes fertilizes a normal ovum, the *XYY syndrome* occurs (Figure 18-15). New research has brought much attention to persons manifesting this syndrome. Tentative results indicate a startling association between the XYY disorder and criminal insanity.[32] Richard Speck, who in 1966 murdered eight Chicago nurses, was found to have the XYY disorder. The XYY chromosomal error is by no means an absolute indicator of criminal behavior. Only a portion of XYY males develop criminal behavior. But it does appear much more commonly in prison populations. Its victims are unusually tall males,[33] often mentally retarded, with histories of aggressive violence. Should they be punished for their crimes? A French court has ruled affirmatively. An Australian court has said ''no'' and acquitted an XYY murderer. In this country, a final decision has yet to be made. Although society must be protected, many suggest that XYY aggressiveness should no more be punished than the genetic gentleness of the Mongoloid is rewarded. Everything possible should be done for the known XYY carrier. With such an individual, environmental conditions that encourage crime take on a special meaning.[34]

[32] Fathers and children of XYY are no more likely to have abnormal chromosomes than the average person in the population. The condition is innate, but not hereditary. Moreover, it should be reemphasized that present scientifically reported associations between human XYY chromosomal structure and criminal behavior are tentative. All that can now be indicated is this: possibly some people with an XYY chromosomal structure may be more susceptible to certain kinds of social stress than people without such a chromosomal structure. However, even this remains theoretical. Widespread and inaccurate news reports about a ''proven'' relationship between XYY chromosomes and criminality have created an unwarranted public stir. In this respect, it is appropriate to quote a distinguished newspaperman of another generation, Heywood Broun: ''For truth,'' he wrote, ''there is no deadline.''

[33] Extraordinary height is not necessarily due to chromosomal abnormality.

[34] An excellent recent review of various aspects of the XYY genotype is Ernest B. Hook, ''Behavioral Implications of the Human XYY Genotype,'' *Science,* Vol. 179, No. 4069 (January 12, 1973), pp. 139–50. Both this article and its extensive bibliography are recommended for the somewhat advanced student.

CONFIGURATIONS WITH THREE, FOUR, OR NO X-CHROMOSOMES Rarely, a person is born with an XXX configuration—the so-called super- or hyper-female. Males with two extra X-chromosomes (XXXY) have also been found. Even more rarely, males and females with four X-chromosomes have been noted by investigators (XXXXY and XXXX). However, these prefixes refer only to the excess number and kind of chromosomes and not to "super-abilities"; such an individual is usually a nonfunctioning mental defective. The complete absence of an X-chromosome in a zygote is lethal.

CHROMOSOMES AND COMPETITION IN ATHLETICS Abnormal chromosome arrangements can become a matter for concern in international female athletic events. In former times, disputes arose when a performance was thought to be due to chromosomal maleness. Microscopic examination of cells usually settled the argument. Most experts disagreed with this superficial approach.[35]

Chromosomal analysis alone does not determine sex. Also to be considered is *nuclear sex.* In the cell nuclei of female mammals (including the human) is a structure not present in males (the *Barr body;* see page 563). Yet, even these two—chromosomal sex and nuclear sex—are not adequate to definitely determine the appropriate sex of some people. Other important criteria include genital appearance, internal reproductive organs, structure of the gonads, influence of other endocrine glands, psychological sex, and social sex.[36] Thus, it was the opinion of some that it was unfair to disqualify the Polish track star Ewa Klobukowska from the 1967 Women's European Athletic Cup competition. In her case, apparently only nuclear and chromosomal sex indicators were used. (Incidentally, there have been instances of males who, disguised as females, won Olympic medals. "Claire," the bronze-medal winner in the 100-meter dash in the 1946 competition at Oslo, today answers to the name of Pierre, is a father, and lives on a farm near Metz, France.)

The differences between male and female performance in athletics is the reason for the concern over chromosomal sex. Fifty years ago (in 1924), Johnny Weismuller won fame and a movie contract (as Tarzan) with his record swim of the 400-meter free style. But since 1924, no fewer than eleven women have surpassed Weismuller's record; among them was Sweden's Jane Cedergvist. "The fact that even Jane can now swim faster than Tarzan is certainly worthy of mention."[37] Today, the only two Olympic events in which men and women compete under the same rules are shooting and equestrian sports. For the other events, it is believed that anatomic differences place women at a disadvantage. Although, in these, the performance of some women equals or betters that of some men, individual records do show a difference. Differences in

18-16 Top: *Nucleus of a human female cell, showing characteristic Barr body (arrow).* Bottom: *Nucleus of a human male cell.*

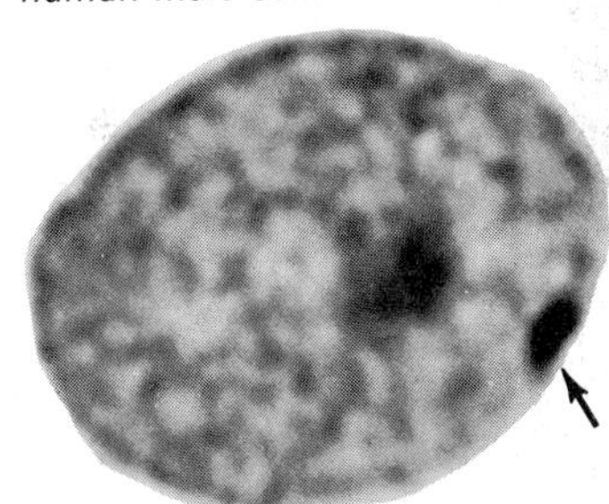

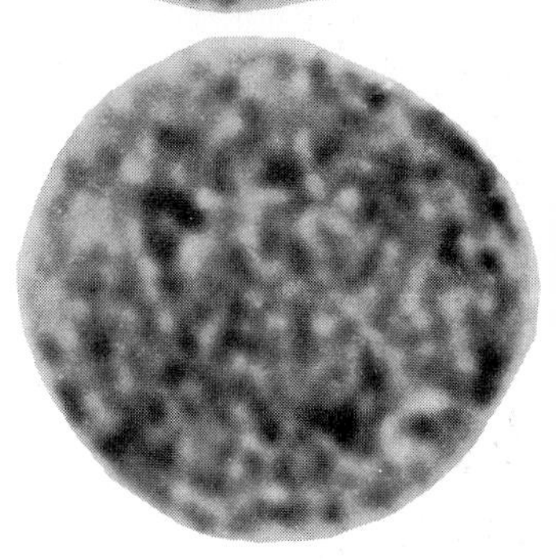

[35] Some tests used in detecting abnormalities in chromosomes are mentioned in the section on genetic counseling on pages 562–68.

[36] Sometimes sex is determined by surgical exploration, but only after all these and other factors have been carefully weighed.

[37] Warren Boroson, "Medicine and the Olympics," *Medical World News,* Vol. 13, No. 31 (August 18, 1972), p. 49.

peak performances in track are between 10 and 18 percent, and in swimming events, 10 percent. Since the breast stroke, butterfly, and backstroke require more muscular effort, the difference in these events rises to 15 percent.

Prior to the competition in the 1972 Olympic Games in Munich, women athletes underwent careful screening. Tests were performed for X- and Y-chromosomes. If these were not decisive, a karyotope (chromosomal map) was constructed and examined. Sample cells were obtained from the mucous membrane of the inner cheek and the hair roots. When an irregularity was apparent, blood tests and gynecologic examinations were indicated. Cases of intersexuality (see page 540) or of hermaphroditism (having sex organs of both sexes) were barred from competition. For each competing female, a "certificate of femininity" was prepared and signed by the President of the Medical Commission of the International Olympic Committee. Some people criticize the entire process as callous and discriminatory. However, it does not presently seem practical to "please everyone" by holding "several Olympic Games . . . to accommodate the different chromosomic groups."[38]

errors during mitosis

Although most abnormalities from nondisjunction occur during meiosis, nondisjunction can also occur during mitosis. A normal sperm fertilizes a normal ovum. But during the early mitotic cellular multiplication following fertilization, two chromosomes may fail to separate. In this way half the body cells of the affected individual have three rather than two of a particular chromosome (forty-seven total) and the other half of his body cells have one instead of the normal two (forty-five total). This is called *mosaicism.* Sometimes three types of cells may occur in one person's body, normal (forty-six chromosomes), trisomic (forty-seven), and monosomic (forty-five). Mosaicism can also result not from failure of chromosomes to separate, but from the loss of a chromosome during the cell division of mitosis. In all these mitotic variables there is the potential for grave illness.

illness and the genes of sex and race

Illness patterns are profoundly influenced by such genetic factors as sex and race.

sex

Fortunately, the union of the human sperm and egg results in about 140 males for every 100 females. Fortunately indeed. The male hold on life is relatively feeble. Even within the safety of the uterus, 50 percent more males than females perish. In all age groups up to the age of eighty, there is a consistent excess of male over female deaths (see Table 18-1). In 1972, almost three times as many males between fifteen and twenty-four died as did females in the same

[38] Eduardo Hay, "Sex Determination in Putative Female Athletics," *Journal of the American Medical Association,* Vol. 221, No. 9 (August 28, 1972), p. 998. It is on this article that most of the material in this section is based.

TABLE 18-1

Male Deaths per 100 Female Deaths by Age Groups, United States, 1972*

AGE	MALE DEATHS PER 100 FEMALE DEATHS
Under 1	132.29
1–4	129.04
5–14	147.23
15–24	282.04
25–34	209.35
35–44	168.86
45–54	176.82
55–59	187.36
60–64	183.99
65–69	162.20
70–74	136.11
75–79	111.23
80–84	86.04
85 and over	62.49
Total all ages	126.38

*These data do not cover deaths of U.S. civilians or members of the armed forces that occurred outside the United States.
Source: National Center for Health Statistics, *Monthly Vital Statistics Report,* Provisional Statistics. Annual Summary for the United States, 1972, Vol. 21, No. 13 (June 27, 1973), p. 19.

age group. Neither U.S. civilians nor members of the armed forces who died outside this country were included in these data. Moreover, the ratios were similar in 1960, a year in which the United States was not engaged in hostilities. For the fragile male, almost all disease categories are more lethal. Death rates from the major heart and blood vessel diseases, as well as those from cancers, accidents, and the more common infections, are considerably higher for males.[39] Aside from the complications of childbirth, it is only in a relatively few disease categories that females die more frequently. Syphilis has been called ''the chivalric disease.'' It surely shows special consideration for the female. For her, the disease is milder and is less likely to involve the heart and central nervous system. Syphilis kills less than half as many females as males. When suitable antibiotics are given to a male child with bacterial meningitis, his chances for survival are less than those of a female child of about the same age and in the same circumstances. Adverse effects of atomic radiation are more frequent in boys than girls.

Why the disparity? There is a good theory. As has been stated, of the forty-six chromosomes in the primordial sex cell of the ovum or sperm, two are sex

[39] National Center for Health Statistics, *Monthly Vital Statistics Report,* Provisional Statistics, Annual Summary for the United States, 1972, Vol. 21, No. 13 (June 27, 1973), p. 19.

chromosomes. The female has two X-chromosomes. These are equal. The male, however, has one X-chromosome and one puny Y-chromosome. Thus, the arrangement of the X- and Y-chromosomes is possibly to the advantage of the female. If something goes wrong with one of her chromosomes, perhaps she can rely on the other. The male is denied such possible insurance. There is evidence, at present inconclusive, that this biological inequality may be gradually equalizing because of the inactivation of one of the female X-chromosomes. Nonetheless, the male is indeed the weaker sex.

about a queen's genes

A rare but deservedly famous disease involving sex chromosomes, in which blood clots slowly or not at all, is *hemophilia.* It is hereditary and sex-linked. Like color blindness (see page 278), the gene for hemophilia is recessive and is carried on the X-chromosome. Since males have only one X-chromosome they are more likely to be "bleeders" than females, who must have two X-chromosomes carrying the hemophilia gene in order to be bleeders. Bleeder fathers transmit the defective gene not to their sons (since a male child does not receive an X-chromosome from his father), but to their daughters. Unless the daughter has also received an X-chromosome carrying the hemophilia gene from her mother, she will not be a bleeder, but she may transmit the disease to her children. In former years, female hemophiliacs did not live to maturity; menstruation was fatal. Modern therapy has corrected this.

The family tree of Queen Victoria was riddled with hemophilia. The son of the last tsar of Russia was a bleeder. This led to the reliance by the royal family on the corrupt quack Rasputin and hastened the decline of the Russian court. The last tsar of Russia shared this tragic situation with the last king of Spain, who also sired a bleeder. Both had married granddaughters of Victoria. "Thus two of the greatest dynasties of European history, the Spanish in the west and the Russian in the east, ended with uncrowned successors who were bleeders."[40]

race

Sickle cell anemia is much more frequent among Negroes than Caucasians. In the United States, tooth decay is more common among Caucasians than Negroes. Among women in Japan, cancer of the breast is rare. One should, however, view with caution the varying frequency of diseases in races. True, heredity helps decide body reactions to disease. But socioeconomics, rather than genes, accounts for the comparatively greater frequency of such illnesses as tuberculosis and syphilis among blacks in this country. Moreover, recent studies emphasize the association between the malnutrition of poverty and mental retardation.

[40] Fritz Kahn, *Man in Structure and Function,* Vol. I, tr. and ed. by George Rosen (New York, 1960), p. 215.

sickle cell disease

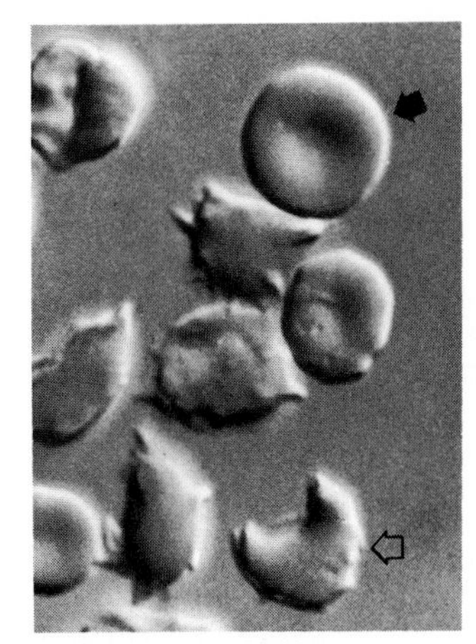

18-17 *Red blood cells showing the sickle-cell trait. The top arrow points to a normal cell; the bottom arrow points to a typical sickle-shaped cell.*

A major abnormality of the red blood cell's hemoglobin is *sickle cell disease.* It is inherited; the only way a person can have the disease is to be born with it. In this condition, there is a genetically transmitted abnormality in the chemical structure of the hemoglobin molecules within the red blood cells. As a result, the hemoglobin molecules can link together to distort the cell. Thus, the ordinarily doughnut-shaped red blood cell is forced into the shape of a sickle. The molecular change is minute; the human suffering caused by it is immense. In this country, sickle cell disease largely affects the Negro population. However, the disease can occur among Caucasians from the Mediterranean area and among the peoples of the Middle East and certain parts of India. More than 2 million U.S. Negroes carry the relatively benign *sickle cell trait;* that is, they have the capacity to pass the disease on to their children. Over fifty thousand U.S. Negroes have the much more serious *sickle cell anemia.*

In some very unusual circumstances, even those individuals with only the trait may become seriously ill. This is because some (although not all) of their red blood cells contain the abnormally structured hemoglobin molecule. In such people, sickling of the affected red blood cells can be brought on by extreme lack of oxygen. This can occur with a severe hemorrhage during a surgical operation, or with exposure to an atmosphere of reduced oxygen tension (as is the case in an unpressurized airplane or on a high mountain). Lack of oxygen during administration of anaesthesia is also a matter of special concern with these individuals. However, in usual situations, people with the sickle cell trait do not have sickle-shaped red blood cells. They are, therefore, generally without symptoms. It is noteworthy that the National Research Council has recommended that people with only the sickle cell trait "should not be excluded from [military] service, even flight duty, except for pilots or copilots," for whom the emergencies of low oxygen pressure may have some ill effects.[41] Moreover, one 1973 study showed that 39 of 579 black players in the National Football League spring training camp carried the sickle cell trait. None of the 39 were frail men.[42]

For the person with sickle cell anemia the situation is much more dangerous. All the red blood cells contain the abnormally structured hemoglobin molecules; all the red blood cells are potential candidates for sickling. A child with this disease can become desperately ill even without the occurrence of a special set of circumstances. Normally, the oxygen tension in the capillaries and small veins is low. In these tiny blood vessels, red blood cells containing abnormally structured hemoglobin will tend to sickle. Worse, the misshapen red blood cells clump together. In this way, they plug the small blood vessels and thus partly or wholly deprive needy tissues of blood and oxygen. Cells die, as do the tissues of which they are a part. Pain, loss of appetite, joint swellings, ulcers—these plague the afflicted child. (The pain is similar to the pain of an acute heart attack

[41] "Defense and Sickle Cells," *Smithsonian,* Vol. 4, No. 2 (May 1973), p. 8.
[42] "Sickle Cell Trait Found in Pro Athletes," *American Medical News,* Vol. 16, No. 33 (August 27, 1973), p. 17.

and occurs for the same reason—lack of oxygen to the tissues.) Normally, red blood cells live more than one hundred days. Sickled, they are destroyed, mostly in the spleen, in ten to twenty-five days. The little patient is exhausted, wan, often desperately anemic. The belabored spleen is not able to provide adequate immunity; there is constant risk from infections such as pneumonia. Periodically, crises of intense sickness imperil life.

Not long ago, it was expected that one-half of these patients would die before they were twenty; the other half would barely survive middle age. Now there is hope. It was first found that a chemical called urea unsickled the affected cells. This was followed by the discovery that it was not the urea, but cyanate, a chemical in the urea solution, that accomplished the beneficial result. By midsummer 1972, intensive work was being done in this area. In addition, several valuable diagnostic tests have been developed for both the sickle cell trait and sickle cell anemia. Those who suffer from the anemia can find hope in renewed research and recent treatments. It has, moreover, been recently reported that it is possible to have sickle cell disease in a mild form. One study of a small group of adults with mild sickle cell disease revealed that they had few or no crises of pain, were actively employed, and led normal lives.[43] How often this type of the illness occurs is undetermined. Those who find that they carry the trait must make their own decision as to whether to risk passing on a tragic genetic legacy to future generations. However, early diagnosis remains essential. It not only makes possible early treatment[44] but also affords the time necessary to make thoughtful decisions about having children. Someday, genetic surgery may be possible to replace the gene responsible for the abnormal hemoglobin with a gene that codes for normal hemoglobin.

the genetic ecosystem: environmental influences on the fertilized ovum

Within the nucleus of the cell, the basic genetic chemicals are arranged in relation to one another. And they are dependent on one another. So, inside the very nucleus there is environment with ecological balance or imbalance.

Within the no longer secret nucleus, the genes contain a pattern set to direct development. But no amount of healthy genetic instruction can bid cytoplasm sickened by an abnormal environment to be normal. Nor can a healthy cyto-

[43] Martin H. Steinberg, Bernard J. Dreiling, Francis S. Morrison, and Thomas F. Necheles, "Mild Sickle Cell Disease," *Journal of the American Medical Association,* Vol. 224, No. 3 (April 16, 1973), pp. 317–21.

[44] Within the uterus, the hemoglobin produced by the normal fetus does not differ from that produced by a fetus with a potential sickle cell problem. Both produce fetal hemoglobin—labeled HbF. For this reason, parents cannot elect abortion to avoid the future problem in their child. Nor does a newborn baby give any indication of the disease. A newborn's hemoglobin is of the fetal variety. Within a few months the normal baby's HbF diminishes and he begins to produce adult hemoglobin—HbA. Babies with sickle cell anemia cannot produce HbA. Instead, they produce sickle cell hemoglobin (HbS). For this reason, the symptoms of HbS-producing children do not usually occur until between the sixth and twelfth month of life. The first manifestation of the disease may be disastrous. Death may occur from overwhelming infection or anemia. Thus, early diagnosis is of critical importance.

plasm receive beneficial patterns of instruction from a gene made deviant by environment. Normal genetic action depends on a normal environment inside and outside the cell. The internal drama of the cell will be disarranged not only when the chromosomal players unaccountably neglect their proper parts but also when they are surrounded by destructive microorganisms, or hostile drugs, or searing radiation. That is why German measles (rubella) and thalidomide and atomic radiation kill and cripple the unborn. Consider now these and other influences.

nutrition

Pregnant women may need extra calories, proteins, minerals, and vitamins. However, this should be decided only by the physician. Deficient maternal diets mean more stillborn babies and more deaths among babies less than one month old. The child is affected by the mother's diet not only during residence in the uterus but also long after birth. Babies born to poorly nourished mothers are more susceptible to infections in early life and have more birth defects. The child who survives the mother's poor nutrition may be smaller at birth and often will grow into a small adolescent and adult. There is a direct relationship between the economic status of the mother and the birth weight of her baby. Children born of poor mothers weigh less.[45] And children with lower-than-normal birth weights have a greater tendency to physical defects in later life.

Should the mother fail to provide enough food for the child within her, will he suffer shortages? Or will he be able to avoid malnourishment by helping himself to whatever is available from his mother's reserve? The availability of the mother's reserve has been overestimated. Daily nourishment for the developing child comes from the daily nourishment of the mother. Even a temporarily inadequate diet, unnoticed by the mother, may wreak irreparable damage to an unborn child. With maternal malnutrition, the unborn infant suffers before, and more than, the mother.

A maternal diet that is poor in calcium may result in a child born with poor bone development and bad teeth. Inadequate iron results in anemia for both mother and child. Severe protein deficiency retards growth and development. Vitamin diseases, such as beriberi, rickets, and scurvy, are seen in the babies of mothers deprived of vitamins B, D, and C respectively. An iodine-deficient maternal diet may result in the birth of a child that will show the distressing signs of cretinism by the sixth to the eighth month of life. Marked by severe physical and mental retardation, cretinism is always a threat when the mother uses plain salt without added iodine.

Many pregnant women, understandably concerned about their figures, embark on a restrictive weight-watching program. To a limited extent this may be good sense; however, it can be seriously overdone. In 1970, the National Research Council Committee on Maternal Nutrition recommended an average weight gain during pregnancy of twenty-four pounds, with a range of between twenty and twenty-five pounds. ''Weight reduction programs and severe caloric

[45]World Health Organization, *Nutrition in Pregnancy and Lactation,* cited in Miriam E. Lowenberg *et al., Food and Man* (New York, 1968).

restrictions should not be undertaken during pregnancy, even for obese women, because of the possibility of adverse effects on the fetus' weight and neurological development."[46] In 1973, the slightly more liberal Committee on Nutrition of the American College of Obstetricians and Gynecologists suggested that an average total weight gain during pregnancy of twenty-two to twenty-seven pounds appeared optimal.[47] Harvard nutritionist Jean Mayer has written that "Ideally, a [pregnant] woman should add two or three pounds a month—somewhere from 18–27 pounds, spread out as evenly as possible over the nine months."[48] For women who were overweight before their pregnancy, a smaller weight gain is recommended; for those who were underweight, the larger weight gain is best. For underweight women and pregnant teen-agers, weight restrictions may be particularly harmful. Moreover, women who smoke during pregnancy deliver babies of significantly lower weights; in their cases, weight restrictions are particularly risky for the child (see pages 396–97).

It used to be thought that weight reduction during pregnancy prevented *toxemia of pregnancy,* a serious and rare metabolic disorder marked by swelling of the body and increased blood pressure. Rarely, toxemia can lead to the more serious *eclampsia.* However, there is no evidence that excessive weight gain, whether it be due to fat or water, causes eclampsia. Nor is there evidence that severe caloric restrictions diminish the chances that the toxemia of pregnancy will occur with a woman who gains too much weight, or that a woman who gains excessively is more prone to toxemia. There is, however, a marked association between low income and deaths due to the toxemia of pregnancy. Women in low-income groups die from this condition at a rate that is about three times that of women in high-income groups.

infection

Women who develop *German measles* (rubella) during the first three months of pregnancy are over five times (15 percent) more likely to give birth to a defective child than women who do not have the disease (2.8 percent). The heart, hearing, and vision (cataracts) are most commonly affected. There is some medical opinion that a woman who contracts *regular measles* (rubeola) also has a greater chance of having a defective child. But many physicians think that this contention is unproved. There are now available effective vaccines to prevent both regular measles and German measles (pages 147–49). There is some evidence that *infectious hepatitis,* a third viral illness, can adversely affect chromosomes. Because *smallpox vaccine* is composed of a living virus, it may affect the unborn child. Consequently, pregnant women are not usually vaccinated against smallpox. *Syphilis* can also be transmitted from mother to unborn child. Adequate treatment of the mother can prevent tragedy for both. Another major infection that may be transmitted from the pregnant woman to the fetus is *cytomegalic inclusion disease* (pages 164–65). This illness, usually noted during the first month of life, is due to a viral infection. It is revealed by

[46] "Pregnant Weight Watchers Risk Harm to Babies," *Public Health Reports,* Vol. 85, No. 11 (November 1970), p. 964. The material in this section concerning the report of the National Research Council Committee on Maternal Nutrition is from this source.

[47] "Weight Gain During Pregnancy," *Briefs,* Vol. 37, No. 8 (October 1973), p. 124.

[48] Jean Mayer, "When You're Eating for Two," *Family Health,* Vol. 5, No. 10 (October 1973), p. 31.

a wide variety and degree of malformations in the child. As with German measles, children with the disease may be contagious for months after delivery. They should, therefore, be isolated, particularly from pregnant women.

direct radiation

Excessive exposure of a pregnant woman to X-rays can result in either fetal death or a malformed child. Women should, therefore, always advise a doctor who plans to X-ray them of a possible, still unapparent, pregnancy.

There have been large-scale experiences with radiation. Seven out of eleven Hiroshima children were born retarded if, within the first twenty weeks of conception, their mothers stood within 1,200 meters of absolute center of the atomic bomb blast. Others, whose mothers were at a greater distance, had malformed hips, eyes, and hearts. Some, symptomless at birth, developed poorly.

In 1954 the United States made a test explosion of a nuclear device at Bikini. An unpredictable wind deposited significant amounts of radioactive material on the residents of four nearby islands as well as on twenty-three Japanese fishermen. Years later, children of the islands who were less than five years old at the time of exposure were found to be retarded in physical growth.

Why does radiation cause abnormal babies? The baby is a triumph of recent cellular multiplication. And radiation has a predilection for multiplying cells. It requires more radiation to kill a fly than a mouse. Why? As a maggot, the fly passes through all its phases of growth and development. As an adult, it has few dividing cells. Adult mice and men have many dividing cells. It is these that are sensitive to radiation.

Radiation reaching the testes or ovaries, and thereby the reproductive cells, can cause changes in the structure of the DNA (genes). Mutation rates are increased by radiation. Since over 99 percent of mutations are harmful and since they do accumulate in man, the threat to future generations is apparent. Depending on the amount, moreover, radiation may cause chromosomal breaks and translocations. So another danger of radiation, more recently recognized, is related to chromosomal aberrations. Thus, radiation may be one of the causes of a wide variety of genetic disorders, ranging from the mental retardation of phenylketonuria to the mental retardation of Mongolism.

chemical pollution

The placenta is no longer considered an effective barrier against environmental pollutants (see Chapters 3 and 4). Large molecules of polluting substances are now thought merely to cross the placenta more slowly than those that are small. Added to this are the constant risks that are taken by prolonged use of chemicals such as food additives without adequate knowledge of the effects they will have. The former use of diethylstilbesterol in meat animals is but one example of this kind of error. Another example is the mercury pollution of water and fish that resulted in the poisoning of numerous Japanese; women who ate the poisoned fish gave birth to blind and paralyzed children (see pages 83–84).[49] A

[49] Neville Grant, "Mercury in Man," *Environment,* Vol. 13, No. 4 (May 1971), p. 3. An excellent account of a recent and tragic outbreak of mercury poisoning in this country is given in Paul E. Pierce, Jon F. Thompson, William H. Likosky, Laurence N. Nickey, William F. Barthel, and Alan R. Hinman, "Alkyl Mercury Poisoning in Humans," *Journal of the American Medical Association,* Vol. 220, No. 11 (June 12, 1972), pp. 1439–41.

third example of the careless chemicalization of the environment is the use of PCBs (polychlorinated biphenyls; see pages 85–86). Little is known of the effects of their prolonged use.[50] Laboratory evidence suggests that a major air pollutant, sulfur dioxide (see page 63), may cause genetic damage.[51] And in 1973, the newly formed federal Consumer Products Safety Division banned the sale of certain spray adhesives, widely used by hobbyists for "foil art"; the reason: a possible link was discovered between use of the adhesives and chromosomal damage.[52]

Since standard test systems for many chemical pollutants are extremely insensitive, it would seem reasonable to take as few chances as possible. Strict regulations should be imposed on chemicals that may possibly affect human beings in an adverse way.[53] And those regulations should be in effect not after, but before human harm occurs.

noise As a pollutant, noise has been attracting increasing attention (see Chapter 4, pages 102–05). It has also been generating understandable irritation. A Canadian hygienist reported the story of a man who "was annoyed by a loud-playing portable radio on a bus. After reasoning with the owner to play the radio more quietly, the man banged her over the head with the radio. He was tried before a jury . . . but was not indicted. In an informal survey, 299 out of 300 persons applauded the act. The 300th person felt he should have waited until the woman got off the bus."[54] That undue noise can have a deleterious effect on animal reproduction is known.[55] The effect it has on the unborn or newborn human is being researched. One recent hospital study found that "under the plastic hood of the incubators the noise spectrum fell well above the recommended acceptance level and, due to the prolonged exposure time, very close to the danger area."[56]

One extraordinary observation has been made by Japanese scientists.[57] Studying 307 babies, they noticed that the way a baby reacted to aircraft noise depended on the length of the mother's stay in Itami City, which is near the Osaka International Airport. When a woman spent the second half of her pregnancy, or the period directly after the birth of the child, in noisy Itami, the child was much more likely to be disturbed by the aircraft noise. When the women moved to Itami before conception, so that the babies spent their entire fetal life near the airport, 58 percent of the babies slept soundly during airplane noise,

[50] "Chemical Pollution: Polychlorinated Biphenyls," *Science,* Vol. 175, No. 4018 (January 14, 1972), p. 156.
[51] "Facts on Pollution's Genetic Hazards," *Medical World News,* Vol. 13, No. 36 (September 29, 1972), p. 10.
[52] "Possible Link to Chromosomal Gaps Leads to Ban on Spray Adhesives," *Journal of the American Medical Association,* Vol. 225, No. 13 (September 24, 1973), pp. 1581–82.
[53] Paul Sampson, "A Warning About Introducing New Teratogens," *Journal of the American Medical Association,* Vol. 221, No. 8 (August 21, 1972), p. 853, quoting Samuel S. Epstein, Professor of Pharmacology at Case Western Reserve University Medical School.
[54] L. K. Smith, "Noise in the News," *Canadian Journal of Public Health,* Vol. 60, No. 8 (August 1969), p. 306.
[55] Krishna B. Singh, "Effect of Noise on the Female Reproductive System," *Journal of Obstetrics and Gynecology,* Vol. 112, No. 7 (April 1, 1972), pp. 981–91.
[56] Frank L. Seleney and Michael Streczyn, "Noise Characteristics in the Baby Compartment of Incubators," *American Journal of Diseases of Children,* Vol. 117, No. 4 (April 1969), p. 450.
[57] "Stick Out the Noise Mums, and Your Kids Will Take It Better," *New Scientist,* Vol. 47, No. 713 (August 6, 1970), p. 270, citing Y. Ando and H. Hattori, "Effects of Intense Noise During Fetal Life upon Postnatal Adaptability," *Journal of the Acoustical Society of America,* Vol. 47 (April 1970), pp. 1128–30.

and only 6 percent awoke and cried. When women moved to the vicinity of the airport during the first five months of pregnancy, 47 percent of their babies slept soundly during airplane noise, and 13 percent awoke and cried. When women moved to Itami City during the second half of their pregnancies or after the birth of their babies, only 9 to 16 percent of the babies slept through airplane noise, and 45 to 50 percent awoke and cried.

During the early months of the baby's development within the uterus, the nervous system (and the hearing mechanism) is relatively undeveloped. It is possible that exposure to intense noise during the earlier months of pregnancy in some way may enable the child's nervous system to adapt to it. Other observers comment that "if Japanese researchers' results are borne out, it does give people living near airports or motorways the dubious satisfaction that, if only they can stick it out, their sons and daughters won't find it so bad."[58] But a likely explanation for the babies who are apparently less disturbed by airplane noise is not amusing: they are born partially deaf.

endocrine influences

Insulin, a product of specific cells within the pancreas (see page 260), regulates carbohydrate metabolism. Without enough insulin, diabetes develops. Diabetes is a genetically transmitted disorder of metabolism. Diabetic mothers have malformed children ten times more frequently than the average. The reasons are undetermined. They may be genetic or endocrine or nutritional or, perhaps, all three.

the Rh factor

In 1969, in this country, about ten thousand babies died of *Rh blood disease.* The condition is also known as *erythroblastosis fetalis* (Greek *erythros,* red + *blastos,* germ + *osis,* increase). The increase in red germ cells refers to the numerous immature primitive red blood cells seen in the circulation of the affected child. Their development in the fetus accounts for the term *fetalis.* Why do they occur? To make up for the normal red cells that are destroyed. Why are the normal red blood cells destroyed? In this the Rh factor is involved. What is Rh?

Rh is a chemical substance. Its exact structure is unknown. It sits on the surface of the red blood cells of 85 percent of all people. They are then Rh positive. The 15 percent who do not carry it are Rh negative. Why is it called Rh? The *Rh*esus monkey also has the factor. Has Rh a known purpose? No. It just causes trouble. How?

One in eight marriages is between an Rh-negative woman and an Rh-positive man. If the child is Rh negative, like the mother, there is no problem. But the child may inherit the Rh-positive factor from the father. The Rh-negative mother thus carries an Rh-positive child. Erythroblastosis fetalis occurs when the Rh-positive blood of the child enters the mother's blood. The baby's Rh-positive factor is a foreigner to the mother. It is an *antigen,* an antibody generator. To neutralize her baby's Rh-positive antigens, the mother produces antibodies in her blood. When these antibodies enter the child, they destroy red

[58] *Ibid.*

blood cells. There are two ways in which the child's antibody-stimulating Rh-positive factor reaches the mother's circulation. One way is through the placenta during pregnancy. Usually only small amounts of baby antigen reach the mother in this fashion. During the time that she is carrying her first child, these minimal amounts are thought to be not enough to cause the mother to manufacture antibodies. The second way that the child's Rh antigen enters the mother occurs during delivery. Indeed, most of the child's Rh-positive blood reaches the mother during delivery, since, at that time, the afterbirth loosens and bleeds. Therefore, it is after delivery that she manufactures antibodies. Once she has manufactured such antibodies, she will be restimulated, in future pregnancies involving an Rh-positive fetus, to produce antibodies with only the small amount of antigen that enters through the placenta. That is why erythroblastosis fetalis usually affects the child of a later pregnancy more severely than an earlier one; a third child, for example, will be more adversely affected than a second; a fourth child, more than a third; and so on.

To repeat, then, in most cases the mother usually does not produce enough antibodies to harm the child during a first pregnancy. During the actual delivery of her first child, however, she receives enough Rh-positive blood to manufacture a high level of antibodies. These antibodies remain in the mother's blood. With the second child, harm is likely. As with the first child, the second may inherit the father's Rh-positive blood factor. The mother's antibodies, formed in response to the Rh-positive antigen of the first baby, now pass through the placenta of the second baby. The antibodies destroy the unborn second child's red blood cells. To recoup, the child hastily makes new cells. These are the primitive red blood cells of erythroblastosis fetalis. But, as immature cells, they do not make up for the destroyed mature red blood cells. Anemia results. Products from the child's red cell destruction seep into the skin. Jaundice occurs.

Well over 90 percent of babies with erythroblastosis are saved. Complete replacement of their blood is necessary. Of the most severely afflicted, only about 25 percent are saved. A relatively new technique has sometimes been helpful. Rh-negative blood is introduced directly into the unborn child. This may maintain life within the uterus long enough to result in a baby who, at delivery, is adequately mature for transfusion. To the baby with erythroblastosis fetalis, the new era of surgery on unborn babies has brought renewed hope. It is now even possible to temporarily remove a child from the uterus, replace the child's blood, and then return that child to the womb to complete the intrauterine life. Although such spectacular fetal surgery is not generally needed in the treatment of erythroblastosis fetalis, the very fact that it has been accomplished opens further the whole new field of surgery on the unborn.

But in some cases erythroblastosis fetalis can now be prevented. Recently, a product containing antibodies against Rh-positive blood has proved successful. Within seventy-two hours of delivery of her first Rh-positive baby, the mother's blood is tested for antibodies. If she already has them in considerable amount, the product is useless. But if she does not have a significant level of antibodies, because not enough of the baby's Rh-positive antigen had passed through the placenta into her circulation, the mother is injected with the medicine containing antibodies against Rh-positive blood. These medicine-antibodies quickly combine with the baby's Rh-positive antigen that had reached the mother's blood during delivery. This happens before the mother has a chance to make her own Rh-positive antibodies. The Rh-positive antigen-antibody mixture is then washed out through the kidney. The mother does not have any antibody against Rh-positive blood to threaten her next baby.

the mother's age

As a rule, young mothers (under thirty) provide a relatively safer intrauterine environment for their children. Perhaps older women do not produce adequate endocrine secretions to guarantee proper development of ova. With increase in the mother's age, for example, the frequency of Mongolism, as well as some other rare abnormalities, increases. It should not be concluded that the younger mother needs less medical attention than the older. Child marriages and pregnancies in this country are but a small percentage of the total, but they are by no means rare. The young–teen-aged mother presents a special problem. She is less likely to obtain early professional care and is more prone to be improperly nourished. Consequently, both her life and that of her baby are at greater risk.

the mother's emotions

Emotional stress, particularly early in pregnancy, may be related to the birth of children with cleft palates. Some emotions cause a hyperactivity of the outer part (*cortex*) of the adrenal glands. This hyperactivity causes the adrenals to produce the hormone hydrocortisone, which can pass through the placenta. If hydrocortisone is injected into mice while their upper palates are being formed, more than 90 percent are born with cleft palates.

Many other factors such as abnormal fetal position or a faulty placenta may adversely affect the environment of the child developing in the uterus. A mother's high blood pressure or hyperactivity of her thyroid gland also detracts from the safety of the embryonic and fetal ecosystem.

drugs

Knowledge about the effect of drugs on the unborn child is incomplete. Sensitivity to various drugs and their combinations may be inherited; an entirely new specialty devoted to studying this problem, called *pharmacogenetics,* has been acknowledged as an increasingly important field in medicine and pharmacology. Animal experiments may be inconclusive, as their results do not always apply to humans. The calamitous crippling of thousands of children, in 1961 and 1962, whose mothers had taken a German-made tranquilizer containing thalidomide early in pregnancy, will long be a mournful reminder of the danger in the use of inadequately tested drugs. How complex such testing can be is illustrated by the facts that humans are 60 times more sensitive to thalidomide than mice, 100 times more sensitive to it than rats, 200 times more than dogs, and 700 times more than hamsters. Thus, enormous doses, given to several species, might not indicate the danger to the human embryo and fetus.[59] (Nevertheless, despite its initial association with tragedy, thalidomide today shows promise in helping people with an ancient disease; it seems to prevent acute

[59] Paul Sampson, "A Warning About Introducing New Teratogens," p. 853.

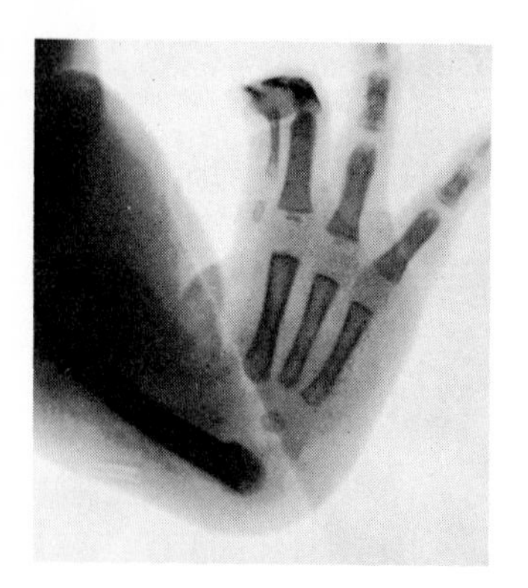

18-18 *X-ray photograph showing the deformed arm of a one-year-old child whose mother had taken the drug thalidomide during early pregnancy.*

reactions of leprosy patients.) When one considers the real scientific problems that exist in establishing toxicity, the sheer foolhardiness of the abuse of illicit, unmeasured, untested, and grossly impure street drugs becomes even more apparent. Yet birth defects may also be due to prolonged licit drug use. One study has revealed correlations between increased birth defects and a wide variety of drugs taken habitually during pregnancy. The most significant correlation was with barbiturates. Others, however, were aspirin, amphetamines, and even antacids.[60]

Whether drugs will affect the unborn child depends on the stage of the child's development. During the first four weeks, the embryo cells undergo extremely rapid proliferation. Food supply and waste elimination are achieved by simple diffusion. Any drug that can diffuse quickly to the rapidly multiplying cells may cause changes that are significant enough to cause loss of the embryo. If this occurs between menstrual periods, the woman does not even know of her pregnancy. Drug action at a more advanced stage (the fifth to the eighth week) can cause abnormal tissue and organ differentiation. There are critical periods in the development of the human embryo in which various structures are being differentiated, and during which some drugs may have the most profoundly deleterious effects. Some of these are: the nervous system, days fifteen to twenty-five; eyes, days twenty-four to forty; heart, days twenty to forty; legs, days twenty-four to thirty-six.[61] By the eighth week of pregnancy, differentiation of these body parts is basically complete. After that, the hazard to the fetus diminishes greatly. It should, however, be understood that some drugs not responsible for immediately apparent effects may nevertheless retard growth and development.

For discussions of the effects of specific drugs on the unborn child, see pages 396–97 (tobacco), 368 (heroin), 410–11 (LSD), and 424-25 (marihuana).

birth defects

More babies die of defective development before they are born than after. Such defective embryos account for most of the million miscarriages in this country every year. Most occur early in pregnancy—the period of greatest vulnerability of the developing child. Some miscarriages occur so early that the woman may never have known she was pregnant. Others occur after a few months. "Many [of such deaths] are nature's way of getting rid of an abnormally developing fetus in order that a new and better one can be started."[62] Of every sixteen babies born alive in this country, one is found to be defective within the first year. (Some birth defects, such as gout and diabetes, may not be apparent for years.) This amounts to about a quarter of a million babies a year. Eighteen thousand of these die in the first year of life.

[60] M. M. Nelson and J. O. Forfar, *British Medical Journal,* Vol. 1 (March 6, 1971), p. 523.

[61] Bernard L. Mirkin, "Effects of Drugs on the Fetus and Neonate," *Postgraduate Medicine,* Vol. 47, No. 1 (January 1970), pp. 91–95.

[62] Edith L. Potter, "Defective Babies Who Die Before Birth," in Morris Fishbein, ed., *Birth Defects* (Philadelphia, 1963), p. 46.

> It may be estimated conservatively that 15 million persons in the United States have one or more congenital defects which affect their daily lives. Included are an estimated 4 million with clinical diabetes, 2,900,000 with mental retardation of prenatal origin, 1 million with congenital orthopedic impairments, 500,000 who were born blind or with serious loss of vision, 750,000 with congenital hearing impairment, at least 350,000 with congenital heart disease, and more than 100,000 with speech defects of prenatal origin.[63]

As the population grows, the number of babies born with birth defects increases. Moreover, modern surgery, newer drugs, and more research combine to keep many defective children alive to adolescence and maturity. Though this kind of effort will always be a basic purpose of medicine, such survival nevertheless means problems.

For too long birth defects have been associated with stigma and superstition. "If a woman gives birth, and the abdomen of the child is open, there will be a dwindling of the suburbs." So predicts an ancient Babylonian tablet. Greek mythology makes frequent reference to half-human, half-animal centaurs and minotaurs. Believing fertility between species to be possible, and birth defect the result, many Greeks were contemptuous of malformed children. In early Judeo-Christian cultures, the parents of defective children were ostracized. Even today, the word *harelip* is used. Mothers of such children were once thought to have been frightened by a rabbit. But modern science has brought mankind a long way from such ignorance.

how to avoid some birth defects

1. A physician should be seen as soon as pregnancy is suspected because (a) the baby is most vulnerable during early pregnancy (the first twenty weeks), and (b) delay increases the chances of premature birth and a defective child.

2. No medication, not even vitamins, should be taken unless prescribed by the family doctor. Drugs may pass through the placenta and the child may be injured.

3. Except in emergencies, abdominal X-rays early in pregnancy should be avoided. Any physician about to X-ray a female patient, therefore, will want to know if she is pregnant.

4. Cigarette smoking should be discontinued. At the very least, excessive cigarette smoking must be avoided. Recent studies show that nicotine injected into a pregnant monkey swiftly crossed the placental barrier. In the monkey fetus the nicotine level declined slowly. Both the heart rate and blood pressure of the monkey fetus were depressed. Potentially harmful disturbances in the unborn monkey's acid–base state and oxygen supply were noted.[64]

5. If possible, elective surgery should be delayed until after pregnancy. Abrupt changes to high altitudes should be avoided. In both instances, even temporary oxygen depletion might injure the embryo. In commercial airliners this is not ordinarily a problem.

[63] V. Apgar and G. Stickle, "Birth Defects: Their Significance as a Public Health Problem," *Journal of the American Medical Association,* Vol. 204, No. 5 (April 29, 1968), pp. 79–82.

[64] Karlis Adamsons *et al.*, "Effects of Nicotine on the Unborn," cited in *Briefs: Footnotes on Maternity Care,* Vol. 33, No. 7 (September 1969), pp. 99–100.

6. An adequate diet must be followed.

7. Relatives should never marry. Even rare hereditary disorders occur much more commonly among the children of such unions. Except in Georgia, state laws forbid a person from marrying a parent, grandparent, child, or grandchild. In Georgia a man may marry his daughter or grandmother. Generally, marriages between persons with a relatedness equivalent to first cousins or closer are not legally sanctioned.[65]

8. Many physicians feel that the relationship between the older mother and the occurrence of Mongolism (and a few other rarer abnormalities) should never alone deter childbearing.

9. Under some circumstances, the advice of a genetic counselor is indicated. The family physician will know if such help is necessary.

10. The mental retardation of the child with untreated phenylketonuria (PKU; see Table 18-2)[66] is always tragically obvious. However, one aspect of the condition has frequently been overlooked. Successful treatment of PKU during infancy and childhood has enabled many women to have normal children. However, treatment is not often maintained into adolescence. Untreated maternal PKU may result in a damaged fetus; indeed, the fetus can be adversely affected even in a woman of normal intelligence with unsuspected PKU. Dietetic treatment of a woman known to have PKU should be begun before the beginning of pregnancy. To discover unknown cases, sisters of all phenylketonuric patients should be examined, regardless of their intelligence. Also, when a woman has had one or more retarded children without obvious cause, PKU must be considered. Some physicians recommend screening for PKU of all antenatal women.[67]

some important relationships

Is there any relationship between survival of a fetus and a child and the spacing of pregnancies? What, if any, are the relationships between fetal and child survivals and the age of parents? In attempting to find answers to these questions, Richard L. Day[68] surveyed the statistical literature. Although his findings by no means necessarily apply to individual cases, they are nonetheless of significance.

1. The ideal time for maternity seemed to be between the ages of twenty and thirty.

2. An interval of about two years between the end of one pregnancy and the beginning of another was associated with the lowest incidence of late fetal and newborn (up to one month of age) mortality as well as prematurity. Since

[65] Michael G. Farrow and Richard C. Juberg, "Genetics and Laws Prohibiting Marriage in the United States," *Journal of the American Medical Association,* Vol. 209, No. 4 (July 28, 1969), p. 534.

[66] An excellent review of PKU is David Yi-Yung Hsia, "A Critical Evaluation of PKU Screening," *Hospital Practice,* Vol. 6, No. 4 (April 1971), pp. 101–12.

[67] "Maternal Phenylketonuria," *British Medical Journal,* Vol. 4, No. 5729 (October 24, 1970), p. 192.

[68] Richard L. Day, "Factors Influencing Offspring," *American Journal of Diseases of Children,* Vol. 113, No. 2 (February 1967), pp. 179–85.

TABLE 18-2

The More Common Birth Defects

TYPE OF DEFECT	APPROXIMATE FREQUENCY	DESCRIPTION	CAUSES AND TREATMENT
Birthmarks	Very common.	The disfiguring ones are red or wine-colored patches of small dilated blood vessels.	Cause unknown. Treatments include plastic surgery, skin grafts, or tattooing of normal skin colors over the purple area.
Cleft lip (harelip)	About 1 in 1,000 babies born in the U.S. has a cleft lip; two-thirds of these also have a cleft palate. Frequency seems lower in blacks than in whites.	If embryonic swellings that will become the upper lip do not fuse at the right time, the gap remains and the baby will have a cleft lip.	Sometimes related to genetic defects. Influence of intrauterine environment and of some drugs given during pregnancy is being studied. Harelip can be repaired in the first few weeks after birth, and cleft palate before age fourteen months in most cases.
Cleft palate	About 1 in every 2,500 babies has a cleft palate without cleft lip. The two conditions are not genetically related.	A cleft palate is a hole in the roof of the mouth.	
Clubfoot	1 in 300.	The foot turns inward (usually) or outward and is fixed in a tip-toe position.	Possibly due to position of child in uterus or to maldevelopment of the limb bud. Treatments include shoe splints, braces, corrective shoes, plaster casts, or surgery. Tends to recur, so treatment must begin early and is often prolonged.
Congenital heart disease	1 in 125.	Some are so slight as to cause little strain on the heart; others are fatal. In some abnormalities, the baby appears blue.	German measles during pregnancy is one cause. Many heart conditions can now be repaired by surgery, saving lives and preventing invalidism.
Congenital urinary tract defects	1 in 250.	May involve kidneys, ureters, bladder, and genitalia. Organs may be absent, fused, or obstructed.	Causes include certain hormones given during pregnancy. Some hereditary tendency. Most conditions are correctable by surgery.
Diabetes	The prevalence of diabetes increases with advancing age, varying from about 1 case per 625 persons under age 25 to 1 in 15 persons age 65 to 75.	A metabolic disorder. The body cannot handle sugar normally, and high glucose levels in the blood and urine result. This familial condition is related in some unknown way to abnormal utilization of insulin. Long-standing diabetics may develop complications involving blood vessels, kidneys, heart, eyes, and peripheral nerves. Obesity predisposes individuals to the disease.	Marked hereditary tendency. Persons with family history of diabetes should seek periodic check-up. Doctors can recognize symptoms, make positive diagnosis, and prescribe specific treatment. Special diets, oral medication, and injections of insulin are measures that will usually keep condition under control and permit normal activity. Good prenatal care is especially important for known or suspected diabetics.

TABLE 18-2 (*continued*)

TYPE OF DEFECT	APPROXIMATE FREQUENCY	DESCRIPTION	CAUSES AND TREATMENT
Erythroblastosis fetalis (see also pages 553–55)	Prior to use of Rh immune globulin, hemolytic disease of the fetus and newborn occurred in 1 in every 150 to 200 pregnancies. About 15 percent of whites and 5 percent of blacks in the United States are Rh negative.	Without Rh immune globulin—and among infants of mothers sensitized during previous deliveries—baby is often yellow soon after birth. Anemia is a common symptom. Mental retardation may be severe. Erythroblastosis is a common cause of stillbirth.	Baby inherits Rh-positive gene from his father, and the mother is Rh negative. Red blood cells of fetus reach mother's blood, causing her blood to form antibodies that pass back through the placenta to the baby and destroy his red cells in varying degrees. First pregnancy is usually uneventful. Rh immune globulin prevents sensitization of mother, if given soon after birth of each baby. Intrauterine or exchange transfusion, replacing baby's blood with compatible blood right after birth, prevents severe damage to babies of sensitized mothers.
Extra fingers and toes (polydactyly)	Extra digits are twice as frequent as fused digits. Incidence is 1 in 100 among blacks; 1 in 600 among whites.	Extra fingers or toes.	Cause unknown; frequently hereditary. Cure is amputation of the extra digits. This can often be done at birth or at about age three.
Fused fingers and toes (syndactyly)	Fused digits do not have such racial variation.	Too few digits.	Surgery can improve the function and appearance of the hand or foot.
Fibrocystic disease (cystic fibrosis)	About 1 in 1,000 births. Rare among blacks; infrequent in Orientals.	A sickly, malnourished child with persistent intestinal difficulties and chronic respiratory problems. Death usually due to pneumonia or other lung complications.	Hereditary. New tests detect carriers. Mucus blocks the exit of digestive juices from the pancreas into the intestinal tract. Excess mucus is also secreted by lungs. Treatments have extended life.
Galactosemia	Somewhat more rare than PKU (see below).	Causes eye cataracts and severe damage to liver and brain, resulting in mental retardation.	Hereditary. Caused by absence of an enzyme required to convert galactose to glucose. Experiments show that early recognition and dietary treatment can arrest the disease. Diagnosis can be made at birth.
Hydrocephaly (water on the brain)	1 in 500.	Enlargement of the head due to excessive fluid within the brain. Fluid's pressure often causes compression of the brain with resulting mental retardation.	Cause unknown. May result from prenatal infection or abnormality in development. Treatment is an operation to lead fluid from brain into blood stream or some other body cavity. Frequently fatal if not treated.
Missing limbs	Very rare.	One to four limbs missing or seriously deformed.	Cause unknown. Recent international outbreak was due to thalidomide used by pregnant mothers. Great strides have been made in prosthetic (artificial) devices.

TABLE 18-2 (*continued*)

TYPE OF DEFECT	APPROXIMATE FREQUENCY	DESCRIPTION	CAUSES AND TREATMENT
Mongolism (Down's syndrome; see also page 540)	1 in 600. Women twenty-five years old have about 1 chance in 2,000 of producing a Mongoloid child. Women of forty-five have about 1 chance in 50.	Short stature, slightly slanted eyes, and varying degrees of mental retardation.	All patients have an extra chromosome or its equivalent. Causes can be hereditary or environmental. No known cure, but IQ can be improved by special training.
Open spine (spina bifida)	Approximately 1 in every 500 births. More common among whites than blacks. About half of the patients are also victims of hydrocephaly (see above).	Failure of the spine to close permits the protrusion of spinal cord or nerves; often leads to total dysfunction of legs, bladder, and rectum. Often the child has other serious defects.	Cause unknown. Sometimes surgery in the early months of life can correct or arrest the condition, preventing other complications. Several new surgical techniques are being used on the bladder, rectum, and spinal cord.
Phenylketonuria (PKU)	Approximately 1 in 20,000 whites. Extremely rare in blacks.	Child appears normal at birth, but his mind stops developing during the first year. Retardation is severe. One-third never learn to walk; two-thirds never learn to talk. Pigment of skin and hair is decreased.	Hereditary metabolic defect. The liver enzyme that changes the protein phenylalanine to tyrosine is inactive or absent; phenylalanine accumulates. PKU can be detected within the first few days of life. Treatment is special low-phenylalanine diet for the infant, which can prevent further retardation. Early treatment important. Some experiments show that after a few years PKU children can be fed normal diets.
Sickle cell anemia	One in 10 American blacks has trait; 1 in 400 has anemia. Low among whites.	Red blood cells of people with this disease periodically become crescent or sickle-shaped, clump together, and prevent transport of needed oxygen to body organs, causing painful sickle cell "crises."	Hereditary. When both parents have the trait, each child has 1 chance in 4 of inheriting sickle cell anemia. Careful management can help prevent crises; research to develop medications is promising.

Source: Adapted from a booklet published by the National Foundation–March of Dimes, White Plains, New York.

prematurely born babies have a higher mortality than those born with a normal weight, this finding takes on added significance.

3. If pregnancy intervals are three years or more, survival through childhood is statistically more likely.

4. If the mother is over thirty-five, the first-born is more likely to be a stillbirth than if she is younger. On the other hand, the very young mother also shows a higher rate of stillborn babies.

5. Children of small families grow taller and weigh more than children of large families.

6. It is the young mother who has already had at least one child and whose baby is at greatest risk from preventable conditions, who is apparently most

likely to profit from medical care (including contraceptive advice). Special efforts to improve her health, particularly if she is poor, would result in a great improvement in statistics that are used to describe the outcome of pregnancy.

7. An older father, regardless of the age of his wife, is statistically more likely to beget a stillborn child than a younger father.

8. Certain birth defects seem to occur more frequently in children with older parents than in those whose parents are young.

genetic counseling

Second cousins want to marry. They share three diabetic parents. What are the genetic dangers? A couple have a second child that is Mongoloid. Can they hope for a normal child? A young man's sister has been incapacitated for ten years with severe muscular dystrophy. He is engaged and deeply troubled. An agency brings a pretty child, the product of an incestuous union. What are the risks to adopting parents? Parents bring their baby. They have been putting it off, but something is wrong. Their family doctor has suggested that they come here.

Such are some of the intensely human problems brought to the genetic counselor. He can help as no one else can. He may discuss risks with those who inquire. In the event a diagnosis of a possible genetic illness is required, more detailed work is necessary. *The International Directory of Genetic Services,* 3rd ed. (September 1971), compiled by Henry T. Lynch, has been published by the National Foundation. It is of great professional value.

At this point, it would be well to differentiate between two frequently confused terms. The word *congenital* does not have the same meaning as *genetic. Congenital* means only "present at birth." It does not signify the cause of a condition. Some congenital conditions are not genetic, and many genetic conditions are not congenital. Huntington's chorea is an illness marked by irregular movements, speech disturbances, and mental deterioration. Although a genetic disease, it is not manifested until adulthood. However, maternal infection with German measles (rubella) virus in the first trimester of pregnancy may result in the infection of the unborn child. The child may then manifest the congenital rubella syndrome.

The mere fact that an illness occurs in more than one member of a family is not necessarily an indication that it is hereditary. Family members often share similar environments and habits; more likely, a combination of environment and genetic predisposition is responsible. During a person's first visit to a geneticist (who is usually, but not necessarily, a physician), a complete family history is taken. In order to obtain a complete family history, more than one family member may have to be interviewed. The geneticist must obtain information about both the paternal and maternal grandparents, parents, siblings, uncles, aunts, and first cousins. Miscarriages, stillbirths, and infant deaths are carefully noted. The inquiry may, but usually does not, extend beyond the first cousins.

From the history the geneticist constructs a *pedigree chart.* Blood samples provide cells for study. These are taken from the patient, both parents, and other relatives likely to be carrying the abnormality. Other procedures besides blood studies are helpful. A few cells scraped from the inside of a patient's mouth can help determine the number of X-chromosomes a patient has. Normal females have a dark area called the *Barr body* in these cells. It is absent in the male. The greatest number of Barr bodies in a buccal cell equals the number of patient's X-chromosomes minus one. Thus abnormal females with no Barr body have only one X-chromosome and abnormal XXY males have one Barr body. Since bone marrow provides most of the circulating blood cells, it also may provide much valuable information.

genetic disorders: the hope in research

It was not until 1956 that scientists discovered that the normal human cell contained forty-six (and not forty-eight) chromosomes. Since then, a whole new era in genetic counseling has taken place. The most significant advances have been made in three major areas. One has to do with the ability to grow cells in culture and to fuse together cells of different origins. The second involves magnificent new staining techniques that reveal hitherto unknown facts about the chromosomes of mankind. The third is a procedure known as *amniocentesis,* in which some of the amniotic fluid in which the fetus floats is withdrawn; both the fluid and the cells within it that are shed by the fetus can reveal the age, sex, some genetic defects, and other valuable information about the unborn child.

human-mouse cell hybrids

As was stated on page 155, scientists have long been able to grow cells in culture. Sick cells are placed in a container of specially prepared "soup." There they are nourished and multiply. As waste collects, some of the cellular growth is transferred to another container of fresh nourishment. These transferred cells multiply in turn. Another transfer is made, and still another. But only abnormal cells live so long in culture. Healthy cells live more briefly. Sick cells derived from various tissues have grown in culture, outside and independent of the organism of their origin, for sixty years. In all that time they lost neither vitality nor reproductive power. Some years ago, cancer cells from a patient's uterine cervix were obtained and, by transfer, repeatedly cultured. Tons of cells, originating from this one person's original cervical cancer cells, have been distributed to virus laboratories throughout the world. (Viruses are grown in them for a variety of technical purposes.)

Laboratory-cultured cells are a basic genetic tool. Long before the microscope was invented, medieval scientists imagined that each human sperm contained a whole, but tiny, person who was just waiting to grow big enough to be born. Today, it is known that each normal body (somatic) cell contains a full set of inherited chromosomes. Thus, the existing genetic differences between entire organisms can be studied from cultured cells gained from those different organisms. When human beings mate, a genetic event takes place. Scientists now know how to mate cells. Such cell fusion was first accomplished between living mouse cells. A third new cell type arose from the fusion; it contained a total number of chromosomes equal to the sum of the chromosomes of the parent cells. Such a cell is called a "hybrid cell"—a hybrid being an animal or plant produced from parents different in kind, such as parents belonging to a different species. In 1967, scientists reported the successful fusion of human and mouse cells. A human-mouse hybrid cell had been obtained. To a public long fed a scary diet of mad scientists in monster movies, this was alarming news. To the geneticist interested in studying chromosomes to prevent untold human suffering, it was a landmark achievement.

Why? Suppose a human being has a genetic illness. Is it due to the lack of an enzyme the presence of which is normally dependent on a certain gene? Cells of the individual lacking the gene can be grown outside the body in a culture medium. They can then be taken from the culture and mated (hybridized) with cells of a mouse that do not contain that gene. The hybrid cells are then grown in culture. As the hybrid human-mouse cells go through mitosis they lose human chromosomes. Human chromosomes seem to be eliminated preferentially. The process by which human chromosomes are selectively eliminated as the cell reproduces is not yet understood. Finally the hybrid cells stabilize; they lose no more human chromosomes. If one human chromosome is retained in the cells of the final hybrid cell culture, then one may regard that entire stabilized culture as a mouse cell culture with one human chromosome. That one human chromosome can be identified. Then the geneticist can test the cell culture for the missing enzyme. If it is not present in the mouse cells and is, indeed, absent in the entire culture, then one can point to the possible failure of the single human chromosome in the culture in making the critical enzyme. This procedure can be carried out in a variety of ways. Does cell hybridization have practical use today? Not yet. Then why is it being carried out and perfected? For the answer to this question one may refer to the reply of Louis Pasteur when, a century ago, he was asked if certain of his experiments had any practical value.

"No," replied the great bacteriologist.

"Then of what use is it?"

"Of what use is a newborn baby?" was the reply.[69]

staining for chromosomal stripes

The elucidation of the human karyotype (see Figure 18-7) spurred study of both normal and abnormal chromosomes. Many genetic conditions became

[69] The relevance of this anecdote to cell hybridization is illustrated by two recent, scientifically provocative discoveries. It is known that some human cells are susceptible to poliovirus because of the presence of a gene that directs the synthesis of poliovirus receptors on their surfaces. This permits the virus to attach itself to the cell's surface. In some human-mouse hybrid cells it has been found that the chromosome bearing the receptor gene is lost. The cells are thus resistant to poliomyelitis. Hybrid cells may become increasingly useful in providing information about the genetic basis of cell sensitivity to virus infection. (Peter Spackman, "Man or Mouse," *Technology Review*, Vol. 74, No. 7 [June 1972], pp. 61–62.) A second discovery revealed that when normal mouse cells were fused to malignant mouse cells, the hybrids were no longer cancerous. However, when most of the chromosomes of the normal mouse cells were lost, the malignancy returned. For a while, however, the cancer had been stopped. (Gail McBride, "Prenatal Diagnosis: Problems and Outlook," *Journal of the American Medical Association*, Vol. 222, No. 2 (October 9, 1972), pp. 135, 138.

better understood. It was demonstrated that some genetic diseases were due to an additional chromosome—for example, the Klinefelter's (see page 540) and XYY syndromes (see page 542). In addition, it was discovered that a chromosomal deficit accounted for some genetic disorders; among these were most cases of Turner's syndrome (see page 540). However, as has been pointed out, there are more subtle errors of the human karyotype that can result in serious illness. These include small deletions and translocations (see page 538) of one portion of a chromosome to another. Until very recently, classification of these disorders was very difficult because the geneticist was unable to consistently identify each chromosome of the normal human karyotype. He was forced to base his identifications on the relative size of the chromosomes and on the position of the clear region where the arms of the chromosome meet (*centromere*).

Now that has changed. Today, newly developed staining techniques permit the accurate identification of every chromosome in the human karyotype. Fluorescing compounds have been discovered that bind to chromosomal DNA. (A fluorescent substance has the property of emitting light after exposure to light.) When treated with the fluorescent substance and placed under a special fluorescent microscope, chromosomes are seen to have a banded appearance; it is as if they had stripes. Certain bands exhibit more fluorescence than others, and the pattern of banding is specific for each chromosome. In addition, not only are the banding patterns characteristic for each pair of the twenty-two autosomes, and for the X- and Y-chromosomes as well, but they are also consistent from cell to cell and from person to person. Thus, in its middle phase of mitosis (metaphase), each chromosome can be identified by its distinctive pattern of fluorescence. The production of bands at specific locations, by bringing out unique chromosomal patterns, will help identify structurally abnormal chromosomes, determine their origins, and provide a means of earlier and more accurate identification of abnormalities. Easy identification of subtle changes, such as extra or missing chromosomal segments, is now feasible. But the banding technique promises to do more. It provides another tool for the gigantic task of "mapping" human chromosomes. The goal of mapping chromosomes is to locate each gene in relation to others and to determine which of the twenty-three pairs of chromosomes carries it. When one considers the many thousands of genes in each chromosome and the significance of each, the size of the task becomes more apparent. But it will be worth the labor. For among the many future possible benefits of chromosome mapping will be the possibility of earlier diagnosis and treatment of genetic disease.

diagnosis of the unborn

Amniocentesis is a procedure in which a needle is inserted through the walls of both the abdomen and the pregnant uterus in order to withdraw amniotic fluid (see page 573), and the cells suspended in it, for examination. It is useful in assessing the maturity as well as the condition of the fetus; it can be of aid in genetic counseling; it is often of assistance in foretelling problems with the

Rh factor (see pages 553–55); combined with X-rays, it may be valuable in determining fetal malformations or the localization of the placenta. As pregnancy advances, the amniotic fluid becomes a rich source of information about the unborn child. Enzymes, amino acids, and a variety of other normal and abnormal products may be added to the fluid as a result of the child's excretion of urine. Among the sources of cells in the amniotic fluid may be the amnion itself, the fetal skin, urine, windpipe, bronchi, and the lining of the gastrointestinal system. The living cells from the fluid proliferate in cell culture. Examination of connective tissue cells from cultured cells of the amniotic fluid can be examined for chromosomal abnormalities. Cells may also be studied for enzyme activity or for the presence (or absence) of various substances.[70]

Thus, the amniotic fluid is useful for diagnosing and possibly preventing a variety of conditions. In a test that requires only an hour of laboratory work, the amniotic fluid, drawn after the thirty-fourth week of pregnancy, can be tested for the maturity of the lungs of the fetus. In this way the physician can determine the likelihood of a serious condition called the respiratory syndrome of the newborn.[71] After the twentieth week of pregnancy, the cells of amniotic fluid may be tested for Rh blood disease (see pages 553–55). The cells of the amniotic fluid inform the geneticists of the genetic sex of the fetus,[72] while both the fluid and the cells within it are useful in determining the age of the unborn child.[73] In addition, amniocentesis is valuable in the diagnosis of a growing number of genetic disorders. Before the fourteenth week of pregnancy the amount of amniotic fluid is small; thus, amniocentesis before the fifteenth week of pregnancy increases the risk of damage to the mother or child. But the diagnosis of serious genetic disorders is a race against time. If abortion is to be contemplated, it must be done as early as possible. To diagnose genetic disorders, amniocentesis might be performed at about the fifteenth week of pregnancy. This may vary, however; the test has been performed as early as the twelfth week. For those in need of genetic counseling it is usually done between the fourteenth and seventeenth weeks. It is believed that the chance of miscarriage is increased when amniocentesis is used early in pregnancy for genetic counseling. At least two to three weeks are required to grow enough cells and to complete the karyotype, or to demonstrate an enzymatic defect.[74] In some cases, an even longer time is required, and the waiting period is a trying time for the anxious parents-to-be.[75]

[70] "Diagnostic Amniocentesis," *Medical Letter on Drugs and Therapeutics,* Vol. 14, No. 15, Issue 353 (July 21, 1972), p. 53.

[71] "Prenatal Test Developed for Respiratory Distress," *Journal of the American Medical Association,* Vol. 220, No. 12 (June 19, 1972), p. 5.

[72] M. E. Ferguson-Smith, M. A. Ferguson-Smith, N. C. Nevin, and M. Stone, "Chromosome Analysis Before Birth and Its Value in Genetic Counselling," *British Medical Journal,* Vol. 4, No. 5779 (October 9, 1971), p. 69; Melvin Gertner, Lillian Y. F. Hsu, Joan Martin, and Kurt Hirschhorn, "The Use of Amniocentesis for Prenatal Genetic Counselling," *Bulletin of the New York Academy of Medicine,* Second Series, Vol. 46, No. 11 (November 1970), p. 916.

[73] "Assessment of Gestational Age from Amniotic Fluid," *Lancet,* Vol. 1, No. 7742 (January 15, 1972), pp. 132–33.

[74] Angel Werch and Paige K. Besch, "Amniocentesis in Daily Obstetrics," *American Family Physician,* Vol. 8, No. 3 (September 1973), pp. 160–64.

[75] Gail McBride, "Prenatal Diagnosis: Problems and Outlook," p. 133.

Amniocentesis has been performed thousands of times. Although in the hands of a trained operator the risk is slight, it is never done unless absolutely necessary. Amniocentesis for the determination of genetic sex, for example, is never done merely to satisfy parental curiosity about whether their child will be a boy or a girl. It may be done so that a woman who is a carrier of an X-linked disorder can elect to permit abortion of a male fetus. Such a woman will transmit the X-linked disorder to only one-half of her sons. Should an abortion be done, a normal as well as an abnormal male fetus could be sacrificed.[76] Unfortunately, the more common X-linked disorders, such as hemophilia, still cannot be diagnosed before birth.

The same is true of genetic disorders that result in abnormal body metabolism. Cystic fibrosis, for example, the greatest killer of white children, cannot be diagnosed before birth. However, research may soon remedy this situation; there is some evidence that a deficiency of a particular component of a certain enzyme may be responsible for cystic fibrosis. It may be possible to diagnose that deficiency before birth.[77] Sickle cell anemia (see pages 547–48) remains among the metabolic genetic disorders that cannot be diagnosed by amniocentesis. (Recent studies, however, suggest that a blood sample obtained from the placenta may provide the material necessary to diagnose this condition, which afflicts and kills so many thousands of black children every year.)[78] An important metabolic genetic disorder that can be diagnosed by amniocentesis is Tay-Sachs disease. This tragic condition, characterized by blindness and severe mental retardation, can be diagnosed as early as the sixteenth week by the detection of the absence of an enzyme. It is most commonly found among this country's Ashkenazic Jews—that is, those Jews who originally settled in northern and central Europe (as distinguished from the Sephardic Jews, who settled in Spain and Portugal). Preliminary results of a recent survey suggest that one of twenty-five U.S. Jews may be a carrier of Tay-Sachs disease.[79]

The most common chromosomal aberration that can be detected by amniocentesis is that causing Down's syndrome (Mongolism; see page 540). The frequency of this disorder increases with the mother's age; between ages thirty-five and thirty-nine, the risk is about 1 in 300; between forty and forty-four, 1 in 100; the risk is 1 in 40 at age forty-five or older. Although only 13 percent of all pregnancies occur in women over thirty-five years old, more than one-half of all Mongoloid children are born to women in this age group. Aside from the suffering and the anxiety that amniocentesis may avert, it is well to mention the economic benefits. About four thousand children with Down's syndrome are born in this country every year. Institutional care for each child who is placed costs about $250,000.[80]

[76] "Diagnostic Amniocentesis," pp. 53–54.

[77] Gail McBride, "Prenatal Diagnosis: Problems and Outlook," p. 134.

[78] Yuet Wai Kan, Andrée M. Dozy, Blanche P. Alter, Frederic D. Frigoletto, and David G. Nathan, "Detection of the Sickle-Cell Gene in the Human Fetus," *New England Journal of Medicine,* Vol. 287, No. 1 (July 6, 1972), pp. 1–5; see also in the same issue Haig H. Kazazian, Jr., "Antenatal Detection of Sickle-Cell Anemia," pp. 41–42.

[79] "Estimates of Tay-Sachs Gene Carriers May Be Low," *Journal of the American Medical Association,* Vol. 220, No. 7 (May 15, 1972), p. 915.

[80] Gerald H. Prescott, R. Ellen Magenis, and Neil R. M. Buist, "Amniocentesis for Antenatal Diagnosis," *Postgraduate Medicine,* Vol. 51, No. 3 (March 1972), pp. 216–17.

There is a continuing possibility that other scientific discoveries helpful to parents-to-be will be made. A 1973 report described techniques that determine the amount of genetic material (DNA) with a precision never before achieved. This work shows great promise; for example, if a woman is suspected of having the X-linked gene for hemophilia, an abnormal amount of X-chromosome material might diagnose her as a carrier of hemophilia. The same technique may turn out to be helpful in determining cancer development.[81] Moreover, an instrument called an *amnioscope* is being developed, which might be used not only to draw blood safely from the placenta or from fetal vessels, but also to inspect the fetus for malformations. Also, ultrasound equipment (which produces sound beyond human hearing) can now deliver more information about the shape of the fetus, while new X-ray techniques are providing more detail about happenings within the pregnant uterus. Even the intrauterine treatment of some genetically diseased fetuses is nearing reality. (See page 763.)

summary

The *cell* is the basic unit of life (page 521). Within the *nucleus* of the cell are the *chromosomes,* which contain the *genes*—the units of heredity (page 521). The *cytoplasm* (the other major portion of the cell in addition to the nucleus) is surrounded by a *plasma membrane* that folds inward at various points, forming the *endoplasmic reticulum* (pages 522–24). The organelles contained within the cytoplasm include *ribosomes,* the *Golgi complex, mitochondria,* and *lysosomes* (page 524). Three chemical substances play important roles in governing the functions of the cell: *cyclic AMP* (pages 525–26), *cyclic GMP* (page 526), and *chalones* (pages 526–27).

There are two basic kinds of human cells: *germ cells,* or gametes (ova and spermatozoa), and *somatic cells,* or body cells. A primordial sex cell divides by *meiosis,* which results in a mature germ cell containing twenty-two *autosomes* and either an *X-chromosome* or a *Y-chromosome*—half the number of chromosomes the original cell had (page 527). A mature ovum carries an X-chromosome; a mature sperm, either an X- or a Y-chromosome. Thus, the *zygote* that results from the fertilization of an ovum by a sperm will contain a full set of forty-six chromosomes (page 528). The zygote and all subsequent somatic cells multiply by *mitosis,* in which the chromosomes duplicate themselves and then separate, with a full set of forty-six chromosomes going to each of the two ''daughter'' cells that result from the division of the original cell (page 529).

Chromosomes are made up mostly of proteins and *deoxyribonucleic acid* (DNA). DNA directs the synthesis of three kinds of *ribonucleic acid* (RNA) from amino acids. Unlike DNA, RNA can leave the nucleus. Once formed, the first kind of RNA leaves the nucleus to become situated on a part of the endoplasmic reticulum as a ribosome, the workbench at which cellular protein will be made. The second type of RNA carries the actual genetic blueprint—the message; as *messenger RNA,* it leaves the nucleus to become associated with a ribosome. The third RNA, *transfer RNA,* is directed by the nuclear DNA to seek out, within the cytoplasm, a specific amino

[81] ''Better Markers for Genetic Diseases,'' *Science News,* Vol. 103, No. 11 (March 17, 1973), p. 166.

acid and bring it to the ribosomal–messenger-RNA complex. There, specific amino acids are linked with other amino acids (brought by other transfer RNAs) to eventually form proteins, the various structures of which will determine various hereditary characteristics (pages 532–35).

Genetic disorders may result either from an error in the *structure* of a chromosome—for example, *spontaneous mutations* (pages 537–38) or *chromosomal translocation and deletion* (page 538)—or from an error in the *number* of chromosomes that occurs during meiosis or early mitosis. The basic error that occurs during meiosis is *meiotic nondisjunction*—the failure of paired chromosomes to separate, so that one cell receives both chromosomes and the other cell receives none (page 538). Some disorders that originate during meiosis are *trisomy 21* (*Mongolism* or *Down's syndrome;* page 540); *Turner's syndrome* (page 540); *Klinefelter's syndrome* (page 540); the *XYY syndrome* (page 542); and configurations with three, four, or no X-chromosomes (page 543). Errors of nondisjunction that occur during mitosis are given the general name *mosaicism* (page 544).

Illness can result from such genetic factors as sex (notably *hemophilia,* page 546) and race (notably *sickle cell disease,* pages 547–48). In addition, the normal genetic development of the fertilized ovum can be profoundly affected by such factors as the mother's nutrition (pages 549–50), infection (pages 550–51), direct radiation (page 551), chemical pollutants (pages 551–52), noise (pages 552–53), endocrine influences (page 553), the Rh factor (pages 553–55), the mother's age (page 555), the mother's emotions (page 555), and drugs (pages 555–56). A number of steps can be taken to avoid some birth defects (pages 557–58). In addition, *genetic counseling,* utilizing new techniques involving human-mouse cell hybrids (pages 563–64), staining for chromosomal stripes (pages 564–65), and *amniocentesis* (pages 565–68), presents possibilities for the prevention of genetic disorders.

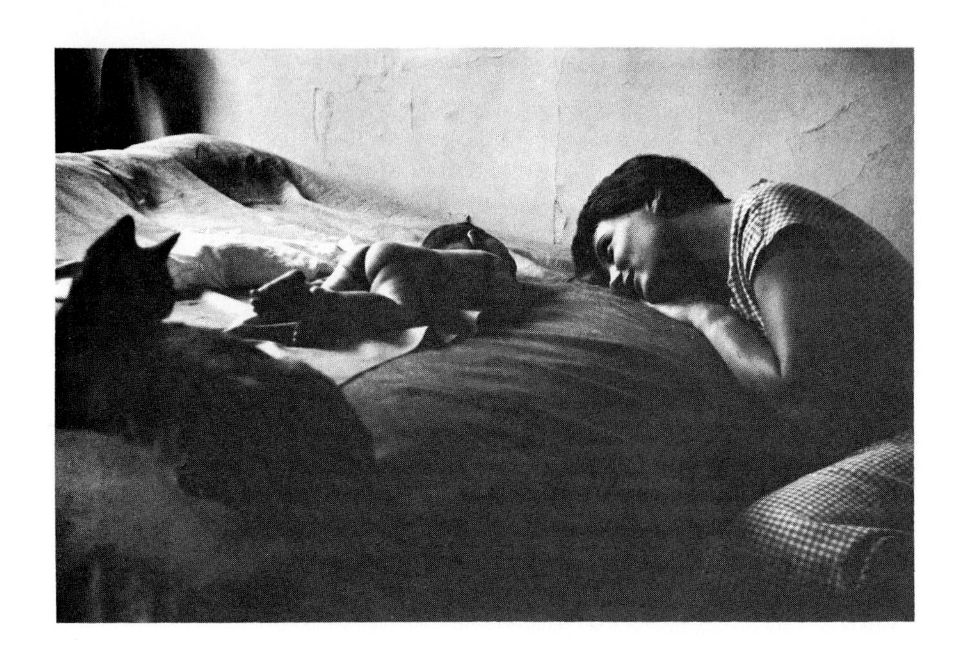

building a family: pregnancy, some infancy problems, subfertility, and adoption

19

pregnancy

The ovum is one of the body's largest cells; the sperm, the smallest. Alone, they are just potential. Together, they can fuse, and the product of their fusion can multiply to form a creature that can wonder. But even in the earliest phases this product is already remarkable. "Every child starts as an invisible unit with a weight of only $\frac{5}{1000}$ of a milligram and gains during the first weeks of life more than a million percent in weight. Which industry, whatever direction or planning boards there may be, can claim such an increase in output?"[1]

the duration of pregnancy

Counting from the time of fertilization of the egg by the sperm (*conception*), the duration of the pregnancy is $9\frac{1}{2}$ lunar months (38 weeks, or 266 days). A "lunar" month is 28 days because there is a full moon every 28 days. Counting from the first day of the last menstrual period, the average pregnancy lasts 10 lunar months (40 weeks, or 280 days).

In calculating the expected date of birth, three months are subtracted from the date of the beginning of the last normal menstrual period. Then seven days are added. For example, if the first day of the last normal period was June 17, the expected date of confinement would be March 24.

But these calculations are only based on averages. Perhaps 10 percent of all pregnancies end 280 days after the beginning of the last menstrual period; less than 50 percent end within one week of the 280th day. The time required for the fetus in the uterus is individual. Extreme but normal variances of 240 days to 300 days in the uterus occur. The calculated expected date of birth is not often exact. There is less than a 50 percent chance that the child will be born within a week of that date and a 10 percent chance that labor will occur about two weeks later.

the child within the uterus

Before pregnancy the uterus weighs one ounce. At the end of pregnancy, the empty uterus weighs 2.2 pounds and its capacity has increased more than five hundred times. (A short time after delivery, it returns to almost its original size.) The remarkable events occurring during the development of the child in the uterus are described in the science of *embryology*—the story of a new person.

The new individual is the zygote—the fertilized egg. It is unique and no larger than the tiniest sand speck. It does not wait long in the uterine tube. While on its two- to four-day, four- to five-inch journey to the uterus, the zygote cleaves daily. When it arrives the uterus is not yet ready for it. About two to four more days pass as the small, continuously multiplying cell mass floats in the uterus. Meanwhile, as described in Chapter 16, the uterine lining continues to prepare for it. At last, as early as day 18 and as late as day 23 of the menstrual cycle and as much as eight days following fertilization, implantation occurs.[2]

When implantation occurs, the cellular mass (*blastocyst*) is a fluid-filled

[1] G. M. H. Veeneklass, cited in *Physicians Bulletin,* Vol. 24, No. 8 (November 15, 1959), p. B/8.
[2] The American College of Obstetricians and Gynecology considers implantation and conception to be synonymous. The reason for this is that implantation cannot be diagnosed unless conception has occurred.

sphere of cells. Cell multiplication continues until, on the internal surface of the blastocyst, a layer of cells separates; this is the *endoderm.* It will contribute heavily to such inner body parts as the digestive and respiratory systems. Cells of the outer layer also multiply. These comprise the *ectoderm* destined for outer structures such as the skin, hair, and nervous tissue. A middle layer of cells multiplies to push in between ectoderm and endoderm. This intermediate *mesoderm* will be muscle and bone, marrow and blood, kidney and gonad. These three layers will further differentiate to become the organized human creature. After the first week of development following fertilization, the cell mass is called an *embryo;* the youngest human embryo is about seven and one-half days old. Not until the beginning of the third month will the embryo be a *fetus.*

the firm establishment of the new life

Not all of the fertilized egg becomes an embryo. Some is destined to be auxiliary embryonic equipment that will not only protect the embryo but also provide means of nourishment, excretion, and respiration. Even in the blastocyst two cell masses differentiate: the *inner cell mass,* which is to become the embryo, and an outer cellular wall, the *trophoblast,* which is the beginning of the auxiliary tissue. (Later in pregnancy the trophoblast is called the *chorion.*) The cells of the trophoblast have the ability to digest or dissolve both the wall of the uterine endometrial lining and the walls of small blood vessels in that area. The multiplying and digesting cells of the trophoblast extend into the endometrium, and around them occur slight uterine bleedings. From the little lakes of mother's blood, seepages of nutriments feed the growing cellular mass. Via these early maternal blood lakes, then, the mother offers the first food to the parasitic cell mass imbedded in the lining of the uterus. Then the inner layer of the trophoblast grows out to push fingerlike projections into the endometrium. These are the *villi;* their encroaching cells continue to digest the cells of uterine endometrium and small adjacent blood vessels.

Some villi extend not only into the endometrium but also into the maternal lakes, in which they float free. Soon the maternal lakes are so crowded by villi that there are now only *intervillous spaces.* It is primarily in these intervillous spaces that the physiological exchanges occur between mother and child during pregnancy. Each mature villus eventually contains fetal blood vessels connected with the circulation of the child.

By a month after fertilization, the inner cell mass that is the embryo is encircled by a *chorionic membrane* and this membrane is surrounded by *chorionic villi.* A fluid-filled sac, or vesicle, has been created. The embryo is attached to the wall of this *chorionic vesicle* by a *body stalk,* which will elongate to become a cable containing blood vessels, the *umbilical cord.* As the last part of the second month of pregnancy approaches, many of the villi on the surface of the chorionic membrane begin to degenerate. Only about 20 percent of the villi remain as the *fetal placenta.* It is apparent that the mother contributes to the placenta and, via her placental arteries, the mother brings oxygen and nourishment to the blood lakes. The placenta is attached to the fetus by the umbilical cord. Within the umbilical cord are two arteries and one vein. Through the arteries, waste-laden blood is carried from the fetus to the villi of the placenta. From the villi, these fetal waste products are then lost to the blood lakes. (The mother will take them up into her placental veins and excrete them with her own venous wastes.) At the same time, oxygen and nourishment are taken up into the villi from the blood lakes. The single umbilical vein carries these from the villi of the placenta to the fetus. At no time will there normally be a direct connection between maternal and fetal blood. The fetal circulation of blood in the placenta is a system that is closed to the mother.

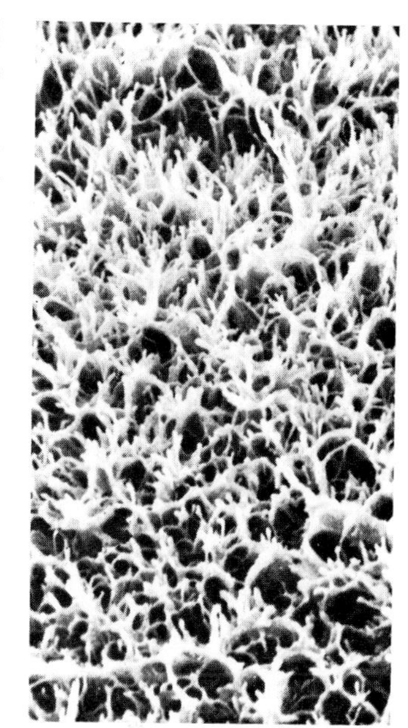

19-1 *The complex surface of the placenta during the twelfth week of pregnancy, as seen through the scanning electron microscope.*

Other extraembryonic equipment is also formed. At the age of two weeks the embryo is tucked beneath the surface of the uterine lining. A hollow beneath it will enlarge to a fluid-filled cavity surrounded by a sac called the *amnion.* This sac is filled with *amniotic fluid;* by the fifth month the fetus is swallowing some amniotic fluid. As long as the fetus remains within this sac in the uterus, it lives the aquatic life of a fish. Also during early development, the extraembryonic membranous *yolk sac* and *allantois* appear. After the second month the yolk sac begins to wither and becomes quite useless, but not until it has contributed to the gut as well as early blood cells and vessels. The allantois becomes the blood vessels in the umbilical cord. It is well to now summarize the functions of the placenta and the amnion.

A versatile temporary organ, the placenta (Figure 19-1) is derived, then, from a fertilized ovum, but the mother contributes too. It serves as a gland, intestine, kidney, lung, and partial barrier. Also, the placenta separates two genetically different individuals. When the placenta is bypassed in laboratory animals, the fetus is rejected.[3] This is not unlike the process that occurs when a recipient rejects a transplanted heart. From the maternal side of the placenta, projections branch into the endometrium and into the mother's blood. By osmosis, nutrients from the mother's blood ooze through the placenta. In a reverse manner, the child eliminates wastes. Attached to the fetal surface of the placenta are an umbilical cord and fused membranes. Through the cord circulation, exchanges are made to and from the placenta. Together, the membranes form a bag or sac, completely encompassing the child. In the bag are the "waters," or amniotic fluid. Throughout intrauterine life the child is submerged in these waters. Like an astronaut in a space capsule, the fetus within the amniotic sac is in a state of weightlessness. Therefore, the child is able to move about without expending energy that is needed for growth and development. In addition, the fluid protects delicate tissues, provides a stable temperature, and is of some help in the dilation of the cervix in early labor.[4] It is not true that a baby born in the membranes of the amniotic sac is lucky. Unless the birth is unattended by a doctor, this does not happen. To enable the baby to breathe immediately at birth, the doctor will, if necessary, rupture the membranes.

[3] Joseph Dancis, Symposium on "Homeostasis of the Intrauterine Patient," cited in "The Purpose of the Placenta," *Briefs: Footnotes on Maternity Care,* Vol. 33, No. 4 (April 1969), pp. 54–55.
[4] Peter J. Huntingford, "The Fetus in Its Aquatic Environment," cited in "Amnion: Protector of the Unborn Baby," *Briefs: Footnotes on Maternity Care,* Vol. 32, No. 9 (November 1968), pp. 131–32.

19-2 the development of human embryonic membranes

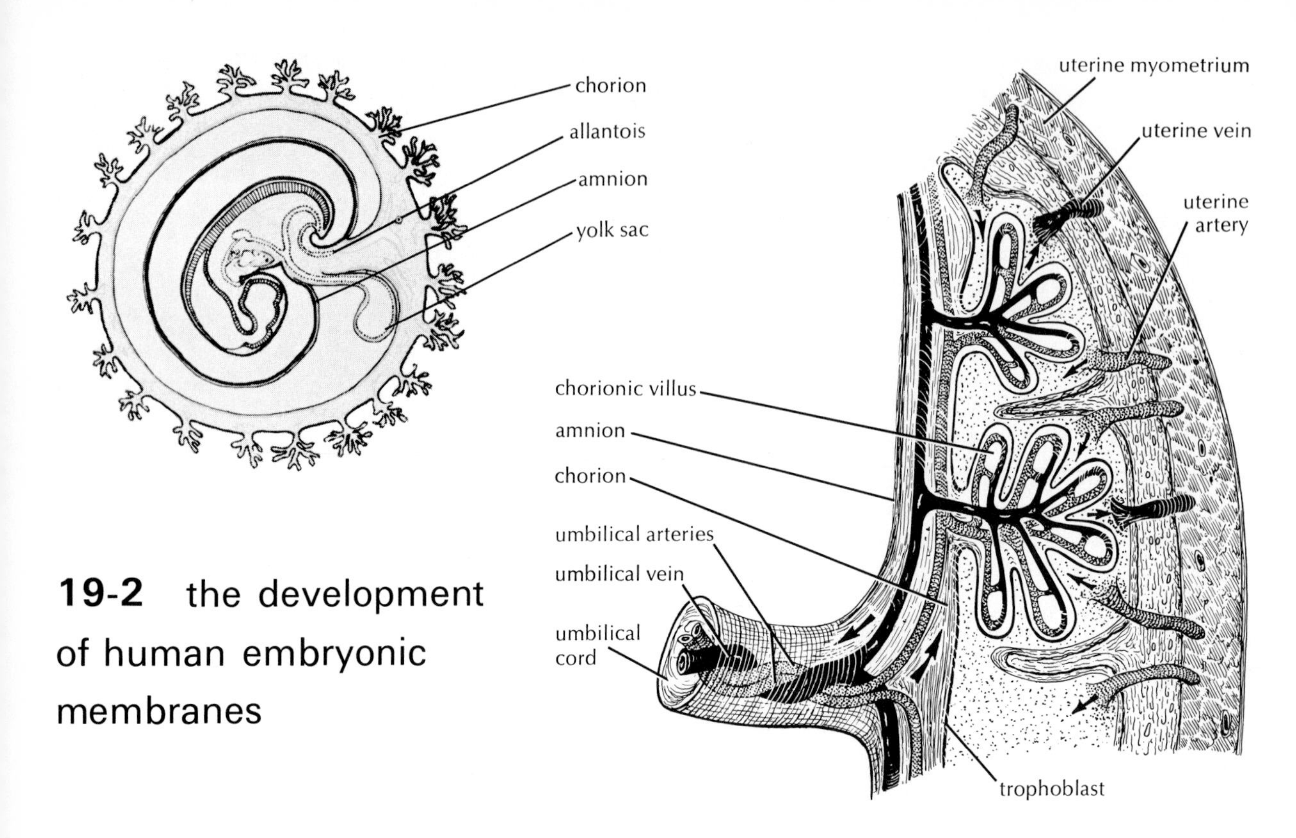

Two stages of embryonic development, showing the interrelationship of embryo and membranes (top left *and* below) *and a cross section of the placenta* (top right).

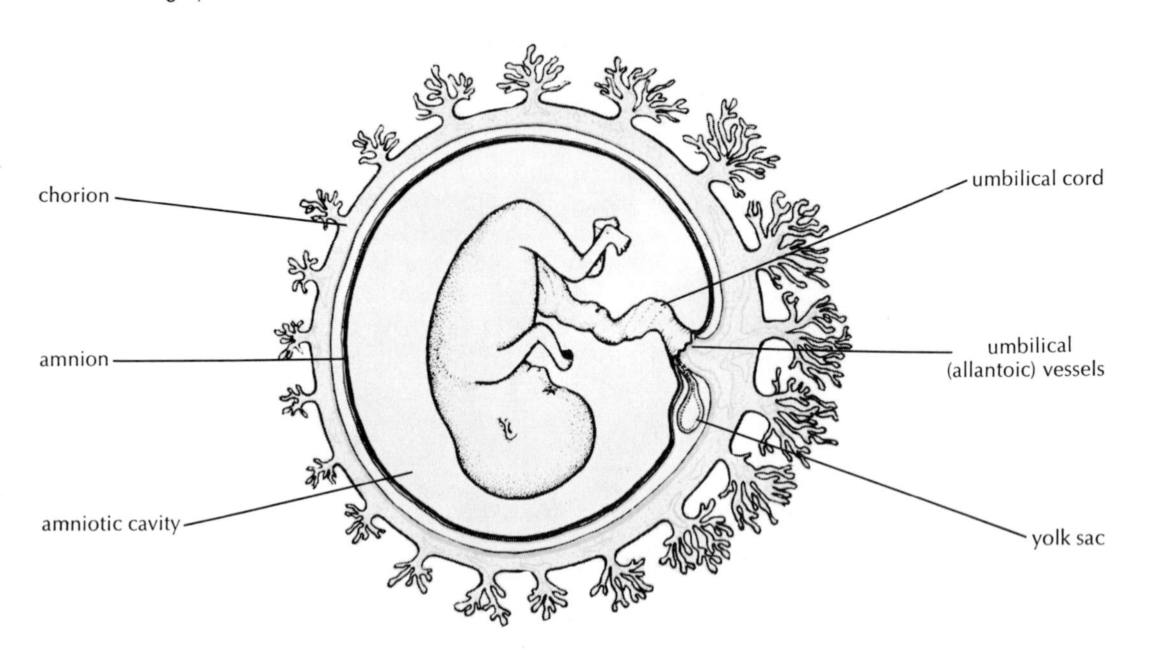

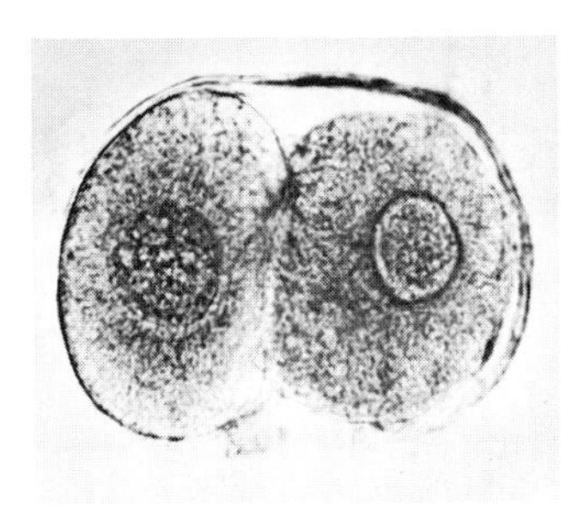

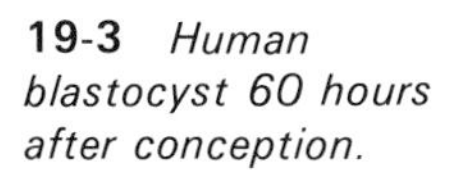

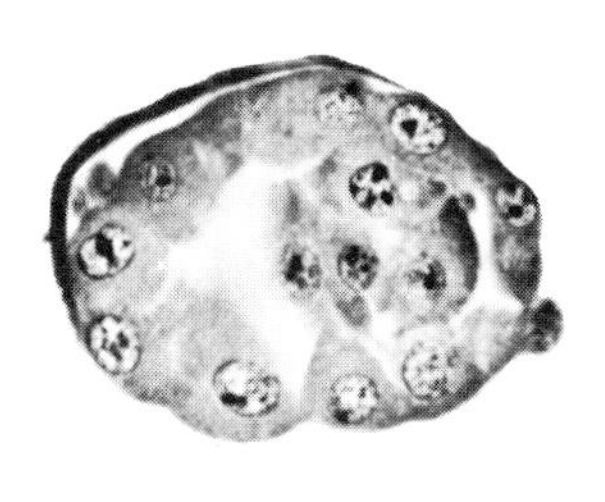

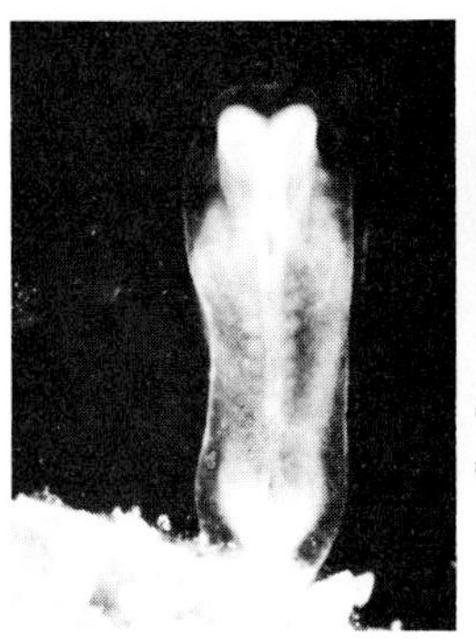

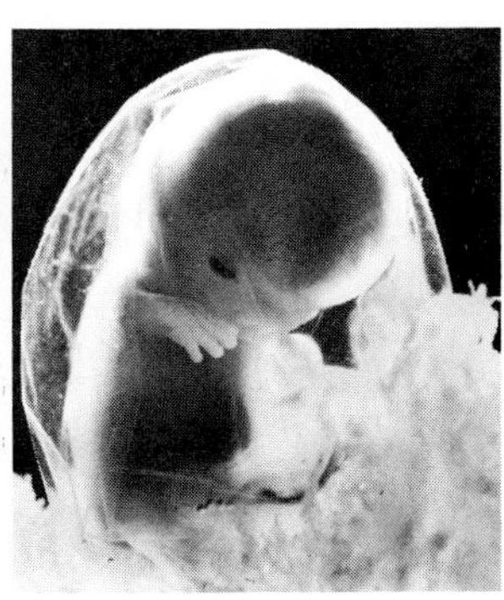

19-3 *Human blastocyst 60 hours after conception.*

Human blastocyst 4 days after conception.

Human embryo at 22 days.

Human embryo at 8 weeks.

The month-by-month changes in the human being during intrauterine residence will now be described.

END OF THE FIRST LUNAR MONTH By the end of the first lunar month, the embryo is about one-quarter of an inch long (about the size of a pea) and resembles a sea urchin. About one-third of the embryo is the head, which almost touches the tail. The bulging, beating heart propels blood through primitive vessels. From a developing mouth leads a tube that will become the digestive tract. Rudiments of eyes, ears, and nose appear, and buds that will become extremities are all visible. Soon the umbilical cord will develop, not as an outgrowth from the baby's body but from accessory tissue.

END OF THE SECOND LUNAR MONTH Every week the embryo has grown one-quarter of an inch and is now a fetus weighing one-thirtieth of an ounce. Sex organs are apparent, but the sex of the fetus is difficult to determine. The developing brain causes the head to be disproportionately large. Pawlike hands have appeared. The half-closed eyes will soon close completely; they remain closed until the end of the seventh month. A few muscles are developing and the feet may kick a few times (but much too feebly to be felt by the mother). The tail begins to regress. At the end of two months, almost all the internal organs have begun to develop. The changes now are mostly related to growth and tissue differentiation.

19-4 *Human fetus at 12 weeks.*

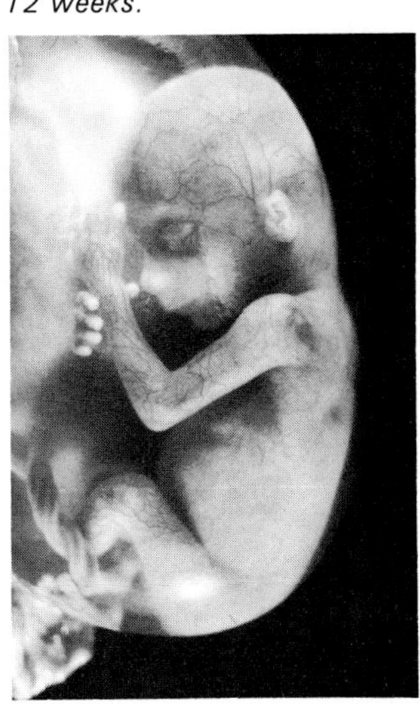

END OF THE THIRD LUNAR MONTH The three-inch fetus weighs about an ounce but the placenta weighs more. The ears rise to the level of the eyes and the eyelids are fused. Soft nails appear on the stubby fingers and toes. Gender sex can be discerned. From rudimentary kidneys, small amounts of urine are excreted into the amniotic fluid. Tooth sockets and buds are apparent. Now the mother's enlarging uterus can be felt below the umbilicus.

END OF THE FOURTH LUNAR MONTH The four-ounce fetus is not quite seven inches long. On the scalp a few hairs may sprout. Soon there will be a fine, downy, whorled growth of hair called *lanugo* covering the whole body. The mother may feel the first subtle movements of the fetus (*quickening*) at the end of this period. Usually, however, these do not occur until the following month.

END OF THE FIFTH LUNAR MONTH The ten-inch fetus weighs about eight ounces. The heart can be heard through the stethoscope. The baby moves actively. Later in pregnancy movements may become quite vigorous but they do not hurt. Since the lungs are not sufficiently developed, babies born prematurely at this time do not survive; they may live but a few minutes.

END OF THE SIXTH LUNAR MONTH Now the fetus weighs a pound and one-half and is about a foot long. The fetus is not idle, sucking an available thumb, swallowing amniotic fluid, exercising developing muscles, even managing an occasional spasmodic chest movement. Noise startles the child in the uterus. When the mother rocks, the child may go to sleep. The child's activity may waken the mother. Intrauterine quarters are crowded and some children are more restless than others. The sebaceous glands and cells that are shed from the wrinkled skin combine to provide a protective *vernix caseosa,* or "cheesy varnish." At birth this may be one-eighth of an inch thick. At the end of this month, the eyelids separate and eyelashes form. If born at this stage, the child is still too undeveloped to survive.

END OF THE SEVENTH LUNAR MONTH The two-and-one-half-pound fetus is about fifteen inches long. The eyes are open and the child can appreciate light. In the male fetus the testicles are usually in the scrotum. Fat begins to

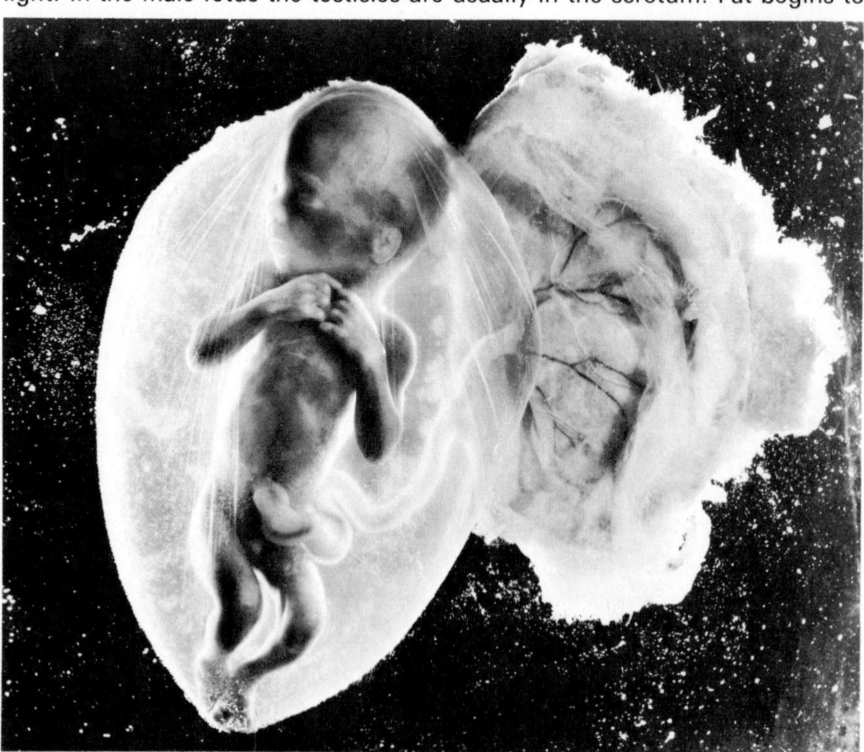

19-5 *Human fetus at 4 months.*

flatten out a few wrinkles. Every day in the uterus at this stage is vital. A baby born at this time has only a fair chance of survival because the lungs and intestinal canal are incompletely developed.

END OF THE EIGHTH LUNAR MONTH The fetus now weighs about four pounds and measures some sixteen and one-half inches. The bones of the head are soft. The fetus looks like a little old man. If provided with good nursing and medical care, a baby born now has a much better chance of surviving than one born in the previous month.

END OF THE NINTH LUNAR MONTH The fetus, weighing about six pounds and measuring about nineteen inches, begins to make ready to leave the weightless watery ecosystem within the uterus. As if to prepare for the new environment, the fetus gains half a pound a week and wrinkles now disappear. The fingernails need cutting and the fetus may be born with harmless scratch marks. If born prematurely during this month, the chances for survival are good.

THE TENTH LUNAR MONTH By about the middle of the tenth lunar month, the full-term twenty-inch fetus is born, weighing about seven pounds (girls) or about seven and one-half pounds (boys). The umbilical cord is about as long as the baby. The placenta weighs about one and one-quarter pounds; it is a disc that is about six to eight inches in diameter. There is from one-half to two quarts of amniotic fluid. Most of the lanugo is gone, although some may remain about the shoulders. The vernix caseosa remains and has to be wiped away. The hormones that cause the mother's breasts to enlarge cause the unborn child's breasts to protrude a little. The newborn may secrete milk (''witch's milk''). Within a few days after birth, the breast enlargement subsides and there is no further secretion of milk. The final hue of the slate-colored eyes cannot be predicted.

the mother

Some married women, perhaps too long denied, eagerly await a first child. Many others want a baby, but not at the moment. Some feel a trifle taken in by their pregnancy. Frequently, a first-time mother may need time to accept the idea. She has about three months to do so. During that time, she weighs herself often. But the scales say little. Her pregnancy is not very real. Nothing much changes.

In the second three months, she grows, and not just physically. The emotional preparations may be more profound than the physical ones.

For many a woman, the last three months of pregnancy drag. A dozen discomforts plague her. This ordeal, she thinks, will be capped by still another. She may wish to be rid of her pregnancy. Yet, she may fear its end. She is weary of glossy magazine pictures of overjoyed women hurrying to the hospital without a care in the world. She wishes she could control her urinary bladder better. And she may worry that her husband, too, is tiring of her pregnant condition.

During pregnancy, some women (not all) are somewhat less interested in sexual intercourse. Knowing this, the husband will not feel rejected. The sensitive husband will, moreover, understand that his wife's emotional state profoundly affects the pregnancy. It is here that his responsibility is so considerable. As never before, she needs his love, patience, and confidence.

about some changes, pregnancy tests, and rules

A regularly menstruating woman's first, most common, sign of pregnancy is a missed menstrual period. The breasts are sensitive. The nipples enlarge and become pigmented. More than one-half of all pregnant women experience nausea. Vomiting is infrequent. This is not necessarily ''morning sickness.'' It may occur at any time of the day. It may never occur at all. It is much less frequent than formerly. Serious vomiting during pregnancy hardly ever occurs anymore.

Within days after the first missed menstrual period, laboratory tests indicating pregnancy are over 95 percent accurate.[5] Following implantation, a hormone is found in the woman's urine. Injection of that urine into immature female mice or rabbits causes ovarian changes. With a male frog, the hormone causes spermatozoa to occur in the urine. Other such biological pregnancy tests are constantly under study. Several nonanimal chemical tests are also being used to diagnose pregnancy. Opinions as to their accuracy vary somewhat. However, they do have the advantage of enabling the laboratory to provide a reading within a matter of hours after receiving the specimen. One disadvantage of the standard urine pregnancy tests is that they do not work until about twelve days after the first missed menstrual period. The most recent advancement in this field is a test that can detect pregnancy before the mother-to-be is aware that she has missed a period. In some cases the pregnancy can be determined within approximately fourteen days of conception. Still another pregnancy test is being tried in Sweden. It gives positive results before implantation into the womb's wall occurs. (Such implantation occurs before the first missed period.) The woman who has a tendency to miscarry will be particularly benefited by such early information about her pregnancy. She can then avoid those activities that may bring about a miscarriage.

Pregnancy has some cosmetic effects. Skin blemishes abate. The complexion glows. But pink stretch marks (*striae*) may appear, mostly on the abdomen. Neither massage nor costly oils prevent them. Most (but not all) will disappear. There is also, temporarily, increased pigment on the abdominal midline, around the nipples, and on the face. The breasts fill. By three months, *colostrum,* the precursor to milk, is secreted. During pregnancy, an average of twenty pounds is gained. Much of this gain occurs in the last two months. The pregnant woman who, as a girl, ate intelligently and exercised, and continues these habits under

[5] Before the days of pregnancy tests ''imaginary'' or ''unconscious'' pregnancy was not uncommon. Young brides hoping for a baby or older women who worried about having one often developed many of the symptoms of pregnancy without actually being pregnant. At thirty-nine, ''Bloody'' Queen Mary Tudor was so anxious for a child by her husband Phillip II of Spain that she developed many signs of pregnancy, including milk-filled breasts. Counting the months, she sewed baby clothes, fitted out a royal cradle, and had announcements made of the birth of her child. Her expected due date was calculated to be between May 23 and June 5, 1555. Surrounding her at Hampton Court were physicians, midwives, and wet nurses who were dismissed when, two months after her expected due date, she failed to deliver. (*M.D., Medical Newsmagazine,* Vol. 13, No. 3 [March 1969], p. 282.)

a physician's direction during and after pregnancy, has the best chance of keeping her figure. Walking is good for her. During the first four months, she may, if she likes, play golf. In the first few months, she may be permitted to swim. Some physicians permit swimming in later months. Surf bathing, horseback riding, and tennis are not advisable. Activities that involve bumping and compression are ill-advised. Only absolutely necessary long trips should be made. Nonfatiguing employment is acceptable. In considering the amount and kind of activity that is best for the patient, the physician always considers the individual. Some pregnant women seem able to do more than others. One recent Olympic swimmer was not much handicapped by her three-and-one-half-month pregnancy; she placed third in her class. It has been reported that of the twenty-six female Soviet Olympic champions of the Sixteenth Olympiad, in Melbourne, Australia, ten were pregnant.[6]

Extra rest is essential. Although showers are preferable in the last month, a daily tepid bath adds to comfort. It is not true that bath water enters the vagina or that vaginal secretions contaminate bath water. Thus, the fear that bath water may infect a pregnant woman is a myth; this was conclusively proved in a 1960 University of Illinois study.[7] The teeth, although more vulnerable, are not demineralized. ''For every pregnancy a tooth'' is an untrue old wives' tale. The kidneys need special attention. The doctor will examine the urine often. Constipation may be relieved by fruits and vegetables; prunes, dates, and figs help.

prenatal care

Two or three weeks after the first missed period, a doctor should be consulted. This marks the beginning of a relationship that, as much as any other single factor, has made pregnancy so safe. Compared to just a generation ago, decreased maternal (and infant) mortality rates in this country have been spectacular.

The pregnant woman must visit her doctor regularly. This *prenatal* (before birth) *care* is essential to her well-being. The whole complex of physical examinations, laboratory examination of the blood (for syphilis, blood types, Rh factor, and anemia), urine tests—all these, and more, create a constancy of communication between patient and doctor that has brought security to mother and child. Problems can be prevented. If trouble threatens, the doctor can then avert it.

Unless special problems arise, visits to the doctor are scheduled every three or four weeks during the first six months. In the next two months, these are usually increased to every two or three weeks. Visits thereafter are usually weekly.

[6] Michael Bruser, ''Sporting Activities During Pregnancy,'' cited in ''Sports and Pregnancy,'' *Briefs: Footnotes on Maternity Care,* Vol. 33, No. 4 (April 1969), pp. 51–53.
[7] A. Herbert Marbach, ''Myths About Feminine Hygiene,'' *Medical Aspects of Human Sexuality,* Vol. 7, No. 6 (June 1973), p. 133.

sexual intercourse during pregnancy[8]

Many women respond to the complex physical, hormonal, and psychological changes of pregnancy with some decline in sexual activity. Some increase their sexual activity. This reflects "the highly individualistic nature of human sensuality and response to pregnancy."[9] Some women experience increased sexual desire particularly during the second three months of their pregnancies. During the last three months, sexual interest may wane. (The same may be true of husbands.) An increasing number of physicians permit their pregnant patients who have no complications to have sexual intercourse throughout the entire period of pregnancy up to the time of the rupture of the membranes. However, not all cases are alike and there are valid reasons for exceptions. The decision must be made by each physician on an individual basis. Three potential hazards concern the physician: uterine contractions, infection, and mechanical injury.[10] Consider these separately.

Some physicians are legitimately concerned that the contractions of the uterus resulting from orgasm might initiate labor. Although definitive data are still unavailable, there are a few small studies that indicate this as a definite risk. Thus, some physicians believe that "while there is no proof that coitus in the second and third trimester induces premature labor, it is undoubtedly safest to abstain from intercourse in the last four weeks of gestation [childbearing]."[11] Similarly competent physicians disagree. They believe that the harm done by forbidding intercourse during the last three months of pregnancy is greater than that done by the unproved risk of uterine contractions resulting from orgasm. It has been pointed out that the hazard resulting from the uterine contractions of sexual stimulation, particularly if carried to orgasm, are significant with women who are more likely to miscarry and who threaten to go into premature labor. "The last factor involves a very small percentage of pregnant women and cannot justify the blanket proscription of sex in the last trimester of an uneventful gestation."[12] Of course, orgasm resulting from masturbation also causes uterine contractions. These contractions are often more intense than those consequent to sexual intercourse. Therefore, concern about uterine contractions would also logically indicate the prohibition of masturbation during the last three months of pregnancy.

There is no longer as much concern as formerly that sexual intercourse during a normal pregnancy will cause infection. It will not occur with an ordinary situation at the opening of the cervix and intact membranes. Should it occur (which is rare), it can usually be easily treated. Moreover, infection of this sort

[8] Much of the material in this section is based on Chapter 4, "Sexual Relations During Pregnancy and the Post-Delivery Period," in *Sexuality and Man,* compiled and edited by the Sex Information and Education Council of the United States (New York, 1970).

[9] Don A. Solberg, Julius Butler, and Nathanial N. Wagner, "Sexual Behavior in Pregnancy," *New England Journal of Medicine,* Vol. 288, No. 21 (May 24, 1973), p. 1098.

[10] Selig Neubardt, "Coitus During Pregnancy," *Medical Aspects of Human Sexuality,* Vol. 7, No. 9 (September 1973), p. 197.

[11] Leonard L. Hyams, "Coital Induction of Labor," *Medical Aspects of Human Sexuality,* Vol. 6, No. 4 (April 1972), p. 90.

[12] Selig Neubardt, "Coitus During Pregnancy," p. 198.

could occur at any time during pregnancy and not just during the last three months.

There are times during pregnancy in which sexual intercourse should be avoided. Abdominal or vaginal discomfort or pain are always reasons to avoid coitus during pregnancy and at any other time. These may be due to a vaginal or cervical wound which coincides with the pregnancy; the penis can mechanically interfere with the healing process. (When the discomfort can be relieved by the physician's care, coitus may sometimes be resumed.) Uterine bleeding during pregnancy is also a valid reason to abstain from coitus. In addition, the pregnant woman should avoid all genital play as well as sexual intercourse after the membranes have ruptured. Inattention to this is dangerous. When the membranes are ruptured the hazard of infection from coitus is greater than at any other time during pregnancy. Infection that occurs from sexual intercourse after the membranes rupture may harm both the mother and the child. There is general agreement among physicians that these three conditions are definite contraindications of sexual intercourse during pregnancy: abdominal or vaginal discomfort, vaginal bleeding, and ruptured membranes. In some cases, other hazards may be defined. These are always the concern of the responsible physician in charge.

It is of importance to note that the fetus is adequately protected in the amniotic sac and that the position of sexual intercourse up to the onset of labor should be determined by the comfort of the husband and wife rather than by fear that the unborn child will be hurt.[13]

labor

A few days before the onset of true labor, ''false labor'' may occur. However, it is the onset of regular, rhythmic contractions that heralds true labor. Discomfort, beginning in the lower abdomen, spreads to the back and thighs. The bag of water may break. (A ''dry birth'' does not prolong labor. Indeed, it may shorten it.) The ''show'' is another common sign of early labor. This pink vaginal discharge occurs with the onset of cervical dilation. Most first-time mothers may start for the hospital when contractions occur every ten minutes. Others should pay no attention to timing. When contractions are regular, they should go to the hospital. Long before, several reliable ways of transportation should have been arranged.

the stages of labor

There are three stages of labor (see Table 19-1). The first stage is the longest. The upper part of the uterus contracts. The lower cervix dilates. To allow passage of the infant into the vagina, dilation of the cervix to four inches must be complete. In this stage the baby, assisted by uterine contractions, does the work. Both mother and doctor must await dilation of the cervix and the descent of the baby into the proper position. To minimize the possibility of infection, the

[13] *Ibid.*

TABLE 19-1
Stages of Labor

STAGE	TASK	DURATION		WHO DOES THE WORK*
		FIRST BABY	SECOND OR LATER BABY	
First stage	Dilation of cervix	8 to 20 hours	3 to 8 hours	Baby
Second stage	Delivery of infant	20 minutes to 2 hours	20 minutes to 2 hours	Mother
Third stage	Delivery of placenta	5 to 20 minutes	5 to 20 minutes	Obstetrician

*In some cases the physician may decide to do a cesarean section during the first stage or to apply forceps during the second.
Source: Adapted from M. Edward Davis and Reva Rubin, *De Lee's Obstetrics for Nurses,* 18th ed. (Philadelphia, 1966), p. 273.

pubic hair will have been shaved. To increase the space in the pelvic cavity, an enema may have been given. As the first stage progresses, the uterine contractions become more frequent and of longer duration. When the cervix is fully dilated, the mother is taken from the labor room to the delivery room. If for any reason the child cannot do his job, if he cannot adequately act as a wedge, the doctor will perform a *cesarean section.* By this safe surgical procedure, the infant is removed through an incision in the abdomen and uterus.

It is in the second stage of labor that the mother works. By bearing down only with each contraction, she adds her fifteen pounds of pressure to the twenty-five pound pressure of the uterine contraction. Very occasionally, for special medical reasons, such as a premature baby, the physician will shorten this stage. For the mother who desires to see her baby born, a mirror can be arranged.

After the birth of the baby, the *afterbirth* (placenta) is delivered. This is the third stage. A drug is then given to further contract the uterus.

about the pain of childbirth

It was 1561. The place: Castle Hill overlooking what is now Princes Street in Edinburgh, Scotland. At the top of the hill a stake had been driven into the ground. Around it had been piled firewood. Up the hill and to the stake was dragged a lovely lady named Eufame Mac Layne. Only a few moments before, her newly born twin babies had been torn from her arms. Now she was chained to the stake. Within an hour she was ashes. Her crime? She had employed "one Agnes Sampson to administer unto her a certain medicine for the relief of pain in childbirth contrary to divine law and contempt of crown."[14]

Labor pain is as old as humanity. As the Bible says: "in sorrow thou shalt

[14] Donald T. Atkinson, *Magic, Myth and Medicine* (New York, 1956), pp. 271–72.

19-6 a child is born

1. A full-term baby, ready to be born.

2. Early first stage. Strong uterine contractions cause the cervix to dilate.

3. Early second stage. Pains every two minutes; membranes rupture; cervix completely dilated; head has begun to extend.

4. End of second stage. Head is born; shoulders have rotated in birth canal.

5. Third stage. Uterus expels placenta and cord.

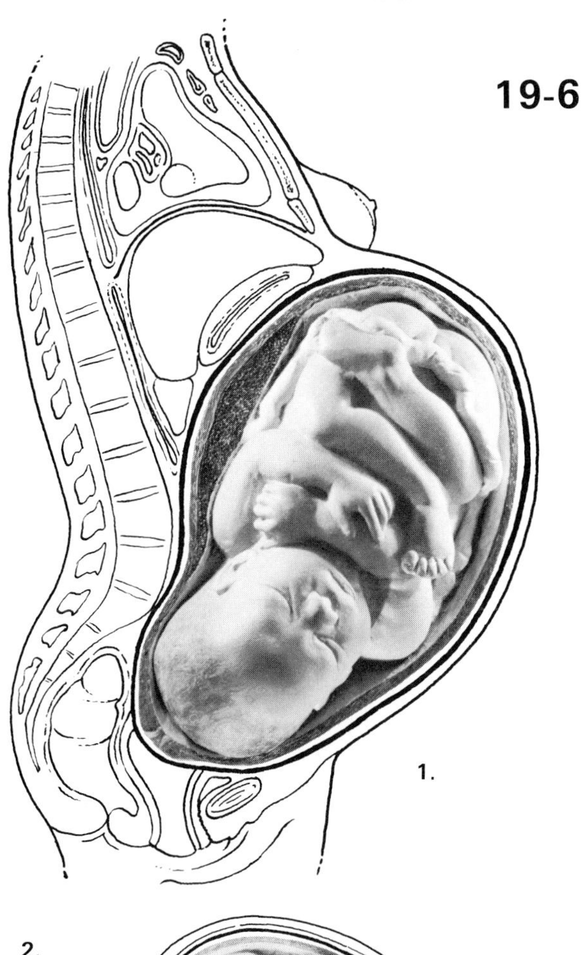

1.

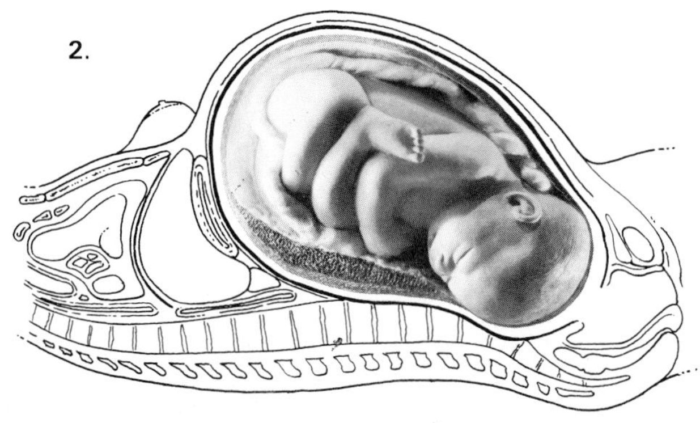

2.

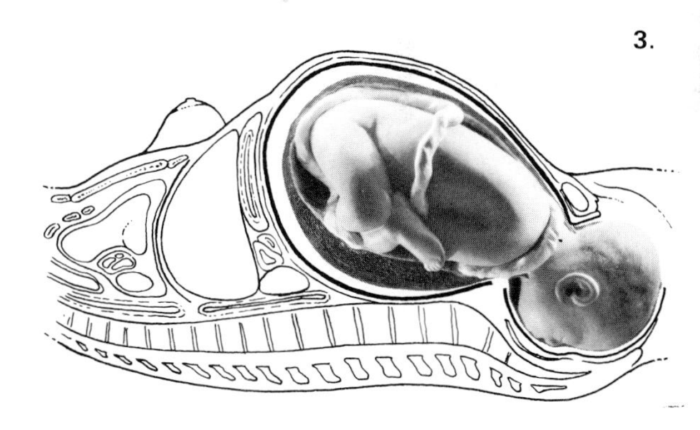

3.

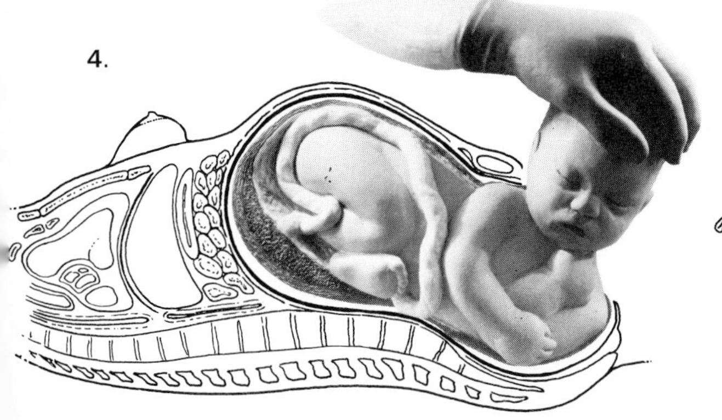

4.

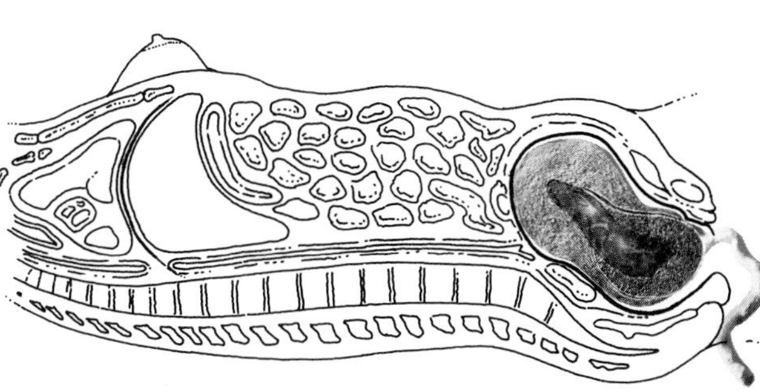

5.

bring forth children'' (Genesis 3:16). Surely it is life's most rewarding sorrow. However, few people today interpret any part of the Bible as meaning that sorrow and pain are not to be relieved.

The human is the only mammal that has pain with the expulsion of the fetus.[15] Uterine contractions do not hurt. What does hurt is the pressure of the descending baby on lower pelvic structures and the stretching of the cervix. In 1857, Queen Victoria was given the anesthetic chloroform for childbirth. A resultant controversy about the morality of this was largely limited to men. Today, most women expect, and receive, relief from the pain of childbirth. No woman need endure more than she can bear. Today, there are adequate safe pharmaceuticals to control pain.

Dr. Grantly Dick Read correctly taught that ignorance breeds fear and fear impedes labor. Although fear is not responsible for all the pain of childbirth, it can cause much of it. The pregnant woman is not helped by those who exaggerate those pains, which, in any case, vary greatly with the individual. Read's concepts of natural childbirth include education, plus exercise in relaxation and breathing. All this is commendable. Pain may occur. Drugs may be used. For some couples, there is much in favor of natural childbirth. Not only the mother but also the expectant father may derive considerable psychological benefit from the experience. There is a long overdue, growing awareness of the father's opportunities to participate in the birth experience.

The past few years have seen an increasing acceptance of the Lamaze method of childbirth, commonly referred to as natural childbirth. Both the pregnancy and the actual childbirth process become a family affair. Together, husband and wife attend prenatal classes to learn the facts about pregnancy, labor, and delivery. The mother-to-be is given breathing and muscle exercises that are useful during labor and delivery. The husband is taught to monitor them correctly. The husband is with his wife during labor and in the delivery room, and he puts his knowledge to good use. Not all physicians approve of this method of childbirth. They believe that childbirth is a surgical procedure with which the father-to-be may interfere.

the ''pregnant'' father

An increasing amount of attention is finally being paid to the ''pregnant'' father. He, too, is expecting. He, too, must adjust to the birth of a baby. One manifestation of this need is the ethnic custom known as *couvade.* According to the custom the husband feigns illness before, during, and after the birth of his child. In the fifth century B.C. the Greek historian Herodotus described couvade among African tribes; in the Middle Ages Marco Polo described couvade among the mountain tribes of China. The custom still exists today among some primitive peoples. During the pregnancy the husband complains of a variety of dis-

[15] Dorothy V. Whipple, *Dynamics of Development: Euthenic Pediatrics* (New York, 1966), p. 74.

comforts, such as nausea and abdominal pain. But it is during the birth of the child that his expressions of discomfort reach their height.

> When the woman gives birth, the man goes to bed sobbingly, writhes with ostensible pains, moans, has warm compresses applied to his body, has himself nursed attentively, and submits to dietary restrictions for days, weeks, or, in exceptional cases, even for months. Until his first bath, he is considered unclean, just as though he had himself given birth to the child.[16]

But couvade is hardly limited to primitive cultures. Certain aspects of it are known to many expectant fathers in industrialized societies. Nausea, diarrhea, constipation, and backache are all common complaints of the father-to-be. In one study of U.S. servicemen it was found that 60 percent of the expectant fathers had some symptoms of pregnancy. Some even went through the "baby blues," the postnatal depression exhibited by some mothers.[17] This has been confirmed by other studies. "Some men experienced the pregnancy as a severe test of their masculinity. Some expressed their envy of pregnancy all the way from vigorously denying it to almost fusing with the wife in an attempt to experience the pregnancy biologically."[18]

Thus the birth of the baby is accompanied by a wide variety of stresses for both parents. It is a time when both husband and wife have to draw from their deepest wellsprings of mutual understanding.

not all human milk is mother's milk

Not all the signs and symptoms usually attributed to the pregnant state occur with pregnancy, nor are they invariably limited to the female. The ancients were aware of this, as can be seen in the biblical observation: "His breasts are full of milk" (Job 21:24). *Prolactin* is the primary hormone responsible for *lactation,* which is the period of milk secretion. As the hormone that stimulates the production of milk in lactating women, it is but one of the several potent products of the anterior lobe of the pituitary gland (see page 255). However, lactation can occur in a wide variety of conditions and situations other than pregnancy. The prolonged use of some tranquilizers and other drugs that influence the hypothalamus may produce lactation. Mechanical trauma, chest or breast burns, herpes zoster (shingles) of the chest wall, are among other conditions that occasionally stimulate lactation. Breast milk may also occur as a result of

[16] Helen Diner, *Mothers and Amazons* (New York, 1965), p. 113. An extremely rare case of false pregnancy, complete with morning sickness, distended abdomen, and a feeling of movement within the abdomen, has been reported in a male. He was delighted with his "condition," took vitamins, and decided he would have to be delivered by cesarean section. (James A. Knight, "Unusual Case: False Pregnancy in a Male," *Medical Aspects of Human Sexuality,* Vol. 5, No. 3 [March 1971], pp. 58, 63–64, 69.)

[17] *Sexuality and Man,* p. 59.

[18] B. Liebenberg, W. H. Trethowan, and M. F. Conlon, "The Couvade Syndrome," *British Journal of Psychiatry* (March 1965) and Illinois State Medical Society, "Expectant Fathers Experience Pregnancy Symptoms Too," Release No. 249 (November 2, 1966), both cited in *Sexuality and Man,* p. 59.

poorly fitting garments or manipulation of the breasts. Lactation has been noted, along with amenorrhea (absence of menstruation), in young women who have never borne a child and who are taking birth control pills. This may theoretically be due to a temporary loss of the hypothalamic control of some aspects of the anterior lobe of the pituitary gland in a certain percentage of women.[19] The occurrence of breast milk has been noted with childless and postmenopausal women who undergo the sucking stimulus. Men who experience a prolonged sucking stimulus may, in time, also lactate. And not only lactation, but also breast enlargement, has been occasionally observed on refeeding severely malnourished prisoners of war.

postnatal concerns

Before leaving the hospital the mother is examined. In six to eight weeks she should be examined again. Of particular interest to the physician are her weight, blood pressure, and the condition of her breasts, uterus, cervix, vagina, and genitalia. He advises her that the first menstruation may normally be somewhat profuse. Some women are troubled by a vaginal discharge. This is easily treated. The busy mother may forget or defer the examination. This is unwise. She cannot adequately take care of anyone else unless she also takes care of herself.

mother love: not always at first sight

It is widely believed that the moment the mother beholds her baby for the first time she feels an immediate love for the child. For many women this is not true. Some mothers apparently love their new babies immediately, but many good mothers do not. During labor the woman usually limits her thoughts to completing the job entailed in the birth process. After the birth many mothers want to see their babies to make certain they are healthy, or simply out of curiosity. A recent study of fifty-four mothers from the middle and upper socioeconomic levels of Washington, D.C., revealed some interesting information in this regard.[20] Thirty-three percent of the mothers reported having no particular feelings upon seeing their babies for the first time. Seven percent had negative feelings. Fifty-nine percent reported positive feelings that were, nevertheless,

[19] Robert B. Greenblatt, ''Inappropriate Lactation in Men and Women,'' *Medical Aspects of Human Sexuality,* Vol. 6, No. 6 (June 1972), p. 33, citing R. D. Gambrell, R. B. Greenblatt, and V. B. Mahesh, ''Post-Pill and Pill-Related Amenorrhea-Galactorrhea'' (in press).

[20] Kenneth S. Robson and Howard Moss, ''Patterns and Determinants of Maternal Attachment,'' *The Journal of Pediatrics,* Vol. 77, No. 6 (December 1970), p. 976. In many U.S. hospitals, newborns are taken from their mothers after a brief initial visit, and the mother-child relationship is continued only at feeding times. Some research has been done to find out if more prolonged contact would result in any changes in the mother. It did. One month after leaving the hospital with their babies, mothers whose early contact with them had been extended ''were more reluctant to leave their infants with someone else, usually stood and watched during the examination, showed greater soothing behavior, and engaged in significantly more eye-to-eye contact and fondling.'' (Marshall H. Klaus, Richard Jerauld, Nancy C. Kreger, William McAlpine, Meredith Steffa, and John H. Kennel, ''Maternal Attachment: Importance of the First Post-Partum Days,'' *New England Journal of Medicine,* Vol. 286, No. 9 [March 2, 1972], p. 460.)

quite impersonal. Most of the mothers did not note the beginnings of positive feelings until the third week following childbirth. With the return of her strength, a growing sense of competence, and a reciprocating baby, the mother's attachment to her child grew. By the end of the third month the attachment had become powerful. Although there is no data, it must be assumed that love for the child evolves at least as slowly in the father as in the mother. For most parents, then, mother love and father love grows slowly; it is not mature upon the birth of the baby. Many parents feel a totally unwarranted sense of guilt for not loving their babies immediately.

sexual intercourse following childbirth

Most women do not desire sexual intercourse for some days following childbirth. This is understandable. The new mother may experience fatigue resulting from delivery. A new baby, moreover, means adjustments for the mother, especially if the child is her first-born. This may be a difficult period for the husband too. A house that was once organized around him may now be organized around the baby. During the first month or so following childbirth, the stresses of motherhood may cause his wife to be less interested in coitus. Her desire for sexual intercourse may be further lessened by postpartum depression. The cause of this ordinarily transient depression is not clear. It may be associated with the return of the menstrual cycle following pregnancy. A profound series of endocrine gland readjustments occur. It would be surprising if the woman did not experience some emotional changes.

Added to all these new stresses is a certain amount of discomfort about the anus and vagina. Incisions and small tears must heal. There may be some vaginal bleeding. When healing has occurred and the bleeding has stopped, sexual intercourse may be resumed. A small amount of brown vaginal discharge may persist for a while, but this is no reason to defer coitus. After the birth of a baby, a woman usually wants to resume sexual intercourse as soon as possible. There is no reason to discourage her if she is comfortable with it; by that time the bleeding usually has stopped. Some women defer sexual activity for an unduly long period of time following childbirth. This may be associated with their own needless fears and misconceptions. In these instances the physician can and will do much to allay apprehensions and correct misapprehensions.

conception during breast-feeding

Contrary to popular notions, sexual intercourse during the time a woman is a nursing mother can result in pregnancy. Breast-feeding tends to prolong the period following childbirth during which the woman does not menstruate (*postpartum amenorrhea*). During this period, conception usually will not occur. But the extent of the prolonged amenorrhea and the delayed conception cannot be accurately estimated in the individual woman. As soon as ovulation occurs, conception can take place, and a woman may ovulate before her first menstrual period following childbirth. About one in twenty women do start another pregnancy without having resumed menstruation following the birth of a baby. It is not known if breast-feeding following the return of menstruation reduces the likelihood of conception.

not all mothers should nurse

By no means should every mother nurse her child. There are medical contraindications to breast-feeding. Some drugs that are prescribed for the mother for a variety of reasons may pass into the breast milk in doses sufficient to harm the child. Breast infections may also make breast-feeding unwise. By late 1973 no human cancer had yet been proved to be caused by a virus. Nevertheless, viruslike particles have been detected in human milk and in tissue specimens of breast cancers; these are known to cause leukemia and breast cancer in mice. For this reason, there is competent medical opinion that "women with a personal or family history of breast cancer should not nurse, since it is possible that the viruslike particles in milk may induce breast cancer or other malignancies later in the life cycle of the nursling."[21]

Various methods have been used to inhibit lactation. Among these are the restriction of fluid intake and the use of a breast-binder or well-fitting brassiere. During this period the breasts should not be manipulated. Sometimes breasts do become painfully engorged; for this condition the physician may recommend the application of an ice pack and, perhaps, judicious use of medication to relieve the pain. Using these procedures, lactation usually stops within a week. Many women who have had more than one child do not do well with these procedures. To avoid painful breast engorgement and the discomfort due to milk leakage, some physicians may wish to administer a single injection of an androgen-estrogen combination toward the end of labor or immediately after delivery. A woman who has had a spontaneous or therapeutic abortion after the sixteenth week of pregnancy, or whose child was stillborn, will usually require help for suppression of lactation.

[21] Helmuth Vorherr, "Suppression of Postpartum Lactation," *Postgraduate Medicine*, Vol. 52, No. 1 (July 1972), p. 145.

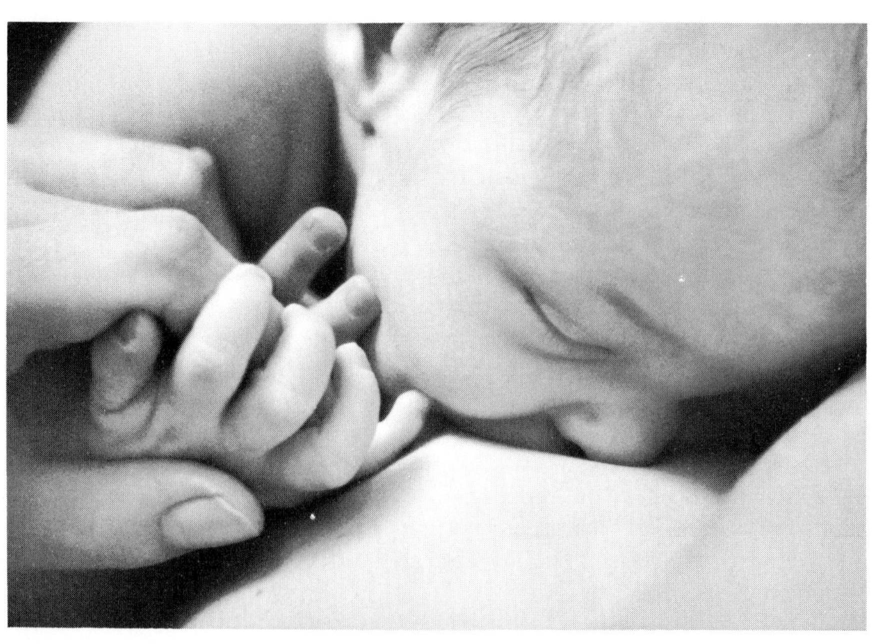

19-7

the sudden infant death syndrome[22]

Each year, some 25,000 to 30,000[23] U.S. babies are put to bed at night and unexpectedly found dead in the morning. Typically, the child is between two and four months old (90 percent are between one and nine months; the average age is 2.8 months).[24] The child had previously been in good health and had given no warning of the tragedy. There may have been some minor symptoms of an upper respiratory infection. This situation is now known as the Sudden Infant Death Syndrome (SIDS).

The agonized parents ask why this has happened.[25] Research has proved the following about the SIDS: (1) it is in no way related to the adequacy of parental care and occurs among the best loved and cared-for babies; (2) it is not hereditary; (3) it does not cause the afflicted child to suffer; (4) it cannot be predicted by even the most competent physician, much less by the watchful parent; it presents no warning symptoms; at this time, it is in no way preventable; (5) it is not caused by vomiting, nor by regurgitating and choking from the last feeding; and (6) it often occurs under conditions in which there is no possibility of smothering.

What, then, causes the Sudden Infant Death Syndrome? One distinguished physician has suggested that "the most convincing hypothesis at this time would tend to suggest that the baby's first experience with respiratory viruses may be overwhelming and that a 'cold of the lungs' is sufficient to interfere with vital and essential ventilation, leading to sharply reduced supplies of oxygen and sudden unexpected death."[26] This conception is somewhat strengthened by recent research. It has been found that during normal sleep the infant may not breathe 5 to 10 percent of the time. During a virus infection, the spells during which the child does not breathe may increase to between 25 and 30 percent of the time. In addition, it has been shown that the reactivity of the autonomic nervous system (which controls involuntary body functions) varies among infants. This division of the nervous system does not mature until the second or third month of life.[27] A mild infection plus an immature nervous system not yet competent to protect the child may be part of the picture. An added bit of evidence leading to the notion that infection is one of the causes of the SIDS is that the deaths occur more frequently during cold weather.

Nevertheless, attempts at isolating viruses and bacteria from afflicted children have not been routinely rewarding. "If infection plays a part it appears

[22] Also called "cot deaths" and "crib deaths."

[23] R. J. Wedgewood and E. P. Benditt, *Proceedings of the Conference on Causes of Sudden Death in Infants.* Public Health Service Publication No. 1412 (Washington, D.C., 1965), pp. 1–9.

[24] Frederick B. Hodges, "Sudden Infant Death Syndrome," *California Medicine,* Vol. 116, No. 1 (January 1972), p. 85.

[25] Only too often parents mistakenly blame themselves for the sudden death of their child. To increase public education about the problem, the National Foundation for Sudden Infant Death, Inc. (NFSID), was formed. The address of its national headquarters is 1501 Broadway, New York, New York 10036. Chapter members, themselves SIDS parents, devote many hours talking to and helping other parents learn to cope with the sudden death of their infant. Recent SIDS families are also often referred to professional help. ("The National Foundation for Sudden Infant Death, Inc.," *Clinical Pediatrics,* Vol. 11, No. 2 [February 1972], p. 83.)

[26] John M. Adams, *Viruses and Colds: The Modern Plague* (New York, 1967), pp. 103–04.

[27] Frederick B. Hodges, "Sudden Infant Death Syndrome," p. 86.

as a trivial affliction rather than as a frank one.''[28] Since some investigations reveal the highest risk to be at night, it may be that body metabolic changes during sleep hinder the ordinary response to respiratory difficulty in some children. Crib deaths have occurred in babies who have been breast-fed all their lives; however, breast-feeding may have some role in preventing such deaths because human breast milk does contain components that ''have positive antiviral and antibacterial activity in the baby, and human milk is believed to be nonallergic to man.''[29] Nevertheless, there is considerable dispute about whether slowly developing milk allergy causes the respiratory distress leading to crib deaths.

One physician suggests that not all reported crib deaths actually occur in the crib. A considerable number occur in the parents' bed. Smothering occurs when a parent accidentally lies over the child. Today, this accident is called ''overlying''; such a tragedy was first reported in the Bible by the woman who tells King Solomon that ''this woman's child died in the night; because she overlaid it'' (I Kings 3:19). ''Parents must be informed that to sleep in the same bed with an infant is to invite disaster which is as ancient as the Temple of Solomon.''[30]

hyaline membrane disease

This condition of the newborn is manifested by respiratory distress. Within the uterus, the child obtained oxygen via the placenta. At birth, it is obtained through the lungs. This dramatic accomplishment depends partly on the mature development of certain lung cells. Ordinarily, these cells mature adequately shortly before birth. If they do not, the lung air spaces collapse and the immature lung cannot retain air. Each baby breath is as difficult as the first gasp. Soon, plasma (the fluid portion of the blood) leaks out into the lung tissue, coating the air spaces. ''This glassy pink coating gives respiratory distress in the newborn the name hyaline membrane disease''[31] (''hyaline'' is from the Greek word *hyalos,* meaning glass).

Just a few years ago, hyaline membrane disease killed some 25,000 babies in this country every year. Today, intensive care, including assistance in breathing, is saving most of them. One method involves providing the newborn with continuous positive airway pressure; this keeps the baby's lung expanded, alveolar air spaces (Figure 13-9, page 390) remain open, and oxygen–carbon dioxide exchange is made possible. Although there is some concern about the long-term effects of this treatment and further study is indicated, preliminary

[28] ''Cot Deaths,'' *British Medical Journal,* Vol. 4, No. 5782 (October 30, 1971), p. 250.
[29] *Ibid.*
[30] J. J. Francisco, ''Smothering in Infancy: Its Relationship to the 'Crib Death Syndrome','' *Southern Medical Journal,* Vol. 63, No. 10 (October 1970), p. 1114.
[31] Mary Ellen Avery, Nai-San Wang, and H. William Taeusch, Jr., ''The Lung of the Newborn Infant,'' *Scientific American,* Vol. 228, No. 4 (April 1973), p. 75. This article is particularly recommended for its lucid explanation of hyaline membrane disease.

results indicate a survival rate as high as 90 percent.[32] Animal research promises still another approach. It has been shown that the use of cortisone for both the fetus and newborn animal does hasten the maturation of those cells essential to proper lung function. In addition, study of amniotic fluid (see page 565) will assist the physician in identifying a fetus that has a greater than average potential for the disorder.

subfertility

How long should it take before a normal couple may expect conception? Usually six months of ordinary cohabitation results in pregnancy. If conception does not occur within a year of marriage, the couple would do well to seek the advice of the family doctor.

Among the married, the threat of childlessness often begins with suspicion, which may grow to anxious doubt, and end in sad resignation. Fully 20 to 25 percent of couples in this country fail to have as many children as they wish. Only 10 percent seek adequate help.

Subfertility refers to a state of being less than normally fertile. It is relative sterility. *Infertility,* or *sterility,* refers to the inability to conceive or to induce conception. In this culture, many people incorrectly consider subfertility to be primarily a fault within the woman. In the Bible, it is the sterile woman who is regarded with pity, if not scorn. The "adversary" of Hannah "provoked her sore, for to make her fret, because the Lord had shut up her womb" (I Samuel 1:6). Of course, the problem occurs almost as often within men.

The cause of subfertility may be easily discovered, or it may require a long investigation. Sometimes it is necessary to consult various medical specialists.

Severe nutritional deficiencies have been known to cause reduced fertility. Both ovulation and menstruation may be impaired in this way. Alcoholism, other drug abuse, chronic infections—all may contribute to a subfertile marriage. Physical problems may range from excess obesity of both marital partners (interfering with actual consummation of the marriage) to an occluded Fallopian tube. It is estimated that malfunction of the Fallopian tube accounts for about 33 percent of all cases of subfertility. A kinked tube, or one blocked as a result of an infection, may be unable to receive the ovum and permit its passage to the uterus. Or it may stop the sperm's ascent to the ovum.

Emotional problems may impede conception. A young wife, forced to live with an interfering mother-in-law, may learn to bide her time. But, while she is biding her time, her vagina, uterus, and tubes tense. She may be unable to conceive. Moving to her own apartment might cure her. Spasm of the vagina and tubes may disappear. The quality of her cervical mucus improves and becomes more receptive of her husband's sperm. She will then more likely conceive. A prolonged sense of guilt over a previous sexual misfortune, such as a

[32] "Putting Pressure on Hyaline," *Medical World News,* Vol. 13, No. 2 (January 14, 1972), pp. 27, 30–32.

venereal infection, combined with lack of knowledge, has resulted not only in subfertility but in serious marital problems. The erroneous idea "VD germs kill sperms" has, at times, been eradicated by showing a husband his own spermatozoa darting about under the microscope.[33] Too many girls, subjected to exaggerated and lurid stories by "well-meaning" mothers and acquaintances, fear both intercourse and childbearing. Resultant tensions may well interfere with fertility. Knowledge of the reassuring facts about both will help. The husband who is sensitive to his wife's sexual needs will enrich his marriage. He is also more likely to enhance her fertility.

The physician usually first investigates the man, since the cause can often be more easily established in the male. After a thorough physical examination, there are several tests to be done. Spermatozoa are examined for numbers, motility, appearance, and other features.

The search for the cause of female subfertility is usually more complex. It may be a persistent, simply treated vaginal inflammation. Or the physician may find that his patient encourages intercourse but once every month or two and then without attention to her ovulation cycle. Some physicians feel that *coitus interruptus* (page 616) sets up a reflex resulting in withdrawal before male ejaculation. The causes of a woman's inability to conceive may be multiple and complex, and patience is needed in investigating them. Only with the discovery of the cause of the problem may a rational approach to its solution be made. When the cause is failure of the woman to ovulate, "fertility drugs" (discussed below) may be considered. However, as has been pointed out, failure to ovulate is not the major cause of subfertility. Approximately 33 percent of all problems of subfertility are due to male dysfunction. Factors involving the uterine cervix account for approximately 20 percent of the cases of infertility, disorders of the Fallopian tubes for 33 percent, and hormonal factors for almost 15 percent.

the sometimes overefficient "fertility drugs"

Gonadotropins are substances that have an affinity for or stimulate the gonads (ovaries and testes). In recent years several have been used to stimulate the ovary to ovulate. Among these is the luteinizing hormone (LH; see page 474). These are the so-called fertility drugs.

A major problem with their use has been their control. Some women become pregnant with more than they bargained for. Not long ago a twenty-nine-year-old Australian woman who had been given a fertility drug gave birth to nine infants. They were twelve weeks premature. None survived. In the winter of 1970, a New Jersey woman who had also received fertility drugs gave birth to quintuplets. Such multiple births should not condemn the use of fertility drugs. For example, the New Jersey woman had become pregnant twice before with the aid of fertility drugs, and both were single pregnancies. To prevent excessive ovulation, fertility specialists are developing new techniques to regulate dosage. Moreover, the recent discovery of the chemical structure and the synthesis of the luteinizing hormone–releasing factor of the hypothalamus (LH-RH; see page 256) may well revolutionize infertility therapy.[34] (It will be

[33] For a discussion of the venereal diseases, see Chapter 7.

[34] For a discussion of the possibilities of LH-RH as a contraceptive, see page 635, footnote 65.

remembered that the luteinizing hormone controls the release of the ovum from the ovary.) The synthesis may result in the production of safe and inexpensive fertility stimulators.

Already some success has been reported in this area. In one woman, egg production was induced by an injection of follicle-stimulating hormone (FSH; see page 474) followed by an injection of natural LH-RH. Not only did she ovulate, but she also had a healthy baby. Single ovulations have also been induced in two women by giving each of them two injections of LH-RH ten days apart. In these two cases, no FSH was used beforehand.[35]

A wide variety of procedures that do not involve drugs that stimulate ovulation are being perfected. Among these are the correction of uterine defects, surgical procedures to reconstruct the Fallopian tubes, and the increased use of artificial insemination. This last procedure offers some hope. Within present limits, improved freezing techniques may make it more possible for newly established semen banks to help solve problems caused by male infertility.

on planning a child's genetic sex

"Throughout antiquity, it was believed that boys were the products of the right testicle, and that girls were the products of the left one."[36] The ancient Hebrews improved on this notion; in the Talmud they apparently appreciated the significance of the time of orgasm and conception in influencing the sex of the offspring.[37] Is it indeed possible to influence the genetic sex of a child? Some interesting (and curious) correlations have been noted that lend credence to the notion that prediction of whether a child will be born a boy or a girl is possible. A few years ago, a U.S. statistician noted that early summer seemed to favor the birth of boys.[38] Also, an English investigator has suggested that couples who have intercourse more frequently are more likely to have boys.[39] His investigation was stimulated by earlier German data showing that more male than

[35] "Correcting Infertility Without Multiple Births," *Science News,* Vol. 101, No. 2 (January 8, 1972), p. 24.

[36] Helen Diner, *Mothers and Amazons,* p. 71. It is further noted that the notion that females were the product of the left testicle may well have been part (or the result) of a male chauvinism that found its way into both language and behavior. Thus, just as the word *black,* in another context, meant "dirty" or implied gloom, so does *left* imply something sinister or clumsy. In French, *gauche* means either "left" or "awkward," and *Les Gauches* refers to the Radical Party. In English, the word *sinister* means "left," but it also signifies evil; a U.S. politician whose philosophy is considered "to the left" has a hard time getting elected. The Spaniards use *siniestro* as an adjective, meaning either "on the left" or "disastrous," and, in German, *links* means "left," but, as slang, it (or *linkstrum*) can also signify homosexual behavior, and *linkisch* means "awkward." In many primitive cultures, the woman serves the man's food from his right, but she eats at his left, even as is often good etiquette in civilized societies. Also, before the days of modern psychology, an attempt was made to train left-handed children to eat and write with their right hands because it was more acceptable socially. And "it seems worth noting that practically all the Madonnas painted or sculptured in the period of real feeling, that is, approximately in the Christian centuries prior to the Renaissance, held the Christ child on their *left* arms." (Helen Diner, *Mothers and Amazons,* p. 71.)

[37] Landrum B. Shettles, "Predetermining Children's Sex," *Medical Aspects of Human Sexuality,* Vol. 5, No. 6 (June 6, 1972), p. 178.

[38] "Early Summer Favors the Birth of a Boy," *New Scientist,* Vol. 45, No. 691 (March 5, 1970), p. 448.

[39] "Why Marital Enthusiasm Upsets the Sex Ratio," *New Scientist and Science Journal,* Vol. 49, No. 735 (January 21, 1971), p. 104, and "Make More Love, Make More Boys," *Canadian Medical Association Journal,* Vol. 104, No. 11 (June 5, 1971), p. 975, both citing William James, "Cycle Day of Insemination, Coital Rate, and Sex Ratio," *Lancet,* Vol. 1, No. 7690 (January 16, 1971), p. 112.

female babies are born if intercourse is engaged in earlier in the menstrual cycle. The observations that more males are born during the usually more active first eighteen months of marriage, and that women under twenty-five years of age have more boys than women over thirty-five, further support this theory. Such a hypothesis may explain why more boys are born after wars, when sex-starved soldiers return to their wives. Still another British researcher has noted a correlation between the ingestion of hard (high mineral content) water and an increased sex ratio; that is, the ratio of boy–girl births increases markedly.[40]

Landrum B. Shettles, of Columbia University's College of Physicians and Surgeons, has studied various factors that might be considered to influence the genetic sex of offspring at fertilization. These factors include the timing of intercourse with respect to the female cycle, the timing and type of douche used, whether or not the woman achieves orgasm, the depth of penile penetration, and the quality of the spermatozoon and ovum. A male offspring is more likely to be conceived if intercourse takes place as close as possible to the moment of ovulation with prior abstinence during a given cycle. This more likely provides a fresh spermatozoon and a fresh ovum. Male offspring are favored by the use of an alkaline douche (two tablespoons of baking soda in one quart of water) immediately preceding intercourse, by the woman's achievement of orgasm, by deep penile penetration, and by the union of a fresh spermatozoon and a fresh ovum. A female offspring is more likely to be conceived if intercourse takes place no later than two to three days before ovulation, and the occurrence of intercourse ceases at that time. This more likely provides a fresh ovum and an older spermatozoon for fertilization. Female offspring are favored by the use of an acid douche (two tablespoons of white vinegar in one quart of water) immediately preceding intercourse, by the woman's failure to achieve orgasm, by shallow penile penetration, and by the union of a fresh ovum and an older sperm.[41] On what basic principles do his suggestions rest?

Human male spermatozoa (those carrying Y-chromosomes) seem to be more efficient at fertilization than the X-spermatozoa resulting in females. Why? The heads of the X-spermatozoa are bulkier because they contain 3 to 4 percent more DNA than do the heads of Y-spermatozoa. This is equivalent to a 1 percent difference in the radius of a sperm head. Thus, the lighter Y-sperm is more efficient in moving against gravitational pull than an X-sperm.[42] In addition, X- and Y-spermatozoa do not occur in approximately equal numbers. Y-spermatozoa greatly outnumber X-spermatozoa. (The reason that more females than males are born is that after fertilization the male nucleus containing the chromosomes is less likely to survive to full term.[43])

To favor the birth of a boy, it would thus seem logical to create an environment in which the smaller, more numerous Y-spermatozoa can outdistance the larger X-spermatozoa. Indeed, conditions favoring conception (fertilization)

[40] W. R. Lyster, "Sex Ratio and Hard Water," *Science Journal,* Vol. 6, No. 11 (November 1970), pp. 61–63.
[41] Landrum B. Shettles, "Predetermining Children's Sex" pp. 172, 177, 178.
[42] "Slimmer Males Win the Race to Self-Perpetuation," *New Scientist,* Vol. 55, No. 807 (August 3, 1972), p. 228.
[43] W. R. Lyster, "Sex Ratio and Hard Water," p. 61.

favor male offspring. Conditions impeding conception favor the birth of a girl. The age (viability) of the spermatozoa and ova are also important factors in determining whether conception occurs. Therefore, the availability of a fresh spermatozoon and a fresh ovum (as near to ovulation as possible) favors a male birth. A fresh ovum and an older spermatozoon would favor a female birth; this is more likely if sexual intercourse occurs two to three days before ovulation. Deep penile penetration during emission results in the deposition of spermatozoa near the favorable alkaline secretions within the cervix. This, combined with the alkaline orgasmal secretions and an alkaline douche that is salubrious for spermatozoa, makes it possible for the Y-spermatozoa to outdistance the X-spermatozoa in the competitive race to the awaiting ovum. On the other hand, the lack of female orgasm adds no alkalinity to a sperm's environment. An acid douche promotes its acidity. (It should be noted, however, that douches should not be used without a physician's advice.) Shallow penile penetration results not only in the emission of the spermatozoa-containing ejaculum into the more hostile acid vaginal environment, but it also increases the distance that the spermatozoa must travel to fertilize the ovum. By using these concepts, it has been reported that couples can select the genetic sex of their children with an 80 to 85 percent chance of success.[44] Not all scientists accept Shettles' suggestions. Nevertheless, they certainly merit consideration.

adoption

The ancient Greeks and Romans adopted children to assure continuance of the family line, thereby protecting property. The child was secondary. Today, he is primary. He needs a secure home and love. Adopting parents must be able to give both.

The depth of relationship between adopted child and parents is no less profound than that with the biological parents. The risk is mutual.

Unfortunately, many an unmarried mother is unaware of the strict privacy available at social welfare agencies. Fearing exposure, she places her child through a "black market" agency. In this way, she puts both herself and her child at a disadvantage. There is yet another problem. There are twice as many nonwhite illegitimate children as white. Yet, most adopted children are white.

A couple considering adoption should seek help from the social welfare agency in their community. They will further profit from conferences with the family attorney and physician.

In this country between 1 and 2 percent of the population is adopted; however, this includes only those children who are brought into families in which neither parent is the biological one. A similar number of children are adopted into families in which one parent is the child's biological parent.[45] It has been observed that adopted children are brought to psychiatric treatment with considerable frequency. This may be due to the greater anxiety of the adopting

[44] Landrum B. Shettles, "Predetermining Children's Sex," p. 178.

[45] Marshall D. Schechter, "Is Adoption a Handicapping Condition?" *Medical Insight,* Vol. 3, No. 8 (August 1971), p. 18.

parents, or to their increased awareness of the psychological problems of an adopted child. Some psychiatrists believe that such problems are somewhat more frequent among adopted children.[46]

Before the adoption takes place, the parents are frequently under stress. During the nine months of pregnancy, natural parents have time in which to build a basic beginning and basic emotional structure for parenthood. For adopting parents, however, the waiting period may be long and filled with anxiety, rather than with pleasurable anticipation. Most adopting parents are, moreover, older than natural parents; they are more set in their ways and may find a new personality in their midst a demanding trial. For some parents, the adopted child may even be a symbol of infertility, which creates an unconscious hostility toward the child. In addition, an errant adopted child may be too severely judged by the parents. His childish transgressions may stimulate the parents into unconscious or even conscious condemning thoughts, such as "bad blood will tell."

The adopted child also has his problems. The need for answering the question "Who am I?" and the difficulties inherent in the search for self-identity, have already been discussed (see pages 339–41). For the adopted child the whole process may become a veritable travail. To the natural child, for example, the parents are powerful and beautiful—for a while at least. During this time (when such a child, as Erik Erikson has written, "hitches his wagon to nothing less than a star") his fantasies about his parents help him to establish his own uniqueness as a person. For the adopted child, however, the fantasy has a measure of reality. He, indeed, does not know who his real parents are. The child's inability to fuse his image of the unknown parents with that of his adopted parents may fill him with anxiety. In an effort to establish continuity in his life, as well as some identity, the adopted child may even run away in search of his real parents. However, this is not common.

What are the risks, to the adopting parents, that drug abuse by the natural parents may have adversely affected the child? A study of one thousand infants who were relinquished for adoption, which included chromosomal analysis of forty-one, revealed that "parental use of illicit drugs does not in itself constitute a valid reason for the refusal to accept or place an infant relinquished for adoption."[47]

Authorities generally agree that the child should be told of the adoption. There is some disagreement as to when. There is no exact time for all children; it should be individualized. There are those who insist that the child should be told as soon as possible and that the information should be affectionately, but consistently, reiterated in a variety of ways. For example, the child could routinely be introduced as one's adopted child. The theory to support this advice is that, in this way, the adopted child becomes desensitized to the knowledge. Later, the theory holds, when the child learns the meaning of adoption, he finds

[46] Henry H. Work and Hans Anderson, "Studies in Adoption: Requests for Psychiatric Treatment," *American Journal of Psychiatry,* Vol. 127, No. 7 (January 1971), pp. 124–25.

[47] Kenneth W. Dumars, "Parental Drug Usage: Effect on Chromosomes of Progeny," *Pediatrics,* Vol. 47, No. 6 (June 1971), p. 1037.

it more acceptable. Others dispute this; they believe that the concept of adoption means little to the very young child. The period between six and ten years of age has been suggested as the best time to tell the child about his adoption; during those years most children are usually less beset by emotional difficulties.[48] To develop a sense of identity, the adopted child will need the opportunity to develop a strong sense of self-esteem. Then, together, child and parents can come to see how they have helped one another while meeting one another's needs.[49] In this, they are like all parents and children. And that they succeed is borne out by the hundreds of thousands of happily adopted children in the United States.

summary

Pregnancy begins with *conception,* the fertilization of an ovum by a sperm, and ordinarily lasts $9\frac{1}{2}$ to 10 lunar months (page 571). During this time, the new individual develops from a *zygote* (at fertilization) to a *blastocyst* (first week after fertilization) to an *embryo* (from about seven and a half days after fertilization to the end of the second month of pregnancy) to a *fetus* (from the beginning of the third month to birth) (pages 571–72). Certain changes take place in the uterus (pages 572–73) and in the new individual (pages 575–77) as pregnancy progresses. The adjustment to changes in physical and emotional states varies with the individual pregnant woman (pages 577–79). Regular prenatal care is essential (page 579). The advisability of sexual intercourse during pregnancy must be decided in consultation with the physician (pages 580–81).

Labor takes place in three stages. During the first stage, the cervix dilates and the baby moves down into the vagina. In the second stage, the child is born. In the third stage, the *placenta,* or *afterbirth,* is delivered (pages 581–82).

The father as well as the mother must make an adjustment to pregnancy and to the birth of the child (pages 584–85). Not all new parents love their baby immediately; initial indifference should not be a source of guilt (pages 586–87). Other postnatal considerations are the resumption of sexual intercourse (page 587), the possibility of conception during breastfeeding (page 587), and whether or not to nurse the child (page 588). Two particularly serious hazards to the newborn infant are the *sudden infant death syndrome* (pages 589–90) and *hyaline membrane disease* (pages 590–91).

Subfertility is the state of being less than normally fertile (page 591). *Infertility,* or *sterility,* is the state of being unable to conceive or to induce conception. Conception may be impeded by such factors as nutritional deficiencies, drug abuse, chronic infection, and physical and emotional problems (pages 591–92). Correction of these conditions, administration of one of the *gonadotropins* ("fertility drugs"), and other procedures (including surgical correction of uterine defects and increased use of artificial insemination), are enabling more subfertile couples to have children (pages 592–93). Despite certain stresses for some parents and child, *adoption* is also a successful means of building a family (pages 595–97).

[48] Marshall D. Schechter, "Is Adoption a Handicapping Condition?" p. 21.
[49] American Academy of Pediatrics: Committee on Adoptions, "Identity Development in Adopted Children," *Pediatrics,* Vol. 47, No. 5 (May 1971), pp. 948–49.

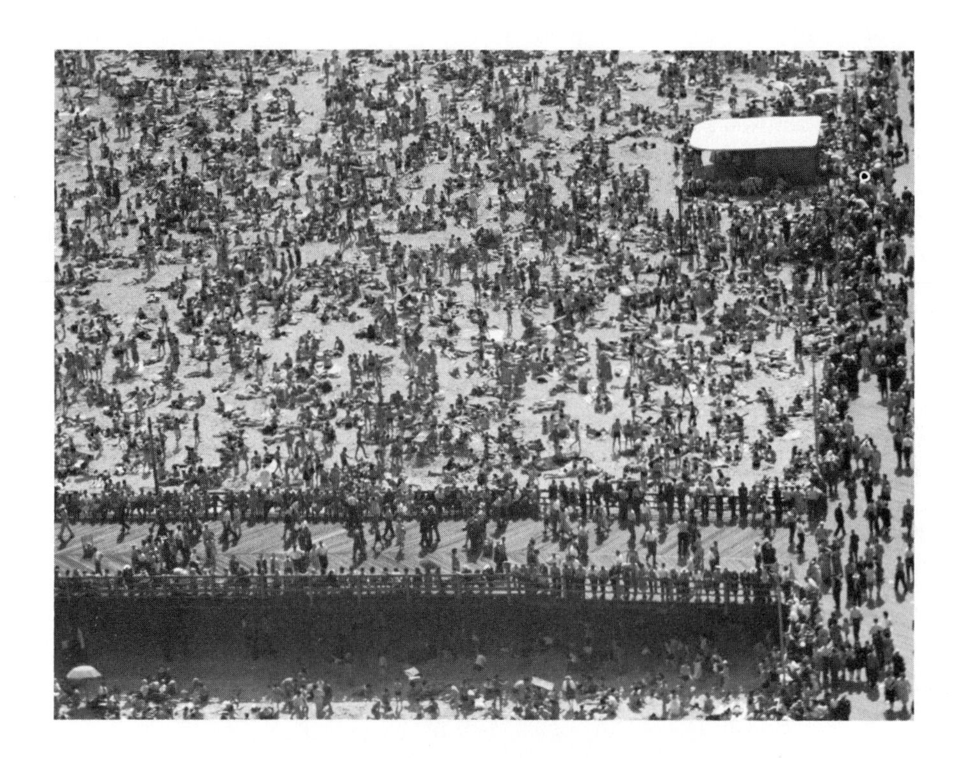

human overproduction

20

introduction

pushers and peelers

Several years ago the following item appeared in the *New York Times:*

> The Japan National Railways has hired 470 more sturdy "pushers" to help cram long-suffering Tokyo commuters into trains already crowded far beyond capacity at the height of the winter crush hour.
>
> The new "oshiya-san" (honorable pushers), mostly students hired on a part-time basis, bring to 2,500 the number stationed at key Tokyo rail points to help move an average of nearly four million commuters daily between their homes and places of work . . .
>
> . . . The "oshiya-san" double as "hagitoriya-san"—pullers or peelers—with the frequently vital job of snatching surplus passengers out of the cars to permit the doors to close and the tight two-minute operating schedules to be maintained.[1]

With this quotation, a central problem of this era is approached. Long ago the prophet Isaiah (5:8) warned against overpopulation. Today the "pushers" and "peelers" of the elegant Japanese symbolize a world threat.

Why is a book on health concerned with the problem? Better health is one cause of the population explosion. In the past, famine, war, and pestilence winnowed mankind. By these three, fertility and mortality ratios were equated. But today communicable disease is under increasing control. The twentieth-century plague in Los Angeles killed fewer than forty people. In the fourteenth century, the same microorganism cost more than 40 million lives. Famine and war still threaten, but there can be only opinionated meditation about their future effect. Those spared today live to propagate tomorrow. Better health promises too large a population and, ironically, threatens health.

It is in a crowded and threatening ecosystem that man competes with other life. Only to the extent that he can maintain his environment and yet best his competitors in environmental control can man hope to prevail. Man is not lacking in the capacity to reproduce. With all his sophistication, he escapes no biological laws. Nature ensures multiplication (and thus survival) of humankind by providing superabundant numbers of reproductive cells. Each human ovary contains about 200,000 primitive, undeveloped eggs. Only one is needed for conception. Each ejaculation of human semen contains 250 to 500 million spermatozoa. Only one is needed for fertilization.

In its abundance, human seed is not unique. If all the progeny of one April mating of houseflies were to live, they would, by August, cover the entire earth with a layer of houseflies forty-seven feet deep. Ruthlessly nature provides for no such endurance. Why do not flies inherit the earth? By limiting space and food, nature prohibits their overmultiplication.

More complex species have more complex methods of population limitation. Populations of Minnesota jack rabbits rise and fall cyclically. After a rise, episodes of mass dying occur. Neither food shortages nor predators account for this. The dead jack rabbits have been examined. Their livers and other glands

20-1 Oshiya-san (*"honorable pushers"*) *in a Tokyo subway station.*

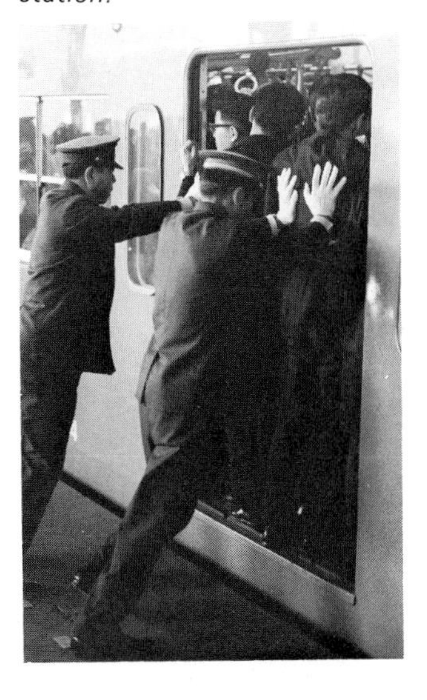

[1]*New York Times,* January 16, 1966, Sect. 1, p. 8.

are diseased. They have signs of high blood pressure. Their arteries are hardened. These result from ''stress sickness'' (see page 717). Similar tensions of crowding have produced this illness in many other animals.

Human overcrowding is being studied. The pituitary-adrenal system of man responds to stress in the same fashion as that of animals. Exactly how does overcrowding contribute to a human stress syndrome? Does it directly cause sickness and death? These remain incompletely answered questions. That overcrowding often contributes to social sickness is, however, undeniable.[2]

Malthus on man

Robert Thomas Malthus was among the first to dramatically portray overpopulation as a social problem. It was an anonymous work that made him famous: *Essay on the Principle of Population as It Affects the Future Improvement of Society, with Remarks on the Speculations of Mr. Godwin, M. Condorcet and Other Writers.* The essay brought bitter attack. A calm, cheerful man, Reverend Malthus was alluded to as a gloomy parson, a prophet of doom. Both Hazlitt and Dickens excoriated him. The former called him a slave to sex. The latter gave the name Malthus Gradgrind to an unpleasant character in *Hard Times.* Karl Marx accused Malthus of a plot to prevent the revolution of the masses by diminishing their numbers. As unkind a cut as any was the opprobrium hurled at him: anti-Cupid! ''It is an utter misconception of my argument,'' he wrote mildly in the 1817 edition of his *Essay,* ''to infer that I am an enemy of population. I am only an enemy of vice and misery.''

The basic thesis of his book was this: human populations, like other species, can increase faster than their means of subsistence.

To support this concept, Malthus postulated that unchecked population growth increases by a geometrical progression, whereas food increases by but an arithmetical progression. In other words, people would increase as do the numbers 1, 2, 4, 8, 16, 32, 64, 128, 256, and so on. Food or subsistence, however, would increase only as the numbers 1, 2, 3, 4, 5, 6, 7, 8, 9, and so on. He theorized that if the population could be assumed to double every twenty-five years, in two centuries the number of people would increase by 256 times, whereas food would increase by only 9 times. In three centuries the ratio of population increase to food increase would be as 4,096 to 13. In time, an astronomical number of people would be fiercely foraging for a dwindling food supply. To forestall this, the Reverend urged late marriage and moral restraint. Malthus was an outspoken foe of contraceptive techniques, labeling them ''im-

[2] There is some evidence to indicate that men and women respond differently to crowding. Under crowded conditions ''men become more competitive, somewhat more severe, and like each other less, whereas women become more cooperative and lenient and like each other more.'' (Paul Ehrlich and Jonathan Freedman, ''Population, Crowding and Human Behavior,'' *New Scientist and Science Journal,* Vol. 50, No. 745 [April 1971], pp. 10–14.) Nor should it be assumed that all people have the same concept of what crowding is. This is amply illustrated by the studies of the U.S. anthropologist Patricia Draper of a hunter-gatherer tribe in southwest Africa. These are the !Kung Bushmen. Although they inhabit an area in which there is an average of one person per ten square miles, they live in crowded conditions that would be intolerable by Western standards. Girls, for example, were in physical contact with at least one other person 57 percent of the time; boys, 35 percent. Draper says, ''As people sit in camp . . . they prefer to gather in clumps or knots, leaning against each other, their arms brushing, their crossed legs overlapping. It's just like 30 people living in one room.'' Do they experience social stress? No, quite the opposite. (''When 30 People to a Room Is Not Overcrowded,'' *New Scientist,* Vol. 60, No. 870 [November 1, 1973], p. 319.)

proper arts to conceal the consequences of irregular connections." Without moral restraint to control population growth, Malthus warned, the miseries of vice, war, and starvation would inevitably ensue.

Many shortcomings weaken the Malthusian theory. For example, he could not recognize the vast untapped resources of the undiscovered agricultural areas of the Americas, Africa, and Oceania. Nor did Malthus consider the possibility of scientific advances increasing food productivity. He failed, moreover, to emphasize that mere reproductive power did not necessarily mean reproduction. Many peoples, including some who do not have access to the modern methods of birth control, successfully limit population.

Nevertheless, Malthus drew serious attention to a spectre.

mankind's limited land[3]

Everything man uses comes from the land. The total land area of the earth is approximately 58 million square miles. Only 25 percent of the earth's total surface is suitable for farming. Impossible climates or unproductive soil, frequently both, force men to forgo cultivating millions of acres of land.

Much high mountain area is uninhabitable. The highest permanent habitations on earth are in Peru (17,100 feet). There, crops are not grown at altitudes over 14,000 feet. People live by grazing sheep, alpacas, and llamas. Some high tropical areas have a friendly climate (Mexico City is more than a mile high). However, earth's mountainous land is only about 5 percent arable.

About 17 percent of the land area of earth is desert. In it lives less than 3 percent of the world's population. Little desert land is now cultivated. Someday, perhaps, desalination and other projects will bend desert areas to man's will. The ingenuity of scientists (such as Israel's Duvdevani) has turned some deserts into gardens. On a more inclusive scale such accomplishment, however, is unlikely. It is estimated that "even when the small 'islands' made productive by irrigation are added, the world's deserts probably have not more than two to five percent of their total areas cultivable."[4]

[3] Langdon White, "Geography and the World's Population," in Stuart Mudd, ed., *The Population Crisis and the Use of World Resources* (The Hague, 1964), pp. 16–25.
[4] *Ibid.*, p. 20.

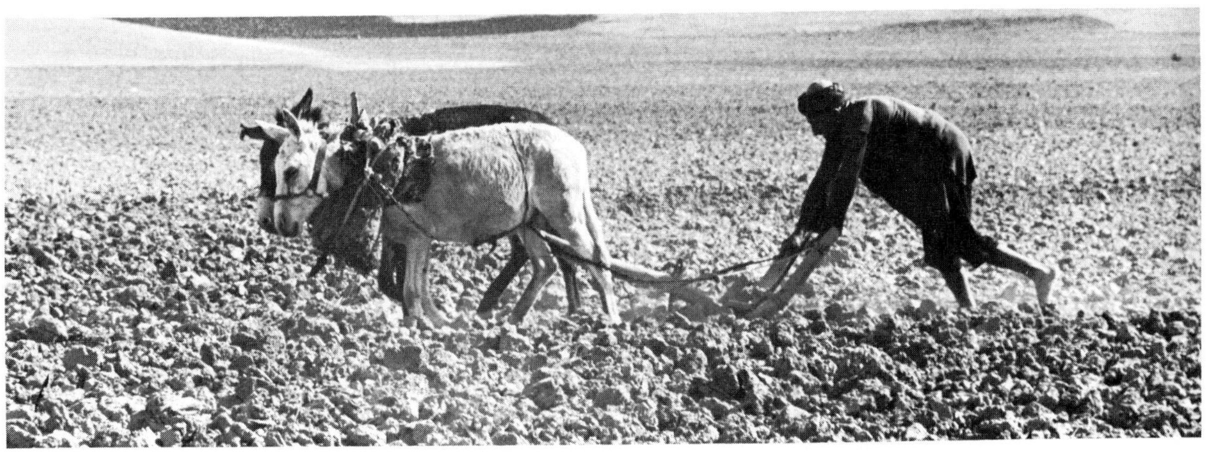

20-2 *An Iranian farmer tills the soil in the same back-breaking way as did countless generations before him. But Iran's economic development plan aims to replace his wooden plow and weary donkeys with modern agricultural equipment, easing his labor and improving his production.*

Cold lands take up about 29 percent of the surface of this planet. Antarctica is almost twice the size of the United States. Not one single human being lives there permanently. Covering millions of square Arctic miles are the frozen, treeless landscapes of the tundras, the world's coldest areas. They offer little hope for food. Seasons without frost are short. The soil is generally infertile. Summer drainage is poor. Russia issues glowing reports of success at the agricultural stations of her tundra, but development of the tundra is still only experimental. Finland, Sweden, and Greenland have grown food in previously unused Arctic areas. But, on a considerable percentage of the world's icy wastes, the day of good crops is not even in the distant future.

Tropical rain forests are not more hospitable. The huge and almost empty Amazon Basin, for example, provides the population with but a bare subsistence. Disease, poor soil, and dense forests combine with an insufferable climate to discourage investment and migration. Exploitation of these vast areas would require more money than is presently available to any government.

Are there other, better, more distant frontiers?

is the solution out of this world?

Much "nonsense arithmetic" about expanding population is, unfortunately, not nonsense. This chilling warning is an example:

> The current rate of [population] growth would lead to an eventual limit of some 60 quadrillion people by the year 2864. This would constitute 220 persons for each square meter of the earth's surface; to house them, the planet would be covered with continuous 2000-story buildings over land and sea alike, providing 7.5 square meters of floor space per person in 1000 stories. . . . As regards emigration to other planets, it would be necessary to send 73 million people a year to maintain the present level of population. Even if this were possible, the solar system's presumably habitable planets would soon be filled. Venus is about the earth's size; with population doubling every thirty-seven years, Venus would reach the earth's population density in that time span. Mercury, Mars and the moon together have half the same area; the excess population of earth and Venus would fill them up in another ten years.[5]

Settlement of other worlds is often mentioned as a possible solution for this world's overpopulation. First stop, the moon. Perhaps a scientific laboratory may someday be built there. It may become an interplanetary bus stop. To the modern geologist, "Earlier concepts of a dead moon have been replaced by that of a dynamic planet."[6] But the recent visits to this interesting cinder revealed little about its ecosystem to seriously invite human colonization.

[5] *M.D., Medical Newsmagazine,* Vol. 10, No. 4 (April 1966), p. 116. A further illustration of this train of thought was provided by Carl E. Taylor: "It is possible to demonstrate mathematically that at present rates of increase we will have standing room only by 2500 A.D. or that in 5,000 years the human race will be expanding so fast that it will form a solid ball of flesh growing out into space at the speed of light." (Quoted in "Crosscurrents of Opinion," *Medical Tribune* [December 18–19, 1965], p. 7.)

But these figures point to the far-distant future. The past is no less instructive. If the current 2 percent per year rate of increase in the world's population "had existed from the time of Christ to the present time . . . there would be over 20 million individuals in place of each person now alive or 100 persons for each square foot." (C. L. Markert, "Biological Limits on Population Growth," cited in William D. McElroy, "Biomedical Aspects of Population Control," *BioScience,* Vol. 19, No. 1 [January 1969], p. 19.)

[6] J. V. Smith and I. M. Steele, "How the Apollo Program Changed the Geology of the Moon," *Science and Public Affairs,* Vol. 29, No. 9 (November 1973), p. 15.

Mars? Oxygen and water are incredibly rare. After nightfall, it is bitter cold. Venus? Vast clouds apparently cover this unfriendly planet. Temperatures would melt lead (800° F). In this harsh ecosystem, the atmosphere is mainly carbon monoxide. Great fog, dust storms, intense heat, bitter cold, and carbon monoxide make of Venus a huge, tropical, poisonous planet of "smog." Mercury has an impossible climate. Pluto is far and dark. Jupiter, Saturn, Uranus, and Neptune freeze. Many hundreds of millions of miles separate them from enough warmth to keep people alive. Countless other planets whirl outside earth's solar system. Some may be paradise. But, for man, no planet can be anything but a hell without a sun to warm it. The nearest sun to earth's is many millions of miles away. To arrive near it would require more years than one lifetime can afford. And the trip would have been in vain. For man's needs that sun warms too weakly. One would not even shiver to death, for to shiver one must first be warm. And so, should an excess of the world's population seek a nourishing home outside of this world, they would have to go on and on, careening past endless, lonely emptiness, occasionally passing faintly glimmering suns that would fail to keep any planet decently warm. Sometimes twin suns would be seen. They maintain deadly heat. After more than a century of travel, the constellation Alpha Aquilae (about 94 million million miles from earth) might be reached. Perhaps it maintains a kindly planet or two for human comfort. Perhaps not. Nobody knows. But it is quite a long, even tiring, journey, and there is always the return trip to be considered.

No, it is on earth that man must seek solutions to his overpopulation problems. And he must always remain cognizant of his environmental limitations, of the confines of his ecosystem.

some general dimensions of overpopulation

the arithmetic of population growth

By 1962 about 77 billion people had been born into this world (Table 20-1). By 1975 about a billion more will have been added. Of the 78 billion people who, by 1975, will have inhabited the earth, over 95 percent will be dead. At the present rate of increase, the 1975 estimated world population will be some 4 billion (see Table 20-2). A medical wag once remarked that statistics are used by some people like a drunk uses a lamp post—more for support than for illumination. So figures must be related to meanings. If the meanings of populations figures signify trouble for mankind, then man must reason a course of action.

The seventy-six centuries from 6000 B.C. to A.D. 1650 began with the New Stone Age, swept through the Bronze and Iron periods, sped past antiquity and the dark medieval era to the Renaissance in the south of Europe and the Reformation in the north. Like a child full of questions, man entered this last age. In seeking and finding answers, he opened a Pandora's box of population problems.

The 23 billion people born during the three centuries following A.D. 1650 were almost half the number born in the seventy-six preceding centuries. In those relatively brief three hundred years, almost twice as many births occurred as

TABLE 20-1
Estimate of Births in Three Periods of Human History

PERIOD	NUMBER OF YEARS IN PERIOD	NUMBER OF BIRTHS IN PERIOD (in billions)	AVERAGE ANNUAL RATE OF INCREASE (per 1,000 population)
600,000 B.C.– 6000 B.C.	594,000	12	0.02
6000 B.C.– A.D. 1650	7,650	42	0.6
A.D. 1650–1962	312	23	4.35

Source: Annabelle Desmond, "How Many People Have Ever Lived on Earth?" from *The Population Crisis and the Use of World Resources* (The Hague, 1964), pp. 45–46.

in the 5,940 centuries of prehistoric times. The surge in world population of the middle seventeenth century continues today. What happened to start the increase?

why did people grow in number?

Because man succeeded in better controlling his ecosystems. One of the most significant marks of his environmental triumph was the invention of the microscope. For, with its magnifications, man identified some of his most persistent predators. Previously invisible, these competitors of man had been totally elusive. Seen, they could be attacked. Such accomplishments quickened a series of epochal revolutions in human history. Men wrought a scientific approach to life—and death. They looked and saw for themselves. Doors were opened to new thought and experiment. Pasteur, Freud, Koch, Ehrlich, Lister, Mendel, Semmelweiss, Noguchi—all built the scientific edifice for the twentieth century. From the back of mankind they lifted a burden of sickness and death; by so doing, they also undermined death control. For a high death rate, albeit cruel, is an efficient control of population growth. The absence of both death control and birth control quickly resulted in vast overpopulation.

With *scientific* revolution came *agricultural* change. Plant breeding, crop rotation, cultivation—these improvements wrested more food from the earth. During prehistory, man ate what was available. In the Old Stone Age he developed tools to farm. In time, his most powerful tool became his mind.

Scientific, agricultural, and industrial changes brought Europe a better life. On that continent today, infant mortality is one-seventh what it was two centuries ago. In the past two centuries, life expectancy in the Western world has increased from thirty years to more than seventy. What does this mean? When babies live to reproductive age, the seed is sown for more population. In industrial nations, almost all children live to have children of their own. Two centuries ago only half of them survived long enough to accomplish this. What is more, most people in developed countries live through the reproductive age. Not only do they live long enough to begin a family, they stay alive to add to it.

TABLE 20-2

Estimated World Population: A.D. 1000–A.D. 2000

CONTINENT	POPULATION AT GIVEN TIMES (in millions)						
	1000	1600	1800	1900	1960	1975 (est.)	2000 (est.)
Asia and Oceania	165	279	599	921	1,700	2,231	3,900
Europe, including Russia	47	102	192	423	641	751	947
Africa	50	90	90	120	244	303	517
Americas	13	15	25	144	407	543	904
Total	275	486	906	1,608	2,992	3,828*	6,268

*More recent projections indicate that world population will pass the 4 billion mark by 1975 (Population Reference Bureau press release, April 1969).

Source: Annabelle Desmond, "How Many People Have Ever Lived on Earth?" from *The Population Crisis and the Use of World Resources* (The Hague, 1964), p. 39, abstracted from *The Future Growth of World Populations; Population Studies, No. 28* (New York, 1958), p. 23.

Today, not only are people increasing in number, but the rate of increase is also accelerating. Every year, mankind reproduces a larger percentage of a larger number. It now takes far less time to double population than formerly. For world population to reach 3 billion took about 600,000 years. To double that number to 6 billion will take less than 40 years. That will be the tenth time the population of mankind has doubled. The first doubling required twenty thousand years. The eleventh could take only twenty years. Among all the creatures of the animal kingdom, such doubling of population is unique to man.

Complicating the population dilemma is the uneven multiplication of peoples (see Table 20-2). In 1960 Asia had 57 percent of the world's peoples. By 1975 that proportion will increase 2 percent. At the present rate of growth, by A.D. 2000 almost two out of every three human beings on earth (62 percent) will be in Asia. Will Asia be ready for them?

some modern meanings of overpopulation

population increase without preparation: Sri Lanka

Since time immemorial, both fly and mosquito buzzed and hummed triumphantly over the prostrate people of Sri Lanka (formerly called Ceylon). Fly-borne diarrhea decimated the child population. Malaria brought daily tragedy to the lives of these gentle people inhabiting the island to India's south.

In 1946 a DDT campaign was introduced. The Western world had two centuries of economic preparation for death control. For Sri Lanka, the knowledge was immediate. She was caught unprepared.

The insects were destroyed in Sri Lanka. In one year the death rate was reduced 40 percent. But the birth rate did not fall. From 1950 to 1960 the number of Sri Lankans increased by 28.9 percent. At this rate the population of Sri Lanka will be doubled about every thirty years. With a limited economy, she now desperately strives to meet her sudden spurt of population.

other areas of crisis

It is not only in Sri Lanka that sudden population increase has resulted from failure to bring high birth rates into line with lower death rates. Already, countless people in underdeveloped countries of South America, Asia, and Africa do not have enough to eat. Most of the malnourished preschool children in the world live in these countries. With one hand, progress gives them life. With the other, it takes it away.

Technical knowledge exists to meet the world's food shortage for some years to come. But arable land is unevenly distributed. Asia is in direst straits. "At present, 400 million human beings in the western industrial nations consume as much protein as 1,300 million of their fellowmen in Asia."[7] The Food and Agriculture Organization of the United Nations estimates that 300 to 500 million people in the developing countries are undernourished. In 1973, the deputy director for nutrition of the World Bank estimated that of the children born at that time, 75 million would die of malnourishment or associated illness. The World Health Organization states that worldwide, about 10 million children under age five are severely malnourished. Such children have smaller than average brains with fewer brain cells—a possibly irreversible effect. Tragically, 1972 world harvests were severely affected by bad weather, and many experts view the future with dismay.[8]

20-3 *"They hold out a skinny hand to a heedless world . . ."*

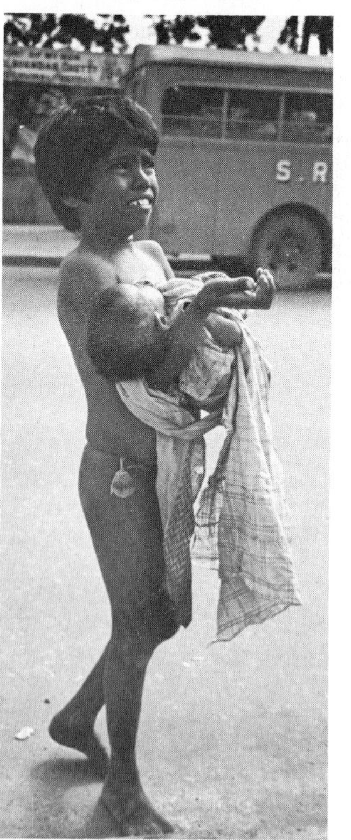

Man can be no more hopeful of soon meeting the housing shortage. In those countries with the largest populations the worst housing exists. Millions in Africa, Asia, and Latin America live in dwellings of mud, straw, or cardboard. Countless others swarm in the streets of crowded cities. They beg, they prostitute, they hold out a skinny hand to a heedless world. Still others have an address of sorts, but the housing is dilapidated beyond description. Fundamental sanitation is a luxury. And in such facilities the population will double in less than a generation. Today, a child born in the West African region of Nigeria will live only to reach his thirty-seventh birthday. A Swedish child can expect to live twice as long.[9]

What are the realistic financial opportunities of these malnourished, inadequately housed peoples of the developing countries? The average per capita income for the modern Asian is about $100 a year. For the Indian and Pakistani it is between $70 and $80 yearly. The average Latin American garners some $300 per year. The future of any nation rests with her children. Excluding mainland China, almost 700 million children under fifteen years of age live in

[7] Robert C. Cook, "Population and Food Supply," in *The Population Crisis and the Use of World Resources,* p. 474.

[8] "World Food Situation: Pessimism Comes Back in Vogue," *Science,* Vol. 181, No. 4100 (August 17, 1973), pp. 634–38.

[9] "The World in Demographic Perspective: A Study in Contrasts," *Newsfeature,* Population Reference Bureau, Inc. (1973), p. 1.

countries with a national per capita income of less than $500 per year; of these, 450 million live in countries where the income is under $100 annually.[10] May one hope to see these incomes rise? A major impediment is the increasing population. In Egypt, for example, the annual population increase (2.7 percent) will negate any economic benefit that might accrue from the completion of the Aswan Dam. It is a tragic fact that of the 120 developing countries in the world, only 31 have policies of encouraging a lower rate of population growth, 28 support family planning to reduce abortion and to enhance maternal and child health, but not for reasons of genuine population control, and 61 are indifferent or actively opposed to family planning.[11]

the U.S. population picture

At the start of 1974, the U.S. population had passed 211.6 million. Will that figure reach 300 million before the turn of the century? That depends on the number of children per family. If the average number of children per family is three, the population will reach 300 million in 1996. If the average is two, that day will be postponed another twenty-five years, to the year 2021. If the average continues as it is at present, between two and three children per family, there will be 300 million people in the United States by about 2008.

But if the average family has only two children, will not the "replacement rate" have been reached? (That rate is 2.11 children per average completed family; it is 2.11, and not the two needed to replace the two parents, because some children die before reaching reproductive age and some never have children.) In this century, a continuous replacement rate is a possibility. Zero population growth (ZPG) is not. Population growth is a legacy of the past. It cannot be brought to an abrupt halt. To achieve ZPG, a replacement level of births would have to be maintained for at least seventy years. Why?

In 1940, the U.S. population was 132 million. Thirty-four years later (1974), that number had been increased by 80 million. During most of the 1950s, there had been a steady rise in the birth rate (births per 1,000 population). Not until 1958, after eight years of steady rise, did the U.S. birth rate begin to descend from its 1957 historic peak of 25.3 per 1,000 people. There had been a baby boom. And those babies are now old enough to have babies of their own. Today, the number of persons moving into childbearing age is much larger than was the case for their parents. In 1975, there will be 5.5 million more people in the prime childbearing years (twenty to twenty-nine) than there were in 1971. By 1985, the number will have increased another 5.5 million.

Despite these projections, there is growing evidence that the baby boom of former times has become a birth dearth. In 1960, the U.S. birth rate was 23.7. In 1971, it was only 17.3. The birth rate in 1972 was 15.6 births per 1,000 population, the lowest annual rate ever observed in this country; this was about 10 percent lower than the 1971 rate—itself a record low. In 1971, however, some states and even regions had shown no birth decline; some had even

[10] United Nations Children's Fund, *Assignment Children,* cited in "The Needs of Children," *Clinical Pediatrics,* Vol. 8, No. 6 (June 1969), p. 6A.

[11] "Population: Target Nations," *Saturday Review/World* (November 6, 1973), p. 39, citing Dorothy Nortman, ed., *Population and Family-Planning Programs: A Factbook,* 5th ed. (New York, 1973).

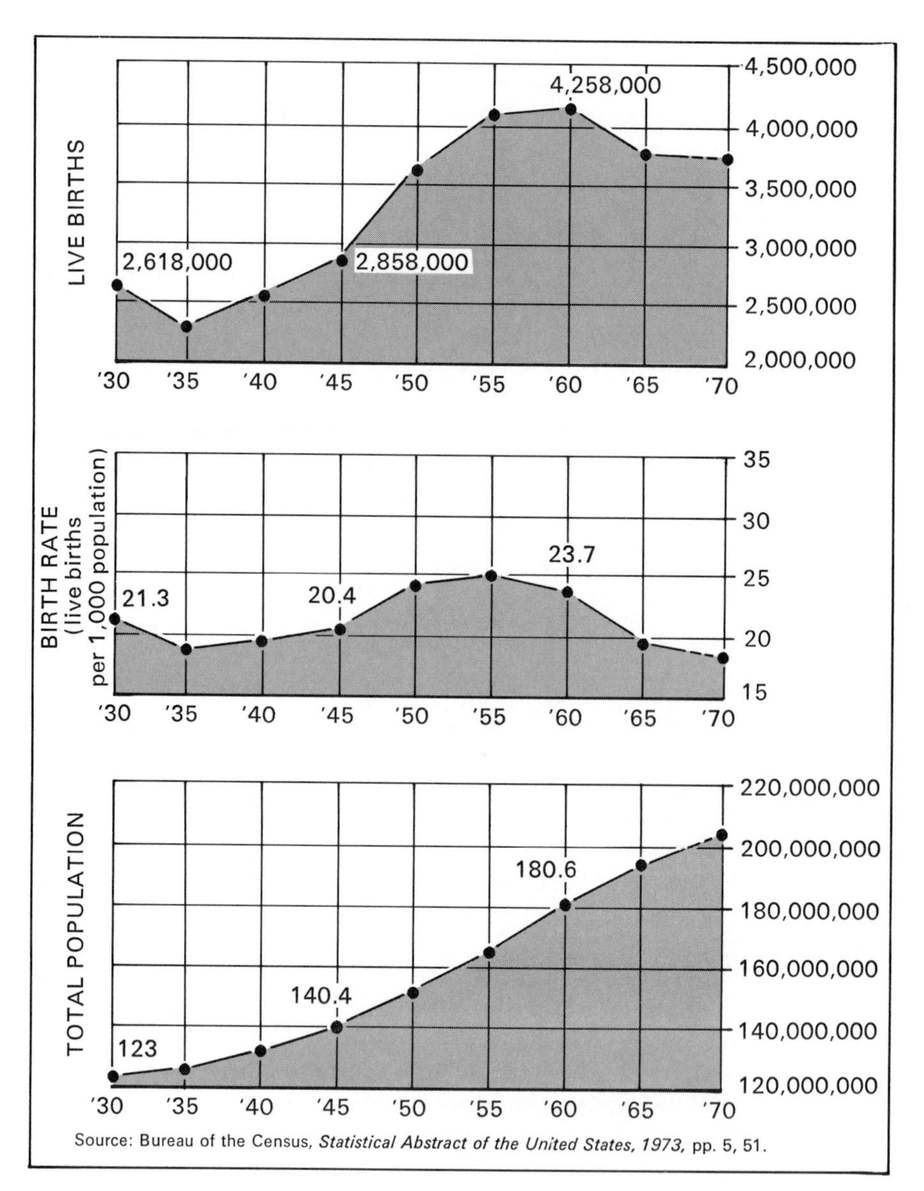

20-4 *U.S. live births, birth rates, and total population: 1930–70.*

shown an increase. In 1972, the number of births declined in every state in the union.

The *general fertility rate* (births per 1,000 women in the reproductive ages of fifteen to forty-four) has also decreased sharply. In 1965 it was 105; in 1970, 87.6; in 1971, 82.3; in 1972, 73.4.[12] The downward trend continued into 1973. For the first seven months of that year there were 3 percent fewer live births than for the same period in 1972. The birth rate was down to 14.8, and

[12] National Center for Health Statistics, U.S. Department of Health, Education, and Welfare, "Births, Marriages, Divorces, and Deaths for 1972," *Monthly Vital Statistics Report,* Vol. 21, No. 12 (March 1973), p. 1.

the fertility rate was 69. These rates were about 5 percent lower than for the first seven months of 1972, when they were 15.5 and 72.7[13]

The *total fertility rate* is the sum of the age-specific birth rates for the female population for any particular year, assuming that the rates do indeed exist. Usually, it is estimated. In 1971 the figure was 2.28. In 1972 it was only 2.03. For the first time fertility had dropped below the replacement level of 2.11 children per family. The U.S. Bureau of the Census recently published population projections to the year 2020 based on four fertility assumptions (see Figure 20-5). Despite the trend toward lowered fertility, all four projections indicate a continued growth of population for many years to come.

some reasons for the decline

Demographers (students of population patterns) are by no means certain why birth and fertility rates have declined. In 1854, a census official estimated that the U.S. population in 1950 would most likely be 150 million. It was actually 150,697,631. Most present-day demographers are reluctant to suggest that they can match that combination of luck and achievement. Liberalized abortion laws (see pages 640–43), increasing numbers of married women working outside the home (40 percent today, compared to 15 percent three decades ago; see pages 329–31), and concern about the environment, are among the reasons given for the present decline in the U.S. birth rate. Moreover, there is a growing tendency for people to marry at an older age. Some demographers suggest that birth rates always fall during periods of economic depression, as occurred in the 1930s. However, fertility rates declined during the prosperous 1920s and 1960s. Perhaps the two most significant reasons for the current decline in birth and fertility rates are changed attitudes about family size and widespread use of more efficient birth control methods.

These latter conclusions were the result of the federally financed 1970 National Fertility Study that was conducted by the Office of Population Research at Princeton University. Between 1965 and 1970, U.S. couples radically changed their reproductive behavior to sharply adjust their fertility goals downward. Interestingly, many Roman Catholic couples are participating in this change. In 1970 they reported that they wanted an average of 9 percent fewer children than did Catholic couples in 1965. Indeed, an increasing number seem to desire two or three children—a number close to the replacement level.[14]

Had there been a marked increase in the proportion of U.S. couples who were using contraceptive devices between 1965 and 1970? No. However, an important change had occurred in the methods used. The most effective contraceptive methods are the oral contraceptive pill, sterilization, and the intra-

[13] National Center for Health Statistics, U.S. Department of Health, Education, and Welfare, "Births, Marriages, Divorces, and Deaths for July 1973," *Monthly Vital Statistics Report,* Vol. 22, No. 7 (September 24, 1973), p. 1.

[14] "Impact of Tumbling Birth Rate: Three Views, "*American Medical News,* Vol. 15, No. 28 (July 17, 1972), pp. 6–7.

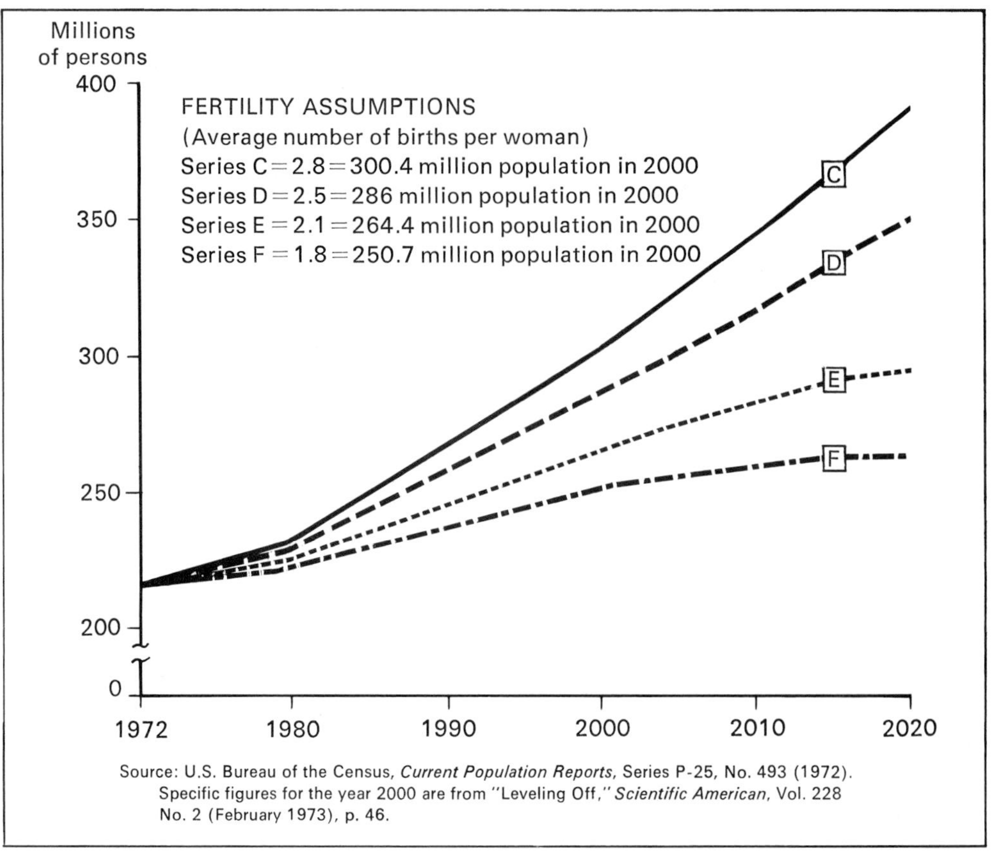

20-5 *Projections of total U.S. population, 1972–2020.*

uterine device (see Table 21-1, pages 618–21). Only 37.2 percent of U.S. couples were using these three in 1965; in 1970 the figure rose to 57.9.[15]

about unplanned and unwanted births

The 1970 National Fertility Study used a national sample of women under age forty-five to measure the number of children women wanted and the number they had borne but did not want. Some revealing estimates were as follows:[16]

1. between 1966 and 1970, 44 percent of all births to married women were unplanned;
2. 15 percent of all births were reported by the parents as having never been wanted; however,
3. only 1 percent of first births were never wanted;
4. two-thirds of all sixth or higher-order births were unwanted;

[15] "Fertility and Contraception," *Scientific American*, Vol. 227, No. 4 (October 1972), p. 46.

[16] *Population and the American Future, The Report of the Commission on Population Growth and the American Future* (New York, 1972), pp. 163–64, citing the 1970 National Fertility Study conducted by the Office of Population Research, Princeton University; Norman B. Ryder and Charles F. Westoff, *Reproduction in the United States: 1965* (Princeton, N.J., 1971).

5. among women with the least education, the percentage of unwanted births was highest.

An unwanted birth does not invariably mean an unwanted child. Love is difficult to measure, but most parents probably love their unplanned children as much as those who were planned. Nevertheless, there is some evidence that an unplanned child is more likely to develop problems of adjustment. One twenty-year Swedish study[17] compared children born to women whose application for abortion had been denied with a control group of other children born at the same time and in the same hospital. The unwanted children eventually needed more psychiatric care and public assistance and engaged in more criminal activities. In addition, a study[18] carried out in this country suggests that unwanted babies do not thrive as well as those who are wanted by their mothers—a not surprising finding (see pages 331–36).

The strain on the parents of an unwanted child can be no less severe. Unwanted births occur more frequently among the poor, and most of them occur in the later years of childbearing. In the past decade, maternal deaths in this country caused by childbearing have declined by 94 percent. However, it is the older mother for whom the risks are greatest. Between the ages of twenty and twenty-four, the risks of dying from childbirth are lowest. For the mother who is between thirty-five and thirty-nine, they are four times greater; between forty and forty-four, eight times greater; at older ages almost twenty times greater. And older mothers have a much greater tendency to give birth to children with certain hereditary diseases (see page 555).[19]

''watch us grow!''

Until recently, ''Watch us grow!'' was the challenge of little cities to the big. Los Angeles grew. And an astronaut gets around the world in less time than one can travel forty miles of the Los Angeles freeways on a busy afternoon. Manhattan grew. At day's end, people flee the island. Rather than live in cities, commuters have forgone the hard-earned eight-hour day. By adding three hours a day for travel to and from the job, they have regressed to a working day of eleven hours. This nation is also short of power, which costs more to distribute than to create. Schools are crowded, air is sewage, water is scanty (millions now drink treated sewage), noise is deafening, housing is short.

But perhaps the most subtle and erosive evil of overpopulation is the loss of personal significance. In his marvelous essay ''Civil Disobedience,'' Thoreau told of his night in jail for failure to pay a poll tax. In prison Thoreau felt free because he felt significant. One can but reflect that this lover of solitude found

[17] *Ibid.*, p. 165, citing Hans Forssman and Inge Thuwe, ''One Hundred and Twenty Children Born After Application for Therapeutic Abortion Refused,'' *Acta Psychiatrica Scandinavica,* 1966.

[18] ''Do Unwanted Babies Fail to Thrive?'' *Family Planning Digest,* Vol. 1, No. 3 (May 1972), p. 7, citing J. Patrick Lavery, ''Neonatal Mortality and Morbidity in a Selectively Controlled Obstetrical Population,'' a paper presented at the fourth annual meeting of the Junior Fellows at the American College of Obstetricians and Gynecologists, San Francisco, May 3–6, 1971. For a consideration of the increased mortality and morbidity of the unwed mother and her child, see pages 349–51.

[19] *Population and the American Future, The Report of the Commission on Population Growth and the American Future,* pp. 165–66.

his original significance in a cabin near Walden Pond, today a polluted watery receptacle for various wastes.

George Washington headed a nation of 4 million people. Today, the President worries about almost 212 million. By 1975 each senator will court 2.25 million people; each representative about 525,000. As population increases, taxes increase, but representation inexorably lessens.

Where can modern man find a Walden Pond? Every year many thousands of acres of lush countryside are bulldozed. Cities stream noisily into one another. A bumper-to-bumper existence in these areas is a valid nightmare. Today, a majority of the U.S. population lives in three great megalopolitan areas. These are the Great Northeastern megalopolis (including the Atlantic Seaboard and the Great Lakes region), the California region, and the Florida region. It has been estimated that, even if the present lower birth and fertility rates should continue, these three major areas will contain more than 143 million people by 1980. In about 1990, these three areas will contain 65 percent of the nation's people—a total population of 170 million.[20]

No, the bumper-to-bumper concept is no exaggeration. By 1975, 120 million vehicles, traveling 1,000 billion miles yearly, will slay close to sixty thousand people a year. For this purpose, roads will be built at about $3.5 million a mile. For each road mile, about forty acres of agricultural land will be sacrificed. Add to this decrease in agricultural land the amount needed for airfields, cities, reservoirs, flood control, and other similar purposes.

Well, Thoreau, at least, found a quiet spot.

if not war, then what solution?

Is war the inevitable "solution"? In the past it has been suggested that man's proclivity for killing other men has helped limit population. Overpopulation promotes war. This generation finds almost 800 million restless Chinese seeking more real estate. Will the next generation find more than one billion Chinese any less restless? Eighty-five percent of the Chinese are now forced to live on but one-third of their land (much of China's territory is uninhabitable desert or high mountains). If China's population goes unchecked, where will her people go?[21] Or those of India? Africa? Latin America? Will the human tragedy that is war be used as a solution?

The tragedy of war's waste is heightened by irony. War does not relieve population growth. If anything, it forces improvements in medicine. And, as occurred after the Second World War, it can create an economic boom that stimulates population growth.

[20] "Where Will the Next 50 Million Americans Live?" *Population Bulletin,* a publication of the Population Reference Bureau, Inc., Vol. 27, No. 5 (October 1971), p. 15.

[21] It is of interest to note that classical Marxists regard the doctrine of Malthus (see pages 600–01) as totally false. Indeed, at the United Nations Conference on the Human Environment, held at Stockholm in June 1972, the Chinese delegation claimed that the root environmental problem was not overpopulation, but social and economic inequity. (*Science News,* Vol. 102, No. 4 [July 22, 1972], p. 51.) Despite this, there is ample evidence that the Chinese government is conducting an intensive birth control program. This, combined with a relatively late age of marriage and the almost universal acceptance of premarital chastity by young people, seems to be resulting in diminished birth and fertility rates among the Chinese people. "The 'liberation' of Chinese women does not extend to the endorsement of free love. All evidence suggests that China's youth continue to pursue the puritanical sexual mores of the past." (Leo A. Orleans, "China: Population in the People's Republic," *Population Bulletin,* a publication of the Population Reference Bureau, Inc., Vol. 27, No. 6 [December 1971], p. 17.) Birth control is heavily promoted by the "barefoot doctors." In that program, promising

Some recommend *abortion* (see pages 636–45). Japan practices it with remarkable success. In 1947 Japan's birth rate was 34.3 percent. The death rate was 14.6 percent. The natural increase (the difference between the two) was 19.7 percent. In 1948 a law authorized the individual physician, on his own responsibility, to induce abortion for physical or financial reasons. By 1957, ten years after the abortion law, the birth rate had dropped to 17.2 percent. The death rate was 8.3 percent. The rate of natural increase was less than half of that of 1947, 8.9 percent. Every year more than 1.25 million abortions are performed in Japan. Since these are done only by physicians, no undue mortality is noted from the procedure.[22]

Abortion, however, is not the only cause of the low Japanese birth rate. Birth control is widely practiced in Japan.

An *economic* solution has been recommended. Can greater efficiency in food production resolve the problem? As long as population numbers outstrip ability to meet needs, this concept remains unrealistic. Today, hundreds of millions starve in miserable housing. Despair is their constant companion. What realistic reason is there to think that the next generation will have solved the overwhelming problem of poverty for twice the number of people who live in poverty today? As one distinguished biologist wrote:

> Some feel that the battle to feed the world population is now lost, and that it is a foregone conclusion that by 1985 we will have world-wide famines in which hundreds of millions of people will starve to death. I must admit I see no major crash program which would lead me to disagree with this conclusion.[23]

The need for such a program is great and urgent.

An *educational* approach has been suggested. As with other public health programs, it should permeate the birth control effort. Directing such programs to maternity services would seem particularly indicated. Of special importance is the education of the mother who has borne her first child. It is she who has the greatest potential for adding to the population. There is, moreover, expert opinion that instruction in population problems and family planning should begin in high school. Indeed, in Baltimore detailed information on family planning and family growth is given to the high school student. The material, incorporated into the social studies and biology courses, has been found to be valuable to both student and parent. Although obtaining competent teachers in this area is a problem, it too can be solved by intensive education.[24]

---

high school graduates are given six months of intensive medical training before being sent to rural areas to operate dispensaries. In addition, registered and practical nurses, as well as midwives, perform many of the procedures that, in the Western world, are limited to physicians. These include tubal ligations and abortions.

[22] Kitaoka Juitso, "How Japan Halved Her Birth Rate in Ten Years," in *The Sixth International Conference on Planned Parenthood* (London, 1959), pp. 27–36.

[23] William D. McElroy, "Biomedical Aspects of Population Control," p. 19.

[24] *Ibid.* However, it has been suggested that essentially only a small proportion of humanity is aware of the population problem, and that birth control programs are most effective where they are least needed. One writer has suggested that research be conducted for a pill favoring the fertilization of the human ovum by a sperm bearing a Y-chromosome. The resulting preponderance of males would quickly limit human reproduction, the theory postulates. It is further claimed that a male child is most desired in many parts of the world; such a pill would thus find wide acceptance. What a large excess of young males would mean to the remaining females is open to speculation, as are other possible consequences. (John Postgate, "Bat's Chance in Hell," *New Scientist,* Vol. 58, No. 840 [April 5, 1973], pp. 12–14, 16.)

The *demographic* solution has been offered. This suggests a reduction of the birth rate to the point where it equals the death rate, so that population growth either slows or stops. Birth control and education are the tools of this solution.

In 1970, Congress passed the Family Planning Services and Population Research Act. Funded for three years with $225 million, the major purpose of the act was to provide 5 million poor women with the ways and knowledge necessary for practicing contraception. It was a beginning. Another major beginning was the establishment by Congress, in March 1970, at the suggestion of President Nixon, of a twenty-four–member Commission on Population Growth and the American Future. Two years later the commission delivered its report to the President and the Congress. Although its numerous recommendations for solving the population problems of the nation did not meet with universal agreement, its thorough and calmly reasoned analyses are an excellent starting point for further discussion and planning.[25]

So a major threat to man's survival is overproduction of his kind. How is this problem being met? This question will be considered in the following chapter.

summary

Overpopulation, paradoxically, is both a result of and a threat to better health (page 599). Robert Thomas Malthus was one of the first to point out the dangers of overpopulation (pages 600–01). The amount of land hospitable to human life is limited (pages 601–02), but human settlement of other planets is a dim possibility (pages 602–03); so humanity must seek solutions to earth's overpopulation problems on earth, within the limits of the present human ecosystem (page 603).

The sudden surge in world population during the past three hundred years resulted from scientific, agricultural, and industrial changes that brought humanity a better life, particularly in the Western world (pages 603–05). Overpopulation is a problem in Western countries, but it has reached crisis proportions in Sri Lanka (pages 605–06) and other underdeveloped nations of Asia, Africa, and South America; for many people in those countries, overpopulation has led to malnourishment, housing shortages, and dire poverty (pages 606–07). In the United States, the population picture (pages 607–12) in recent years has been characterized by a decline in birth and fertility rates.

A number of measures have been put forth as solutions to the overpopulation problem, including *war, abortion, economic programs* involving more efficient food production, *educational programs* urging limitation of family size, and a *demographic solution* involving birth control and education to bring the birth rate down to a level equal to the death rate (pages 612–14).

[25] An official version of the lengthy report of the commission is published by the United States Government Printing Office, Public Documents Department, Washington, D.C. 20402. An advance edition was published in March 1972 by the New American Library, Inc., 1301 Avenue of the Americas, New York, New York 10019. In April 1972, the Population Reference Bureau, Inc., 1755 Massachusetts Avenue, Washington, D.C. 20036, published a twenty-nine–page summary of the report: "Population: The Future Is Now," *Population Bulletin,* Vol. 28, No. 2 (April 1972).

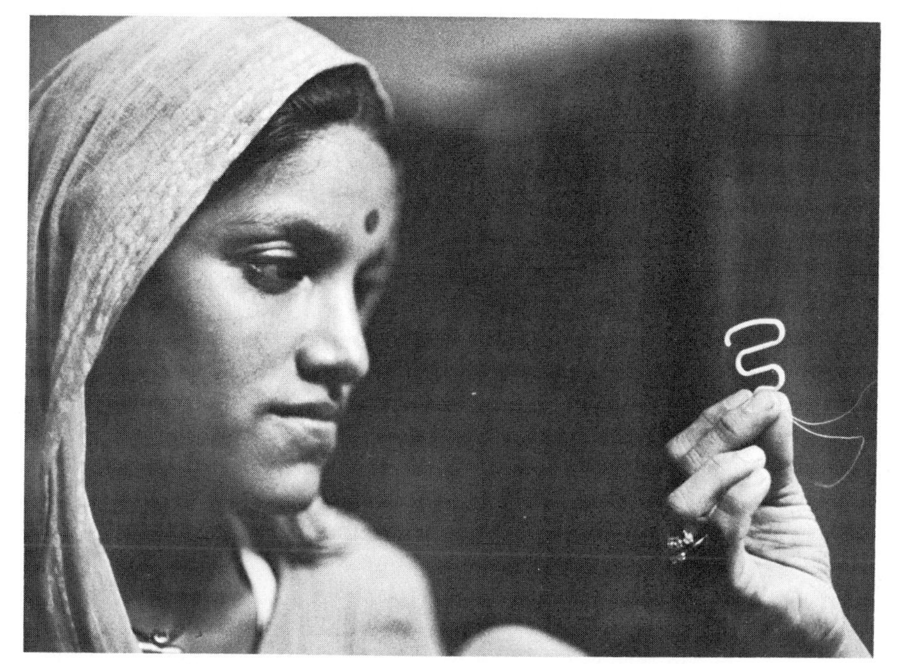

Will this Indian woman use the intrauterine device? Many factors, among them tradition and belief, will influence her decision.

controlling human reproduction

21

birth control

Birth control is not a modern development of a civilized society. Nevertheless, that it has become both civilized and modern is undeniable. In this country, by mid-1972, thirty-nine of the fifty states had affirmed the right of unmarried women over the age of eighteen to arrange for their own contraceptive care, and in nineteen states they could do so at a considerably younger age.[1] Primitive societies have always limited their numbers in various ways. Although less common than formerly, *infanticide* still occurs. Some African tribes practice *coitus interruptus* (coitus in which the penis is withdrawn from the vagina before ejaculation). The primitive Achinese of Sumatra use a vaginal suppository containing tannic acid. This primitive group has hit upon a valid scientific principle; tannic acid is an effective spermicide.[2]

Ancient writings are replete with instructions on birth control. In the Petri papyrus (1850 B.C.), crocodile dung is recommended. Twenty-seven hundred years later, the Arabian physician Qusta ibn Tuqa substituted elephant dung for that of the crocodile. Few if any prescriptions, contraceptive or otherwise, persisted for as many years as did dung.[3]

Coitus interruptus is described in the Bible (Genesis 38:9). It was practiced by the ancient Hebrews. Infanticide is also mentioned in the Bible.[4] It was condemned by Jew and Christian alike.[5] Nevertheless, in eighteenth- and nineteenth-century Europe, infanticide was practiced. "It was not an uncommon spectacle to see the corpses of infants lying in the streets or on the dung hills of London and other large cities."[6]

The views of Saint Thomas Aquinas have been vastly influential. In the *Summa Theologica,* he wrote: "In so far as the generation of offspring is impeded, it is a vice against nature which happens in every carnal act from which generation cannot follow."

> Nevertheless, by 1970, two-thirds of all Catholic women were using [contraceptive] methods disapproved by their Church; this figure reached three-quarters for

[1] "Girls Under 18 Can Consent to Birth Control Services in Two-Fifths of the States," *Family Planning Digest,* Vol. 1, No. 6 (November 1972), p. 1. For a further consideration of this subject see Judith Blake, "The Teenage Birth Control Dilemma and Public Opinion," *Science,* Vol. 180, No. 4087 (May 18, 1973), pp. 708–12.

[2] Norman E. Himes, *Medical History of Contraception* (Baltimore, 1936), p. 63.

[3] *Ibid.*

[4] See, for example, Leviticus 18:21; Deuteronomy 12:31; II Kings 3:27, 16:3; II Chronicles 28:3, 33:6; Psalms 106:38; Isaiah 57:5; Jeremiah 19:5; Ezekiel 16:21.

[5] In China's first official document against infanticide, in 1659, Choen Tche (1633–62) wrote: "I have heard that the sad cry uttered by these girl babies as they plunged into a vase of water and drowned is inexpressible. Alas! that the heart of a father or mother should be so cruel." (Fielding H. Garrison, "History of Pediatrics," in Arthur Frederick Abt and Fielding H. Garrison, *History of Pediatrics* [Philadelphia, 1965], p. 3.)

[6] William L. Langer, "Checks on Population Growth—1750 to 1850," *Scientific American,* Vol. 226, No. 2 (February 1972), p. 95.

21-1 *A portion of the Petri papyrus (1850 B.C.), which prescribes the use of crocodile dung as a contraceptive.*

women under age thirty. The change between 1965 and 1970 was especially striking for Catholic women who had attended college . . . Perhaps the most significant finding is that the defection has been most pronounced among the women who receive Communion at least once a month. Even among this group, the majority now deviates from Church teaching on birth control; among the younger women in this group the proportion not conforming reaches two-thirds.[7]

Moreover, it is worth noting that in 1973 about 5.7 million U.S. women of childbearing age were in "low income" brackets; another 3.4 million were in "marginal income" brackets.[8] Such data indicate the need for family planning; they do not indicate that most children of mothers on welfare are illegitimate, nor that most welfare families are black, nor that most people on welfare are able-bodied loafers, nor that most welfare families have many children, many of whom were conceived to obtain more welfare payments. All these notions have been disproved by data compiled by the Social and Rehabilitation Service of the Department of Health, Education, and Welfare.[9]

birth control for the female

oral contraceptives and clots

Table 21-1 presents the most common birth control methods available today. Because they are used by millions of women and have been associated with serious illness, oral contraceptives merit special discussion. Most of the currently marketed oral contraceptive pills are composed of synthetic estrogens and synthetic progesterone (progestin).[10] They are administered in one of two ways, either in combination or in a sequential fashion.

Each of the combination oral contraceptive pills is identical; each contains synthetic estrogens and progestins. There are different kinds of estrogens and progestins and the kind and the amount of estrogens and progestins in an oral contraceptive pill varies with the brand. Most combination pills are taken for twenty-one days, then discontinued for a week before beginning a new cycle. However, some brands add seven "sugar pills" to be taken at the end of the cycle so that a pill is taken every day of the month. The sequential oral contraceptive pills are not identical. The first fifteen or sixteen pills in a cycle contain only synthetic estrogens; the last five pills contain estrogens and progestins. Like the combination type, the amount and kind of the synthetic hormones and the dosage taken in a monthly series varies with the brand. Oral contraceptives should never be used without the advice of a physician, and he will prescribe the brand he thinks is most advisable for the individual patient. In most cases he will prescribe one of the brands of pills that has the lowest dosage of estrogen (not more than .05 milligrams of estrogen in each pill). Why? The answer requires some understanding of thromboembolic disease.

A *thrombus* is a clot in a blood vessel (or in the heart) that is formed by the

[7] Charles F. Westoff and Larry Bumpass, "The Revolution in Birth Control Practices of U.S. Roman Catholics," *Science,* Vol. 179, No. 4068 (January 5, 1973), p. 44.

[8] "A Formula for the 1970's: Estimated Need for Subsidized Family Planning Services," *Family Planning Perspectives,* Vol. 5, No. 3 (Summer 1973), p. 147.

[9] "Myths About Welfare Births Are Refuted," *Family Planning Digest,* Vol. 1, No. 4 (July 1972), p. 3.

[10] For a discussion of estrogen and progesterone, see pages 474 and 478.

coagulation of blood. It remains at the site of its formation. An *embolus* is a clot that has left the site of its formation. It is carried by the blood stream from a vessel and forced into a smaller one, where it obstructs circulation and may cut off the blood supply to a part of the body. Thromboembolic disease has always been a serious medical concern. That concern has increased with the widespread use of oral contraceptives. In one major study, death from pulmonary embolism[11] occurred in fifteen women who took oral contraceptives. This was four times the expected number for women of their age.[12] Other investigators reported that "in the absence of other predisposing causes the risk of developing deep vein thrombosis, pulmonary embolism, or cerebral thrombosis is increased about eight times by the use of oral contraceptives, while the risk of developing coronary thrombosis[13] is apparently unchanged."[14]

By 1970, the Food and Drug Administration of the U.S. Department of Health, Education, and Welfare had published the results of a survey of the available data concerning the connection between oral contraceptives and thromboembolic disorders.[15]

The association between thromboembolism and the use of oral contraceptives was confirmed, and the sequential type of oral contraceptives seemed to be associated with more risk than the combination type. Since contraceptives containing relatively higher doses of estrogen seemed to be connected with a greater risk of thromboembolic disease, "good therapeutics would indicate the use of the lowest effective dose of estrogen."[16] On January 12, 1970, these findings were made available in the form of a newsletter to almost all the physicians in the United States. Considering the widespread use of oral contraceptives, it must be pointed out that the risks are of a low order of magnitude. Indeed, the risk of death from the use of oral contraceptives is even lower than the extremely low (and decreasing) risk of death from pregnancy.

There has been some expressed concern that the use of contraceptive pills is linked to cancers of the breast or cervix. Both British and U.S. studies have failed to demonstrate such a risk.[17] Experiments with rats and mice, however, remain inconclusive.[18] It might be well here to recall the classic caution made

[11] Pulmonary embolism refers to a clot obstructing the pulmonary artery (or one of its branches), which brings blood to the lungs.

[12] W. H. N. Inman and M. P. Vessey, "Investigation of Deaths from Pulmonary, Coronary, and Cerebral Thrombosis and Embolism in Women of Child-bearing Age," *British Medical Journal,* Vol. 2, No. 5599 (April 27, 1968), p. 193.

[13] Coronary thrombosis refers to the formation of a clot in a coronary artery which supplies blood to the heart. With blood supply to the heart blocked, the heart suffers a lack of oxygen and is thus damaged.

[14] R. Doll, cited in the *Second Report of the Advisory Committee on Obstetrics and Gynecology,* Food and Drug Administration (August 1969), Chairman's Summary, Louis M. Hellman, M.D.

[15] John J. Schrogie, "Oral Contraceptives: A Status Report," *FDA Papers,* Vol. 4, No. 4 (May 1970), pp. 23–25.

[16] "Oral Contraceptives and Thromboembolic Disorders," *FDA Current Drug Information* (April 24, 1970). Late in 1973, the FDA approved a combination oral contraceptive containing a progestin and only .02 milligrams of estrogen. Theoretically, the lower amount of estrogen will reduce serious side effects, such as thromboembolic disease. However, irregular bleeding patterns are more frequent, and for this reason many women discontinue these pills. Other low-estrogen pills are being tested both here and in Britain. ("FDA Approves Pill with Least Estrogen," *Family Planning Digest,* Vol. 2, No. 5 [September 1973], p. 16, citing P. G. T. Bye and M. Elstein, "Clinical Assessment of a Low-Oestrogen Combined Oral Contraceptive," *British Medical Journal,* Vol. 2 [1973], p. 389.)

[17] "British, U.S. Studies Find No Link Between Pill Use and Breast and Cervical Cancer," *Family Planning Digest,* Vol. 2, No. 1 (January 1973), pp. 3–4.

[18] *Ibid.,* p. 5.

TABLE 21-1

A Summary of Birth Control Methods

METHOD	WHAT IT IS AND HOW IT WORKS	EFFECTIVENESS AND ACCEPTABILITY
Oral contraceptives (the pill)	It is generally accepted that the synthetic hormones contained in oral contraceptives (estrogens and progestins) inhibit ovulation. There are two contraceptive pill methods. The most commonly used method is often referred to as the "combination" or "balanced progestin–estrogen" method. This method is by far the one most commonly prescribed (more than 90 percent). Each pill contains a combination of both synthetic estrogen and progestin to assure inhibition of ovulation. When no egg is released from an ovary, a woman cannot become pregnant. In the other one, called the "sequential" method, two different pills are used each month. When this method is used, a pill containing synthetic estrogen is taken daily for the first 14, 15, or 16 days of the cycle. This pill inhibits ovulation. The second pill, containing a mixture of synthetic estrogen and progestin, is then taken for 4, 5, or 6 days to assure orderly bleeding within 3 to 5 days after the last pill is taken in each cycle. The pills are usually taken for 21 or 28 consecutive days in each menstrual cycle.	Except for total abstinence or surgical sterilization, the combination pill is the most effective contraceptive known. Failures, even when occasional pills are omitted, are extremely rare, numbering less than 1 per 100 women per year. The sequential pill method, when used correctly, is only slightly less effective, with a failure rate of about 1.4 per 100 women per year. No woman should take the pill until she has had a physical examination by a physician who knows her medical history and has approved its use. Reexaminations are usually performed at 6- to 12-month intervals. Initial and refill prescriptions must be authorized to obtain the pills from a pharmacy or clinic. There are definite contraindications, important warnings, and precautions to both the user and the prescriber, as well as a number of side reactions reported to be associated with the use of the pill. The pill is by far the most acceptable method in terms of numbers because it is reliably effective and its nonmessy, convenient use is unrelated to the timing of sexual play and coitus. It does not interfere with the spontaneity and passion of lovemaking.
Intrauterine devices (IUD)	Objects of different shapes made of plastic or stainless steel are inserted into the uterus by a physician. They may be left in place indefinitely. How the devices prevent pregnancy is not completely understood. They do not prevent the ovary from releasing eggs. At the moment the evidence suggests they probably speed descent of the egg or the egg may reach the uterus at a time when it cannot nest there. (There is also some evidence that they stimulate the production of macrophages, which attack and destroy spermatozoa; see page 631).	The protection afforded by the IUD is superseded only by that of the pill. Protection with the IUD is greater than with such "traditional" methods as the diaphragm or condom, even when these methods are used without any deviation in their regular use. Failures are about 2.7 per 100 women per year. Some women cannot satisfactorily use the devices because of expulsion, bleeding, or discomfort. Contraindications to insertion include pregnancy or suspected pregnancy, abnormalities that distort the uterine cavity, infection or inflammation of the uterus or adnexa, a history of postpartum endometritis, or of infection with abortion within the past three months, and endometrial disease (hyperplasia, carcinoma, polyps, or suspected malignancy). Serious problems reported to be associated with the IUD are pelvic inflammatory disease and perforation of the uterus. Pregnancy can occur with the device in place. Insertion in nulliparous women is restricted because of their narrow cervical canals. Expulsions limit

TABLE 21-1 (*continued*)

METHOD	WHAT IT IS AND HOW IT WORKS	EFFECTIVENESS AND ACCEPTABILITY
		immediate postpartum insertions. IUDs are now inserted in about 7 percent of an obstetrician's contraceptive users. Few general practitioners insert them. IUDs are very acceptable when sustained motivation is lacking, when the user is fearful of using the pill, or when other methods cannot be used successfully.
Diaphragm*	A flexible hemispherical rubber dome, used in combination with cream or jelly which women insert into the vagina to cover the cervix, provides a barrier to spermatozoa. It must be left in place at least 6 hours after intercourse and may be left in place as long as 24 hours. It must be fitted by a physician; refitted every 2 years and after each pregnancy.	Offers a high level of protection, although occasional failures may be expected because of improper insertion or displacement of the diaphragm during sexual intercourse. A rate of 2 to 3 pregnancies per 100 women per year would seem to be a generous estimate for meticulously consistent users. If motivation or self-control is weak, much higher pregnancy rates must be expected. On the average, therefore, failures are about 17.5 per 100 women per year. Many women use the diaphragm successfully. Others have difficulty inserting it correctly, or dislike the procedure required.
Rhythm	This depends on abstinence from intercourse during the time of month when a woman is fertile. Due to menstrual irregularity in many women and the inability to accurately determine the time of ovulation, success with this method may require abstinence for as long as half of every month. While some couples have successfully worked out this system for themselves, most couples will require assistance from a doctor or rhythm clinic.	Self-taught "rhythm," haphazardly practiced, is one of the least effective methods of family planning. For most couples the practice of rhythm is a guessing game. Failures are to be expected in at least 24 per 100 women per year. However, the effectiveness of the rhythm method may approach that of the diaphragm and condom when it is correctly taught, understood, and practiced. Rhythm is generally an unacceptable method, not only because it is unreliable but also because success requires that the woman have regular menstrual cycles (few have) and that both partners accept long periods of abstinence each month.
Surgery: *Vasectomy*	A vasectomy involves a relatively simple operation to prevent the spermatozoa from entering the ejaculate through the tubes (vas deferens) leading from the testes to the urethra in the male. Cutting and tying or ligating of the vas deferens can be done under local anesthesia and usually in less than 30 minutes in the doctor's office or hospital. Ligation of the vas deferens should be considered a permanent procedure since there is no guarantee that fertility will be regained with the tubes reopened.	Once the spermatozoa have been prevented from entering the ejaculate after a vasectomy, the male is considered sterile and his sperm can no longer fertilize the female egg. Many men find this method highly acceptable since it decreases neither the desire or the ability for sexual intercourse nor the amount of ejaculate. Some men, however, experience psychologic effects from a feeling of guilt or fear of lost manhood after this surgical procedure.

*For an excellent review and several expert commentaries about the diaphragm see Aquiles J. Sobrero, "Vaginal Diaphragms," *Medical Aspects of Human Sexuality,* Vol. 75, No. 3 (March 1973), pp. 23, 26–28, 34–35, 37.

TABLE 21-1 (*continued*)		
METHOD	WHAT IT IS AND HOW IT WORKS	EFFECTIVENESS AND ACCEPTABILITY
Tubal ligation	Tubal ligation involves blocking the Fallopian tubes through which the fertilized egg travels from the ovary to the uterus. This procedure, which involves cutting, separating, and tying the tubes, can be done primarily through the abdominal wall or sometimes vaginally and is often performed just after childbirth. Reuniting the tubes is a major surgical procedure, and success may be defined by the fact that the tubes are reopened, but this does not necessarily mean that fertility is restored.	A tubal ligation is virtually 100 percent effective, but failures with this method have been reported. While a tubal ligation is more involved than a vasectomy and must be performed in a hospital, it has become more acceptable to more women who desire permanent sterilization.
Condom	This is a thin, strong sheath or cover, made of rubber or similar material, worn by the man to prevent spermatozoa from entering the vagina. (The woman may also use a vaginal foam, cream, or jelly to provide added protection and lubrication.)	A high degree of protection is offered if the man uses it correctly and consistently. Some couples find the use of condoms objectionable. Failures are due to tearing of the sheath or its slipping off after climax. The condom rates in effectiveness with the diaphragm. There are approximately 16 failures per 100 women per year. The condom is universally accepted as one of the best preventives against venereal disease. A distinct advantage is that it can be purchased without a prescription.
Chemical methods:	These products are inserted into the vagina. Their purpose is to coat vaginal surfaces and cervical opening, and to destroy sperm cells; these products may act as mechanical barriers as well. They provide protection for about 1 hour.	The effectiveness of these vaginal chemical contraceptives used alone is lower than if they are used in combination with a diaphragm or a condom. Nevertheless, significant reductions in pregnancy rates may be obtained by the use of these simple methods. Among these contraceptives the vaginal foams are the most effective, followed by the jellies and creams. Foaming tablets and suppositories are the least effective. Failures with the foam, the best of these methods, are about 28 per 100 women per year. Drainage of the chemical materials from the vagina is objectionable to some couples. Foaming tablets may cause a temporary burning sensation. The foam is acceptable to many women primarily because it is available to them without a prescription.
Vaginal foams	The foam is packed under pressure (like foaming shaving cream); it is inserted with an applicator.	

TABLE 21-1 (continued)		
METHOD	**WHAT IT IS AND HOW IT WORKS**	**EFFECTIVENESS AND ACCEPTABILITY**
Vaginal jellies and creams	These are inserted into the vagina with an applicator.	
Vaginal suppositories	These small cone-shaped objects melt in the vagina. They must be inserted in sufficient time to melt before sexual intercourse.	
Vaginal tablets	The tablets are moistened slightly and inserted into the vagina; foam is produced. They must be inserted in sufficient time for the tablets to disintegrate before sexual intercourse.	

Source: Adapted from "Contraceptive Methods Requiring Consultation with Physician," Searle & Co., San Juan, Puerto Rico.

by one of the greatest researchers who ever lived. "Never forget, gentlemen," said bacteriologist Robert Koch (1843–1910), "that mice are not human beings."

Research on other possible side effects of oral contraceptives indicates that the risk of stroke from a thrombus is about nine times greater than in women who do not use them. It should be emphasized, however, that the risk to the individual woman is very small. In addition, there are reports of a slight rise in blood pressure among users of contraceptive pills. And recent research indicates that oral contraceptives containing estrogen diminish the amount of nutrient protein, fat, and calcium in the milk of the nursing mother. There appears to be no association between use of the contraceptive pill and depression.[19]

The recognized adverse effects of the pill certainly do not warrant its removal from the market at this time.[20] The best insurance is for the woman to follow

[19] "Stroke, High Blood Pressure, Changes in Blood Sugar, Milk Are Pill-Related; No Association with Benign Breast Disease, Mood," *Family Planning Digest,* Vol. 2, No. 5 (September 1973), pp. 12–15.

[20] Philip E. Sartwell, "Oral Contraceptives and Thromboembolic Disease," *Journal of the American Medical Association,* Vol. 220, No. 3 (April 17, 1972), p. 416. This remains true despite several additional reports pointing to problems associated with the use of birth control pills. An ophthalmologist (eye specialist) writes that "dry eyes from oral contraceptives are a . . . fairly frequent finding in refitting contact lenses in our office. If the patient decides to discontinue the medication, it is our clinical impression that adequate tears for wearing contact lenses may not return for a year. Some patients taking the pill develop symptoms of burning and photophobia" (abnormal intolerance to light). This intolerance to light may occur with patients taking the pill even when they do not wear contact lenses. Relief is obtained by the installation of artificial tears or other eye drops. (" 'The Pill' Can Dry Up Contacts," *California Medicine,* Vol. 115, No. 1 [July 1971], p. 33, citing Paul R. Honan, extracted from *Audio-Digest Ophthalmology,* Vol. 7, No. 24, in the Audio-Digest Foundation's Subscription Series of tape-recorded programs.)

A second report indicates that women using birth control pills experience bodily depletion of vitamin C. Previous animal experiments had shown that estrogens (a major component of the contraceptive pill) increase the breakdown of vitamin C. Studied were eighty-eight women: thirty-one were controls; eighteen were pregnant; and thirty-nine were taking oral contraceptives. In each group were European, Asian, and African women. The findings showed that when compared with the controls and the pregnant women, the women who were taking the contraceptive pill had significantly lower vitamin C levels. Apparently, the pill partially inhibits the breakdown of vitamin C for body use. The investigators suggest that the induced deficiency of vitamin C due to the pill may account for some of the reported side effects attributed to oral contraceptive medication. Consequently, they recommend that consideration be given to the use of supplementary vitamins for women the advice of her physician—advice that is tailored to her individual requirements. One requirement is indeed individual. Because of the prolonged bed rest needed to simulate weightlessness, female nurses who volunteered to undergo space flight test conditions could not use oral contraceptives for at least ninety days before the study began. The prolonged bed rest combined with the oral contraceptives might have increased the risk of thromboembolic disease. Nevertheless, the ''nursetronauts'' were found to be just as able as men to withstand the rigors of space. There were a few adjustments in equipment. For example: cardiac monitoring of the women was accomplished through electrodes sewn into their brassieres. Daily fluctuations in body temperature were recorded with the aid of a vaginal capsule that radioed temperatures to laboratory recording devices. Male volunteers had to swallow their temperature recording devices.[21]

tubal ligation

Tubal ligation is an effective method of birth control.[22] By a surgical procedure, the Fallopian tubes are tied and cut or cauterized. So as to avoid another time-consuming and expensive hospitalization, the operation is best performed immediately after the woman has had a child. If the ligation is done after vaginal delivery, an extra day may be required for recovery. If the child is born by cesarean section, no extra time is required for recuperation. Although the struc-

---

taking oral contraceptives. Interestingly, the injected contraceptive that was studied did not appear to influence vitamin C levels. (Michael Briggs and Maxine Briggs, ''Vitamin C requirements and Oral Contraceptives,'' *Nature,* Vol. 238, No. 5362 [August 4, 1972], p. 277.) It is not known whether women taking oral contraceptives suffer more episodes of upper respiratory infections than women who do not (see Chapter 22, pages 652–53, and Chapter 6, footnote 7, page 163).

The contraceptive pill has been noted to have other effects pertaining to nutrition. Exclusive of the fetus, membranes, and amniotic fluid, the weight gain of a woman during pregnancy is about ten pounds; most women gain about six pounds when they begin to take oral contraceptives. In both instances the weight gain may be due to fluid retention, breast enlargement, and some impairment of carbohydrate metabolism. Moreover, there may be an increased need for one of the components of the vitamin B complex called *pyridoxine.* ''Clinical investigators have already reported that women who have annoying headaches or depression as a result of the pill often obtain marked or complete relief when they take supplements of pyridoxine. Some have experienced relief from nausea and vomiting, but it is important to note that [controlled] studies must be performed for firm conclusions.'' (Robert E. Hodges, ''Nutrition and the Pill,'' *Journal of the American Dietetic Association,* Vol. 59, No. 3 [September 1971], pp. 215–16, citing M. Baumblatt and F. Winston, ''Pyridoxine and the Pill,'' Letters to the Editor, *Lancet,* Vol. 1, No. 7651 [April 18, 1970], p. 832; D. P. Rose and I. P. Braidman, ''Oral Contraceptives, Depression, and Amino-Acid Metabolism,'' Letters to the Editor, *Lancet,* Vol. 1, No. 7656 [May 23, 1970], p. 1117; and A. L. Luhby, P. Davis, M. Murphy, and M. Gordon, ''Pyridoxine and Oral Contraceptives,'' Letters to the Editor, *Lancet,* Vol. 2, No. 7682 [November 21, 1970], p. 1083.) It is of interest to note that pyridoxine is sometimes used in the treatment of nausea and vomiting during pregnancy. Reports about its benefits vary.

Still another observation concerning the contraceptive pill has been reported by a Baylor College of Medicine gynecologist. ''The most frequent cause today for copious vaginal discharge unrelated to vaginal pathogens [any disease-producing microbe or material causing vaginal disease] is the taking of birth control pills.'' The chief source of this type of functional secretion is the cervix. He believes that the sequential type of contraceptive pill causes more secretion than the low estrogen dosage combined type. This is due to its relatively high dosage of estrogen. However, a profuse vaginal discharge may be due to a variety of causes. The diagnosis includes laboratory analysis of both normal and possibly abnormal vaginal microbes. (Herman L. Gardner, ''Unexplained Leukorrhea,'' *Medical Aspects of Human Sexuality,* Vol. 6, No. 5 [May 1972], p. 181.)

There is excellent reason for using birth control pills for the treatment of acne. They are often quite helpful and the risks are small. (Albert M. Kligman, ''Oral Contraceptive Therapy for Severe Acne in a Woman,'' *Journal of the American Medical Association,* Vol. 224, No. 2 [April 9, 1973], p. 257.)

[21] ''Space Medicine: Nursetronauts,'' *Medical World News,* Vol. 14, No. 41 (November 9, 1973), p. 5.

[22] Contraception allows intercourse between fertile partners while preventing conception. Since a tubal ligation renders the female infertile, it is not a contraceptive method, although it is a method of birth control.

tures may sometimes be rejoined later, tubal ligation is usually irreversible. A new method of tubal ligation that can be performed with local anesthesia is now being tried. Only one abdominal incision is necessary, and the operation can be an outpatient procedure. An instrument is inserted into an incision that is approximately the diameter of a finger. The instrument has a light so that the Fallopian tubes can be located and cauterized. Also being developed is an instrument that will apply a clip around the tubes rather than cauterize them.

The majority of women who have had tubal ligations suffer no emotional problems as a result. Many, totally freed from the nagging fear of pregnancy, report enhanced coital enjoyment. As is the case with vasectomy in men (see the following section), the incidence of emotional problems following tubal ligation varies with the individual and with circumstances. A woman who previously has had a difficult pregnancy, or whose husband's earning power is inadequate, or who fears that her child might have a hereditary defect, may find that the tubal ligation increases her sexual pleasure. However, a woman who considers the operation to violate her religious beliefs, or who feels that her feminine image depends on her fertility, may regret the ligation and experience diminished sexual enjoyment.[23]

birth control for the male[24]

There are fewer contraceptive methods available to the male than to the female. Aside from condoms (see Table 21-1) and coitus interruptus, the only male birth control method currently in use is vasectomy.[25] Vasectomy is the surgical removal of a portion of the vas deferens (see page 469). When the operation is complete, the spermatozoa that are formed in the testes no longer reach the ejaculatory ducts (which lie on each side of the prostatic urethra) via the seminal vesicles. Therefore newly formed spermatozoa cannot become part of the semen. However, after vasectomy, residual spermatozoa are left in that part of the vas deferens on each side that remains connected to the seminal vesicles. It requires several ejaculations for the residual spermatozoa to leave the body. During that time the man remains fertile. In one series of 1,000 vasectomies, it was not until ten weeks after surgery that 94.5 percent of the patients were considered sterile. The overall complication rate was 7.6 percent. These varied from swelling due to effusion of blood to inflammation of various tissues in the area.[26] Several postoperative microscopic examinations of the semen for spermatozoa are necessary to ascertain sterility.

Vasectomy is legal in all fifty states, although in Utah it may be performed only if medically indicated. In 1972, the Utah statue was being challenged in the courts. Usually only local anesthesia is required. Two very small incisions are made in the scrotum. The vas deferens is then easily exposed and cut. A tiny section of each vas deferens is removed. The cut ends are then sutured. A few stitches close the skin incision. By the day after the operation, about

[23] Eleanor B. Easley, "Sexual Effect of Female Sterilization," *Medical Aspects of Human Sexuality,* Vol. 6, No. 2 (February 1972), p. 58.

[24] For an excellent review of this subject see Joan Solomon, "The Second Reproducers," *The Sciences,* Vol. 13, No. 6 (July–August 1973), pp. 11–15.

[25] Like a tubal ligation, a vasectomy is not a contraceptive method, although it is a method of birth control.

[26] "Vasectomy Complications Aplenty," *Medical World News,* Vol. 13, No. 41 (November 3, 1972), p. 19.

two-thirds of all patients can move about normally. The rest require a day or two longer to recuperate. Approximately one man in four has moderate pain at the operative site or some swelling of the testicles. Neither is usually cause for concern, and they subside in a week or two. Failures are uncommon. The vas deferens may recanalize itself, and the patient again become fertile. This is rare. In some cases the operation can be reversed; however, this possibility cannot be predicted. The man who is considering a vasectomy at this time should consider the possibility that he may never again be fertile. For some men, this realization may have adverse psychological effects. There are surgical procedures for reversing a vasectomy. The operation is prolonged (about two hours) and expensive, with about a 25 percent chance of success. Sufficient repair of the originally interrupted nerve and blood supplies is one of the difficulties faced by the surgeon.[27]

Antibodies to spermatozoa have been identified in the blood of some men who have had vasectomies. The blocked-up sperm may act as an antigen (antibody generator; see page 142). The antibodies have remained in the blood stream for at least a year, and they may further diminish the chances of reversing the effects of the operation.[28] Even if the operation were successfully reversed, the man might be producing an immunity to his own spermatozoa that could prolong his infertility.[29]

The problem of the irreversible vasectomy is being investigated. Now under study is a mechanical device made of gold and stainless steel. It is permanently implanted in the vas deferens and has a tiny faucetlike valve that may be set on or off. A second operation is necessary to change the position of the valve. Other experimental instruments that may make vasectomies reversible employ clips, threads, chemicals, and catheters as blocking mechanisms.

Vasectomy does not affect erection, climax, ejaculation, or volume of ejaculation. Thus it usually does not affect the man's response during sexual intercourse. Moreover, the operation has no demonstrated effect on the production of spermatozoa or of the male sex hormone testosterone (see page 467). Almost all patients report both no change in physical health and a significant increase in coital frequency following the operation. They claim to feel freer and more satisfied with sexual intercourse, and report little change in "duration of ejaculation, control of ejaculation," and ease and "strength of erection." In the opinion of most husbands, "wives seem less restrained in intercourse and . . . over half of them obtain climax more easily."[30] It is emphasized that these are patient opinions.

[27] "Regaining Fertility—Tough Road," *Medical World News,* Vol. 13, No. 41 (November 3, 1972), pp. 17–18.

[28] "Antibodies to Sperm May Form After Vasectomy," *Journal of the American Medical Association,* Vol. 217, No. 10 (September 6, 1971), p. 1310.

[29] Harold Lear, "Vasectomy—A Note of Concern," *Journal of the American Medical Association,* Vol. 219, No. 9 (February 28, 1972), p. 1207, citing A. M. Phadke and K. Padukone, "Presence and Significance of Autoantibodies Against Spermatozoa in the Blood of Men with Obstructed Vas Deferens," *Journal of Reproduction and Fertility,* Vol. 7 (1964), pp. 163–70. For two brief but excellent answers to a question about the immunological effects of vasectomy, see the reviews of John Bernard Henry and Fletcher C. Derrick, Jr., in the "Questions and Answers" section of the *Journal of the American Medical Association,* Vol. 225, No. 6 (August 6, 1973), p. 642.

[30] Andrew Ferber and William L. Ferber, "Vasectomy," *Medical Aspects of Human Sexuality,* Vol. 2, No. 6 (June 1968), p. 34.

> Interestingly, careful psychological study does not entirely support the opinions of the patients . . . Although the effects were not dramatic . . . adverse changes in psychological functioning following vasectomy were confirmed . . . The data suggest that the operation is responded to as though it had [a] demasculinizing potential, with a result that the behavior of the man after vasectomy is more likely to be scrutinized by himself and others for evidence of unmasculine features.[31]

Sometimes the operation led to self-scrutiny that was actually beneficial. Some men were able to improve their formerly immature and indecisive behavior pattern. In others, however, the operation was followed by an increased level of anxiety that interfered with marital harmony. This observation has been confirmed by other studies that suggest that "vasectomized men, their friends, their relatives, and their physicians equate vasectomy with castration and masculine inferiority"[32] and that "other couples denigrated those who chose vasectomy as a method of birth control."[33]

How frequent are postvasectomy psychological problems? "The most optimistic surveys indicate a potential three percent casualty rate, and others report a much higher incidence of psychological implications."[34] Such difficulties occur much more frequently in men who have experienced sexual dysfunctions or emotional problems before vasectomy, who have not sought and obtained wholehearted agreement from their wives, and who have not rationally considered all the implications of the operation, including its probable permanence. If a man divorces and remarries, he meets with a new marital situation that may cause him to bitterly regret his vasectomy. The same may be true should he become a widower. Vasectomy should not be considered casually. The decision is best made in a conference between the physician and both marital partners.[35]

[31] F. J. Ziegler, D. A. Rogers, and S. A. Kriegsman, "Effect of Vasectomy on Psychological Functioning," *Psychosomatic Medicine,* Vol. 28 (1966), p. 50.

[32] A. S. Ferber, C. Tietze, and S. Lewit, "Men with Vasectomies: A Study of Medical, Sexual, and Psychosocial Changes," *Psychosomatic Medicine,* Vol. 29, No. 4 (July-August 1967), p. 354.

[33] D. A. Rogers, F. J. Ziegler, and N. Levy, "Prevailing Cultural Attitudes About Vasectomy: Possible Explanation of Postoperative Psychological Response," *Psychosomatic Medicine,* Vol. 29 (1967), p. 367. Note, however, that vasectomy has become much more socially approved; the rate of psychological problems may have lessened greatly since 1967.

[34] Harold Lear, "Vasectomy—A Note of Concern," p. 1207, citing *Vasectomy: Follow-up of 1,000 Cases, Simon Population Trust Sterilization Project* (Cambridge, England, 1969), and H. Wolfers, "Psychological Aspects of Vasectomy," *British Medical Journal,* Vol. 4, No. 5730 (October 31, 1970), pp. 297, 300.

[35] Pauline Jackson, Betson Phillips, Elizabeth Prosser, H. O. Jones, V. R. Tindall, D. L. Crosby, I. D. Cooke, J. M. McGarry, and R. R. Rees, "A Male Sterilization Clinic," *British Medical Journal,* Vol. 4, No. 5730 (October 31, 1970), pp. 295–97. Vasectomies are essentially easier and safer than tubal ligations. One psychiatrist has noted that when a couple chooses a ligation, it may be a sign of marital discord. The man may believe that his wife should have the ligation because it is she who bears the children; this may imply that he considers her to be merely a sex object. Or he may think that he will want to have children with another woman in the future; this may suggest a lack of permanent commitment to his wife. Third, the man may feel that vasectomy will make him less of a man; thus, he erroneously equates vasectomy with castration. Examination and recognition of these feelings may be helpful in resolving some marital difficulties. ("When You Get a Vasectomy . . .," *Science News,* Vol. 103, No. 10 [March 10, 1973], p. 152.)

By no means, however, should it be assumed that the choice of sterilization depends mostly on marital discord. The prevalence of sterilization increases as the woman gets older and also as the number of children in the family increases. Race also plays a role. In 1970, vasectomy was extremely rare among blacks (1 percent of the risk population, compared to 9 percent of the white risk population). In that year, on the other hand, tubal ligations were twice as prevalent among black women as among white women. As of 1970, women of low educational levels were much more inclined to have tubal ligations than their husbands a vasectomy. Religion is also a factor; in 1970 the percentage of Protestant couples who were sterilized was more than twice that of Catholic couples (22 versus 10 percent). Among all couples sterilized between 1965 and 1970, the wife averaged 31.8 years of age; the husband averaged 35.1 years of age. They had been married 11.5 years

Studies with immature rats whose vas deferens were cut have shown both a significant rate of shrinkage of the testes and reduction of testosterone.[36] This occurred in young, growing animals. This experiment must be repeated in other laboratories with special attention to varying surgical procedures. Whether operations on mature tissues have the same results demands urgent investigation.[37]

There is no proof that vasectomized men are more prone to disease later in life. Nor is there, as yet, adequate proof that they are not. Pointing to this gap, researcher Nancy Alexander recently said, "Vasectomy is probably not detrimental for most individuals, but it may well be for some . . . We can't identify which is which, in our present state of knowledge."[38] She opposes discontinuance of vasectomy, but calls for more extensive long-term studies of the procedure. And, although "valid social ends do not justify unscientific means,"[39] results with laboratory animals can by no means always be applied to human beings. Between 1969 and 1972, an estimated 2.5 million U.S. men had vasectomies. Serious reactions have been in the minority. How significant vasectomy risks are on a long-term basis only time will tell. For those who accept the possibility of future complications, vasectomy remains an effective method of birth control in selected cases.

semen banks: fertility insurance?

Competent medical authorities have advised against relying on spermatozoa banks for long-term fertility insurance.[40] Long-term storage of spermatozoa apparently diminishes their viability. Freezing and thawing an average specimen of spermatozoa reduces their motility by half. After three years, additional deterioration occurs that further reduces the number of live spermatozoa in a semen specimen. A large number of motile spermatozoa is essential for successful long-term storage. However, after three years of freezing, seven samples often provide spermatozoa of which only 25 percent are motile. Few women have been successfully inseminated and carried pregnancies to term as a result of the use of semen specimens stored longer than one year. Even short-term freezing of semen may have some deleterious effect.[41] By 1972, the longest well-documented time in which thawed spermatozoa had been suc-

---

and had an averge of 2.8 children. They had waited 3.9 years after the birth of their last wanted child before seeking sterilization. ("One in Six Couples Who Want No More Children Have Contraceptive Sterilizations," *Family Planning Digest,* Vol. 2, No. 2 [March 1973], pp. 8–9.)

[36] Arthur M. Sackler, A. Stanley Weltman, Vijay Pandhi, and Ralph Schwartz, "Gonadal Effects of Vasectomy and Vasoligation," *Science,* Vol. 179, No. 4070 (January 19, 1973), pp. 293–95.

[37] "Fresh Anxiety Over the Consequences of Vasectomy," *New Scientist,* Vol. 57, No. 830 (January 25, 1973), p. 172.

[38] "Experts Stress Need for Vasectomy Studies," *Hospital Tribune,* Vol. 7, No. 6 (February 12, 1973), p. 4.

[39] Arthur M. Sackler, A. Stanley Weltman, Vijay Pandhi, and Ralph Schwartz, "Gonadal Effects of Vasectomy and Vasoligation," p. 293.

[40] "MD Groups Caution Men on Semen Banks," *Family Planning Digest,* Vol. 1, No. 5 (September 1972), p. 14.

[41] "Study Shows Freezing Sperm Decreases Conception Rate; Continued Research Urged," *Family Planning Digest,* Vol. 2, No. 3 (May 1973), pp. 1–2, citing K. D. Smith and E. Steinberger, "Survival of Spermatozoa in a Human Sperm Bank," *Journal of the American Medical Association,* Vol. 223 (1973), p. 774, and E. Steinberger and K. D. Smith, "Artificial Insemination with Fresh or Frozen Semen," *Journal of the American Medical Association,* Vol. 223 (1973), p. 778.

cessfully used for insemination was sixteen months after freezing. As of that year, approximately four hundred children in the world had been born as a result of impregnation with thawed spermatozoa; the oldest child was sixteen. To date, no undue increase in genetic problems has been noted; however, longer-term studies are necessary.[42]

research on contraceptives

Extensive research on contraceptives is being conducted both in this country and abroad. In mid-1971, no fewer than fifteen experimental methods were being tested on consenting men and women.

> The list includes: daily, weekly, and monthly pills for use by women; semi-permanent under-skin capsules for men or women; intermittently-used vaginal inserts or chronically used intrauterine inserts which act as carriers of . . . infertility agents; pills taken intermittently by women on the basis of coital exposure—before or after; intravenous infusion to terminate an early pregnancy . . . a remarkable foreign body placed in the vas deferens to impair male fertility; vaginal tablets to induce menstrual flow—whether or not a fertilization has occurred, or to cause abortion at a later stage.[43]

One new method, requiring the oral ingestion of small, daily doses of progestin (the synthetic form of the hormone released by the corpus luteum; see page 478) has already been approved by the FDA. Known as the minipill, it is taken daily throughout the year. It is safer but not quite as effective as the other two kinds of oral contraceptives and, moreover, is often associated with irregular bleeding patterns.[44]

Another promising method also involves the use of progestin. The synthetic hormone is stored in a small Silastic container that is inserted under the skin. Minute doses of progestin are released into the blood stream. Studies of this contraceptive method are being conducted in the United States, India, Chile, Brazil, and Italy. With its use, the risk of forgetting to take the daily pill is averted. Still another product containing a synthetic progesterone can be injected intramuscularly and remain in place as a depot. From this focal point, measured amounts of the hormone are released into the blood. By midsummer 1968 ''a long-acting contraceptive administered to women by injection once every three months . . . proved effective during three years of clinical trial.[45] Late in 1973, the Food and Drug Administration approved the limited use of an injectable contraceptive called Depo Provera (its chemical name is medroxy-

[42] ''Vasectomy Patients Multiply, but Doubts Linger,'' *American Medical News,* Vol. 15, No. 6 (April 24, 1972), pp. 8–9.

[43] Sheldon J. Segal, ''Beyond the Laboratory: Recent Research Advances in Fertility Regulation,'' *Family Planning Perspectives,* Vol. 3, No. 3 (July 1971), pp. 17–21.

[44] U.S. Department of Health, Education, and Welfare, Public Health Service, *FDA Drug Bulletin* (December 1972), p. 3. The FDA notes that, although the new minipill is a pure synthetic progesterone (progestin), it has a built-in estrogenic component. Up to 8 percent of the minipills' degradation products becomes biologically active estrogen. What significance this has is unknown. Studies have yet to be done to determine whether the progestin-only pill is associated with thromboembolic disease. (''Minipills: Progestin-Only Orals Approved by FDA,'' *Family Planning Digest,* Vol. 2, No. 3 [May 1973], p. 4. See also ''Bleeding, Pregnancy Problems Found in Five Minipills Tested,'' *Family Planning Digest,* Vol. 2, No. 1 [January 1973], pp. 10–11.)

[45] ''The Long-Acting Contraceptives: Quarterly Injections Pass Three-Year Trials,'' *Journal of the American Medical Association,* Vol. 204, No. 11 (June 10, 1968), p. 35.

progesterone acetate). It is recommended not for the general population, but for certain women who refuse oral contraceptives, are unable to accept the responsibility of taking them, cannot tolerate their side effects, or have had no success with the use of other contraceptive methods. The drug is injected at three-month intervals. Its major drawback: present evidence indicates that most women can become pregnant after discontinuing the drug, but only after some months; some women apparently cannot become pregnant. Moreover, although there is no evidence that the drug causes an increase of breast cancer in women, it may do so in dogs. Use of this drug will be carefully controlled by the FDA.[46]

A nine-year study of 907 Mexican women between nineteen and forty-five years old of proven fertility provides encouraging data about the acceptability of contraceptive injections despite their sometimes disagreeable side effects. The study population comprised one group of 839 low-income women in Mexico City and a second group of 68 women who lived in a remote rural area. The rural women received only injectable contraceptives. The city women had a choice between injectable and oral contraceptives. One-half of the city women chose the injections. One of the reasons for this was the women's belief that injections were more effective than oral medication. Three injectable contraceptives were used. Side effects included irregular periods of bleeding, headache, dizziness, and nervousness. Only a very small percentage of the women discontinued the injections for these reasons. The majority of the women were pleased to be relieved of the need to take a daily pill and were grateful for the long-acting (up to eighty-four days) injectable contraceptives. The most serious of the complications was occasional severe bleeding, which could be a problem with women suffering malnutritional anemia.[47] The ability of Silastic to store and gradually release birth control drugs is being used in still another way. Progestin is being incorporated into Silastic vaginal rings. When placed in the vagina, the rings release a small amount of progestin that is absorbed by the blood via the vaginal mucous membrane.

Morning-after pills are also under investigation. A recent study demonstrated their effectiveness. "One thousand women of child-bearing age were given, within 72 hours of sexual exposure, 25 mg [milligrams] of diethylstilbesterol twice daily for five days. No pregnancies resulted and there were no serious adverse reactions."[48] Diethylstilbesterol (DES) is one of the synthetic estrogens. The hormone apparently acts on the uterine lining, making implantation unlikely. It may also increase the speed of the descent of the ovum. Since the probability of conception from a single unprotected coitus is between 1 in 50 and 1 in 25, these results are indeed promising.[49] The effects of their long-

[46] "FDA Okays Limited Used of Injectable Contraceptive," *Journal of the American Medical Association,* Vol. 226, No. 7 (November 12, 1973), pp. 734–35.

[47] "Contraceptive 'Shots' Prove to Be Effective," *Journal of the American Medical Association,* Vol. 220, No. 8 (May 22, 1972), pp. 1061–65.

[48] Lucile Kirtland Kuchera, "Postcoital Contraception with Diethylstilbesterol," *Journal of the American Medical Association,* Vol. 218, No. 4 (October 25, 1971), p. 562. See also Lucile Kirtland Kuchera, "Stilbesterol as a 'Morning After' Pill," *Medical Aspects of Human Sexuality,* Vol. 6, No. 10 (October 1972), pp. 169, 173, 177.

[49] *Ibid.,* citing C. Tietze, "Problems of Pregnancy Resulting from a Single Unprotected Coitus," *Fertility and Sterility,* Vol. 11 (September–October 1960), pp. 485–88.

term or frequent use have yet to be intensively studied, nor has the significance of their disagreeable aftereffects in some persons been ascertained.

In May 1973, the Federal Food and Drug Administration approved, under restricted conditions, postcoital contraceptive use of DES as an emergency measure. Situations warranting its use were rape, incest, or where, in the physician's judgment, the patient's physical or emotional well-being was in jeopardy. The FDA explicity warned against its routine or frequent use as a contraceptive. Pregnancy was to be ruled out by appropriate tests before DES was administered. "Failure of postcoital treatment with DES deserves serious consideration of voluntary abortion."[50] The following paragraph explains why.

In very small single doses, diethylstilbesterol was widely used between 1945 and 1965 as an accepted treatment of spontaneous abortion (see page 636) and as a prophylactic in asymptomatic patients. Recent studies suggest an association between a woman's ingestion of stilbesterol during pregnancy and the development, years later, of a type of cancer of the vagina in her daughters.[51] In November 1971, the Food and Drug Administration warned physicians of this statistically significant association.[52] Throughout the nation physicians are examining their records to find "stilbesterol offspring." Such efforts are not unwarranted. By the end of 1973, about one hundred "DES babies" had been found to have vaginal malignancies. But further studies showed more. They indicated that a considerable proportion of patients with a history of *in utero* exposure to DES and similar agents had other, nonmalignant lesions of the vagina and the cervix. Although it has not been proved that these lesions become cancerous, it cannot be denied that there is a risk. Early diagnosis and treatment give excellent results.[53] On the basis of data obtained from animal experiments, diethylstilbesterol is now thought to be a carcinogen; it should not be added to chicken feeds or be present in beef for human consumption.[54]

A family of body chemicals that may be used to control fertility are the *prostaglandins.* These hormonelike substances are found in many tissues and fluids of the body. Prostaglandins are an important component of human semi-

[50] "Postcoital Diethylstilbesterol," *FDA Drug Bulletin,* U.S. Department of Health, Education, and Welfare (May 1973), p. 1.

[51] A. L. Herbst, H. Ulfelder, and D. C. Poskanzer, "Adenocarcinoma of the Vagina: Association of Maternal Stilbesterol Therapy with Tumor Appearance in Young Women," *New England Journal of Medicine,* Vol. 284, No. 16 (April 22, 1971), pp. 878–81. P. Greenwald, J. J. Barlow, P. C. Nasca, *et al.,* "Vaginal Cancer After Maternal Treatment with Synthetic Estrogens," *New England Journal of Medicine,* Vol. 285, No. 7 (August 12, 1971), pp. 390–92.

[52] "Diethylstilbesterol Contraindicated in Pregnancy: Drugs Used Linked to Adenocarcinoma in the Offspring," *FDA Drug Bulletin,* U.S. Department of Health, Education, and Welfare (November 1971).

[53] "Nine Out of Ten 'DES' Babies Have Vaginal Adenosis," *Medical World News,* Vol. 14, No. 4 (November 9, 1973), pp. 17–19.

[54] Frederick B. Hodges, "Diethylstilbesterol: Problems of Unusual Drug Dosage and Administration," Public Health Reports, *California Medicine,* Vol. 116, No. 2 (February 1972), p. 84. Nevertheless, it was not until late summer of 1972 that the Food and Drug Administration reversed its previous defense of DES. The ban on its use did not become effective until April 27, 1973; until then, the use of this cancer-causing substance with meat animals was permitted in the form of a pellet implanted in the animal's ear. This caused considerable concern among scientists, who considered the FDA's change of position belated. "On the day following its ban, the Senate health subcommittee passed a bill proposing a complete and immediate ban on DES. Maybe the FDA decided to act against the carcinogen before Congress did it for them." (Nicholas Wade, "FDA Invents More Tales About DES," *Science,* Vol. 177, No. 4048 [August 11, 1972], p. 503.)

nal fluid and are also found in menstrual fluid. Despite their name, they are formed in the seminal vesicles (see page 469), and not the prostate.[55] The effect of the prostaglandins on the body is astonishingly versatile. For example, they are involved in the regulation of blood pressure and the stimulation and relaxation of smooth muscle. The extent of their action is just beginning to be understood. Since the prostaglandins stimulate contractions of the uterus, they have been found effective in inducing labor and terminating unwanted pregnancies. They are also being tried as an ''after-the-fact'' method of birth control. The contracting uterus brings on menstruation; the ovum is expelled, whether or not it has been fertilized. The mechanism by which menstruation is induced is not yet known.[56] In addition, the prostaglandins have been suggested as a possibly effective means of inducing menstruation in cases of menstrual failure. Although much research remains to be done, the use of prostaglandins is considered by some researchers to be the most important advance in fertility control since the introduction of oral contraceptives.

Since surgical abortions after the first trimester are not as safe as those performed earlier, the prostaglandins eventually may be used to induce abortions at a later stage of pregnancy. In December 1973, the Food and Drug Administration approved the commerical medical use of prostaglandins to induce abortion in the second trimester of pregnancy.[57] But at present, they do not seem to be always effective. Several prostaglandins have already been synthesized in the laboratory. It should be emphasized that prostaglandins act on almost all body systems. Much needs to be learned not only about their side effects, but also about how they are metabolized in the body. Present prospects for an effective oral form of prostaglandins (that might be used as a method of birth control) are dim because of the very rapid destruction of natural prostaglandins in the body. The development of a synthetic prostaglandin analogue ''could not be expected before the next decade at the earliest.''[58]

some precautions about the use of IUDs

Intrauterine devices are being used for birth control by more than 3 million women in this country. Their mechanism is believed to depend on the foreign-body reaction they produce. An estimated 10 percent of IUDs are expelled during the first year after insertion; this occurs most frequently among younger women and during menstruation. Adverse reactions include excessive bleeding, inflammatory disease within the pelvis, and perforation of the uterus. Less serious adverse reactions are irregular bleeding, uterine cramps, pelvic pain, and backache (see Table 21-1, page 619). The FDA has received numerous

21-2 *How the IUD is believed to work: macrophages (see page 143) attack the IUD and thus also attack and destroy spermatozoa* (arrow).

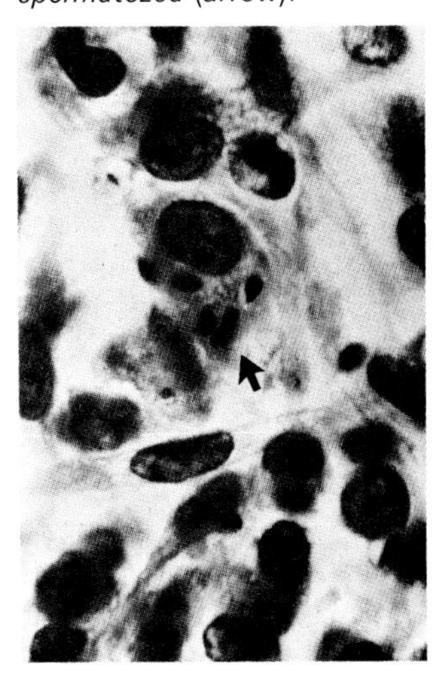

[55] John E. Pike, ''Prostaglandins,'' *Scientific American*, Vol. 225, No. 5 (November 1971), p. 84.

[56] ''Birth Control Method Tried 'After-the-Fact,' '' *HSMHA Health Reports*, Vol. 87, No. 1 (January 1972), p. 84.

[57] ''Prostaglandins: Legal for Abortion,'' *Medical World News*, Vol. 14, No. 48 (December 28, 1973), pp. 4–5.

[58] Carl Djerassi, ''Fertility Control Through Abortion: An Assessment of the Period 1950–1980,'' *Science and Public Affairs: Bulletin of the Atomic Scientists*, Vol. 28, No. 1 (January 1972), p. 44. For a discussion of the potential of LH–RH as a contraceptive see page 635, footnote 65.

complaints about an IUD known as the Majzlin Spring. "The danger of the device imbedding in the walls of the uterus increases the longer it is left in place."[59] Women using this particular IUD should have their physicians remove it. The FDA is preparing to establish appropriate controls over IUDs. At the present time this agency believes they are safe and effective, provided adequate precautions are taken.

possible improvements on the rhythm method

Several new methods of predicting the "safe period" for coitus are presently being investigated that are of particular interest to those who wish to use the rhythm method (see Table 21-1 and pages 472–76). It has recently been discovered that the amount in the saliva of an enzyme called alkaline phosphatase increases just before ovulation. Every day the woman places in her mouth a paper strip containing a chemical that reacts to a high level of alkaline phosphatase. When the paper strip turns blue, the woman is ovulating. The woman can then avoid intercourse accordingly.

Another method of determining the safe period depends on the changing quality of the mucus in the vagina during the menstrual cycle.[60] Studies have indicated that following menstrual bleeding there is a variable number of days in which there is no vaginal discharge. Then an increasing amount of a cloudy, sticky secretion becomes noticeable. The duration of this, too, is variable. Before ovulation, the consistency of the mucus changes. It becomes clear and slippery, has the characteristics of raw egg white, and produces a feeling of lubrication. This lasts from one to two days; the last day of its occurrence is called the "peak mucus symptom" and is closely correlated with the day of ovulation. After ovulation, the mucus becomes thick and opaque for a variable number of days. It has been suggested that conception may be avoided by abstaining from intercourse during the peak of mucus symptom and for four days afterward. One advantage of the method is that under a physician's supervision it can be easily learned. Women are advised not to have intercourse during the first menstrual cycle in which they are learning the method. Disadvantages of the method include the irregularity of ovulation in some women and the confusion of the ordinary mucous discharge with one that requires treatment. This procedure, which is of doubtful reliability, is being further studied.

why no male pill?

"1984 appears to be an exceedingly optimistic target date for development of a male contraceptive pill ready for use by the public."[61] Why? First, the basic knowledge of male reproductive biology is even less advanced than that of female. To improve on that knowledge would require extensive research with

[59] "Intrauterine Devices: Precautions During Use," *FDA Drug Bulletin,* U.S. Department of Health, Education, and Welfare (August 1973), p. 1.
[60] E. L. Billings, J. J. Billings, J. B. Brown, and H. G. Burger, "Symptoms and Hormonal Changes Accompanying Ovulation," *Lancet,* Vol. 1, No. 7745 (February 5, 1972). p. 282.
[61] Carl Djerassi, "Birth Control After 1984," *Science,* Vol. 169, No. 3949 (September 1970), p. 946.

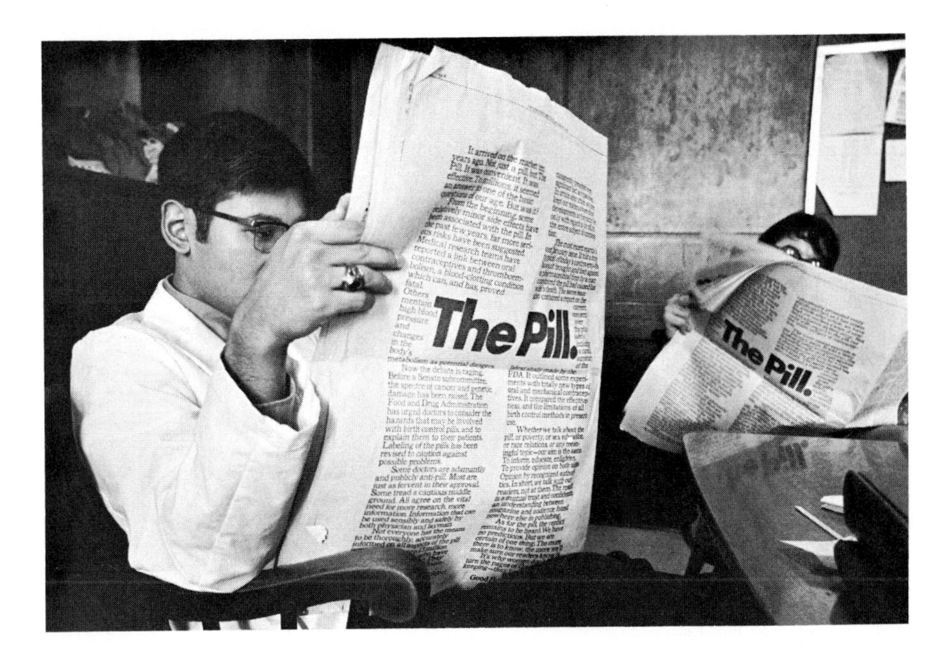

21-3

exceedingly expensive and still relatively unavailable infrahuman primates, such as chimpanzees.[62] This obstacle will take years to overcome. Second, the presently known variety of chemical agents that affect the fertility of male animals such as the rat are either toxic or potentially poisonous to man.[63] Third, evolutionary changes necessary to ensure human survival have occurred much more frequently with the female. One example of such a change is the limited production of ova by the human female that are capable of being fertilized—about four hundred in a lifetime. The human male still produces millions of spermatozoa. However, the human female usually releases but one egg at a time, and each egg is nourished singly to come to maturity in its own elaborately ripened follicular abode. Fourth, the male has fewer steps in his reproductive cycle that are vulnerable to controlled interference. The maturation of the ovum, ovulation, the pick-up and beginning transport of the ovum down the Fallopian tube, its fertilization, the continued transport down the tube of the beginning life in the resulting zygote, and the eventual implantation in the prepared uterine endometrium—these are some episodes in the woman's re-

[62] Carl Djerassi, "Fertility Control Through Abortion: An Assessment of the Period 1950–1980," p. 41. This article is also essential for learning more about the female's reproductive process.

[63] Carl Djerassi, "Birth Control After 1984," p. 947, citing "Developments in Fertility Control," *World Health Organization Technical Reprint Series,* No. 424 (1969). This research should not be confused with the discovery in Germany of a new drug called cyproterone acetate, which, it is reported, chemically castrates men. It counters the effect of androgen, but does not produce feminizing effects. Since it blocks testosterone, it reduces sexual desire and the capacity to have an erection and orgasm, and prevents sexual fantasies. Its action is believed to be reversible. That it may be used in prisoners with long histories of sexual offenses is causing considerable disquiet among European scientists. There should be more widespread information about this and similar drugs, and a code of ethics to govern their use—if such use can be justified. ("Chemical Castration," *New Scientist,* Vol. 57, No. 836 [March 8, 1973], pp. 523–24.)

productive history that are possibly amenable to scientific interference. Added to these are conditions that influence the possibilities of fertilization, such as the penetrability of the cervical mucus to spermatozoa, and the changing state of the endometrium. In contrast, the male reproductive cycle is vulnerable at only its three basic steps: the production of spermatozoa in the testes, the storage and maturation of spermatozoa in the epididymis, and the transportation of spermatozoa via the vas deferens. Along with these areas of interference, scientists have thought of the possibility of changing the chemical composition of the seminal fluid. Research is presently being directed into all these possibilities. "The future of research in male fertility control should not be viewed with gloom. . . . There seems good reason to expect the eventual development of successful methods."[64]

brain chemicals: the ultimate control of reproduction

On a late midsummer afternoon in 1971, Andrew V. Schally, of Tulane University's School of Medicine, rose to deliver a paper at a meeting of the American Endocrine Society. What he had to say made worldwide scientific headlines. In the laboratory, his group had successfully synthesized the ultimate control in the reproductive hormone network. That control is in the form of a releasing factor (or hormone) generated in the brain's hypothalamus. This factor is now known as the *luteinizing hormone–releasing hormone* (*LH–RH*). It has not yet been shown that the follicle-stimulating hormone has its own releasing factor. However, it is known that the hypothalamic hormone LH–RH induces not only the release of luteinizing hormone (LH) but of follicle-stimulating hormone (FSH) as well. (For this reason some scientists refer to the hormone as a single entity, calling it LH–RH/FSH–RH.)

Specific signals from the central nervous system are decoded and the hypothalamus produces the releasing factor. Upon reaching the anterior lobe of the pituitary, LH–RH is responsible for the release of luteinizing hormone (LH) and, apparently, follicle-stimulating hormone too. In the female, FSH stimulates the growth and maturation of the follicles in the ovaries (see page 474). But of the two to thirty-two follicles that begin to mature in each cycle only one will usually come to complete maturity. LH, helped by FSH, promotes the maturation of that single follicle and, following its maturation, LH causes the rupture of the follicular wall and the release of the ovum (*ovulation;* see page 475). Moreover, in the human being, LH also stimulates the corpus luteum to release progesterone (see page 478). The male hypothalamus generates the same releasing factor as that of the female; in addition, the anterior lobe of his pituitary gland releases the same follicle-stimulating and luteinizing hormones. In the pubescent male, however, FSH acts to open the testicular tubules, to enlarge the testes, and to initiate the production of spermatozoa (*spermatogenesis*). Male LH stimulates testosterone (a male sex hormone) production. Thus, the differences between

[64] Harold Jackson, "Chemical Methods of Male Contraception," *American Scientist,* Vol. 61, No. 2 (March–April 1973), p. 193.

the male and female, in these respects, is not in the chemical structure of the factor generated by the hypothalamus or the hormones produced and released by the anterior lobe of the pituitary. The difference lies in their action and in their timing. In the female, the hormonal production and action is cyclic. In the male, it is not (see pages 500–01).

Research begets research. Schally's announcement of the synthesis of the chemicals generated and used by the hypothalamus of the brain to communicate with the anterior lobe of the pituitary, and by means of which the elaborate reproductive system is controlled, paves the way for a better understanding of conception and contraception. As examples: it is known that there is a mechanism whereby estrogens and progesterone feed back to the hypothalamus to control the production of FSH and LH by the anterior lobe of the pituitary gland. This feedback mechanism (see page 255) accounts for the periodicity of ovulation and the efficacy of the more recent contraceptive pill. A basic component of the contraceptive pill is estrogen. Whether both FSH and LH are suppressed depends on the level of estrogen in the blood. This has been useful in determining the dosage of estrogen in the new contraceptive pill. Twenty micrograms of estrogen suppress only FSH; a dosage of fifty micrograms (.05 milligrams) suppresses both FSH and LH and is also relatively safe (see page 617). Furthermore, it has been learned that FSH and LH peaks indicate that a woman will ovulate within forty-eight hours. This correlation may some day lead to a single pill (or only a few) that will suppress FSH and LH only during the established period of ovulation. Or better still, rather than depend on the presently practiced risky rhythm method, the woman may be able to abstain from sexual intercourse during an ovulatory period that is based on scientifically precise laboratory measurements.

It has also been discovered that there is a feedback mechanism between anterior pituitary LH and FSH and the male hormone testosterone. Thus, the level of testosterone in the male seems to be monitored by the amounts of LH and FSH in the anterior lobe of the pituitary. That the subfertility of some men may be due to inadequate levels of the executive hormones in the anterior pituitary is further demonstrated by the discovery that, via an unknown substance, there is also a feedback mechanism between sperm maturation and FSH. It is possible to measure FSH levels in human beings; these may now be correlated with a type of subfertility that occurs because something is amiss in one of the stages of spermatogenesis. Finally, the work of Schally and his group may yet lead to fertility and subfertility controls at the hypothalamic level, rather than at the level of the pituitary, or at the target ovaries, or even at the testes.[65]

[65] Joan Arehart-Treichel, "Sperm and Eggs on the Go," *Science News*, Vol. 102, No. 7 (August 12, 1972), pp. 108–09. In the future LH–RH may also be used as a contraceptive. By inducing ovulation, the hormone could make the rhythm method of contraception more reliable. Use of the drug could establish the exact date of ovulation, and the woman could have sexual intercourse accordingly. ("Giving Reason to Rhythm: Inducing Ovulation," *Science News*, Vol. 100. No. 19 [November 6, 1971], p. 310.) In addition, the development of an LH-RH antagonist is imminent. "The antagonist, which could be given to block the release of luteinizing hormone [and consequent ovulation], could be the first contraceptive free of side effects . . . It might someday be used as a long term 'inoculation' against conception." ("Synthetic Hormone Could Improve Fertility Control," *Journal of the American Medical Association*, Vol. 217, No. 6 [August 9, 1971], p. 757.)

abortion

some definitions

A viable fetus is one that has reached such a stage of development that life can continue outside of the uterus. This prompts questions. For how long? How old must the fetus be? How big? Medical opinions have varied. Generally, a viable fetus can be thought of as one that had lived *in utero* for at least twenty-eight weeks, or weighed at least 1,000 grams (1 pound = 453.59 grams), or was 35 centimeters or more in length (1 centimeter = 0.3937 inches). Today, with rapid changes in the legal approach to abortion, some new state legislation has arbitrarily set viability at twenty weeks *in utero.* The premature expulsion from the uterus of a nonviable fetus or an embryo is considered an abortion.

Abortions may be *spontaneous, illegal* (*criminal*), or *therapeutic-legal.* Lay people refer to a spontaneous abortion as a miscarriage. It is estimated that between 10 and 15 percent of pregnancies end in miscarriage. The causes of spontaneous abortions are numerous and frequently unknown. A defective germ plasm, such as will occur with an abnormal sperm or ovum, may be a major cause. Maternal illness, such as German measles (see pages 148 and 164) or those due to malnourishment (see pages 549–50), may also be causative.

Even the most liberal abortion laws do not protect illegal practitioners. The untrained person who attempts to abort a friend (or herself) with a coat hanger or a knitting needle risks uterine perforation, hemorrhage, peritonitis, and death. The indiscriminate use of caustics or such drugs as ergot can result in serious illness and death. Nor do laws protect "fly-by-night" practitioners, who prey upon public ignorance and fear, with little regard for patient safety.

Therapeutic-legal abortions are those approved by state law. They are carried out under approved conditions, in approved hospitals or clinics, and by persons licensed to perform them. The number of strictly medical-therapeutic indications for abortion is diminishing. Heart disease, for example, was once a common reason for medical termination of pregnancy. Advances in heart surgery have made that reason less frequent. Nevertheless, many cases of chronic hypertension and kidney disease as well as breast and uterine cancers are reasons for most physicians to advise abortion.

changing ideas about legal abortion

Only a generation ago, abortion, like contraception, was rarely discussed in public. There are ample reasons for this change. First, *the sheer number of abortions* makes the procedure a major concern. Throughout the world, every year, some 25 million legal and illegal abortions are performed. Illegal abortions remain a major cause of maternal deaths. In Latin America half of all pregnancies end in illegal abortions. The resultant cost of women's lives is a shocking tragedy. It is fully four times greater than in countries in which abortions are legal. Formerly, about 1 million abortions a year in this country killed more than ten thousand women. For many women, extensive infection, the most common complication of illegal abortions, resulted in death. Only too often, the criminal abortionist is an incompetent, operating in atrociously unsanitary conditions. Second, *medical knowledge now warns of possible abnormal babies.* Maternal infection with German measles (rubella) virus in the first trimester, for example, results in a high percentage (20 percent) of abnormal babies. Such information has stimulated interest in legal abortion. Third, *the failure of contraception in overpopulated countries* has brought about a reevaluation of abortion. Fourth, some think restrictive *abortion laws* penalize the poor, are unenforceable, and are less applicable to married than to unmarried women.[66] Fifth, in this country, a growing number of people vigorously expressed their conviction that it was their right, as individuals, to make responsible decisions about the spacing and number of their children, should a chosen method of birth control fail. The statement, in 1971, by a physician-member of the Maternal Mortality Committee of Wisconsin's medical society, that assistance in fertility control "could have prevented" thirty-two of the last forty-eight deaths reviewed by the committee, stimulated much professional discussion (twelve of the dead women left a total of seventy children).[67] Lastly, the civil rights movement emphasizing individual rights, and an increasingly frank approach to human sexuality, encouraged widespread discussion about abortion.

Numerous ethical and theological problems arise when fallible men attempt to define indications for abortion. One of these is the scientific limitation in predicting abnormal births. Another lies in the variable interpretation of "health" of the mother. The family of a poor woman would suffer more, perhaps, with the addition of another child. Her health might thus be adversely affected. Should she be more eligible for abortion than the wealthy woman? Complicating the issue even more is the present gulf between some scientists and some theologians.

"Life is a continuum," the scientists say,

> it has evolved and survived over billions of years by the provision of fantastic margins of safety in terms of excess sperms and ova; the particular conjunction of sperm and ovum that leads to conception is not a unique event but is rather a matter of chance, the development of the individual from conception to full humanity is an unbroken process—who is to say when "life" began?[68]

Opponents of abortion place a sacred and infinite value on each separate beginning, on each potential life. Many consider that this value must be protected even beyond the mother's life. Threats to this concept, such as selfishness, irresponsibility, and sexual promiscuity, are especially condemned.

Both theologians and scientists revere life. To the responsible, both concepts surely have much to offer.

the most common legal methods of inducing abortion

There are several ways by which most abortions are today legally performed by competent physicians. Like all strictly medical procedures, their safety depends on the presence of an experienced and knowledgeable physician. The two most common methods are vacuum aspiration and dilation and curettage.

[66] *M.D., Medical Newsmagazine,* Vol. 12, No. 2 (February 1968), p. 105.
[67] "Maternal Deaths Laid to Lack of Family Planning, Abortion," *Obstetrical and Gynecological News,* Vol. 7, No. 19 (October 1, 1971), p. 46.
[68] "Abortion and the Doctor," *Annals of Internal Medicine,* Vol. 67, No. 5 (November 1967), pp. 1111–13.

vacuum aspiration (or suction)

This method is similar to dilation and curettage. However, it employs suction rather than the hand-manipulated curette. It is somewhat more expeditious than the D and C, and it usually results in less blood loss. As with all surgical procedures, there is some risk associated with this technique. This is because "the powerful suction needed to accomplish the procedure does pose a serious hazard to neighboring viscera in the event of uterine or cervical perforation."[69] In the hands of an experienced operator, such risks are minimal, and they very rarely occur. The vacuum aspiration technique is now used most frequently for the termination of early pregnancies.

dilation and curettage (D and C)

In this procedure, the opening in the cervix (see Figure 16-4, page 473) is slightly dilated. A hand-instrument called a curette, a metal loop on the end of a long, thin handle, is inserted into the uterus through the cervical opening. With hand manipulation of the curette the physician gently scrapes the pregnancy tissue from the surface wall of the uterus and then removes it. Most physicians prefer to limit dilation and curettage to about the ninth week of pregnancy. Beyond this time complications occur somewhat more frequently.

saline injection into the amniotic sac

In this procedure, a hypodermic needle approximately six to eight inches long is inserted through the abdominal wall into the amniotic sac (see Figure 19-2, page 574), and some of the amniotic fluid is withdrawn. This fluid is then replaced by a strong saline solution. The saline solution upsets the delicate water and chemical balance within the sac, placenta, and fetus. Fetal death is almost immediate and is hastened by the placental damage, which results in sharply diminished oxygen and food supplies to the fetus. In addition, the hormonal balance, so necessary to maintaining the pregnancy, is disrupted. The hormone oxytocin is released from the pituitary gland; it stimulates contraction of uterine musculature. Prostaglandins (see page 630) may also be released. From six to twelve hours after the saline injection, the uterus begins to contract. The placenta and fetus are expelled from twenty-four to thirty-six hours after the injection. Most operators prefer the saline technique for pregnancies of sixteen to twenty weeks because, before that time, the amniotic sac is small and difficult to locate.

In the United States, this method has largely replaced hysterotomy (see below) for abortions beyond the first trimester of pregnancy. In one study it was used to terminate almost 95 percent of pregnancies at seventeen weeks or later, with a median of 18.5 weeks. The procedure is not without complications, but in that study only three deaths occurred among 14,690 patients aborted by

[69] D. P. Swartz and M. K. Paranjpe, "Abortion: Medical Aspects in a Municipal Hospital," *Bulletin of the New York Academy of Medicine,* Vol. 47, No. 8 (August 1971), p. 848.

saline.[70] Pelvic infections, as well as disturbances in blood coagulation and hemorrhage, also occur, but competent operators are prepared to deal with these risks. Blood coagulation problems may occur because the replacement of fluid in the amniotic sac by the salt solution may disturb the clotting mechanism of the blood. With most women, this mechanism returns to normal by the time of expulsion.[71]

hysterotomy

With a hysterotomy an incision is made in the abdomen and then through the uterus, and the fetus is removed. This is obviously a major surgical procedure requiring hospitalization. Hysterotomy does not impair the woman's reproductive system, unlike a hysterectomy, or removal of the uterus, with which it is often confused.

oxytocin stimulation

Oxytocin is one of the hormones produced in the hypothalamus. It is stored in the posterior lobe of the pituitary gland. Upon being injected, oxytocin stimulates contraction of the muscles of the uterus. It is used to induce active labor or to cause contraction of the uterus after the afterbirth (placenta) has been delivered. In the expert hands of a physician it is safe. Its use to terminate pregnancy may require several administrations over several days.

trends in abortion techniques

In 1966 there were an estimated 6,000 legal abortions performed in the United States; it has been estimated that by the mid-1970s, the demand for legal abortions will reach about 2 million a year.[72] This increase has been accompanied by a rapid change in abortion procedures. The traditional method of dilation and curettage is being abandoned for the vacuum aspiration technique. Although vacuum aspiration is primarily used in the first trimester of pregnancy, it is also being employed as late as the sixteenth week from the last menstrual period.

During the Bangladesh civil war, mass rapings led to the opening of outpatient emergency abortion clinics. "Lady family planning visitors," rather than physicians, performed aspiration procedures under medical supervision. A U.S. physician in Bangladesh recently demonstrated a relatively simple abortion technique; it employs a length of polyethylene tubing adapted for the purpose and a suction device. It has been reported that with proper patient relaxation, six- to ten-week pregnancies can be terminated in a few minutes with little pain or blood loss. The dilation and curettage procedure requires forty-three instruments; polyethylene-tubing aspiration requires only two. The recent Supreme

[70] Christopher Tietze and Sarah Lewit, "Early Medical Complications of Abortion by Saline: Joint Program for the Study of Abortion (JPSA)," *Studies in Family Planning,* Vol. 4, No. 6 (June 1973), pp. 133–38.
[71] "Salt Abortion—Changes in Blood May Spell Danger," *Medical World News,* Vol. 13, No. 33 (September 8, 1972), pp. 15–17.
[72] "Abortion Statistics: Mortality, Morbidity in Legal Abortions Drop as Women Learn Earlier Procedures Safer," *Family Planning Digest,* Vol. 2, No. 3 (May 1973), p. 9.

Court decision on abortion laws (discussed below) will no doubt have a profound effect on the legal status of outpatient procedures, which had been illegal in most states. They are being supported by some leading medical authorities, as is the use of nonphysician paramedical personnel to do the actual abortion.

Still another trend is ''menstrual induction''; this is also called ''menses extraction,'' ''minisuction,'' ''menstrual regulation,'' and ''endometrial aspiration.'' In this procedure the uterus is evacuated with a vacuum aspiration tube of small diameter. In one study[73] of 1,108 terminations of suspected early pregnancies, in 315 cases either there was no pregnancy or pregnancy was unconfirmed. As a form of early abortion, the procedure is best done when the pregnancy test is positive; then the patient knows that she is undergoing a procedure she needs and wants.

Also being studied is a ''Supercoil'' as a substitute for the saline induction of a second-trimester abortion. The ''Supercoil'' is formed by inserting a series of up to eight coiled intrauterine devices. When they are removed in sixteen to twenty-four hours, fetal and placental tissue may then be removed by suction or curette. Some of the simpler abortion techniques present the danger of inviting self-abortion or abortions done by untrained individuals. This can only result in an increase in infections and other serious complications.[74]

U.S. abortion laws are liberalized

On January 24, 1906, President Theodore Roosevelt wrote a long and blistering letter to Reverend Franklin C. Smith, pastor of Christ Church Rectory, Central City, Nebraska.

> I feel that no man who is both intelligent and decent can differ with me . . . It is not a debatable subject . . . The attitude you seem tentatively inclined to favor is one of astounding folly as well as of astounding immorality. To advocate artificially keeping families small, with its inevitable attendants of pre-natal infanticide, of abortion, with its pandering to self-indulgence, its shirking of duties, and its enervation of character, is quite as immoral as to advocate theft or prostitution, and is even more hurtful in its folly, from the standpoint of the ultimate welfare of the race and the nation . . . [This] theory of conduct . . . if adopted, would mean the speedy collapse of this republic and of western civilization.[75]

Sixty-seven years later, on January 22, 1973, the U.S. Supreme Court overturned all state laws prohibiting or restricting a woman's right to obtain an abortion during the first twelve weeks of pregnancy. The court held that the ''right of privacy . . . founded in the Fourteenth Amendment's concept of personal liberty . . . is broad enough to encompass a woman's decision whether or not to terminate her pregnancy.'' In effect, the decision was left to the individual woman and her physician.[76] The court considered that after about the first trimester, abortion could endanger the woman's health. Thus, the state

[73] ''Menstrual Induction Experience Reported,'' *Family Planning Digest,* Vol. 2, No. 4 (July 1973), pp. 13–14.

[74] ''Two-Minute Abortion Is Here—Are We Ready?'' *Medical World News,* Vol. 13, No. 19 (May 12, 1972), pp. 15–17.

[75] Quoted in Charles Hamilton Auction Catalogue, No. 65, New York City, February 15, 1973, lot no. 258, p. 55.

[76] The court emphasized that ''the fetus, at most, represents only the potentiality of life . . . The unborn have never been recognized in the law as persons in the whole sense.''

could regulate abortions during the twelve to sixteen weeks following the first trimester, but only to protect maternal health.[77] During the final weeks of pregnancy, the state could prohibit abortion except when necessary to preserve the life or health of the woman.

By no means did the court's decision meet with universal agreement. Many U.S. citizens opposed it (and other methods of "keeping families small") just as strongly as had President Roosevelt two generations before. But the court's sweeping and historic action did reflect an increasing tendency among the states to liberalize abortion laws. In 1967, Colorado, California, and North Carolina adopted abortion laws suggested by the American Law Institute: abortions could be performed to preserve a woman's life or health, in cases of rape or incest, or in cases where the fetus was considered to be possibly defective. They were soon followed by thirteen other states. In 1970, the state of Washington adopted a law that essentially made abortion available on request. In that year, Hawaii, Alaska, and New York passed legislation with the same purpose.[78] What has been the effect of such legislation? As an example, consider the experience of New York.

the New York experience with abortion

In April 1970, the New York State abortion law was amended from extremely conservative to extremely liberal. The new law became effective on July 1, 1970. Formerly abortions were permitted only if a physician judged that the pregnancy endangered a woman's health or life. The new law permitted abortions on the request of a woman, with the consent of her physician, within twenty-four weeks of conception. It made no stipulation as to the place of the abortion, nor were there any residency requirements. An Obstetric Advisory Committee helped the Health Department to establish standards, which included a stipulation that pregnancies that had progressed beyond the twelfth week had to be terminated in a hospital. Those of twelve weeks or less could be done in an outpatient facility if conditions permitted. If the outpatient facility was outside the hospital building, it had to be supported by a hospital located within ten minutes travel time. This requirement could be waived if the outpatient facility had available all the equipment of a minihospital, such as operating rooms and X-ray equipment.

[77] The court said that as of "approximately the end of the first trimester . . . a state may regulate the abortion procedure to the extent that the regulation reasonably relates to the preservation and protection of maternal health." Among the "permissible" regulations were requirements as to: medical licensure; whether an abortion may be performed in a clinic as well as a hospital; and whether abortion facilities must be licensed. However, it specifically struck down requirements in the Georgia law that abortion be done only in accredited hospitals and that the decision be approved by a hospital committee and by two licensed physicians in addition to the pregnant woman's own physician. In addition, the court ruled that Georgia's residence requirement for abortion was unconstitutional.

[78] The Supreme Court decision left thirty-one states that prohibited abortion except in life-threatening situations, without effective legislation. Even the liberalized abortion laws based on the American Law Institute model (which were in effect in fifteen states and the District of Columbia) were invalid, in that they limited the grounds for abortion during the first trimester. Many of these states also had unconstitutional residency and other requirements. And, although the abortion laws of Alaska, Hawaii, New York, and Washington were largely consistent with the Supreme Court decision, they too were unenforceable in some respects. For example, their restrictions as to where abortions could be performed were no longer supportable. Even New York, which prohibited all abortions after twenty-four weeks except to preserve the woman's *life,* did not meet with the Supreme Court wording, which held that an exception could also be made to preserve the woman's *health.*

data on abortions in New York City[79]

Within the first two years after the new law took effect (July 1, 1970–June 30, 1972), 334,865 abortions were reported to have been performed in New York City. Almost two-thirds (65.7 percent) were performed on women who were not residents of New York City. However, it is believed that about 16.7 percent of abortions are not reported; thus, it is conservatively estimated that 402,000 abortions were actually performed in the two-year period. In the second year the total number of abortions increased by 41 percent, with the increase greater for nonresidents. Most women who came to New York for abortions were from New Jersey, Illinois, Michigan, Ohio, Pennsylvania, Florida, Massachusetts, and Connecticut.

By far the majority of abortions were performed at less than thirteen weeks of pregnancy. The suction method of abortion was the most commonly used technique. The greatest proportion of women seeking abortion were between the ages of twenty and twenty-nine. During the first year, teen-agers had 16.5 percent of the resident abortions; this increased to 18.1 percent during the second year.[80] Among nonresidents, the teen-aged proportion rose from 18.1 percent in the first year to 33.9 percent during the second. During the first year, the youngest person to receive an abortion was ten years old; she had already given birth to one live infant.[81] By the second year, an increasing percentage of abortion patients (almost two-thirds) had already had at least one pregnancy; among the nonresident groups, however, almost two-thirds were experiencing a first pregnancy.

How did the patients fare in regard to complications? During the second year all reported complications declined from 8.5 to 7.2 per 1,000 abortions. However, although the complication rate declined for early terminations, they increased for late terminations. Indeed, for the two years combined, the complication rate for late terminations was no less than seven times that of early terminations. And for the second year, the saline method of abortion had a

[79] Data from Jean Patker, Donna O'Hare, Frieda Nelson, and Martin Svigir, "Two Years Experience in New York City with the Liberalized Abortion Law—Progress and Problems," *American Journal of Public Health,* Vol. 63, No. 6 (June 1973), pp. 524–35. Since the law went into effect, several New York City hospitals have noted a reduction in the number of abandoned infants and immature births. One group of five Brooklyn hospitals reported a 5,800 percent increase in the number of elective abortions. ("Abortion Cuts Numbers of Abandoned Infants, Immature Births," *Journal of the American Medical Association,* Vol. 224, No. 13 [June 25, 1973], pp. 1697–98). In the first three years under the liberalized law (July 1, 1970–June 30, 1973), a total of 598,283 abortions were performed in New York City, more than half of them on women from out of state.

[80] The greater risk of the teen-age pregnancy is often not realized. Mothers under twenty have a 30 percent higher death rate than mothers aged twenty to twenty-four. Maternal deaths associated with toxic complications and those due to uterine infections consequent to illegal abortions are 50 percent higher for the pregnant teen-aged girl. Nor are their babies spared. Late fetal deaths and prematurity are higher with teen-aged pregnancies. Moreover, the babies have a 30 percent greater risk of dying before their first birthday than the babies of mothers aged twenty to twenty-four. ("MD Cites Dangers of Teenage Pregnancy," *Family Planning Digest,* Vol. 2, No. 2 [March 1973], pp. 2–3.)

[81] Jean Pakter, David Harris, and Frieda Nelson, "Surveillance of Abortion Program in New York City," *Bulletin of the New York Academy of Medicine,* Vol. 47, No. 8 (August 1971), pp. 853–74. In an extensive study of 42,598 patients conducted between mid-1970 and mid-1971 by the Joint Program for the Study of Abortions, which involved sixty hospitals and four independent clinics in twelve states, it was found that the most common patient was a young, single, white woman pregnant for the first time. The most common procedure was the vacuum aspiration technique (69.5 percent) compared to the once standard dilation and curettage (5.4 percent). ("Who Gets Abortions, How, and When," *Medical World News,* Vol. 12, No. 45 [December 3, 1971], p. 52.)

complication rate more than ten times that of the suction or dilation and curettage method. During the two-year period, twenty-nine women were known to have died from causes associated with abortion; of these sixteen followed legal and thirteen illegal abortions. Of the sixteen deaths from legal abortions eight followed the saline method; five, hysterotomy; two, dilation and curettage; and one, the suction method.[82]

data on abortions nationwide[83]

By May 1973, *nationwide* figures on abortion were available for 1971 from twenty-four states and the District of Columbia. In that year, 480,259 legal abortions had been performed. Twenty-nine percent were performed on women less than twenty years old; 79.2 percent of the women were white, 18.9 percent nonwhite, and 1.9 percent, unknown. About two-thirds of legal abortions were performed on single, widowed, separated, or divorced women. About 84 percent were performed by suction or D and C. Almost 80 percent were performed during the first trimester. In 1971, two states reported more than 79 percent of the total number of legal abortions (New York 55 percent and California 24.3 percent). Moreover, 38.7 percent of reported abortions were performed outside the woman's state of residence. In this country, almost all first-trimester abortions are done by the vaginal route (suction or D and C). Most abortions at sixteen weeks or later are performed by saline injection. During the intervening three weeks, hysterotomy is almost always the method used.

what has been learned so far?

The principal factors responsible for death associated with legal abortions are the length of time that the woman has been pregnant and the method used to terminate the pregnancy. Since the method used depends largely upon the duration of the pregnancy, prolonged illness or death from abortion will drop when women seek abortion early—before the twelfth week of pregnancy. This is the experience not only in this country but in other countries as well. Elective abortion in Hungary and Czechoslovakia is limited to the first trimester; in 1969–1970 they had the lowest mortality rates of eight countries and two places in the U.S. that were studied. During that period, Sweden, England, and Wales had the highest percentage of second-trimester abortions; their mortality ratios were seven to fifteen times those of eastern European countries and Japan (where 95 percent of elective abortions were done during the first trimester[84]).

With regard to the psychological effects of abortion, limited objective studies so far indicate that "there was little new psychiatric illness that appeared

[82] Theresa van der Vlugt and P. T. Piotrow, "Uterine Aspiration Techniques," *Population Report,* Department of Medical and Public Affairs, George Washington University Medical Center, Ser. F, No. 3 (June 1973), p. F38.

[83] Data from "Abortion Statistics: Mortality, Morbidity in Legal Abortions Drop as Women Learn Early Pregnancy Procedures Safer," *Family Planning Digest,* Vol. 2, No. 3 (May 1973), p. 9.

[84] Today, Japan's abortion law, liberalized in 1948, is causing some misgivings. There is concern that Japan's 1.5 million annual abortions has resulted in a disregard for the unborn, that abortion is replacing contraception more than is generally realized, and that there are too few young people to care for the increasing population over sixty-five years of age. ("Abortion in Japan After 25 Years," *Medical World News,* Vol. 14, No. 41 [November 9, 1973], p. 37.)

after the abortion that could be related to the abortion."[85]

It has been emphasized that family planning should be stressed to reduce the number of abortions and "repeaters." How soon after abortion should a woman begin contraception? Recent studies indicate that many women ovulate before they resume menstruation. It has therefore been suggested that contraception should be started as early as two weeks after abortion.[86] It is also urged that abortion services be broadened to include all the states. This, it is believed, would not only spare the woman who desires an abortion the added physical, emotional, and financial stress incurred by the need to travel, but also reduce the crucial time factor. There is little question that abortion has resulted in an enormous decline of live births in New York City. It has been estimated that over the two years from 1970 to 1972, the annual number of live births declined by from 17,000 to 21,000. Other changes in reproductive behavior accounted for a considerable further decline.[87] Of paramount importance in this entire picture is the need for constant surveillance and the cooperation of the medical profession to assure high quality in all aspects of family planning, for surely the costly, illegal, and dangerous abortion practices of the past had cost the lives of many women.[88] It is important to note that the New York City Department of Health offers free pregnancy tests in the health centers in which prenatal and family planning services are provided. This increases the number of newly pregnant patients seeking either earlier prenatal care or an earlier abortion. It also increases the demand for family planning services.[89]

Finally, there is a growing conviction of the advantages of uterine aspiration over dilation and curettage. These include:[90]

1. A shorter time required for the procedure
2. A more complete removal of uterine contents
3. Fewer perforations of the uterus
4. Less blood loss
5. Fewer major complications
6. Well-suited for local rather than general anesthesia
7. Appropriate for performance by supervised, well-trained paraprofessionals
8. Easily adapted to outpatient facilities
9. Less costly for the patient

[85] R. Bruce Sloane, "The Unwanted Pregnancy," *New England Journal of Medicine,* Vol. 280, No. 22 (May 29, 1969), p. 1209.

[86] "Six Week Check Late for Contraception?" *Family Planning Digest,* Vol. 1, No. 6 (November 1972), pp. 12–13, citing E. F. Boyd and E. G. Holmstrom, "Ovulation following Therapeutic Abortion," *American Journal of Obstetrics and Gynecology,* Vol. 113 (1972), p. 469. Of the 402,059 legal abortions performed in New York City between July 1, 1970, and June 30, 1972, only 2 percent (6,936) were repeat abortions. However, with time, the number appears to be increasing. (Edwin F. Daily, Nick Nicholas, Frieda Nelson, and Jean Patker, "Repeat Abortions in New York City: 1970–1972," *Family Planning Perspectives,* Vol. 5, No. 2 (Spring 1973), pp. 89–93.

[87] Christopher Tietze, "Two Years Experience with a Liberal Abortion Law: Its Impact on Fertility Trends in New York City," *Family Planning Perspectives,* Vol. 5, No. 1 (Winter 1973), pp. 36–41.

[88] For an excellent discussion of Hawaii's experience with liberalized abortion laws, see Milton Diamond, James A. Palmore, Roy G. Smith, and Patricia G. Steinhoff, "Abortion in Hawaii," *Family Planning Perspectives,* Vol. 5, No. 1 (Winter 1973), pp. 54–60.

[89] Edwin F. Daily and Nick Nicholas, "A Free Pregnancy Testing Service," *Family Planning Perspectives,* Vol. 5, No. 1 (Winter 1973), p. 6.

[90] Theresa van der Vlugt and P. T. Piotrow, "Uterine Aspiration Techniques," p. 2.

abortions: caution!

There is little question that the recent changes in abortion laws in the United States have been enacted as a result of public pressure. Nor are physicians averse to changing their minds in this respect. A 1967 study noted that only 23.5 percent of 5,289 members of the American Psychiatric Association favored laws allowing abortion on request. By 1969, 72 percent of 2,041 psychiatrists polled favored such action.[91] Moreover, it is not necessarily true that abortion-on-request laws are accompanied by a decline in the use of contraceptive methods. It is claimed that this occurred neither in Japan nor in various European countries. Indeed, there is the belief that, in these countries, an increased number of abortions has resulted in an increase in the use of contraceptives.[92]

Nevertheless, there are hazards to abortion-on-request laws. One danger is that many young women may regard an abortion too casually. Another is that the availability of inexpensive abortions may reduce the individual use of contraceptives. ''Why use a contraceptive this time?'' a young wife may ask herself. ''Abortions are quick and easy and cheap and no trouble.'' But abortions can be trouble. An induced abortion temporarily interferes with the body's hormonal system. Although return to normal is the rule, postabortion medical help may be needed. Moreover, even skillfully induced abortions may be unavoidably connected with future problems. There is reliable opinion that the physical trauma of repeated induced abortions may be associated with a later inability to conceive or to carry a child to full term.[93] In Hungary, Rumania, and the Soviet Union the most recently available records show a higher number of induced abortions than live births.[94] In Hungary the rate of premature births is also rising, and that country now has the highest rate in Europe. ''It is widely felt that this change is the result of the free recourse to abortion possible in Hungary and particularly to the termination of first pregnancies.''[95] This opinion may be applicable to the experience in this country. In the early years in both California and Delaware, the first pregnancies in single women were the ones most frequently terminated. During the first two years of California's revised abortion law, girls younger than twenty years of age constituted almost 33 percent of all abortion cases. Fifty-three percent of all abortions were performed on childless women. In Colorado by 1970, more than half of abortions were performed on women who had yet to bear their first child.[96] Physicians are concerned about the one-child-sterility syndrome—couples are unable to have a second child. Although not proven, it has been theorized that this may be due to low-grade infection.[97] Such infections can occur following abortion.

Although most abortions are surely justifiable, they should never be regarded as a substitute for a reliable contraceptive.

[91] E. Pfeiffer, ''Psychiatric Indications or Psychiatric Justification of Therapeutic Abortion,'' *Archives of General Psychiatry,* Vol. 23 (1970), pp. 402–07, cited in ''About Abortion,'' *Journal of the American Medical Association,* Vol. 215, No. 2 (January 11, 1971), p. 286.

[92] ''About Abortion,'' *Briefs: Footnotes on Maternity Care,* Vol. 35, No. 6 (Summer 1971), p. 91.

[93] Melita C. Gesche and Donald G. Dickinson, ''Abortion and the Young,'' *Health News,* Vol. 47, No. 8 (August 1970), p. 6.

[94] Carl Djerassi, ''Fertility Control Through Abortion: An Assessment of the Period 1950–1980,'' p. 12.

[95] Melita C. Gesche and Donald G. Dickinson, ''Abortion and the Young,'' p. 6.

[96] *Ibid.,* p. 13.

[97] *Ibid.,* p. 14.

summary

The two major ways in which the problem of overpopulation (discussed in Chapter 20) is being met are *birth control* and *abortion.*

The most common methods of *birth control* are presented in Table 21-1 (pages 619–22). Despite their recognized adverse effects, the *oral contraceptives* are used safely and effectively by millions of women (pages 617–23). The only birth control methods currently available to men are *condoms, coitus interruptus,* and *vasectomy* (pages 624–27); vasectomy is similar to *tubal ligation* in women (pages 623–24). Research is under way on additional contraceptives, including the synthetic hormone *progestin* (pages 628–29), *diethylstilbesterol* (the "morning-after" pill; page 629), and *prostaglandins* (pages 630–31). Recent research has also revealed information on the possible dangers of intrauterine devices (pages 631–32); on possible improvements on the rhythm method (page 632); on oral contraceptives for men (pages 632–34); and on the contraceptive possibilities of synthetic brain chemicals (pages 634–35).

Abortion is the premature expulsion from the uterus of a nonviable fetus or an embryo (page 636). Abortions may be *spontaneous* (*miscarriage*), *illegal* (criminal), or *therapeutic-legal* (page 636). Attitudes toward abortion have changed markedly in the past generation, for a number of medical, social, and political reasons (pages 636–37). The two most common legal methods of inducing abortion are *vacuum aspiration* (page 638) and *dilation and curettage* (page 638). Other legal methods are *saline injection* (pages 638–39), *hysterotomy* (page 639), and *oxytocin stimulation* (page 639). Recent trends in abortion techniques include: abandonment of dilation and curettage in favor of vacuum aspiration (page 639); increasing numbers of abortions performed as outpatient procedures (pages 639–40); use of the "menstrual induction" procedure (page 640); and use of the "Supercoil" as a substitute for saline induction of second-trimester abortion (page 640).

In 1973 the U.S. Supreme Court ruled unconstitutional all state laws prohibiting or restricting abortion during the first twelve weeks of pregnancy (page 640). A few states had previously liberalized their abortion laws, notably New York in 1970 (pages 641–43). Subsequent data indicate that although abortion should not be casually regarded as a substitute for a reliable contraceptive, legal abortion (preferably during the early months of pregnancy) is safe for the vast majority of women (pages 643–45).

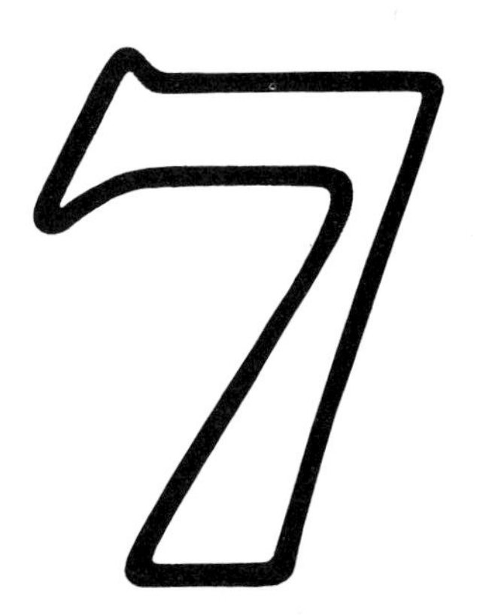

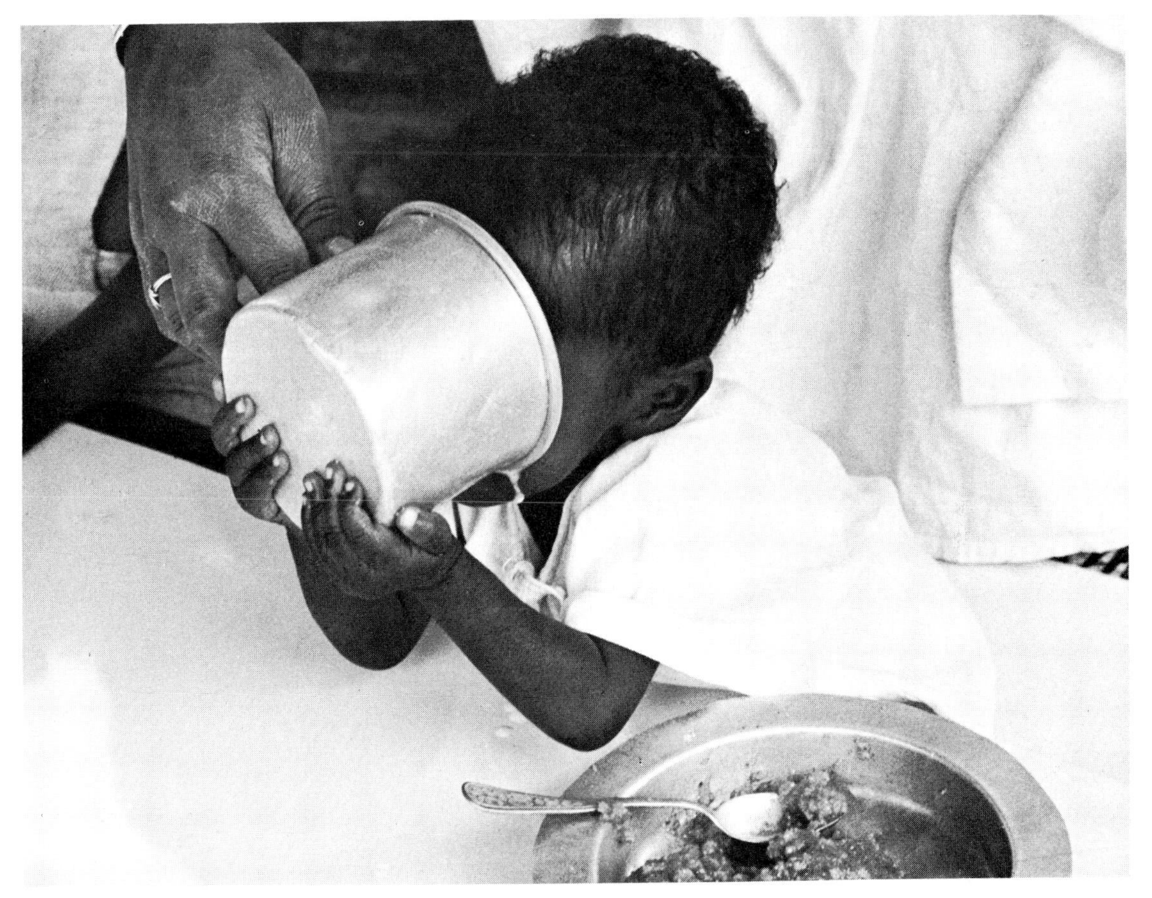

health maintenance, illness prevention

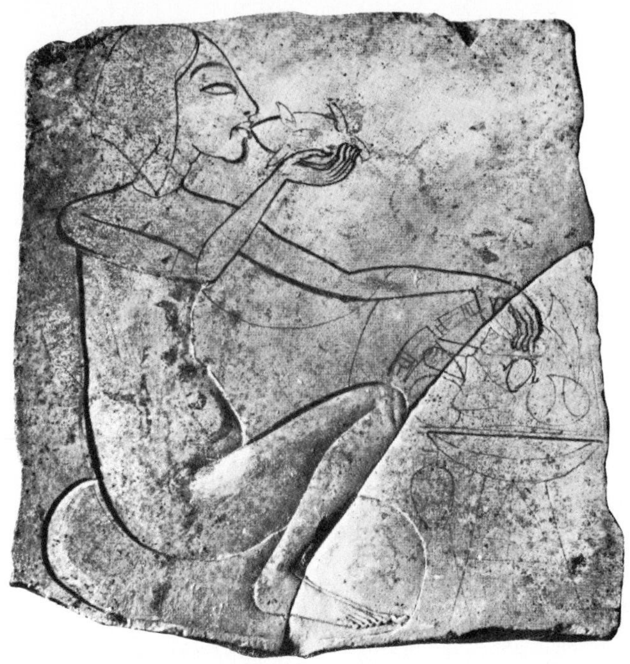

Ancient Egyptian relief showing a princess eating a bird, which had probably been roasted or grilled.

nourishment

22

taste, for which there is some accounting

In that year, 1959, a lot of the citizens of Peoria, Illinois, were shocked, even revolted by the deed. To make matters worse, it had been perpetrated by an officer of the U.S. Army. What had Lieutenant Andrew O'Meara done to so arouse his community?

To demonstrate a means of military survival to some friends, he had killed and skinned a stray dog, and then put it on a spit. The lieutenant was prosecuted, and a judge—under considerable public pressure—fined him the maximum $200 for cruelty to animals. The animal had been killed not cruelly, but by a sudden blow. The lieutenant could have pleaded innocent, but the furor resulting from his demonstration that dogmeat could prevent starvation was too intense. He did not contest the case.[1]

Food taboos have a long history. Hebrew biblical instruction forbidding swine, for example, is specific. "Of their flesh shall ye not eat, and their carcase shall ye not touch: they are unclean to you" (Leviticus 11:8).[2] It was doubtless man's affectionate domestication of the dog that led to strong feelings against consuming the meat of the family pet. Members of Judeo-Christian cultures have had over twenty centuries to learn to abominate dogmeat. The ancient Zoroastrians of Iran considered dogs holy and the eating of them a sin. Moslems also reject dogmeat. But in some cultures puppyhams are a delicacy. Those who consider eating "man's best friend" a savage act should know that, until recently, dogflesh was relished among the Chinese, and their great culture extends over fifty centuries. (Dog breeding for human feeding was urged by one Man Lan-Chun, in an advertisement published in the July 19, 1962, edition of a Peking newspaper. It brought forth little enthusiasm. It seems there was a dog shortage.)[3]

Some religions have banned meat-eating altogether on certain days. On March 18, 1552, the Lord Mayor of London sentenced "a wyfe of Hammersmith . . . and a simple carpenter to public disgrace" for eating meat on "fysshe days." They were forced to "ryde on 2 horses with panelles of strawe about the markettes of the Citie, having eche of them a garland of theyr heades of pyges . . . toes, and a pygge hanging on . . . theyr breastes."[4] Charles IX of France (1550–74) ran no such risks. His marriage to Elizabeth of Austria fell on a meatless Friday. His guests were fed two barrels of oysters, fifty pounds of whale meat, two hundred crawfish, four hundred herring, and eleven hundred pairs of frog's legs.[5]

22-1 *A trichina larva (×180) encapsulated in muscle tissue of a swine, which may have been fed uncooked garbage. For this reason, trichinosis (see footnote 2) is sometimes called "the garbage sickness."*

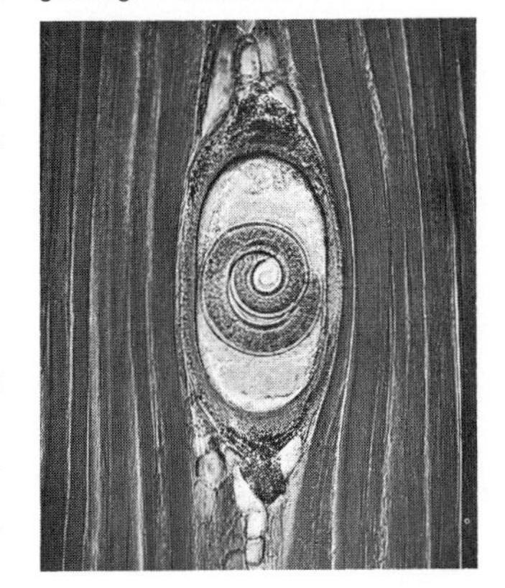

[1] *Wisconsin State Journal* (August 11, 1959), cited in Frederick J. Simoons, *Eat Not This Flesh* (Madison, Wis., 1961), p. 91.

[2] This may have been due to the infestation of pork meat with a parasite that still causes a disease called *trichinosis.* In its early stages the disease is manifested by nausea, diarrhea, and fever; in its later stages, by swelling and pain of the muscles. It is produced by eating undercooked pork containing the parasite.

[3] Jacques Marcuse, *The Peking Papers* (New York, 1967), pp. 60–62.

[4] *A Chronicle of Engleand, 1485–1559,* Vol. II, cited in J. C. Drummond and Anne Wilbraham, *The Englishman's Food* (London, 1939), p. 63.

[5] William Harlan Hale and the editors of *Horizon* magazine, *The Horizon Cookbook and Illustrated History of Eating and Drinking Through the Ages* (Garden City, N.Y., 1968), pp. 126–27.

Food choices have not only been influenced by religion but have also been peppered with politics. Over two hundred years ago, John Adams tartly observed that the English (''absurd masters'') had taught the colonists to dislike Parisian cookery.[6] Nevertheless, Thomas Jefferson brought a French cook to the White House. Patrick Henry bitterly attacked Jefferson's affection for French foods.[7]

Even the painfully hungry often reject food to which they are unaccustomed. The Arctic explorer Vilhjalmur Stefansson related that the Eskimos ate berries only when on the verge of starvation, before eating their dogs and, finally, one another.[8] Yet many Eskimos are fond of raw birds (bones, feathers, intestines—everything but the bills and feet);[9] they also enjoy caribou dung and the stomach contents of various animals.

Poorly prepared foods are long remembered. Spoiled food provoked the Harvard Butter Rebellion of 1766 and the students wrote a biblical parody, which read in part:

> And it came to pass in the ninth month of the 23rd day of the Month, that the Sons of Harvard murmured and said
>
> Behold! Bad and unwholesome butter is served out unto us daily; now therefore let us depute Asa the Scribe, to go out unto our Rulers and seek redress
>
> Then arose Asa, the Scribe, and went unto Belcher, the Ruler and said behold our butter stinketh and we cannot eat thereof; now give us, we pray thee, butter that stinketh not.[10]

But no matter how fresh the food is, many inhabitants of developing countries reject food because of taboos. The Hindu will not eat beef, since the cow is sacred to him. To the Moslem the pig is unclean. He refuses pork.[11] Milk is the favorite food of men in the U.S. Army.[12] To the Dravidians of Southern India it is a nauseating excrement.[13]

So a multitude of factors—rooted in fear, poverty, religion, and habit—decide a person's food choices. Nobody decides his diet alone. Influencing cultural dietary patterns, moreover, are individual emotions. Few people realize the degree to which food intakes are responses to emotional stresses. Ice cream may be associated with parental reward, spinach with rebellion over parental punishment or authority, coffee with growing up, milk with mother and security. Some people may eat rattlesnake to gain attention. A single food may evoke different responses at various times. Milk, for example, may be both a ''reward'' and a ''security'' food.

[6] Charles Francis Adams, ed., *Familiar Letters of John Adams and His Wife, Abigail Adams,* cited in Richard Osborn Cummings, *The American and His Food* (Chicago, 1941), p. 30.

[7] James Schouler, *Americans of 1776,* cited in Richard Osborn Cummings, *The American and His Food,* p. 22.

[8] *World Health,* Vol. 15, No. 5 (September–October 1962), p. 10.

[9] Meyer Klatsky, ''Studies in the Dietaries of Contemporary Primitive Peoples,'' *Journal of the American Dental Association,* Vol. 36, Nos. 4 and 5 (April–May 1948), pp. 385–91.

[10] Quoted in C. A. Wagner, *Harvard—Four Centuries and Freedoms,* cited in Adelia M. Beeuwkes, E. Neige Todhunter, and Emma Seifert Weigley, eds., *Essays on History of Nutrition and Dietetics* (Chicago, 1967), p. 154.

[11] W. R. Aykroyd, *Food for Man* (New York, 1964), p. 51.

[12] Charlotte M. Young, ''Food Habits and Faddism,'' in Abraham E. Nizel, ed., *The Science of Nutrition and Its Application to Clinical Dentistry,* 2nd ed. (Philadelphia, 1966), p. 224.

[13] H. D. Renner, *The Origin of Food Habits* (London, 1944), p. 73.

Mingled with the vast array of cultural and individual emotional factors deciding food tastes are the endlessly subtle sensory perceptions of food. Man smacks his lips over coffee with ''body.'' It provides a pleasurable resistance in his mouth. He also relishes color. Hence, the sprig of green parsley on the plate. Food without salt is deplored by Job. ''Can that which is unsavory be eaten without salt?'' (Job 6:6). Creamy substances mixed with air are smoothly delicious. A ''rough'' chocolate insults exquisitely sensitive mucous membranes. Crisp biscuits are tastier than tough meat. Good bread pleases the palate. There is more to food than eating.

The digestive process is often described in terms of combustion machines and hydraulic pressures. As book illustrations, these are useful. But digestion is profoundly influenced by the mind. Hunger is not the same as appetite. And food can cause physiological effects totally unrelated to either hunger or appetite. ''Mine eyes smell onions,'' old Lafew remarks in Shakespeare's *All's Well That Ends Well* (V.iii.325). Centuries before Pavlov's drooling dogs, the playwright, in four short words, thus defined the conditional reflex. Yet he well understood the effect of the mind on digestion. ''Unquiet meals make ill digestions,'' says the Abbess in *The Comedy of Errors* (V.i.74). The bard clearly saw the difference between mere hunger and appetite. Macbeth speaks: ''Now good digestion wait on appetite, / And health on both!'' (III.iv.38–39).

Appetite is a human quality. Animals enjoy food but do not savor sharing meals. ''The infant cannot be fed by food alone,'' writes Dorothy V. Whipple, ''he needs to dine . . . He cannot eat until the conditions of dining have been met . . . the infant relaxes and is eager to eat when picked up by gentle, warm, comfortable arms.''[14] These are the observations of a pediatrician, but the emotional needs of dining have also been recorded by those who treat the aged—the geriatricians. The aged person who forgets to eat because he is alone is all too common. From the first infant intimacy of mother's warmth to the last suppers of the aged, humans learn this: man eats alone, but dines with others.

the basic constituents of foods

The basic constituents of foods are six—*carbohydrates, fats, proteins, vitamins, minerals,* and *water.* In health, all work together. A healthy body is a delicately balanced ecosystem, and a balanced diet helps to maintain that balance. The major nutritional uses and sources of the most important nutrients are outlined in Table 22-1 (pages 658–59).

''all flesh is grass'' (Isaiah 40:6)—carbohydrates, fats, proteins

All human food is ultimately derived from green plants. From the air, plants take carbon dioxide, which is carbon and oxygen. From the soil, plants take water, which is hydrogen and oxygen. From the sun, they get energy. Chlorophyll in the leaves of green plants uses carbon dioxide, water, and the energy from the

[14] Dorothy V. Whipple, *Dynamics of Development: Euthenic Pediatrics* (New York, 1966), pp. 368–69.

sun to form formaldehyde and its related acids. (These acids account for the sour taste of unripe fruit.) With continued synthesis, with ripening, acids become sweet sugars. These, in turn, combine into starches. Then starches combine to form cellulose. These three—sugars, starches, and cellulose—are the most important forms of food *carbohydrates.* Cellulose and maple sugar are found in the leaves, wood, and bark of trees; grains contain starch, cellulose, and some sugars; fruits and vegetables contain all three carbohydrates.

But not all carbon dioxide and water in plants becomes carbohydrate. Some combine to form complex acids, the *fatty acids.* These are the chief constituents of *fats.*[15] Unlike carbohydrates and fats, *proteins* contain nitrogen. The nitrogen originally comes from air, which is essentially a mixture of oxygen, nitrogen, a small amount of carbon dioxide, and some rare gases. Twenty-three nitrogen-bearing acids, the *amino acids,* are the constituents of body proteins. According to DNA instructions (Chapter 18), these twenty-three known amino acids are arranged in hundreds to thousands of ways to become the thousands of body proteins. Of these twenty-three, ten cannot be synthesized in the human body. Since they must be provided in the diet so that the body can make the proteins essential to life, these ten are called the *essential amino acids.* From these ten the body is able to build the remaining thirteen. As sources of the ten essential amino acids, a variety of animal proteins are generally superior to the vegetable proteins.

Carbohydrates, fats, proteins—the three basic food constituents—are, then, all synthesized by green plants. Normally, when consumed, carbohydrates and fats combine with body oxygen (oxidation) to produce life-supporting energy. With a diet deficient in these, the body must resort to using proteins for energy instead of using them for body growth and maintenance. Growth—indeed, basic health—is then impeded. Present in adequate amounts, carbohydrates and fats free the proteins from energy-producing duty and save them for body-building.

Before an animal can begin to use the carbohydrate, fat, or protein of another plant or animal, it must break it down or *digest* it. Why? For two reasons. First, ingested food must be reduced to a size small enough to enter body cells. Second, within the far-flung billions of cell factories, the raw material must be reconstructed to resemble more closely the tissues to be rebuilt.

And so the processes of nutrition can become quite complex. However, one fact remains simple: all flesh is grass.

the vital amines

vitamin C

''My company,'' wrote Sir Richard Hawkins almost four centuries ago, ''began to fall sick, of a disease which Sea-men are wont to call the Scurvy . . . The cause . . . some attribute to sloth; some to conceit [imagination] . . . That which I have seen most fruitful for this sickness is sour Oranges and Lemons.''[16] In

[15] *Cholesterol,* which is involved in fat digestion, is thought to be related to certain diseases of certain arteries, as was noted in Chapter 9.

[16] Sir Richard Hawkins, *Observations in His Voyage to the South Seas* (1593), quoted in F. E. Shideman, ed., *Take as diRected* (Cleveland, 1967), p. 36.

scurvy, a disease of dietary deficiency, there is bleeding of the gums as well as under the skin surfaces and into the exquisitely tender joints. Observations such as Hawkins' led to a requirement that British sailors drink lemon and lime juices. Hence their nickname ''limeys.'' Prevention and treatment of scurvy are accomplished by the use of vitamin C (ascorbic acid). The commonly used fruits and vegetables are rich in this vitamin. If a mother's intake of vitamin C is inadequate, her milk will be poor in the substance. Among infants, scurvy is manifested early by poor growth or brittle bones that fracture easily. Symptoms of mild vitamin C deficiency in babies are frequently reported. However, they also occur in adults.

The human body cannot manufacture an adequate supply of vitamin C, so humans must depend on their diets for this vitamin. Unfortunately, vitamin C is unstable, easily destroyed. To prevent its being destroyed in the cooking process, a person cooking vegetables should drop the vegetables (undamaged) into a minimal amount of already boiling water and immediately cover the pot, so that air will be kept out (and oxidation reduced). Since even slight alkalinity destroys vitamin C, soda should not be added to food that is being cooked. Modern food canning and freezing procedures retain most of the vitamin C.

On page 163, footnote 37, the possibility was discussed that large doses of vitamin C help to lessen the duration and complications of the common cold. Experiments with animals indicate that vitamin C may also be helpful in the treatment of diabetes,[17] the blocking of the cancer-causing effects of certain chemicals,[18] the prevention of coronary heart disease,[19] and more rapid recovery from anesthesia and faster rates of scab formation.[20] It must be emphasized, however, that large doses of vitamin C may be hazardous for some people. For example, long-term ingestion of large doses of vitamin C may have a deleterious effect ''on the metabolism of either bone or calcium and phosphorous in humans, especially children.''[21]

vitamin B

In the 1870s, a disaster struck the newly created Japanese Navy. Almost half the sailors suffered a painful and crippling disease that paralyzed their legs, affected their hearts, and was accompanied by marked manifestations of impaired digestive function, such as loss of appetite and severe constipation. Kanehiro Takaki, a surgeon in the Japanese Navy, related the disease, *beriberi* (from the Singhakese, ''I cannot''), to the sailors' diet of polished rice. Less rice but more wheat, meat, and vegetables were made available. The result: in 1886, there were only three cases of beriberi; in 1879, there had been 1,789.

[17] ''Vitamin C Reduces the Need for Insulin by Diabetics,'' *New Scientist,* Vol. 57, No. 835 (March 1973), p. 471.

[18] ''Chemical Carcinogen Adversaries?'' *Medical World News,* Vol. 14, No. 20 (May 18, 1973), p. 23.

[19] ''Vitamin C May Reduce Coronary Heart Disease,'' *New Scientist,* Vol. 57, No. 834 (February 22, 1973), p. 413, citing Emil Ginter, ''Cholesterol: Vitamin C Controls Its Transformation to Bile Acids,'' *Science,* Vol. 179, No. 4074 (February 16, 1973), pp. 702–04.

[20] ''Do We Need a Lot More Vitamin C?'' *New Scientist,* Vol. 58, No. 846 (May 17, 1973), p. 401, citing Man-Li Yew in *Proceedings of the National Academy of Sciences,* U.S.A., Vol. 70 (1973), p. 969.

[21] R. G. Brown, ''Possible Problems of Large Intakes of Ascorbic Acid,'' *Journal of the American Medical Association,* Vol. 224, No. 11 (June 11, 1973), p. 1530.

But Takaki erred in attributing the disease to protein deficiency. At the turn of the century, two Dutch doctors stationed in Java noted a curious coincidence in a prison yard. Prisoners and some hens in the prison yard shared both a diet of milled rice and beriberi. A series of classic experiments proved that the "rice polishings," the germ and outer layer of rice, removed by milling, prevented the disease. It is now known that the outer husky portion of the rice grain contains B vitamins, particularly thiamine (vitamin B_1). Infantile beriberi is so rapidly fatal that an afflicted child may die only a few hours after being seemingly well. Even today beriberi is common among breast-fed children in Thailand, Malaysia, and Vietnam. When the mothers are given thiamine, recovery is dramatic.

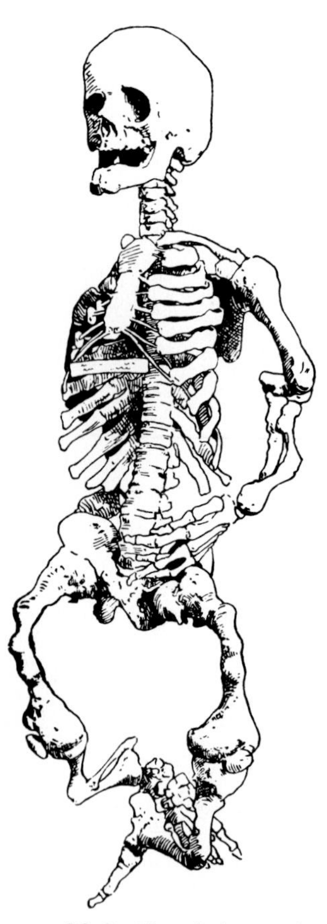

22-2 *The skeleton of a twenty-one–year–old American Indian, severely deformed by rickets.*

vitamin D

As dietary deficiency diseases, scurvy and beriberi are hardly alone. The first few decades of this century saw science illuminate more old dietary mysteries. The softening of children's bones from *rickets* had long been noted. The relationship of the illness to inadequate sunlight and its cure by cod-liver oil therapy was established many years before 1918, when an antirickets vitamin was first described. It required more years to prove that this vitamin—vitamin D—is manufactured in the skin that is exposed to sunlight. Now it is known that vitamin D is essential to maintaining the correct balance of calcium in the body. Calcium is important not only in the manufacture of bone, but in normal nerve function and in many important enzyme reactions. When vitamin D is ingested, both the liver and kidneys take part in the complex process of maintaining the body's calcium balance. This helps to explain why people with diseased kidneys lose bone calcium and fail to absorb calcium from the intestine.[22]

niacin

In 1914, an American, Joseph Goldberger, turned his attention to *pellagra* (Italian *pelle,* skin + *agra,* rough). He proved that this disease, which was debilitating many people in the southern United States, is due to the deficiency in the diet of a factor later named *niacin,* a member of the vitamin B complex. Opponents of Goldberger's dietary concept of pellagra insisted that the disease was infectious. In a series of human experiments begun on April 25, 1916, twenty men and two women swallowed capsules of infectious concoctions of blood, feces, and urine of pellagra patients. Dr. and Mrs. Goldberger were among them. None of the human volunteers developed pellagra.

vitamin E

Discovered more than half a century ago, vitamin E was noted to be necessary in the diet of female rats if they were to reproduce normally. It was identified

[22] Roger Lewin, "Vitamin D Changes Its Clothes," *New Scientist,* Vol. 57, No. 833 (February 15, 1973), pp. 371–75.

as an alcohol and given the name *tocopherol* (Greek *tokos,* childbirth + *phero,* to bring). It is an essential nutrient, but in normal people whose diet is average, disease from vitamin E deficiency does not occur spontaneously. Despite this fact, and despite the presently incomplete knowledge about the action of vitamin E in the human body, sales of it as a veritable cure-all are enormous. It is claimed that vitamin E improves the complexion and sexual potency, protects against miscarriage, pollution, and heart disease, and performs a host of other miracles. But as of spring 1973, there was no definitive evidence to support such claims; a lot of people were wasting a lot of money. (For a discussion of quackery, see pages 753–57.)[23]

vitamin K

Vitamin K is essential for the manufacture of substances necessary for normal blood clotting. Much of it is made by bacteria in the large intestine, and it is then absorbed into the circulation. When oral antibiotics are ingested, the intestinal ecosystem of these vitamin K–producing bacteria changes, so they may not survive. The termination of the beneficial action of these bacteria in the human intestine can result in vitamin K deficiency—a potent argument against self-medication.

more about vitamins

In 1912 the Polish biochemist Casimir Funk summed up what was known about vitamins at that time. There were four substances containing nitrogen, *amines,* that were vital to life, he postulated. These vital amines he called *vitamines.* Each specifically prevented beriberi, scurvy, rickets, or pellagra. He was right, as far as he went. Now it is known that there are more than four such vital substances. Since new factors have been discovered, the "e" has been dropped in "vitamines."

Each vitamin is either water- or fat-soluble. The water-soluble vitamins are the B complex vitamins and vitamin C. The fat-soluble vitamins are A, D, E, and K, two of which (A and D) are presented in Table 22-1 (pages 658–59).

Vitamin pills never make up for an inadequate diet. Furthermore, their indiscriminate use can be harmful. Folic acid (one of the B vitamins) and vitamin B_{12} are both needed by the bone marrow to make red blood cells. Used in high doses, folic acid relieves some of the symptoms of pernicious anemia. But folic acid does not halt the progressive deterioration of the nervous system caused by pernicious anemia. For a while, a self-medicating individual with the disease may feel better. But he has been lulled into a false sense of security. By the time he seeks medical care it may be too late to correct the error. The toxicity of excessive doses of vitamin D provides another example of the hazards of self-medication. A host of disagreeable symptoms, including nausea, vomiting, and

[23] Three excellent discussions of vitamin E are *Consumer Reports* (January 1973), pp. 60–65; Ellen E. Rodert and Jesse C. Obert, "Controversial Vitamin E," *Morbidity and Mortality,* County of Los Angeles Community Health Services (March 1973), p. 1; and Robert E. Hodges and Roslyn B. Alfin-Slater, "Vitamin E: A Review," *Nutrah,* Vol. 1, No. 3 (January 1972), pp. 1–3.

diarrhea, may occur. Intake of too much vitamin A may cause serious toxic signs and symptoms, including loss of appetite, irritability, abnormal skin pigmentation, dry skin, loss of hair, and bone and joint pains. It is the family physician who should decide about the use of vitamin pills.

necessary elements

Disintegrating rocks provide minerals for soil. From soil, growing plants take needed minerals. Man obtains minerals from plants, from animals that consume plants, and from such animal products as milk and eggs. Twenty-five of the ninety naturally occurring earth's elements have been proven essential to mammalian and avian nutrition. Of these, eleven are *major:* carbon, nitrogen, hydrogen, oxygen, sodium, potassium, calcium, phosphorus, sulfur, chlorine, and magnesium. Fourteen occur in minute traces. These *trace* elements are: iron, iodine,[24] zinc, copper, cobalt, molybdenum, selenium, manganese, chromium, vanadium, nickel, tin, silicon, and fluorine.[25]

The amount of essential minerals in the human body varies greatly. An average-sized man has about two and three-fourths pounds of calcium in his body but a mere trace of iron. Although human requirements of most of the trace elements have not yet been established, tiny amounts are known to exert an enormous influence. Zinc deficiencies, for example, have resulted in retarded adolescent growth and sexual maturation.[26] Some trace elements, though essential to life, may be harmful in larger amounts. This is of particular importance in considering pollution problems (see pages 82–88).

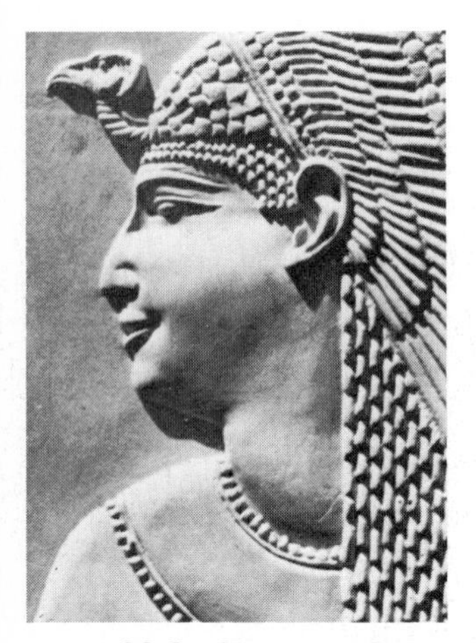

22-3 *Cleopatra, Queen of the Nile, and her goiter (see footnote 24).*

Unlike proteins, fats, and carbohydrates, but like water and vitamins, mineral elements are not directly acted upon by digestive juices. Freed from foods by digestion, they are absorbed, used in body building and regulation, and then excreted. To make up for their constant loss, they must, therefore, be regularly supplied in the diet.

It is in calcium and iron that the diet of this nation's people is often poor. Foods with enough protein and calcium usually contain adequate phosphates too. Some foods (milk, for example) contain more calcium than others (such as eggs); some (milk again) contain calcium that is more readily absorbed than the calcium in other foods (such as spinach).

Women need more iron than men. Periodic blood loss and the needs of a baby during pregnancy account for greater iron requirements of women. Iron deficiency among women is common. Also, during the growth years from infancy to adolescence the need for iron is particularly great.

water

Man can live for weeks without food but only for days without water. Slightly more than half of the adult body weight is water. It is the medium in which all

[24] Iodine is essential for the adequate production of thyroxine and triiodothyronine, hormones manufactured by the thyroid gland. With reduced thyroid hormones in the serum, the pituitary gland causes the thyroid to produce more cells to manufacture hormone. This abnormal enlargement of the thyroid is *goiter.* Common goiter is primarily an iodine-deficiency disease.

[25] Fluorine is a gaseous element, and although it has not been proven essential to life, fluorides are important to prevention of cavities (see pages 682–83).

[26] Michael Hambidge and Donough O'Brien, "On Developmental Nutrition: Trace Metals," *Ross Laboratories,* No. 7 (March 1973), citing J. A. Halsted, H. A. Ronaghy, P. Abadi, M. Haghshenass, G. H. Amirhakemi, R. M. Barakat, and J. G. Reinhold, "Zinc Deficiency in Man," *American Journal of Medicine,* Vol. 53 (1972), pp. 277–84.

chemical reactions of the body take place. As the most important of all solvents, water brings enzymes (footnote 56) into the digestive tract. As a carrier, water is essential to digestion, circulation, absorption, and excretion. Cells waiting to receive food are bathed in water. Two-thirds of body water is inside the cells, and one-third is outside. Nutrients are brought to the cells by the blood, which is about 80 percent water. After food has been used by the cells, there are waste products. These are transferred through watery solutions to the blood and excreted via the kidney in the urine, which is about 97 percent water. In the discussion of water pollution (in Chapter 3), it was pointed out that man is now recycling waste water and using it again after making it pure. The normal kidney has always done this efficiently. Large volumes of water carry waste to the kidney, but in passing through the kidney most of the water is reabsorbed and reused. The urine that is excreted is a concentrated watery solution of the body's waste products (see pages 243–45). Water has even more functions. In its involvement with the movements of the internal organs of the abdomen, and in the lubrication of the joints, water is essential to body mechanics. Too, water helps regulate body temperature.

some measures of nutrition

calories

In 1794, the elegant aristocrat and great scientist Antoine Laurent Lavoisier was ordered guillotined by a judge of the French Revolution. Begged to spare his valuable head, the judge curtly answered, "The Republic has no need of scientists." After the execution, Lagrange, an old friend of Lavoisier, whispered wiser words. "It took but a second to cut off his head; a hundred years will not suffice to produce one like it."[27] One of Lavoisier's contributions was to point out that ingested food is burned in a chemical reaction (oxidation) to yield heat and energy. From this "body fuel" concept comes the idea of the *calorie.*

A calorie is the amount of heat required to raise the temperature of one gram of water one degree Centigrade. This is truly a tiny unit of heat. What nutritionists really use is the large kilocalorie, which is a thousand times greater. The term "calorie" is now so commonly used, however, that the "kilo" is dropped in ordinary usage.

Caloric contents of food vary enormously. A given weight of fat contains over twice as many calories as an equal weight of carbohydrates or proteins. Proteins and carbohydrates each have four calories per gram. In a gram of fat there are nine calories.

What is adequate nutrition for the normal, nondieting person? One may rely on the food groups. Table 22-2 provides caloric values in single servings of representative samples of the basic four—the milk, meat, vegetable-fruit, and bread-cereal groups. It also includes representative fats and sweets. Table 22-3 gives the caloric values of some snacks. (Table 22-4 provides another measure of adequate nutrition—the U.S. Food and Drug Administration's recommended daily allowances of certain nutrients.)

[27] Quoted in Graham Lusk, *Nutrition* (New York, 1964), p. 63.

TABLE 22-1

A Dozen Leading Nutrients

NAME	IMPORTANT FOOD SOURCES	WHY NEEDED
CARBOHYDRATES (Sugars and starches)	Breads and cereals Potatoes and corn Bananas Dried fruits and sweetened fruits Sugar, syrup, jelly, honey	To supply energy. To carry other nutrients present in the food.
FATS	Butter and cream Salad oils and dressings Cooking fats Fat meats	To supply a large amount of energy in a small amount of food. To help keep skin smooth and healthy by supplying "essential fatty acids."
PROTEINS	Meat, fish, poultry, eggs All kinds of cheese Milk Breads and cereals Dried beans and peas Peanut butter and nuts	To build and repair all tissues in the body. Cellular proteins provide most of the cell's structure and are the enzymes controlling the cell's chemical reactions. To help form antibodies in the blood for fighting infection. To supply energy.

NAME	IMPORTANT FOOD SOURCES	WHY NEEDED	STABILITY TO HANDLING
VITAMINS Vitamin A	Yellow fruits and dark green and yellow vegetables Butter, whole milk, cream, Cheddar-type cheese, ice cream Liver	To help keep skin smooth and soft. To help keep mucous membranes firm and resistant to infection. To protect against night-blindness.	Stable to ordinary cooking temperatures. Unstable to long exposure in warm air. Not dissolved in cooking water.
Vitamin B_1 (Thiamine)	Meat (especially pork), fish, poultry, eggs Enriched and whole-grain breads, cereals Milk White potatoes	To keep appetite and digestion normal. To keep nervous system healthy. To help prevent irritability. To help body release energy from food.	Unstable to heat, especially in alkaline solutions (soda). Dissolved in cooking water.
Vitamin B_2 (Riboflavin)	Milk All kinds of cheese Ice cream Meat, fish, poultry, eggs	To help cells use oxygen. To help keep vision clear. To help prevent cracking at the corners of the mouth. To help keep skin and tongue smooth. To help prevent scaly, greasy skin around mouth and nose.	Fairly stable to ordinary cooking temperatures, especially in acid solutions. Unstable to ultraviolet light (direct sunlight). Dissolved in cooking water.

TABLE 22-1 (*continued*)

NAME	IMPORTANT FOOD SOURCES	WHY NEEDED	STABILITY TO HANDLING
Vitamin C (Ascorbic acid)	Citrus fruits—lemon, orange, grapefruit, lime Strawberries and cantaloupe Tomatoes Green peppers and broccoli Raw greens and cabbage White potatoes	To make cementing materials that hold body cells together. To make walls of blood vessels firm. To help resist infection. To help prevent fatigue. To help in healing wounds and broken bones.	Stable in acid. Unstable: destroyed by oxidation which is hastened by warm temperature, long, slow cooking, exposure to alkali and copper. Dissolved in cooking water.
Vitamin D	Vitamin D milk Butter Fish liver oil (also reaches man in sunshine)	To help maintain a correct balance of calcium in the body and thereby to help build bones and also to help in normal functioning of nerves and certain enzyme reactions.	Stable to heating, aging, and storage. Destroyed by excess ultraviolet light.

NAME	IMPORTANT FOOD SOURCES	WHY NEEDED
MINERALS		
Calcium	Milk Cheese Ice cream Turnip and mustard greens Collards and kale	To help build bones and teeth. To help make blood clot. To help muscles react normally. To delay fatigue and help tired muscles recover.
Iron	Liver Meat and eggs Green leafy vegetables Raisins and dried apricots	To combine with protein to make hemoglobin, the red substance in the blood that carries oxygen to the cells. About two-thirds of the body's iron is in the hemoglobin of the blood. (The minerals copper and cobalt also affect the red blood cell formation.)
Copper	Essentially the same foods that provide iron	To act in the process by which iron is used in the synthesis of hemoglobin. Also, an essential constituent of many enzymes that function in tissue metabolism.
Iodine	Iodized salt Salt-water fishes Foods grown in iodine-rich soil Water in nongoiterous regions	To enable the thyroid gland to produce enough of its hormones (thyroxine and triiodothyronine).

Sources: Adapted from Ruth M. Leverton, *A Girl and Her Figure,* National Dairy Council (Chicago, 1955), and Ethel A. Martin, *Nutrition in Action,* 2nd ed. (New York, 1965), pp. 116, 164–65.

TABLE 22-2

Caloric Values for Representative Foods, Classified by Food Groups

FOOD*	WEIGHT OR APPROX. MEASURE	CALORIES
MILK GROUP		
Cheese, Cheddar	1⅛ in. cube	115
Cheese, cottage, creamed	¼ cup	60
Cream	1 tbsp.	35
Milk, fluid, skim (buttermilk)	1 cup	90
Milk, fluid, whole	1 cup	165
MEAT GROUP		
Beans, dry, canned	¾ cup	250
Beef, pot roast	3 oz.	245
Chicken	¼ small broiler	185
Egg	1 medium	80
Frankfurter	1 medium	155
Haddock	1 fillet	135
Ham, luncheon meat	2 oz.	170
Liver, beef	2 oz.	120
Peanut butter	1 tbsp.	90
Pork chop	1 chop	260
Salmon, canned	½ cup	120
Sausage, salami	1 slice	135
VEGETABLE GROUP		
Beans, snap, green	½ cup	15
Broccoli	½ cup	20
Cabbage, shredded, raw	½ cup	10
Carrots, diced	½ cup	20
Corn, canned	½ cup	85
Lettuce leaves	2 large or 4 small	5
Peas, green	½ cup	55
Potato, white	1 medium	90
Spinach	½ cup	20
Squash, winter	½ cup	50
Sweet potato	1 medium	155
Tomato juice, canned	½ cup (small glass)	25
FRUIT GROUP		
Apple, raw	1 medium	70
Apricots, dried, cooked	½ cup	135
Banana, raw	1 small	85
Cantaloupe	½ melon	40
Grapefruit	½ medium	50
Orange	1 medium	70
Orange juice, fresh	½ cup (small glass)	60
Peaches, canned	2 halves with juice	90
Pineapple juice, canned	½ cup (small glass)	60
Prunes, dried, cooked	5 with juice	160
Strawberries, raw	½ cup	30
BREAD-CEREAL GROUP		
Bread, white, enriched	1 slice	60
Cornflakes, fortified	1⅓ cup	110
Macaroni, enriched, cooked	¾ cup	115
Oatmeal, cooked	⅔ cup	100
Rice, cooked	¾ cup	150
FATS GROUP		
Bacon, crisp	2 strips	95
Butter or fortified margarine	1 tbsp.	100
Oils, salad or cooking	1 tbsp.	125
SWEETS GROUP		
Beverages, cola type	6 oz.	80
Sugar, granulated	1 tbsp.	50

*Foods on this list are in forms ready to eat. All meats and vegetables are cooked unless otherwise indicated.
Source: Adapted from Ethel A. Martin, *Nutrition in Action,* 2nd ed. (New York, 1965), p. 61.

TABLE 22-3

Caloric Values for Common Snacks

FOOD	AMOUNT OR AVERAGE SERVING	CALORIES	FOOD	AMOUNT OR AVERAGE SERVING	CALORIES
SANDWICHES	With bread:		CANDIES		
Hamburger	3-in. patty	330	Chocolate bars:		
Peanut butter	1 tbsp.	330	Plain, sweet milk	1 bar (1 oz.)	155
Cheese	1 oz.	280	With almonds	1 bar (1 oz.)	140
Ham	1 oz.	320	Chocolate-covered bar	1 bar	270
Pizza, cheese	$\frac{1}{8}$ pie	180	Chocolate fudge	1 piece 1-in. sq.	90–120
BEVERAGES			Caramels, plain	2 medium	85
Carbonated drinks,			Lifesavers	1 roll	95
soda, root beer, etc.	6-oz. glass	80	Peanut brittle	1 piece $2\frac{1}{2} \times 2\frac{1}{2} \times \frac{3}{8}$ in.	110
Pepsi-Cola	12-oz. glass	150			
Club soda	8-oz. glass	5	DESSERTS		
Chocolate malted			Pie:		
milk	10-oz. glass	500	Fruit	$\frac{1}{6}$ pie	375
Ginger ale	6-oz. glass	60	Custard	$\frac{1}{6}$ pie	265
Tea or coffee, black	1 cup	0	Mince	$\frac{1}{6}$ pie	400
Tea or coffee, with			Pumpkin with		
2 tbsp. cream and			whipped cream	$\frac{1}{6}$ pie	460
2 tsp. sugar	1 cup	90	Cake:		
ALCOHOLIC DRINKS			Chocolate layer	3-in. section	350
Ale	8-oz. glass	155	Doughnut, sugared	1 average	150
Beer	8-oz. glass	110	SWEETS		
Highball (with ginger			Ice cream:		
ale)	8-oz. glass	185	Plain vanilla	$\frac{1}{6}$ qt.	200
Manhattan	average	165	Other flavors	$\frac{1}{6}$ qt.	260
Martini	average	140	Orange sherbet	$\frac{1}{2}$ cup	120
Wine (muscatel, port)	2-oz. glass	95	Sundaes, small choco-		
Sherry	2-oz. glass	75	late nut with		
Scotch, bourbon, rye	$1\frac{1}{2}$-oz. jigger	130	whipped cream	average	400
FRUITS			Ice-cream sodas,		
Apple	1 medium	70	chocolate	10-oz. glass	270
Banana	1 small	85	MIDNIGHT SNACKS		
Grapes	30 medium	75	Cold potato	$\frac{1}{2}$ medium	65
Orange	1 medium	70	Chicken leg	1 average	88
Pear	1	65	Milk	7-oz. glass	140
SALTED NUTS AND			Roast beef	$\frac{1}{2}$ in. $\times$ 2 in. $\times$ 3 in. piece	130
POTATO CHIPS					
Almonds, filberts,			Cheese	$\frac{1}{4}$ in. $\times$ 2 in. $\times$ 3 in. piece	120
hazelnuts	12–15	95	Leftover beans	$\frac{1}{2}$ cup	105
Cashews	6–8	90	Brownie	$\frac{3}{4}$ in. $\times$ $1\frac{3}{4}$ in. $\times$ $2\frac{1}{4}$ in.	140
Peanuts	15–17	85			
Pecans, walnuts	10–15 halves	100			
Potato chips	1 serving	108	Cream puff	4 in. diam.	450

Source: Adapted from Helen S. Mitchell *et al., Cooper's Nutrition in Health and Disease,* 15th ed. (Philadelphia, 1968), pp. 282–83. Data provided by Smith, Kline, and French Laboratories.

TABLE 22-4

U.S. Food and Drug Administration Recommended Daily Allowances for Certain Vitamins and Minerals

VITAMIN OR MINERAL	UNIT	INFANTS (0–12 MONTHS)	CHILDREN UNDER 4 YEARS	ADULTS AND CHILDREN 4 OR MORE YEARS	PREGNANT OR LACTATING WOMEN
Vitamin A	IU	1500	2500	5000	8000
Vitamin D	IU	400	400	400	400
Vitamin E	IU	5	10	30	30
Vitamin C	mg	35	40	60	60
Folic acid	mg	0.1	0.2	0.4	0.8
Thiamine (B_1)	mg	0.5	0.7	1.5	1.7
Riboflavin (B_2)	mg	0.6	0.8	1.7	2.0
Niacin	mg	8	9	20	20
Vitamin B_6	mg	0.4	0.7	2	2.5
Vitamin B_{12}	mcg	2	3	6	8
Biotin	mg	0.05	0.15	0.3	0.3
Pantothenic acid	mg	3	5	10	10
Calcium	g	0.6	0.8	1.0	1.3
Phosphorus	g	0.5	0.8	1.0	1.3
Iodine	mcg	45	70	150	150
Iron	mg	15	10	18	18
Magnesium	mg	70	200	400	450
Copper	mg	0.6	1.0	2.0	2.0
Zinc	mg	5	8	15	15

Source: *FDA Drug Bulletin*, December 1973.

With physical activity, calorie requirements increase (Table 22-5). But age, sex, body size, and climate also influence the number of calories a person uses. Because of growth requirements, adolescents need relatively more calories than adults. The aged need fewer calories than the young. Women usually need fewer calories than men. Pregnancy and lactation increase caloric demands. A hot day, mostly because it decreases activity, decreases caloric needs.

TABLE 22-5

A Typical Female College Student's Activities for One Day

ACTIVITY	HOURS SPENT IN ACTIVITY	CALORIES PER POUND PER HOUR	TOTAL CALORIES PER POUND (Calories × Hours)
Asleep	8	.4	3.2
Lying still, awake	1	.5	.5
Dressing and undressing	1	.9	.9
Sitting in class, eating, studying, talking	8	.7	5.6
Walking	1	1.5	1.5
Standing	1	.8	.8
Driving a car	1	1.0	1.0
Running	½	4.0	2.0
Playing ping-pong	½	2.7	1.3
Writing	2	.7	1.4
Total	24		18.2

Total calories used per pound	18.2
Weight in pounds	×115.0
Total calories expended for the day	2,093

Source: Adapted from Helen S. Mitchell *et al.*, *Cooper's Nutrition in Health and Disease*, 15th ed. (Philadelphia, 1968), pp. 50–51.

Nutritive values of foods, moreover, depend in part on the way the foods are prepared. Fried potatoes, for example, contain much more fat than baked potatoes. In addition, some sick people are unable to digest some foods. Fats are poorly digested by some people with disease of the pancreas (see page 687). Fatigue also impedes the labor of digestion, as do tension and rapid eating. That is why, insofar as possible, one should rest before and after dinner. Thus, the number of calories on a calorie chart may not always be the number of calories eventually used by the eater.

weights and measures

It has been found that people who are of average or slightly less than average weight at twenty-five are healthier and live longer if they maintain that weight for the rest of their lives. In addition, after one's maximum height is achieved, there is no need to gain more weight. Moreover, fat, muscles, organs, bones, and fluid all contribute to weight. Thus, a muscular athlete may weigh more than is recommended because of the weight of his larger muscles. He is heavy

TABLE 22-6

Desirable Weights in Pounds for People Twenty-five or Over*

MEN				WOMEN			
HEIGHT† Ft. In.	SMALL FRAME	MEDIUM FRAME	LARGE FRAME	HEIGHT† Ft. In.	SMALL FRAME	MEDIUM FRAME	LARGE FRAME
5 2	112–120	118–129	126- 141	4 10	92– 98	96–107	104–119
5 3	115–123	121–133	129–144	4 11	94–101	98–110	106–122
5 4	118–126	124–136	132–148	5 0	96–104	101–113	109–125
5 5	121–129	127–139	135–152	5 1	99–107	104–116	112–128
5 6	124–133	130–143	138–156	5 2	102–110	107–119	115–131
5 7	128–137	134–147	142–161	5 3	105–113	110–122	118–134
5 8	132–141	138–152	147–166	5 4	108–116	113–126	121–138
5 9	136–145	142–156	151–170	5 5	111–119	116–130	125–142
5 10	140–150	146–160	155–174	5 6	114–123	120–135	129–146
5 11	144–154	150–165	159–179	5 7	118–127	124–139	133–150
6 0	148–158	154–170	164–184	5 8	122–131	128–143	137–154
6 1	152–162	158–175	168–189	5 9	126–135	132–147	141–158
6 2	156–167	162–180	173–194	5 10	130–140	136–151	145–163
6 3	160–171	167–185	178–199	5 11	134–144	140–155	149–168
6 4	164–175	172–190	182–204	6 0	138–148	144–159	153–173

*These figures are based on the person's wearing indoor clothing. For nude weight, women should subtract two to four pounds; men, five to seven pounds. Girls between the ages of eighteen and twenty-five should subtract one pound for each year under twenty-five.

†Height is measured with shoes on: one-inch heels for men, two-inch heels for women.

Source: Metropolitan Life Insurance Company. Derived primarily from data of the Build and Blood Pressure Study, Society of Actuaries, 1959.

but his problem is not excessive fat. Although modern charts attempt to correct this by adding body build to weight charts (Table 22-6), the best way to determine actual body fatness is by measuring skinfold thickness with *calipers.* Norms for this measurement have yet to be completely agreed upon.

What is meant by overweight? The term does not directly connote excessive fat. A better term might be over-heaviness. However, many nutritionists would agree that someone who weighs 10 to 20 percent over the desirable body weight is overweight. *Obesity* is a general term, commonly denoting 20 percent or more above the desirable weight. It results from an increase in the amount of fatty tissue. A person who is obese has three to five times more fat cells than one who is not. In addition, the fat cells of an obese person are greater in size. Fat cells of obese children six years old have been observed to have attained adult size.[28] By proper dieting and exercise, an obese person can lose weight. This is accomplished not by reducing the number of fat cells, but by decreasing the fat content within these cells. It is believed that most fat cells are laid down during three different stages of life: first, during the late fetal stage; second,

[28] "Control of Hypercellularity Held 'Best Hope' in Obesity," *Pediatric Currents* (Ross Timesaver), Vol. 22, No. 5 (May 1973), p. 1, citing J. L. Knittle, *Journal of Pediatrics,* Vol. 81 (1972), p. 1048.

in the first year of life; and third, during early adolescence. Pinpointing, through research, the time of greatest multiplication of fat cells will make more likely the prevention or early treatment of obesity.[29] However, dietary limitations during these periods of fat-cell multiplication must be approached with great caution. It must be remembered that these are periods of significant growth; unwise dietary practices during these times can cause irreversible harm (see pages 670–71).

Harvard nutritionist Jean Mayer describes some "unscientific" yet worthwhile methods of assessing fatness. "If you *look* fat," he writes, in suggesting the *mirror test,* "you probably *are* fat." The *pinch test* involves lifting free a fold of skin and its underlying fat from various body areas such as the back of the upper arm or the abdomen. If the fold is markedly greater than one inch, excessive body fat is indicated. (If the fold is thinner than one-half inch, the individual is probably too thin.) When the *ruler test* is used, the individual lies flat on his back. "If he or she is not too fat, the surface of the abdomen between the flare of the ribs and the front of the pelvis is normally flat or slightly concave and a ruler placed on the abdomen along the midline of the body should touch both the ribs and the pelvic area." In the *belt-line test,* Mayer points out that a man has too much abdominal fat if the circumference of the abdomen at the navel exceeds the circumference of the chest at the nipples. Ordinarily the circumference of the chest exceeds that of the abdomen.[30]

weighing too much

why do people weigh too much?

A relatively small number of people are obese because of an endocrine gland (see page 254) disturbance. Such obesity may be genetically transmitted.[31] (Specific tests help make such a diagnosis.) There are others who, although spared an actual endocrine dysfunction, nevertheless have a genetic predisposition to being fat. It should be added that much about the problem of overweight remains an enigma. It is surely true that some people can eat gluttonously without putting on weight; others, exercising just as little (or as much), gain weight on a relatively modest diet. The glutton's body metabolism is such that he handles food differently.[32]

However, for a good many people, the problem is simpler. Their overweight is due to overeating and lack of exercise. Caloric intake exceeds energy needs. The excess is stored as fat, and excess fat is detrimental to health. Labor-saving devices have eased life, but the food intake of the U.S. citizen has not decreased with his energy needs. A typist who uses a manual typewriter rather than an electric one burns seventy-five more calories in five hours. That is equal to a slice of bread. "This is the kind of trade-off we're going to have to make if we

[29] Jules Hirsch, "Can We Modify the Number of Adipose Cells?" *Postgraduate Medicine,* Vol. 51, No. 5.
[30] Jean Mayer, *Overweight* (Englewood Cliffs, N.J., 1968), pp. 29–30.
[31] Edgar S. Gordon, "Obesity: Gluttony or Genes?" *Postgraduate Medicine,* Vol. 45, No. 2 (June 1969), pp. 95–100.
[32] Jerry Cowhig, "Is There More to Obesity Than Food?" *New Scientist* (July 6, 1972), p. 32.

want to avoid obesity in our sedentary lives."[33] The customary snack between meals has added to the problem of weight control for the people of this nation. Small children and teen-agers may need between-meal fuel to help meet their growth needs. But it should be remembered that snacks represent calories and that calories do count.

Sheer boredom often accounts for overeating. For some people there seems to be little to do but eat and watch old movies on television. Emotional problems are often associated with this cause of overeating. These may originate in the mother who compensates for her rejection of a child by lavishing him with food and other physical comforts. The mother may compound the problem by restricting the child's physical activity so that he will not hurt himself. The child learns that eating earns approval and brings affection. Years later, when feeling disapproval or lack of love, he eats excessively. And his basic training in inactivity does not help him burn up excess calories.

Doubtless this is one reason why obesity tends to be familial. But there are other reasons. A gastronomic family atmosphere may be a symbol of wealth. Time was when the size of the meal and the circumference of the paunch were measures of success. Queen Victoria was once served a dinner of seventy dishes, including four soups, four fish, a haunch of venison, and six roasts.[34] Unlike her husband, she ate sparingly. He had a huge paunch. Perhaps not coincidentally, she lived almost twice as long as he.

Today, obesity caused by overeating is usually intemperance. A vegetarian, the dramatist George Bernard Shaw was tall and thin. Greeting him on a London street one day, the short, stout writer G. K. Chesterton said, "From the looks of you, George, one would think there was a famine in England."

"And from the looks of you," replied Shaw, "one would think you had caused it."

obesity: a heavy load for mind and body

Intemperance is often concealable. One can, for example, get drunk and then sober up, and (at least for a while) no one will be the wiser. But people who eat too much carry their mark of intemperance with them constantly. So it was with Chesterton.

Sometimes people who are moderately overweight and, more commonly, people who are obese suffer distortions of body image. This refers to the idea one has of oneself as an independent object in space. Such distortion can take the form of an overwhelming concern with obesity. For those with this problem, fat is all that matters. People are not better or worse; they are thinner or fatter. Importantly, body image disturbances occur almost exclusively among persons who were obese during adolescence. (If the onset of obesity occurs later in life, body image distortions are rare.) Derogation by parents of obese children later results in body image distortion problems.[35]

To the emotional stress of the obese, one must add physical hazards. Fat people are more susceptible than the thin to sickness and death from heart

[33] Doris Calloway, quoted in *California's Health,* Vol. 30, No. 3 (September 1972), p. 10.
[34] John Burnett, *Plenty and Want* (London, 1966), p. 68.
[35] Albert J. Stunkard, "Body Image Disturbance in Obesity," *Feelings and Their Medical Significance,* Vol. 10, No. 1 (January–February 1968), pp. 1–4.

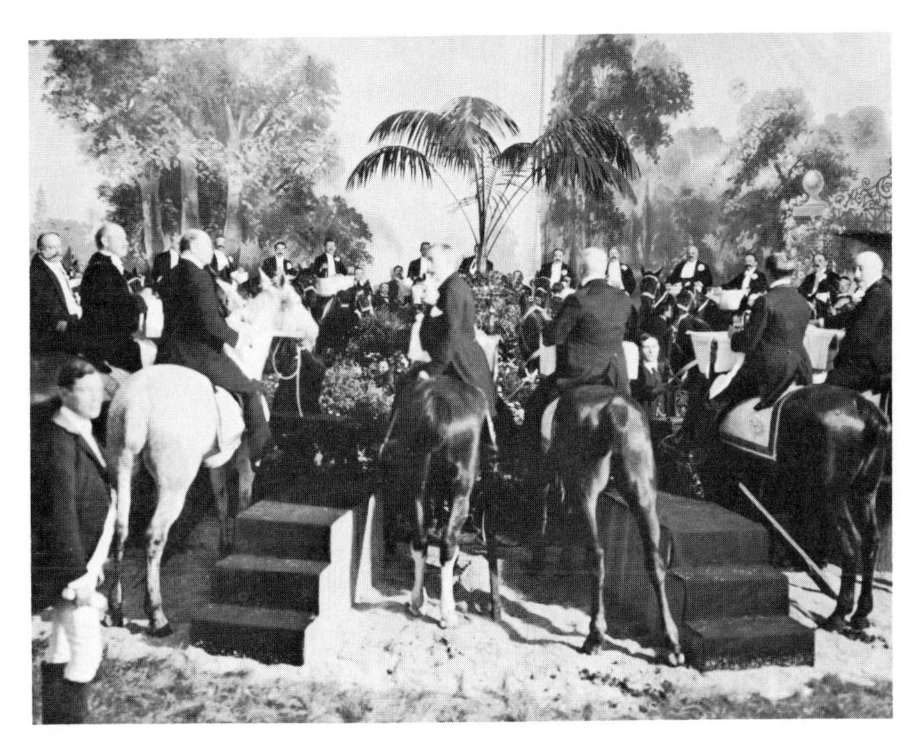

22-4 *A banquet served on horseback in 1903. Given by a millionaire to celebrate the completion of his private stable, the banquet was held in the Grand Ballroom of Sherry's, an elegant New York City restaurant.*

disease, stroke, nephritis, diabetes, cancers, and various diseases of the digestive system such as gallstones and a variety of liver conditions. And the fat do not live as long as the lean. It is, moreover, noteworthy that "At the moment the only agent known to be capable of doubling rodent lifespan is caloric restriction."[36]

how to reduce weight problems

exercise

The child's training in weight control begins at home and may continue at school. School people do well to realize the importance of an overall program of physical activity. Winning football teams are fun but take little weight off the whole student body. People settling into the routines of their late twenties and early thirties soon find themselves fitting tightly into their clothes. It is then that fewer calories are needed to maintain usual weight. Exercise should have been woven into the lifetime pattern long before this. It is never too late to begin walking to the drugstore and taking the steps instead of the elevator.

Moderate exercise *over a prolonged period* is an excellent reducer. Half an hour a day of vigorous handball or squash burns up, in a year, the equivalent of sixteen pounds of fat. (Table 22-5 provides the caloric loss per hour resulting from various common activities.) That exercise increases appetite is a mistaken notion. Indeed, the reverse is true, and, moreover, physical fitness improves

[36] Alex Comfort, "Eat Less, Live Longer," *New Scientist,* Vol. 53, No. 789 (March 30, 1972), p. 689.

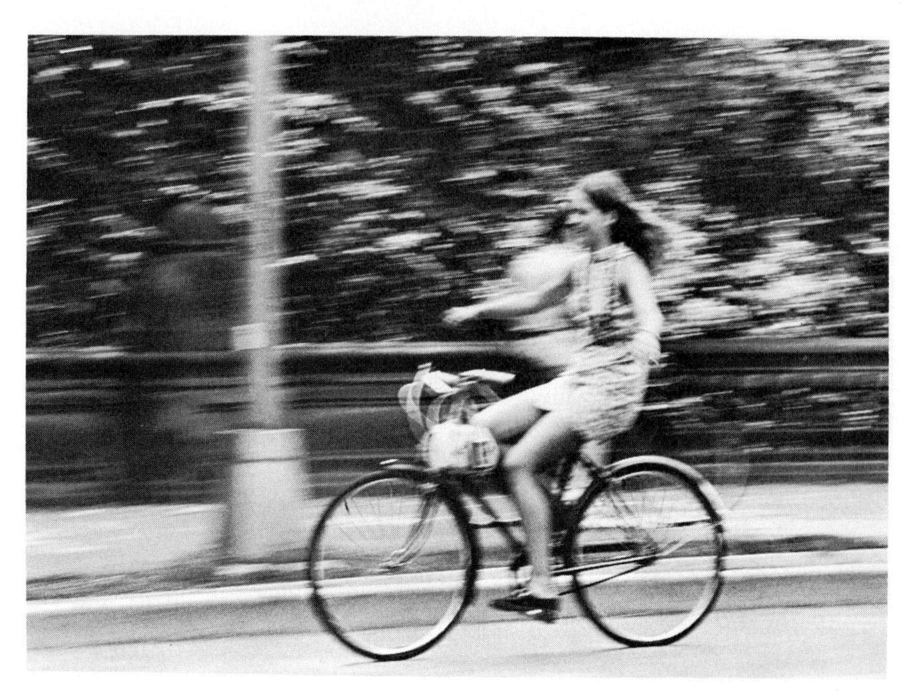

22-5 *Bicycling, an effective and enjoyable aerobic exercise.*

the way the body handles food. Not all exercise is equally effective. Far superior to weight-lifting and sit-ups are swimming, bicycling, jogging, and walking.

Sadly, those needing exercise most may get it least. Yet, does this not suggest the role of inactivity in obesity? In one study of normal and obese girls playing volleyball, it was found that "normal weight girls were motionless, on the average, 50 percent of the time, obese girls 85 percent . . . in tennis normal girls were motionless 15 percent of the time, obese girls, 60."[37]

Exercise is discussed in more detail in Chapter 23.

dieting

The would-be dieter is often exposed to a barrage of poor advice. Reliance on quacks, diet fads, and self-medication may all end disastrously. For many people, calorie counting ought to become a way of life.[38] Nothing is more discouraging than repeated weight losses followed by repeated gains. One study revealed "that 69 of 91 girls who dieted to lose weight in the ninth grade were

[37] Jean Mayer, quoted in Herbert L. Jones, Margaret B. Schutt, and Ann L. Shelton, eds., *Science and Theory of Health* (Dubuque, Iowa, 1966), p. 185.

[38] The Council on Foods and Nutrition of the American Medical Association has suggested several simple formulae to help the dieter. To maintain their present weight, most normally active people need 15 calories per pound of weight per day. Assume that an individual weighs and wishes to stay at 150 pounds. To maintain this desired weight, he may consume

$$150 \times 15 = 2{,}250 \text{ calories per day}$$

However, consider the individual who wishes to reduce his weight to 150 pounds. He wants to lose one pound still trying to lose weight in grade 12."[39] Nevertheless, there are those who find it difficult to understand that, for many growing children, weight loss may be undesirable. During the growing period, good weight control may mean either maintaining the same weight for several months or decreasing the weight gain. The success of dieting, at that time, should not be measured by actual weight loss.[40] Dramatic weight losses during this stage of life are fraught with danger and should not be expected. But what is learned about overweight in the learning, growing years can later be put to good use.

Normal water retention prior to menstruation makes daily weighing meaningless for some women. In other people, early weight loss is loss of fluid, not fat. Weight checks once weekly are quite enough. A varied, tastefully prepared diet is essential to morale. A snack an hour before a meal may be helpful to the dieter in reducing his appetite for the large meal. A lot of energy is required to use up relatively few calories (see Tables 22-4 and 22-5). As was pointed out above, for the dieter, exercise is essential. Moderation in both dieting and exercise is basic. Vitamin supplements are necessary for adults on weight reduction diets.[41]

It should be reemphasized that adolescent and adult overweight are not based on the same problem. "All adolescents gain weight while growing. Increased adipose tissue [see page 691] is the problem."[42] The average growing teen-ager should not expect large amounts of fat to be lost. It is more realistic in early and middle adolescence to prevent further gain of body fat by eating what the rest of the family eats, whether it be pizza or potatoes, but *in smaller portions.* Nobody should embark on a strict diet without first consulting a physician. Without close supervision, losing two pounds a week may be hazardous. Patients on diets of less than 1,000 calories per day are often admitted into a hospital for supervision of their diet.[43]

---

a week. In each stored pound of fat there are 3,500 calories. Every day he must do with 500 calories less to lose one pound a week. The formula:

150	pounds (the desired weight)
× 15	calories
2,250	calories per day needed to maintain present weight
− 500	calories per day to lose 3,500 calories (1 pound) per week
1,750	total calories permitted per day to lose one pound per week

To lose *two* pounds a week, the same dieter would have to reduce his caloric intake by twice as much, or by 1,000 calories per day, which means he would be permitted to consume 1,250 calories per day. (From *The Healthy Way to Weigh Less,* Council on Foods and Nutrition, American Medical Association, cited in Mort Weisinger, "How to Stick to Your Diet," *Today's Health,* Vol. 51, No. 7 [July 1973], p. 35.)

[39] Ruth L. Huenemann, "Food Habits of Obese and Nonobese Adolescents," *Postgraduate Medicine,* Vol. 51, No. 5 (May 1972), p. 105.

[40] Johanna T. Dwyer, Caroline V. Blonde, and Jean Mayer, "Treating Obesity in Growing Children," *Postgraduate Medicine,* Vol. 51, No. 5 (May 1972), p. 93.

[41] George A. Bray, "Clinical Management of the Obese Adult," *Postgraduate Medicine,* Vol. 51, No. 5 (May 1972), p. 126.

[42] Felix P. Heald, "Treatment of Obesity in Adolescence," *Postgraduate Medicine,* Vol. 51, No. 5 (May 1972), p. 112.

[43] Particular care must be exercised in treating the obesity of the child. "Many obese children are anemic; thus, foods providing vitamins and minerals such as iron should not be restricted unduly . . . [Moreover,] growth and maturation depend in great part on energy intake, and caloric restriction must not be so severe as to halt or retard growth. Calorie restriction of a degree acceptable for mature adults may adversely affect linear growth in children." (Johanna T. Dwyer, Caroline V. Blonde, and Jean Mayer, "Treating Obesity in Growing Children," *Postgraduate Medicine,* Vol. 51, No. 7 [June 1972], pp. 112–13.)

weighing too little

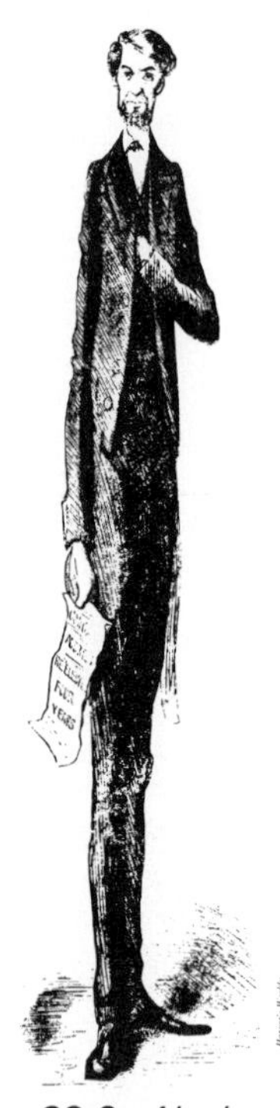

22-6 *Abraham Lincoln—a thin man made even thinner by a cartoonist.*

Justified concern with obesity has made the social life of the underweight individual much more pleasant than it was in former days. Poorly eating infants often suffer from their tense response to an unhappy mother. When an adult is more than 10 percent underweight, particularly if he is in his twenties, a physician's advice is indicated. By increasing their attention to some details, moderately underweight people usually gain weight. Among these details are elimination of infections, particularly of the appendix, teeth, and tonsils. Overactivity of the thyroid gland may need correction. Increased rest or a job change involving less tension may be indicated. Appetite-dulling tobacco is contraindicated. Frequent, extra-high-caloric snacks are better than overeating at mealtimes. Malted milks and milk shakes, cream with cereals, milk instead of soft drinks, extra butter, rich desserts, eggs, and meat—all these increase caloric intake. Vitamin supplements, especially thiamine, stimulate the appetite and improve digestion. Using a drug called *cyproheptadine,* a group of researchers was able to increase the appetites, weights, and growth rates of a small group of children.[44]

In this country, severe malnutrition (as differentiated from a moderate underweight problem) is much less common a problem than obesity. Moreover, genetics plays some role in body build. Genetic factors resulting in a stout build are dominant; those making for leanness are recessive. One study showed that "progeny from lean matings resulted in 90.0 percent leans and 9.1 percent stouts, while the matings of stouts showed 73 percent stout progeny and 27 percent lean . . . Compared with persons of average weight, the thin man has better resistance to cardiovascular and renal diseases, to diabetes and . . . accidents."[45]

the hurt of hunger

Retardation—whether physical, mental, or both—has multiple causes varying from hazards within the uterus to those within the slums. The brain of a three-year-old weighs 80 percent of what it will weigh in adulthood. At that time the body weight is 20 percent that of maturity. It is postulated that during the early years of life malnourishment can do its greatest irrevocable damage.[46] If the malnutrition of poverty can be one of the causes of childhood retardation, the tragedy is double, for the retarded child is unequipped to someday better his circumstances. Adult malnutrition results in inefficiency but is not thought to cause mental retardation.

[44] "Cyproheptadine Helps Children Gain in Size," *Journal of the American Medical Association,* Vol. 223, No. 6 (February 5, 1973), p. 611.

[45] "The Thin Man," *M.D., Medical Newsmagazine,* Vol. 15. No. 7 (July 1971), pp. 160 and 156.

[46] Philip H. Abelson, "Malnutrition, Learning, and Behavior," *Science,* Vol. 164, No. 3875 (April 4, 1969), p. 17.

At the second Western Hemisphere Nutrition Congress, evidence was presented to show that "brain growth of infants subject to severe protein malnutrition from the first months of life is markedly impaired."[47] Another writer says that "apathy typical of chronic protein deficiency, an apathy which translates into diminished learning potential, is estimated to affect 350 million children, 7 out of every 10 children under the age of 6 in the entire world."[48]

Are children in this country affected? Early in 1969, the U.S. Senate Select Committee on Nutrition and Related Human Needs heard a startling report. Preliminary findings of the first federal nutrition survey in the United States "clearly indicates an alarming prevalence of those characteristics that are associated with undernourished groups." Indeed, 10 to 15 percent of all the children examined showed retarded growth levels and were, therefore, "a high risk in retardation of mental and physical performance."[49] This richest nation, which finds the means to war and explore, cannot afford to permit millions of its children to be permanently crippled by malnutrition and hunger, yet government programs to solve this problem are grievously inadequate.

food fads and fancies

organic foods

Organic, natural, and *health foods* are not identical. *Organic foods* are those grown in soil that has been treated with organic matter, such as manure, vegetable compost, or natural and mineral fertilizers. Pesticides, antibiotics, and hormones are not used. Such foods are not processed; that is, they are prepared without the use of artificial food additives.[50] Sometimes, however, processed foods are sold as organic because they were grown with the use of organic fertilizers and without pesticides. *Natural foods* are not necessarily organically grown; they are merely neither refined nor processed, and thus contain no

[47] "Malnutrition and Innate Capacity," an editorial in *Hospital Tribune* (May 5, 1969), p. 11.

[48] Francis Keppel, "Food for Thought," in Nevin S. Scrimshaw and John E. Gordon, eds., *Malnutrition, Learning, and Behavior* (Cambridge, Mass., 1968), p. 6. Research promises hope for these hungry millions. A kind of cereal called sorghum is the basic diet of 300 million poor and hungry Asians and Africans. In South America, sorghum is a livestock feed. While a graduate student at Purdue, Rameshwar Singh, a plant geneticist, identified two superior sorghum strains containing 30 to 40 percent more protein than ordinary sorghums; these new sorghums also ensure a balance of essential amino acids necessary for absorption of the protein by the body. Although various technical problems remain, it is believed that the improved sorghum strains will be available for human consumption between 1976 and 1978. ("New Improved Sorghum: 'Scientific Achievement of the First Magnitude,' " *Science News,* Vol. 104, No. 14 [October 6, 1973], p. 212.)

[49] "Malnutrition and Innate Capacity," p. 11.

[50] Food additives were used thousands of years ago by the Eqyptians and Chinese. Modern chemistry has added to the number of natural additives; today some 2,500 natural and synthetic chemicals are added to foods to maintain or improve their flavor, freshness, coloring, and texture. It is estimated that flavoring agents alone number as high as 1,400. The importance of preservatives is emphasized by the World Health Organization, which estimates that 20 percent of the world's food supply is lost through spoilage. Sometimes, new information leads to a ban on a formerly approved additive. For example, in this country in 1969, the Food and Drug Administration banned cyclamates, a group of artificial sweeteners, when it was shown that massive doses caused bladder cancer in mice. An excellent review of food additives is G. O. Kermode, "Food Additives," *Scientific American,* Vol. 226, No. 3 (March 1972), pp. 15–21.

additives; examples are honey, molasses, brown (unpolished) rice, and grains, whole or ground into flour. The meaning of the term *health foods* is both unclear and misleading. This doubtless helps make them so profitable. Many buyers believe that products sold as health foods are both organic and natural and are therefore more healthful than other foods. This is not necessarily true.

Much of the current interest in organic foods is based on fears that conventionally grown foods are nutritionally inferior and dangerously contaminated by pesticides. What claims are made for organic foods? And what are the facts?

1. *The nutritional value of organic foods is higher than that of similar foods produced under ordinary conditions.* The nutrient content of a plant is controlled not by soil conditions or type of fertilizer, but by its genetic structure. Soil that is deficient in essential nutrients simply will not support plant growth. Fertilizers increase crop size, not nutrient value. Organic fertilizers often do contain more trace minerals than inorganic fertilizers. But a plant absorbs what it needs, and the kinds of minerals in a plant are determined by its DNA. Moreover, organic fertilizers must first be decomposed by bacteria in the soil before their elements can be absorbed by the plant, and these elements are inorganic. Thus, organic fertilizers are eventually used by the plant in an inorganic form. In addition, inorganic fertilizers are more efficient, because bacterial conversion prior to plant use is unnecessary.

2. *The use of pesticides makes consumption of inorganically grown foods dangerous.* Pesticides are sprayed on foods, not in them. They are easily washed or peeled off. Moreover, there is no scientific evidence that the pesticide level on foods in this country is approaching dangerous levels.

3. *Organic foods are always freer of contaminants such as bacteria, pesticides, natural toxins, and heavy metals (lead and mercury).* This belief is scientifically invalid. Moreover, organic foods may have pesticides on them that were blown over from neighboring orchards and farms. So, although the buyer pays one-third to two times more for foods purported to be organic, he has no way of knowing whether he has the genuine product. Foods grown without pesticides are quite likely to have insect markings; therefore, damaged produce grown under ordinary conditions can easily be sold as organic. In addition, the customer cannot be certain whether a washed or peeled product was actually grown under pesticide-free conditions. It is worth noting that long-established labeling and inspection standards regulate the quality of conventionally grown foods, but no such standards yet apply to the $100 million organic food industry that supplies more than 3,500 stores in the nation.

4. *Organic foods can supply most of the nation's population.* This impractical notion fails to consider that most people live in cities and that they desire foods grown in different climates. Such foods must be harvested before ripening, protected by pesticides, processed, and shipped great distances in order to make a variety of foods available year-round.

5. *"Natural" or "organic" vitamins are superior to those manufactured by a reliable pharmaceutical company.* This claim is fraudulent. Whether extracted from a natural product, as is ascorbic acid (vitamin C; see pages 652–53 and footnote 37, page 163) from rose hips, or synthesized in the laboratory, the vita-

min acts exactly the same in the body. Any particular vitamin has only one chemical structure. In one case, "Rose Hips Vitamin C Tablets" actually contained 20–25 percent chemical ascorbic acid added to the natural base. Had this not been done, the tablet "would have been as large as a golf ball."[51] Such labeling of a synthetic vitamin as "natural" or "organic" is illegal. Unfortunately, most local health agencies do not have the resources to handle these misrepresentations to the consumer.

vegetarianism[52]

"Oh, how criminal it is," wrote the Roman poet Ovid (43 B.C.–A.D. 18), "for one greedy body to grow fat with food . . . through the destruction of another living thing!" He urged people to eat only "the food which Earth, the best of mothers, has produced." One of the countless millions who failed to follow his advice was the English dandy Beau Brummel. Asked if he ever ate vegetables, he replied, "I once ate a pea." Nevertheless, vegetarians abound in this and other cultures. Their reasons vary. For Bible Christians and Seventh Day Adventists, the reasons are religious. For Mahatma Gandhi, vegetarianism was a means of "calming the spirit and allaying animal passion." Others believe that a vegetable diet promotes intellectual capacity.

Vegetarians must endure considerable spoofing. Glancing at one of George Bernard Shaw's meals of vegetables drowned in oil, an observer once inquired of the dramatist whether he was going to eat it or had already eaten it. A more serious problem for vegetarians is that of finding alternative sources of protein. Meats ordinarily contain ten essential amino acids; a single vegetable is rarely adequate in this respect. To meet daily protein needs, vegetarians must add other foodstuffs to their diets, such as milk, cheese, enriched corn and wheat, Brazil nuts, and soybean products. Soybeans are a particularly valuable source of protein, are also rich in phosphorus, iron, and calcium, and contain substantial amounts of vitamins A, B_1, and B_2. Calcium and iron are abundant in milk, cheese, fruits, and vegetables. Kidney beans, lima beans, whole wheat, peanut butter, and leafy vegetables are good sources of iron. There is no shortage of vitamin sources for the vegetarian: spinach, turnips, dandelion greens, and broccoli are rich in vitamin A; soybeans, lima beans, peas, wheat germ, and salad greens provide B_1; B_2 can be obtained from milk, soybeans, spinach, and asparagus; a medium-sized orange or grapefruit supplies more than the presently accepted daily requirement of vitamin C.

Thus, there is considerable reason to believe that a well-balanced vegetarian diet can be adequate for health. Millions of the earth's inhabitants, however, are vegetarians not by choice, but by economic necessity. They suffer chronic protein shortages. Modern nutrition research leading to protein-enriched food products and high-protein strains of wheat, corn, and rice promises to make their diets adequate.

[51] Margarita Nagy, "Natural vs. Synthetic Vitamins," *Journal of the American Medical Association,* Vol. 225, No. 1 (July 2, 1973), p. 73, citing A. Kamil, "How Natural Are Those 'Natural' Vitamins?" *Journal of Nutrition Education,* Vol. 4 (1972), p. 92.

[52] An excellent review of this subject is Sanat K. Majumder, "Vegetarianism: Fad, Faith, or Fact?" *American Scientist,* Vol. 60, No. 2 (March–April 1972), pp. 175–79.

the Zen-macrobiotic diet The Zen-macrobiotic diet (Greek *makros,* long + *bios,* life) was developed by a Japanese-born writer named George Ohsawa. Each of its allowable foods is assigned to either yin or yang, which in one system of Chinese philosophy are the active and passive forces of balance in the universe. Yin is the passive "female" element associated with silence, cold, and darkness; supposedly relaxing vegetables, as well as sweet, sour, and spicy foods are assigned to it. Yang, the active "male" element, is associated with energy, such as sound, heat, and light; its foods, such as cereals and meat, are supposed to cause one to contract and be more active.[53] The macrobiotic diet shrewdly appeals to the emotional aspects of eating. Analyzing his own temperament, as well as the seasons, weather, and geographic location, the macrobiotic dieter seeks a balance between his yin and yang foods. Starting with a fairly well-balanced diet of meats, vegetables, and fruits, he aims for an "ideal" diet consisting only of cereals and severely restricted quantities of fluid and salt.

Fortunately, for most people food fads are of brief duration. Unfortunately, their consequences often persist. Already reported have been scurvy, rickets, anemia, low protein and calcium blood levels, emaciation from sheer starvation, and loss of kidney function. Macrobiotic diets have killed some people. They are purported to create a spiritual awakening. Excluded, apparently, are the small children of macrobiotic dieters. An inadequate diet during early childhood diminishes the number and size of cells. Added to the danger of childhood rickets and scurvy is the serious risk of mental retardation. But the possible cruelties of macrobiotic dieting do not end there. Consider this statement by Ohsawa: "No illness is more simple to cure than cancer (this also applies to mental disease and heart trouble) through a return to the most natural eating and drinking: Diet No. 7."[54] A similar recommendation is given for appendicitis. Following such advice will delay proper diagnosis and treatment. It may cost the life of a macrobiotic dieter. It is of interest to note that the diet has been rejected by Zen Buddhists.

the process of nourishment

Nourishment depends on an intricate interplay of many organs and body chemicals. A special area in the hypothalamus of the brain tells a person whether he is hungry or full (see body chart 8 in the color section). Destroy the satiety center in an animal, and it will gorge itself to obesity; damage the area signaling hunger, and the animal will die of starvation. However, the functions of nutrition begin even before food is ingested. It is now known, for example, that hunger is rarely the stimulus causing an ordinarily obese person to eat. It is his "hungry eye or nose."

[53] Dale Erhard, "Nutrition Education for the 'Now' Generation," *Journal of Nutrition Education* (Spring 1971), pp. 135–39.

[54] Quoted in Council on Foods and Nutrition of the American Medical Association, "Zen Macrobiotic Diets," *Journal of the American Medical Association,* Vol. 218, No. 3 (October 18, 1971), p. 397.

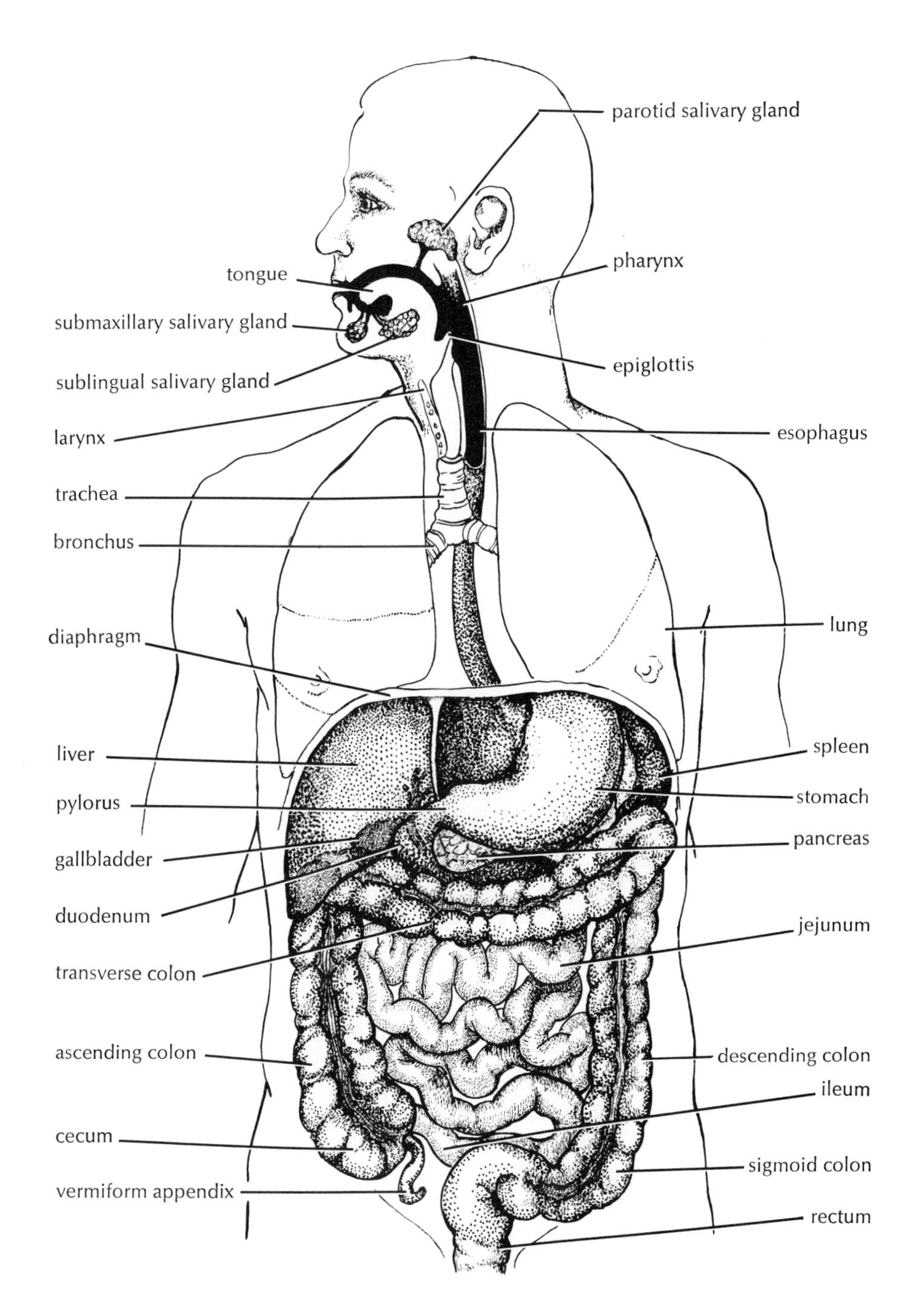

22-7 *The digestive system. Parts of the respiratory system are also labeled here. See also body chart 13 in the color section.*

Once food is ingested it enters the *digestive system,*[55] so the mouth and its associated structures contribute to the *digestive process.* For the moment, skip the first part of the digestive system and consider food in the small intestine. Nerves stimulate the contraction of the outer layers of muscle of the small intestine. This *mechanical* process propels the food within it and breaks it down into finer particles. Stimulated by nerves and hormones, intestinal glands in the lining of the inside of the small intestine produce *enzymes.*[56] The enzymes attack the food, breaking it down into even finer particles. This is a *chemical* reaction. So *digestion* is both a mechanical and chemical process by which nutrients are broken down into smaller units. The digestive process makes possible the transfer of nutrients primarily from the small intestine into the blood and lymph channels. This transfer is called *absorption* and, like digestion, it is part of the nourishment process. After absorption, nutrients must be *transported* by the blood to the tissue cells. By means of a complex activity within the tissue cells called *metabolism,* nutrients are converted into energy and are used to create new molecules for tissue. But not all nutrients are immediately used. Some, such as fat and vitamin A, are *stored* within specific cells. Other nutrients (proteins) are held in *reserve.* The difference between reserve and storage is that reserves are body-wide. Some ingested nutrients are never used; they are evacuated as feces or excreted with the urine.

digestive activity in the mouth

Even on the first day of life, the newborn drinks sugar water or his mother's early milk, making good use of his lips. Composed of muscle fibers, the lips are surrounded by a circular band of still more muscle, the *orbicularis oris.* The ''little circle around the mouth'' (translated from the Latin) curls the lips snugly about the nipple, sealing off air, making sucking possible. The *orbicularis oris* is a sphincter muscle. ''Sphincter'' is Greek for ''that which binds tight.'' Body sphincters do just that. By constricting a passage, the sphincter keeps it closed. It relaxes temporarily to permit some material to continue through the passage. For example, a constricted sphincter prevents food from prematurely leaving the stomach for the small intestine. When the sphincter relaxes, it helps to govern the amount of food that goes from one part of the passage to the next.

One cannot help admiring the constant labor of the heart. Consider, however, the *mouth.* It is used in talking, breathing, chewing, singing, whistling, coughing, vomiting, laughing, kissing, yawning, spitting, and other activities. But, through it all, one function is constant. The adult human mouth is not diverted from being the receptacle for a daily total of about two pints of saliva.

Food is taken into the mouth, passing under the nostrils. Then taste begins. Taste is partly smell. Eliminate vision and smell and one cannot differentiate between wine and lemonade or between apples and potatoes.

[55] The *digestive system* includes the mouth and its associated structures, the pharynx, the components of the digestive tube, and the organs and glands associated with digestion. The *alimentary tract* or *canal* is that part of the digestive tract formed by the esophagus, stomach, and small and large intestines. The *gastrointestinal tract* includes the stomach and intestines. *Gastric* pertains only to the stomach.

[56] All plants and animals produce thousands of *enzymes.* They are proteins that increase the rate of a reaction without becoming a part of the products of the reaction. Since they are used up in the body's chemical processes, enzymes are continuously produced by the living cells.

The muscular *tongue* is covered with a great many fine, wartlike *papillae.* Within the walls of the papillae are the *taste buds.* The buds at the back of the tongue are sensitive to bitter; at the tip, sweet; at the sides, sour. In the tongue's center, the "zone of silence," there is no taste. Man makes much of his cultivated taste. Compared to the cow's thirty-five thousand taste buds, his three thousand buds are few. Nevertheless, the tastes of man (including intermingled smell) are refined enough to recognize the finest size of grains, the subtlest body of liquids, the most piquant wines.

Skillfully guided by the muscular, shoveling, kneading tongue, the incisors cut, the canine teeth tear, and the molars masticate (chew) the solid food (see Figure 22-8). In this maceration and fragmentation, the *salivary glands* (see Figure 22-7) have already begun to help. The mere thought of tasty food sets the brain to instruct the salivary glands to increase secretory activity. There are many salivary glands about the lips, cheeks, and tongue. Three pairs of them have been named: the largest of these are the *parotid glands* (in front of and below the ears); the others are the *sublingual glands* (in the floor of the mouth, beneath the tongue) and the *submaxillary glands* (under the jaw). (See Figure 22-7.) All their ducts empty into the mouth.

Since fish eat moist food, they neither have nor need salivary glands. But in one day, a drooling cow, confronted with a dry feed, can muster two hundred quarts of softening saliva. For dry toast man needs, and so produces, more saliva than for milk. In the human, to replace swallowed saliva, and thus to keep the mouth moist, salivary secretion is continuous. In one ordinary lifetime, the specialized microscopic salivary cells secrete over fifty thousand pints of saliva—more than enough to fill two large swimming pools. This secretory activity, like all other body activities, requires energy available only through food.

Glands throughout the entire lining of the gastrointestinal tract secrete a slimy substance called *mucus.* Its chief chemical constituent is called *mucin.* Mucus lubricates the lining of the gastrointestinal tract in order to facilitate the passage of its contents. In so doing it protects the inner lining of the tract from damage. Moreover, it can neutralize both acids and bases. Its value, for example, in protecting the stomach from the erosive action of the hydrochloric acid liberated there is obvious. About half of the saliva is mucus, and its mucin makes it sticky. The lubricative action of salivary mucus makes possible the swallowing of food. The other half of the saliva is a solution of a protein enzyme, *ptyalin.* This enzyme breaks down starch into simple sugars (maltose and dextrins). Thus does digestion begin in the mouth. It is in the mouth that food is rendered into a liquid or semiliquid.

The mouth is an anatomic exception. All other body structures or cavities are lined with an unbroken layer of skin or mucous membrane. But in the mouth that protective mucosal layer is penetrated by the erupted teeth. Also, nowhere else but in the mouth are there such singular anatomic connections as there are between tooth and soft tissue or between tooth and bone. Nor does the oral ecosystem promote tooth health. Swarming with microorganisms, often containing a bewildering variety of food chemicals, tolerating wildly fluctuating temperatures ranging from hot soup to frozen ice cream, containing gold, silver, cements, and plastics, enduring endless pollution and even small electric currents between dissimilar metals in the electricity-conducting saliva, the oral ecosystem is a challenge to dental survival. The teeth profoundly affect nourishment and health, and they merit discussion.

the teeth and gums

an old problem

> For there was never yet philosopher
> That could endure the toothache patiently.[57]

At twenty-four, George Washington had his first tooth extracted; at fifty-seven, he lost his last tooth. In the United States today, half of all persons over fifty have lost their natural teeth. For all ages, the ratio is one of eight. The Colonial General would feel at home with this: ''For every 100 inductees entering the military service today there are needed 20 dentures, 25 bridges, 80 extractions''[58] and 450 fillings. These figures describe the soldiers not of Washington's day but of today.

Washington's dental sufferance included more than concern for his speech, chewing, and swallowing. A year before his death, he wrote his dentist of needed ''alterations'' to his false teeth so they would not ''have the effect of forcing the lip out just under the nose.''[59] It was said that Washington suffered more from his ''patent masticators'' than from the winter at Valley Forge.[60] However, when they are properly fitted, false teeth at least do not hurt. The ''cures'' for aching teeth have sometimes been no less dreadful than the aches. Suggested treatments have included biting off the head of a live mouse,[61] filling the tooth hollow with raven dung,[62] and touching the tooth with the hand of a corpse.[63] The Slovenes wryly advise filling the mouth with cold water and sitting on a hot stove. As the water boils, the tooth is forgotten.[64]

Some people have purposely parted with healthy teeth. In 1862, French soldiers had to bite off the cartridges for their guns. Inadequate dentition meant exemption from military duty. Extracting the teeth became a method of draft evasion.[65] Others sold their teeth. A 1782 advertisement, placed by George

[57] William Shakespheare, *Much Ado About Nothing,* V.i.35–36.

[58] John W. Knutson, ''Prevention of Dental Disease,'' in Duncan W. Clark and Brian MacMahon, eds., *Preventive Medicine* (Boston, 1967), p. 229.

[59] Arthur Ward Lufkin, *A History of Dentistry,* 2nd ed. (Philadelphia, 1948), p. 171.

[60] ''Reliever of Pain,'' *M.D., Medical Newsmagazine,* Vol. 12, No. 1 (January 1968), p. 194. Washington's false ivories were a source of constant distress to him. They ''generated foul odors by rotting in his mouth, and had a depressing effect on his appearance due to lack of support for his sagging mouth and surrounding tissues . . . The false teeth he began wearing after 1789—a full upper and lower set carved from hippopotamus tusks—were also not satisfactory.'' Not only did they fit improperly, but port wine turned the ivory black. In other cultures of the time, however, black teeth were a sign of beauty; Japanese geishas stained their teeth black. From a Western viewpoint, however, this was not so radical as the custom among the Kilao Chinese. On her wedding day, a young bride was taken from her house and two of her incisors were knocked out. This identified her as married. Later, it became a sign of beauty. (Charles I. Stoloft, ''The Fashionable Tooth,'' *Natural History,* Vol. 81, No. 2 [February 1972], pp. 12, 14–16, 18–22.)

[61] Leo Kanner, *Folklore of the Teeth* (New York, 1928), p. 141.

[62] Arthur Ward Lufkin, *A History of Dentistry,* 2nd ed., p. 78.

[63] Leo Kanner, *Folklore of the Teeth,* p. 145.

[64] *Ibid.,* p. 149.

[65] *Ibid.,* p. 217.

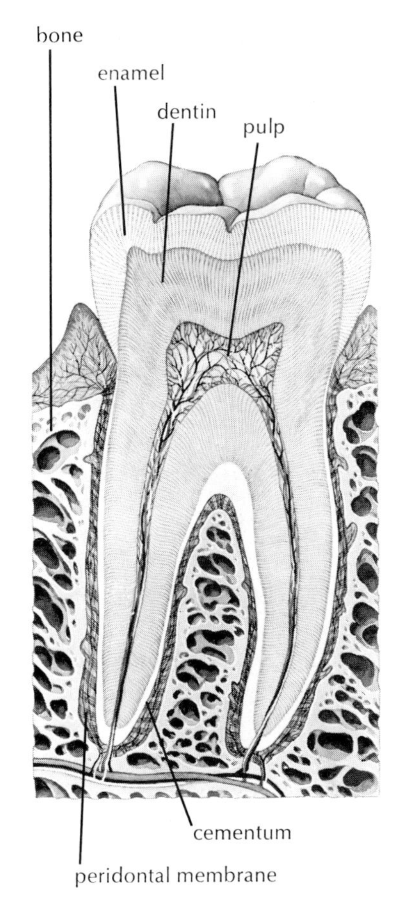

second permanent molars
first permanent molars
permanent teeth
deciduous teeth
permanent teeth

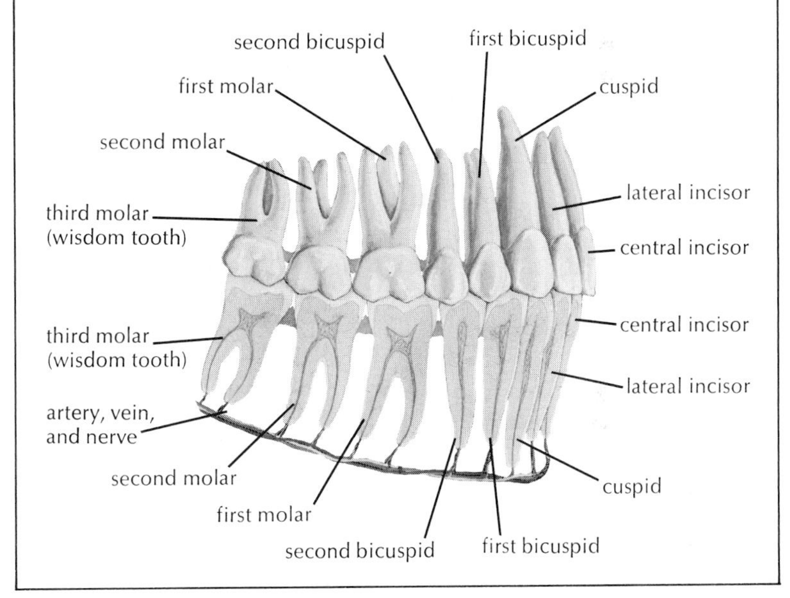

22-8 *Teeth: a longitudinal section of a molar* (above), *the dentition of a six–year–old child* (top right), *and the dentition of an adult* (bottom right).

Washington's dentist in *Rivington's Royal Gazette,* offered four guineas for each front tooth.[66]

One might conclude this brief historical review of dentistry with some lines published almost a century ago:

> View this gravestone with all gravity,
> Jones is filling his last cavity.[67]

[66] J. A. Taylor, *History of Dentistry* (Philadelphia, 1922), p. 75. The seventeenth-century English king James I, on the other hand, paid not for teeth, but for the sheer pleasure of extracting them. Thus did Kunnard the barber earn eighteen shillings for "twa teith drawin furth of his heid by the King." (Quoted in Arthur Ward Lufkin, *A History of Dentistry,* 2nd ed., p. 136.)

[67] "Southern California Practitioner," cited in Henry Harris, *California's Medical Story* (San Francisco, 1932), p. 292.

growth and structure

Teeth are almost indestructible. They survive fire and decompose slowly, Ancient skulls are studded with diseased dentition. Teeth are arranged in a highly individual way from person to person. An "oral fingerprint" has been evidence enough to convict more than one murderer who, having set his victim on fire, left nothing behind but a few teeth and, perhaps, a few unincriminating gallstones.

Anchoring the tooth (see Figure 22-8) in the jawbone is the *root.* The portion of the tooth that one sees in the mouth is the *crown.* Where root and crown meet is the *neck.* Four tissues make up a tooth. The *enamel,* hardest of all body tissues, covers the crown; the bonelike *cementum* covers the root. The ivorylike *dentin,* harder than bone but softer than enamel, forms the body of the tooth. The pulp contains the nerves, blood vessels, and lymphatics. Covering the root of the tooth and extending to line its socket is the *periodontal membrane.* It helps to hold the tooth in place. It is also a shock absorber.

At six weeks, the human embryo begins to form tooth buds for the twenty temporary *deciduous teeth.* Shortly thereafter, the buds of the thirty-two *permanent teeth* begin to form. At birth the unerupted deciduous teeth are almost complete. Beneath the deciduous teeth some permanent teeth begin to calcify.

At about six months, the baby shows the first tooth. Before his third birthday, he has a mouthful of deciduous teeth. These will be shed at various times. Neglect of temporary teeth may result in permanent problems. The temporary teeth guide the permanent dentition beneath them. Loss or decay of temporary deciduous teeth may result in crooked permanent teeth, chewing and speech problems, and psychological wounds. Between the ages of two and one-half and three years, a child should see the dentist for the first time.

Usually the first or "six-year" molars are the first permanent teeth to erupt (see Figure 22-8). At about this time, the child is losing his front deciduous teeth. The position of the first molars helps determine the position of the other teeth and the shape of the whole lower face. The entire future of the individual's dentition is profoundly influenced by the first molars. "A mouth without grinders," mourned Don Quixote to Sancho, "is like a mill without a stone; and a diamond is not so precious as a tooth."[68] So wrote Cervantes over four centuries ago. As soon as the first molar erupts, this tooth, the "keystone of the dental arch," should be examined by the dentist.

some major dental problems

Dental cavities (or *caries*) share with the common cold the distinction of being the most common human ailments. How does a cavity form in a tooth? Three things are necessary: a susceptible tooth, sugar, and certain bacteria.

Most teeth are usually covered by a filmy *dental plaque.* This slimy coating collects and holds together an untidy agglomeration of mucus, food debris, and bacteria. The plaque is the same color as the teeth. Some, but not all, of the

[68] Miguel De Cervantes, *Don Quixote de La Mancha,* tr. by Charles Jarvis (London, 1842), p. 188.

dental plaque may be temporarily removed by brushing. But it is the plaque that provides the medium for tooth decay. It is within and around it that the bacteria live and are protected.

From simple sugars formed by the breakdown of food in the mouth, some of these mouth bacteria, certain of the *streptococci,* synthesize complex sugars (polysaccharides) and store them. Between feedings, the streptococci derive energy by converting the stored polysaccharides to destructive acids (the most important of which is lactic acid). How much time do the streptococci need to transform sugar to erosive acid? Within fifteen or twenty minutes most of the damage is done. That is why rinsing or brushing the teeth immediately after eating is so helpful. Another microorganism that is involved in tooth decay is the *lactobacillus.* Joining the streptococcus in destructive acid formation, it is a common component of dental plaque. Emotions may be involved in cavity formation. The rate of salivary flow is influenced by suggestion. A diminished rate of salivary flow encourages cavities. Why? The acid concentration in the mouth rises, and this helps to destroy teeth. Even heredity may play a role in the tendency to cavity formation.

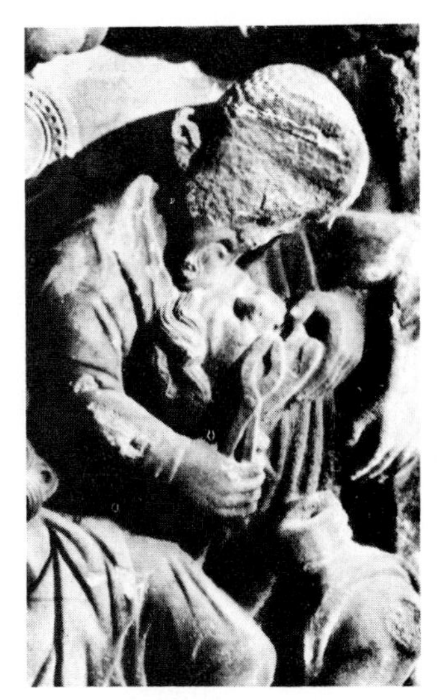

22-9 *A 13th-century Italian sculpture showing a barber-surgeon extracting a tooth.*

If the tooth-bathing saliva has enough buffers to neutralize acids formed by bacteria, tooth decay can be prevented. If not, the chemical process of decalcification begins. The acid in the saliva, formed by bacterial action on sugar, first destroys the tooth enamel. At this stage there is usually no warning pain. Only later, when destruction has reached the dentin, is there toothache. An unchecked cavity may get to the pulp. Infection sometimes travels from the pulp towards the tissues surrounding the root. Abscess formation may occur. Pus may spread through the blood vessels, causing a swelling of the adjacent soft tissues.

what can be done?

PERSONAL CARE 1. If at all possible, teeth should be brushed after each meal. Even rinsing with a warm drink helps remove food particles. Mouthwashes are not substitutes for brushing. Many dentists recommend water-under-pressure equipment to be used after (but not instead of) brushing. Except for the handicapped, electric toothbrushes are not more effective than the manual kind. Many dentists urge the use of dental floss after each meal.

2. To find cavities and arrest their progress, prompt and continuous care by a dentist is essential.

3. During the intrauterine period and first eight years of life, nutrition is critically important. The mother's diet provides minerals for the developing teeth of the child within her. Should her diet be lacking, the child obtains minerals not from the mother's teeth, but from her bones. It is after birth that permanent teeth are calcified. So the child's diet should include foods rich in calcuim and phosphorus as well as vitamins A, C, and D (see pages 652–56). Moreover, all living tissue needs and contains protein. An adequate diet, so essential for general health, is also an absolute necessity for development of normal tooth structure.

Do adult teeth, permanent and calcified, need calcium? No, but the bone, by which teeth are held in place, cannot remain healthy without calcium. Does adult dental health require an adequate diet? Indeed it does. Without enough protein for tissue replacement, for example, mouth structures would quickly suffer. And the deleterious effect on adult oral health of shortages of vitamin B and C has long been recognized.

4. For centuries in the Western world sugar was a luxury, available only to the rich and sold to them by apothecaries by the ounce. It has been a significant part of the U.S. diet for less than a century. Today, the average person in this country consumes about two pounds of sugar (sucrose) every week.[69] Sucrose is the villain in modern caries. It is the way in which sucrose is used by oral streptococci that causes caries. In the United States, two-thirds of a person's weekly consumption of sucrose is not in the form of table sugar, but in jams and jellies, cakes and cookies, frozen and canned fruits, frozen and packaged desserts, and bottled beverages. For the prevention of caries, avoidance of these sweet foods is essential. Of particular importance is the frequency and duration of exposure to sucrose. Thus sucrose-containing foods that stick to the teeth are particularly harmful. A piece of chocolate cake is not quite as caries-inducing as a candy caramel, but it is best to avoid them both. Modification of the diet, so that carbohydrates would be obtained from starchy foods instead of sweets, would surely help to reduce the incidence of caries in this country.[70] Unfortunately, "sweetness is the only one of the four primary tastes (sweet, sour, salty, bitter) that is always pleasant to man."[71] What is needed is a sweetener that has been proved to be totally harmless.

FLUORIDATION For more than thirty years the effect of fluoride on human health in general, and dental health in particular, has been carefully investigated. Beginning in the 1930s massive studies have been carried out in communities over the entire North American continent. The results are summarized here:

> All studies made prior to 1945, when the first controlled water fluoridation projects were instituted, as well as studies conducted since that time, have added support to the conclusion that optimally fluoridated drinking water in a range of 0.7 to 1.3 parts per million is a safe, relatively simple, and practical health measure that effects a two-thirds reduction in the incidence of tooth decay, with a concomitant and significant reduction in the loss of teeth from dental caries.[72]

[69] Frederic W. Nordsiek, "The Sweet Tooth," *American Scientist* (January–February 1972), p. 41. There is no evidence whatsoever to support the claim that either raw or brown sugar, honey, or maple syrup contribute less to caries than products with similar amounts of refined sucrose. (James H. Shaw, "Diet Regulations for Caries Prevention," *Nutrition News,* Vol. 36, No. 1 [February 1973], p. 4.)

[70] Henry W. Scherp, "Dental Caries: Prospects for Prevention," *Science,* Vol. 173, No. 4003 (September 24, 1971), p. 1200.

[71] Frederic W. Nordsiek, "The Sweet Tooth," p. 41. Some dieters using saccharin fear that it might be a cancer-causing agent. Recent animal experiments indicate that almost all saccharin is cleared from most tissues after three days of a saccharin-free diet. Thus the recommendation: "It might be beneficial if regular users of saccharin would occasionally discontinue its use for several days and thus allow for tissue clearance." ("Saccharin: At Last, Normal Doses," *Medical World News,* Vol. 14, No. 40 [November 2, 1973], pp. 6–7.)

[72] John W. Knutson, "Prevention of Dental Disease," in Philip E. Sartwell, ed., *Preventive Medicine and Public Health,* 9th ed. (New York, 1965), p. 236.

Today, in this country, some four thousand communities, populated by over 83 million people, have fluoride fed into water supplies. Two-thirds of the major cities in the United States, including New York, Chicago, Philadelphia, and Detroit, have adopted controlled fluoridation. In some cities a vocal minority has succeeded in confusing enough people to delay fluoridation of the water supply. By their misguided action, they condemn millions to needless pain, expense, and disability. Over one-fifth of the U.S. population (about 44 million people) have no access to a public water supply. For them, it would be advisable to add fluoride to such widely consumed foods as salt, flour, milk, and, of course, sugar. Fluoride *solutions* applied to the teeth of children have resulted in a reduction of from 75 to 80 percent of cavities. These treatments are more expensive and time-consuming than water fluoridation. Intensively and properly applied, one topical application of fluoride has an anticaries effect that lasts at least twenty-three months. Fluoride *tablets* and *drops* taken during the early years of life can be ingested only if prescribed. The beneficial results of tablet- and drop-taking are comparable to those obtained from water fluoridation. However, a regimen involving the ingestion of fluoride tablets or drops does not provide a reliable method of cavity prevention. Few people can be expected to cooperate on such a long-term basis. Stannous fluoride dentifrices may help.

SEALING Despite fluoridation, some caries will occur in the pits and fissure that are normally found on the grinding surfaces of the molars and bicuspids. This can be prevented by sealing these surfaces with a newly developed adhesive substance.[73] Sealing should be done soon after the eruption of a tooth, whether it be deciduous or permanent. As a result of the sealing procedure, caries reduction in deciduous teeth has been reported to be 87 percent and in permanent teeth, 99 percent.[74]

periodontal diseases

Disorders of the tissues surrounding and holding the teeth in their sockets are called *periodontal diseases.* For people under thirty-five, cavities cause most tooth loss. After thirty-five, periodontal disease is the major cause. It can vary from a mild gum inflammation to actual bone destruction.

Periodontal disease can have several manifestations. The initial signs of inflammation of the gums (*gingivitis*), such as redness, swelling, and bleeding, are usually painless. Poor oral hygiene, tartar or calculus accumulation, and malocclusions are common causes. Less ordinary evidences of periodontal disease are systemic conditions such as diabetes, leukemia, and deficiencies of vitamins B and C. *Vincent's angina* (''trench mouth''), caused by two different bacteria, is amenable to penicillin and good dental hygiene. *Periodontitis* (pyorrhea) can be related to the presence of calculus. Calculus appears when bacteria-loaded plaque calcifies and hardens. The subsequent irritation and infection can promote periodontal disease. *Improper alignment* (*malocclusion*) of

[73] Henry W. Scherp, ''Dental Caries: Prospects for Prevention.'' p. 1200, citing M. G. Buonocore, *Journal of the American Dental Association,* Vol. 75 (1967), p. 121.
[74] *Ibid.*

the teeth, such as occurs when upper and lower teeth fail to meet efficiently, promotes periodontitis. This can be corrected by an orthodontist. Periodontitis may also be initiated by *improper brushing* or by the trauma of *toothpicks.*[75] In the *Babies Book* of about 1475, children were enjoined "youre nose, youre teeth, youre naylles from pykynge."[76] That advice is still good today.

Good mouth hygiene is essential in preventing periodontal disease. Proper brushing is helpful. Professional scaling and polishing of the teeth are important.

research

Modern dental research involves numerous disciplines. For example, in periodontal disease, the normal connective tissue protein (collagen) breaks down. The enzyme collagenase may be involved. It catalyzes the destruction of collagen. In periodontal disorders, the secretion of this enzyme markedly increases. Biochemists are researching this aspect of periodontal disease. Geneticists and microbiologists have found that minor dietary changes make resistant animals more susceptible to cavities. And, if nursed by susceptible foster mothers, resistant-bred animals become susceptible, too. Moreover, streptococci from decayed teeth of laboratory animals will cause decay in teeth of germ-free animals. People who must take daily oral penicillin for prolonged periods in order to prevent recurrences of rheumatic fever, have less tooth decay than other people; this has stimulated research on the use of oral antibiotics to reduce caries. However, because of allergies, and the development of resistance by microbes, oral penicillin is not recommended for the prevention of caries. From the materials experts comes other help. Implanted into a baboon, a plastic tooth has lasted six years. From rocket engineers and metallurgists has come a powerful light steel suitable for tooth bridges and caps. Using one another's knowledge and ability, scientists are together attacking this nation's enormous dental problems.

swallowing

Having been cut and ground to a pulp by the teeth, moistened by the saliva, and partly digested by salivary enzymes, the soft food mass is ready to be swallowed. *Swallowing,* or *deglutition,* is the last voluntary digestive act. When the food is slid by the tongue into the *pharynx* (see Figure 22-7), digestion becomes involuntary, automatic. The pharynx is in the neck, as is a small portion of its continuation, the muscular *esophagus* (see Figure 22-7). The pharynx is a muscular passageway for both food and air. Above, it opens into the nasal passages; below, into the larynx. During swallowing, both of these openings, above and below, must be shut off. The *soft palate* and *uvula* (Latin, little grape) shut off the upper nasal part of the pharynx. The *epiglottis* covers the larynx. Thus,

[75] There is some evidence to suggest that *prostaglandins* (see pages 630–31) may also be implicated in periodontitis. Animal experiments indicate that the local application of prostaglandins can destroy bone. Moreover, mouth bacteria, which are involved in dental disease, may produce prostaglandins. Prostaglandins are produced with inflammatory processes in other parts of the body; thus it is possible that the bone sockets in which the roots of the teeth are imbedded produce their own prostaglandin. This response may also be true of inflamed gums. ("Prostaglandins: Involved in Dental Disease," *Science News,* Vol. 101, No. 14, pp. 215–16.)

[76] J. Menzies Campbell, *From a Trade to a Profession: Byways in Dental History* (London, 1958), p. 59.

without being forced back into the nose or into the larynx and bronchi,[77] swallowed food safely reaches the esophagus. This organ also secretes and is protected by mucus.

Food, even liquid, does not swiftly drop down the ten-inch esophagus. The food dilates it, causing muscular contractions, or *peristalses.* Unless food is too hot or large, it is not felt in the esophagus. The esophagus travels down the chest behind the heart, between the lungs, and through the *diaphragm* into the abdomen, where it empties into the stomach (see Figure 22-7). Normally it takes about seven seconds for food to pass from the mouth through the esophagus and into the stomach.

the stomach and duodenum

The often abused *stomach* is a muscular, distensible, bottle-shaped tube in the left abdomen (see Figure 22-7). It is separated from the major chest contents (heart and lungs) by the diaphragm. Its usually empty upper portion, the *cardia* (Greek *kardia,* heart), may fill with gas, which can be expelled by belching. The stomach is closed off from the esophagus by the cardiac sphincter and from the small intestine by the pyloric (Greek *pylouros,* gatekeeper) sphincter.

Before leaving the stomach for the small intestine, some food may remain in the stomach for three to four hours. Other foods are fed into the small intestine within a few minutes. What determines this? The nature of the food. In their early digestive stages, meats tarry in the stomach. Soft drinks bubble on into the small intestine. For this reason, meats provide a greater sense of satiety or fullness than do soft drinks.

The inner mucous lining of the stomach contains millions of microscopic *gastric glands.* Their juice contains three enzymes—*rennin, pepsin,* and *lipase.*[78] *Hydrochloric acid*[79] is also a constituent of gastric juice, as is a substance named the *intrinsic factor.* Without this factor, vitamin B_{12} would not be absorbed. This vitamin is necessary for red blood cell formation. (Rennin is found in the human infant, but not the adult.)

The entrance of liquid and semiliquid food from the esophagus (through the open cardiac sphincter) into the stomach is the signal for the gastric glands to produce their juice. This secretion, in turn, stimulates the muscular stomach walls to begin peristaltic waves. Food is then slowly and thoroughly churned with the acid gastric juice. During this process, trapped gas in the stomach may move about, causing the stomach to rumble. (Peristalsis may also occur when the stomach is empty.) Gas pressure against the stomach wall causes ''hunger pangs.'' It is in the stomach that an ironic and paradoxical problem of nature occurs. It is this: how can the stomach secretions carry out their basic function of beginning the digestion of proteins without also digesting the protein stomach lining? Part of the answer lies in the great amount of protective mucus secreted by the stomach. When its production is inadequate to deal with an increase of acid, ulcer soon develops (see below). Another reason for the

[77] The *bronchi* are the larger air passages in the lungs and are continuations of the windpipe (Chapter 13).
[78] Enzymes were defined on page 676.
[79] The normal stomach is insensitive to the acid in the gastric juice. However, the ''heart burn'' that occurs with regurgitation of hydrochloric acid proves the esophagus to be only too sensitive.

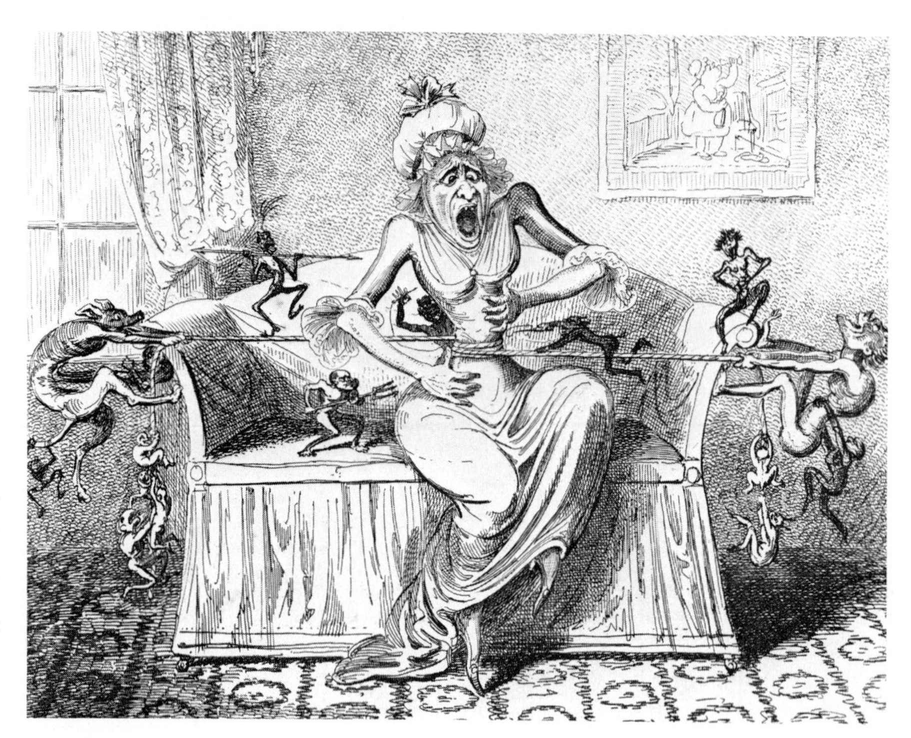

22-10 *A cartoon by George Cruikshank (1792–1878) caricaturing the acute pain of adult colic, which is usually caused by spasm of the smooth muscle of the stomach and intestines.*

resistance of the stomach lining to digestion by its own secretions lies in its microscopic cellular structure.

So the food is prepared in the stomach for its intermittent entrance into the approximately foot-long *duodenum,* the upper part of the small intestine. The opening of the stomach leading to the duodenum is called the *pylorus.* Only a small amount of food at a time is passed into the duodenal section of the small intestine. Food that is adequately mixed with acid gastric juice causes the pyloric sphincter to open. As soon as food touches the alkaline intestine, the pyloric sphincter closes. Such regulation from acid stomach and alkaline intestine provides for intermittent opening and closing of the pyloric sphincter. Extra mucin made at the top part of the duodenum protects its lining from the acid stomach contents.

peptic ulcer

A *gastric ulcer* is an eroded lesion in the stomach lining. Much more common but similar is the *duodenal ulcer.* Both are referred to as *peptic ulcers,* and they are treated similarly. Either ulcer may erode a blood vessel, causing hemorrhage. Either may penetrate the wall of the involved organ, necessitating emergency surgery. Because gastric ulcers are more likely to be cancers than duodenal ulcers, they can be particularly dangerous.

Peptic ulcers may occur at any age. Usually a peptic ulcer is first noted in the early thirties. Men suffer them four times more frequently than women. However, the increasing number of women exposed to the stresses of the competitive business world is changing this ratio. Although these ulcers do occur in relatively phlegmatic people, they are more common in conflict-ridden, striving individuals. For this reason peptic ulcer is called the ''executive's'' disease. Stress seems to increase greatly the acid secreted by the lining of the stomach. The stomach and duodenal linings (rarely the lower esophageal) are eroded by the high concentration of acid. Significantly, ulcers occur only in those areas of the digestive tract that come in contact with hydrochloric acid—the stomach, the duodenum, and the lower esophagus. The burning or gnawing abdominal pain of peptic ulcer usually begins two or three hours after meals. Occasionally pain will awaken an individual during the night. Milk, alkali, or food relieves the pain. Several hours after eating there is no food in the stomach to neutralize the excess acid secreted by the mucous membrane of the stomach. The free excess acid acts upon the ulcer, causing the pain. An X-ray usually reveals the ulcer, and laboratory analysis of the gastric juice shows abnormally high levels of acid. A much less stressful environment, frequent feedings of a bland diet emphasizing milk and milk products, and complete abstinence from tobacco, alcohol, and coffee contribute to recovery.

the pancreas

The head of the *pancreas* (Greek *pan,* all + *kreas,* flesh) nestles in the duodenal loop, and its long body lies beneath the stomach (see Figure 22-7). Although it is the second largest body gland, the pancreas weighs only one-twentieth as much as the largest gland, the liver. Along with the duct from the liver, the *pancreatic duct* opens into the duodenal part of the small intestine. Through the pancreatic duct pour the alkaline enzymes produced by the pancreas, *trypsin, amylase,* and *lipase.* Specialized cells of the pancreas also produce a carbohydrate-regulating protein called *insulin* (Latin *insula,* island). These cells are scattered throughout the tail of the pancreas as islands, and they are called the *islets of Langerhans* (see page 260). They do not secrete into the pancreatic duct. Insulin is secreted directly into the blood. Thus, the pancreas is both an *exocrine* (*ductal*) and an *endocrine* gland (see page 254). Failure of the islets of Langerhans to secrete insulin results in *diabetes mellitus* (see pages 260–61).

the four-lobed liver

The multipurpose human liver fits under the diaphragm and occupies most of the upper abdomen, particularly on the right. It is a veritable chemical factory. Not only does it produce bile, it also chemically treats carbohydrates, proteins, and fats, preparing them for human cellular use. It detoxicates poisons, such as alchohol[80] and caffeine. It destroys bacilli. Like the muscles, it stores glycogen, a sugar. It manufactures carbohydrates from fats. It is also influenced by

[80] An excess of alcohol (or other liver toxin) gradually poisons liver cells. This, combined with poor nutrition, causes the cells to die. They are replaced by fibrous scar tissue. To make up for the loss of liver cells, the remaining liver cells multiply. Finally fibrous scar tissue permeates the liver tissue. Due to local cell multiplication the remainder of the liver becomes knobby. Poor liver function may cause yellow jaundice. The sick liver structure also interferes with the flow of blood from the liver to the heart. It backs up into the veins of the stomach and esophagus. These may rupture and there will be vomiting of blood. With this condition far advanced, fluid from the blood will leak into body tissues, causing the swelling of *edema.* This liver sickness is *cirrhosis,* or the ''hob-nailed'' or ''gin-drinker's'' liver.

the emotions. Anger may temporarily stop the flow of bile, robbing one of an essential body juice. Infections, such as *infectious* and *serum hepatitis* (see pages 166–67), may threaten liver function.

the sometimes troublesome gallbladder

A secretion of the liver is yellow, bitter *bile.* Another name for it is *gall.* Before reaching the duodenum, bile stops to be stored and concentrated in a two- or three-inch pouch located under the right side of the liver. This is the *gallbladder* (see Figure 22-7). Concentration of bile in the gallbladder is accomplished when part of its water is absorbed by the mucous membrane of the gallbladder and returned to the bloodstream.

With entrance of food into the duodenum, the fat in the food stimulates the duodenal wall to liberate a hormone (see page 254) into the bloodstream. This hormone, in turn, causes the muscular gallbladder to contract. Bile is thus forced from the gallbladder into its duct (*cystic duct*) and via the continuation of the cystic duct into the *common bile duct.* From it, bile enters the duodenum. Just before the common bile duct enters the duodenum, it is joined by the *pancreatic duct.* Thus one duct carries both bile and pancreatic juice into the duodenum.

Bile contains three major constituents: *bile salts, cholesterol,* and *lecithin.* Bile salts hasten fat digestion by helping the moving intestine to break up (*emulsify*) large fat globules in the duodenum. The smaller, broken-up fat globules have more surface. This increased surface makes the fat more susceptible to the digestive action of the pancreatic enzyme, *lipase.* Cholesterol is a fat like substance found in all animal fats; it is, therefore, a constituent of the normal diet. Moreover, certain body tissues synthesize cholesterol. Thus, there is a normal level of cholesterol in the human body. It is when the dietary intake of cholesterol is high that concern about it as a cause of atherosclerosis occurs (see pages 226–27). Lecithin is found not only in bile but also in nerve tissue, semen, and blood. A pigment called *bilirubin* gives bile its golden-yellow color. Bilirubin is produced as the result of the ordinary destruction of worn-out red blood cells. The normal amount of bile pigment in the blood gives urine its characteristic straw color.

gallstones

Some animals, such as the elephant, whale, horse, camel, and rat do not have a gallbladder. Both man and mouse have cause to envy them. Normal human gallbladder bile is 85 percent aqueous (prepared in watery solution). This aqueous solution of bile can ordinarily carry the solid 15 percent of bile salts, lecithin, and cholesterol in solution. However, the bile's ability to dissolve cholesterol (and thus keep it in solution) depends on the relative concentrations of bile salts and lecithin. Perhaps for genetic reasons, in many people this delicate metabolic balance functions inadequately. The excess cholesterol precipitates into tiny crystals, which adhere to one another, forming gallstones.

Most gallstones do not cause symptoms. They may pass harmlessly from the gallbladder into its duct and, via the continuation of the cystic duct into the

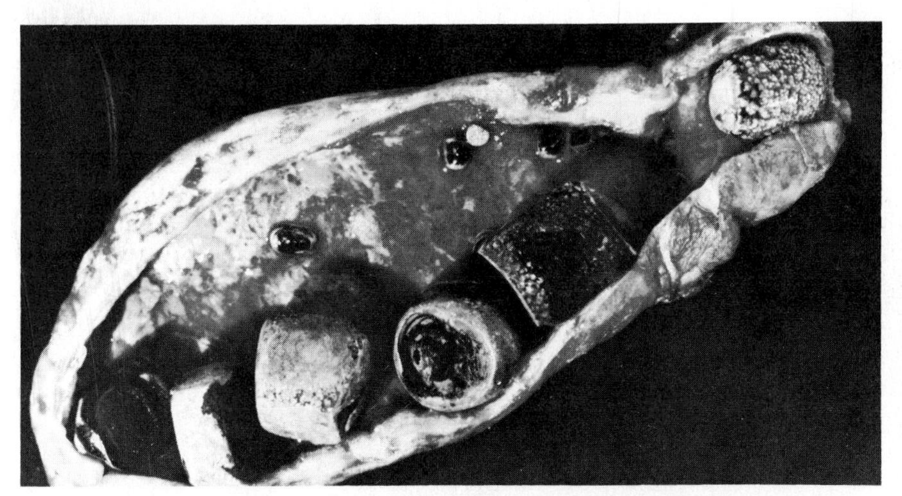

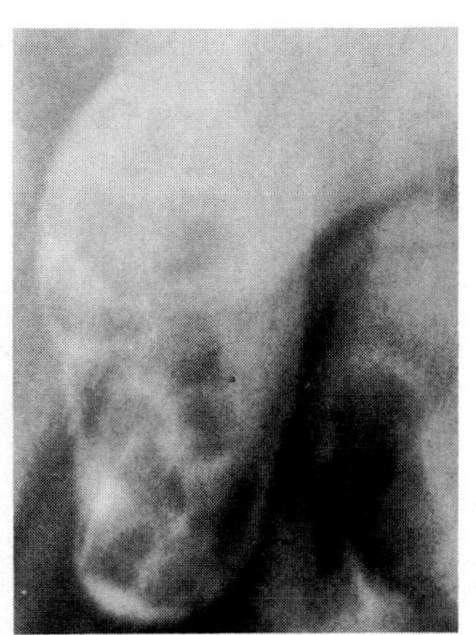

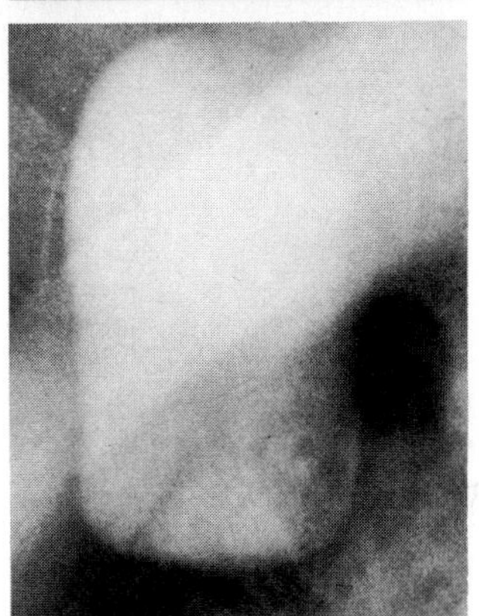

22-11 Above: *Gallstones within a surgically removed gallbladder.* Top right: *X–ray of a gallbladder showing numerous gallstones.* Bottom right: *X–ray of the same gallbladder after a year of drug therapy that "dissolved" the gallstones.*

common bile duct, into the duodenum. They will then proceed down the intestine without incident. Often, however, they cannot pass through the ducts. The ensuing pain is agonizing.

Until recently, the only cure for symptomatic gallstones was surgical removal of both gallbladder and stones. The gallbladder is not an essential organ. A person who has been surgically parted from his gallbladder is still able to adequately digest a fatty meal. It is estimated that about 16 million people in the United States have gallstones. They are twice as common in women as in men, and occur most frequently in middle age. Early in 1973, it was estimated that some 400,000 operations for the removal of gallbladder and stones are performed yearly in the United States and about six thousand people die postoperatively.[81] For selected patients, chemical treatment may replace surgery. In an attempt to increase the bile's ability to dissolve stones, the use of a compound named chenodeoxycholic acid (CDCA) is being tried. Results at Minnesota's Mayo Clinic and in London are encouraging. Given before symptoms occur, CDCA has been known to dissolve gallstones within one or two years. After symptoms appear, however, surgery is necessary because CDCA requires so much time to be effective. Also, phenobarbital (see page 374), which enhances the conversion of cholesterol into bile salts, is being tested.

the tortuously coiled intestine

The *intestine* (see Figure 22-7) is divided into the long, narrow *small intestine* and the shorter, but wider, *large intestine.* Below the point of entrance of the small intestine into the large intestine is the dilated intestinal pouch, the *cecum.*

[81] "Tracing the Rise of Gallstones Points the Way to Future Therapies," *Medical World News,* Vol. 14, No. 13 (March 30, 1973), p. 18.

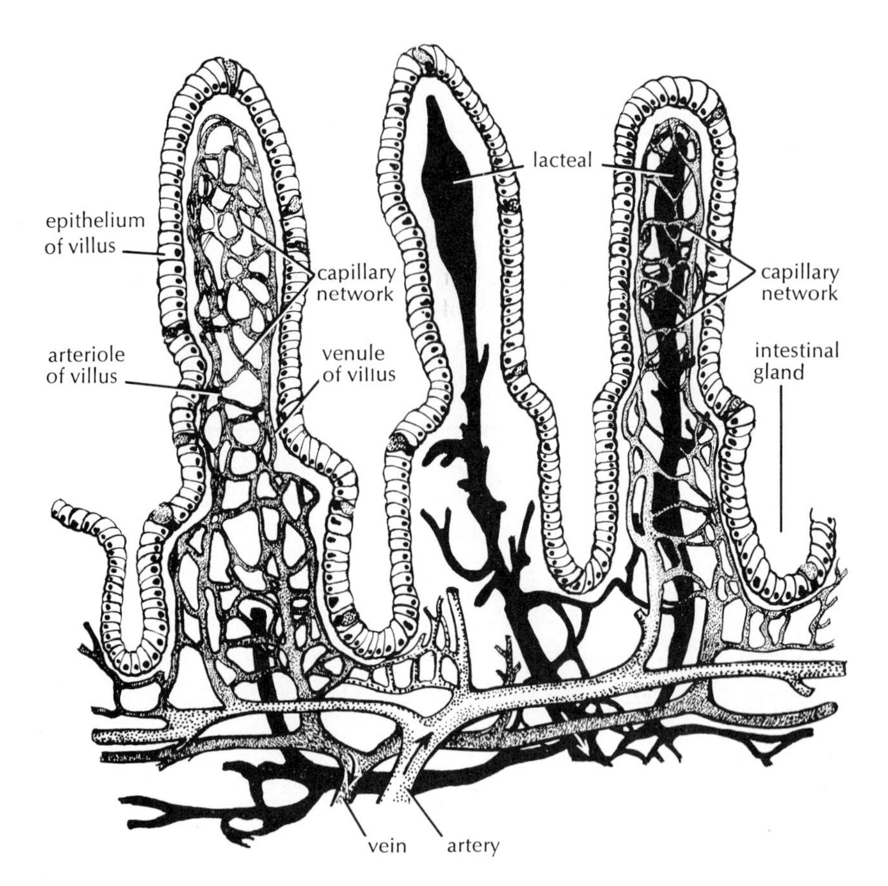

22-12 *Villi in the small intestine. The villus at the left shows only the blood vessels; the villus in the center, only the lymph vessel (the lacteal); the one at the right is complete, showing both the blood and lymph vessels.*

From the cecum projects a narrow tube, the *vermiform appendix.*[82] The entire intestine of a dead human is about twenty-eight feet long. However, the muscle tonus of life shortens the intestine to about ten feet. The large intestine, or *colon,* terminates in the four or five inches of *rectum.*

the small intestine

This is the major digestive organ. Within it, digestion is completed. In its lower portion, absorption of the products of digestion into the bloodstream takes place. Encouraged by intestinal peristalsis, food morsels from the duodenum are mixed with pancreatic juice and bile. They are then pushed into the *jejunum* and then to the *ileum,* the final three-fifths of the small intestine.

Covering the inner lining of the small intestine are millions of *villi* (Latin *villus,* tuft of hair). Villi are tiny fingerlike projections extending into the intestinal canal (see Figure 22-12). It has been estimated that the total surface of the

[82] The opening from the cecum to the appendix is usually small. Cecal contents are ejected into the intestine with difficulty. The appendix may become plugged. Then its wall ulcerates. Inflammation (*appendicitis*) progresses. Eventually, the appendix may rupture. If this occurs, its spilled, bacteria-laden contents cause *peritonitis*—inflammation of the peritoneum. (The peritoneum is the membrane lining the walls of the abdomen and pelvis. Peritonitis also occurs with a perforated peptic ulcer.) To prevent all this, it is essential that a diseased appendix be surgically removed (*appendectomy*) as soon as possible. Appendicitis occurs more often in children than in adults, but the disease is more serious in adults.

villi is about three thousand square feet. Combined with the intestinal folds and coiling, the villi enormously increase the digestive and absorptive surface of the small intestine. But that is not all. The surface of each villus is further increased by *microvilli,* which are visible under the electron microscope. These further increase the effective absorptive surface of the intestine thirty-fold. At the base of each villus, the *intestinal glands* secrete the intestinal juices. Carbohydrate-digesting enzymes, as well as enzymes for fat and protein digestion, are secreted in the small intestine. And along the entire inner surface of the small intestine is secreted a protective film of mucus.

It is from this remarkable inner surface of the small intestine that food is absorbed into the blood and lymph vessels. The ingested food has been broken down. It can now be transported by the blood and lymph to the liver and from there, via the blood, to the body cells to be built up again into the carbohydrates, fats, and proteins of the human type. The products of carbohydrate and protein digestion first go directly to the liver and then to the other body cells. Not all the products of fat digestion follow this route. About 60 percent of the fat is first absorbed into the lymphatic system and then travels on to tissue (see page 223). The rest goes directly to the liver. As droplets, fat may be stored in connective tissue cells. This is called *adipose* tissue.

About 20 million glands in the small intestine secrete an average of a gallon and a half of intestinal juice daily. Every day about 10 percent of the body's total water and salt enters the small intestine. Ninety percent of the total secretion is reabsorbed by the body tissues. What is lost is easily replaced. Thus not only digestion and absorption of food take place in the small intestine but also reabsorption of fluid.

In from three to four hours food usually passes through the small intestine into the large intestine.

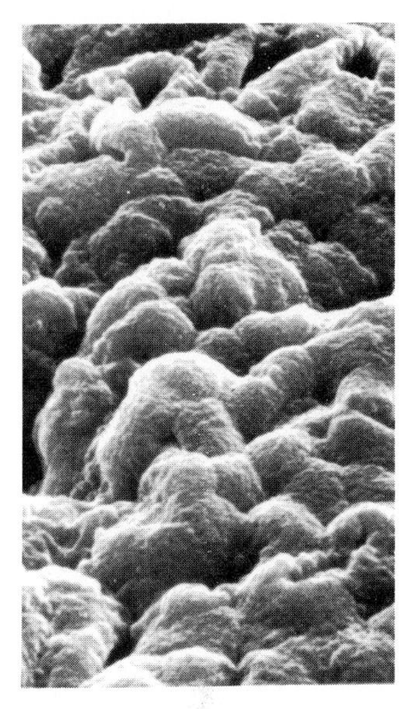

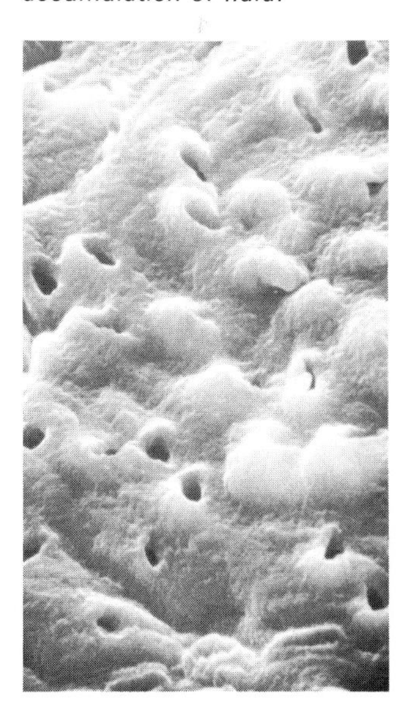

22-13 Above: *A normal colon, showing the characteristic cobbled surface and microvilli* (× *1400*). Below: *An irritated colon* (× *1300*); *the mucosal surface is swollen, and the microvilli are less apparent due to accumulation of fluid.*

the large intestine

Entering the *large intestine,* or the *colon* (see Figure 22-7), from the small intestine, through the ileo-colic sphincter, is a semifluid material.[83] Bereft of nutrient, it is waste—largely water. However, salt, bile, and undissolved (even undigested) food are contained in it. As in the esophagus, digestion does not occur in the large intestine. Water absorption in the large intestine causes the contents to solidify and to form *feces* (Latin *faeces,* refuse).

Fecal material should be soft and formed like a column. Consistently fluid adult feces (*diarrhea*) or small pieces expelled with difficulty (*constipation*) merit investigation by the physician. If severe diarrhea occurs, digestive enzymes enter the large intestine. Since they do not normally belong there, they are irritating. Here again the protective mucus secreted by the large intestine is helpful. Feces are expelled from the rectum through the rectal opening, the *anus* (Latin for "ring"). Regulating this passage of waste material from the body is the anal sphincter. With this, the process of digestion is completed.

[83] A chronic ulceration of the colon (*ulcerative colitis*) occurs in both children and adults. Its cause remains unclear. Many physicians consider it of psychosomatic origin.

summary

There are six basic constituents of foods. Three are synthesized by plants: *carbohydrates* (sugars, starches, and cellulose), *fats,* and *proteins* (pages 651–52). Among the most important *vitamins* are vitamin C (pages 652–53), vitamin B (pages 653–54), vitamin D (page 654), niacin (one of the B vitamins; page 654), vitamin E (pages 654–55), and vitamin K (page 655). *Minerals* (page 656) and *water* (pages 656–57) are also essential.

The basic measurement of nutrition is the *calorie,* the amount of heat required to raise the temperature of one gram of water one degree Centigrade (pages 657–63). *Obesity* generally denotes 20 percent or more over the desirable weight; it results from an increase in the amount of fatty tissue (page 664). Most overweight and obese persons can lose weight by sensible exercise (pages 667–68) and dieting (pages 668–69). There are also some measures that underweight persons can take to gain weight (page 670). Malnourishment can cause severe damage, especially to children (pages 670–71). Concern with proper nutrition sometimes results in food fads such as eating only *organic, natural,* and *health foods* (pages 671–73); *vegetarianism* (page 673); and the *Zen-macrobiotic diet* (page 674).

The process of nourishment begins in the *mouth,* where solid food is broken into smaller particles by the *teeth* (pages 674–78); thus, the teeth and gums are of critical importance to nourishment and health (pages 678–84). Having been ground by the teeth and moistened by *saliva* (page 677), the food is swallowed and moved along the *pharynx* and *esophagus* by involuntary muscular contractions called *peristalses* (pages 684–85) to the *stomach* (pages 685–86). The food is released at intervals into the upper part of the small intestine, the *duodenum* (page 686), where it is mixed with juice from the *pancreas* (page 687) and *bile* from the *liver* (pages 687–88) that has been stored in the *gallbladder* (pages 688–89). Digestion is completed in the *small intestine,* where the products of digestion are absorbed into the blood stream (pages 689–91). Waste materials are formed into feces and eliminated by the *large intestine* (page 691).

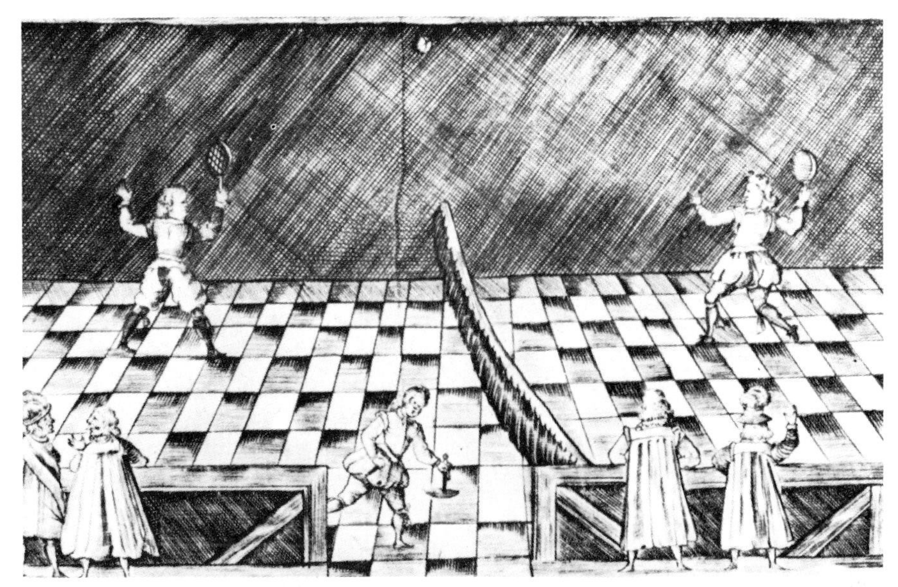

Indoor tennis in 16th-century England.

physical fitness

23

some historical notes and observations

> I thank God I am endued with such qualities that, if I were turned out of my realm in my petticoat, I were able to live in any place in Christendom.[1]

With these forthright words, the young Queen Elizabeth I faced her restless parliament more than four centuries ago. At that time she may well have felt fit enough to do her complex job. And, if she did not, she was at least fit enough not to admit it to a roomful of ambitious plotters. That she might do well to begin and follow some regimen of regular activity to maintain, or even improve, her sense of fitness doubtless never occurred to her. Elizabethans shunned swimming, for example, as a perilous sport (for generations Cambridge University undergraduates were warned against it).[2] The fact that Elizabeth even risked a watery bath once a month "whether she needed it or no,"[3] was considered but further evidence of her royal courage. Indeed, except for some mincing dance steps, ladies of quality during that era engaged in little exercise. The supposedly less refined rural English girls were happily less inhibited. "Smock races" were often held among them, and by the eighteenth century had even become a spectator sport. Some cricketers of the time were reported to "have subscribed for a Holland smock of one guinea value, which will be run by two jolly wenches, one known by the name of The Little Bit of Blue (the handsome Broom Girl) at the fag end of Kent Street, and Black Bess, of the Mint. They are to run in drawers only, and there is excellent sport expected."[4]

[1] Denis Brailsford, *Sport and Society, Elizabeth to Anne* (London and Toronto, 1969), p. 7, citing Address to the Lords and Commons, 1566, quoted in Sir John Neale, *Elizabeth I and Her Parliaments* (1953), p. 149.
[2] *Ibid.*, citing *ibid.*, p. 176.
[3] *Ibid.*, citing Lawrence Wright, *Clean and Decent: The Fascinating History of the Bathroom and the Water-Closet* (Toronto, 1960), p. 75.
[4] *Ibid.*, p. 240, citing G. B. Buckley, *Fresh Light on Eighteenth Century Cricket* (1935), p. 18.

23-1 *Golf has long been a popular form of exercise. This drawing is from the 14th century. Eighteenth-century golfers "butted" the ball with a "butter," but when Czar Nicholas I of Russia played King George IV of England in 1797, he pronounced "butt" as "putt"; the king politely did not correct him. The term "tee off" also originated in the 18th century, when English aristocrats usually drank a cup of tea before playing each hole. The players came to realize that as many as eighteen cups of tea were adversely affecting their game; the custom was gradually abandoned, and "tea" became "tee."*

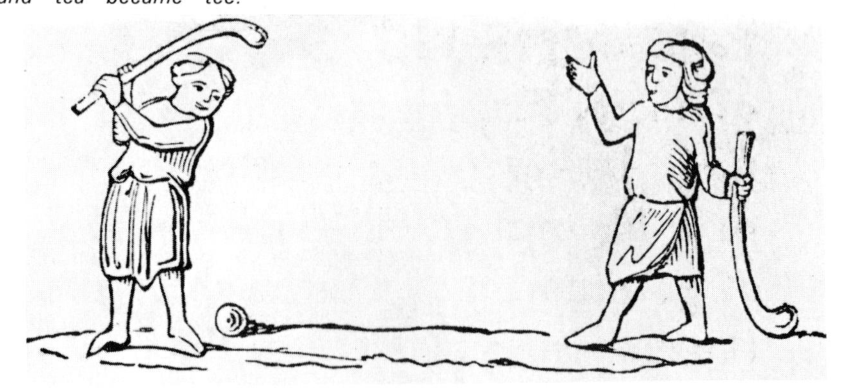

It is apparent that Bloomer girls were about long before the nineteenth-century U.S. feminist Amelia Bloomer shocked many people by urging that women wear loose trousers instead of dresses.[5] As for the winner of the race—if fitness can be related to a task to be done and an individual's relative ability to do it—the spoils doubtless went to the fitter of the "two jolly wenches." There are degrees of fitness; though both girls could run, presumably one could run faster. Imagine, however, that the Little Bit of Blue lost the race. Could she have won it with some weeks of preparatory training? If so, was not her potential degree of fitness, both in general and of the kind specifically needed for the race (such as sturdy legs within those drawers), equal to winning the Holland smock? And, to carry the question further, could not some training have helped Queen Elizabeth to carry her heavy burdens?

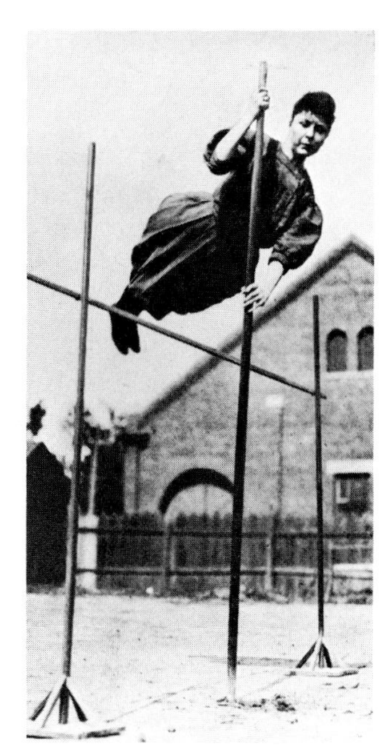

23-2 *At the turn of the century, a bloomer-clad pole vaulter at the University of Nebraska sails coolly over a four-foot bar.*

That physical training could be helpful for other activities was not ignored during Elizabeth's time. In 1541 an act was passed forbidding commoners to play bowls and ordering them to practice archery instead.[6] Archers were necessary to protect England. The military usefulness of physical fitness had long ago reached its greatest recognition in the ancient Greek state of Sparta. Drafted by the state on his seventh birthday, the son of a Spartan couple was rigorously trained to be a soldier. Boys were gathered into herds, and each herd was put through regular gymnastic classes. As they grew older, the exercises gradually became more demanding. As will be seen, modern man has devised some tests for the physical and emotional endurance aspects of fitness. The Spartan test was brutally simple. At a religious altar, the boys were flogged; the honors went to the boy who could longest endure the flogging. He earned the title of "altar-conqueror"; for the rest of his life he could carry that title (presumably along with his scars). Frequently, a boy died rather than utter a cry.[7] If he survived, he continued his training: ball playing, javelin throwing, bareback riding, running, wrestling, and boxing. The girls of Sparta also wrestled, hurled the javelin and discus, and ran races. Jumping and kicking one's buttocks with one's heels was a favorite leg exercise; one Spartan woman accomplished this "one thousand times in succession, a feat which was recorded on her tombstone."[8] That all this exercise resulted in bodily changes can be inferred from these lines spoken to a Spartan girl by Lysistrata, the heroine of a comedy by that name written by the Greek comic dramatist Aristophanes in 411 B.C.:

> O welcome, welcome, Lampito, my love.
> O the sweet girl! how hale and bright she looks!
> Here's nerve! here's muscle! here's an arm could fairly
> Throttle a bull![9]

[5] Let it not be assumed that in the New World, all women rejected vigorous exercise. In New Orleans, "In January, 1858, three women overlooked polite society's opposition to female athleticism and joined the ranks of professional runners. Mademoiselle Eugenie La Fosse of Paris, Miss Lucy Reynolds of Liverpool, and the fleet and celebrated Indian squaw Ba-tu-uh-o-ua-ra, of the Cherokee tribe, agreed to race in Jackson Square for a set of jewelry." (Dale A. Somers, *The Rise of Sports in New Orleans, 1850–1900* [Baton Rouge, 1972], p. 62, citing the *New Orleans Daily Picayune,* January 9, 1858.)

[6] Denis Brailsford, *Sport and Society, Elizabeth to Anne,* p. 7, citing G. B. Buckley, *Fresh Light on Eighteenth Century Cricket,* p. 31.

[7] Clarence A. Forbes, *Greek Physical Education* (New York, 1971), p. 24.

[8] *Ibid.,* p. 30.

[9] Aristophanes, *Lysistrata,* ll. 78–81, quoted in *ibid.,* p. 41.

motivation and courage

During his cruel flogging, the Spartan boy's parents stood by, urging him to endure, motivating him. To bear a son and see him raised to know Spartan courage was the motivation for the training of the Spartan girl. The Greek biographer Plutarch (46?–120? A.D.) wrote of the tart comment by a foreign woman: "You Spartan women are the only ones who rule over your men." "Ah yes," was the reply, "that is because we alone among women give birth to *men*."[10] Nevertheless, Sparta deteriorated, and the wise Aristotle clearly saw what man has yet to learn: "Most of these military states," he wrote, "are safe only when they are at war, but fall when they have acquired their empire; like unused iron they lose their edge in time of peace. And for this the legislator is to blame, because he never taught them to lead a life of peace."[11] Part of Aristotle's meaning is that peace often requires as much courage as war. In *Paradise Lost,* the English poet John Milton (1608–1674) extolled courage:

> And courage never to submit or yield:
> And what is else not to be overcome?[12]

Competitive sports (which will not be the main concern of this chapter) require a peak of special fitness; in such enterprises much is correctly made of motivations associated with courage. There are other kinds of physical fitness that do not necessarily involve competition but yet demand courage. (These will be the main concern of this chapter.) "There are civil occupations," wrote George Bernard Shaw, "which many successful prize-fighters would fail in or fear to enter for want of nerve."[13] Doubtless there is some truth to this, but it must be emphasized that motivations vary. A Russian scientist recently observed of the Spartan behavior of some Russian soldiers: "During the march on Kazan [in 1552] the 150,000 men army of Ivan the Terrible travelled a distance of 900 kilometers [562.5 miles] in 43 days with a long string of carts and there were no roads!"[14] Now, Ivan IV (1530–1584) richly deserved to be called "the Terrible." In one of his sadistic rages, he slew his own son and heir. Could it not be that his soldiers feared the ferocity of their leader more than that of their opponents, and thus were motivated to march under such harsh circumstances? Fear of failure is not a good motivating factor, but it is certainly a common one. The battlefield, the football field, the dance stage, the tennis court, the baseball field, the executive suite, the classroom—all have their own motivating factors and their unique elements of courage. Fear of failure should not be one of them.[15]

[10] Plutarch's *Life of Lycurgus,* xiv.8, quoted in *ibid.,* p. 28.

[11] Aristotle, *Politics,* vii. 15, tr. by Benjamin Jowett, quoted in *ibid.,* p. 43.

[12] John Milton, *Paradise Lost,* Book I, ll. 108–09.

[13] Quoted in *The Noble Art: A Boxing Anthology,* comp. by T. B. Shepherd (London, 1950), p. 26.

[14] From the translation of the chapter entitled "Endurance in Military Action" in the Russian-language booklet entitled *Fixicheskaya Vynnslivost Cheloveka i Puti Yeye Razvitiya* by Doctor of Medical Sciences Professor Yakov Anariyevich Yegolinskiy, Moscow, 1966. This booklet, published by the Ministry of Defense, U.S.S.R., was edited and revised by V. I. Pahkov, N. N. Kokina, and G. I. Chernakova, pp. 15–17. In the U.S. published by the U.S. Department of Commerce, Clearinghouse for Federal Scientific and Technical Information, Joint Publications Research Service, titled *Man's Physical Endurance and Its Development* (June, 19, 1967), p. 14.

[15] Referring to the Little League, one psychiatrist has said: "Anything that makes a failure of nine-year-old boy, I'm against." And another physician has tartly observed: "The only four-letter word not permitted in this culture is 'fail.'"

Much has been made of the difficulty of motivating today's U.S. citizen to engage in some regimen of training to promote fitness. The physical body is but part of the entire person, adjusting in a stressful environment. In this respect, it is well to recall the wise words of a noted U.S. psychoanalyst: "Fortunately analysis is not the only way to resolve inner conflicts. Life itself still remains a very effective therapist."[16] To the enormous extent that the search for fitness can increase life's effectivity, it, too, can be an effective therapist. For many people, that is motivation enough. And often it is a motivation that also requires courage to bring about positive action.

fitness: meaning of the term

"The term physical fitness defies exact definition or measurement."[17] So wrote, in 1973, Forrest H. Adams of the UCLA School of Medicine. He was not the first to reach this conclusion. It is difficult enough just to define "fitness," without adding the problems of defining its physical aspects. A few years before, a Canadian expert wrote that when he was a student, his professor considered the term "fitness" to be "so vague as to be void of scientific meaning and . . . prohibited its use."[18] That expert was a member of a 1968 committee of the World Health Organization charged with defining fitness. Six laboriously prepared drafts brought no agreement. Some measure of agreement was finally reached with the seventh draft, but "mainly because the time available for discussion was exhausted!"[19]

In the broadest sense of "fitness," most people want to be fit enough to adjust dynamically to their various ecosystems—physical, psychological, and social. But each person is a whole made of many parts. In considering movement, for example, one must consider the central nervous system, which transmits nerve impulses, causing muscular contractions, which transmit forces to responding bones. For the sake of simplicity, fitness may be approached from its mechanical aspects. But it must never be forgotten that different people have different desires, needs, tasks, rhythms, requirements for relaxation, and levels of fatigue; they also vary in age, gender, occupation, emotional makeup, and numerous other ways. To some extent, then, fitness is an individual matter. And it can be either specific or general.

specific fitness

Specific fitness refers to the degree of fitness required to perform a specific task. Even slight anatomical differences can make one person more fit for a particular task than another. Differences in bone length or attachment of tendons to bones, for example, will make one person an excellent sprinter, another person a poor sprinter. But the second person may be an excellent jumper or weight lifter. On the other hand, an understanding of the mechanics of movement, of

[16] Karen Horney, quoted in *Medical World News,* Vol. 14, No. 36 (October 5, 1973), p. 89.
[17] Forrest H. Adams, "Factors Affecting the Working Capacity of Children and Adolescents," in G. Lawrence Rarick, ed., *Physical Activity: Human Growth and Development* (New York, 1973), p. 81.
[18] Roy J. Shephard, *Endurance Fitness* (Toronto, 1969), p. 1.
[19] *Ibid.*

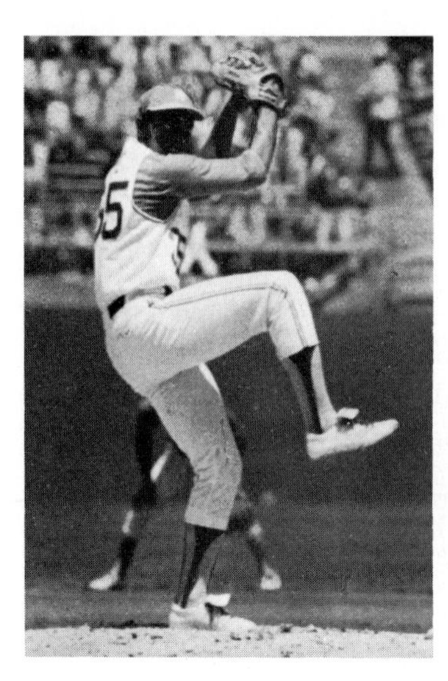

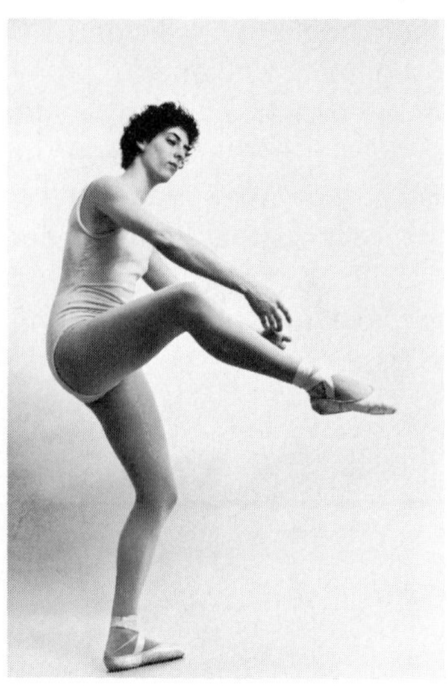

23-3 *The movements—and the physical training—of the baseball player (here, Vida Blue of the Oakland Athletics) and the ballet dancer are very similar.*

the prerequisites for its greatest efficiency, combined with graduated attempts to improve that efficiency, can yield satisfying results. ''The most beautiful motion,'' Plato wrote, ''is that which accomplishes the greatest result with the least amount of effort.''

As examples, consider two athletes, the ballet dancer and the baseball pitcher. Their functions are not so disparate as they might seem (see Figure 23-3). Both are athletes whose bodies are trained to perform specific tasks. For the dancer, leaping in the air, completing two 360° turns, and landing on one foot in a perfect arabesque is one form of physical and psychological tension; carrying a 115-pound woman at arm's length above shoulder height as though she were a floating leaf—this, too, is a feat not easily achieved. Or consider the baseball pitcher, a less elegant character, perhaps, a ball of gum pouching his cheek and sweat running down his back, standing out there alone on the rubber, fighting to keep from being sent to the showers. Sports writers discuss his ''control'' and his ''pitching arm.'' What they often fail to mention is the training that had to go into that arm and into the body to which it is attached. Consider, for example: in what position must his arm exert its greatest strength? When his hand is arm-distant in front of his body? No. He must train the muscles of his arm so that they reach their greatest strength, their peak control, just before the ball leaves his hand. That is long before the automatic follow-through motion that propels his arm forward. The average person will not be a great athlete, perhaps not even a good one. But he can seek the greatest efficiency of movement within his limitations and often surprise himself at the greater ease of movement and his lessened fatigue.

general fitness General fitness implies the ability to meet with all the tasks of life, including its emergencies. Moreover, a person who is generally fit has enough residual energy at the end of a work day to enjoy his or her ways of relaxation. And with those pleasures passed, such a person is not too tired or tense to enjoy a night of refreshing sleep. It is doubtful that a perfect level of general fitness is ever reached by the average person. But a practical level of general fitness is within the reach of most people. How? The answers to that question will be explored in this chapter.

posture, movement, and their involved tissues

People do not often think of posture as movement, yet they rarely stand completely still. One researcher concluded that "even standing is not static but rather it is 'movement upon a stationary base.'"[20] People, she discovered, sway constantly, if slightly. Thus their center of gravity is constantly changing. Such swaying is involuntary (not done consciously) and is of assistance in both returning venous blood to the heart and in bringing sufficient blood to the brain. From the evolutionary point of view, relatively soft cartilage is enough for the watery ecosystems of fishlike creatures; they do not need hard, bony support. Venturing from the seas, early land creatures clung to the ground, and that ground had to be muddy; their soft-bending skeletons and short limbs could permit no more. Hundreds of millions of years passed. Elizabeth Bowen aptly wrote in *A Time in Rome* that "Time is one kind of space; it creates distance." Evolving creatures waddled from the watery edges. For the fittest to survive, bones had to harden, extremities had to lengthen, and other profound changes had to take place. Eventually, perhaps to escape predators or to find enough food, some animals took to the trees. Tree-living primates stood erect part of the time; this was a major evolutionary change. During this time, postural weight was largely suspended from the forward extremities. At last, man stood, and fully erect. Then he bore his weight, instead of suspending it. For this accomplishment he needed connective and supportive tissues as well as muscles.

connective and supportive tissues

These are *fibroelastic tissue, adipose tissue* (from the Latin *adiposus,* "fatty"), *cartilage,* and *bone.* All these have the same embryonic origin. Unlike muscle cells, the cells of these four do not themselves carry out the function of the tissues of which they are a part. They maintain and repair these tissues, but they do not do the work of the organ. In contrast, muscle cells do the work of the tissues of which they are a part. This is significant because connective and supportive tissue can be replaced by repair when injured or destroyed. But once injured or destroyed, muscle can never be replaced by more muscle. Only scar tissue takes its place.

Since *fibroelastic tissue* holds the parts of the body together, they can be found throughout its entire structure. Fibroelastic tissue can be more elastic than fibrous where the body needs flexibility and mobility, as with the muscles and blood vessels; it can be tougher (more fibrous) where necessary, as in the *periosteum,* the membranes covering the bones (see body chart 6 in the color

[20] Quoted in Marion Broer, *Efficiency of Human Movement* (Philadelphia, 1973), p. 129.

section). Fibroelastic tissue is not limited to the grossly observable parts of the body. It exists in the most elegantly structured organs, among the minuscule ovarian follicles, among the tiny alveoli of the lung, and between the microscopic glomeruli and tubules of the kidney. As for *adipose cells,* it is only in them that body fat is deposited. The amount of body fat therefore depends on the number of adipose cells. Where there are no fat cells (such as in the eyelids), there is no fat storage. Unfortunately, most people have an abundant number of adipose cells in the abdominal wall. From the point of view of physical fitness (and survival), however, matters could have been worse; fat cells might have been more abundant in the soles of the feet. For some discussion of *bone* and *cartilage,* see body charts 1 and 2. During embryonic development the differentiation among soft connective tissue, harder cartilage, and hardest bone begins and continues. Throughout the entire period of human growth, bone continues to form new bone.

This is not the case with muscles. Almost all the individual muscle fibers a person will ever have are formed before birth. Muscle growth, then, is due to an increase not in the number, but in the size of individual muscle fibers. All muscle is involved in movement. For a brief statement of the various types of muscle, see body charts 3 and 4. At this point, attention is turned to *striated muscle,* the type of muscle involved in voluntary physical activity.

striated muscles

There are more than four hundred skeletal, or striated, muscles in the human body. They account for about 42 percent of its weight. They are called skeletal because they are attached to bone (see body chart 5 in the color section). They are also referred to as striated because under a microscope they are seen to have alternating light and dark stripes (see Figure 23-4). When muscles contract, they force two regions of the skeleton closer together, thus moving a joint (see body charts 5 and 6). Each muscle is a unit; that is, it has its own supply of nerves, arteries, veins, and lymphatic channels. Nevertheless, muscles usually contract in groups, rarely alone. And they contract in response to stimuli from the central nervous system (see pages 265–66).

muscles: a microscopic view

Each striated muscle consists of numerous cylindrical cells with many nuclei. These cells are called *muscle fibers;* under an ordinary microscope they appear to be striated. Muscle fibers are composed of *myofibrils,* which contain nuclei and mitochondria. It is the high-powered electron microscope that has revealed the long-secret miniature world of myofibrils and, in so doing, provided new knowledge about the way striated muscle contracts. The electron microscope has revealed the myofibril as a striking pattern of alternating light and dark bands. This banded pattern of the myofibrils is due to the presence within them of two kinds of filaments, thick and thin. For parts of their lengths, these two overlap; it is this overlapping that gives a striated appearance to the myofibril

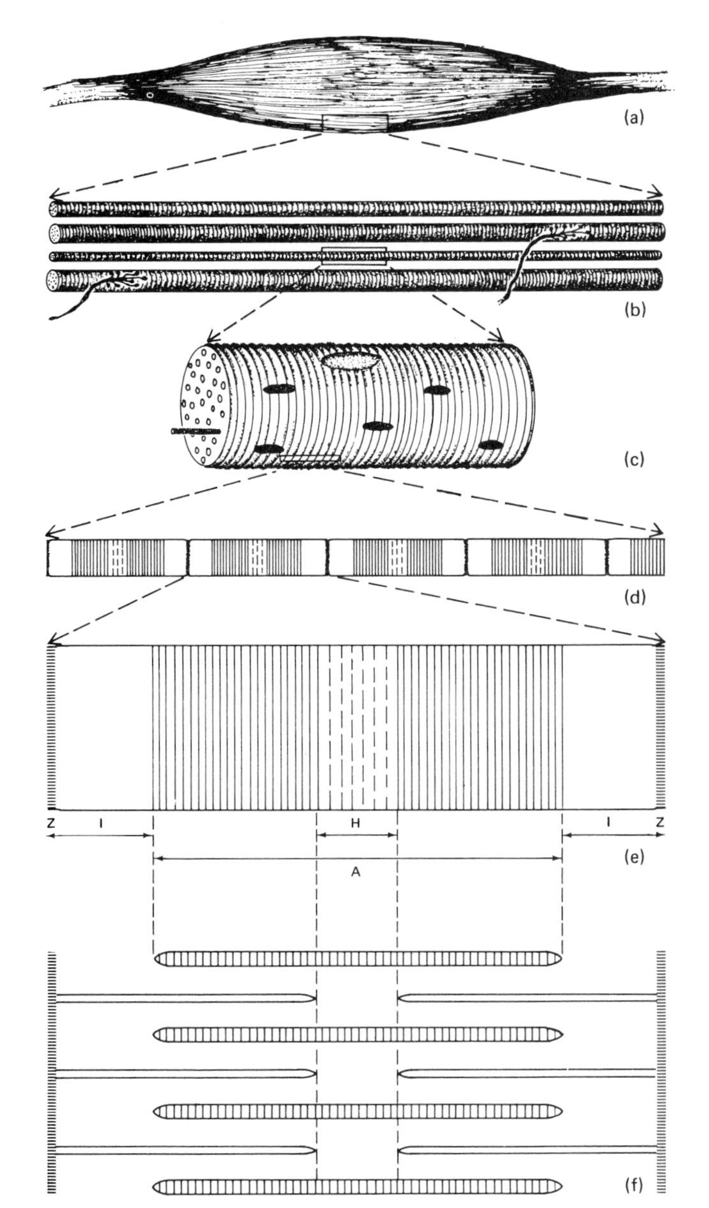

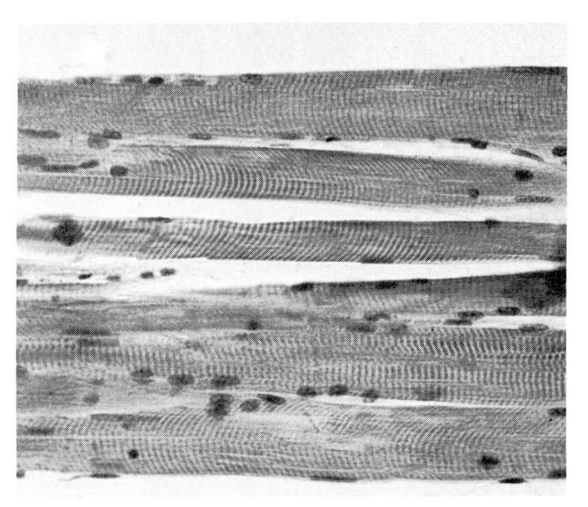

23-4 Above: *Striated muscle fibers (each of which is equivalent to c in diagram at left).* Left: *Schematic dissection of skeletal muscle. A muscle (a) is made up of muscle fibers (b), which appear striated under the microscope. The small branching structures at the surface of the fibers are the "end-plates" of motor nerves, which signal the fibers to contract. A single muscle fiber (c) is made up of myofibrils. In a single myofibril (d), the striations are resolved into a repeating pattern of light and dark bands. A single unit of this pattern (e) consists of a "Z-line," then an "I-band," then an "A-band," which is interrupted by an "H-zone," then the next I-band, and finally the next Z-line. Electron micrographs have shown that the repeating band pattern is due to the overlapping of thick and thin filaments (f).*

and thus to the muscle fibers. What is more, there is a remarkable order to the arrangement of the filaments (see Figure 23-4). Study of a dense part of the "A band" reveals the astonishing fact that each thick filament is surrounded by six thin filaments; each thin filament is surrounded by three thin ones. (This is not shown in Figure 23-4.) In addition (also not shown), the two kinds of filaments are connected by a complex system of cross-bridges. When a muscle contracts, neither type of filament changes in length, as was once thought; instead, it is believed that the thick and thin filaments slide over one another.

When muscles are reduced to their tiniest anatomic elements, one fact becomes clear: muscles were made for movement. That is why, with prolonged inaction, they wither.

But where does the muscle obtain its capacity to contract, to do its work? Like all operative engines, it needs a source of energy, of fuel. Muscles have several different energy sources. When a muscle runs out of a fuel it needs, it is capable of generating that fuel itself. How does this occur?

muscles: a chemical view[21]

Chemical compounds within the muscle cells, called *phosphagens,* are the two basic and direct sources of energy provided to the muscle so that it can contract. First, the phosphagen called *adenosine triphosphate* (ATP; see page 717) breaks down into two compounds, adenosine diphosphate (ADP) and phosphoric acid. This releases the energy needed for contraction. But there is a hitch. ATP is not stored continuously in the muscle; it must be constantly resynthesized from the products of its own breakdown. And for these products—ADP and phosphoric acid—to recombine into ATP, yet another source of energy is needed. This energy is supplied by the splitting of a second phosphagen in the cell called *creatinine phosphate.* Since creatinine phosphate is also not stored in the cell continuously, it too must be almost immediately resynthesized. To make possible this second recombination (and thus the recombination of the phosphagens), there are two ultimate sources of energy. The first is the combustion of food; the amount of this energy can be measured by the amount of oxygen consumed by the body. The second is the breakdown into lactic acid of a carbohydrate called *glycogen* that is stored in the muscle. This breakdown of glycogen into lactic acid (*glycolysis*) is reversible. When oxidation occurs during food combustion, lactic acid is reconstituted to glycogen. ''The system, then, consists of five reactions, three of which [phosphagen-splitting, food combustion, and glycolysis] yield energy and two of which [phosphagen and glycogen resynthesis] absorb energy.''[22] (See Table 23-1.) Careful study of this system and of the time relationships of the five reactions suggests that ''proper pacing of . . . work . . . and intervals of rest [enable] a person [to] produce more work than by driving himself relentlessly.''[23] This finding is applicable to physical exercise—such as walking and running—as well as to work.

strength, flexibility, and endurance

The basic elements of physical fitness have been considered to include *strength, flexibility,* and *endurance.*[24] These three will be the basic subjects to be discussed in the remainder of this chapter. However, it should not be assumed that they are isolated, noninterconnected aspects of physical fitness. To a marked degree, one influences the other. And they are each influenced by a variety of

[21] This section is based on Rodolfo Margaria, ''The Sources of Muscular Energy,'' *Scientific American,* Vol. 226, No. 3 (1973), pp. 84–91.
[22] *Ibid.,* p. 84.
[23] *Ibid.,* p. 91.
[24] Harold B. Falls, Earl L. Wallis, and Gene A. Logan, *Foundations of Conditioning* (New York, 1970), p. viii.

TABLE 23-1

Energy Expenditures for Various Everyday Activities

ACTIVITY	CALORIES PER POUND PER HOUR	ACTIVITY	CALORIES PER POUND PER HOUR
Asleep	.4	Playing ping-pong	2.7
Bicycling, moderate speed	1.7	Reading aloud	.7
Cello playing	1.1	Running	4.0
Dancing, mildly active	2.2	Sewing, on a machine or by hand	.7
Dishwashing	1.0	Sitting quietly, watching TV	.6
Dressing and undressing	.9	Skating	2.2
Driving a car	1.0	Standing	.8
Eating a meal	.7	Sweeping, vacuum cleaner	1.9
Horseback riding, trot	2.6	Swimming, 2 m.p.h.	4.5
Ironing	1.0	Tailoring	1.0
Laundry, light	1.1	Typing rapidly	1.0
Lying still, awake	.5	Walking, 3 m.p.h.	1.5
Painting furniture	1.3	Walking, 4 m.p.h.	2.2
Piano playing, moderate	1.2	Writing	.7

Source: Adapted from C. M. Taylor, Grace MacLeod, and M. D. S. Rose, *Foundations of Nutrition,* 5th ed. (New York, 1956).

other factors, such as body build, reaction time, physical acuity of the senses, and emotional states.[25] Reaction time is hardly as important in weight lifting as it is in tennis. And endurance is surely helpful in long-distance running, but if one runs to avoid a car, acuity of the senses and quick reaction time can be life-saving.

strength: through isometrics, isotonics, or both?

Refer again to body chart 5 in the color section. Note that, in order to function, a striated muscle can never be attached to only one bone; whether contracting or relaxing, it invariably crosses a joint and is attached to another bone by means of a *tendon.* (*Ligaments* are the tissues that attach bones to other bones.) Moreover, muscles tend to be arranged in pairs on opposite sides of joints; one of the pair bends the joint, the other extends or straightens it. When there is no interfering resistance, this *antagonistic action* between a pair of performing muscles affords joint leverage. Each muscle of the pair, when called upon to contract, performs its basic function. It develops tension within itself. It exerts equal force at each of its two ends. It pulls its fibers toward its center, bunching them there. All this contraction can occur only because the muscle is part of a *neuromuscular unity;* it ultimately acts under the direction of impulses from the central nervous system.

When a striated muscle contracts, however, it may do so in either of two

[25] Marion Broer, *Efficiency of Human Movement,* p. 33. This invaluable book is highly recommended for its lucid and thorough coverage.

ways, *isometric* or *isotonic.* ''Isometric'' is from the Greek *isos,* ''equal'' or ''constant,'' and *metron,* ''measure''; it can, thus, refer to length. Isometrically contracting muscles would, then, maintain a constant length. How does this come about? To the concept of antagonistic action (that, for example, there are muscles that bend or flex the elbow and other muscles, antagonistic to them, that straighten or extend it), add an outside force in the form of some work. With equal force press the palms together so that they do not move. The muscles exert themselves against this force. Tension has been created in them, but as long as the opposing forces are equal the muscles will contract isometrically, and their length will remain unchanged. Moreover, body levers will not move; there will be no joint action. And the strength of the isometrically acting muscle can be measured only through its tension.

Now press the palms together unequally, so that one hand forcefully overcomes the other. Again, tension is created in the involved muscles. But now joint leverage does occur. One elbow will straighten, or extend; the other will flex, or bend. The straightening extension of a joint, such as the elbow, is accomplished by dynamic lengthening of the involved muscles (a lengthening contraction). The flexing or bending of a joint occurs because the necessary muscles shorten by contraction. This is *isotonic contraction* as opposed to isometric contraction. It is derived from the Greek word *tonikos,* which refers to tension and connotes movement. Walking and running are among the numerous isotonic exercises.

In programs to develop strength it is believed that both isometric and isotonic exercises may be useful.[26] As has been seen, isometric exercises cause muscle contraction when there is an exertion against an immovable object. This may be done by pushing or pulling at the object. Thus, little equipment is needed. ''All that is needed is a firm resistance against which the muscles can push or pull. Even one's own muscle can be used—one group pulling or pushing against the other.'' Another advantage may be the satisfaction that comes with the ability to see oneself overcome ''fixed amounts of resistance.''[27]

Other possible reasons for the wide popularity of isometric exercises are that, assiduously performed, they will produce muscles that will bulge on the beach and will produce considerable muscle tension during isometric contractions. But it is emphasized that

> only repeated maximal or near maximal contractions produce measureable results . . . and both the number of daily contractions and their magnitude must be large . . . to obtain measureable increases in muscular strength . . . The question is only: For what use? . . . For performing certain tasks in labor or sport, isometric training probably is rather worthless . . . because the obtained isometric strength apparently cannot be transferred directly to other forms of activity where the muscles are to be used under other conditions. Furthermore, . . . even strong and long-lasting isometric contractions put only very light demands on the cardiorespiratory and vascular systems and, therefore, are a very poor training for endurance.[28]

[26] Harold B. Falls, Earl L. Wallis, and Gene A. Logan, *Foundations of Conditioning,* p. 66.
[27] *Ibid.,* p. 68.
[28] Erling Asmussen, ''The Neuromuscular System and Exercise,'' in *Exercise Physiology,* ed. by Harold B. Falls (New York, 1968), p. 36.

Thus, for most people and purposes, the exercises of choice should be isotonic—those that involve movement.[29]

flexibility: bending readily without breaking

In his *Just So Stories,* the English writer Rudyard Kipling (1865–1936) rhymed:

> The Camel's hump is an ugly lump
> which well you may see at the Zoo;
> But uglier yet is the hump we get
> From having too little to do.

Kipling's little poem may be applied to adults whom the ancient Roman orator Cicero (106–43 B.C.) described as "in perpetual repose."[30] It is noteworthy that one of the most prolonged natural periods of repose is one of flexion, and it occurs within the narrow confines of the uterus. Therein curls the fetus, backbone flexed, head bent onto the chest, and extremities flexed at the shoulder and hip joints. The fetus can accommodate so easily to the limited living space because of the elasticity of fetal tendons and connective tissue and the pliability of a largely cartilaginous skeleton. Upon release from the watery ecosystem of the uterus, the newborn is in a less buoyant environment. Gravity pulls upon the infant, so that the head and back lie flat, although the extremities remain flexible for some months.

> Much of the skeleton of the infant is still pliable and will take on the shape of constantly held positions. In early infancy, the baby's position needs to be changed for him, so that undue molding of the bone does not take place. This is especially true of the feet. An infant who lies always on his abdomen everts his feet and stretches the ligaments, holding the feet at right angles to the leg. This has a tendency to produce pronation [a turning outward] when weight bearing is accomplished.[31]

23-5 *Flexibility: Zinaïda Drujinina, one of the top women gymnasts in the Soviet Union.*

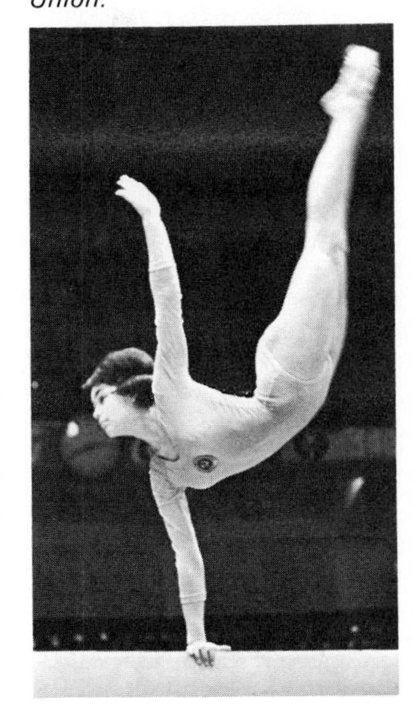

With increasing control of his striated muscles, the infant soon can bring his head upward, then his back, pulling, straining. Next he sits, temporarily supporting the shift of weight on his arms. Growing stronger, the child crawls, and at last, never idle, stands and walks. There are few exercises of which he is capable that the toddler will not attempt. His is a life not of "perpetual repose," but of seemingly perpetual motion. Unfortunately, his weary mother may not find space and equipment for his exercise. Too often, the toddler spends long hours sitting motionless in front of the television screen. Nor is much physical exertion demanded of a child during the school years. To aggravate the situation, the inherent mimicry of childhood ensures that children will copy the exercise habits and posture of the adults around them. Even cursory observations of student postures on high school and college campuses suggest that all too often, the imitation has been deplorably accurate.

[29] An excellent discussion of isotonic conditioning exercises is Chapter 5 of Harold B. Falls, Earl L. Wallis, and Gene A. Logan, *Foundations of Conditioning.*
[30] Cicero, *De Finibus,* Bk. V, Ch. 20, Sec. 55.
[31] Dorothy V. Whipple, *Dynamics of Development: Euthenic Pediatrics* (New York, 1966), p. 238.

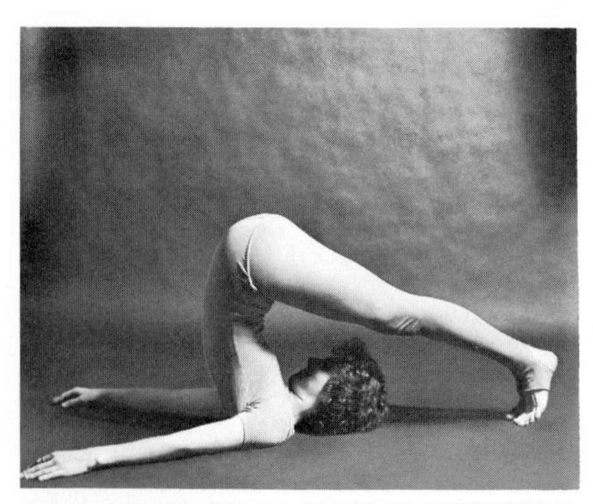

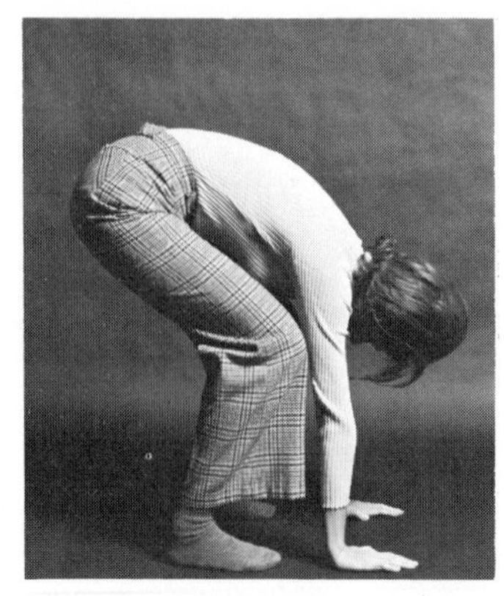

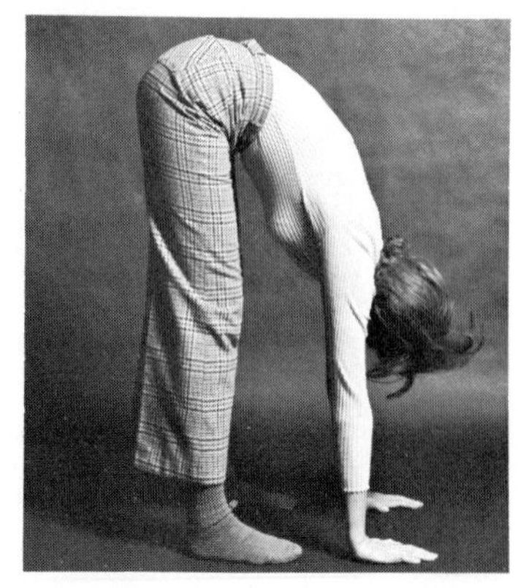

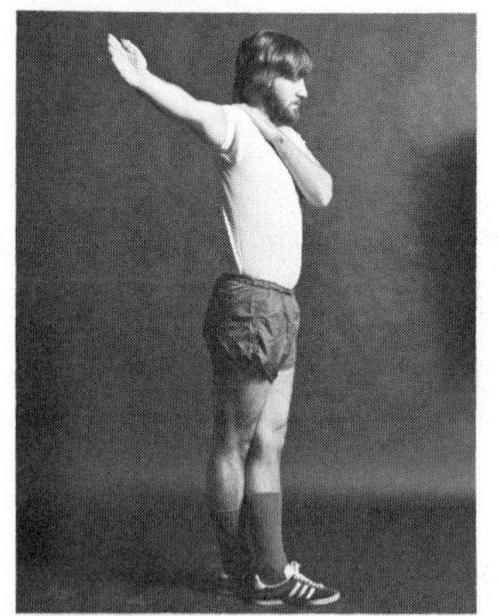

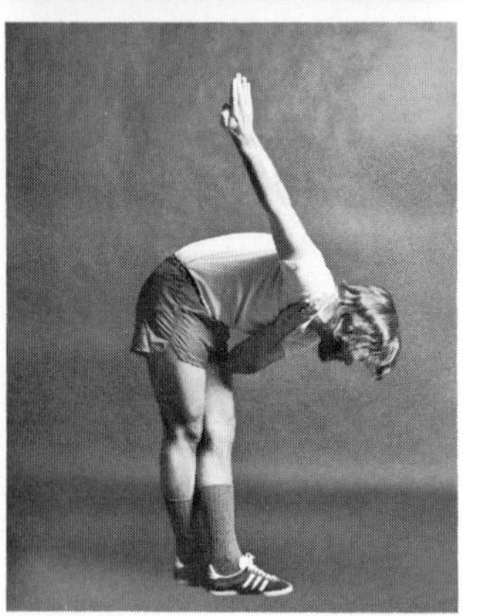

23-6 *Three good stretching exercises—all of which should be done slowly.* Left: *The hamstring, or Billig, stretch, which increases flexibility of the lower back and hips. The first photograph shows the starting position, and the second shows the forward flex position. The stretch should be repeated to the opposite side. The position of the arms provides balance.* Above left: *A stretch that increases flexibility of the upper spine. The hands should be pressed against the floor, and the abdominal muscles should be strongly contracted.* Above right: *Another stretch that increases flexibility of the lower back and hips. This exercise begins with the position shown in the first photograph, with hips and knees flexed; then, as shown in the second photograph, the legs are straightened slowly while the hands and arms remain in the same position.*

Inactivity breeds inflexibility—an insufficient range of motion. Flexer muscles cause a joint to bend, but only if the opposing muscles lengthen sufficiently. If they cannot, bending (or flexion) is limited. Ligaments and other connective tissue must also be extensible in order to facilitate adequate range of motion. Due to variations in body structure, not all people have equal ranges of motion. Moreover, flexibility varies enormously in the various joints of the normal body. However, when an individual's range of motion is inadequate, flexibility can be regained by specialized exercises. Slow, controlled, stretching procedures entail less energy expenditure, possibly less muscle soreness, and more relief from muscle pain. Recommended exercises involve stretching slowly to the point of mild discomfort—then stretching a little more. Moreover, during the flexibility exercise, the opposing muscles should be actively stretched. No form of exercise demands more help from a specialist than those designed to increase flexibility. Two persistent myths should be laid to rest at this point. The notion of the "muscle-bound" person who loses flexibility as strength is gained, is false, and so is the Victorian idea that exercise will transform a "feminine" woman into a muscle-bound, manlike creature.

endurance: aerobics and anaerobics

"The over-all determinant of endurance fitness is the ability of the body to transfer oxygen from the atmosphere to the sites of biochemical activity in the working tissues."[32] As has been seen, chemical sources of energy are required so that microscopic muscle filaments can slide over one another during contraction. But energy is also necessary so that the phosphagens (which by their very

[32] Roy J. Shephard, *Endurance Fitness*, p. 29.

act of splitting supply the energy for the filaments to slide) can be resynthesized. It is from the energy resulting from the oxidation of food materials that phosphagen resynthesis occurs. But the body cannot keep an unlimited supply of oxygen available. Why not? After all, is there not more than sufficient oxygen available in the ordinary atmosphere? Normal lungs surely have more than enough capacity for oxygen diffusion. And a healthy heart muscle certainly has sufficient strength to pump enough oxygen-carrying blood to the muscles. That oxygen gets to the muscle cells via the red blood cells in the capillaries. And it is at the capillary-cell level[33] that the hitch occurs. For oxygenated blood to reach the capillaries, energy must be expended. For the oxygen to leave the red blood cells, pass through the capillary, and enter the cell through its watery medium, no energy is required. This gaseous exchange is a passive movement. It cannot be hastened. Moreover, when a muscle contracts, the pressure within it increases. Blood vessels are compressed. Blood flow to the muscle is hindered. When the muscle relaxes, blood flow to it is increased. In this way, a steady state is reached: oxygen and nutrients are brought to the muscle as rapidly as they are needed.

A young man runs a long-distance race. His effort is intense but measured and rhythmic. As he nears the end of the distance, his energy requirements become maximal; his oxygen intake is also maximal. This maximal oxygen intake, the amount of oxygen he can take from the air under the most extreme circumstances, is known as his *aerobic capacity* (from the Greek *aer,* ''air'' or ''gas''). The greater his aerobic capacity is, the greater will be his endurance. And the regular exercise that contributes the most to his endurance fitness is the one that most benefits his cardiorespiratory function—*aerobic exercise.* To be of value, the exercise must make demands on the cardiorespiratory system. Isotonic, not isometric, exercise accomplishes this. A leisurely stroll down a long-forgotten wooded path may produce a nostalgic sigh but it will not exercise the lungs; it may warm the heart but it will do little to exercise it. For a normal person, the motion of isotonic exercise should increase the heart rate to about 130 to 135 beats a minute. Swimming, long-distance running, rowing, bicycling, and rapid walking—these are among the best isotonic exercises.

What is *anaerobic* exercise? Anaerobic refers to the absence of oxygen. Suppose a young man attempts to run the hundred-yard dash in less than ten seconds. For a brief time his excess need for oxygen cannot be met. This is called ''oxygen debt.'' This oxygen-debt exercise is anaerobic. More oxygen is being used than is readily available through the aerobic process. In such circumstances, where does the energy come from to resynthesize phosphagens? Through an anaerobic mechanism in which glycogen is broken down to lactic acid. But lactic acid is a fatigue-producing toxin. When glycogen has been broken down to the extent that the muscle can no longer tolerate the toxic lactic acid, activity must be slowed until the process stops. If it is not, the individual will collapse; he can exercise no longer. No man or woman has the endurance to run at top speed, using full energy, for very long. After the exercise stops, the individual consumes more oxygen and pays the oxygen debt.

23-7 *''To men, rich and poor, the bicycle is an unmixed blessing; but to woman it is deliverance, revolution, salvation. It is well nigh impossible to overestimate . . . its influence in the matters of dress and social reform''* (Cosmopolitan *magazine, 1895*).

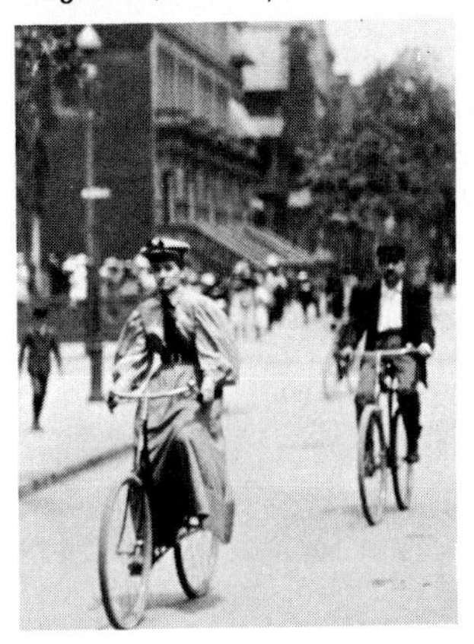

[33] For a discussion of the respiratory-circulatory processes, see pages 221–23 and 388–91.

on some measurements of physical fitness

Measurements of physical fitness are often made, but sometimes unscientifically. The story is told of a world-famous symphony conductor who insisted that his heart rate was normal. This despite a life full of stress, incessant cigar smoking, constant traveling and, except for conducting, relatively complete inactivity. How could his heart be abnormal? he asked his physicians. His heart rate was synchronous with the tempo of the Scherzo of Beethoven's Second Symphony. The conductor died at a relatively young age after suffering his fourth heart attack. A check of the tempo of the Scherzo showed it to be about 116 beats per minute[34]—considerably above the normal heart rate. Another case of an inaccurate measurement of physical fitness was fortunately corrected in time. An enthusiastic horsewoman wanted to know of Kenneth H. Cooper, the originator of the Aerobic Exercise Method (see the following section) how much aerobic credit she earned by riding for one hour. "You don't get any credit," he told her. "It all goes to the horse."[35]

Sometimes even scientific efforts at measuring physical fitness can be misleading at first. Some years ago the entire Philadelphia 76ers professional basketball team became disheartened and despondent when it was learned that its great star player, 7-foot-2-inch Wilt Chamberlain, showed signs and symptoms of a heart attack. He complained of severe chest pain; his electrocardiogram and blood studies suggested heart damage due to a lack of blood supply to the heart. However, a review of Chamberlain's past electrocardiographic heart tracings revealed that they were a stable characteristic of his particular heart pattern. His abnormal blood chemistries were apparently due not to heart damage, but to inflammatory damage of the pancreas. Like most of his teammates, Chamberlain has a heart rate of only 50 beats per minute—considerably below the average. To raise it to the average level, he had to run up several flights of stairs. After violent exercise, his electrocardiogram also reverted to an ordinary picture. All this indicated that one of the greatest of all basketball players was not, at the time, suffering from a heart ailment.[36]

Cooper's aerobic measurements: testing toward fitness

Accurate measurement of endurance fitness—maximum oxygen consumption—is a laboratory procedure. Fortunately, Kenneth H. Cooper has developed a method whereby an individual can measure his maximum oxygen consumption merely by determining how far he can go by running and walking in twelve minutes. The individual taking the test usually begins by running; when he gets short of breath, he walks; as soon as he is able, he begins to run again. Cooper has established the standards shown in Table 23-2 to establish fitness as it relates to various ages of the adult male population.

After determining his physical fitness category, the man begins graded ex-

[34] Hans Kraus and Wilhelm Raab, *Hypokinetic Disease: Diseases Produced by Lack of Exercise* (Springfield, Ill., 1961), pp. 71–72.
[35] Mildred Cooper and Kenneth H. Cooper, *Aerobics for Women* (New York, 1972), p. 37.
[36] "Family Physicians to the 76ers," *Roche Medical Image,* Vol. 10, No. 2 (April 1968), p. 33.

TABLE 23-2

Standards at Various Ages for Cooper's Twelve-Minute Field Test for Men

FITNESS CATEGORY	DISTANCE IN MILES WALKED AND RUN IN TWELVE MINUTES AT VARIOUS AGES			
	UNDER 30	30–39	40–49	50+
I. Very poor	Less than 1.0	Less than .95	Less than .85	Less than .80
II. Poor	1.0–1.24	.95–1.14	.85–1.04	.80–.99
III. Fair	1.25–1.49	1.15–1.39	1.05–1.29	1.0–1.24
IV. Good	1.50–1.74	1.40–1.64	1.30–1.54	1.25–1.49
V. Excellent	1.75 or more	1.65 or more	1.55 or more	1.50 or more

Source: Kenneth H. Cooper, *The New Aerobics* (New York, 1970), p. 30.

ercises. As his fitness increases and he progresses to categories higher on the scale, his oxygen consumption increases. However, the exercise that is selected must be vigorous enough to produce a "training effect." In this respect Cooper's research has led him to establish two principles:

1. If the exercise is vigorous enough to produce a sustained heart rate of 150 beats per minute or more, the training-effect benefits begin about five minutes after the exercise starts and continue as long as the exercise is performed.

2. If the exercise is not vigorous enough to produce or sustain a heart rate of 150 beats per minute, but still demands oxygen, the exercise must be continued considerably longer than five minutes, the total amount of time depending on the oxygen consumed.[37]

Thus, activities that are sustained for longer than five minutes demand more of the body's oxygen-transporting system (the cardiovascular system) than do short bursts of energy. This is why the hundred-yard dash, for example, cannot offer the same endurance-training effect that can be gained from long-distance running. One of the singular advantages of the Cooper Aerobic System of exercise is that it presents a goal toward which the out-of-condition person can strive. In order to earn 30 points a week (5 points for each of six days a week), a man must be able to run a mile in less than eight minutes six days a week. This places him in category IV or V—good or excellent.

Because the average woman's size and aerobic capacity are smaller than the average man's, Cooper's aerobic test for women is not the same as that for men. The average woman has a lesser amount of circulating blood and, thus, fewer red blood cells and less hemoglobin. Cooper does not believe that the twelve-minute test is essential for the average woman; all she need do to achieve physical fitness is earn twenty-four points a week. Nevertheless, he does present an optional twelve-minute test for women, shown in Table 23-3.

[37] Kenneth H. Cooper, *Aerobics* (New York, 1968), p. 40.

TABLE 23-3
Standards for Cooper's Optional Twelve-Minute Field Test for Women

FITNESS CATEGORY	DISTANCE IN MILES WALKED AND RUN IN TWELVE MINUTES AT VARIOUS AGES				
	UNDER 30	30–39	40–49	50–59	60+
I. Very Poor	Less than .95	Less than .85	Less than .75	Less than .65	Not recommended
II. Poor	.95–1.14	.85–1.04	.75–.94	.65–.84	
III. Fair	1.15–1.34	1.05–1.24	.95–1.14	.85–1.04	
IV. Good	1.35–1.64	1.25–1.54	1.15–1.44	1.05–1.34	
V. Excellent	1.65 or more	1.55 or more	1.45 or more	1.35 or more	

Source: Mildred Cooper and Kenneth H. Cooper, *Aerobics for Women* (New York, 1972), p. 52.

the two doctors

Perhaps the most convenient, least costly, and yet least practiced of all aerobic isometric exercises is walking. "I have two doctors," the English writer G. M. Trevelyan wrote long ago, "my left leg and my right."[38] But Joseph Wood Krutch was only partially right when he wrote, a decade ago, that "the modern male lost interest in his own legs about the time that he developed an ardent concern with those of his female companions."[39] Nowadays, modern man has forsaken his legs for his automobile. Unfortunately, so have many modern women. There are those who cannot go to the corner drugstore without the family car; a common sight on city streets is hitchhikers for whom a two-mile walk is as unthinkable as one from Los Angeles to San Francisco (some four hundred miles). Yet there is abundant evidence to indicate that a two-hour daily brisk walk can be more than healthful. It can be life-saving. It should be incorporated into one's daily life and time must be set aside for it. Those who simply cannot find the time might at least consider this question: "What do you usually do with the time you save?"

the feet and shoes The foot of the U.S. citizen is usually in bad shape. It has endured much mistreatment. Overweight, poor posture, lack of exercise, high heels, and pointed toes—all these have taken a toll that the barefoot or moccasined Indian never had to pay. Some foot problems need the attention of an orthopedist. A long walk will tire normal feet, but will not hurt them. A tepid (not hot) footbath will relieve aching muscles. Moreover, dancers and other athletes advise that, after

[38] Quoted in Aaron Sussman and Ruth Goode, *The Magic of Walking* (New York, 1967), p. 15. This book, available in paperback, is one volume that belongs on every bookshelf. Unless otherwise noted, this section is based on that work.

[39] Joseph Wood Krutch, "Is Walking the New Status Symbol?" *The American Scholar,* Vol. 33, No. 4 (August 1964), quoted in Aaron Sussman and Ruth Goode, *The Magic of Walking,* p. 314.

long periods of inactivity, foot use should at first be moderate. Conditioning is important.

Everyday clothes and comfortable shoes are enough for the man who briskly walks a few miles to and from work every day. The problem for working women is somewhat more complex but generally solvable. Fortunately, one no longer often sees the working woman tottering to her job on high heels. Today's low-heeled shoes are better and attractive. But often the soles are too thin and not protective enough against the unyielding pavement. Callouses and joint pain result. The prevention: cushioned insoles or metatarsal insoles. No more acceptable than the atrocious cripplers forced on women by fashion a generation ago are modern platform shoes (see Figure 23-8). In the concluding months of 1973, these elevators that lifted the wearer three to seven inches off the ground had thrown so many people back onto the ground that they had caused a 30 percent increase in injuries varying from painfully skinned knees and elbows to sprained ankles and broken bones.[40] More expensive than an ordinary shoe, but a good investment, are those that are individually molded to the foot. One caution about them, however. They can be heavy and, therefore, tiring. What does the walking woman wear to work? In this, the suburban homemaker led the way. Stylish slacks, pants suits, and enviably comfortable shoes have long been part of her wardrobe.

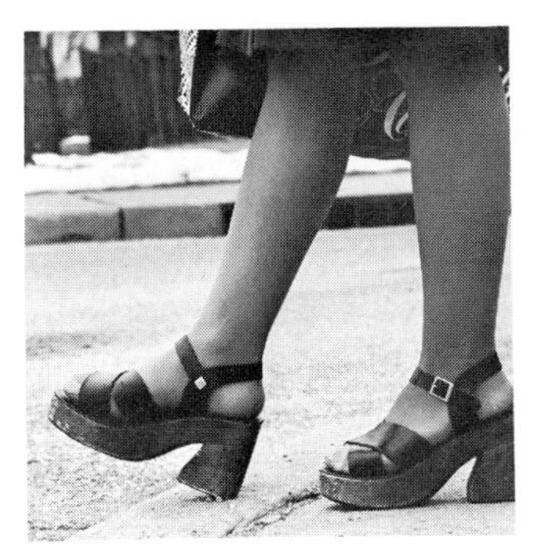

23-8 *The wearer of platform shoes always risks injury, even when she—or he—is merely stepping off a curb.*

handbags

For women, handbags are a special problem. The strap must be held by a hand attached to an almost immobilized arm, and this interferes with the rhythm of walking. A constantly slipping shoulder strap or a thigh-slapping or too-heavy bag is even worse.

climate and clothing

Consider climate at the opposite ends of the country. Summer walkers of both sexes in New York and California may pretty well solve their problem equally. Even when it rains, one need not be deprived of one's walk. Sports shops sell hooded waterproof and water-repellent parkas that weigh less than a pound, and rainsuits are also available. Also, one can Scotchgard one's ordinary clothes, and there are silicone sprays for shoes. Those making a transition from a warm climate to a cold one will discover that modern thermal underwear is well-designed and comfortable. In warm weather, light-colored clothes are cooler because they reflect both heat and light waves. A brimmed hat will do as well as sunglasses; it should also shade the back of the neck. (Very prolonged skin exposure to the sun promotes wrinkling of the skin; in the case of blonds, such exposure may hasten skin cancer.) Besides, the eyes are usually equipped to handle light and shade, and the eye muscle needs exercise too. Exposure to glare from snow or sand, however, does necessitate good sunglasses.

Winter walking requires some personal adjustment wherever it is done. For example, it rarely snows in southern California, but a sunny, warm morning can turn into a chilly afternoon and evening. Shirts, long- or short-sleeved sweaters, and a light windbreaker can take care of most situations. Heavier layered-

[40] "Platform Shoes Raise More Than Feet: Injuries Up 30%," *AMA Health Education Service,* Vol. 13, No. 10 (December 1973), pp. 1–2, citing *Platform Shoes,* AMA News Release, October 22, 1972.

clothing combinations can be made for winter walking in colder climates. What are some essential parts of the body to keep warm? The extremities and the head and neck. "You can keep your whole body warm if you wear gloves . . . cover your head and neck, and keep your thighs warm."[41] So a hat, scarf, warm sleeves, and thermal underwear under warm slacks or trousers are insurance against the cold. Two pairs of socks have been recommended for serious walkers—a thin inner pair of cotton (or even silk) and a thicker outer pair of wool or textured cotton. Nylon is nonabsorbent and is not as flexible as silk or cotton. The outer wool or thick cotton hose are both sweat-absorbers and cushioning agents; some walkers prefer a blend of nylon and either cotton or wool. Knee-high socks are now available for men as they always have been for women. They are a warm comfort against inhospitable cold. And it should not be forgotten that walking itself helps keep the body warm.

setting the pace

A mile is exactly 5,280 feet. An average man's walking stride is two feet per step. Thus, 2,640 steps will carry him a mile. Moreover, the average man will walk three miles an hour. The smaller woman of perhaps 5 feet, 2 or 3 inches will find that speed hard going. Her legs are shorter. But most women can walk as fast as most men, unless the man is unusually tall. Former New York Mayor John Lindsay is 6 feet, 3 inches tall. During the transit strike in 1966 he walked to City Hall every morning. Average-height newspeople were frequently exhausted by the briskly walking mayor. And their problem was aggravated not only by the height–stride factor; they were also working for an interview. That makes a huge difference. There are others. A girl has an appointment with her boyfriend at noon. He arrives at 12:15. "You're an hour late," she tells him, and means it. To her, the time seemed much longer. So it is with walking. Psychologically, there can be a long, dull mile or a short, interesting one. Everybody develops his or her own technique for making walking time pass quickly. One infantry soldier clipped a few pages out of his Bible every day and stuffed them into his helmet. When the walks seemed long, he would ponder, even memorize a passage or two. "And he found that the rolling King James rhythms made remarkably fine marching music."[42]

How can one increase one's walking pace without increasing fatigue? Lengthen the stride and increase the speed. But do these gradually. Soon, tense muscles and stiff joints will loosen, the body's flexibility will improve, and so will one's negotiations with the down-pulling force of gravity. All this will help to prevent the fatigue and the aches and pains so common with the inexperienced walker. There is a rhythm, a beat to walking. That beat is part of the joy of walking, and it comes with experience.

Also to be considered is the placement of the feet. This can be determined by walking in the sand or wet-footed on the bedroom rug, or by stopping while walking to observe which way the toes point. Interestingly, if the toes point out, so do the hands. Ballerinas walk with their toes pointed out. But the blistered, bleeding feet of their student days are problems of the past. Now their feet are

[41] Aaron Sussman and Ruth Goode, *The Magic of Walking,* pp. 120–21.
[42] *Ibid.,* p. 83.

incredibly strong. Other people will do well to point the toes neither in nor out. They should be pointed in the direction of the body's movement. This does not mean a tightrope walk. The good walker swings a trifle to one side as the corresponding foot takes a forward step, and the opposite arm swings forward to keep the body from moving too far from the center line. "A good walking stride on a level surface could be diagrammed as two parallel lines, one line for each foot, with a third line running between them."[43] The good walker does not waddle. He does not walk a tightrope. "And the toes point neither in nor out, but straight ahead."[44]

jogging

With attention to these details, a good walk can be enough fun to make one break into a jog. As with walking, there is some individuality to jogging. But there are some worthwhile suggestions to follow: one should stand up straight; the back should be kept as straight as is naturally comfortable; the head should be kept erect and the eyes not focused on the feet; the arms should be held a bit away from the body; the elbow should be bent so that elbow and hand are about the same distance from the ground. Occasionally the arms and shoulders should be shaken and relaxed while running. This helps to reduce the tightness that may develop while jogging. The best way for the foot to hit the ground is to first land on the heel, then rock forward to take off from the ball of the foot on the next step. This might be uncomfortable; one might land with most of the weight on the ball of the foot. Landing *all* the weight on the ball of the foot will cause soreness of both foot and leg. Hard surfaces are not for beginning joggers. Ungiving cement or asphalt may cause muscle strain.[45]

why exercise?

In their excellent review of the answers to this question, Falls, Wallis, and Logan referred to two investigators who, "writing on the concept of function and structure as it relates to growth of muscle and bones, indicated that the kinetic stimulus ["kinetic" pertains to motion] is indispensable for life and that lack of this stimulus results in underdevelopment."[46]

Almost two centuries ago, William Cowper (1731–1800) emphasized the same principle in his long descriptive poem, *Task:*

> By ceaseless action, all that is subsists;
> Constant rotation of the unwearied wheel
> That Nature rides upon, maintains her health,
> Her beauty, her fertility. She dreads an instant's pause,
> And lives but while she moves.[47]

[43] *Ibid.,* p. 73.
[44] *Ibid.*
[45] "Jolting Sport," *M.D.*, Vol. 15, No. 1 (January 1973), pp. 228, 230.
[46] Harold B. Falls, Earl L. Wallis, and Gene A. Logan, *Foundations of Conditioning,* p. 11, citing H. W. Knipping and H. Valentin, "Sports in Medicine," in *Therapeutic Exercise,* ed. by S. Licht (New Haven, 1961), pp. 354–74.
[47] Quoted in William Kitchinev, *The Art of Invigorating and Prolonging Life, by Food, Clothes, Air, Exercise, Wine, Sleep, &c. and Peptic Precepts, Pointing Out Agreeable, and Effectual Methods to Prevent and Relieve Indigestion and to Regulate and Strengthen the Action of the Stomach and Bowels, to Which Is Added, the Pleasure of Making a Will* (London, 1822), p. 122.

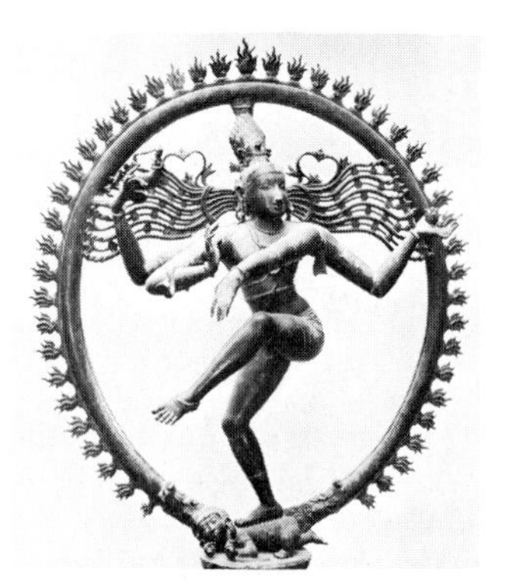

23-9 *The Hindu god Siva as Lord of the Dance.*

But the essential principle of movement goes even deeper than that. The very stuff of life, chemicals, move too. The ammonia molecule, for example, consists of three atoms of hydrogen and one of nitrogen. The vibration of the nitrogen atom is an up-and-down movement, the exactness of which has been measured. It moves up and down 23,870,100 times per second.[48] Scientists have postulated an ''atomic clock'' based on these precise movements.

Biology teaches that matter that is invested with life has specific properties or powers—reproduction, growth and repair, derivation of energy from food, response to stimuli, self-regulation, and—not the least of these—movement.[49] In Indian mythology this last power takes the form of dancing; Hindu mythology says that the universe was in total darkness until Siva, in his role of god of the dance, performed a dance of such vitality that he sent sound waves into space and all matter began to dance by his rhythm. Ancient Hindu writings of Siva glorify him, therefore, in this way:

> The movement of whose body is the world, whose speech is the sum of all language,
> Whose jewels are the moon and stars—to that pure Siva I bow.[50]

Thus do the exactitudes of science and the mysticisms of a religion agree on the quality of movement in life. It is a quality in physical fitness, too.

growing toward better posture

Exercise facilitates growth. As has been seen, even early controls of striated muscle are signals for infant exercise. Every muscle is used in growing. As the child grows taller, the muscles will increase in length. If exercise is inadequate, the muscles will grow anyway, but they will be thin and underdeveloped. The child will not have the muscle strength to hold the body erect in its most efficient posture. Moreover, the bones are not yet mature. Pliable, they are still capable of being shaped and molded. Poor posture is more than a sign of inadequate exercise during childhood. It is unattractive. Whether casual or not, clothes fit better on a body whose segments are well aligned. Good posture adds to self-confidence and to the first impression made on others. When the body segments sag—head and shoulders drooping, hips forward, upper back rounded and trunk listing backward—it is as if the person would fall were he not held together by bone and ligaments. Indeed, one expert refers to this posture of fatigue as ''hanging on the ligaments.''[51] So stretched are both muscles and ligaments that much body adjustments must be made before efficient movement can be achieved. Moreover, prolonged poor posture can eventually cause pain due either to pressure of a firm structure such as bone or a taut muscle on part of a nerve, or to severe tension on a structure such as a tendon or ligament.

[48] Albert Piltz and Roger Van Bever, *Time Without Clocks* (New York, 1970), p. 21.

[49] Alan Dale, *An Introduction to Social Biology* (London, 1953), p. 2.

[50] *The Mirror of Gesture,* tr. by A. K. Coomaraswamy and Duggirala Gopalakrishnayya (New York, 1936), p. 31, quoted in *A Treasury of Traditional Wisdom,* ed. by Whitall N. Perry (New York, 1971), p. 688.

[51] Marion Broer, *Efficiency of Human Movement,* p. 129, citing Katherine F. Wells, *Kinesiology* (Philadelphia, 1971), p. 382.

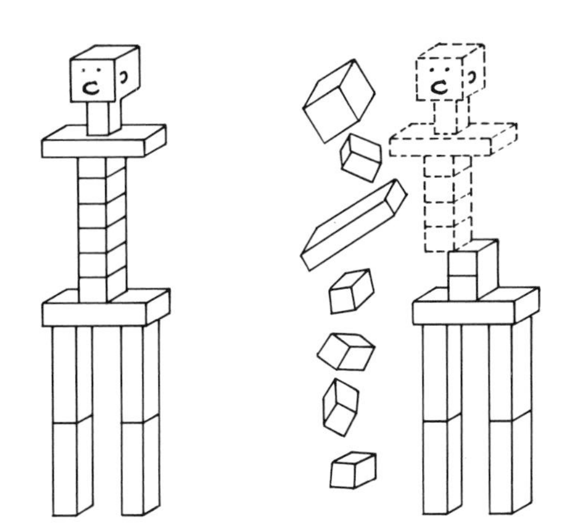

23-10 *Like this figure of blocks, the human body is made up of segments. The blocks will stand as long as they are centered on top of one another* (left). *Move one block, however, and its center is no longer over the blocks below. The figure of blocks collapses* (right). *When a person's posture is good, then, each body segment is centered over the base that supports it. When a person's posture is poor, the body does not collapse because muscles and ligaments hold the segments together; rather, the body sags, which promotes fatigue.*

> Since the body is made up of segments, assuming an upright position can be likened to building a man of blocks [see Figure 23-10]. . . . Good posture [is] that position in which the center of gravity of each body segment is centered over its supporting base [the segment immediately below]. In this position the force of gravity is used to advantage . . . in keeping the alignment in the weight-bearing joints.[52]

Other writers have emphasized this by pointing out that the force of gravity has a tendency to cause the skeletal framework of the body to collapse, to buckle at the ankle, knee, and hip. To counteract these buckling tendencies, certain muscle groups are at work. Exercise of these muscle groups is of primary importance in any body-conditioning program.[53]

physical conditioning and coronary artery disease[54]

Before the Second World War, the prescription for a patient who had survived the initial assault of a coronary thrombosis (see Chapter 9) was prolonged bed rest, followed by the adoption of an entirely new way of life devoid of responsibility. This led many people into a life of utter stagnation beclouded by the ever-present fear of impending death. Worse, it did nothing to prevent further heart attacks. Following the war, investigators, led primarily by two U.S. physicians, Samuel A. Levine and Bernard Lown, demonstrated the error of this approach. A patient who had recovered from an acute coronary thrombosis could resume a way of life similar to the one he had led before the attack without undue risk.[55] At about this time, studies of the occurrence and distribution among various population groups of heart disease indicated that it caused less sickness and death among people in active, nonsedentary occupations.[56] In-

[52] *Ibid.,* pp. 130–31.
[53] Harold B. Falls, Earl L. Wallis, and Gene A. Logan, *Foundations of Conditioning,* pp. 9–10.
[54] For the advanced student only, the American Heart Association journal *Modern Concepts of Heart Disease* recently published four excellent articles on exercise as it affects the heart and blood vessels: Donald O. Nutter, Robert C. Schlant, and J. Willis Hurst, "Isometric Exercise and the Cardiovascular System," Vol. 41, No. 3 (March 1972); Samuel M. Fox III, John P. Naughton, and Patrick A. Gorman, "Physical Activity and Cardiovascular Health," Parts I, II, and III, Vol. 41, Nos. 4, 5, 6 (April, May, June 1972).
[55] Eugene Z. Hirsch, Herman K. Hellerstein, and Cathel A. MacLeod, "Physical Training and Coronary Artery Disease," Chapter 8 in *Exercise and the Heart,* comp. and ed. by Robert L. Morse (Springfield, Ill., 1972), p. 106.
[56] *Ibid.,* p. 107.

activity came to be believed to be a factor causing coronary thrombosis.[57] The human cost of heart disease has already been discussed in Chapter 9. But it is worth reemphasizing that considerable numbers of the U.S. population in their twenties and thirties are prone to coronary heart disease. Moreover, exercise-stress testing of people who are apparently healthy has revealed an alarming percentage to be particularly vulnerable to heart attacks.

These findings have led to two questions. They are here presented with the answers that can be provided on the basis of evidence as of 1973:

1. Can physical conditioning be of value in the treatment of patients who have coronary artery disease? The answer: Yes.[58]

2. Can physical conditioning be helpful in preventing a heart attack in normal people who are prone to develop coronary artery disease? The answer: It may be.[59]

Consider further the first question and its answer. Present studies suggest that medically supervised physical training is not detrimental to selected patients. It can be used as a medicine—that is, for treatment. As with any medication, there are cautions to be observed. A few of these are: the fitness program must suit the individual patient;[60] the spouse should be involved; competition and faddism are to be avoided. The majority of heart specialists consider graded, controlled, appropriate activity to be among the major advances in the treatment and rehabilitation of the patient who has recovered from an acute coronary thrombosis.[61]

But, to turn to the second question, can physical conditioning actually prevent heart attacks in people who have a tendency to them? There is much evidence to indicate that physical inactivity does shorten the life span and predispose the individual to coronary disease. Nevertheless, scientifically adequate studies to answer this question have not been made; a clear cause-and-effect relationship has not been conclusively established. Moreover, "the nature of the problem is such that a definitive answer, acceptable to everyone, will require decades."[62] "Nonetheless," three specialists have written, "in the absence of such definitive studies we can advocate physical fitness enhancement on the basis of the *likelihood* of reducing a risk factor . . . One cannot claim at the present time that fitness will *extend* life or *prevent* a heart attack."[63] And

[57] "The Longshoreman's Life," *Lancet,* Vol. 2, No. 7663 (July 11, 1970), p. 87.

[58] Eugene Z. Hirsch, Herman K. Hellerstein, and Cathel A. MacLeod, "Physical Training and Coronary Artery Disease," p. 107.

[59] *Ibid.*

[60] One group of middle-aged men undergoing walking, running, or bicycle training improved markedly in cardiovascular and body-composition measures regardless of their mode of training. ("Walking, Running, Bicycling Bring Similar Improvements," *Hospital Tribune,* Vol. 7, No. 16 [April 23, 1973], p. 31.)

[61] A 1972 report stated that "Physical training . . . seems to improve exercise performance consistently," and the data also suggested that delivery of oxygen to the heart might be enhanced. (David R. Redwood, Douglas R. Rosing, and Stephen E. Epstein, "Circulatory and Symptomatic Effects of Physical Training in Patients with Coronary-Artery Disease and Angina Pectoris," *New England Journal of Medicine,* Vol. 286, No. 18 [May 4, 1972], pp. 959–65.)

[62] Carleton B. Chapman, "Keynote Address," in *Exercise and the Heart,* ed. by Robert L. Morse, p. xv.

[63] Eugene Z. Hirsch, Herman K. Hellerstein, and Cathel A. MacLeod, "Physical Training and Coronary Artery Disease," p. 150. Such a claim was made in 1973 by investigators at the London School of Hygiene and Tropical Medicine. Comparing the weekend exercise habits of almost 17,000 men from 1968 through 1970, they reported that rigorous exercise appeared to help prevent heart attacks regardless of the man's age. This effect may be due, they believe, to enlargement of the coronary and smaller blood vessels. ("Vigorous Exercise and the Physically Fit Heart," *Science News,* Vol. 10, No. 13 [March 31, 1973].)

to this a warning is added: "Unsupervised jogging as a physical training activity must be considered out of the question for unfit men over thirty years of age unless effort testing has established that the subject can tolerate this energy requirement without untoward effect."[64]

heart disease, stress, and exercise

An increasing number of physicians are convinced that the constant stress of modern life is a major contributor to heart attacks. The person who is a slave to his watch, who is overly competitive, who subjects himself to a frenzy of social and economic pressures, soon finds that he is not living but suffering.[65] And it is a suffering that too often leads to a myocardial infarct. Recent animal experiments at the Harvard School of Public Health indicate that environmental "psychologic factors can predispose to electrical instability of the heart, which can account for the mechanism of sudden death."[66]

Is all stress damaging? No. (See Chapter 12, pages 323–24.) "Stress is the nonspecific response of the body to any demand made upon it."[67] Shivering from cold is a response to stress. Running up a flight of stairs at full speed causes such responses to stress as an increase in heart rate and blood pressure. "Normal activities—a game of tennis or even a passionate kiss—can produce considerable stress without causing conspicuous damage."[68] Thus, it is not stress, per se, that is potentially harmful, but the kind of stress and the ways of adapting to it that may be deleterious.[69] It is possible to enjoy and benefit

[64] *Ibid.*, p. 172.

[65] People leading lives of stress are often told to slow down. "Be lazy," they are advised. "Be more slothful." And indeed, the furry sloth is among the world's slowest animals. They cannot be made to jump, and, when, dropped, they just fall to the ground in a heap, making no effort to right themselves. And the sloth's meal takes two long weeks to travel the short length from his mouth to his anus. But one cannot compare the sloth to the human. His muscle arrangements make him slow and ATPase (the enzyme that breaks down molecules supplying the energy for contractions; see page 702) is in extremely short supply in the sloth's slothful muscle cells. So, unlike man, the sloth is slow both muscularly and biochemically. ("Sloth Is in Muscle As Well As in Mind," *New Scientist*, Vol. 59, No. 854 [July 12, 1973], p. 64.) Not only is it hazardous to compare animals to man, but such matters among people are not always what they seem. Primitive man, it is claimed, is a hunter, and his activities keep him fit. But studies of the hunting patterns of aborigines show that they spend most of their time being slothful. And the evidence that modern man is more sedentary than his grandfather is rather weak. (S. S. B. Gilder, "London Letter: The Changing Pattern of Human Activity," *Canadian Medical Association Journal*, Vol. 104, No. 11 [June 5, 1971], p. 972.)

[66] Bernard Lown, Richard Verrier, and Ramon Corbalan, "Psychologic Stress and Threshold for Repetitive Ventricular Response," *Science*, Vol. 182, No. 4114 (November 23, 1973), p. 834.

[67] Hans Selye, "The Evolution of the Stress Concept," *American Scientist*, Vol. 61, No. 6 (November–December 1973), p. 692. This article is highly recommended.

[68] *Ibid.*, p. 693, citing H. Selye, *The Stress of Life* (New York, 1956).

[69] In this regard, Selye has formulated a personal philosophy exemplified by this jingle:

> Fight for the highest attainable aim
> But do not put up resistance in vain.
> (Hans Selye, "The Evolution of the Stress Concept," p. 699.)

This is not unlike the bit of Oriental philosophy:

> For three things I pray:
> The serenity to accept that which cannot be changed;
> The courage to change that which can be changed;
> And the wisdom to tell the one from the other.

In these changeful times it may be said that the philosophies of both Selye and the Oriental sage require plenty of wisdom and prayer. Both are easier to write than accomplish.

from the stress of a judicious exercise program; it is possible to risk one's life with an injudicious program. It has been suggested that tension and anxiety may often be relieved by a few minutes of vigorous exercise.[70] "Emotions are best dissipated in the form of activity."[71] What that activity should be depends on the age and health of the individual.

some words of caution

Nobody should engage in a regular exercise program without a thorough prior examination by the family physician. Not all physical limitations are immediately apparent, and some need more investigation than others to be discovered. The obese person will need one kind of exercise program, the individual with a heart problem will need another, the hypertensive person still another. Also, the type and extent of exercise may need to be adjusted to the individual's age. Here again, there are considerable variations. One person at forty may be as fit for certain exercises as another at twenty-five. Cooper tells of a 102-year-old man, a regular jogger since eighty, who celebrated his 102nd birthday by running the hundred-yard dash in 17.3 seconds. This was 0.5 seconds faster than he had run the distance at 101.[72] Not all people can achieve so much improvement in one short year, but a regular exercise program, medically supervised, can help the average person achieve some measure of improvement.

There is no reason why an adequate program of physical fitness should be expensive. Cooper points out, for example, that his methods are free as the air. A program that proves too costly will often be discontinued. Nor should the individual choose an activity that he finds boring. A brisk walk pleases many people (see pages 710–13). Others enjoy a swim; still others, tennis. A joyless exercise program is soon abandoned. Moreover, the exercise program should not be limited by the seasons. This may seem easier for Californians to accomplish than for New Yorkers. Nevertheless, few cities are without convenient indoor swimming pools and gymnasiums. After one leaves college, the pressures of earning a living may interfere with a regular schedule of exercise and, further, the common complaint may be made, "There's nobody to exercise with." But exercise to the point of physical fitness is a life-giving procedure. One's day must be arranged to include enjoyable exercise. True, the team members of one's college days are dispersed, but there are always new friends to be found. Too, exercise can become a family affair.

Physical fitness phonies have been enriched by the gullible. Indeed, physical fitness may rival the intestinal tract as a lucrative source of income for the quack. Many devices are sold by mail. Electric energizers, vibrating machines, and the like have hoodwinked millions. Some are of ancient vintage; they were not meant to defraud, but were merely the result of much well-intentioned work and confusion. And there have even been patented devices designed to prevent even a small amount of exercise (Figure 23-11).

can exercise be harmful?

If done without proper regard to body mechanics, yes (see Figures 23-6 and

[70] Roy J. Shephard, *Endurance Fitness,* p. 182.
[71] Harold B. Falls, Earl L. Wallis, and Gene A. Logan, *Foundations of Conditioning,* p. 15.
[72] Kenneth H. Cooper, *The New Aerobics,* p. 26.

23-10). Although formal studies are lacking, there are plenty of examples of people for whom sports participation seems to delay the deterioration of advancing age. However, other factors may be involved in such examples: being born of hardy, long-lived parents is but one. Nevertheless, elderly people are joining the young in physical fitness programs. One New Jersey cardiologist, a former college runner returning to his youthful sport, completed the twenty-six–mile Boston marathon in 1972 at age fifty-three. There are other, even more striking examples (see page 718). But the average person should start slowly, and seek his physician's advice about an appropriately individualized exercise program.

Rigorous training may produce some untoward results. Mark Spitz, who won seven gold medals in the 1972 Olympics, began grueling training at about six. This kind of rigorous early training could discourage other children, causing them to desert physical training permanently. One expert recommends that strenuous training be delayed until about twelve or thirteen, and then be undertaken only if the child is interested. Also, recent animal experiments suggest that early sports training in childhood must be studied in detail. Forced to swim strenuously on a regular basis, young rats showed some indication of growth retardation as well as bone and kidney abnormalities. In noncontact sports, it is of interest to note that strenuous physical exertion uncommonly results in a transient occurrence of blood and protein in the urine. This is usually without symptoms and not considered serious. It is probably due to forceful bending and endocrinological effects of stress that, in turn, cause microscopic trauma. The fact is that young athletes are demonstrating their prowess before scientific investigation has discovered how they do it.[73]

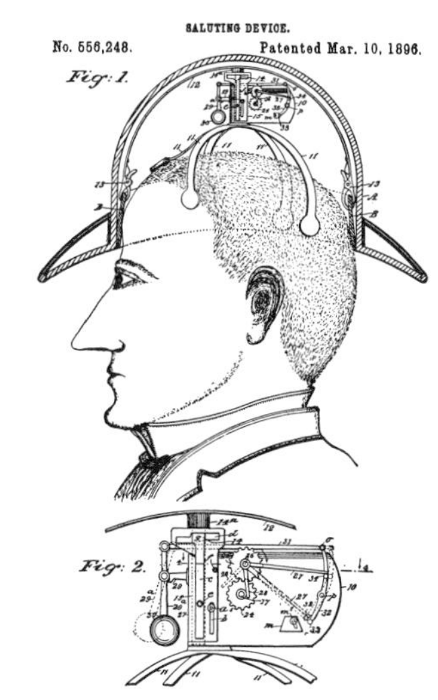

23-11 *Even in earlier days, there were people who sought ways to avoid the slightest exercise. This is a device for tipping the hat without using the hands, patented in 1896.*

exercise and health: concluding considerations

The value of exercise to various aspects of health has been discussed in other sections of this book. Its relationship to weight control, for example, is considered in the preceding chapter. There has been some sense and much nonsense written about the diet best suited for athletics. One ancient myth is that successful athletes train on a diet of meat. The Greek wrestler Milo of Croton, who won the wrestling matches at seven successive Olympiads, is reported to have "once carried a 4-year-old bull around the stadium at Olympia on his shoulders, killed it with a single blow of his fist, and then ate the whole animal in one day."[74] One wonders what people will think 2500 years from now when they read that at least one U.S. Olympic superstar, Mark Spitz, apparently had a preference for milk. There is no valid reason why the diet of a successful athlete should vary from that recommended for the rest of the population.[75]

[73] "Today's Rigorous Training of Young Athletes," *Medical World News,* Vol. 14, No. 15 (April 13, 1973), pp. 51–57.

[74] Geoffrey H. Bowne, "Nutrition and Exercise," Chapter 5 in *Exercise Physiology,* ed. by Harold B. Falls (New York, 1968), p. 157.

[75] *Ibid.,* p. 170.

The significance of exercise during and after pregnancy is discussed on pages 578–79. Exercise doubtless also has a beneficial effect on the diabetic by indirectly promoting weight control.[76] There is insufficient evidence that exercise will reduce the severity of hypertension.[77] Very limited data indicate that moderate exercise is helpful to those suffering from asthma or emphysema; however, it is very doubtful that it helps to cure the underlying disease; possibly, exercise within the individual's capacities helps him to adapt to the discomforts of the ailment.[78] Some people are convinced—wrongly—that regular deep-breathing exercises are helpful. The breathing reflex is governed by the demands made upon it; there is no increased oxygenation of blood by forced inspiration, the capacity of the lung is not greatly affected, and respiratory diseases are not prevented in this manner.[79]

Exercise programs are of value not only in accident prevention but in the rehabilitation of a worker after an injury; it has been suggested that exercises, in the form of "active gymnastic pauses, are more effective in relieving fatigue than passive pauses, particularly in light or sedentary work."[80] There have been scores of studies seeking an association between academic achievement and participation in athletics. However, "there seems no great future in the equation of exercise and intelligence; if we feel a need to justify physical activity, better ammunition will be obtained from studies of obesity and of cardiovascular disease."[81] That exercise does, however, play a positive role in relieving tension for many people cannot be disputed; this, in itself, might benefit academic performance. Interestingly, an increasing number of psychiatrists urge exercise as part of their therapeutic program. Are drugs of value in improving athletic performance? This is an old question. In Nordic legend, the warriors called Berserkers used the constituents of a fungus to stimulate themselves for battle, and during their Olympic games the Greeks tried mushrooms. In 1865, canal swimmers at Amsterdam used drugs in the hope that they would be helped to win. Almost a century ago, sugar cubes dipped in ether and nitroglycerin were among the favorite drugs used for this purpose. And in 1866 an English cyclist died during a race from Paris to Bordeaux; the cause: an excessive dose of a stimulant reportedly fed him by his coach. Cyclists were apparently using amphetamines during the 1960 Olympic Games, and one of them, Knute Jensen, died after a race.

The American Pediatric Society Joint Committee on Physical Fitness, Recreation, and Sports Medicine concluded after careful study that "There is no scientific basis for any such practices."[82] Moreover, use of drugs could impede rather than enhance athletic performance, in addition to being generally haz-

[76] James S. Skinner, "Longevity, General Health, and Exercise," Chapter 8 in *Exercise Physiology,* ed. by Harold B. Falls, p. 230.

[77] *Ibid.,* pp. 225–26. In a relatively small study at New York Infirmary, isometric exercises have been used with some success to reduce blood pressure. ("Isometrics to Reduce Pressure," *Hospital Tribune Hypertensive Bulletin,* Vol. 7, No. 18 [May 14, 1973], p. 18.)

[78] *Ibid.,* pp. 231–32.

[79] Harold B. Falls, Earl L. Wallis, and Gene A. Logan, *Foundations of Conditioning,* p. 18.

[80] Roy J. Shephard, *Endurance Fitness,* p. 159.

[81] *Ibid.,* p. 156.

[82] "Athletes Need Drugs? Not So, Report States," *Los Angeles County Medical Association Bulletin,* Vol. 103, No. 19 (October 4, 1973), p. 19.

ardous (see Chapters 13 and 14). Tobacco is particularly detrimental to athletic performance. "Clinical studies in healthy, young men have shown that cigarette smoking impairs exercise performance, especially for many types of athletic events and activities involving maximal work capacity. Some of these effects are mediated by reduced oxygen transport and reduced cardiac and pulmonary function."[83]

The point of this chapter can be summed up with two words: Get moving. Exercise, especially in the company of family or friends, will provide more pleasant memories than television ever will. And exercise will improve health to enable one to enjoy such memories all the more. Some physicians emphasize that the quality of life has too often been sacrificed to the mere extension of life.[84] The ideal is a long life of high quality. For this aim, the words of John Locke (1632–1704) in his essay *On Politics and Education* remain valid:

> It would be none of the least secrets of education to make the exercises of the body and the mind the recreation one to another.

summary

Motivation and a certain degree of courage are required to maintain a program of training to promote physical fitness (pages 696–97). Broadly, *fitness* is the ability to adjust dynamically to one's various ecosystems—physical, psychological, and social (page 697). *Physical fitness* may be either *specific*—the ability to perform a particular task (pages 697–98)—or *general*—the ability to perform all the tasks of one's life, including its emergencies (pages 698–99).

Of central importance to physical fitness are *posture* and *movement* (page 699), and the tissues involved in both (pages 699–700)—especially the striated (voluntary) *muscles* (pages 700–02).

The basic, interrelated elements of physical fitness include

1. *strength,* which may be improved through *isometric* or (preferably) *isotonic exercises* (pages 703–05);
2. *flexibility,* a sufficient range of movement (pages 705–06); and
3. *endurance,* which relates to the body's ability under maximal exertion to take a maximal amount of oxygen from the air (its *aerobic capacity*) to be used in the production of energy (pages 706–07).

Aerobic exercise best promotes endurance fitness (page 707). This type of exercise is the basis of tests devised by Kenneth H. Cooper, which are useful measurements of physical fitness (pages 708–10). Two convenient, inexpensive, and beneficial aerobic exercises are *walking* and *jogging* (pages 710–13).

The reasons for exercising regularly are many: it facilitates growth and better posture (pages 714–15); it may help to prevent—and to recover from—heart attacks (pages 715–18); and it promotes overall body health and a sense of well-being (pages 719–21).

[83] U.S. Department of Health, Education, and Welfare, Public Health Service, *The Health Consequences of Smoking* (January 1973), p. 247.

[84] Samuel M. Fox III, then president of the American College of Cardiology, cited in "Improving Life, Not Prolonging It, Main Benefit of Exercising," *Internal Medicine News,* Vol. 6, No. 4 (February 15, 1973), pp. 1, 33.

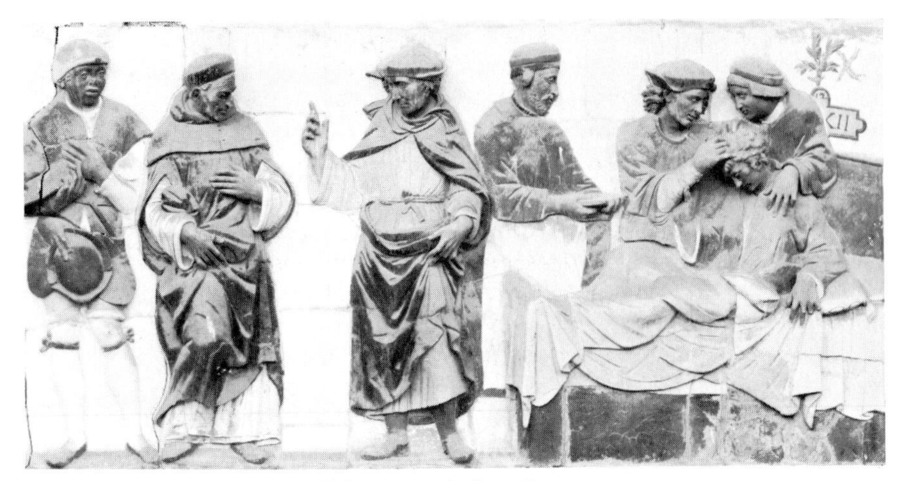

A 16th-century Italian dispensary.

the U.S. health care industry

24

the past as prologue

"The first cry of pain in the primitive jungle was the first call for a physician."[1] Whether that first call was ever answered will never be known, but the tribal witch doctor has long maintained a primitive medical practice. Sometimes the fee for his services was a weapon or some poultry. It has been known to be a daughter.[2] Primitive peoples have also had some form of health insurance. A witch doctor often receives gifts in advance, not only from those who will want his services but also from those who fear his art.[3] Sometimes the primitive physician would rather do without payment. For failing to cure his patient, he may be put to death.[4] However, such rough treatment of physicians is not limited to primitives. Four thousand years ago, the Babylonians were paying ten shekels of silver for a major operation on a freeman and two shekels on a slave. If the freeman died, the surgeon's hands were cut off; if the slave died, the surgeon merely had to replace him.[5] As late as the fifteenth century, Pope John XXII had an unsuccessful physician burned alive, and when this pope died, his physician was flayed alive.[6] During the medieval era, teaching medicine could also be risky. A candidate for examinations in medicine at the University of Paris had to swear he would not avenge himself on his teachers if he failed.[7]

Citizens in ancient times had government health insurance. The Greek historian Diodorus wrote in the first century before Christ that, in Egypt, "all [the sick] are taken care of without giving pay privately. For the physicians receive support from the community."[8] During the Middle Ages groups of workers banded together in guilds to help one another in case of sickness. Thus, the guild of Birmingham provided a rent-free home to "the common midewyffe" in return for obstetrical care.[9]

Early European hospitals were most often built by the healthy to protect themselves from the sick. People did not go to them to get well. During the seventeenth century, in the French hospital Hôtel-Dieu, three or four persons occupied each bed while as many lay on the floor beside it. Every six hours, those on the floor exchanged places with those in the bed.[10] In a single bed, one person might be ill, another dying, a third dead. "By 1787 the practice was to put two or three at the head of a bed, while between their faces were two or three pairs of reciprocal feet."[11] The English were more considerate; at

24-1 *An ancient Greek tablet showing a physician examining a child.*

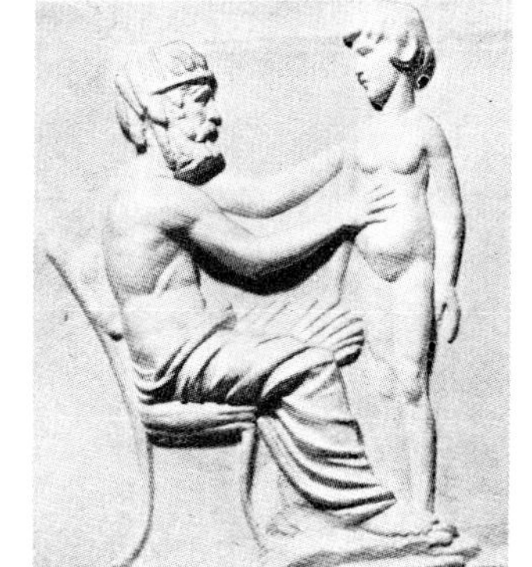

[1] Victor Robinson, *The Story of Medicine* (New York, 1931), p. 1.
[2] Jonathan Wright, "Medical Fees Among Primitive Man," *New York Medical Journal* (December 16, 1916), p. 4.
[3] *Ibid.*, p. 6.
[4] Jonathan Wright, "The Responsibilities and the Dangers of Medical Practice Among Primitive Men," *New York Medical Journal* (February 24, 1917), p. 4.
[5] Sir Weldon Dalrymple-Champneys, "An Examination of the Place of the Doctor in the State from Ancient Times to the Present Day," *Royal Society of Medicine Proceedings,* Vol. 37 (January 1944), pp. 89–100, in *Free Medical Care,* comp. by Clarence A. Peters (New York, 1946), p. 12.
[6] *Ibid.*
[7] David Reisman, *The Story of Medicine in the Middle Ages* (New York, 1935), p. 155.
[8] *Ibid.*, pp. 12–13, citing Diodorus Siculus, *History,* tr. by C. H. Oldfather *et al.* (London, 1935), Vol. 1, p. 82.
[9] J. Toulmin Smith, *English Guilds* (London, 1870), p. 249.
[10] E. B. Hoag, "Diseases as Regarded by the Ancients," *Los Angeles Medical Journal* (May 1904), p. 5.
[11] Lawrence Wright, *Warm and Snug* (London, 1962), pp. 292–93.

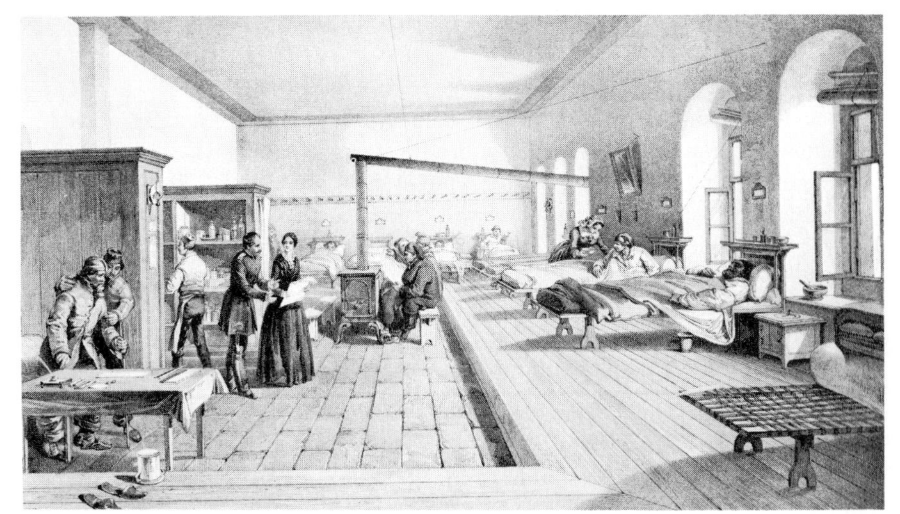

24-2 *A hospital for soldiers wounded in the Crimean War (1854–1856). It is clean, well-ventilated, light, and spacious—largely as a result of the efforts of Florence Nightingale to improve hospital conditions.*

the Manchester Infirmary, in 1771, strict regulations required that "every new admission had clean sheets, to be changed every three weeks."[12]

In this country, medical care did not get off to a particularly good start. True, the Massachusetts Bay Colony hired a tax-paid physician to care for the sick poor, and, almost a century later, Benjamin Franklin helped establish the first general hospital,[13] but the people seemed to prefer quacks and cultists.[14] The general suspicion of physicians was demonstrated by the "Doctor's Riot" that occurred in New York on April 13–15, 1788, after a human arm or leg tumbled out of a hospital window onto some people in the street. "The cry of barbarity &c was soon spread," and the Doctor's Riot ensued. "An innocent Person got beat & abused, for being *only dressed in black.*"[15] As a result of the riot four people died.

In those days, most physicians were trained in Europe. As medical schools began to open in this country, medical teachers were developed. One of the greatest nineteenth-century teachers was Oliver Wendell Holmes. He could be remarkably direct. In 1860, in an address before the Massachusetts Medical Society, he tartly observed that, with a few exceptions, "if the whole *materia medica,* as now used, could be sunk to the bottom of the sea, it would be all the better for mankind—and all the worse for the fishes." Such forthright self-criticism set the stage for what followed. U.S. medicine began a long and laborious journey of achievement that was to make it among the most respected in the world. Yet its benefits have not been equitably available to everyone. That is the basic paradox of today's health care industry in the United States, and it is the subject of this chapter.

[12] *Ibid.,* p. 293.
[13] Wilson G. Smillie, *Public Health: Its Promise for the Future,* (New York, 1955), pp. 87–89.
[14] Rosemary Stevens, *American Medicine and the Public Interest* (New Haven, Conn., 1971), p. 21.
[15] Letter written by William Heth to Edmund Randolph, New York, 1788, in the Executive Papers, Box 53, Folio April 11–20, 1788, Virginia State Library, quoted in Wilbur J. Bell, Jr., "Doctor's Riot, New York, 1788," *Bulletin of the New York Academy of Medicine,* Vol. 47, No. 12 (December 1971), p. 1502.

the U.S. health care industry: size and structure

The health care industry is this nation's third largest. Between 1960 and 1972, the amount spent for health services rose from $26.4 billion to $83 billion. An increasing proportion of this amount is being spent by the federal government. In 1972 it contributed 24.7 percent of the nation's spending in this area.[16] By 1971, the number of people employed in health services was about 4½ million—an increase of more than 25 percent in ten years. One of the fastest-growing of the health occupations was nursing.[17]

The Program Area Committee on Medical Care Administration of the American Public Health Association has classified medical care programs in the United States into three general types.[18] These are:

1. programs that organize to provide health services,
2. programs that finance health services, and
3. programs that both organize and finance health services.[19]

These categories comprise the basic structure of this chapter.

programs that organize to provide health services

Material resources (hospitals, nursing homes, equipment) and health personnel (such as physicians, nurses, and technicians) are organized in such a way as to provide services directly to those who need them. These services are provided on an outpatient (ambulatory) or inpatient basis, or they may be provided in the home or elsewhere.

hospitals: a vast U.S. investment

In 1971, hospitals in the United States numbered 7,733, contained more than 1½ million beds, and had assets of more than $34 billion. The scope of their activity was similarly huge: in 1971, more than 2½ million hospital employees were involved in handling more than 32½ million admissions as well as millions of outpatient visits.

Hospitals are either public or private. Somewhat more than a third (37 percent) of all hospitals are publicly owned; of these, federal hospitals receive most of their funds from government agencies; to a lesser extent this is true of state and local government hospitals. On the other hand, private hospitals generally receive their funds from patients, third parties (insurance carriers), and government programs such as Medicare and Medicaid (see pages 739–40). By far the greatest majority (86 percent) of the private hospitals in the United States are

[16] Committee for Economic Development, *Building a National Health-Care System* (New York, 1973), p. 29.
[17] *Health Manpower and Health Facilities, 1972–73: Health Resources Statistics,* National Center for Health Statistics, Washington, D.C. (1974), p. 8.
[18] *A Guide to Medical Care Administration, Vol. I: Concepts and Principles,* prepared by Beverlee A. Myers for the Program Area Committee on Medical Care Administration, American Public Health Association, revised 1969, pp. 42, 43.
[19] One such program, the health maintenance organization, became part of the U.S. health care picture after this classification was prepared. HMOs are discussed on pages 743–44.

operated on a nonprofit basis. Thus, their profits are reinvested in improvement of services and facilities. The remaining 14 percent of the private hospitals are run for profit. In 1969, the profit-making hospitals netted an average of $5.30 per patient day; nonprofit hospitals netted only $2.34 per patient day. Profit-making hospitals are smaller institutions and "are the cause of most of the concern regarding the quality of . . . hospital care."[20]

the Hill-Burton Act

Since 1946, the federal government has assisted local areas in the building of hospitals. This was made possible by passage of the Hill-Burton Hospital Survey and Construction Act. The original purpose of this act was to improve the distribution of hospitals, with particular emphasis on needy rural areas. However, rural populations have diminished in the past quarter-century. It may be that the more than $6 billion spent in providing 300,000 hospital beds has resulted in too many rural hospitals. Because old urban hospitals were not much helped by the original act, it was amended to provide the states with federal money for the improvement of urban hospitals.

accreditation of hospitals

Accreditation is the mechanism by which U.S. medicine seeks to establish high standards of hospital care. Hospitals are accredited by a Joint Commission on Accreditation of Hospitals sponsored by the American Medical Association, the American Hospital Association, the American College of Surgeons, and the American College of Physicians. The commission judges a hospital on the basis of its physical plant, governing body, administration, staff, and the extent and types of service. Accreditation is sought by most hospitals; today, about two-thirds of U.S. hospitals, containing well over three-fourths of the nation's hospital beds, are accredited. Accreditation is one means by which a prospective patient can choose a hospital.

nursing homes Nursing homes are institutions that provide health services for people, particularly the elderly, who must be inpatients but who do not need hospital care. Nursing homes developed as a result of the 1935 Social Security Act. Understandably, the framers of the act did not wish to perpetuate the grim public poorhouses of the time. Consequently, public institutions were originally excluded from the act, and privately owned nursing homes became immensely profitable. Today there are more than 13,000 nursing homes in the United States.

Some nursing homes provide excellent services in a good environment and add to the dignity of old age. Many are sad places. Old age can be a rich and fruitful experience (see pages 777–81). It can also be a prolonged nightmare,

[20] Arnold J. Kisch, "Medical Care," in *Mustard's Introduction to Public Health,* ed. by Lenor S. Goerke and Ernest L. Stebbins (New York, 1968), p. 140. The 1969 data were the most recent available at the time of writing.

"more to be feared than death."[21] In his poem *The Old Men Admiring Themselves in the Water,* the Irish poet W. B. Yeats (1865–1939) wrote of the despair of many an aged person:

> I heard the old, old men say,
> "All that's beautiful drifts away
> Like the waters."

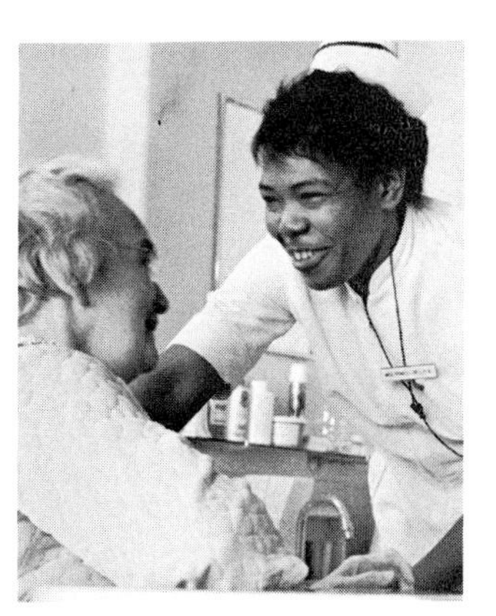

24-3 *The best of nursing-home care.*

So it is today with many aged patients in many of this most wealthy nation's nursing homes. Their average age is eighty. Often the medical and nursing care they receive is minimal. They spend their wintry years surviving feebly in drab and cheerless surroundings. Recently passed Medicare legislation (page 739), by stipulating that funds be withheld unless certain standards are met, has had a beneficial effect on nursing homes. Medicare has also stimulated the formation of the Joint Committee on Accreditation of Nursing Homes.

the physician

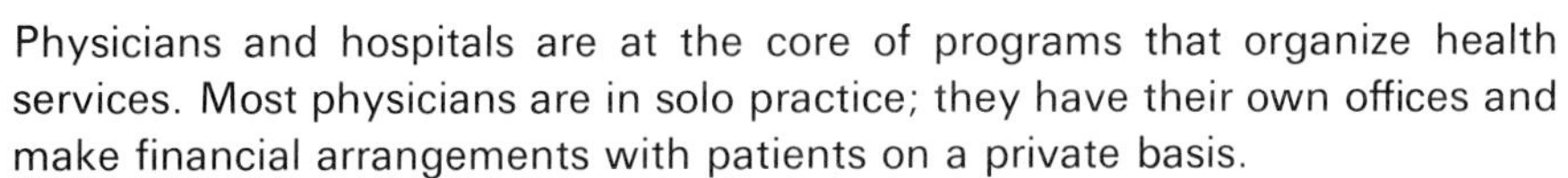

Physicians and hospitals are at the core of programs that organize health services. Most physicians are in solo practice; they have their own offices and make financial arrangements with patients on a private basis.

A *doctor of medicine* (M.D.) is a graduate of an accredited medical school (see below). He cannot legally practice in a state until he has passed the state board examination and has been licensed by the state.

the generalist: a family doctor

Engaging in general medical practice as family physicians, generalists care for all family members, of all ages and conditions. It is they who will recommend a specialist when needed. Fortunately, a great deal of postgraduate training is available to family physicians. In this technological age the modern physician without such training does not remain modern very long.

U.S. medicine is modernized—and specialized

In this country medical schools must meet the rigid requirements of the Committee on Medical Education representing both the American Medical Association and the Association of American Medical Colleges. It was not always so. At the turn of this century, most medical instruction was wretched. Medical diploma mills were common.[22] This situation became generally known as a result of the Flexner Report of 1910.[23] Abraham Flexner's advice revolutionized medical teaching for the better in this country. One of his recommendations, however, changed the picture of medical care. Flexner recommended that the medical curriculum be divided into its major specialty areas and that intensive education be given in each area. This concept was adopted, and new knowl-

[21] Juvenal, *Satires,* Satire XI, l. 45.
[22] Rosemary Stevens, *American Medicine and the Public Interest,* p. 67, citing *Medical Education in the United States and Canada,* Carnegie Foundation for the Advancement of Teaching, Bulletin No. 4 (New York, 1910).
[23] *Ibid.,* citing *Medical Education in the United States and Canada.*

edge that developed in each medical area was eagerly applied to the appropriate specialty.

Inevitably, this system of medical education, based on technological advance, began to produce an increasing number of specialists. This development served a purpose; the physician could hardly continue to practice out of a little black bag. After the Second World War, the emphasis on specialization was accelerated. Through the National Institutes of Health, the federal government poured millions of dollars into an attack on health problems that required the services of specialists. In 1931, four out of five physicians in this nation were general practitioners. Today, only about one out of five is a generalist.[24] Pediatricians, internists, and general practitioners are now called "primary physicians." In numbers, the primary physicians are steadily losing ground to the specialists.

Unfortunately, such intensive specialization is not what the people of this nation need. The overwhelming majority need, not more specialists, but more primary physicians through whom they can gain entrance into a medical care system. Given the opportunity, people will go to a primary physician twice as often as to all the specialists combined.[25]

Nevertheless, specialist physicians will surely continue to be major providers of health care in the future—as they were in the past. Even in ancient times, physicians specialized. In the fifth century B.C., the Greek father of history, Herodotus, wrote that the Egyptians had "a treater of the teeth, and a guardian of the colon." In this country, modern specialty training is a far cry from what it was in the 1890s. Writing about some of the abdominal and pelvic surgeons of that time, the *Journal of the American Medical Association* editorialized that they were "as restless and ambitious a throng as ever fought for fame on the battlefield."[26] Today, U.S. specialty training ranks with the world's best.

To become a specialist, the physician must undertake three to five years of extra training in a hospital that is approved for that purpose. Upon completion of the rigorous residency, the physician may be certified as a specialist by passing a written and oral examination that takes several days. The burden of proof of special competence is upon the applicant. The American Examining Board for each specialty must be approved by the Council on Medical Education of the Department of Medical Education of the American Medical Association and the Advisory Board for Medical Specialists. If a high school student of eighteen decides to become a certified medical specialist, he or she may not accomplish this mission until past the age of thirty. Specialty training is not for those who have great difficulty in deferring gratification.

Physicians may engage in *medical* or *surgical* specialties or in others that are allied to either or both. Moreover, various subspecialties have been created.

[24] Donald L. Madison, "The Structure of American Health Care Services," *Public Administration Review,* Vol. 31, No. 5 (September 1971), pp. 518–19, and citing J. N. Haug *et al., Distribution of Physicians, Hospitals, and Hospital Beds in the U.S., 1968* (Chicago, 1970), p. 13.

[25] *Ibid.,* p. 519, citing Jocelyn Chamberlain, "Selected Data on Group Practice Prepayment Plan Services," *Group Health and Welfare News,* Special Supplement (June 1967).

[26] *Journal of the American Medical Association,* Vol. 17 (1891), p. 947, quoted in Rosemary Stevens, *American Medicine and the Public Interest,* p. 50.

For example, treatment of allergies has become a subspecialty of internal medicine. A list of medical specialties and subspecialties appears in the Glossary under "Specialties."

help for the harried physician

One way in which some physicians have been trying to ensure efficient and effective patient care is by using a physician's assistant. Though the idea of having lay assistants perform some of a physician's functions is an old one, dating back to the seventh century B.C. in Greece, the recent upsurge of interest was sparked in 1965 by Dr. Eugene A. Stead, Jr., former chairman of medicine at Duke University Medical Center. Tapped for the program were newly discharged Army and Navy corpsmen. They had already had two years of training in patient care. In 1967 four ex-Navy corpsmen graduated; in 1968, twelve graduated. They did not diagnose or determine treatment, but they served their physicians and communities in a variety of other ways, such as taking medical histories, giving injections, taking X-rays, doing preliminary physical examinations, repairing sensitive electronic equipment, and suturing minor wounds.

The idea took hold. In 1968, the World Health Organization issued its Technical Report No. 385 on the training of medical assistants and similar personnel. It became a model for many later programs.[27] In 1969, the University of Washington initiated the Medex Project, in which practicing physicians taught medical corpsmen. Here, three months of university training were followed by a nine- to twelve-month preceptorship under the trainee's future employer. At the end of 1972, some two hundred Medex were practicing in twenty-four states. By 1973, well over a hundred physician's-assistant training programs had been authorized in twenty-three states. In Alabama, surgeon's associates were being trained; Grady Memorial Hospital in Atlanta was training coronary-care physician's assistants; Case Western Reserve University in Ohio had a program for anesthesia associates; at the Marshfield Clinic in Wisconsin, assistant physicians were being trained to help with general surgery and neurosurgery, treatment of diabetes, and other specialties; at the University of Colorado, child health associates were being certified.

PROBLEMS Physician's assistant programs have made some mistakes and have been the target of some criticism and apprehension. There is some question as to which type of physician's assistant is more desirable—the preceptorial (Medex) or the practical.[28] Others think there should be both. Some physicians express concern that if such assistants were trained in sufficient numbers, they would displace physicians. Others are concerned that, particularly in rural areas, physician's assistants will assume too much responsibility. The 200,000-member American Nurses' Association considers that physician's assistants do have a valid place on health care teams. However, they are concerned that the assistants will assume functions for which nurses are more

[27] Edwin F. Rosinski, "'Doctor's Assistant' Has Grown to Be a World-Wide Skill with Various Degrees of Responsibilities," *California's Health,* Vol. 30, No. 4 (October 1972), pp. 15–16, citing *World Health* (June 1972).
[28] "Casting a Mold for Doctors' Helpers," *Medical World News,* Vol. 12, No. 39 (October 22, 1971), pp. 15–18.

qualified; they also point to the higher salaries of physician's assistants as discriminatory to women.

Many nurses are interested in similar training programs, such as those at the City University of New York's Herbert Lehman College, Montefiore Hospital and Medical Center, and Cornell Medical Center, all in New York, and the University of North Carolina Nursing School.[29] (The nursing profession has long had programs to broaden nurses' responsibilities. An example: the excellent Psychosocial Department at the University of Washington School of Nursing. Training in that department is designed to recognize the interdependence of social and emotional illness. Moreover, a few nurses are in private practice, helping patients with health problems that they are educationally and legally qualified to treat.) Nevertheless, the American Nurses' Association, composed of less than one half of U.S. nurses, is believed to be concerned that physician's assistant programs will cost them membership. They also deplore what they consider to be a lack of adequate guidelines for training, certification, and utilization of physician's assistants. There are, however, two groups who seem to find relatively little fault with physician's assistants: the physicians and patients they serve.

group practice

Group practice has been defined as "any group of three or more physicians (full-time or part-time) formally organized to provide medical services, with income distributed according to some prearranged plan."[30] Most group practitioners are specialists in the various fields of medicine; occasionally one or more family physicians may be included in a group.

The history of group medical practice in the United States is not without significance. In 1932, the Committee on the Costs of Medical Care published its disturbing findings about the unavailability of medical care to vast segments of the population. Among the recommendations made by the majority of the committee was that medical personnel be organized into units. Each unit would include physicians, dentists, nurses, and other technical personnel, and each would preferably be focused on a hospital.[31] This proposal met with bitter hostility from the American Medical Association. In an editorial, its official journal referred to those who had made the recommendation as "medical soviets."[32] A week later another editorial read: "There is the question of Americanism versus sovietism for the American people."[33] (Interestingly, physicians have begun to unionize in increasing numbers. Recently thirty private physicians formed the Nevada Physicians Union, Local 676 of the Service Workers International Union [AFL–CIO].[34])

[29] "Nurses, Too, Learn Primary Care," *Medical World News,* Vol. 12, No. 39 (October 22, 1971), p. 19.

[30] *A Guide to Medical Care Administration, Vol. I: Concepts and Principles,* p. 42.

[31] *Medical Care for the American People: The Final Report of the Committee on the Costs of Medical Care* (Chicago, 1932).

[32] *Journal of the American Medical Association,* Vol. 99, No. 23 (December 3, 1932), p. 1950.

[33] "The Report of the Committee on the Costs of Medical Care," an editorial in the *Journal of the American Medical Association,* Vol. 99, No. 24 (December 10, 1932), p. 2035.

[34] "Doctor's New Bag Out West Is Unionism," *Medical World News,* Vol. 13, No. 15 (April 14, 1972), pp. 17–18. Although their legal bargaining status is open to question, similar organizations were considered in

Group practice has not thus far proved to be without drawbacks:

> The results of group practice for the patient have not been as impressive as the advantages enjoyed by the group; frequently the patients do not receive the benefits of reduced medical costs. Many groups have been drawn together by their professional, economic, and intellectual interests rather than by a desire to meet the diversified needs of the clientele. Of the 6,400 groups existing in 1969, only slightly more than a third provided multispecialty care, one-half were devoted to a single specialty, and the remainder were in general practice. A minority of the groups (about a fifth) were hospital-based, and only 385 groups were directly associated with prepayment and offering care to a subscribing population.[35]

free clinics: ambulatory care for the alienated

More than two hundred free clinics have been opened in major cities throughout the nation; a few serve people in rural areas. They occupy abandoned homes, storefronts—any place where the rent is cheap and the location convenient. Most of the costs of a free clinic are borne by private donations, and most of the help is voluntary. Perhaps the first of these was San Francisco's Haight-Ashbury Free Medical Clinic. In 1967, that city's "hippie invasion" created an emergency medical care crisis of huge dimensions. Within three months, more than twenty thousand young people sought help from the clinic. "Sickness and drugs were two things they all had in common."[36] Three years later the "flower children" were gone. Most of them had returned home and gone back to school; some left for other parts of town; others went wandering and were hallucinating along the Pacific coast. A few were in communes. Today, though there are plans for improving it, "the Haight" is a rat-infested, crime-ridden disaster area. The free clinic is still there, however. It is still a busy place. Nowadays, one of the major illnesses that its physicians see is heroin abuse.

In January 1970, the Illinois Black Panther Party opened the Spurgeon

---

Florida, San Francisco, and San Antonio, Texas. In Chicago, a group of physicians were considering affiliation with the AFL–CIO Amalgamated Meat Cutters and Butcher Workmen of North America. ("Physician Union-Guilds," *California Medicine,* Vol. 117, No. 3 [September 1972], p. 92.) "The physician has long ceased to be an independent entrepreneur," wrote the president of the Union of American Physicians. "He has . . . become an employee, either of insurance companies or of government. His compensation, either by salary or on a piecework basis, has been determined for him, and the government has acknowledged his status as an employee by including the medical profession under Social Security coverage . . . Long years of training have shortened his earning life span, inflation has eroded his chance of providing for his own security . . . now is the time to stand and fight, or to witness as an alternative the destruction of the world's finest medical community." (Sanford A. Marcus, "Physicians Unions: Can They Shore Up a Falling Idol?" *Medical Dimensions: The Magazine for the Young Doctor,* Vol. 2, No. 1 [January 1973], p. 31.) This article is suggested as a forthright statement of a point of view. The physicians-union movement appears to be growing despite AMA opposition. Its future will be interesting to follow. Another article recommended for reading in this general area is Anne R. Sommers, "Who's in Charge Here?—Or Alice Searches for a King in Mediland," *New England Journal of Medicine,* Vol. 287, No. 7 [1972], pp. 849–55. "Five groups share major responsibility—for both our current problems and their solution: consumers, doctors, hospitals, private health-insurance carriers and the government. Within this shared responsibility, the pre-eminent role will probably go to the group demonstrating greatest capacity for leadership, which, paradoxically, may mean greatest capacity for self discipline." Sommers ended her article with these words: "Ten years ago (on June 14, 1962), the *New England Journal of Medicine* carried an article by my husband and me entitled, 'The Paradox of Medical Progress.' We concluded with these words:

"'It is essential not to be bemused by simple notions that single or permanent solutions can be found. The problems are multifaceted and enduring. One can steadily seek progress in change while accepting the realism of John Galsworthy's dictum: "Nothing is so sure to change as the *status quo,* and nothing so unlikely to arrive as the millennium."'"

[35] Committee for Economic Development, *Building a National Health-Care System,* p. 49.

[36] David E. Smith, John Luce, and Ernest A. Dernburg, "The Health of Haight-Ashbury," *Transaction,* Vol. 7, No. 6, Whole No. 56 (April 1970), p. 43.

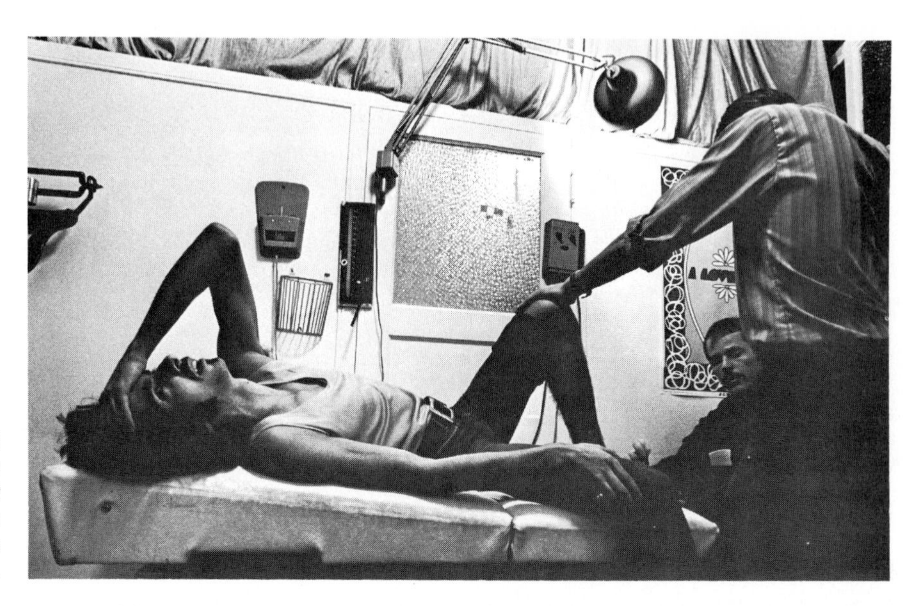

24-4 *A young man receives treatment for a painful foot infection at San Francisco's Haight-Ashbury Free Clinic.*

''Jake'' Winters People's Free Medical Care Center in Chicago's West Side black ghetto. ''This is a free clinic,'' a sign read, ''but if you would like to give us some money, it would be taken with love and used to improve your clinic even if it's a dime or less. Thank you and power to the people.''[37] Inside the building were photographs of Black Panther leaders and printed political messages. Along with the propaganda, nevertheless, went an effort to provide some medical care to an alienated and needy community.

Not all free clinics are at loggerheads with community resources that are considered ''establishment.'' Some receive aid from health departments in the form of equipment and certain drugs.[38] Others request and receive advice from local physicians.[39]

Some people see free clinics as a temporary and ineffective way of providing medical care of poor quality. Others consider some free clinics to be an effort to sell a slanted political point of view to the disadvantaged by offering the lure of free, albeit necessary, medical service. To many of those who go to a free clinic, it is neither of these. For them the free clinic fills a health care vacuum in a comfortable setting. Some governmental units have taken the broad hint. For example, for several years the County of Los Angeles Department of Health Services has allocated hundreds of thousands of dollars to its youth clinics.[40]

[37] ''The Free Clinics: Ghetto Care Centers Struggle to Survive,'' *American Medical News,* Vol. 15, No. 7 (February 21, 1972), p. 12.

[38] Gordon T. Stewart, ''Health Care in America—Privilege or Right?'' *The Lancet,* Vol. 22, No. 7737 (December 11, 1971), p. 1305.

[39] J. David Curb and Joel Trujillo, ''Medical Problems Among Rural Hippies,'' *Rocky Mountain Medical Journal,* Vol. 68, No. 9 (September 1971), pp. 37–38.

[40] Such governmental activity is long overdue. In one study of the health problems and practices of youth preparatory to opening a youth clinic, it was found that ''A surprising number use the services of pseudo-medical men,'' such as practitioners of folk medicine, chiropractors, and naturopaths (a form of therapy making use of physical forces such as air, light, water, heat, and massage—hardly adequate for the treatment of most of the sickness of the young). (Jack J. Sternlieb and Louis Munan, ''A Survey of Health Problems, Practices, and Needs of Youth,'' *Pediatrics,* Vol. 49, No. 2 [February 1972], p. 177.)

Here, too, the traditional aseptic clinic environment has been dispensed with in favor of an appropriate decor and personnel chosen to make the patient feel at home. Thus, these youth clinics are more than a place to go to be treated; for some, they are a place to go to be understood.

the dentist

The academic requirements for the degrees of Doctor of Dental Surgery (D.D.S.) and Doctor of Dental Medicine (D.D.M.) are essentially the same. Dental training is not limited to study of the teeth. Since dental health is part of body health, the introductory years of dental school are today quite similar to those of medical school. Most of the fifty-two U.S. dental schools are attached to a major university. Dental schools must be approved by the Council on Dental Education of the American Dental Association. Upon completion of dental school, the graduate must pass a state board examination before he or she can practice. A list of dental specialties appears in the Glossary under "Specialties."

the dentists' plan for comprehensive dental health care

A recent (1971) report[41] of a five-committee Task Force of the American Dental Association stated that:

> The average child is a dental cripple by the time he graduates from high school. . . . The time has come for the nation to apply the dental knowledge and technology at hand through an organized national dental health program. . . . The most efficient and economic approach to improving the status of the nation's dental health is to prevent and control dental disease beginning with children.[42]

The Task Force made numerous recommendations, most of which had not been implemented as of April 1974. Two of the most important were:

1. *comprehensive dental care for children,* beginning with preschool-age children and progressively expanding the program by age groups until all children through the age of seventeen are included.

2. *the provision of emergency dental services to all persons.* This would include control and treatment of serious bleeding, acute infections, injuries, severe pain, and other grave conditions such as cancer of the mouth.

This program would be continued for ten years. After that time, those persons already in the program would be continued in it and all persons over sixty-five years of age would be added.

The Task Force membership favored patient participation in costs, preferably through copayment (see page 735). The cost of dental care for the indigent who would eventually be included in the program would be met by general tax revenues. For the nonindigent, the Task Force recommended employer-employee payroll deductions into a fund administered by nongovernmental agencies.

[41] "Task Force/Priorities," *Journal of the American Dental Association,* Vol. 83, No. 9 (September 1971), pp. 573–89.
[42] *Ibid.,* p. 577.

programs that finance health services: profit and nonprofit

People cannot predict when they will be ill; consequently, they cannot know in advance when they will need money for medical care, nor how much they will need. Health insurance programs are based on the concept that the amount of money that a large group of people will need to pay for health services can be predicted reasonably accurately. Therefore, money is collected from the individuals of the group. These pooled funds are then used to pay part or all of the costs of the unpredictable individual illnesses of the group. Thus, in effect, the individuals of the group budget for sickness in advance, and they share the risk. Such financing is done through the private health insurance industry or through the federal government, as with Medicare.

the private health insurance industry

The private health insurance industry is made up of three broad categories: (1) Blue Cross and Blue Shield, (2) independent insurance plans, and (3) commercial insurance companies.

Blue Cross and Blue Shield

Seventy-five *Blue Cross* plans provide health insurance for about 71 million people in all the states. Insurance plans that wish to use the Blue Cross symbol must meet the approval of the American Hospital Association's Blue Cross Commission. One requirement that a plan must meet in order to be approved by the Commission is a nonprofit method of operating—that is, profits must go into improving the plan. Blue Cross plans pay a large proportion of hospital, surgical, laboratory, and other medical costs.

Seventy-two *Blue Shield* plans in the fifty states insure about 63 million people. Like Blue Cross plans, they are nonprofit and provide free choice of physician. The amount paid depends on family income level. Family income levels vary for different Blue Shield plans; usually they are set at $4200 to $7500 yearly. People whose family income is at or below the level set by their particular plan, are completely covered if their physician accepts the Blue Shield fee schedule. If their income is above the established level, they are obligated to pay any surcharge added by the physician. Blue Shield plans must be approved by local medical societies. Like Blue Cross plans, Blue Shield plans operate outside the regular insurance laws in most states. Both Blue Cross and Blue Shield plans are sold to individuals as well as to groups. Their benefits and provisions vary in different states.

independent insurance plans

Eight million people are enrolled in the five hundred independent insurance plans in the nation. Some are joint ventures between unions and management. Others provide benefits through comprehensive prepaid group practice plans (see pages 742–43). Also among these are nonprofit service corporations which permit a free choice of dentists and also provide service benefits.

commercial insurance plans

In the United States, about a thousand profit-making commercial insurance companies write group and individual health insurance policies covering about 122 million persons for hospital care. Some of these companies offer "package insurance." Added to hospital coverage are life and disability insurance as well as other benefits. Another innovation made by these companies is *major medical insurance.* Major medical policies are not designed to pay for sickness costs that can be handled by ordinary insurance. Instead they cover the costs of illnesses that run into thousands of dollars. The section below suggests how a major medical insurance claim may be computed.

ON COMPUTING MAJOR MEDICAL INSURANCE BENEFITS[43] Major medical policies have maximum benefits that range from $2000 to ten or even twenty times that figure. Usually they contain both a *deductible* and a *coinsurance* clause. As with most automobile insurance, the insured pays the deductible amount before the company pays anything. The cost of the premium affects the size of the deductible; a higher deductible means a lower premium. A coinsurance clause provides that a stated percentage of the cost must be borne by the insured *after* the deductible amount has been subtracted.

For example: A man has two types of sickness insurance policies. One pays total basic hospital and surgical benefits up to $1200. The second is a major medical policy paying a maximum benefit of $10,000, with a deductible clause of $500 and a coinsurance clause of 20 percent. The man is diagnosed as having an operable brain tumor. Costly surgery and months of aftercare bring his total expenses to $9700. His calculated benefits would be as follows:

Total cost of the illness	$9700
Total benefit paid by basic plan	−1200
Balance covered by major medical	8500
Minus the deductible amount	− 500
Balance subject to coinsurance (20 percent)	8000
Minus coinsurance	−1600
Amount paid by major medical	$6400

So:

The basic insurance paid	$1200
The major medical insurance paid	6400
The patient paid ($9700 − $7600)	$2100

Of course, these figures are theoretical and would be higher or lower depending on the premiums paid.

[43]The discussion in this section is based on Fred T. Wilhelms, Raymond P. Heimerl, and Herbert M. Jelley, *Consumer Economics,* 3rd ed. (New York, 1966), pp. 278–79.

disability insurance

In circumstances such as those of this hypothetical patient, disability (loss-of-income) insurance would be most helpful. During such a protracted illness, months without employment means that money is being spent but none is being earned. The patient may have accumulated sick leave with pay, but that source of income is limited. Family security is thus threatened. With the exception of death benefits, no insurance has a longer history than that covering loss of income. For example, the ordinances of the fourteenth-century Gild[44] of the Smiths of Chesterfield in England provided that "If any brother is sick, and needs help, he shall have a half penny daily from the common fund of the gild until he has got well."[45]

Today, premiums are paid to insurance companies, which in the event of disability may pay as much as 75 percent of the insured person's monthly income. Usually there is a waiting period. Why? Some unscrupulous individuals might fake an illness or an accident. Investigations of these possibilities would be so costly that the company would be forced to discontinue this type of insurance. Loss-of-income policies may also contain lump-sum benefits paid to the insured person if he or she loses a limb, part of a limb, or an eye, or to survivors if he or she suffers an accidental death.

on knowing what one is buying

Whether an individual buys medical expense or disability insurance, it is his responsibility to know what is in his policy and to review it annually. He must select the company with care. If he does not understand the "fine print" in the policy, he should, before investing in it, ask for and receive clarification in writing from the company. He should also compare a particular policy with others and ask some basic questions: What risks are covered? Which are specifically excluded? Some policies cost very little, which may well be because they offer so little; they exclude all but the most unusual risks. Referring to this type of policy, a comedian once joked: "I have health insurance. If a giraffe bites me on the shoulder, I get $18, provided I am pregnant at the time."[46] The risks that should be covered are those that are most likely to happen and to cost the most. Among other questions to ask about insurance coverage are these: Is the policy cancellable by the company during the life of the contract? Does the company have the right to refuse renewal of the contract? If so, when? At what age of the insured may the policy be canceled? Do the premium costs increase as the insured gets older? By how much? In the event the insured becomes ill and collects benefits, must he continue to pay premiums during the time he is disabled? Is there a waiting period before benefits are paid? If so, how long is it? If the insured becomes ill and collects benefits, and in the same year (or any other time) falls ill again with the same or another illness, will the company continue to pay benefits? If so, for how long? If the insured is hurt and then

[44] The modern spelling is "guild."

[45] J. Toulmin Smith, *English Guilds,* p. 169.

[46] Rosemary Stevens, *American Medicine and the Public Interest,* p. 427, citing Richard Carter, *The Doctor Business* (New York, 1958), p. 96, quoting Phil Leeds.

dies, how much time must elapse before the company pays a death benefit? Does the policy cover complete or partial disability or both, and, in any case, for how long? Exactly what does the policy pay for, and how does it compare with policies that cost slightly less or more? Are all the costly benefits in the policy really needed now? Might they be needed later? Are there less expensive policies with a more practical list of benefits? Can the policy be changed to meet the changing needs of the insured?

shortcomings of private insurance plans[47]

This nation's private health insurance industry does not meet the needs of great numbers of people. Although by 1970 about 80 percent of the U.S. population was covered by some form of health insurance, in many cases the amount and type of coverage were inadequate. Although the vast majority of the people had at least some hospital-associated coverage, nonhospital-associated coverage (such as nursing home care) was held by a much smaller percentage.

In addition, for many people private health insurance is too expensive. The lower a person's income, the less likely he is to be insured. Yet it is the poor who are most likely to be sick. Poor children are particularly disadvantaged. In 1968, less than 25 percent of the poor children in this country had hospital insurance protection.

public health insurance and Wilbur Mills

The passage, in 1965, of Medicare legislation for the aged was largely due to the political astuteness of the very man who had blocked it for eight years. In 1957, a forerunner of Medicare had been introduced by Representative Aime J. Forand, Democrat from Rhode Island. That plan, and subsequent ones, were scuttled by Wilbur Mills, a Democrat from Arkansas and Chairman of the powerful House Ways and Means Committee. Mills is a practical politician. Whenever a new version of a plan for old-age health insurance reached the committee, Mills tested the political winds from four directions—from the people, from the Congress, from his own committee, and finally from the White House. Until 1965, the voters were divided. So was Congress. Mills knew that his own support was essential to favorable consideration of the bill by his committee. He withheld that support. During the Eisenhower years, White House interest in compulsory health insurance for the aged was, at best, lukewarm. President Kennedy wanted Medicare, but he did not have enough support for it either in the Ways and Means Committee or on the floor of the House. Nor did he live long enough to push effectively for the program.

Then came the overwhelming Johnson landslide. Again, Mills looked to the people. They were no longer divided. The past three election campaigns had built up vast support for old-age health insurance. The tragic death of President Kennedy had particularly stimulated widespread sentiment for his legislative program.[48] In the Congress, thirty-eight Democrats had been added to the

[47] *Basic Facts on the Health Industry,* Staff of the Committee on Ways and Means (1971), pp. 94–112.

[48] Peter A. Corning, *The Evolution of Medicare . . . from Idea to Law,* U.S. Department of Health, Education, and Welfare, Social Security Administration, Office of Research and Statistics, Research Report No. 29 (Washington, D.C., 1969), p. 106.

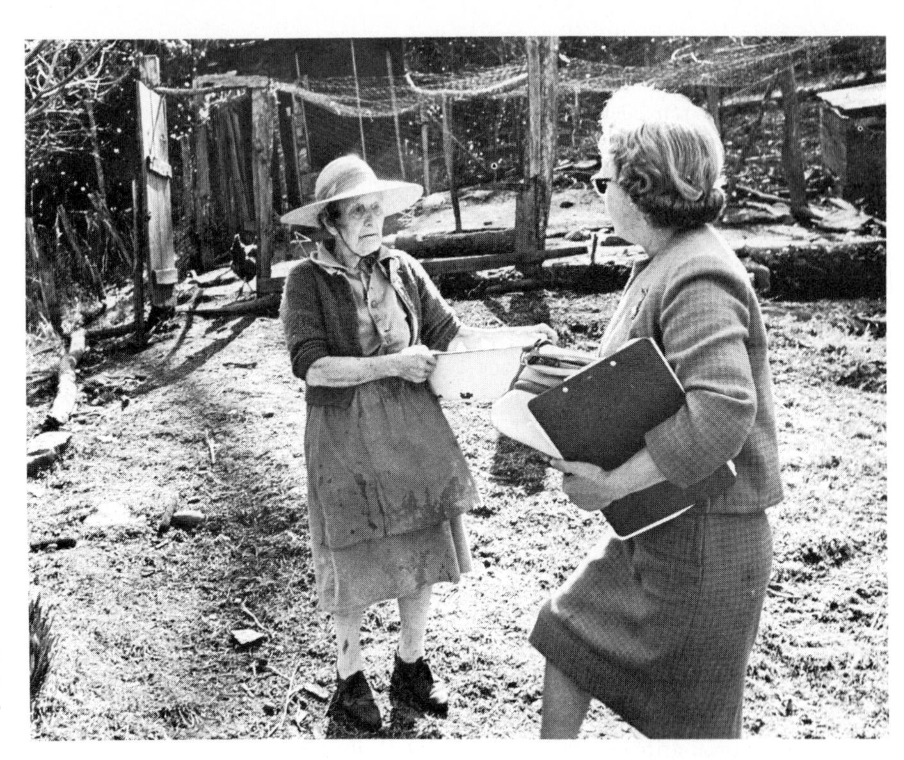

24-5 *A North Carolina mountain woman is signed up for Medicare benefits.*

House and two to the Senate, giving the Democrats greater majorities in both houses. To impede Medicare legislation would invite their rebellion. Mills' own Ways and Means Committee was no more reassuring: old members had retired or had been defeated; new men sat in their places, and they wanted Medicare. And in the White House now lived the persuasive Lyndon Johnson, at the peak of his enormous power and in no mood to be denied. For Wilbur Mills, the political winds had changed direction. To attempt to block old-age health insurance might mean defeat and possibly the end of his own influence. It was no longer whether, but how, to engineer passage of health insurance for the aged.

How indeed? Bitterly opposing Medicare was the American Medical Association. Since the government's plan depended on compulsory tax deductions, the AMA lobby labeled it un-American. Second, said the AMA, Medicare was a fraud; it was an expensive insurance scheme that did not even offer payment for doctor bills. A third objection made even avid supporters of Medicare waver. Health insurance claims would be paid out of existing Social Security funds. Overpayments were inevitable, it was said, and eventually the entire Social Security structure would crumble. Then the senior Republican member of the House Ways and Means Committee, Representative John Byrnes of Wisconsin, presented an alternative bill that was somewhat more to the AMA's liking. It was voluntary—that is, people sixty-five years of age or older could decide for themselves whether or not to buy the insurance; it would pay a large share of doctor bills; it had nothing to do with the Social Security system and so could not imperil it.

It was an appealing alternative—so appealing that the adroit Mills could not resist it. He executed a masterpiece of political dexterity. To the government-sponsored, tax-supported, compulsory bill offering hospital and nursing care, he simply added Byrnes's AMA-approved voluntary bill that paid a large share of doctor bills. With the doctor's bill insurance, the aged would receive much more than the government had originally offered. But now, of course, the whole package was credited to the government. How was Social Security protected? The compulsory hospital benefits were to be paid out of a separate trust fund. It would be financed by its own share of the Social Security payroll tax. The Social Security financial structure was totally unaffected; it was merely an administrative means of collecting federal insurance premiums.

Medicare and Medicaid

In 1965, Congress amended the Social Security Act to include Title 18 (Medicare), which provided a program of health insurance for persons sixty-five years of age or older. Title 18 established two programs:

1. *compulsory hospital insurance* financed by Social Security taxes paid by workers and their employers. The hospital insurance program helps to pay the costs of hospital care, extended-care facilities (such as nursing homes), and outpatient diagnostic services.

2. *voluntary medical insurance* financed by the voluntarily paid premiums of the insured and matching funds from the government's general revenues. The medical insurance program helps to pay for doctor bills and certain other services not covered by the hospital insurance.

Congress also amended the Social Security Act to include Title 19 (Medicaid). This provides for federal grants to the states to:

1. operate a medical assistance program for those persons who were already receiving public assistance from the federal government; included in this group were the aged, blind, disabled, and families with dependent children;

2. help those who had enough money to live on, but not enough to pay for medical expenses;

3. provide assistance for all children under the age of twenty-one whose parents were unable to pay their medical bills.

Medicaid was thus an expansion of already existing federal aid. It was Medicare that was the true landmark in medical care history in the United States. As was explained above, its unique feature is the combination by the government of both compulsory and voluntary methods of payment.

Today, both Medicare and Medicaid are in serious financial trouble. Part of the problem arises from failure to accurately estimate future costs. The House Ways and Means Committee, Wilbur Mills later confessed, had been "seriously misled about future cost increases, in 1965, when [it] was considering the Medicare and Medicaid legislation. The actual cost projections at that time were greatly underestimated."[49] Thus, "pouring more money into the health care

[49] Quoted in Eugene G. McCarthy, "Reorganizing the Delivery and Payment of Health Care in the United States," *The Lancet,* Vol. 22, No. 7737 (December 11, 1971), p. 1303.

industry without either increasing the supply of services, regulating prices, or creating incentives to increase productivity will exacerbate the problem of costs."[50]

professional standards review organizations (PSROs): peer review

In 1972 a significant amendment to the Social Security Act mandated review by physicians of the quality of another physician's services and the reasonableness of his fees for institutional Medicaid and Medicare services. To take effect in 1975, this legislation has prompted much discussion among physicians. Some evaluation of the quality of a physician's services had long been a part of the medical scene. Physicians whose quality of service was deemed low or whose fees were outrageous were "talked to" privately by a committee of their fellow physicians. Punitive action was a possibility; it could, for example, take the form of loss of hospital privileges—a disaster for any modern medical practitioner. Peer review had even become an essential part of the accreditation program of hospitals. A 1972 survey had showed that forty-five state medical societies had professional review organizations or other programs to evaluate professional care, and 71 percent of county medical societies had similar programs.[51] Most physicians in organized medicine seemed prepared to accept peer review of their professional care; it was peer review of their fees that brought about powerful opposition. A host of questions were raised: Would there be more paperwork? Who should judge the judged—practitioners in the same specialty, of the same age, similar amount of experience, of the same location, with similar clientele?[52]

Other physician groups saw possible benefits to the legislation. Editorialized the *Rocky Mountain Medical Journal:* "Our peers will come much nearer to providing equity and justice in judgment of professional performance and its compensation than any other individual or groups . . . Effective peer review can be obtained by government or any third party only by utilizing the practicing physician . . . Peer review is our most powerful weapon in the relentless struggle to preserve private enterprise in the practice of medicine. Peer review is a trump card. Don't knock it."[53] During early 1974, the position of the powerful House of Delegates of the American Medical Association was essentially this: (1) In principle, peer review under professional direction was supported. (2) The Professional Standards Review Organization law ought to be repealed.

The AMA group realized the difficulties in repealing the law. It suggested a long-range goal of public education; in this way it was hoped by some that people would be sent to Congress who would support their position. Meanwhile, "while the law remains on the books, professional leadership would have

[50] Basil J. F. Mott, "The Changing Health Care Scene," *Public Administration Review,* Vol. 31, No. 5 (September–October 1971), pp. 502–03.

[51] "Medicine and PSROs," *American Medical News,* Vol. 16, No. 13 (April 2, 1973), p. 4.

[52] "The MD's Vital Role in Peer Review," *American Medical News,* Vol. 15, No. 49 (December 11, 1972), p. 4.

[53] Quoted in *ibid.*

to be exerted to assure that its deleterious effects be kept at a minimum.[54] In March 1974, the U.S. Department of Health, Education, and Welfare established 203 PSRO areas throughout the nation.

compulsory national health insurance

That the 1970s will witness some form of compulsory national health insurance for the people of the United States now seems inevitable. The popularity (despite its problems) of Medicare, the spiraling costs of health care, the unequal distribution of health care personnel and facilities, the inaccessibility and unavailability of health care for millions of the most needy citizens, the wasteful emphasis on diagnosis and treatment rather than the more sensible and economical prevention of sickness, the lack of continuity of health care for the individual, the disproportionately high sickness and death rates among the poor, the disgracefully high national sickness and death rates in this country as compared to other industrialized countries—all these are health problems that will be discussed below (pages 744–53). They are among the stimuli that are causing an increasingly educated population to demand that serious consideration be given to compulsory national health insurance.

criteria for a new venture

It is beginning to receive that consideration. From the conservative American Medical Association to the somewhat more liberal labor unions, various groups have put forth a profusion of avidly discussed plans. Their very number has led to confusion. It is well, therefore, to consider this basic question: What criteria may be used in evaluating national health insurance proposals? The criteria may change with the times. However, they represent concepts that will need to be considered by the Congress before it passes further national health insurance legislation.[55]

Eilers[56] has suggested the following criteria for evaluating a national health insurance proposal:

1. The program must guarantee that adequate health coverage will be within financial reach for everyone.

2. Arrangements for the delivery of health services should be understandable and acceptable to the consumer.

3. The program should provide for the most comprehensive health care with the most efficient use of resources.

4. Whether by taxation or coinsurance payments, most of the consumers

[54] "The AMA Charts Its Course for PSRO," *American Medical News,* Vol. 16, No. 48 (December 10, 1973), p. 4.

[55] On December 10, 1973, the Health, Education, and Welfare Secretary of the Nixon Administration briefed reporters on some of the provisions in a national health insurance bill that was being considered and was to be submitted to President Nixon within several weeks and sent to Congress very early in 1974. Some of the points of the proposed bill: employers would be required to provide a health insurance policy to employees on a cost-sharing basis. The government would pay the premiums for low income premiums. Other features included catastrophic protection, preventive services such as children's dental care, and an option for coverage through HMOs (pages 743–44). ("Administration NIH Proposal Nearing Completion," *PMA Newsletter,* published by the Pharmaceutical Manufacturers Association, Vol. 15, No. 50 [December 14, 1973], p. 4.)

[56] Robert D. Eilers, "National Health Insurance: What Kind and How Much?" *New England Journal of Medicine,* Vol. 284, No. 16 (April 22, 1971), pp. 881–86, and Vol. 284, No. 17 (April 29, 1971), pp. 945–54.

covered by national health insurance should help pay for it. This cannot include those below the poverty level, who must, nevertheless, be covered.

5. The program should include and impose standards for the quality of care. These should be reviewed periodically. Consumers as well as professional people should be involved in establishing and maintaining high standards of care.

a variety of plans

Health Planning, 1972

Planners generate projections,
Doctor-critics make corrections.
Outcome? Programs, targets, ranges—
But patients don't see any changes.[57]

On March 29, 1972, a bill "to establish a Department of Health" was simultaneously introduced in both the House of Representatives and the Senate of the United States Congress (92d Congress, 2d Session, S 3432, and HR 14199). Its basic purpose was to coordinate the widely distributed, fragmented health activities of the federal government. It was long overdue. Numerous health activities are being carried out by dozens of federal agencies that hardly communicate with one another. Section 5 (a) of the bill proposed the establishment of a National Advisory Committee on Health Planning. One of its charges would be to "set forth national goals and priorities for making comprehensive high quality care and treatment available at reasonable cost to any person in the United States."

In seeking to meet this charge the commission would not be short of ideas. Among the plans presented to the public were those proposed by President Nixon, by Senator Edward Kennedy, by the American Medical Association (Medi-credit), the American Hospital Association (Ameriplan), the Health Insurance Association of America (HIAA), and the Committee for National Health Insurance. Any health insurance legislation would require immediate taxation. For this reason the Constitution requires that its consideration begin in the House of Representatives. Thus, it would first go to the Committee on Ways and Means. At the beginning of 1974, the chairman of that committee was still Congressman Wilbur Mills.

programs that both organize and finance health services

comprehensive prepaid group practice plans

People who enroll in a comprehensive prepaid group practice plan purchase the assurance that they will receive complete medical care, including hospitalization. Comprehensive care is obtained by the payment of a fixed annual amount. If the costs of the program are greater than anticipated, the physicians in the group absorb the excess. If costs are smaller, the physicians share a bonus.

[57] Dr. Michael M. Stewart, *Hospital Tribune,* Vol. 7, No. 1 (January 1, 1973), p. 22.

Thus, two factors are at work: the incentive to economize and the responsibility for providing complete care to its clientele. For this reason, expensive specialists are consulted only when necessary; primary physicians (general practitioners, internists, and pediatricians) provide the basic medical skills.

For members of the Kaiser Foundation Medical Care Program in California, Hawaii, and the Portland-Vancouver area, the cost of comprehensive care is between 20 and 30 percent less than the private physicians' fee-for-service system.[58] The Health Insurance Plan of New York is another example of a comprehensive prepaid group practice plan, as are the Ross-Loos Medical Group in Los Angeles, the Community Health Organization of Detroit, the Group Health Association in Washington, D.C., and the Group Health Cooperative of Puget Sound.

neighborhood health centers

The purpose of a neighborhood health center is to bring comprehensive health services to people in low-income urban areas. The person does not need to go from one place to another to receive care for more than one organ or ailment. Diagnosis and treatment of disease are but part of comprehensive health care. Also included is an active program for the prevention of illness.

Neighborhood health centers are federally supported; by 1972 about seventy such centers were in operation throughout the country. Representatives of the community have an important voice in the planning, development, and management of neighborhood health centers. Some people claim that the poor are not knowledgeable enough to contribute to so sophisticated a project. They forget two things: first, that many of this nation's greatest hospital and beneficial health societies were founded by poor immigrants who were imbued with a proud desire to help their own; second, without the active participation of community representatives, the people of the community do not think of the health center as their own. Instead, they resent it as just another humiliating project, planned by outsiders who have no real feeling for their needs.

health maintenance organizations

Conceived in 1970 and established by law in 1973 by the Nixon administration, a health maintenance organization (HMO) is one that delivers comprehensive health care to a voluntarily enrolled population at a prenegotiated *annual rate.* The HMO concept developed from the proven success of prepaid group practice plans such as the Kaiser Foundation program (noted above). Such organizations meet the definition of an HMO most completely. However, other kinds of groups may form HMOs. These include either providers of health services, such as physicians, hospitals, medical societies, or consumers of health services, such as labor unions or business firms.

Any HMO must meet the four basic requirements that are inherent in the definition: that is, it must be (1) a system of health care (including personnel and facilities) organized to serve all the health needs of (2) a defined population that chooses to enroll, and for which the HMO assumes responsibility twenty-four hours a day, seven days a week, in return for (3) payment for total services

[58] Donald L. Madison, "The Structure of American Health Care Services," *Public Administration Review,* Vol. 31, No. 5 (September–October 1971), p. 522, and footnote 25, p. 527.

that is made on a previously established, prepaid, per-person or per-family basis and that is handled by (4) an adequate managing organization.

Because the annually prepaid amount is fixed, the HMO is economically motivated to maintain the subscriber's health, to expedite his recovery when sick, and to perform these services with maximum efficiency. Added costs of inefficient service are not borne by the subscriber. Since HMOs compete with one another for subscribers, the consumer is in a bargaining position to receive the most for his money. In that case, however, might not HMOs tend to curtail costs by decreasing services and serving only low-risk populations? To avoid this, the federal government's plans for HMOs include a system of controls. If, for example, an HMO contracts with the federal government under Medicare, its management must provide mechanisms for government monitoring. Federal financial help, in the form of loans, grants, and contracts, is now expanding existing HMOs and establishing new ones. On December 30, 1973, for example, President Nixon signed a bill providing $375 million to encourage the formation of Health Maintenance Organizations. By that time there were about 115 of these group plans in the nation. It was hoped that the legislation might help establish three hundred more. The new law was intended to demonstrate the feasibility of the prepaid HMOs over five years. Aside from the allocation of funds, the bill required employers of twenty-five or more persons to offer an HMO option in addition to private insurance in their negotiations of health benefits with their employees.

some health care problems

the rising costs of medical care[59]

In 1970, the average health bill for each person in this country was $324. Ten years before it was less than half that amount ($145). In 1950, the average health bill was only $79. One reason for this enormous increase is medical progress. Technological advances have made possible a costly array of new diagnostic and treatment facilities that were unheard of a generation ago. An example: hospital intensive-care units for heart attack patients have saved thousands of lives; the equipment and highly trained personnel they require are tremendously expensive.

A second reason for the spiraling costs of medical care may be found in the changing nature of the population. An increasingly urbanized and educated populace is demanding better preventive, curative, and rehabilitative care. No longer is this considered a privilege; it is a right. And this changed population is now being attacked by a host of illnesses that were not so common a generation ago. With increased control of communicable disease, people are living longer than ever before; thus they survive to develop chronic ailments (see page 193). Since the turn of the century, the proportion of the elderly to the rest of the population has more than quadrupled.

The cost of chronic sickness is high. For an aged person the average hospital

[59]The data in this section are from *Basic Facts on the Health Industry*, pp. 32–38.

expenditure in 1970 was $372—more than eleven times that of a youth ($33), and more than twice that of a middle-aged patient. Doctor bills for the elderly are three times those for the young, and twice those for the middle-aged. Moreover, people over sixty-five years of are twice as likely to suffer chronic diseases as are those under sixty-five; they are admitted to hospitals more often and stay longer. On the one hand, hospitals are faced with increased demands for more expensive and prolonged care; on the other hand, they are forced to meet increased payroll and other expenses. The results: hospital bills have skyrocketed, and so have health insurance premiums. Unfortunately, increased costs have not been translated into more medical care. "Medical costs are rising twice as fast as the cost of living. The resultant inflation in health expenditure has meant that 60% of the growth in expenditure between 1960 and 1970 purchased no additional service."[60]

the unavailability of health care

The present organization and method of distributing health care in the United States is, like any business, based on competition. Physicians in private practice compete with one another for the consumer who can afford to pay. The physician is an entrepreneur who relishes his independence. The same is true of the private hospital. An independent institution, it is responsible only to a board of trustees. Both private physicians and hospitals go where the money is and, aside from much charity work, serve those with money. Those without money must seek care in charity hospitals.[61] Are charity hospitals as desirable as private hospitals? The medical care they offer may be as good. Nevertheless, those who have enough money do not ordinarily go to them.

In addition, hospital beds are not distributed according to population needs. North Dakota has 6.3 hospital beds per 1,000 residents—more hospital beds per person than any other state; yet that is an average of less than 0.8 hospital beds per 1,000 square miles. The discouraging inconvenience to the sick is obvious. Massachusetts has twice as many hospital beds per 1,000 square miles.

Physicians are also unevenly distributed. In Mississippi, there are only 69 physicians for every 100,000 people; in New York, the ratio is 200 physicians for every 100,000 people.[62] In 1969, nearly half a million people in the United States lived in counties without a single practicing physician. An example: in Missouri, 96,300 people in fifteen counties had no physician.[63] It is becoming

[60] Eugene G. McCarthy, "Reorganizing the Delivery and Payment of Health Care in the United States," p. 1302.

[61] Milton Terris, "The Need for a National Health Program," *Bulletin of the New York Academy of Medicine,* Vol. 48, No. 1 (January 1972), p. 25.

[62] For good primary medical care one study indicated a need of 133 physicians per 100,000 people; the present supply is about half that many. To overcome this, various procedures need to be considered such as increasing the number of medical students, reevaluating the number of years needed for their training, and accelerating the development of group practice. (Hyman K. Schonfeld, Jean F. Heston, and Isidore S. Falk, "Number of Physicians Required for Primary Care," *New England Journal of Medicine,* Vol. 286, No. 11 [March 16, 1972], pp. 571, 576.) Particularly important are plans to transfer some tasks that have traditionally been the province of the physician to the specially trained extended-role nurse. ("Extending the Scope of Nursing Practice," *Journal of the American Medical Association,* Vol. 220, No. 9 [May 29, 1972], pp. 1231–36.) There is also an acute shortage of dentists. In the seventeen years from 1953 to 1970, the number of dental school graduates increased by only 1.9 percent. During the past few years this rate has improved somewhat. Since the cost of dental education is high, federal plans are to increase financial aid to dental schools so that more dentists may be graduated.

[63] *Basic Facts on the Health Industry,* pp. 76–78.

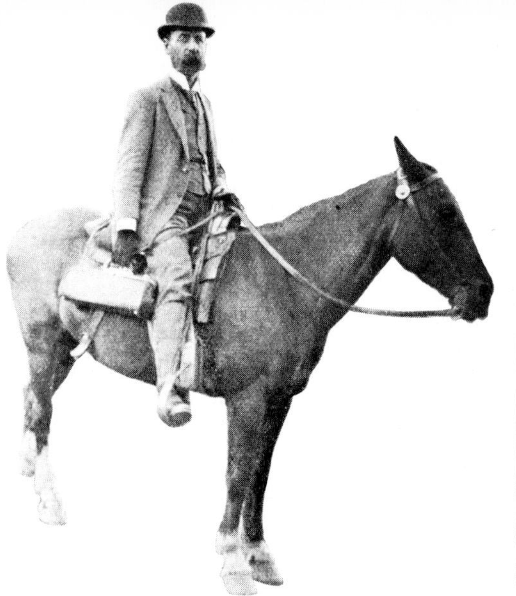

A 19th-century frontier U.S. physician making his rounds on horseback.

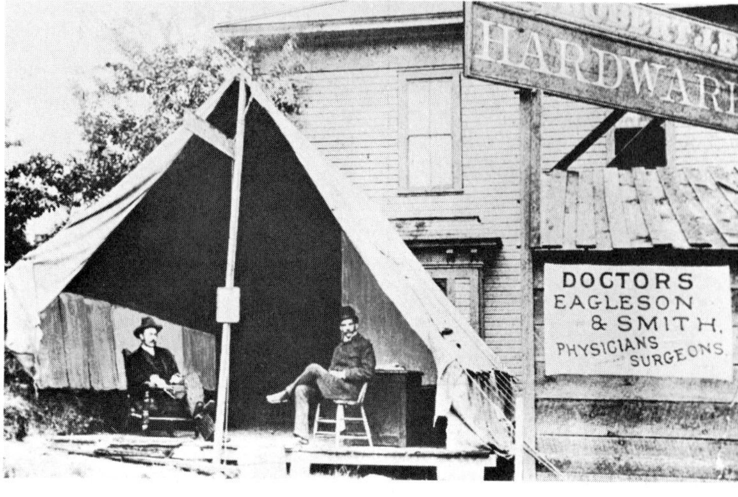

Two physicians set up a group practice in the front yard of a house in Seattle in 1889.

24-6

U.S. health care, yesterday and today

$175
150
125
100
75
50
25
0
Hospital care
Physicians' services
1950 1967 1972

Per-capita expenditures for hospital care and physicians' services, 1950–1972.

A burn-treatment unit in a modern hospital.

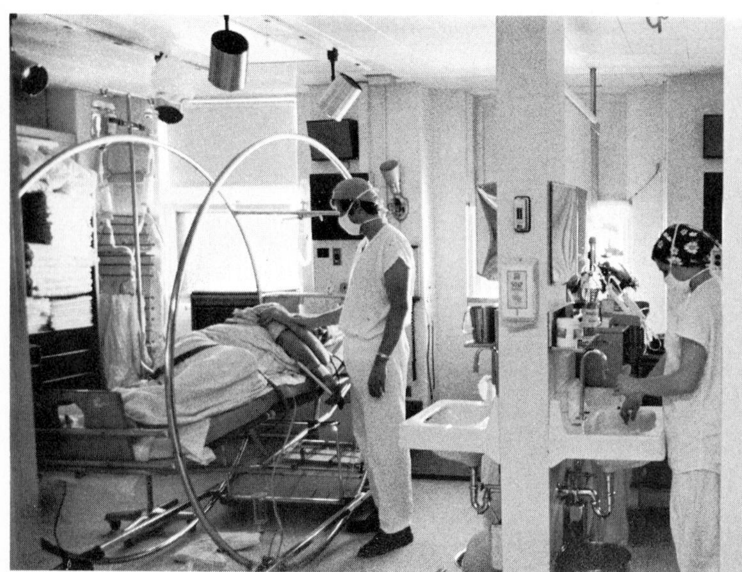

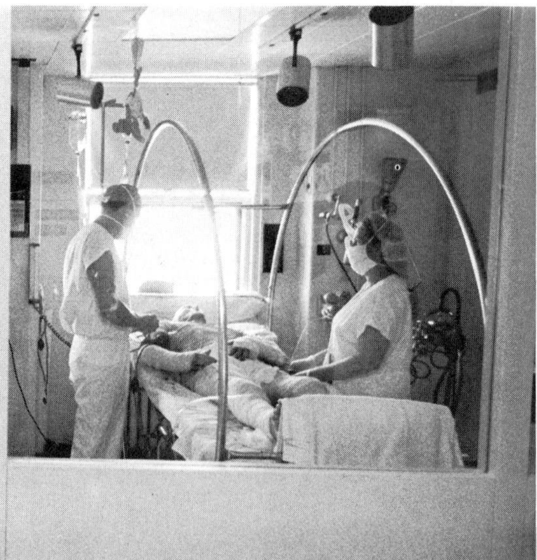

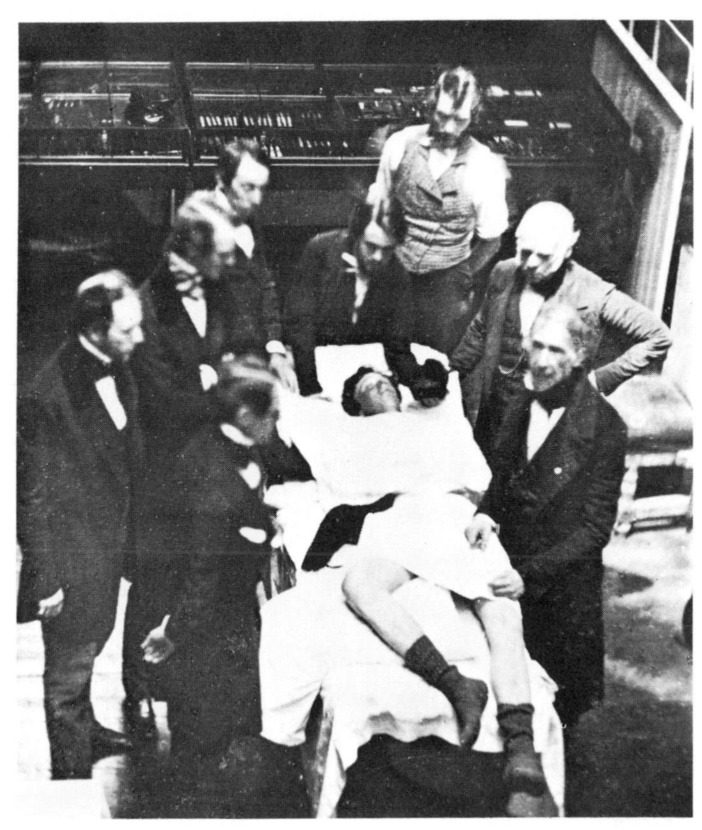

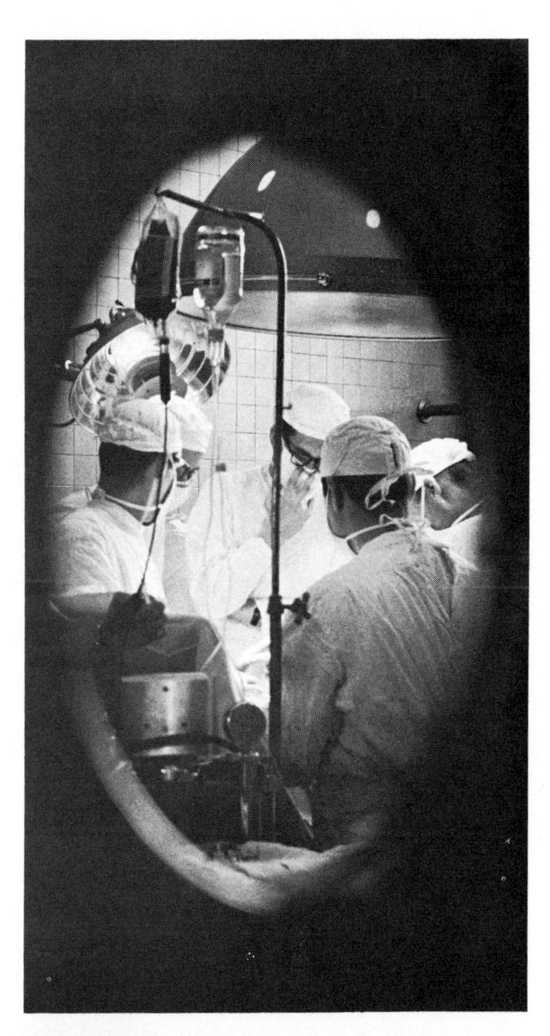

Surgery in the 19th century (*above*) and today (*right*).

MONEY BACK
FOUND NOT GUILTY
CERTIFICATE OF PURITY
KEY STONE

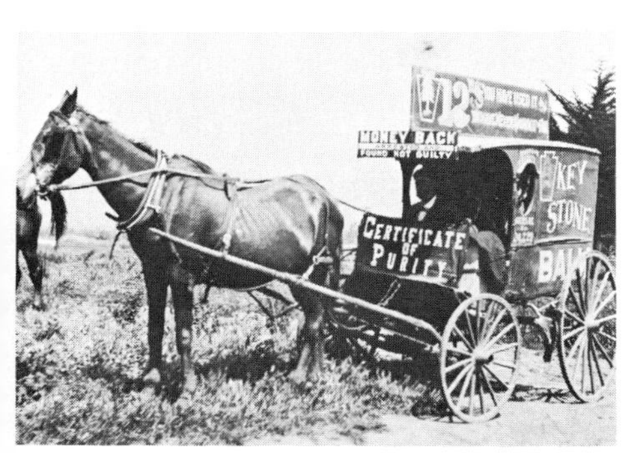

Above: This medicine-show wagon served as a pharmacy in Pasadena, California, in 1900.

APOTHECARY · IMPORTED SOAPS
THE STORY OF:
PREVENTIVE MEDICINE
STRANG CLINIC
55 EAST 34th STREET
OPEN
SUNDAYS
MU3-3838
OUR NEW YEARS RESOLUTION:
BECAUSE OF THE OVERWHELMING EVIDENCE OF THE EFFECT OF SMOKING ON ONES HEALTH, PASTEUR PHARMACY IS DISCONTINUING THE SALE OF ALL TOBACCO PRODUCTS. ALTHOUGH THIS DECISION WILL REFLECT IN OUR TOTAL SALES, WE FEEL THAT THIS CONTRIBUTION TO OUR COMMUNITY'S HEALTH IS IT'S OWN REWARD.

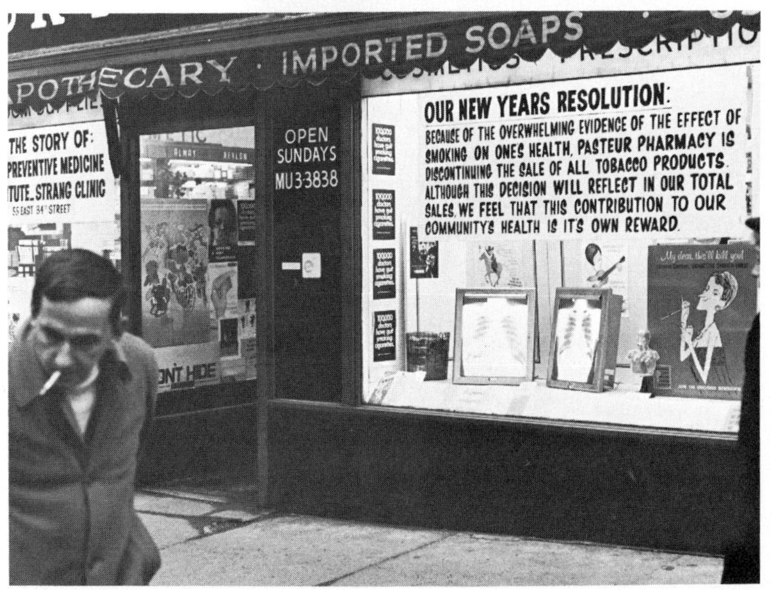

Right: A modern pharmacy—with a message.

increasingly difficult to entice physicians, nurses, and other medical personnel to rural parts of the country. How serious is this situation? ''The rates of infant and postnatal mortality are higher in rural than in urban areas, the number of draftees rejected on health grounds is much higher, and some 19 percent of the adults on farms suffer from such chronic ailments as hypertension, arthritis and heart disease to an extent that limits their capacity to work.''[64]

the quality of health care

The overspecialization, high cost, and maldistribution of health care cannot help affecting its quality. Comprehensive care and continuity of service are increasingly difficult to obtain. Patient service is fragmented. It has been wryly remarked that many an ambulatory patient avoids entering the front door of a hospital for fear of getting lost in a maze of specialists' offices. It is only in the emergency room that patients can be sure of obtaining medical care at all times. Between 1955 and 1965, visits to emergency rooms of short-term general hospitals in the United States increased by 186 percent.[65] However, only a small proportion of these could be classified as true emergencies.[66] Nevertheless, emergency room visits continue to increase.

Hospital emergency rooms are equipped to handle only urgent problems. They may provide provisional diagnoses leading to admission to the hospital for firm diagnoses and treatment. Nevertheless, for most patients hurried treatment in a crowded emergency room is a poor substitute for a thorough, time-consuming approach to each patient as a whole person with interrelated problems. Preventive medicine and follow-up care are not generally practiced in emergency rooms. Thus, emergency room care for the ambulatory patient is seldom more than medical piecework. Continuity of care, so desirable for both physician and patient, is rarely achieved.

could the U.S. health dollar buy more?[67]

In 1949, an average male child born in the United States could be expected to live 65.2 years; a female, 70.7. In this statistical measure of longevity, the *average remaining lifetime at birth,*[68] the U.S. male ranked fourteenth among males of other nations; the female, ninth.

In 1973, an average male child born in the United States could be expected to live 67 years; a female, 75. The 1949–73 improvement: an increase of 1.8 and 4.3 years respectively. But, compared to other nations, in those twenty-four years the U.S. male longevity slipped to twenty-second place and the female rose to seventh place.[69]

[64] ''Country Blues,'' *Scientific American,* Vol. 226, No. 4 (April 1972), p. 56.

[65] Donald L. Madison, ''The Structure of American Health Care Services,'' p. 520, citing ''Hospital Statistics,'' *Hospitals,* Guide Issue, Vol. 30 (August 1, 1956), p. 62, and ''Hospital Statistics,'' *Hospitals,* Guide Issue, Vol. 40 (August 1, 1966), p. 474.

[66] Paul Torrens and Donna Yedvab, ''Variations Among Emergency Room Populations: A Comparison of Four Hospitals in New York City,'' *Medical Care,* Vol. 8 (January–February 1970), pp. 60–75. For many physicians, emergency medical care is becoming a career, and there is a considerable effort to make emergency medicine a specialty. (*Medical World News,* Vol. 15, No. 5 [February 1, 1974], pp. 38–42.)

[66] Paul Torrens and Donna Yedvab, ''Variations Among Emergency Room Populations: A Comparison of Four Hospitals in New York City,'' *Medical Care,* Vol. 8 (January–February 1970), pp. 60–75.

[67] Much of this section is based on an article by William H. Forbes, ''Longevity and Medical Costs,'' *New England Journal of Medicine,* Vol. 277, No. 2 (July 13, 1967), pp. 71–78.

[68] *Longevity* refers to the average remaining lifetime at various ages. For example, in 1962, the average remaining lifetime for the newborn male in Sweden was 71.32 years. For ten-year-old Swedish males it was 63.05 years. In the United States in 1964, it was 66.9 and 59.2 for the two ages respectively.

[69] Data for 1973 are from Population Reference Bureau, Inc., *1973 World Population Data Sheet.*

A few more figures: in 1955, the average remaining lifetime at birth for U.S. males was 66.6 years; for females, 72.7. Thus, in the period 1955–73, a statistically insignificant 0.4 years had been added to male life expectancy at birth. A more significant 2.3 years had been added to the U.S. female expectancy.

In the United States, the life expectancy of the female is eight years more than that of the male. That is also true of Finland; in the Soviet Union the difference is nine years; and the figure for Hungary is ten years. But that gap is narrower in the fifty-nine other countries for which comparative 1973 data are available. In those other nations, the average difference between male and female life expectancy is 4.3 years.[70]

What do these data mean? U.S. health expenditures rose from $12 billion a year in 1949 to $83 billion in 1972. So, despite an enormous annual increase of health expenditures extending over twenty-three years, male longevity failed to increase remarkably, and female longevity improved somewhat more. Is longevity at least a partial measure of health? Yes. There are exceptions—a healthy child killed in an auto accident, for example. But, generally, healthy people live longer.

In this affluent nation can one correlate sheer expenditure with better health? More than one expert thinks not. Forbes wrote:

> In the United States there is no longer any significant relation between the money spent on health and the results achieved . . . the main determinants of longevity are cultural rather than medical . . . That is why the undoubted progress of medicine in the last fifteen years has had such a very small effect on longevity in this country and why many countries with less highly developed medicine have greater life expectancy than the United States.[71]

That this statement could come from so reliable a source is, in itself, remarkable. Correlation between expenditure and health was not always so questionable. At the turn of this century human life was abbreviated, mostly by communicable disease. Leading the list of lethal ailments were influenza, pneumonia, tuberculosis, and gastroenteritis. Arrayed against these costly killers were vast monies and efforts. Sewage systems routed danger away from human beings. Water, food, and milk were purified. Too, more effective medicines and surgical procedures were developed. Prevention of communicable illness became a way of life. An outbreak of typhoid, for example, was preventable. Its occurrence was a correctable failure. A death from tuberculosis was needless. Not even the existence of one case of tuberculosis was excusable. And pneumonia? To cure many cases of pneumonia, what was necessary? A few cents' worth of penicillin? Or Aureomycin? Or Terramycin? The money was spent. Whether by prevention or cure, communicable disease was curtailed. If a disease could not be prevented or cured, death from it was delayed. Longevity increased. And, while all these benefits were happening, health, in terms of longevity, could be equated with expenditures. In developing countries, this is still possi-

[70] *Ibid.*

[71] William H. Forbes, "Longevity and Medical Costs," *New England Journal of Medicine,* Vol. 277, No. 2 (July 13, 1967), p. 78.

ble. In the United States, according to some experts, this statistical correlation no longer seems possible. Why? The answer lies in the changed nature of the U.S. health problem.

Communicable diseases still sap the nation's strength (see Chapters 6 and 7). "In fact, flu is such a thief of life among the elderly that the National Center for Health Statistics attributed a .3 of a year increase in life expectancy between 1963 and 1964 largely to the fact that there was no influenza epidemic in the latter year."[72] As the major executioners, however, the communicable diseases have been replaced by heart disease, cancer, and stroke. All need research. But even now it is apparent to some experts that this deadly trio will not be conquered by the same kind of expenditures as in the past. By the separation of man from his microbes, typhoid fever has been almost eliminated in this country. But lung cancer is another matter. Methods of diagnosing and treating lung cancer have improved. Yet it kills more than ever before. In fifteen years it has increased almost 90 percent. Today, it accounts for more than 2.5 percent of all deaths. There is no gainsaying that routine physical examinations, early diagnosis, and more efficient organization and delivery of medical care will help reduce its death rate. But more effort must surely be expended in behavioral science. Why do people smoke? What can be done to induce them to stop this fatal dependency? Another example of the need to study behavioral science is accidents. As a cause of death in this nation, they rank fourth. For people under the age of twenty-five, they are the leading cause of death. Like lung cancer, they are responsible for more than 2.5 percent of all fatalities. How may they be reduced? By education? Yes. But behavioral science can reveal many a secret about causes of accidents and their prevention.

Increased knowledge in the behavioral sciences will hardly provide all the answers needed to increase U.S. longevity. Money for research is essential. The unequal distribution of health services must be corrected. Constant improvement of health service organization and delivery to those in greatest need—these are prime priorities.[73] (One would wish that organization and delivery of health were as efficient as that of automobiles!) But if the average longevity of the people of this nation is to be increased, more study of their behavior in their complex ecosystem is essential.

It is not only in the longevity of its citizens that the United States compares poorly with other industrial countries. In sixteen industrial nations, infant mortality rates are lower than those in the United States. Thus do data from life's opposites—infant mortality and longevity—indicate to this nation's health workers that there is much work to do.

[72] Hollis S. Ingraham, "Long Life and Good Health," a paper presented at the symposium on "Advances in Medical Care of the Aging," State Medical Society, February 17, 1966, New York. Indeed the fluctuations in U.S. death rates between 1963 (9.6) and 1973 (9.4) are attributed to the presence or absence of epidemic influenza. Influenza epidemics invariably increase death rates.

[73] The importance of these should be stressed. "Now we are waking up to the fact that emphasis on financing research, although desirable in itself, has been at the expense of equal attention to the training and other health manpower to deliver, to a growing and more demanding population, the medical knowledge and skills already existing." (Greer Williams, "Needed: A New Strategy for Health Promotion," *New England Journal of Medicine,* Vol. 279, No. 19 [November 7, 1968], p. 1033.)

on being penny-wise and pound-foolish

Some years ago a physician addressed the regular meeting of the city council of a large Midwestern city. A deliberate man, he developed his theme carefully: to cure a child cost more than to prevent his disease. His audience, largely composed of businessmen, regarded him with curious interest. Unaccustomed to this approach, some listeners were not sure they liked it. They were more comfortable with sentiment. Someone had brought a crippled child of seven to the previous meeting. The child's eyes were enormous and reproachful. A lot of money had been raised that afternoon for a crippled children's clinic.

Now the physician told them that contributions were needed to support a psychiatrist for the crippled children's clinic. Treatment was needed for the mental limp. A child, benefited by such treatment, would be less likely to inhabit costly psychiatric wards, would be less prone to populate prisons, would more likely work and pay taxes someday. Such a child would cost now but repay later. Health was an investment. Contributions to it, deductible from personal income tax this year, would lower taxes in the future. They did not need to be told of their obligations to children, the physician told them. But had they realized that health was good business? It was a bargain.

His theme was not new, he admitted. At the turn of the century, summer was the season of death in the New York tenements. Thousands of babies died of summer diarrhea. Physicians, hurrying to beat the undertaker to the tenement baby, had a slogan: "It costs $25 to save a baby, but $75 to bury it."

"Let us take another example you all know about," the physician continued. "Recently, we vaccinated 100,000 children against measles. At $1.50 per vaccination, the cost was $150,000. This means, however, that 100,000 children won't get the disease. But without the vaccine, just about all the children would have contracted measles. One measles case out of 1,000 develops encephalitis.[74] This is a brain inflammation. Had we not vaccinated the 100,000 children, we would have had 100 cases of measles encephalitis. Of these, 25 children would have died and 40 would have been permanently retarded physically and mentally, or both. We won't talk now about the 25 children that would have been lost. But to care for one retarded child during his lifetime costs $200,000. It is simple arithmetic. Forty children times $200,000 equals $8,000,000. Subtract the $150,000 cost of the vaccination program from the $8,000,000. The net profit: $7,850,000."

The speaker sat down. There was a pause and then a murmur of approval. The chairman asked for comments. One after another the businessmen rose to support the speaker. Saving a child appealed to their emotions; saving a dollar, to their business sense. It was a good way to be good.

The physician's talk had convinced the businessmen of the community that preventive health measures were indeed good business. By unanimous vote, adequate funds for the psychiatrist were made available.[75]

[74] Saul Krugman and Robert Ward, *Infectious Diseases of Children,* 4th ed. (St. Louis, 1968), p. 140.

[75] At times, government spending seems less businesslike—even incongruous. "We hear health-care costs that in their size and growth stagger everyone, but yet Washington is hesitant to allocate $\frac{1}{4000}$ of the $80 billion [Health, Education, and Welfare budget] to obtain facts that would help decide whether this huge sum is being spent appropriately." (F. J. Ingelfinger, "National Center for Health Statistics," *New England Journal of Medicine,* Vol. 289, No. 21 [November 22, 1973], p. 1143, citing "Congress Votes Bigger HEW Budget," *Medical World News,* Vol. 19, No. 38 [1973], pp. 18–19.)

In such instances, the facts are clear, the arithmetic obvious. Preventive action will save money and lives. But sometimes money is spent to support scientific research that does not seem to be beneficial. Consider this example. At an eastern university a bespectacled professor spends long hours in his laboratory studying microbes in soil. He is obeying the ancient exhortation of Job: "Speak to the earth, and it shall teach thee" (12:8). It is enough work for a lifetime. "A handful of soil contains as many microorganisms as there are human beings in the world."[76] The scientist's budget is small; he is more interested in microbes than money—and particularly in a certain microbe called *Streptomyces griseus.* He discovers that this microbe produces an antibiotic substance. It is *streptomycin,* and it is effective against the bacillus that causes tuberculosis. For the scientist, words uttered long ago in the Book of Ben Sirach in the Apocrypha have come true: "The Lord created medicines out of the earth and he that is wise shall not abhor them."

Soon streptomycin is being widely used. In the United States, many tuberculosis sanatoria close. Thousands of tuberculosis patients can go home and be treated on an ambulatory basis. In fifteen years (1954–69), "savings in hospitalization costs . . . are estimated conservatively at $3.77 billion." With streptomycin (and other drugs subsequently discovered), cured tuberculosis patients get well faster and can return to work earlier. Thus, "savings due to elimination of decreased productivity . . . are $1.2 billion."[77]

Basic research is good economics. It may begin with curiosity about a fruit fly or a forgotten microbe in a heap of soil. But it often ends with the prevention of human suffering and death, and the saving of vast amounts of money.

confusion about generic drugs

Drugs are approved by the Food and Drug Administration under *generic* names. *Trade* names are given to generic medicines by manufacturers so that they may be readily identified by buyers. Thus, *meprobamate* is the generic name for a drug named Miltown and Equanil by its two different manufacturers. Sometimes generic medicines are sold at prices much lower than those quoted by the original manufacturer. They are purported to contain exactly the same amount and kind of active principle as their more expensive counterparts. In spring 1974, for example, a pharmaceutical firm offered a generic antibiotic tablet at a cost of $6.95 per hundred; the original manufacturer's price for the same number of similar, trade-named tablets was $14.95.

They are similar but not necessarily the same. It is doubtless true that a generic drug does contain the same amount of active principle as the more expensive trade-named product. But the question that must be asked is: Does "generic equivalency" have the same meaning as "equal effectiveness"? Sometimes the answer is no. The action of a drug on an individual may be altered in a variety of ways, depending on how it is prepared. Numerous factors, other than the active medicinal principle, may affect the action of a drug. The metal

[76] Kenneth V. Thimann, *The Life of Bacteria* (New York, 1963), p. 3.

[77] H. H. Fudenberg, "The Dollar Benefits of Biomedical Research: A Cost Analysis," *Journal of Laboratory and Clinical Medicine,* Vol. 79, No. 2 (March 1972), p. 355, citing V. Hauk, "The Trend in Hospitalization Beds Available and Occupied for Tuberculosis," *Journal of Infectious Diseases,* Vol. 121 (1970), pp. 572–75.

of the cap covering the container may react with the drug, making it harmful rather than helpful. Among the other factors are the vehicle, or chemical medium, in which the drug is contained, the buffering agents, and the substances used to stabilize the drug.

What is cheapest is not always best for treatment. "Generic equivalency is frequently a fable without basis in fact; chemical equivalency of the primary agent or agents is *not* necessarily clinical nor pharmacological equivalency."[78]

fakers and phonies

> For the mind of man is far from the nature of a clear and equal glass, wherein the beams of things should reflect according to their true incidence; nay, it is rather like an enchanted glass, full of superstition and imposture.[79]

To this point, this chapter has been concerned with a variety of financial problems draining the health and pocketbooks of many people of this nation. There is yet another health care issue that has not so much to do with economy as with gullibility. Each year, millions of citizens ruin their health as they waste their money on a variety of cruel medical hoaxes. The ancient Roman writer Martial said that to deceive was "to sell smoke" (*Epigrams,* Bk. IV. epig. 5). Quacks sell nothing more substantial. It is to their costly deceptions that attention is now turned, for no health care program can help those who permit themselves to be deceived about health.

early medicine shows

Show biz and fake medicine share hardy ancestors. The medieval mountebank would mount a bench and, by act and costume, strive to gain the attention of the market populace. His medicine show drew gullible crowds, who then bought his phony remedies. Quackery[80] rolled on in tandem with performance, and in the eighteenth century, London actor-author David Garrick immortalized the playwright-quack John Hill this way: "For physic and farces, his equal there scarce is / His farce is his physic, his physic a farce is."[81]

In the New World, early California quacks also playacted. During the Gold Rush days, "they bought diplomas from physicians' widows, thereafter assuming the name of the deceased as a professional alias . . . the tip-off of an abortionist was a medication advertised . . . *not* for pregnant women."[82]

Such widely disparate Americans as "The Hoosier Poet" James Whitcomb Riley and William Avery Rockefeller (the father of the financier) spent years as traveling medicine men. Billed as the "Hoosier Wizard," Riley did everything from playing the violin and drums to giving poetic readings.[83] An engaging

[78] Max S. Sadove, Ronald Rosenberg, Floyd Heller, and Morton Shulman, "What Is a Generic Equivalent?" *American Professional Pharmacist,* Vol. 31, No. 2 (February 1965), p. 29.

[79] Francis Bacon, "Advancement of Learning," Basil Montague, ed., *The Works of Francis Bacon,* Vol. 1 (Philadelphia, 1844), p. 211.

[80] "Quacksalver" is an old word for a medical phony; the word "quack" is an abbreviation of the term and dates from 1638.

[81] Quoted in C. J. S. Thompson, *The Quacks of Old London* (New York, 1928), p. 325.

[82] George W. Groh, *Gold Fever* (New York, 1966), p. 285.

[83] James Harvey Young, *The Toadstool Millionaires* (Princeton, N.J., 1961), p. 194.

entrepreneur, Rockefeller often feigned being deaf and dumb. He attracted crowds by using his talents as a marksman.[84]

modern showmen of nutrition

P. T. Barnum said, "There's a sucker born every minute." He was not short of followers. Many a modern-day showman has parlayed the digestive system into a successful financial enterprise. Among the most unabashed of these were Bernarr Macfadden and Gaylord Hauser. Both Eleanor Roosevelt and George Bernard Shaw contributed to Macfadden publications. Shaw, a vegetarian, perhaps was at home with the Macfadden diets of carrot strips and nuts and fruits. Macfadden had, incidentally, borrowed his philosophy of chewing from a predecessor food faddist, Horace Fletcher. Thirty-two teeth inhabit the human mouth. It followed that food had to be chewed no fewer than thirty-two times. So Fletcher rhymed: "Nature will castigate / Those who don't masticate."[85]

The Duchess of Windsor wrote the introduction to the French edition of a Gaylord Hauser book.[86] What prompted her? Certainly not poverty. Was it the lure of show biz? Did she not, after all, merely join such other luminaries of the day as Greta Garbo and Paulette Goddard? They, too, were Hauser fans.[87] How were they to know the use of blackstrap molasses was nutritional nonsense? And that the M.D. on Hauser's stationery was a mistake?

> Hauser took a degree in naturopathy early in his career; a typographic error that transformed "N.D." into "M.D." on his stationery led to understandable difficulties with the American Medical Association; in recent years he has been careful to disclaim medical status and to state that his "wonder foods" are to be regarded only as diet supplements.[88]

[84] Allan Nevins, *John D. Rockefeller,* Vol. 1 (New York, 1940), Chapters 2 and 3.
[85] Ronald M. Deutsch, *The Nuts Among the Berries* (New York, 1961), p. 91.
[86] *Ibid.,* p. 163.
[87] *Ibid.,* p. 167.
[88] *M.D., Medical Newsmagazine,* Vol. 3, No. 5 (May 1959), p. 160.

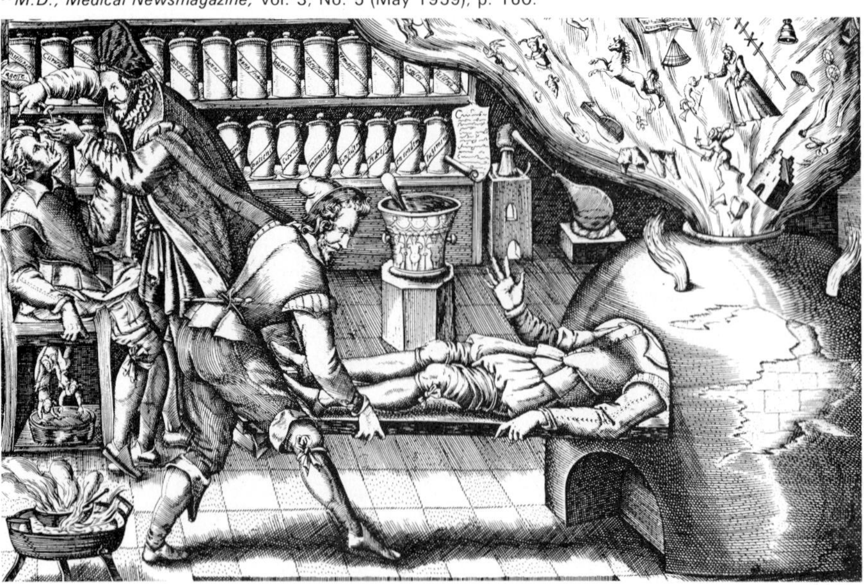

24-7 *A satire on early quackery. A 16th-century physician cures a patient of "phantasies" by baking his head. A colleague pours medicine through a funnel down another patient's throat.*

Long before Hauser, during the nineteenth century, a stream of medicines had flooded the market, concocted to "open men's purses by opening their bowels."[89] Arnold Ehret, the "professor," claimed that "every disease is constipation." He urged a rigorous regimen of fruits and nuts, fasting, and air bathing. This regimen, he claimed, offered the added dividends of relief from sterility, impotence, masturbation, and prostitution. Women followers were even offered immaculate conception. As Barnum would have predicted, there were plenty of takers.

MORPHINE!
EASY, PAINLESS, PERMANENT HOME CURE.
We will send any one addicted to MORPHINE, OPIUM, LAUDANUM, or other DRUG HABIT, a trial treatment, FREE OF CHARGE, of the most remarkable remedy for this purpose ever discovered. Containing the GREAT VITAL PRINCIPLE lacking in all other remedies. Confidential correspondence invited from all, especially PHYSICIANS.
ST. JAMES SOCIETY, 1181 BROADWAY, N. Y. CITY

....CANCER....
The following and many other reliable persons testify to my scientific treatment of cancer without the knife. T. E. C. Brinly, Louisville, Ky., noted plow manufacturer, cured 10 years ago. Prof. H. McDiarmid, Hiram College, Hiram, Ohio, cured 7 years ago. Address Dr. C. Weber, 121 W. 9th St., Cincinnati, O., for further particulars and free book.

24-8 *Perilous 19th-century quackery.*

It was the sheer absorptive qualities of the gut that alcohol peddlers found so useful—that, and human taste. At her death in 1883, Lydia Pinkham was a respected member of the Woman's Christian Temperance Union. Little, if anything, was said of the 18 percent alcohol content of her "vegetable compound." (Most present-day wines are 13 percent alcohol.) Was it not, after all, "added solely as a solvent and preservative"? The recommended dosage was, nevertheless, more than generous. A full, even overflowing, tablespoon, four times daily, was not too much for "a falling of the womb." For Lydia's devoted customers, prohibition was no hardship. The Pinkham people were part of a pattern. For seventy years, Kansas voted for prohibition, meanwhile merrily tippling such spirited drink as Wild Cherry Tonic and Dr. Worme's Gesundheit Bitters.[90] Another cure-all, called Hostetter's Bitters, originally contained 39 percent alcohol. It was often dispensed in saloons by the shot.[91]

There were quacks who were mechanically inclined, and they did not limit their machines to the gut. Perhaps inspired by the Industrial Revolution, many got off to an early start in this country. By the end of the eighteenth century, the Chief Justice of the Supreme Court, numerous legislators, and even George Washington had been hoodwinked. From a Colonial medical humbug, Elisha Perkins, they all bought a pair of brass and iron rods that was supposed to cure all ills. Such wholehearted governmental support helped Perkins become rich.[92] He was but one of the first of a long line. Not long ago, for example, Dinsha P. Ghadiali, the man with "fifteen college degrees," invented the Spectro-Chrome. It was a metal box housing a one-thousand-watt bulb. In front of the bulb, he could slide panes of colored glass. For each disease, he had a different colored glass. Ruth Drowns fixed herself the Drowns' Radio Vision Instrument. A drop of blood (any drop would do) was all she needed for a diagnosis. The patient could be miles away. The tragedy of all such fraud remains with the sick. By phony tests and treatment, individuals with early treatable disease, such as operable cancer, may be delayed into a hopeless stage of their disease.

kidney quacks

The kidney rivals the intestine for the number of quacks who have exploited it. If not an actual kidney quack, Ann Moore, the "Fasting Woman of Tutburg," certainly gave the phonies of her time something to think about. She solemnly swore, in 1809, to have neither eaten nor drunk a thing for five years. Many

[89] James Harvey Young, *The Medical Messiahs* (Princeton, N.J., 1967), p. 21.
[90] Gerald Carson, *One for a Man, Two for a Horse* (Garden City, N.Y., 1961), p. 44.
[91] Hostetter V. Sommers, cited in James Harvey Young, *The Toadstool Millionaires,* p. 130.
[92] Morris Fishbein, *Fads and Quackery in Healing* (New York, 1932), p. 12.

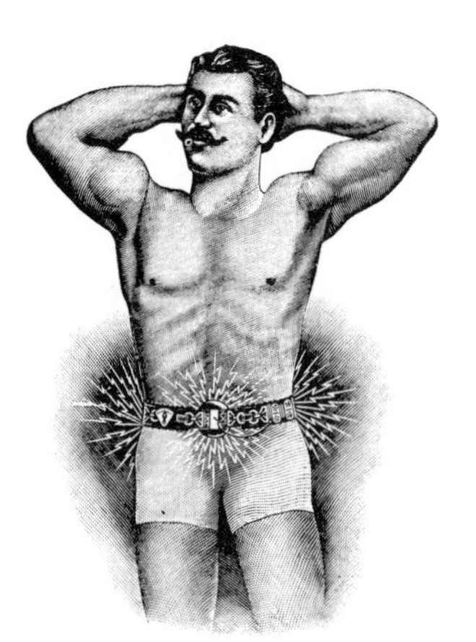

24-9 *This "Giant Power Heidelberg Electric Belt" was sold through a mail-order catalog for $18, and promised "quick cure of all nervous and organic disorders."*

a credulous Englishman believed her. A doubting Dr. Alexander Henderson revealed the fraud when he noted her sweating skin. Nor did he help Ann Moore's claim when "chance contact of his foot with an earthenware vessel hidden under the bed left him in no doubt that her kidneys were functioning very much as other people's."[93]

Quacks used to diagnose illness not by examining the patient, but merely by inspecting the urine. "What says the doctor to my water?" asks Sir John Falstaff in Shakespeare's *The Second Part of King Henry the Fourth.* His page answers: "He said, sir, the water itself was a good healthy water, but for the party that owned it, he might have moe diseases than he knew for" (I.ii.1–5).

The seventeenth-century English enriched several quacks who claimed to know the secret of turning urine to gold. The injection of a woman's urine into an immature rabbit can now provide a useful pregnancy test. A character in a seventeenth-century English play obtains this diagnosis without a rabbit: "I was once sicke and I tooke my water . . . to a doctors . . . The doctor told me I was with child."[94]

Modern quacks have been no less imaginative than their predecessors. But the kidneys are a grim choice for quackery. Chronic kidney disease affects the entire body. Heart disease and hypertension often accompany the kidney's inefficiencies. "Bones can break, muscles can atrophy, glands can loaf, even the brain can go to sleep, without immediately endangering our survival; but should the kidneys fail to manufacture the proper kind of blood, neither bone, muscle, gland nor brain could carry on."[95]

why are quacks so successful?

In *A Black Job,* the English poet Robert Hood wrote more than a century ago that

> A certain portion of the human race
> Has certainly a taste for being diddled.

However, it is more than merely a desire to be cheated that prompts people to seek out modern mountebanks. Quacks succeed primarily by exploiting susceptibility and fear of death and disability. Latent in humankind, too, is "a primitive craving for the supernatural . . . here primitive medicine and quackery are at one."[96]

Others who seek quacks do so out of hostile rebellion against the omnipotent parent-physician figure. He is remembered, resented, and cloaked in suspicion. To all this must be added the unfortunate approach of some physicians. Always busy, some are at times unable to take time to listen. A quack always listens.

Particularly vulnerable is the chronically ill person. Some illnesses are char-

[93] Alexander Henderson, *An Examination of the Imposture of Ann Moore,* quoted in J. C. Drummond and Anne Wilbraham, *The Englishman's Food* (London, 1939), pp. 343–44.

[94] Thomas Dekker, *North-ward Hoe,* quoted in Herbert Silvette, *The Doctor on the Stage* (Knoxville, Tenn., 1967), p. 22.

[95] Homer W. Smith, *From Fish to Philosopher* (Boston, 1953), p. 4.

[96] Fielding H. Garrison, "On Quackery as a Reversion to Primitive Medicine," quoted in *Bulletin of the New York Academy of Medicine, 1925–35* (New York, 1966), p. 602.

acterized by spontaneous episodes of temporary improvement (remission). An individual with multiple sclerosis, for example, may improve for short periods during the progressive downhill course of the disease. Wandering from quack to quack, the patients find renewed but false hope with each new remission, sinking, in the end, into cruel despondency.

how to identify quacks

One distinguished nutritionist offers these pointers:[97]

1. They always have something to sell.
2. They offer quick cures on a money-back basis.
3. They proclaim themselves experts with vastly important "professional" associations.
4. Testimonials and phony case histories, rather than responsible studies published in reputable journals, are their stock in trade.
5. Scientific data are distorted rather than reported.
6. They always condemn one's present way of eating.
7. They claim that such institutions as the American Medical Association and the Food and Drug Administration are "corrupted" by "big business" and conspire to persecute them to hide the "truths" that they alone possess.

how may the quack be defeated?

How may the quack be defeated? By dispelling the fear on which he breeds. And this can best be accomplished through enlightenment and understanding. In an entirely different context, a distinguished physicist recently quoted still another scientist in a manner singularly appropriate to the present subject. "Maria Sklodowska-Curie said: 'Nothing in life is to be feared—it is only to be understood! Now is the time to understand more—so that we may fear less.'"[98]

summary

Health care programs in the United States may be classified into three types:

1. programs that *organize* to provide health services, including *hospitals* (pages 725–26), *nursing homes* (pages 726–27), *physicians* (pages 727–31), *free clinics* (pages 731–33), and *dentists* (page 733).

2. programs that *finance* health services. Such programs may be profit-making *private* organizations such as Blue Cross–Blue Shield (page 734), independent insurance plans (page 734), or commercial insurance plans offering hospitalization, life, disability, and major medical insurance (pages 735–36). The first system of nonprofit *public* health insurance in the United States was Medicare and Medicaid (pages 737–40). In 1972, a law was enacted establishing professional standards review organizations (PSROs) to review the performance of physicians receiving Medicare and Medicaid funds (page 740). An increasing number of proposals have been made in recent years for a system of compulsory national health insurance (pages 741–42).

3. programs that both *organize* and *finance* health services, including compre-

[97] Frederick J. Stare, *Eating for Good Health* (New York, 1964), pp. 154–55.
[98] Glenn T. Seaborg, "Need We Fear Our Nuclear Future?" *Bulletin of the Atomic Scientists*, Vol. 24, No. 1 (January 1968), p. 42.

hensive prepaid group practice plans (pages 742–43), neighborhood health centers (page 743), and health maintenance organizations (HMOs; pages 743–44).

Health care problems in the United States include rising costs (pages 744–45), unavailability in some areas (page 745), and uneven quality (page 748). Despite enormous and ever-increasing expenditures for health care, the United States compares unfavorably with other industrial nations in such areas as life expectancy and infant mortality (pages 748–50). Another problem affecting health care is a widespread refusal to acknowledge that basic research and prevention of illness are generally less costly than treatment (pages 751–52). Confusion also arises over the question of using drugs under their *generic* or their *trade* names (pages 752–53). Another major health care problem is *quackery* (pages 753–57), which deters many sick people from seeking legitimate medical care—sometimes until it is too late, as in cancer.

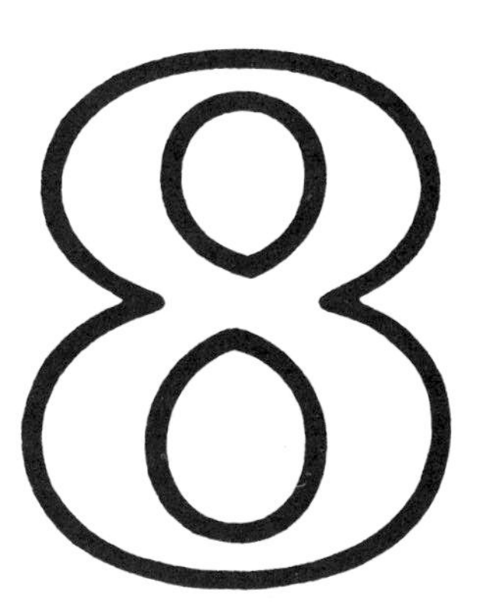

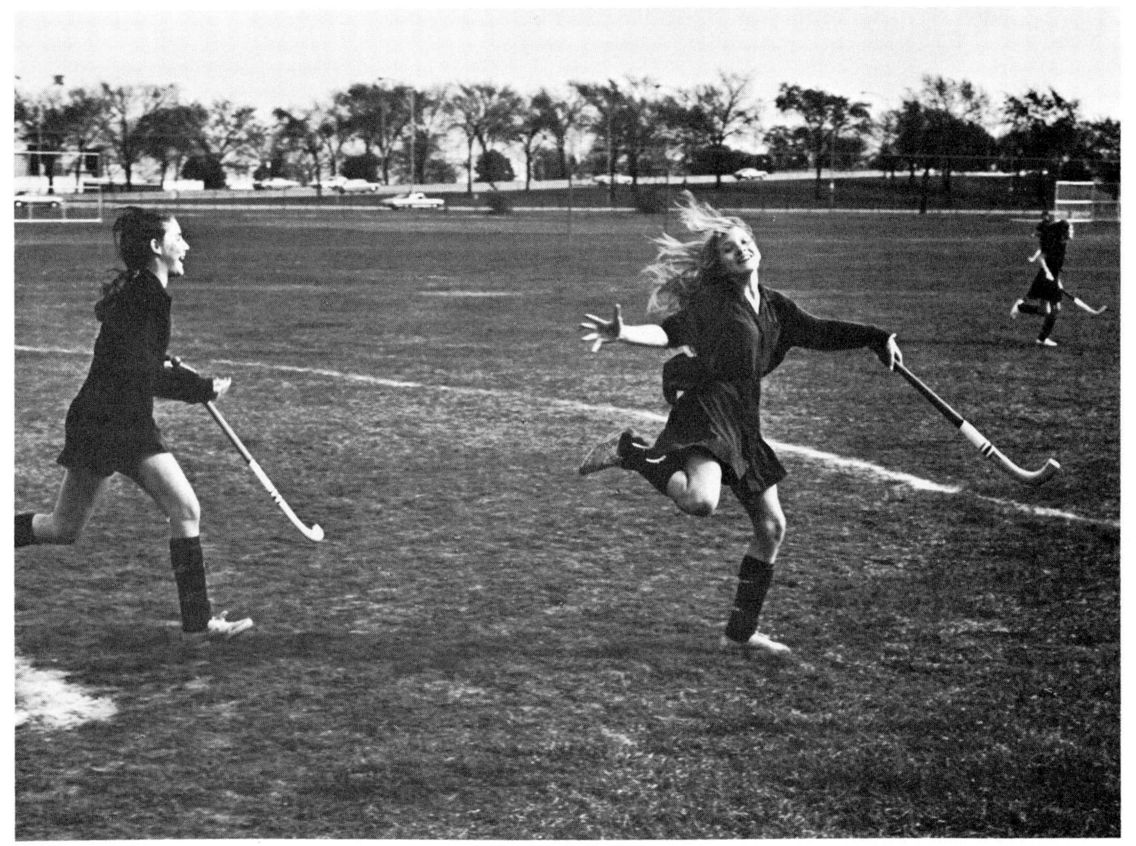

"I must laugh and dance and sing, / Youth is such a lovely thing" (*Aline Thomas, "A Song of Youth"*)

epilogue

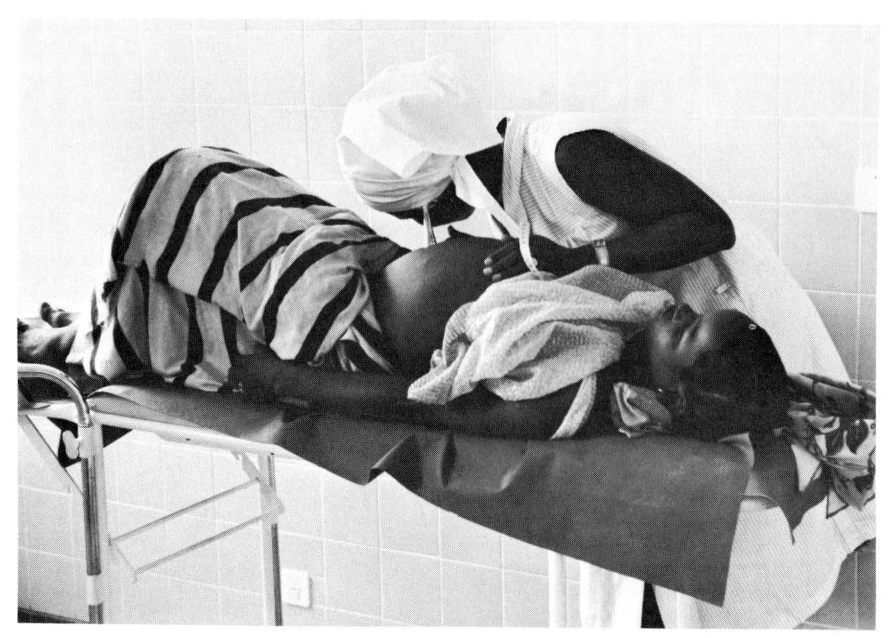

A trained midwife in central Africa examining a patient.

the last chapter: health for the freeman

25

In health there is freedom.
Health is the first of all liberties.[1]

modern miracles

engineers join the health team

In a San Francisco hospital, a young patient intently watches a television screen. Beside him sits his psychiatrist. There is a close-up of hands gesticulating jerkily, then of eyes, troubled and suspicious. The camera lengthens the shot and includes the entire figure of the main character. Almost oblivious to other people seated in the room, he talks incessantly. Slowly, the camera picks up the expressions of the silent onlookers. The patient watches, absorbed. For it is he who is the main character. Only a few moments before he was in the waiting room. Instant replay television is showing him himself.

After two centuries the wish of an eighteenth-century poet becomes reality: "Oh wad some power the giftie gie us/ To see oursels as others see us!/ It wad frae monie a blunder free us."[2] Uninvolved, the electronic device has involved the patient. And yet the patient sees himself apart from himself and as others see him. He confronts himself. Now, with his view uncluttered, he may improve.[3]

Four hundred miles to the south, in Los Angeles, a medical specialist ponders a patient's heart problem. To improve the heart muscle tone, to strengthen the heart's action, the drug digitalis has been prescribed. But digitalis tends to accumulate in body tissues. Now the patient complains of a loss of appetite—one sign of early digitalis intoxication. Of critical importance is how well the kidneys function. Impaired kidney function means diminished digitalis excretion. Consequently, within the body, the drug rises to poisonous levels.

Carefully, the internist reviews the patient's chart. Finally, he telephones the University of California at Los Angeles Medical Center. He tells a physician there about the type of digitalis used and results of the patient's kidney function tests. The information is fed into a computer. Previously, the machine had been programmed to receive and correlate such information. Within moments it has computed the ability of this particular patient's kidneys to eliminate this particular kind of digitalis. Then it tells how much digitalis accumulates in his body. From this information the doctor decides the best level of digitalis for the patient. "The computer then prints a suggested dose program, tailored to the patient's kidney function, to achieve and maintain that level."[4]

The technology developed in the space programs has proved to have many applications to medicine. Doubtless it will have many more. Medical discoveries have often followed the physical sciences. The ancient Greeks knew about the

[1] Henri Frédéric Amiel, quoted in *M.D., Medical Newsmagazine,* Vol. 7, No. 4 (April 1963), p. 109. In his *Journal,* the Swiss philosopher wrote on Easter Monday, April 14, 1879: "Sickness makes one dependent . . . sickness is a blow to our freedom and our dignity." (*The Private Journal of Henri Frédéric Amiel,* tr. by Van Wyck Brooks and Charles Wyck Brooks [New York, 1935], p. 569.)
[2] Robert Burns, "To a Louse."
[3] Harry A. Wilmer, "Innovative Uses of Videotape on a Psychiatric Ward," cited in "Videotaping in Psychiatric Evaluation," *Modern Medicine,* Vol. 36, No. 23 (November 4, 1968), p. 88.
[4] "Clicking Clinicians," *M.D., Medical Newsmagazine,* Vol. 12, No. 11 (November 1968), p. 91.

heart and blood vessels, but it was not until the development of the water pump that Harvey was able to understand how the heart circulates blood through vessels (see pages 215–16). Physical optics enabled Leeuwenhoek to invent the microscope and open the whole field of the germ theory of disease.

The flywheel, an ancient device, is merely a spinning wheel that stores mechanical energy. "Advances in materials and mechanical design make it possible to use giant flywheels for the storage of energy in electric-power systems and smaller ones for the propulsion of automobiles, trucks and buses."[5] The hope here for a new, clean energy source is obvious. In the near future, better methods of predicting weather patterns will result in better management of agricultural and mineral resources as mankind monitors day-to-day inventories of various crops and the distribution of plant disease, water, and mineral resources. Space exploration will bring a better understanding of air and water pollution. Weather satellites have already saved many lives. At the turn of this century, a hurricane in Galveston, Texas, killed more than five thousand people. In the summer of 1971, a hurricane of similar intensity almost destroyed Corpus Christi, Texas. But almost two days of warning, provided by a weather satellite, made possible mass evacuations.

Human care satellites[6] have been useful in emergencies on more than one occasion. In a remote Alaska village, in March 1972, eleven-year-old Sally Sam lay critically ill. By means of the Applications Technology Satellite, contact was made with a physician in Tanana. The diagnosis: acute appendicitis. "Within fifteen minutes the girl was picked up by an aircraft and taken to a hospital."[7] Since 1971, the experimental communications satellite has provided daily two-way radio contact between trained native health aides in remote Alaska communities and a Public Health Service physician. Doctor-to-doctor communication is also possible. The satellite radio also provides an opportunity for villagers to consult an expert regarding their problems: for example, a veterinarian has discussed how to keep dogs healthy with the driver of a dog team. Health-education matters are also discussed, such as the importance of well-baby clinics and the building of wells and outhouses. The launching of another satellite was planned for April 1974.[8]

Use of the satellite does not stop here. As 1973 drew to a close, plans were being made to launch a space satellite as another step in the development of a national biomedical communications network, to be used for such purposes as the training of medical students, continuing medical training, consultation between specialists and isolated physicians, and the transmission of X-rays, medical records, and other medical information. It is said that a clinic, hospital, or medical school would need only a television set and a dish-type antenna (at a cost of about $3,000) to receive satellite-relayed information. Being planned

[5] Richard F. Post and Stephen F. Post, "Flywheels," *Scientific American,* Vol. 229, No. 6 (December 1973), p. 17.

[6] A term suggested by Kenneth T. Bird, an internist at Massachusetts General Hospital, who has been intimately involved in health education "telemedicine."

[7] "Diagnosis by Satellite: Doctors Hail Alaska Test," *Science News,* Vol. 102, No. 2 (July 8, 1972), p. 22.

[8] Heather E. Hudson and Edwin B. Parker, "Medical Communication in Alaska by Satellite," *New England Journal of Medicine,* Vol. 289, No. 25 (December 20, 1973), pp. 1351–53.

for launch in October 1975 is a two-way educational television link between the United States and Canada.

By 1974, telemedicine networks had been established in various states. The day is foreseen "when the contents of the physician's little black bag will include a little black box."[9] It, in turn, will contain electronic circuits and tiny television tubes. Coded messages will be unscrambled from distant telemedicine stations by means of standard telephone lines. Indeed, at a cost of $2.50 a minute plus $10 monthly for the terminal, U.S. scientists can now immediately exchange research information with the Soviet Union. It is the first communications link with the U.S.S.R. since the White House–Kremlin "hot line." Two-week delays can thus be avoided, so researchers need not be bogged down waiting for a few pieces of information. Moreover, patients involved in the two nations' joint drug treatment program for cancer need not suffer the serious reactions that might result from delay.[10] (See also page 132.)

The marriage of medicine and engineering has produced a variety of useful offspring. Surgery, teletype, television, satellite, ultrasound, and computer—all combine to bring a new era in health care. In a Swedish hospital a man's cancerous lung is removed. In his recovery room is an input terminal. Via the input terminal, the nurse promptly feeds vital information—temperature, blood pressure, laboratory test results—into a computer. In the doctor's office, or his home, there is an output terminal, which is connected to a television screen. The doctor receives information immediately. Perhaps a laboratory test indicates that a certain medication might help the patient. Into his computer connection the doctor feeds certain specific information. From it he expects an organized answer. "What," for example, he may ask, "is the hospital experience with this new drug?" Within moments the answer is formulated on his screen. From his office he relays instructions to the hospital room. In an emergency, time is the enemy. Computers speed accurate help to the sick.[11]

Yet another diagnostic advance: The physician suspects that a pregnant patient is carrying a grossly abnormal fetus. Ultrasonics (an echo reflection technique) will tell him the truth. As one physician has put it: "The womb is a perfect water tank. Sound travels beautifully through it."[12] Also being developed is a scope that can be inserted into the uterus, as (and perhaps with) an amniotic needle. It is less than .08 inch in diameter, yet it is so precise that by inserting it into only one place, the operator will be able to count the fetus's fingernails. It is now being used experimentally in animals and should be available for human use in a few years.[13]

From all these innovations a new and urgent discipline has developed—*biomedical engineering.* Just as there are engineering systems, there are also

[9] "Small Hospitals Get T.V. Link to Medical Center," *Journal of the American Medical Association,* Vol. 226, No. 12 (December 17, 1973), p. 1408.

[10] This discussion of the medical uses of television is based in part on a series of investigations by the associate editor of the *Journal of the American Medical Association,* Vol. 226, No. 12 (December 17, 1973), pp. 1401–09.

[11] A. Marcus, "The Computer Comes to the Patient's Bedside," *World Health* (August 1968), pp. 8–15.

[12] Joan Lynn Arehart, "Sounding Out the Womb," *Science News,* Vol. 100, No. 26 (December 25, 1971), pp. 424–25. This article briefly describes the technique and its values and is recommended.

[13] Janet Kreiling, "Genetic Manipulation: A Fresh Problem Brings Fears and Questions," *Technology Review,* Vol. 75, No. 5 (March–April 1973), pp. 60–61.

biological systems. The diffusion of a fluid, for example, through a semipermeable membrane resulting in pressure equalization on both sides is *osmosis*. That basic bioengineering fact is being put to good experimental use. By osmosis some anesthetics may seep through tubes into the blood. Many patients will eventually receive anesthetics in this way. Pain relief without sleep is a possibility.[14] Body repair will be easier. And miraculous, too. Consider this case.

replanting, replacing, repairing

The date: April 10, 1965. Near Denver, a twenty-one-month-old girl is picked from a car-train wreck. She is still conscious. Her entire left arm is severed. A state patrolman looks for the arm and finds it alongside the track. In twenty minutes both the child and her amputated arm are at the University of Colorado Medical Center. With deliberate speed surgeons work to replant the arm. Much later they will report, "Recirculation of the extremity was instituted 4 hours and fifty minutes after the accident and resulted in return of color to the arm," and, in 18 months, the child "would use her left hand to . . . comb a doll's hair."[15]

It was not the first successful replantation of a human arm. That had been done in 1962.[16] But in 1967, an even more startling surgical first was performed.

A team of surgeons in Cape Town, South Africa, had completed a singularly taxing operation. While relaxing with a postoperative cup of tea, one of them said, "Perhaps we should tell someone what we've done."

It was agreed to tell the hospital superintendent.

"Was it on a dog?" the superintendent asked.

"No, on a human," was the reply.[17]

Thus did Christiaan Barnard announce the first heart transplant.[18]

Throughout the world physicians read about it in this scientific reference:

> Barnard, C. N.: A Human Cardiac Transplant: An Interim Report of a Successful Operation Performed at Grotte Schuur Hospital, Cape Town, *S. Afr. Med. J.*, 41:1271–74 (Dec. 30) 1967.

25-1 *This Chinese woman's arm, blown off by an explosion, was successfully replanted.*

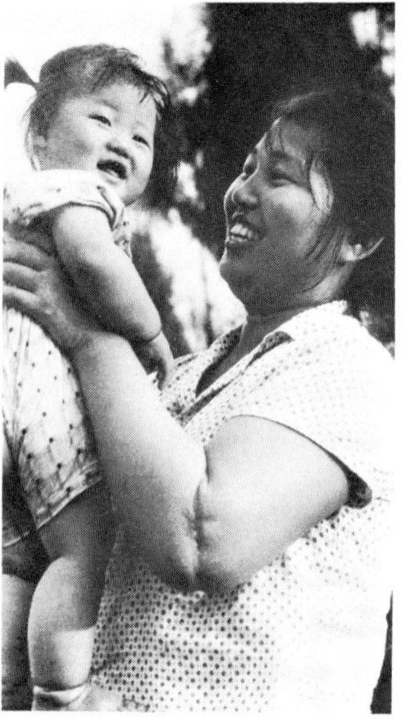

[14] "Engineering the Body," *Science News*, Vol. 94, No. 20 (November 16, 1968), p. 493.

[15] Jens G. Rosenkrantz, Robert G. Sullivan, Keasley Welch, James S. Miles, Keith M. Sadler, and Bruce C. Paton, "Replantation of an Infant's Arm," *New England Journal of Medicine*, Vol. 277, No. 11 (March 16, 1967), pp. 609–11. Before the accident the little girl's mother considered her to be left-handed.

[16] Ten years after that, a workman named Russell Stratton accidentally severed his left hand with an electric saw. Somewhat "taken aback," as he later recalled, he nevertheless calmly shut off the saw, fished his hand out of the scrap box, put it in his carpenter's apron, found his foreman, twice revived the fainting foreman who was finally able to help him with a tourniquet, got to a nearby hospital, and had his hand successfully replanted. ("Calm Accident Victim 'Saves' His Severed Hand," *Journal of the American Medical Association*, Vol. 216, No. 2 [April 12, 1971], pp. 233, 238.) In another instance, a toe was used to replace a right thumb that had been lost in an accident. (Arthur S. Freese, "What's the Future for Human Transplants?" *Science Digest*, Vol. 71, No. 6 [June 1972], p. 12.) It was a valuable exchange. Without a thumb, the hand is but a hook. For advanced premedical students, a recommended review of limb replantations is William R. Vath, "A Decade of Limb Transplantations," *Journal of the American Medical Association*, Vol. 233, No. 2 (January 8, 1973), pp. 121–26, 131.

[17] *Medical Tribune*, Vol. 10, No. 68 (August 25, 1969), p. 2.

[18] A number of heart transplants have since been done, with varying degrees of success (see page 765). They have emphasized the need for a precise legal definition of death. On September 10, 1973, one man shot another in the head. Two days later, physicians declared the victim neurologically dead. After the consent of the victim's wife and mother was obtained, his heart was removed and used as a transplant. California state law requires that a potential heart donor must be pronounced dead by a physician before a transplant can be performed. However, the law does not define death. The assailant's defense at his trial: the victim's heart was still beating when it was removed, therefore he had not caused the death. ("Transplant Is Issue in Murder Trial: Death Due to Gunshot or Removal of Victim's Heart?" *American Medical News*, Vol. 16, No. 14 [November 12, 1973], p. 11.)

Today's success is tomorrow's commonplace. Tissue banks (which are distinct from organ-sharing programs) have made possible the storage of connective and structural tissues such as bone, dura (the outermost of the membranes covering the brain and spinal cord; see page 265), heart valves, and fascia (the fibrous tissue investing the muscles and various body organs). Thousands of patients have received tissues from such banks, resulting in the "salvage of many young members of our society who would otherwise face a lifetime of disability."[19] Even an animal brain-tissue transplant has become a reality. It has long been believed that once they have been specifically formed and positioned, brain cells do not divide and, therefore, neither regenerate nor heal.[20] Using brain cells of week-old rats that were not yet completely organized, surgeons have, at last, successfully transplanted rat brain tissue.[21] Surgical techniques have also been developed to transplant a uterus in the rhesus monkey.[22] And, for the first time, pregnancy recently occurred from a transplanted ovary. The genetic characteristics of the child born from such a pregnancy would be that of the donor, not of the recipient. Whether this would create psychological problems for both women—or for the child—remains to be seen.[23]

Of the 184 human heart transplants performed between January 1, 1968, and January 1, 1972, the longest time that a surviving recipient lived with a functioning graft was forty months; of the 155 liver transplants, the longest surviving recipient lived forty-one months; of 28 lung transplants, ten months; of 131 bone marrow transplants,[24] forty months; and of 8,256 kidney recipi-

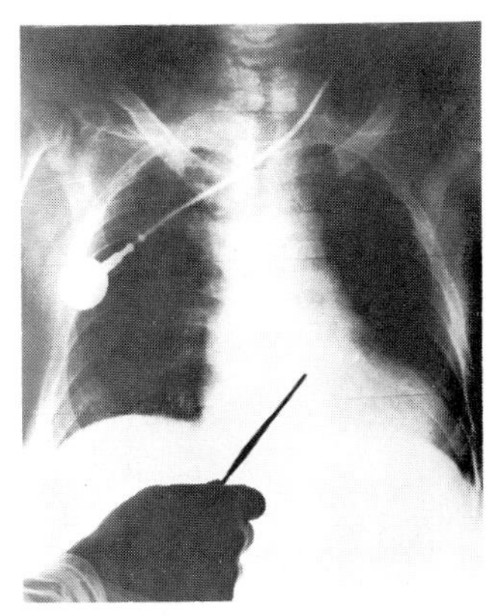

25-2 *The first X-ray photograph of the chest area of Louis Washkansky, the first recipient of a heart transplant. The pointer indicates the location of the transplanted heart. The cylindrical object at the left is the electrode of the cardiograph monitor attached to his chest.*

[19] Kenneth W. Sell, "Long-Term Tissue and Organ Preservation," *Transplantation Proceedings*, Vol. 3, No. 1 (March 1971), p. 274.

[20] Why some amphibians like the salamander, and crustaceans like the lobster, can repair or grow back (regenerate) missing parts has long mystified man. The lobster, for example, can catch its claw and, when unable to free it, leave it behind. Another claw will form in its place. (It has been suggested that this capacity could be most useful for pickpockets.) One theory is that man lost most of his regenerative ability when, during evolution, most of the body's electrical activity came to occur in the brain. The only truly regenerative growth process left to man is in fracture healing (see caption of body chart 2 in the color section). Recently some limb regeneration has been accomplished with rats. The regeneration is sparked by an electrical current. The current causes cells to reverse their differentiation process and to form cell masses which redifferentiate into the missing part. The strength of the electric current is critical; too little results in no regeneration; too much destroys tissue. (Someday, this may be useful in slowing down or reversing tumor growth.) It has been found that electrical stimulation by direct current can promote faster healing of such tissues as bone and ulcerated or burned skin. One expert feels that widespread use of these procedures is premature because they tamper with the basic materials and organization of life; moreover, administration of direct current to bone marrow leads to structural changes similar to those associated with bone cancer. He also cautions that applying direct electric current to the central nervous system might produce changes in behavior and understanding abilities that may not become evident for years. ("Electric Current Sparks Mammalian Tissue Regeneration," *Journal of the American Medical Association;* Vol. 223, No. 5 [January 29, 1973], pp. 483–84, 494.)

[21] "Transplanted Brains and Sprouting Nerves," *New Scientist,* Vol. 54, No. 792 (April 20, 1972), p. 118.

[22] "Transplant of Uterus in Monkeys," *Science News,* Vol. 100, No. 1 (July 3, 1971), p. 11.

[23] "Pregnancy from Transplanted Ovary," *Science News,* Vol. 102, No. 22 (November 22, 1972), p. 345.

[24] Bone marrow transplants have been performed to provide immune systems to people who were born without them. In 1973, for example, a Copenhagen boy was being provided with life-saving lymphocytes as the result of a bone marrow transplant from his uncle. By April 1973, at least sixteen youngsters in the world had immune systems because of successful bone marrow transplants. When only T cells (see page 142) are missing, only a thymus graft is necessary. Some years ago a Miami baby was born without a thymus. It was decided to try a fetal thymus transplant. Why fetal? Because it was hoped that the cells of a fetal thymus would be too immature to be rejected (see pages 144–45). In London, a researcher was known to maintain a tissue bank of fetal organs. From Miami came an urgent request for a fetal thymus. From London came the laconic telegraphed reply: "Thymus arriving Miami BOAC flight 661." Within hours the thymus was transplanted into the six-month-old boy's abdominal muscle. In 1973, at the age of six, his immune system was normal. Bone marrow and thymus transplants are not always successful, but progress in this area is undeniable and remarkable. (Barbara J. Culliton, "Restoring Immunity: Thymus and Marrow Transplants May Do It," *Science,* Vol. 180, No. 4082 [April 13, 1973], pp. 168–70.)

ents, the longest survivor was a monozygotic twin (see page 246)—seventeen years.[25]

Artificial heart valves and portions of blood vessels have brought a healthier life to scores of the otherwise disabled. Figure 25-3 shows an aneurysm of the abdominal aorta and a Dacron graft that has replaced and taken over the work of the damaged segment. Those photographs were taken at Baylor University, where, too, an artificial heart pump temporarily assumes the vital function of an ailing, failing heart. The exhausted organ rests and heals. Then the artificial pump is removed. In a few weeks the rescued patient goes home, his lease on life renewed. At times another technique may be indicated. To control an erratic heart, a pacemaker may need to be inserted beneath the skin. Its impulses bring regularity to the heart beat, life to its beneficiary. Every four or five years, batteries for the electric pacemaker have to be replaced. Recently a new radioisotope battery was developed. For a decade or more this battery—a small nuclear power plant—may safely generate electrical impulses. Still another electrical unit, worn by the selected heart patient, brings relief from the suffocating pain of angina pectoris.[26] When he feels the impending attack, the patient presses a button. Electrical stimulation of certain nerves brings almost instant relief.

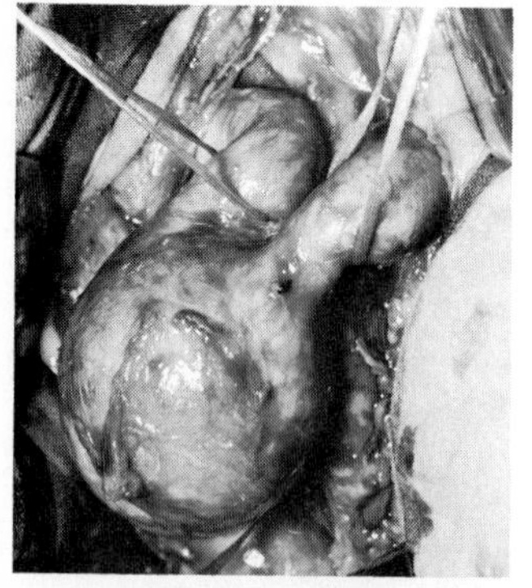

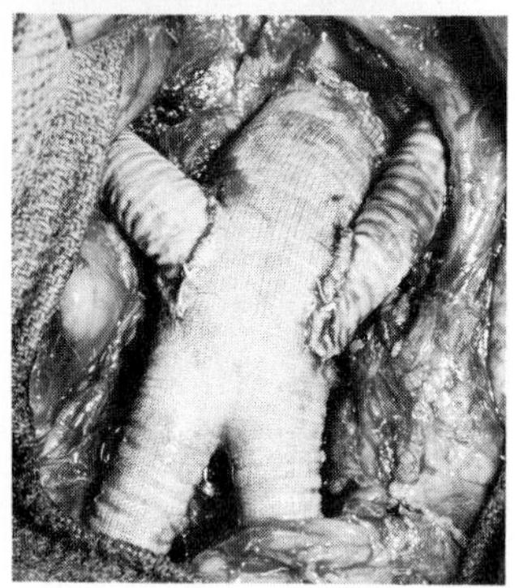

25-3 *An aneurysm of the abdominal aorta* (top) *and a Dacron graft* (bottom), *which has replaced portions of the abdominal aorta* (*the large tube*), *the iliac arteries* (*the bottom branches*), *and the renal arteries* (*the top branches*). *An aneurysm is the sac formed by abnormal dilation of the weakened wall of a blood-filled blood vessel. The wall is impaired by disease, such as advanced atherosclerosis or syphilis.*

wiring the brain

Nor have the possibilities of electrical stimulation been neglected elsewhere. Electrodes have been placed in the pleasure centers of the brain. So intense is the pleasure obtained by pressing the connected lever that starving animals have preferred it to eating.[27] Upon stimulating the pleasure centers of his brain via similar electrodes, one man had the sensation of "building up to a sexual orgasm. He was unable to achieve the orgastic end point, however, and explained that his frequent, sometimes frantic, pushing of the . . . button was an attempt to reach a 'climax.' "[28] Another patient became "more communicative and flirtatious and she ended by openly expressing her desire to marry the therapist."[29] Several physicians have recently reported the successful use of brain stimulation to relieve the pain of inoperable cancer. One patient described the effect of stimulation as resembling that of "two martinis."[30] For a variety of valid therapeutic reasons wires have been left in the thinking brains of many patients. The presence of electrical conductors in their heads has produced no discomfort. "Some women have shown their feminine adaptability . . . by

[25] Arthur S. Freese, "What's the Future for Human Transplants?" p. 10.

[26] Angina pectoris is a pain in the chest, accompanied by a feeling of suffocation, due to a lack of blood supply (and therefore oxygen) to the heart muscle (see Chapter 9).

[27] Leon R. Kass, "The New Biology: What Price Relieving Man's Estate?" *Science,* Vol. 174, No. 4011 (November 19, 1971), p. 781. Electrical stimulation of a certain portion of the brain can stimulate not only pleasurable sensations, but also the desire to kill. Carbachol is a substance that mimics the behavior of a chemical nerve transmitter called acetylcholine. Application of carbachol to a specific part of the brain of a rat turned it into a vicious killer. "The killing elicited by carbachol is . . . specific for the chemical and for the site of action, leading to the obvious hypothesis that the natural killing behavior of rats is mediated by the action of acetylcholine." ("A Chemical Control of Killing," *New Scientist,* Vol. 45, No. 689 [February 19, 1970], p. 342.)

[28] Peter Nathan, *The Nervous System* (Philadelphia and New York, 1969), p. 243.

[29] Leon R. Kass, "The New Biology: What Price Relieving Man's Estate?" citing J. M. Delgado, *Physical Control of the Mind: Towards a Psychocivilized Society* (New York, 1969), p. 185.

[30] "Striatal Influence on Facial Pain," cited in Donald B. Louria, "Some Aspects of the Current Drug Scene," *Pediatrics,* Vol. 42, No. 6 (December 1968), pp. 904–11.

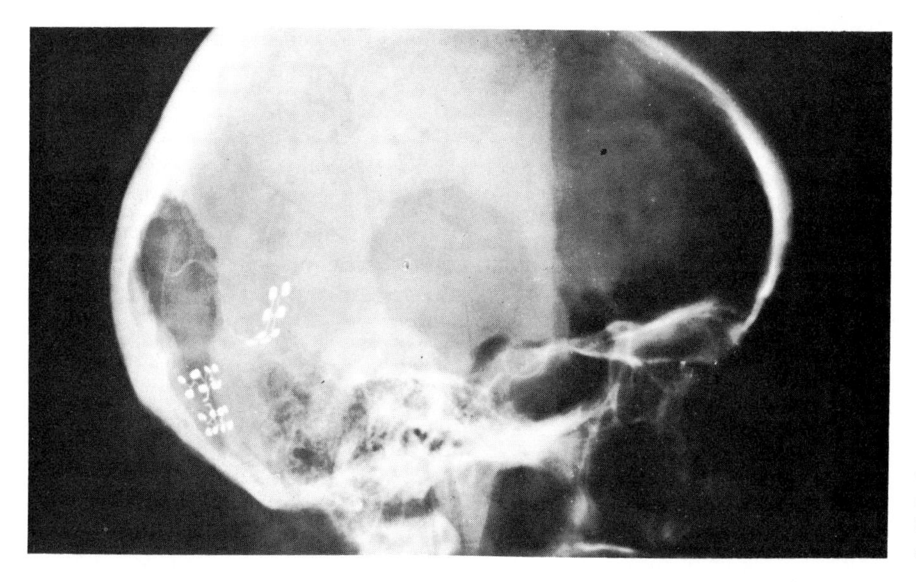

25-4 *X-ray showing electrodes implanted on the surface of the cerebellum of the brain. Electrical stimulation of the area controls epilepsy.*

wearing attractive hats or wigs to conceal their electrical headgear."[31] One of the most remarkable recent accomplishments involving the insertion of electrode arrays into the brain has enabled one totally blind man to see a pattern of light that he can reproduce (see the Preface).[32]

Do these remarkable surgical events threaten to produce an electrically controlled society? How is the electrical threat related to the drug threat? Creating, if not answering, such basic societal enigmas, the scientific quest for new knowledge continues. Kidney transplants? They are almost common. So are artificial kidneys. In this country several thousand people depend on them to survive.

acupuncture: needles in a haystack?

Acupuncture is an ancient Chinese method of relieving pain or treating illness by inserting needles into certain parts of the body. Some have dismissed it as sorcery, sleight of hand, hypnotism, and merely a tool of national propaganda. Others have called it a cure for ailments of all kinds, from cancer to chilblains. It is neither. Chinese scientists do not consider all acupuncture to be the same. Acupuncture has been used for anesthesia during some surgical procedures for less than twenty years; it has been in use as a folk medicine for treatment for more than twenty centuries. Western-trained Chinese physicians doubt the treatment claims made for acupuncture much more than the claims that are made for it as an anesthetic. Some acupuncture anesthesia has been shown to be effective; its use for treatment has not.[33] Acupuncture anesthesia cannot be hypnotism, unless one can accept the unacceptable notion of hypnotism of newborn infants and animals.

[31] Leon R. Kass, "The New Biology: What Price Relieving Man's Estate?" citing J. M. Delgado, *Physical Control of the Mind: Towards a Psychocivilized Society*, p. 88.

[32] W. H. Dobelle, M. G. Mladejovsky, and J. P. Girvin, "Artificial Vision for the Blind: Electrical Stimulation of Visual Cortex Offers Hope for a Functional Prosthesis," *Science*, Vol. 183, No. 4123 (February 1, 1974), pp. 440–43.

[33] H. Jack Geiger, "How Acupuncture Anesthetizes: The Chinese Explanation," *Medical World News*, Vol. 14, No. 27 (July 13, 1973), p. 53.

For three thousand years the Chinese have been studying *meridian points;* these are certain points in the body surface that correspond specifically to a particular diseased organ. "Many of these meridian points correspond to areas where nerves appear to surface from a muscle, or an area where vessels and nerves are located rather superficially, such as areas between muscle and bone or between bone and joint."[34] Moreover, some of these points are less electrically resistant than other areas.[35] "The introduction of electrical current for the purpose of local or regional anesthesia, as practiced in China, is an entirely new concept of anesthesia . . . the application of electrical current to acupuncture needles placed in the meridian points increases the efficacy of acupuncture in controlling pain."[36] In the words of the chairman of anesthesiology at the University of Washington, "Preliminary results indicate that it [acupuncture anesthesia] might be useful in pain problems and may be effective in producing anesthesia for some surgical procedures."[37]

saving high-risk babies

> But what am I?
> An infant crying in the night:
> An infant crying for the light:
> And with no language but a cry.

There is a time during which the threat to the infant's life is greatest. It is the *perinatal* (from the Greek *peri,* about, and *natal,* birth) period, the period of childbirth and shortly thereafter. The above lines from Alfred Lord Tennyson's "In Memoriam" are especially appropriate to this period. In medical statistics, the perinatal period is generally considered to begin with the birth of a fetus after twenty weeks or more of pregnancy and to end seven to twenty-eight days later. In this country, more babies die during the perinatal period than during the remaining first two years of life. Consequently, a new field has developed: *perinatal medicine,* or *perinatology.* Special laboratory studies and special equipment have been developed for it. For example, by determining the level of a certain chemical in the amniotic fluid by means of amniocentesis (see page 565), it has become possible to determine more accurately whether a fetus's respiratory tract is mature. Monitoring devices, which give the observer continued reports about the baby's health during labor and delivery, combined with the availability of positive pressure equipment (which introduces a suitable gas mixture into the lungs at a pressure above that of circulating air on the outside of the baby's chest) have prevented the deaths of numerous newborns with immature respiratory tracts. When a specialist is present in the delivery unit, infant death rates have been reduced to less than 10 per 1,000 live births, down from 15 to 17 deaths.[38]

At the Lying-In Hospital of the University of Chicago, fetal heart beats are

[34] Teruo Matsumoto, "Acupunctures and U.S. Medicine," *Journal of the American Medical Association,* Vol. 220, No. 7 (May 15, 1972), p. 1010.
[35] *Ibid.,* citing M. Hiyodo, *New Management of Pain* (Tokyo, 1970).
[36] *Ibid.* There is evidence to support this; see J. F. Fulton, *A Textbook of Physiology* (Philadelphia, 1955).
[37] "Injecting Science into the Acupuncture Picture," *Medical World News,* Vol. 14, No. 12 (March 23, 1973), p. 27.
[38] Robert J. Luby, "What's New and Important in Perinatal Medicine?" *Hospital Tribune,* Vol. 7, No. 33 (October 1, 1973), p. 9.

monitored in the case of high-risk pregnancies, such as pregnancies that must be terminated by cesarian section (see page 582) and pregnancies complicated by diabetes (see page 260) or by the Rh problem (see pages 553–55). Such monitoring has brought the survival rate of monitored fetuses up to that of unmonitored infants born at the hospital of low-risk mothers. Intensive care does not stop with the birth of the monitored baby, however. It continues until the perinatal specialist feels certain that the baby is out of danger. And so the helpless infant, with no language but a cry, is beginning to be better heard and understood.

Triumphs vie with one another.[39] Perhaps the greatest are occurring in the laboratories of the molecular biologists.

[39] Many other devices and procedures for replanting, replacing, and repairing are helping the sick, prolonging life, or holding out the promise of better health. Only a few of these will be mentioned here.

An implantable prosthetic device is relieving people who have lost the ability to contain their urine. ("Prosthetic Device Aids Incontinent," *Hospital Tribune,* Vol. 7, No. 42 [December 10, 1973], pp. 1, 15.) At the University of Alabama, a portable oxygen system contained in canisters the size of beer cans is being tried to increase the physical activity of patients with heart and respiratory problems. (*Journal of the American Medical Association,* Vol. 220, No. 2 [April 10, 1972], p. 187.) New approaches to the treatment of burns (see footnote 20) are saving lives that would have been lost just a few years ago. In 1973, for example, eight-year-old Sherry White was the first person in medical history to survive burns over more than 90 percent of her body. ("Two 'Miracles' of Burn Treatment," *Medical World News,* Vol. 14, No. 35 [September 28, 1973], p. 19.) On December 18, 1971, Wayne Lindblom, a construction worker, was caught by a heavy piece of earth-moving equipment. His body was pounded to a bloody pulp. But the San Francisco Trauma Team saved his life, using new equipment and methods of treatment. (Stewart Coulter, "Trauma," *California's Health,* Vol. 30, No. 6 [February 1973], pp. 1–4.)

There was a time when damage to the spinal cord was a guarantee of crippling. Today, work directed toward cooling the cord at the injury site and chemically reversing the damage has been done with promising results. ("Fighting Crippling Spinal Cord Injury," *Medical World News,* Vol. 13, No. 42 [November 10, 1972], pp. 51–53.) Some paraplegics (people stricken with various degrees of paralysis) can walk with the aid of crutches and a new cloth garment that, when filled with air, supports the patient in an upright position. The garment can be worn under street clothing. ("Inflatable Orthesis Helps Paraplegics Walk Again," *Journal of the American Medical Association,* Vol. 226, No. 11 [December 10, 1973), pp. 1293–94.) Coil springs are now being used to manage some spinal fractures; the fractured spine is supported and aligned by springs hooked over the spinal vertebrae above and below the damaged area. (*Medical World News,* Vol. 13, No. 42 [November 10, 1972].) A new procedure for stimulating the leg's peroneal nerve electrically aids stroke patients to walk with greater ease. ("Device Aids Stroke Patients," *Bulletin of the Los Angeles County Medical Association,* Vol. 102, No. 13 [July 20, 1972], p. 12.) And there are now, as a result of new implantation procedures, a variety of artificial substitutes for joints lost through damage or disease. These substitutes are called *prostheses.* Prosthesis has been proving valuable, for example, when knee cartilage and bone are lost because of arthritis. ("Arthritic Knee Prosthesis: When Bone and Cartilage Are Lost," *Roche Medical Image,* cited in *Hospital Tribune,* Vol. 7, No. 24, p. 13.)

Unique investigations also promise to contribute to the prevention and treatment of heart disease. Eating excessive saturated fat has been linked to high cholesterol levels and heart disease. Beef and lamb contain relatively high amounts of saturated fatty acids. Lambs are now being raised on a diet that reduces the amount of the saturated fatty acids by as much as ten times. ("Polyunsaturated Lamb Chops," *Chemistry,* Vol. 46, No. 9 [October 1973], p. 33.) And heart damage can be more accurately assessed by sophisticated X-rays of the coronary arteries; the specialist can evaluate the function of the cardiac muscle during cardiac catheterization (the passage of a soft rubber tube through blood vessels of the heart, or even into the heart itself) while the patient is exercising. (Joseph W. Linhart, "What's New and Important in the Diagnosis and Treatment of Coronary Artery Disease?" *Hospital Tribune* [April 2, 1973].) There is even a catheter pacemaker—a temporary or permanent device that, inserted in the tip of the intracardiac catheter, can stimulate the heart electrically. Even some newborn hearts with congenital defects can benefit from the results of cardiac catheterization. The lack of a prosthetic material that is compatible with blood is the greatest impediment to a mechanical device to aid the failing heart. Discovery of such a material may be a reality in ten years, and from it can come pumps, conduits, oxygenators, heart valves, and better grafts of blood vessels. New electronic devices promise to provide a better continuous record of heart function during ordinary daily activities. The ability to measure the tiny amounts of hormones in the blood has opened whole new vistas for human health (see pages 254–59).

The elimination of diseased bone marrow and improvements in transplants of healthy marrow are but two procedures that can incalculably benefit man. The effect of chemicals such as lactate on anxiety neuroses (page 301) is but the beginning of a trend, as is the use of lithium in the manic phase of manic-depression (page 299). Nuclear medicine is still in its infancy, yet it has already helped humanity enormously (see page 95). (Jack W. Baker, "The Horizons of Medicine," *Bulletin of the Los Angeles County Medical Society: Centennial of the Society* [1971], pp. 30–35, 38.)

"for nothing is secret, that shall not be made manifest" (Luke 8:17)

In the laboratories of the world, researchers have been learning about DNA and RNA. In 1961, at the National Institutes of Health, Marshall Nirenberg learned to read the code, the message that DNA imparts to RNA. It is the RNA, carrying the DNA instruction, that prescribes new protein manufacture at the ribosomes in cellular cytoplasm (Chapter 18, page 532). Limitless possibilities tantalize the inquisitive scientists. Will they not someday make genetic materials, which are, after all, only complex chemical compounds? Will it not then be possible to manipulate DNA and to modify living cells? Perhaps chromosomal error can then be corrected before it warps cellular harmony. Or the malignant messages of cancer DNA may be thwarted and replaced by man-made DNA. However, scientists issue a warning: "When man becomes capable of instructing his own cells, he must refrain from doing so until he has sufficient wisdom to use his knowledge for the benefit of mankind."[40]

At Stanford University researchers labored to create an artificial DNA—the code-containing genetic instructor of the cell. It might be done by making a DNA virus. In the laboratories at the University of Illinois, biologically active RNA virus had already been synthesized. Magnificent as this accomplishment was, the synthesis of DNA virus would overshadow it because RNA genes occur in a limited group of specialized cells, while DNA genes are found in many known viruses and living cells.

On December 15, 1967, the Stanford scientists made a startling announcement: after eleven years of work, they had succeeded in producing biologically active DNA from inert chemicals (see Figure 25-5). This DNA was, indeed, the genetic material, the inner core, of a virus. And, like the genetic material of ordinary natural virus, the synthetic DNA infected cells and caused them to participate in making more DNA virus. Some scientists do not consider viruses living particles. Viruses cannot reproduce themselves. To reproduce they depend on living cells. But one of the manifestations of virus existence is the ability to infect. Another is the capacity to seduce cells into helping make more virus. These criteria the Stanford University laboratory-created virus met. A long step had been taken toward creating life in the test tube.

25-5 *This biologically active DNA virus was synthesized from inert test-tube chemicals.*

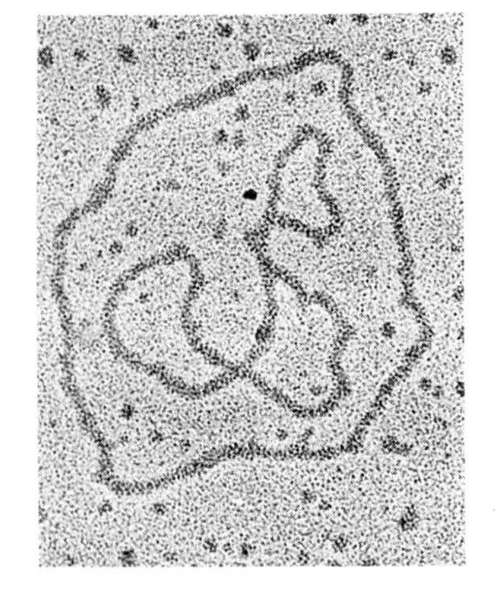

Within a few years there were more steps, and they were becoming shorter. In 1970, while at the University of Wisconsin, Indian-born Nobel laureate Har Gobind Khorana and his group (which included nine young scientists from seven nations) created the first artificial gene from basic chemical materials.[41] Since one gene could now be made to order, it had become technically possible to make other, more complex genes. Possible also was the eventual production of variations of natural genes. These could have profound, and not necessarily desirable, effects on the cells containing them. In short, man-made mutants were now in sight. In 1971, Khorana and his group, now at the Massachusetts Institute of Technology, synthesized the first wholly artificial gene with the potential for functioning inside a living cell.[42] It was yet another step toward

[40] "Nobel Prizes in Medicine: Geneticists Rewarded," *Science News,* Vol. 94, No. 17 (October 26, 1968), p. 411.

[41] "First Total Gene Synthesis Achieved by Wisconsin Team," *Medical Tribune,* Vol. 11, No. 35 (June 15, 1970), p. 26.

[42] Thomas H. Maugh II, "Molecular Biology: A Better Artificial Gene," *Science,* Vol. 181, No. 4106 (September 28, 1973), p. 1235.

the distant day when a biochemical cure for some genetic defects would be possible. These discoveries emphasized once again the need for the wisdom that "giveth life to them that have it" (Ecclesiastes 8:2).

Such work has given rise to the possibility of introducing new and functional genes into mammalian cells. In order to show how such genetic knowledge may someday be engineered to help mankind, consider, as an example, diabetes mellitus (see page 260). Rectifying the genetic defect in the production of insulin by the pancreas that results in this disease, one scientist has written,

> would first require identification of the exact structure of the insulin molecule, which is a proteinaceous hormone—a gene product. This has already been done. Next we would have to know the genetic code words for each component of the molecule; the code has been deciphered and the genetic dictionary is complete. Next we would have to be able to synthesize a segment of DNA representing the specific genetic code for the insulin molecule. Man-made DNA has become a reality, although refinement of the technique is needed before a specified gene can be artificially synthesized. Alternatively, technique for isolating a specific gene from simple organisms such as bacteria opens the possibility of selecting a "ready made" gene with the desired function. In either case, the specified gene will ultimately have to be put into the cells of the pancreas where the production of insulin occurs. A mechanism for accomplishing this step exists and current research is aimed at "domesticating" the process for human use. The mechanism is viral infection. . . . A virus with the requisite DNA for insulin (naturally occurring or man-made) should be able to treat diabetes.[43]

On the other hand, the limitations and hazards of gene therapy must be considered. Genetic disorders are numerous, but only a small proportion could even hopefully be helped by gene therapy. The majority of genetic disorders, the "inborn errors of metabolism" (see page 537), occur in about 1 person per 1,000. Only a small fraction of these might be helped by gene therapy. Moreover, both known and unknown hazards accompany notions of gene therapy. The changes induced by gene therapy may be harmful to the cell. Alteration of the regulatory process in the cell by means of a possible tumor-producing virus in an attempt to alleviate a genetic disorder is, of course, senseless. Thus, it is well to remember that although much has been accomplished in genetics, there are years of hard work ahead.[44]

experimenting with the unborn

Yet, scientists are edging toward realities undreamed of a generation ago. The following experiment has been performed:[45] Using a powerful microscope and minute surgical tools, the nucleus is extracted from a skin cell of a frog. With ultraviolet radiation the nucleus in an unfertilized egg of a second frog is destroyed. The naked nucleus from the first frog's skin cell is transplanted into the denucleated frog egg. Originally the unfertilized frog egg had had only half the number of chromosomes as the skin cell nucleus now residing in it. Now containing a full set of chromosomes, the egg is tricked. The transplanted skin

[43] James J. Nagle, "Genetic Engineering," *Science and Public Affairs: Bulletin of the Atomic Scientists,* Vol. 27, No. 10 (December 1971), p. 44.

[44] Maurice S. Fox and John W. Littlefield, "Reservations Concerning Gene Therapy," *Science,* Vol. 173, No. 3993 (July 16, 1971), p. 195.

[45] Anthony Blackler, quoted in "Protecting Man from Man," *Science News,* Vol. 95, No. 2 (January 11, 1969), p. 32.

cell nucleus causes the frog egg to behave as if it had been fertilized. The result: from the egg develops a new frog that is exactly like the frog whose skin nucleus was transplanted. No sperm was necessary. This kind of cell division in tissue culture (see pages 155–56) is called "cloning."

Such work with higher animals is in progress. A transplant scientist has said, "An Einstein could literally be made immortal. One may envision a transplant generation" composed of "individuals born from eggs fertilized by nuclei transplanted from body cells rather than by sperm."[46] As yet, the techniques that are essential to insert a nucleus into a frog's ovum are not applicable to the much smaller mammalian egg. But it has been estimated that "A human being born of clonal reproduction . . . will most likely appear on the earth within the next twenty to fifty years."[47] Thus, perhaps the next generation will experience this not necessarily beneficial scientific event.

Experiments on the unconceived and the unborn are proceeding at a rapid rate.[48] Test-tube fertilization of human ova by human sperm has been accomplished. The difficulty of recovering mature ova after their release from the ovary was surmounted by surgically removing them directly from the ovarian follicle before they were released. In an appropriate culture medium, the human zygote has gone on to divide into a blastocyst (see page 478).[49] Implantation into the uterine endometrium of a test-tube human blastocyst has yet to be accomplished. It would be a chancy experiment. However, successful implantations of such rabbit and mouse blastocysts have been reported.[50] Moreover, in both the mouse and the rabbit, the implanted blastocysts have developed into full-term normal progeny.[51] Both males and females have been conceived, implanted, and born in this fashion.[52] Indeed, three-day-old mouse embryos

[46] *Ibid.*, pp. 31–33.

[47] James D. Watson, "The Future of Asexual Reproduction," *Intellectual Digest*, Vol. 2, No. 2 (October 1971), p. 72.

[48] For a recent review of this subject, see Joan Arehart-Treichel, "Test-Tube Babies in the Making," *Science News*, Vol. 103, No. 8 (February 24, 1973), pp. 124–26.

[49] Leon R. Kass, "Babies by Means of In-Vitro Fertilization: Unethical Experiments on the Unborn?" *New England Journal of Medicine*, Vol. 285, No. 21, p. 1175, citing R. G. Edwards, B. D. Bavister, and P. C. Steptoe, "Early Stages of Fertilization 'in Vitro' of Human Oocytes Matured 'in Vitro,'" *Nature*, Vol. 221 (1969), pp. 632–35; R. G. Edwards, P. C. Steptoe, and J. M. Purdy, "Fertilization and Cleavage 'in Vitro' of Preovulator Human Oocytes," *Nature*, Vol. 227 (1970), pp. 1307–09; P. C. Steptoe, R. G. Edwards, and J. M. Purdy, "Human Blastocysts Grown in Culture," *Nature*, Vol. 229 (1971), pp. 132–33; L. B. Shettles, "Human Blastocysts Grown 'in Vitro' in Ovulation Cervical Mucus," *Nature*, Vol. 229 (1971), p. 343; C. B. Jacobson, J. G. Sites, and L. F. Arias-Bernal, "'In Vitro' Maturation and Fertilization of Human Follicular Oocytes," *International Journal of Fertility*, Vol. 15 (1970), pp. 103–14; and P. C. Steptoe and R. G. Edwards, "Laparoscopic Recovery of Preovulatory Human Oocytes After Priming of Ovaries with Gonadotropins," *Lancet*, Vol. 1 (1970), pp. 683–89.

[50] "Implanted Ova Produce Live Rabbits," *Journal of the American Medical Association*, Vol. 220, No. 2 (April 10, 1972), p. 179.

[51] Leon R. Kass, "Babies by Means of In-Vitro Fertilization: Unethical Experiments on the Unborn?" p. 1175, citing M. C. Chang, "Fertilization of Rabbit Ova 'in Vitro,'" *Nature*, Vol. 184 (1959), pp. 466–67; D. G. Whittingham, "Fertilization of Mouse Eggs 'in Vitro,'" *Nature*, Vol. 220 (1968), pp. 592–93; and A. B. Mukherjee and M. M. Cohen, "Development of Normal Mice by 'in Vitro' Fertilization," *Nature*, Vol. 228 (1970), pp. 472–73.

[52] A variation of this was experiments with frozen embryos. Before 1971, mammalian ova had been difficult to preserve in a frozen state. But that problem was solved that year by an English scientist at Cambridge. (D. G. Whittingham, "Survival of Mouse Embryos After Freezing and Thawing," *Nature*, Vol. 233, No. 5315 [September 10, 1971], pp. 125–26, and "Frozen Embryos," *Lancet*, Vol. 2, No. 7728 [October 8, 1971], p. 806.) In mid-1973, a deep-frozen calf embryo was thawed and implanted in a foster mother. It was carried to term and was born to become a healthy calf. Such research holds great promise for the commercial livestock industry.

have been successfully implanted, not in uterine endometrium, but in a test tube. This was accomplished by using rat-tail collagen in the test tube (collagen is the main supportive protein of connective tissue, bone, tendon, cartilage, and skin).[53]

Although such experiments may not be applicable to humans for many years, it is interesting to contemplate the situation when they are. Birth certificates of the future may have to contain information about "as many as five parents: the legal father and mother, who raise the child; the proxy mother, who incubated the child; and the biological father and mother, who contributed the genetic material to the child."[54] Test-tube fertilization of human ova followed by implantation into a biological or other mother promises to someday solve some infertility problems. However, "in an overcrowded world infertility is an individual problem, not a great social issue."[55] Experiments yielding apparently normal rabbits and mice are not directly applicable to humans without risk. The danger of producing abnormal humans must be critically considered. Defects of reproduction are not uncommon results of cloning amphibian eggs. It is disconcerting to note that these experiments have gone from frogs to rodents to man. Little or no work with primates other than man has been carried out.

When one considers the implications of these experiments, scientifically altered genes seem but a part of the whole biological revolution. To alter the chemical structure of DNA, to create artificial genes so as to correct genetic defects, to eventually modify tumor DNA with alternate DNA, to bring about human birth by clonal reproduction and extrauterine fertilization—these are not fanciful visions of science. They are likelihoods. And, since they will bring to one generation of man untold powers over succeeding generations (see page 520), they pose ethical problems of enormous magnitude.[56]

on the need for scientific wisdom

Some research of this nature has become a source of dispute in the scientific world. The Harvard student group that first isolated a simple gene from a common intestinal bacterium (see Figure 18-3, page 523) shocked both laymen and their fellow scientists when they expressed concern (in the famous "Beckwith letter") about the implications of their own work. In essence, they pointed out that scientific achievements have usually outstripped human wisdom. Their observation was not new. Two centuries before them, the English writer Samuel Johnson had noted in *Rasselas* that "Integrity without knowledge is weak and useless . . . Knowledge without integrity is dangerous and dreadful." And almost two centuries before that, the great English essayist and statesman Francis Bacon (1561–1626) had observed in *Advancement of Learning: Civil Knowledge* that "There is no great concurrence between learning and wisdom."

In 1971, Nobel laureate Sir Macfarlane Burnet, one of the world's most

[53] "An Embryo Implants in a Test Tube," *New Scientist and Science Journal,* Vol. 50, No. 747 (April 15, 1971), p. 137.

[54] James J. Nagle, "Genetic Engineering," p. 45.

[55] "Rules and Regulations for Test-Tube Babies," *Nature,* Vol. 231, No. 5298 (May 14, 1971), p. 69.

[56] A recommended article regarding the ethical aspects of research in human embryology is Robert G. Edwards and David J. Sharpe, "Social Values and Research in Human Embryology," *Nature,* Vol. 231, No. 5298 (May 14, 1971), pp. 87–90. A later editorial, "Should Reproductive Biology Be Encouraged?" appeared in *Nature,* Vol. 233, No. 5322 (October 29, 1971), p. 579.

distinguished microbiologists, decried the experimental study of the genetics of viruses that could potentially cause illness in man. "It is simply a question of balancing a small probability of an appalling catastrophe against an equally small likelihood of something useful emerging, such as a trivial improvement in virus vaccines," he said. "There is nowadays only one source from which new infectious diseases could come. If they come they will come from deliberate or accidental manipulations dealing in the microbial genetics."[57] Prominent biologists throughout the world disagreed. From Sweden came the opinion that laboratory-changed microorganisms had little chance of survival in nature. From a scientist at Germany's Max Planck Institute came the reminder that all knowledge of DNA and RNA, the genetic code, and the mechanism of antibiotics was generated by such research. More to the point, he said, would be discontinuance of research on bacteriological warfare (a move completed by the United States in 1971). Other distinguished biologists (from Paris) considered Sir Burnet's analysis one-sided and (from Japan) theoretical.

But the concern among scientists would not go away. Late in 1973, a writer for the prestigious journal of the American Association for the Advancement of Science pointed to some 3,500 cases of laboratory-acquired infections since the turn of the century; 150 people had died as a result. "Besides the risk to scientists themselves, there are also dangers posed by the new kinds of viruses that are now being created in the laboratory and which, if they escape, might constitute a threat to public health."[58] One distinguished researcher in the field "guessed" that the risk of infection by tumor viruses is small. Another found the guess unimpressive. Said he, "We're in a pre-Hiroshima situation; it would be a real disaster if one of the agents now being handled in research should in fact be a real human cancer agent."[59]

More threatening than the hazards of the tumor viruses are those arising from research with hybrid viruses designed to produce a better influenza vaccine (see pages 149–51). Why? A new combination, a new hybrid of viruses might escape from the laboratory via an infected employee and spread to a nonimmune population. Said one researcher of the National Institute of Allergy and Infectious Diseases, "This could recreate the conditions for an influenza pandemic [worldwide epidemic] like that of 1918."[60]

What can be done? The problem must be further studied. In June 1973, a group of scientists sent a letter to the president of the National Academy of Sciences urging that a committee be established to study the hazards of laboratory hybrid virus molecules. Safety precautions must be tightened in all laboratories working with potentially dangerous viral combinations. Technical handling of such virus molecules should be limited to those best equipped to do so. The public and its representative politicians must be kept educated and

[57] Quoted in "Genetic Studies of Viruses Called Danger by Nobelist," *Hospital Tribune,* Vol. 5, No. 24 (December 13, 1971), p. 1.

[58] Nicholas Wade, "Microbiology: Hazardous Profession Faces New Uncertainties," *Science,* Vol. 182, No. 4112 (November 9, 1973), pp. 566–67.

[59] *Ibid.,* p. 567. For a further discussion of the possible health hazards of manipulating strands of DNA to produce hybrids, see Edward Ziff, "Benefits and Hazards of Manipulating DNA," *New Scientist,* Vol. 50, No. 869 (October 25, 1973), pp. 274–75.

[60] *Ibid.*

informed (the atomic bombs were dropped on Hiroshima and Nagasaki without adequate communication between scientists and politicians[61]). And in the last analysis, much will depend on the wisdom of the scientist.

problems: a price of progress

searching space above and space below

The exploration of outer space and the exploration of the oceans are complex undertakings. But scientists can be concerned about simple problems even under the most esoteric circumstances. Before actual space flights were made, they were worried about details that might affect the astronauts' health. Every ninety minutes astronauts would be subjected to a day and night. Ordinary intercontinental travelers are often sickened by interference with their normal circadian rhythms (see Chapter 1, pages 6–8). What grave consequences might ensue when astronauts endured forty-five minutes of day followed by forty-five minutes of night? How, for example, could they sleep? How could this threat to their health be diminished?

The solution? Like a cloth over a birdcage, "the spacecraft was artificially darkened by covering the windows, and, as far as the crew was concerned, it was night."[62] Few health problems are so easily solved. The efforts to avoid contamination of the moon by germ-laden earthly spacecraft are more complicated. Spacecraft sterilization is now under study. The problem goes both ways. Upon returning from its moon landing, the Apollo 11 spacecraft, its astronauts, and moon samples needed to undergo a period of quarantine and testing to safeguard against the possibility of introducing stowaway, immigrant moon organisms to earth.

There remains another vast ecosystem to explore. It lies beneath the ocean. "Do you know," says one fish to another, "that over a quarter of the earth is covered by land?" Beneath the seas, the mountains are greater and the canyons are deeper than those above. But inner space is even less hospitable than outer space. Astronauts feel freer, see vast distances, are moved by overwhelming beauties, and can easily communicate with earthlings. But under just two hundred feet of water, human life is miserable. Visibility is almost zero. At great depths, radio waves do not travel far. Communication with the world above remains impossible. Astronauts and aquanauts share some problems. Pressure, weightlessness, cold—these hazards vary with the ecology. In space, the astronaut is weightless. In deep water, the aquanaut is nearly so. The astronaut works in a vacuum. Every square inch of the aquanaut's body is under enormous pressure. Yet one can feel secure that science will solve these problems. (It is the ruination of man's natural environment that causes concern.)

For various reasons the space above and the space below are being explored. Man's need to penetrate the unknown, to solve the mystery of his life

[61] Lord Ritchie-Calder, "Mortgaging the Old Homestead," *Foreign Affairs*, Vol. 48 (January 1970), pp. 207–20.

[62] Charles A. Berry, "Space Medicine in Perspective," *Journal of the American Medical Association*, Vol. 201, No. 4 (July 24, 1967), p. 234.

on earth, to understand his relationship with all else—these drive him to search. He seeks unity, to be part of a greater whole, to fit into an encompassing order and purpose. Jedáleddin wrote: "All that is not One must ever suffer with the wound of Absence." [63] It is this wound that man needs to heal. He seeks one unified idea of himself. Thus, reflected Einstein, "the story goes on until we have arrived at a system of the greatest conceivable unity." [64] Man wants order. Without it, he is not quite well.

And in his search there is serendipity. In "serendipity," there is meaning that merits digression. In 1754, the English writer and wit Horace Walpole told a tale of three travelers, *The Three Princes of Serendip.* Being blessed with a mixture of luck and keen observation, the three made all sorts of valuable discoveries they were not looking for. So the word *serendipity* refers to the faculty of happening on valuable findings when not searching for them. But as Louis Pasteur succinctly said, "Chance favors the prepared mind."

Formidable indeed are the serendipitous results of oceanography. Submarine rescue (pitifully inadequate in 1963, when the nuclear submarine *Thresher* disappeared) is now a realistic hope. From the surfaces and crevices of the ocean floor come minerals. But that sea farming will soon result in limitless food is a false belief. True, sea studies have helped somewhat. Between water depths ranging from thirty to nine hundred feet there live succulent sea plants. These are consumed by minute animal organisms, which are in turn consumed by flesh-eating fish. By using new understandings of sea science, oceanographers can now help the world's fishermen find their catch. But the concept of the seas as a vast, untapped food source is unsubstantiated. To a world expecting a population of more than 6 billion in a generation, this is bitter news. Its impact is lessened by the possibility that the oceans contain vast sources of medicines. Nevertheless, much work is still needed in this area.

in the United States, more health for more people; more problems with progress

Regular measles (and poliomyelitis too) has become a relatively rare disease. A hopefully improved vaccine for German measles (rubella) may render that crippler of the unborn a melancholy memory. Drugs (streptomycin, rifampin, and isoniazid) have helped to cut the tuberculosis death rate tremendously. And antibiotics have reduced the death rates from pneumonia and rheumatic fever. Nor have these victories been limited to infectious diseases. The control of infectious diseases has provided longer life in which to develop chronic ailments. Nevertheless, drugs have lowered death rates from hypertensive heart disease. Strokes kill fewer people. Deaths from stomach and duodenal ulcers have been greatly lessened. Infant death rates[65] have fallen. Maternal mortality is decreasing. All these declines are continuing. They tell a story of hard-won success. But, since more people now live to an advanced age, they bring into relief the problems of the aged. How are older people faring?

[63] Quoted in John M. Dorsey, *Illness or Allness* (Detroit, 1965), p. 540.

[64] Albert Einstein, "Physics and Reality," *Out of My Later Years* (New York, 1950), p. 63.

[65] The infant mortality rate is the number of deaths occurring among children less than one year of age, divided by the number of births. In the United States, the 1960 infant mortality rate was 26.0 per 1,000 live births. In 1966, it was 23.7. (Myron E. Wegman, "Annual Summary of Vital Statistics," *Pediatrics,* Vol. 42, No. 6 [December 1968], pp. 1005–09.) In 1973, the rate was 18.5. Although the nonwhite infant mortality rate has declined substantially, it remains much higher than the white rate.

aging: man's common denominator

Once upon a time in Asia Minor, it was the custom for people who had reached the age of sixty to be taken away to a cave. There they might live in peace the rest of their lives, and, of course, would be out of people's way.

It was considered most proper that when the time came for a man to leave for the cave, his son should contribute the necessary food and "chull," a goat-haired woven blanket.

One day a middle-aged man asked his own little boy to take the chull and come with him and grandpa, for they were taking the latter to the cave from which none returned. Though the grandson was brokenhearted at his grandfather's departure, he was about to shoulder the chull obediently when suddenly he was struck by an idea. Cutting the chull in half, he took one part with him and left the other part at home. When the grandfather had been deposited with due filial piety in the cave, son and grandson returned home.

Then it was that the son discovered what had happened to the chull. He scolded the boy severely. "Look what you've done. Everyone would say we were too stingy to give grandpa the whole blanket!" "No, father," the boy replied, "I wasn't being stingy, but I thought it was better to give grandpa only half . . . Then I could keep the other half for you."[66]

If mankind has failed to escape eventual aging, it has not been for want of trying. By drinking the warm blood of dying gladiators, elderly Romans sought to partake of youth. Others bathed in young people's blood. Those violent Roman emperors, Nero and Caligula, hopefully ingested male gland preparations.[67] In the twentieth century, Serge Voronoff made a fortune by surgically implanting monkey glands. John Brinkman got rich by transplanting goat glands. His profits helped pay for an almost successful campaign to a governor's chair. There have been phony pills, creams, and "serums." But man continues to age.

Science has now entered the quest for prolonged youth. The process of growing old (*senescence*) is being avidly studied. *Gerontology* is the science of the physical and psychological changes incident to old age. *Geriatrics* is concerned with the treatment of the problems of the aged.

Why do people age? In the 1930s, Nobelist Alexis Carrel reported that cells from a chicken embryo's heart could be kept alive indefinitely in tissue culture. His results are now disputed. Some believe that Carrel had unwittingly added new, living embryonic cells to the chicken embryo extract he used as a nutrient. This error was compounded when it was noted that mouse and other animal cells would go on dividing indefinitely. But these cells are always abnormal. Normal cells die after a limited number of divisions. For example, animal tumor cells can be transplanted and divide indefinitely; but normal cells transplanted from one animal to another cannot. Some animal cells stop dividing after about fifty divisions, but various cells from the human body stop dividing after a lesser number. In adult humans, for example, certain lung cells were found to slow down and stop dividing after about twenty doublings. Also, when certain cells were frozen at a stage of their doubling and then thawed years later, they "remembered" how many times they had divided and took up again where they had left off. Will chilling a sleeper someday be a way of increasing age?

[66] George Lawton, ed., *New Goals for Old Age* (New York, 1943), p. v.
[67] "Quest for Youth," *M.D., Medical Newsmagazine,* Vol. 2, No. 8 (August 1958), p. 86.

Perhaps the determinants of aging lie in the chromosomal pattern. This pattern possibly dictates the time schedule of cellular aging. Maybe this is why the heart and blood vessels wear out more often and earlier than other body parts. If (as has been theorized) aging speed is predetermined in the configuration of genetic structure, perhaps the chemical program can be changed. Already scientists have transplanted DNA (genes) from one bacterial cell to another. Those bacteria that received transplanted DNA transmitted the new genetic characteristics to their progeny.[68] Can DNA transplants be accomplished in man? Can young genes be transplanted into old cells? Those who peremptorily dismiss this possibility are out of step with the scientific strides of the past twenty years.

To increase the life span, to bring more people to older age—these are agelong efforts by civilized communities. As has been seen, in the latter decades of this century longevity has leveled off. Nevertheless, the number of people attaining old age continues to multiply. In 1900, only 4 percent of the U.S. population was sixty-five years of age or older. In 1968, about 9.5 percent were. In 1973, that proportion was 10 percent.

In various cultures age has had various meanings. Among the Ainos of Japan, it was recorded that the "old women show themselves the most vigorous and wildest dancers."[69] Montaigne wrote that "there is nothing more notable in Socrates than that he found time, when he was an old man, to learn music and dancing, and thought it time well spent."[70]

Some members of the youth-oriented society of today have a harsh view of age. It is the image described by the Chief Justice, addressing the old rogue Sir John Falstaff, in Shakespeare's *The Second Part of King Henry the Fourth* (I.ii.204–12):

> Do you set down your name in the scroll of youth, that are written down old with all the characters of age? Have you not a moist eye? A dry hand? A yellow cheek? A white beard? A decreasing leg? An increasing belly? Is not your voice broken? Your wind short? Your chin double? Your wit single? And every part about you blasted with antiquity? And will you yet call yourself young? Fie, fie, fie, Sir John!

Perhaps the greatest pain of the aged is thinking that this is youth's view of them.

the extra gift

In 1940, the great painter Henri Matisse lay dying. He was then seventy-one. But he did not die. Confined to his bed or to a chair, he could sit up for only brief periods. Yet he lived to create some of his greatest work. About his illness he said this:

> I was extremely ill and had to have an operation. I had hardly regained consciousness, and still seemed to be sleeping, when I heard the doctors gathered

[68] "Scientist Says Senility May Be Controlled," *Geriatric Focus,* Vol. 4, No. 10 (June 15, 1965), pp. 1–6.

[69] R. Hitchcock, "The Ainos of Yezo, Japan," quoted in Leo W. Simmons, *The Role of the Aged in Primitive Society* (New Haven, Conn., 1945), p. 97.

[70] Michel de Montaigne, "Living to the Point," quoted in J. Donald Adams, ed., *The New Treasure Chest* (New York, 1953), p. 2.

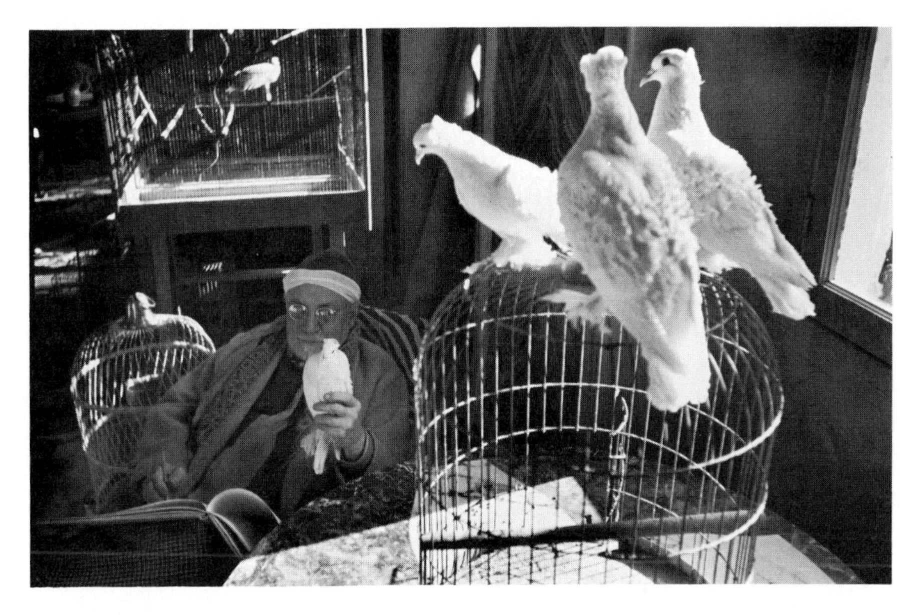

25-6 *Henri Matisse during the years of his "extra gift."*

at the foot of my bed, speaking among themselves: "We cannot do any more for him; if he gets over this, he has himself to thank for it; all depends on the way his body reacts." I did get over it. Since that day I have had the impression of having started a new life. My previous life was terminated at the moment when theoretically I was going to die. The life I am now enjoying is an extra gift; I have the right to do as I please, to try any experience, no longer seeking a link with a completed past. Moreover, I have a sense of total liberty in my experiments.[71]

The extra gift also came to Oliver Wendell Holmes, Jr. He had fought in the Civil War. He had fought for civil rights. In 1882, at forty-one, he had been made a Justice of the Supreme Court. There, for more than half a century, he fought for the law as a living instrument. In 1931, he was ninety years old. This was his birthday message to the nation:

In this symposium my part is only to sit in silence. To express one's feelings as the end draws near is too intimate a task.

But I may mention one thought that comes to me as a listener-in. The riders in a race do not stop short when they reach the goal. There is a little finishing canter before coming to a standstill. There is time to hear the kind voice of friends and to say to one's self: "The work is done."

But just as one says that, the answer comes: "The race is over, but the work never is done while the power to work remains."

The canter that brings you to a standstill need not be only coming to rest. It cannot be while you still live. For to live is to function. That is all there is to living.

And so I end with a line from a Latin poet who uttered the message more than fifteen hundred years ago:

"Death plucks my ears and says, Live—I am coming."[72]

[71] Quoted in Raymond Cogniat, "Art and Longevity," *Abbottempo,* Vol. 1, No. 1 (March 22, 1963), pp. 9–13.

[72] Oliver Wendell Holmes, Jr., a radio talk on the occasion of a national celebration of his ninetieth birthday, quoted in Max Lerner, ed., *The Mind and Faith of Justice Holmes* (Boston, 1943), p. 451.

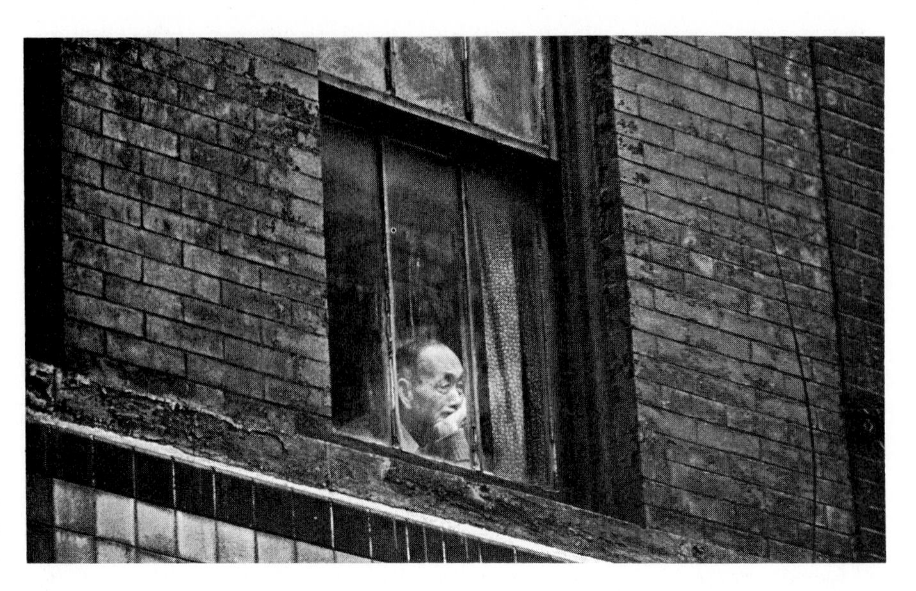

25-7 *For too many people, aging means loneliness.*

But what about the average man? As he survives, he has a predictable chance of a longer life. In this country, retiring at sixty-five, a man has a 50–50 chance of living twelve more years. Today, Western man experiences both a prolonged period of learning and a prolonged retirement. It is during the first that preparation should begin for the second. This is not to say that youth should be haunted by the spectre of old age. But it is during youth that the foundation for age is built. In the *Republic,* Plato puts these thoughts into the conversation of Cephalus with Socrates:

> How well do I remember the aged poet Sophocles, when in answer to the question, How does love suit with age, Sophocles,—are you still the man you were? Peace, he replied; most gladly have I escaped that, and I feel as if I had escaped from a mad and furious master . . . And of these regrets, as well as of the complaint about relations, Socrates, the cause is to be sought, not in men's ages, but in their characters and tempers; for he who is of a calm and happy nature will hardly feel the pressure of age, but he who is of an opposite disposition will find youth and age equally a burden.[73]

the plight of the poor everywhere

> Upon this gifted age, in its dark hour,
> Rains from the sky a meteoric shower
> Of facts . . . they lie unquestioned, uncombined.
> Wisdom enough to leech us of our ill
> Is daily spun, but there exists no loom
> To weave it into fabric . . .[74]

To the poor of this nation sickness and death come sooner and oftener. Lack of prenatal care, for example, kills the poor infant a third more often than the

[73] *Dialogues of Plato,* tr. by Benjamin Jowett (Oxford, Eng., 1897), p. 14.
[74] Edna St. Vincent Millay, "Huntsman, What Quarry?" cited in F. J. Inglefinger, "National Center for Health Statistics," *New England Journal of Medicine,* Vol. 289, No. 21 (November 22, 1973), p. 1142.

baby born to parents in nonpoverty areas. Premature birth and malnutrition are but two of the prices of poverty paid by the helpless infant.

Other statistics add to this totally unacceptable picture. The white infant mortality rate is dropping more sharply than the nonwhite. Moreover, the poverty of racial inequality kills almost four times as many pregnant black women as white. And there is the inequality not only of race, but also of place. The intimate relationship between poverty areas and high maternal and infant mortality rates is a chronic concern of health workers. This is further evidence of the need for more equal distribution of medical care (see Chapter 24).

For many a nation, aging people are no issue. Not enough people live to be old. True, U.S. data give little reason for complacency. But the information on sickness from developing countries provides even less. Compared to the rates in industrial nations, infant mortality rates in developing countries are two to eight times greater. Yet, even in these struggling areas, infant mortality rates portray but a part of the childhood calamity. "Mortality for children 1 to 4 years of age is from 20 to 30 times higher, sometimes much more in underdeveloped nations."[75] Affliction is piled on affliction. In the developing countries:

Every year the 20 million people with active cases of *tuberculosis* infect 2½ million people. Two million die of the disease.

Twelve million people suffer *leprosy,* and the number is increasing.

Plague, an ancient enemy, is on the rise (see Chapter 5).[76]

Despite the major efforts of the World Health Organization, *malaria* continues to be a major problem.

Diarrheal diseases, perpetuated by three tragic factors—poor sanitation, low economic development, and inadequate nutrition—afflict so many of the globe's inhabitants as to defy estimation. In many areas, for example, *typhoid fever* (rare in this country) is common. Other parasitic diseases, such as anemia-causing *hookworm* and the colic-producing *ascariasis* (a roundworm infestation) torment more than a billion and a half sufferers.[77] *Cholera,* that scourge of mankind, was a major world public health problem in 1970 and 1971 (see page 126 and Figure 25-8). By mid-1973 the disease was beginning to abate. But there is no room for complacency. The conditions that promote the spread of the disease remain, and indeed the disease has become entrenched in many a community.[78]

[75] Nevin S. Scrimshaw, "The Death Rate of One-Year-Old Children in Underdeveloped Countries," *Archives of Environmental Health,* Vol. 17, No. 5 (November 1968), p. 692.

[76] In Vietnam, for example, defoliation bombing in the mid-1960s deprived many a wild rodent of its natural habitat. Scurrying from the devastated woodlands, wild rats have made their way to the devastated cities. There, war has unbalanced the human ecosystem, but not that of the domestic rat. In the disorder of war, the latter thrives. It, however, becomes plague-infested by its immigrant country cousins. The incidence of human plague in Vietnam has therefore increased. (Alexander Alland, Jr., "War and Disease: An Anthropological Perspective," *Bulletin of the Atomic Scientists,* Vol. 24, No. 6 [June 1968], p. 29.) Due to U.S. interest in the reporting of plague, some of the dramatic rise was more apparent than real. (J. D. Marshall, Jr., *et al.,* "Plague in Vietnam 1965–1966," *American Journal of Epidemiology,* Vol. 86, No. 3 [November 1967], p. 616.)

[77] "The Second Ten Years of the World Health Organization," *WHO Chronicle,* Vol. 22, No. 7 (July 1968), pp. 267–312.

[78] "Surveillance Summary: Cholera—Worldwide 1973." *Morbidity and Mortality Weekly Reports,* U.S. Department of Health, Education, and Welfare, Public Health Service, Vol. 22, No. 28, for week ending July 14, 1973, p. 1.

Oral vaccination to prevent *poliomyelitis,* so successful in this and other countries, is not meeting with adequate protective immunity among infants and young children in some parts of the world.[79]

And, throughout the world, those who survive these endure cardiovascular illness, cancer, emotional disabilities, malnutrition, and dental problems.

There is work to do. Who does it?

organized participants in health work

Organized health work is done by *official* and *voluntary agencies.* Official agencies are governmental, have legal health responsibilities, and are tax-supported. Voluntary health agencies are not part of governmental structure, are not responsible for carrying out health laws, and are supported by voluntary contributions. Both types of agencies have paid staffs. Millions of unpaid workers help voluntary agencies. Without volunteers, official health agencies could function, albeit not so comprehensively. Without volunteers, voluntary agencies would not exist.

official agencies

who's WHO in health?

The World Health Organization is an agency of the United Nations. Today, more than a quarter of a century after it was founded in 1948, it includes more than 130 member states. In WHO's governing body, the *World Health Assembly,* each member state has one vote. Not often in history have so many nations labored together so long and so harmoniously. Each WHO worker is witness to a world of woe. Yet hope, not despair, is his image. Clearly he sees his purpose and his vision in these lines:

> And hold Humanity one man, whose universal agony
> Still strains and strives to gain the goal, where agonies shall cease to be.[80]

Meeting annually, the World Health Assembly establishes its policy, program, and budget. It also selects the rotating membership of its executive arm—the *Executive Board.* This twenty-four–member group, the representatives of twenty-four nations, effectuates assembly decisions. In case of an emergency plea—prompted perhaps by national trials such as earthquake, flood, or epidemic—the board is empowered to give immediate help. But it is through six regional field offices of WHO (in Brazzaville, Alexandria, Copenhagen, New Delhi, Manila, and Washington, D.C.) that most of the work of WHO reaches the people. Member nations apply to these offices for help, and from these offices field workers are assigned. The nerve center of WHO—its central headquarters—is located in Geneva.

[79] Maxwell Finland, "Global Epidemiology—Stocktaking at WHO." *New England Journal of Medicine,* Vol. 287, No. 11 (September 14, 1972), p. 566.

[80] Richard Francis Burton, *The Kasîdah of Hâjî Abdû El-Yezdi,* Part 9, verse 31 (Portland, Me., 1896), p. 56.

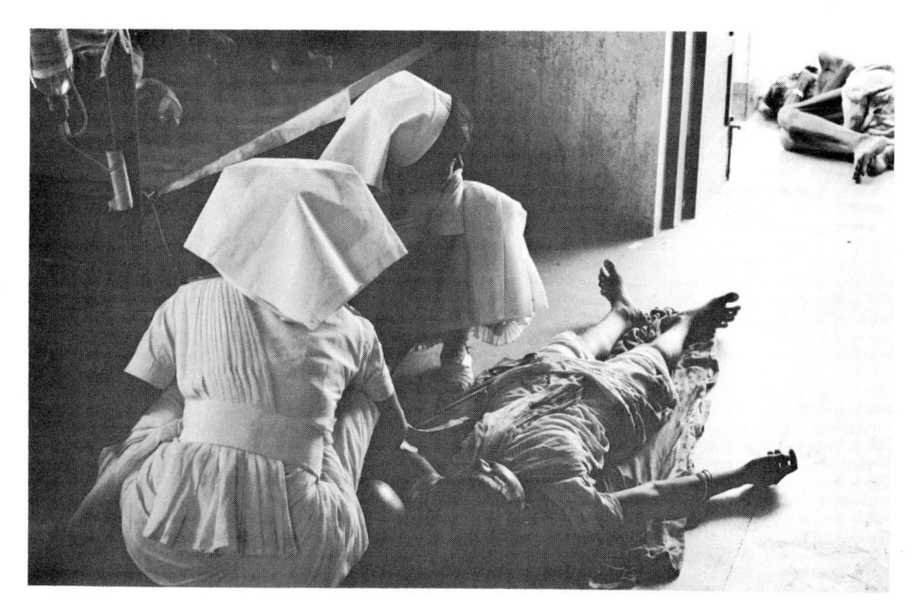

25-8 *WHO nurses tend to victims of a cholera epidemic a few years ago.*

WHO's basic purpose is to help applicant nations help themselves. Thus WHO assists nations in planning basic health services as an integral part of local development. Expert consultants on forty-four panels include 12,000 scientists, educators, and administrators. A permanent staff of 3,500 includes physicians, nurses, engineers, and other personnel. With WHO's worldwide intelligence system, world communicable disease control is a practical reality. It helps set international standards on foods, vaccines, drugs, diagnoses, and disease classifications. It is part of the counterspy system against the international drug racketeer. Its participation in training health personnel and in research is vast. It directs enormous campaigns against drug abuse, smallpox, malaria, tuberculosis, syphilis, and other plagues of mankind. It combats maternal and infant death. To old countries it has brought new concepts for dealing with water, soil, and air pollution; mental disease; accidents; heart disease; and cancer.

Its annual budget is less than the cost of a battleship.[81]

federal health work

It is from a broad interpretation of the Constitution that the federal government derives public health powers. The Constitutional phrase ''promote the general welfare'' establishes the basic philosophy. More specific is the federal *power to tax.* For example, the physician's annual $1 tax for his narcotic license provides the government with one way of checking on drug use. Or federal tax monies may eventually be used for local health programs. By its *controls over foreign commerce,* other problems are contained, such as the exclusion of dangerous drugs (thalidomide, for example) or people (such as unvaccinated aliens

[81] ''Twenty-fourth World Health Assembly—2,'' *WHO Chronicle,* Vol. 25, No. 8 (August 1971), pp. 337–42.

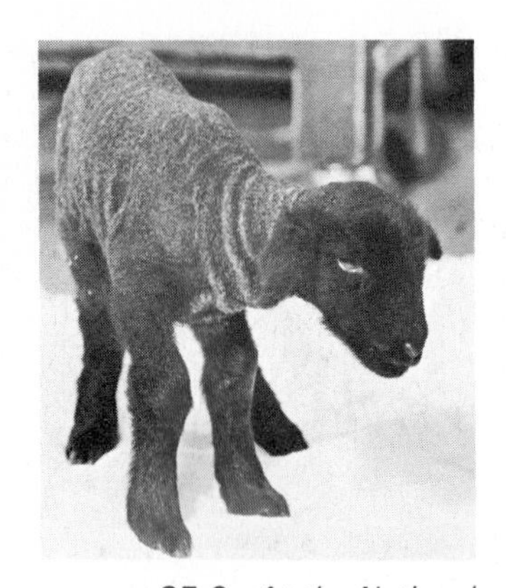

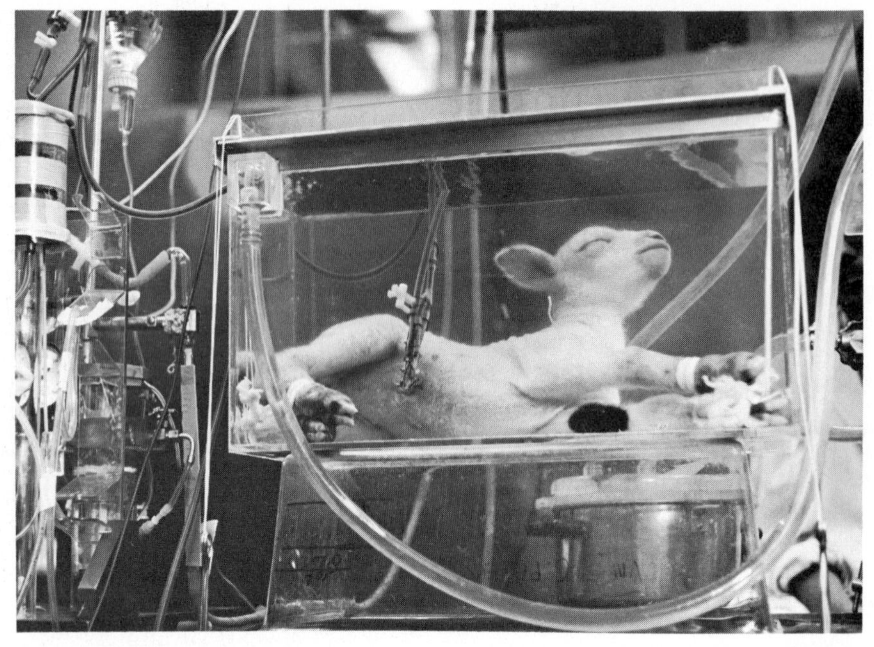

25-9 *At the National Heart Institute, fetal lambs have been sustained for up to fifty-five hours in a womblike tank of synthetic amniotic fluid. The artificial "placenta" is the apparatus shown at right. The healthy lamb* (above) *was weaned from such an apparatus. Human premature babies, who need respiratory support while their lungs finish developing, and patients with serious lung problems may be among those who eventually profit from these experiments.*

from smallpox areas). *Interstate commerce regulations* empower the federal government to exert controls over food and drugs transported from one state to another. *The federal right to raise armies* makes possible medical care for soldiers and veterans. *Control over federal territories* (Indian reservations, the District of Columbia) and the *Postal Service* include extensive federal health powers. In making treaties (as with Canada and Mexico) the United States exerts wide public health influence. Recent years have seen much international health activity abroad without treaty involvement. Much U.S. health work abroad is done via the World Health Organization, Public Health Service, State Department Agency for International Development, Peace Corps, and the military. All have done distinguished work.

In various agencies throughout the federal establishment, a wide variety of health activities are dispersed. Examples: the provision of medical services to federal prisoners by the Department of Justice and the interest in industrial safety of the Department of Labor. There are many more. These have their counterparts in state and local government. But it is in the *Department of Health, Education, and Welfare* that the nation's greatest concentration of health program activity occurs. Table 25-1, depicting the organizational structure of this department, reveals the extraordinary extent of its effort. Its projected budget for 1975 would commit $11 billion "for human resources programs."[82] Its major interest: health.

[82] Secretary of Health, Education, and Welfare Caspar Weinberger, quoted in Barbara J. Culliton, "Health, from a News and Comment Discussion of the 'Budget of the U.S. Government,'" *Science,* Vol. 183, No. 4125 (February 15, 1974), p. 638.

TABLE 25-1

Organization of the U.S. Department of Health, Education, and Welfare*

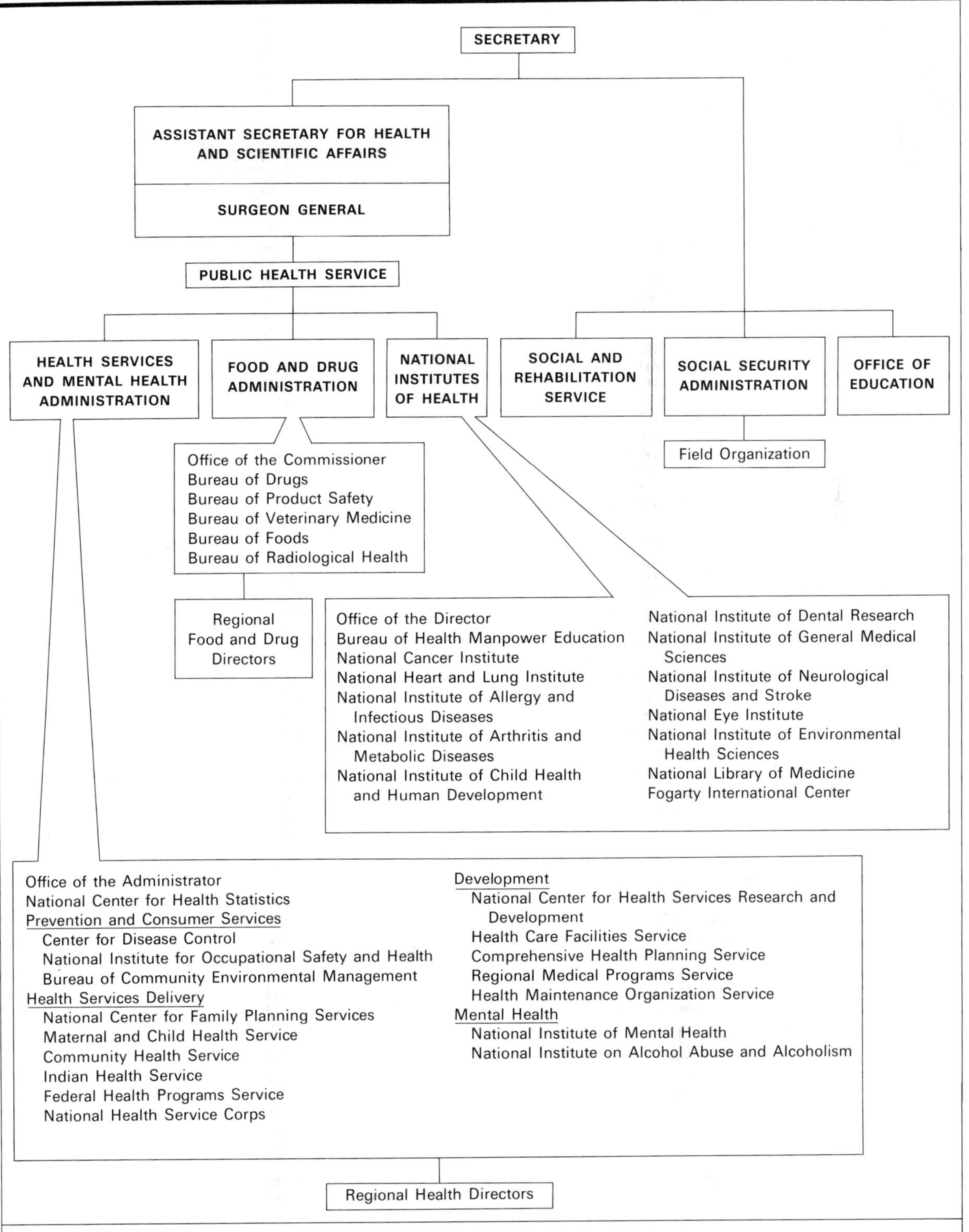

*Partial listing, highlighting certain health and health-related activities. Organization as of January 1972.
Source: U.S. Department of Health, Education, and Welfare, Office of the Secretary, as reprinted in Daniel M. Wilner, Rosabelle Price Walkley, and Lenor S. Goerke, *Introduction to Public Health,* 6th ed. (New York, 1973), pp. 36, 40.

Table 25-1, also presenting the basic structure of the *Public Health Service,* provides a general concept of its activities. Its functions include education and research, assistance to state health departments, and provision of medical and hospital services to eligible persons. It is, moreover, responsible for protecting U.S. borders against the entry of communicable diseases. The *Bureau of Health Manpower Education* is particularly interested in training health personnel. Education and research are, however, common denominators of the service. Among the agencies concerned with research are the *National Institutes of Health,* the *Center for Disease Control,* and the *National Institute of Mental Health.* And they are assisted in this work by the largest and most comprehensive collection of medical literature in the world: the collection located in the *National Library of Medicine.*

state and local health departments

Protection of the public's health is part of the legal obligation of each state. The federal government may interfere only when it is invited or when problems between states occur. Examples: a state has an outbreak of viral encephalitis. The governor requests federal Public Health Service help. Or a contaminated vaccine manufactured in one state is sold in another. This offense is federal and action is taken by federal agents. Similarly, it is only by state authority that a local city or county health department exists. Should a local department fail in its duty, the state can assume control. This almost never happens.

The basic job of the state health department is to help the local health departments do a better job. State departments, consequently, are more concerned with health legislation, planning, and policy. They are consultants, helping to set the standards of city and county health departments. And, since local health departments provide the services detailed in their organization charts (Table 25-2), state health departments, to advise them best, are organized to help them.

Examine the organization chart of Milwaukee's Health Department (Table 25-2). It may seem complex and the different bureaus may seem to have little connection with each other. Yet, during a few duty hours, a public health nurse may perform functions directly related to every bureau, indeed every division. Before leaving her assigned district office for a home visit, she notes her mileage. Eventually relayed to the Bureau of Administration, this information makes possible her reimbursement. During her home call she sees a child with whooping cough. The Division of Acute Contagious Diseases (within the Bureau of Preventable Disease) is interested. And so is the Bureau of Maternal and Child Health. The child's mother is pregnant. "I can't afford the doctor," she tells the nurse. Mindful that delay in prenatal care means increased risks to both mother and child, the nurse arranges a health department prenatal clinic appointment. "I've got a rat problem," the mother may tell the nurse. This information will go to the Bureau of Environmental Sanitation. From that office a trained sanitarian will come to help. Within a few days, the mother-to-be will be seen by a department medical social worker. They will discuss such matters

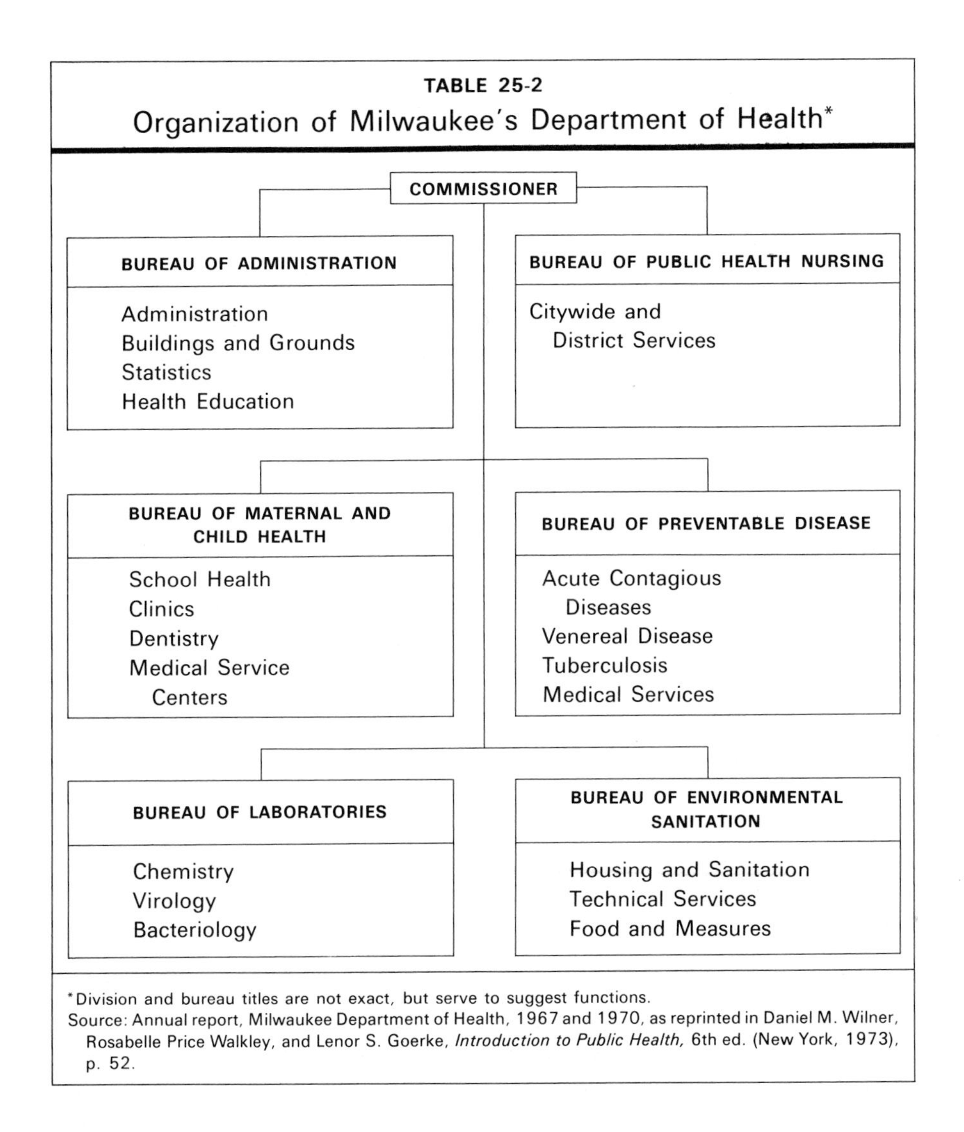

TABLE 25-2
Organization of Milwaukee's Department of Health*

*Division and bureau titles are not exact, but serve to suggest functions.
Source: Annual report, Milwaukee Department of Health, 1967 and 1970, as reprinted in Daniel M. Wilner, Rosabelle Price Walkley, and Lenor S. Goerke, *Introduction to Public Health,* 6th ed. (New York, 1973), p. 52.

as her hospitalization and her husband's employment. Part of the examination period in the prenatal clinic will be given to obtaining a blood specimen. It will be tested for syphilis by the Bureau of Laboratories. Thus is the local health department organized to give service. But its basic purpose is health education. Modern health departments employ health education specialists. But that does not relieve the obligation of every health department professional to teach health. A recent trend in some cities is to amalgamate the health department with other local official health agencies to form one "super-agency." For example, the Department of Health Services of the County of Los Angeles now includes the former Departments of Public Health, Veterinary Medicine, Mental Health, and Hospitals.

It is clear that official agencies perform a variety of vital services. But they are not alone in attempting to meet the health needs of the public; major contributions are made by the voluntary health agencies.

people care—and organize

During the long trial of his convalescence from tuberculosis, Lawrence Flick conceived an idea that led to the establishment of the first voluntary health agency in this country. Recovered at last from his illness, he set to work. Gathering together a small group of medical and lay people, he fired them with his own zeal. He told them this: a volunteer army, an organized community, could conquer consumption. Thus the Pennsylvania Society for the Prevention of Tuberculosis was founded in 1892 and later developed into the National Tuberculosis Association. And from its small beginnings came the whole voluntary health agency movement.

Other personal pain quickened similar activity against other problems. From the psychic sufferings of Clifford Beers, as told in his book *A Mind That Found Itself,* came a Connecticut mental health association and then one for the country. The loss of a son lent purpose to Edgar F. Allen's efforts to create a lasting memorial—the National Society for Crippled Children and Adults. The plight of Franklin Delano Roosevelt brought millions of dollars to a poliomyelitis foundation. That money helped Salk and Sabin to develop their vaccines. And Mrs. Rose Kennedy's quiet public reminder that she bore not only brilliant children but also a retarded child has brought wide citizen support for a society founded to attack that problem. Not the least important feature of the voluntary health agency movement is the willingness of these agencies to tackle seemingly insoluble problems. This gives hope to those afflicted with muscular dystrophy, multiple sclerosis, and a host of other robbers of human health and life.

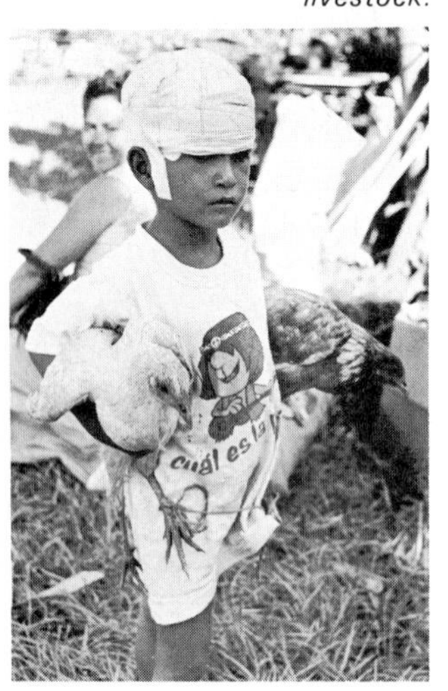

25-10 *A voluntary agency (the Red Cross) and an official U.S. agency (the Public Health Service) worked together after a 1973 earthquake in Nicaragua to help people like this injured boy—who has not forgotten the family livestock.*

In the United States today there are some seventy-five national voluntary health agencies. To their more than 25,000 local chapters millions of citizens donate both time and money. So numerous are they that they have been classified according to their interest in:

1. *specific diseases* (American Cancer Society, American Diabetes Association);
2. *special organs or structures* (American Heart Association, National Society for the Prevention of Blindness);
3. *special groups or society as a whole* (Planned Parenthood Federation of America, Ford Foundation, Alcoholics Anonymous, National Safety Council).

Like official agencies, volunteer health agencies are organized on four levels. They are international, national, state, and local.

Of both national and international import are such volunteer philanthropies as the Rockefeller, Ford, W. K. Kellogg, and Markle Foundations, as well as the Commonwealth and Milbank Memorial Funds. And justly famed are the dedicated contributions of Seventh-Day Adventist, Roman Catholic, and other church groups. These usually offer direct service. A newer development of international service is the private physicians who volunteer for short-term service abroad. Their contributions are great, but they receive much, too. They return with changed concepts and values that enable them to better deal with the social conditions that are at the root of disease at home.[83]

Some voluntary health agencies have been bitterly assailed for competitiveness over donations, others for high administrative costs, still others for overlapping functions. Their enduring contributions, however, are not to be denied. As health educators, as stimulators of official agencies and supplementors of their programs, as demonstrators of newer, better ways to health, as compaigners for improved health legislation, and as contributors to productive research, volunteer health agencies make a bright light. And they prove something important.

People care.

epilogue: health—whose responsibility?

But people must care as individuals, as active participants. Without enough individual participation, the best health organization is enfeebled. In the individual lies the basic responsibility for health. That is what this book has to say. A parable from the Talmud, very old and completely modern, sums it up.

> There was once a rabbi who had the reputation for knowing what was in a man's mind by reading his thoughts. A wicked boy came to see him and said: "Rabbi, I have in my hand a small bird. Is it alive, or is it dead?" And the boy thought to himself: If he says it is dead, I will open my hand and let it fly away; if he says it is alive, I will quickly squeeze it and show him it is dead. And the boy repeated the question: "Rabbi, I have in my hand a small bird. Is it alive, or is it dead?" And the rabbi gazed steadily at him, and said, quietly: "Whatever you will; whatever you will."[84]

Man is neither a victim nor an innocent bystander. He is more than a casual collection of chromosomes. Sartre has written that man is "condemned to be free."[85] "Everything," Sartre continued, "takes place as if I were compelled to be responsible . . . engaged in a world for which I bear the whole responsibility without being able, whatever I do, to tear myself away from this responsibility for an instant. For I am responsible for my very desire of fleeing responsibilities."[86] So freedom means responsibility. This is the freeman's paradox, his reality, and his health.

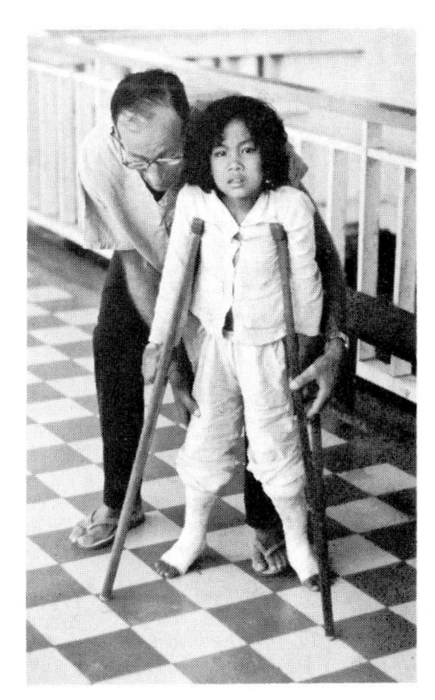

25-11 *A volunteer U.S. physician in Vietnam with one of his patients, a polio victim whose bent legs are being straightened by a series of casts.*

[83] Carl E. Taylor, "International Health: Getting More Than We Give," *Roche Medical Image,* Vol. 12, No. 4 (April 1970), p. 3.
[84] Quoted in Daniel Bell, "The Year 2000—The Trajectory of an Idea," *Daedalus,* Vol. 96, No. 3 (Summer 1967), p. 697.
[85] Jean-Paul Sartre, *Of Human Freedom,* ed. by Wade Baskin (New York, 1966), p. 94.
[86] *Ibid.,* p. 97.

summary

In recent years, advances have been made in health care that can truly be described as ''modern miracles.'' *Engineering technology* has made possible the medical use of closed-circuit television, computers, space satellites, telemedicine networks, ultrasound, and other innovations (pages 761–64). Advances in *surgical techniques* now permit successful replanting of severed limbs, transplanting of organs, and repair of diseased or damaged tissue (pages 764–67). Other areas of medicine that offer possibilities for revolutionary advances are *acupuncture* (pages 767–68), *perinatal medicine* (pages 768–69), *molecular biology* (pages 770–71), and *genetics* (pages 771–73). Some aspects of research in these and other fields present major ethical problems (pages 773–75).

Despite such dramatic achievements, many health care problems remain. Space travel and exploration of the oceans provide hope for remedying some of humanity's ills, while at the same time presenting their own special, complex problems (pages 775–76). Better health care now permits more people to live longer; the physical and emotional problems of aging are thus receiving more attention (pages 777–80). The poor of the world, and especially the children of the poor, are still beset by disease (pages 780–82).

Some organizations that perform health services are *official*—for example, the World Health Organization (pages 782–83), agencies of the U.S. government (notably the Department of Health, Education, and Welfare) (pages 783–86), and state and local health departments (pages 786–88). Other health organizations are *voluntary,* staffed largely by unpaid volunteers and supported largely by citizens' contributions (pages 788–89). In such individual participation and concern rests the essential responsibility for health (page 789).

glossary

A

abdomen The front part of the body between the chest and the pelvis.

abortion The premature expulsion from the uterus of a nonviable fetus or embryo.

abscess A focus of pus formation within a tissue, caused by an infection.

abstinence The refraining from sexual intercourse or from the ingestion of food or drugs.

abstinence syndrome A group of temporary symptoms caused by the lack of a drug in the body of a person who is physically dependent on that drug.

accreditation The mechanism by which health institutions seek to establish quality of care. To be accredited, a program or facility must meet approved standards set up by an accrediting body.

acne A skin disease common among adolescents and young adults, characterized by chronic inflammation of the sebaceous glands of the skin, usually causing pimples on the face, chest, and back.

acromegaly A condition characterized primarily by abnormal growth of hands and feet, nose, and jaw; it is caused by overproduction of growth-stimulating hormone from the anterior lobe of the pituitary gland.

active immunity Long-lasting resistance to infection acquired either through the production of antibodies by the body after invasion by disease-causing organisms or through injection of a vaccine composed of organisms that have been weakened or killed.

acupuncture An ancient Chinese method of relieving pain or treating illness by inserting needles into meridian points, certain points in the body surface that correspond to a particular diseased organ.

acute Having a rapid onset, a short course, and definite symptoms.

adenoids An increase in the amount of tissue containing white blood cells, often situated (particularly in children) at the back of the nose and above the throat.

adenosine diphosphate (ADP) A product that results from the release of energy by the breakdown of adenosine triphosphate.

adenosine triphosphate (ATP) A phosphagen that contains high-energy chemicals which when broken down yield the energy necessary for muscular contractions, production of proteins, maintenance of body heat, and other energy-requiring reactions. The other phosphagen is creatinine.

adipose Fat; of a fatty nature.

adolescence The time of life beginning with puberty (when secondary sex characteristics appear) and ending with adulthood (when major body growth stops); usually culturally determined.

adrenal gland One of two small ductless glands situated on the upper part of each kidney. Its inner portion (medulla) secretes epinephrine and norepinephrine in response to stress. Its outer portion (cortex) secretes steroids that regulate sugar and salt metabolism.

aerobic Occurring in or requiring the presence of oxygen.

aerobic capacity The maximal amount of oxygen an exercising person can take from the air.

afferent Conveying toward a center. An afferent nerve is one that transmits impulses from an outside body surface toward the central nervous system.

agglutinin An antibody that causes red blood corpuscles, or any specific bacteria it touches, to come together into clumps.

alcoholism The chronic abuse of alcohol to the extent that it interferes with the drinker's health or social functioning, or dependency on the drug to avoid withdrawal symptoms.

allergy A specific and acquired overreaction of the immune response that begins with exposure to a specific substance and then, upon later exposures to the same substance, is marked by release of a chemical substance called histamine. Also called *hypersensitivity*.

ambulatory care Any type of health service that may be provided on an outpatient basis. The term implies that the patient comes to a facility to receive services.

amebic dysentery Infection of the lower intestine by a protozoon (one-celled animal), resulting in abdominal pain and diarrhea. It is usually transmitted through water contaminated by sewage or through food contaminated by infected persons or insects. Also called *amebiasis*.

amino acid One of a group of nitrogenous organic compounds that serve as the basic units of proteins.

amotivational syndrome A group of characteristics manifested by a disinterest in self, in social improvement, and in the purposeful pursuit of goals. It is believed by some to be a result of chronic marihuana use.

anaerobic Occurring in or requiring the absence of oxygen.

androgen A hormone that produces male secondary sex characteristics and structures.

androsterone A male sex hormone, or androgen, excreted in the urine of both men and women.

anemia A condition characterized by a lower than normal number of red blood cells, and by a reduction below normal of hemoglobin.

aneurysm Abnormal dilation of the weakened wall of a blood-filled artery or a communicating blood-filled sac, such as the heart.

angina pectoris A condition characterized by recurring and intensified chest pain, often radiating to the left shoulder or arm, with a feeling of suffocation and impending death, usually due to anoxia (lack of oxygen) of the heart muscle. It may be precipitated by exertion or excitement.

antagonistic action In this text, the action by which muscles tend to be arranged on opposite sides of joints in pairs: one of the pairs bonds the joint; the other, antagonistic to it, extends the joint.

antibiotic A chemical or drug that has the ability to inhibit the growth of or to destroy bacteria and other organisms.

antibody A protein substance produced by plasma cells in response to a specific antigen; it combines with and, in effect, neutralizes the antigen.

antibody immune response A bodily reaction to microbial invasion; it involves both B and T lymphocytes, but B lymphocytes play the major role.

antigen A substance, usually protein, that when foreign to the body stimulates the formation of a specific antibody.

antigenic shift The production of a new or different strain or subtype of a virus through a spontaneous change in the chemical structure of its genes.

antihistamine A chemical substance that inhibits the production of histamine by the body.

antitoxin Antibody formed in response to the poison (toxin) of a microorganism, usually of a bacterium.

aorta The artery that transports oxygenated blood from the left ventricle of the heart to the body.

aqueous fluid (aqueous humor) The fluid filling the front and rear chambers of the eye. It is secreted by the ciliary body.

arteriosclerosis A degenerative change in an artery, resulting in thickening of the walls of the artery, loss of elasticity, and usually deposits of calcium.

artery A tubular vessel through which the blood passes away from the heart to the parts of the body.

asthma Respiratory symptoms that result from particle irritation, infection, or an allergic reaction. These symptoms include recurrent attacks of labored breathing, wheezing, coughing, and a sense of constriction in the chest.

astigmatism A visual defect that results when two adjacent portions of the cornea of the eye have different curvatures, preventing the image from being clearly focused on the retina.

atherosclerosis A circulatory disease process of large and medium-sized arteries, marked by deposits of yellow plaques containing cholesterol and other fatty substances.

atrioventricular node A very small collection of specialized heart muscle fibers situated beneath the right atrium. It is part of the heart's electrical mechanism and sends impulses received from the pacemaker to the ventricles.

atrium (pl. **atria**) One of the pair of smaller chambers of the heart, with thin muscular walls, which receives blood from the veins and passes blood to the ventricles.

atrophy Wasting away or lessening in size of a tissue, organ, or part.

auditory nerve The nerve that transmits hearing impulses from the organ of Corti to the auditory centers of the brain.

autonomic nervous system The part of the nervous system concerned with regulation of body functions over which it was formerly thought the individual had no control; its nerves extend into smooth muscle, such as of the arteries, heart, blood vessels, and glands. See also *parasympathetic nervous system, sympathetic nervous system.*

autosome A chromosome that is not a sex chromosome. In humans there are forty-four autosomes (twenty-two pairs). See also *sex chromosome.*

aversion therapy A method used in the treatment of alcoholism, smoking dependency, and some psychological problems. An alcoholic, for example, is given a drug that causes nausea, then drinks alcohol. When this is done repeatedly, the alcoholic eventually comes to associate alcohol with nausea.

B

bacterium (pl. **bacteria**) Any microorganism of the order *Eubacteriales.*

barbiturate A depressant drug used as a hypnotic (causing sleep) or a sedative (producing a quieting effect on the central nervous system).

Barr body A dark area in the nuclei of the cells of normal female mammals; sex chromatin (the chromosomal material in a nucleus that stains readily for microscopic examination).

Bartholin's gland One of the two small bodies embedded in the labia minora on either side of the opening of the vagina; they produce a lubricating material during prolonged sexual stimulation.

BCG (Bacille-Calmette-Guerin) vaccine An effective preparation for vaccination against tuberculosis; it is made from weakened cow tubercle bacilli.

benign Not malignant; not recurrent.

bile A fluid secreted by the liver into the small intestine via the gallbladder; it aids in the emulsification and absorption of fats.

birth control Intentional limitation of the number of children by preventing conception through such means as contraceptives, the rhythm method, tubal ligation, and vasectomy.

bladder A membranous sac that serves as a receptacle for the temporary retention of a body secretion, such as urine.

blastocyst The tiny mass of cells resulting from the continued division of a fertilized ovum (zygote).

blood The fluid tissue that travels through the circulatory system (heart, arteries, capillaries, and veins), carrying nutrients and oxygen to the body cells. The microscopically visible elements are red blood cells (erythrocytes), white blood cells (leukocytes), and blood platelets.

blood plasma The fluid part of the blood.

blood pressure The pressure that the blood exerts on the walls of the blood vessels or of the heart.

blood serum The clear fluid that separates from the blood when it is allowed to clot. It is blood plasma from which fibrinogen (the protein clotting factor) has been removed during the clotting process.

blood type The phenotype (the visible expression of the genotype) of the red blood cells; it is determined by one or more antigenic properties.

bowel The intestine.

brain The mass of nerve tissue contained within the skeleton of the head (cranium), including the cerebellum, cerebrum, pons, and medulla oblongata.

brain stem All of the brain except the cerebrum, cerebellum, and the white matter associated with them; it includes the sensory and motor tracts and cranial nerve centers.

bronchiole One of the small subdivisions of the branched bronchial tree of the lung.

bronchus (pl. **bronchi**) One of the large air passages within the lungs that transport air between the alveoli and the windpipe.

bursa A small sac lined with synovial membrane and filled with synovial fluid; it is found between parts that move upon each other. Example: the bursa above the bone in front of the knee (patella).

C

calorie The amount of heat necessary to raise the temperature of one kilogram of water one degree Centigrade. Also called *large calorie* or *kilocalorie.*

cancer A malignant cellular tumor.

candidiasis See *moniliasis.*

carbohydrate Any of certain organic compounds, including starches, sugars, and cellulose, that are made up of carbon, hydrogen, and oxygen.

carbon dioxide A colorless, odorless gas that is formed as waste in body cells and is eventually excreted by the lungs.

carbon monoxide A colorless, odorless, poisonous gas that causes suffocation when irreversibly combined with blood hemoglobin.

carcinogen A cancer-producing substance.

carcinoma A cancer of epithelial cells such as those in glands, skin, and the lining membranes of organs. It tends to infiltrate surrounding tissues and to spread to other parts of the body.

cardiovascular system That part of the body's circulatory system composed of the heart and blood vessels.

carrier An individual whose body harbors the organisms of an infectious disease but has none of its symptoms. Thus, a carrier may inadvertently spread the infection to others.

cartilage A specialized, fibrous connective tissue. It exists in several types, forming most of the temporary embryonic skeleton and providing a model from which most bones develop.

cataract Opacity or cloudiness of the lens of the eye.

cell A minute, bounded mass of protoplasm containing a nucleus. It is the basic unit of life and makes up all tissue.

cell-mediated immune response A bodily reaction to microbial invasion; it is carried on by ''killer'' cell T lymphocytes aided by macrophages. B lymphocytes may also be involved in this type of resistance, but how is as yet unclear.

central nervous system The brain and spinal cord.

cerebrum The main portion of the brain, located in the upper cranium and forming the largest part of the human central nervous system. It is believed to control conscious and voluntary processes.

cesarean section, cesarean delivery A surgical operation for the delivery of a fetus performed when birth by natural means is dangerous or impossible. It is accomplished by means of an incision through the walls of the abdomen and uterus.

chancre The primary sore or ulcer that is the first sign of syphilis.

chancroid A venereal disease caused by bacteria; it begins as a pustule on the genitalia and develops rapidly into a lesion that eventually becomes an open sore discharging pus.

chalones Protein-like substances that are synthesized within the mature cells of various tissues. They are widely distributed and inhibit mitosis. They may be a balancing factor between the production and loss of cells in tissues. They may someday play a role in the treatment of cancer.

chickenpox A viral disease, usually of children, caused by the same virus responsible for shingles. It is characterized by small, discolored spots on the skin. Also called *varicella.*

cholera A severe bacterial infection of the small intestine characterized by severe diarrhea, vomiting, cramps, loss of body fluids, prostration, and loss of kidney function. It is chiefly epidemic, but may also be pandemic. It is most often found in temperate, underdeveloped countries such as India.

cholesterol A chemical substance found in the fatty parts of animal tissue. It may be involved in atherosclerosis.

chromosome One of the several, more or less rod-shaped bodies that appear in the nucleus of a cell. They are constant in number for each species and contain the genes or hereditary factors; the normal number in humans is forty-six: twenty-two pairs of autosomes, and two sex chromosomes.

chronic Lasting or persisting over a long period of time.

cilia Extremely small, hairlike structures located in the bronchi and other body passages that serve to transport fluids by wavelike motions.

circadian Pertaining to the cyclic repetition of

certain phenomena in living organisms at about the same time every twenty-four hours.

circulatory system Broadly, the channels through which flow the nutrient and other vital needs of the body.

cirrhosis of the liver A disease characterized by progressive destruction of liver cells and accompanied by an increase of connective tissue. It is common among alcoholics.

climacteric The bodily, glandular, and sometimes emotional changes that occur at the end of the reproductive period in the woman and that usually result in some diminution of sexual activity in the man. In the woman, menstruation ceases; in both sexes, there is a reduction in the production of sex hormones.

cocaine A stimulant derived from coca leaves that causes powerful psychological dependence.

cochlea The spirally wound portion of the dense part of the bone of the temple containing the inner ear. Resembling a snail shell, it contains the essential structures of hearing.

coinsurance A provision in health insurance policies under which the insured individual pays part of the medical costs, usually according to a fixed percentage. For example, the insured may have to pay 20 percent of the charges in excess of $100, with the insuror paying the remainder.

coitus Sexual union in which the penis is inserted into the vagina; sexual intercourse.

coitus interruptus Sexual intercourse in which the penis is withdrawn from the vagina before ejaculation occurs; often used as a method of birth control.

comprehensive health care A type of health care delivery in which the patient can receive attention for all or most ailments in one place.

comprehensive prepaid group practice plan A type of health care plan in which the individual purchases the assurance that he or she will receive all medical care needed, including hospitalization.

conception The fertilization of an ovum by a spermatozoon.

conductive deafness Partial or total deafness due to interference with transmission of sound through the outer or middle ear.

cone One of the specialized light receptor cells of the retina of the eye that distinguish color and bright light. See also *rod*.

congenital A condition existing at birth, regardless of its cause; resulting from or developing in the prenatal environment.

congestion Excessive or abnormal accumulation of blood in a body part.

congestive heart failure An impairment of the ability of the heart to keep up an adequate flow of blood to the tissues; there is thus circulatory congestion due to heart failure.

connective tissue The tissues of an organ that support the specialized parts of that organ; for example, adipose (fatty), osseous (bony), elastic, fibrous, and cartilagenous (gristle-like) tissue.

contact dermatitis An allergic inflammation of the skin resulting from contact with causative substances.

contraception The prevention of the fertilization of an ovum by a spermatozoon.

contraceptive A device or method designed to prevent conception.

coordination The control by the nerves of muscle contractions in the performance of an act.

copulation Sexual intercourse; coitus.

coronary occlusion Hindrance of the flow of blood through an artery to the heart, resulting from a spasm of the vessel or the presence of a plug or clot.

coronary thrombosis The formation of a clot or plug in a coronary artery or one of its branches, which obstructs the flow of blood to the heart and thus leads to a heart attack.

corpus luteum A yellow body on the ovary formed by an ovarian follicle that has matured and released its ovum; it secretes the hormone progesterone.

cowpox A viral disease of cattle; the virus is genetically so closely related to smallpox virus that it can provide some immunity to smallpox.

cranium The skeleton of the head.

creatinine A phosphagen that is one of the basic sources of energy needed for muscle contraction. The other is adenosine triphosphate.

cretinism A chronic condition due to lack of thyroid secretion; it is characterized by retarded physical and mental development.

cross-tolerance The decreased susceptibility that individuals who have acquired a tolerance for one drug may exhibit toward another drug, usually a similar one. Example: LSD has a cross-tolerance to psilocybin but not to marihuana.

cunnilinction Using the mouth and tongue to stimulate the external female sex organs.

curettage The removal, by scraping, of material lining the walls of the uterus (or any other body cavity).

cyclic AMP (cyclic adenosine monophosphate) A chemical that acts as an intermediary in the release of energy for muscular work and possibly for other types of cellular work. Its mediating action in certain cells is unique; for example, as a "second messenger" within the cell it acts as a mediator of the action of many hormones (such as epinephrine).

cyclic GMP (cyclic nucleotide, quanosine 3′, 5′-monophosphate) A chemical that is apparently present in all living cells. One widely held theory about its action is that it interacts with cyclic AMP in those body cells in which occur strongly contrasting events, such as contraction–relaxation.

cystic fibrosis A chronic, hereditary disease of children marked by the malformation or the absence of the excretory duct of any or several of the exocrine glands. Organs commonly affected are the liver, pancreas, sweat glands, testicles, and mucus-producing glands of the lung and the throat.

cytomegalic inclusion disease A disease of newborns, characterized by mental and motor retardation, enlargement of the liver and spleen, and abnormal smallness of the head. It is due to a cytomegalovirus infection, often congenitally acquired.

cytoplasm All the protoplasm (the essential substance of the cell) contained within a cell except the nucleus.

D

decibel A unit of sound measurement, or of loudness.

deductibles Sums that must be paid by an insured person before health insurance benefits are payable. They are usually intended as deterrents to over-utilization of the health insurance.

degeneration Change from a higher to a lower level, especially change of tissue to a lower or functionally less active form.

delirium An emotionally disturbed state characterized by sudden onset, illusions, hallucinations, delusions, excitement, restlessness, and incoherence, and usually lasting a comparatively short time. It may be associated with severe fever, alcoholic or other drug poisoning, head injury, and other brain illnesses.

delirium tremens Delirium with a variety of signs and symptoms such as constant trembling, excitement, anxiety, and insomnia. It is associated with sudden withdrawal from alcohol and with some brain disorders.

depersonalization Loss of the sense of personal ownership of one's body.

depressant A drug that depresses the central nervous system.

detumescence The more or less gradual subsiding of swelling of the body's erectile tissue, as occurs following orgasm; it is due to the diminished congestion of the blood vessels.

diabetes mellitus An inherited chronic disorder of sugar metabolism. It is usually due to improper functioning of the pancreas, especially of its islets of Langerhans, and the resulting disturbance of the normal insulin mechanism.

diastole The rhythmic period of relaxation and dilation of a heart chamber as it fills with blood. Compare *systole*.

differentiation The progressive specialization and modification of cells into tissues and organs.

digestive system The structures related to the ingestion and digestion of food; these include the mouth and its associated structures, the pharynx, the parts of the digestive tube, and the associated glands and organs.

digitalis The dried leaf of the foxglove plant. It is used to stimulate the heart and indirectly acts as a diuretic, increasing the volume of urine.

dilation and curettage (D and C) A procedure used to perform abortions; the opening of the cervix is slightly dilated, a curette is inserted into the uterus through the cervical opening, and the pregnancy tissue is gently scraped from the wall of the uterus.

diphtheria An acute upper respiratory bacterial infection characterized by the production of a toxin, which, released into the blood stream, causes a variety of signs and symptoms. Sometimes the heart is affected.

diploid Having two sets of chromosomes, as is normal in the nucleus of the body cells of the human being.

disability insurance Usually, loss-of-income insurance, which pays a percentage of the insured individual's income while disabled.

diuretic A drug that removes water from the body by causing increased excretion of urine.

DMT (dimethyltryptamine) A potent hallucinogen. It is a common adulterant of marihuana.

DNA (deoxyribonucleic acid) A chemical substance found in the nucleus of cells; it is the material of the gene and, thus, of heredity; along with proteins, it makes up the chromosomes. DNA is also found in mitochondria and in cytoplasm.

Down's syndrome A congenital condition associated with a chromosomal abnormality; it is characterized by a somewhat flattened skull and nose, slanted eyes, and other physical abnormalities; there is usually moderate to severe mental retardation. Also called *Mongolism, trisomy 21 syndrome.*

drug Any chemical substance that is foreign to the body and is intentionally ingested to affect body function.

drug abuse According to the World Health Organization, "persistent or sporadic excessive drug use inconsistent with or unrelated to acceptable medical practice."

drug dependence A state of dependence—physical, psychological, or both—on a drug, arising from ingestion of that drug on a continuous and periodic basis.

dysfunction Any abnormality or impairment of function.

dystrophy A disorder arising from faulty or insufficient nutrition. Also, defective development, degeneration.

E

ecdemic Pertaining to a disease brought to a region from another place; for example, malaria brought to the United States from Vietnam. Compare *endemic.*

ecology The study of the relationships between living organisms and their environment.

ecosystem The fundamental unit in ecology, made up of living organisms and nonliving elements, all of which interact within a defined area in a systematic way.

ectopic pregnancy A pregnancy in which the fertilized ovum is implanted and develops outside the uterus, usually in the Fallopian tube.

eczema An inflammatory skin disease of unknown cause, marked by redness, blisters, itching, and the development of scales and crusts.

edema The swelling of tissues due to the abnormal accumulation of excess fluids.

efferent Conveying away from a center. An efferent nerve is one that transmits impulses from the central nervous system to the muscles, glands, or blood vessels.

ego-identity A term used by Erikson and other psychologists to describe the sense of self-identity that develops as a result of continuous interaction with the environment.

ejaculation The expulsion of semen that usually occurs at the climax of sexual stimulation; it is accomplished by peristaltic contractions of parts of the male genital system.

Electra complex A conscious or unconscious emotional and psychological attachment of a daughter to her father. See also *Oedipus complex.*

electrocardiogram (ECG) The graphic recording of electrical activity produced by contraction of the heart.

electroencephalogram (EEG) The graphic recording of the electrical wave patterns of the brain.

electron Any of the nonnuclear, negatively charged particles that are a part of all atoms.

electron microscope An instrument that uses rays of electrons instead of light rays to magnify an object.

embolism The blockage of a blood vessel by a clot or other obstruction that has been brought to its position by the blood flow.

embolus A clot or other obstruction that travels through the blood stream until it lodges in a blood vessel and plugs it.

embryo The early stage of development of an organism in the uterus. In the human, the term describes the period of development from one week after fertilization to the end of the second month of pregnancy.

emphysema A lung condition marked by abnormal increase in size of the air spaces farthest from the terminal bronchioles. The walls of the alveoli (air sacs) of the lungs are also destroyed.

encephalitis Inflammation of the brain.

endemic Pertaining to a disease that is peculiar to a certain region or people, and persists in a region without sudden variation.

endocrine gland A gland that secretes its hormone directly into the blood stream rather than into a duct, as does an exocrine gland.

endoplasm The inner portion of the cytoplasm of a cell.

endoplasmic reticulum A membranous transportation system of canals within the cytoplasm of cells, which are formed by inward folds of the plasma cell membrane that surrounds the cell. Materials needed by the cell move through these canals. The endoplasmic reticulum also connects with the nuclear membrane.

engorgement Congestion, usually by blood.

enzyme An organic compound, usually a protein, that acts as a catalyst, speeding up specific chemical reactions of other compounds without itself taking part in those reactions.

epidemic Pertaining to a disease that attacks many individuals in an area within a short time; an unusual outbreak of a disease.

epilepsy A chronic condition of the nervous system, marked by widely varying signs and symptoms, which may include convulsions, loss of consciousness, and psychic or sensory disturbances.

epithelium The sheetlike tissue that lines the internal and external surfaces of the body, including the surface of the skin, the vessels, and the digestive, respiratory, and genital tracts.

erogenous zone An area of the body that is especially sensitive to sexual stimulation. Some of these are the mouth, lips, tongue, breasts and nipples, buttocks, and genitals.

erythroblastosis fetalis An anemia of the newborn infant or fetus, caused by transfer through the placenta of maternal antibodies that are usually formed because of an incompatibility between the blood group of the mother and the child. Also called *Rh blood disease.*

erythrocyte See *red blood cell.*

estrogen The female sex hormone. Also, a general term for compounds produced by ovarian hormonal activity resulting in secondary sex characteristics and cyclic genital changes.

etiology The study of the cause or causes of a disease.

exocrine gland A gland that secretes its products into a duct rather than directly into the blood stream, as does an endocrine gland.

F

Fallopian tube See *oviduct.*

family physician A physician engaged in family practice, who assumes continuing responsibility for all the health matters of all family members, regardless of age, seeking the aid of a specialist when necessary.

farsightedness A visual disorder marked by the ability to see far objects more clearly than near ones and caused by a loss of elasticity in the lens that causes images to fall in back of the retina. Also called *hyperopia.*

fatigue A lessened capacity for physical activity caused by previous activity.

fats Substances high in caloric value and found in some form in most foods.

feces The solid waste products of digestion excreted from the intestine.

feedback mechanism The means by which hormone production is controlled. The target organ sends back a chemical message to the gland, signaling it to halt production and release of its hormone.

fee-for-service The payment of a specified fee to the provider of health services for each item of service performed.

fellation Oral stimulation of the penis.

fertile Capable of producing young.

fetus In humans, the developing child in the uterus from the beginning of the third month of pregnancy until birth.

fibrillation Rapid, nonrhythmic, ineffective contractions of the heart or any other muscle.

fibrinogen The protein that enables the blood to clot.

flexibility Range of motion.

flexion Bending of one part of the body upon another part.

follicle See *Graafian follicle.*

follicle-stimulating hormone (FSH) One of the gonadotropic (gonad-stimulating) hormones produced by the anterior lobe of the pituitary gland under the direction of the hypothalamus of the brain. FSH promotes the maturation of the Graafian follicle in the female and stimulates the formation of spermatozoa in the testes of the male.

foreplay The preliminary stages of sexual intercourse, in which the individuals stimulate each other by kissing and caressing.

foreskin See *prepuce*.

fovea A tiny pit in the retina that is the area of clearest vision because the layers of the retina are spread aside, allowing light to fall directly on the cones.

Frolich's syndrome A condition caused by impaired function of the hypothalamus and pituitary gland. It is characterized by deposits of fat, incomplete or abnormal genital development, metabolic disturbances, and retarded development of the gonads. Also called *adiposogenital dystrophy*.

fungus (pl. **fungi**) A parasitic low form of plant life that lacks chlorophyll.

G

gamete A secondary sex cell. In humans, either a male spermatozoon or a female ovum. See also *primordial germ (sex) cell*.

gamma globulin A general term referring to blood proteins, many of which contain antibodies.

ganglion (pl. **ganglia**) A group of nerve cell bodies that are usually located outside of the central nervous system.

gastric Pertaining to the stomach.

gastric ulcer An ulcer of the mucous lining of the stomach.

gastritis An inflammation of the stomach.

gastroenteritis A term for a variety of inflammations of the stomach and intestine that may be caused by a number of viral or bacterial infectious agents.

gastrointestinal Pertaining to the stomach and intestine.

gene The basic unit of heredity and genetic information. Each gene is self-reproducing and is located at a specific place on a chromosome.

generalist A physician, such as a family physician, who engages in general medical practice, caring for all members of a family, regardless of age, and seeking the aid of a specialist when necessary.

generic drug A drug not registered or protected by a trademark.

genetic code The hereditary instructions contained in DNA; structurally, the arrangement of four chemicals (called the nitrogenous bases) that determines the formation of proteins.

genital Pertaining to reproduction or to the reproductive organs.

genital herpes A viral genital infection in which blisters form; these may become ulcers that, in turn, become infected.

genital louse The "crab louse," a small parasitic insect that usually infests the pubic region but can spread to other hairy parts of the body.

genitals, genitalia The reproductive organs.

genital wart A benign viral tumor that may be transmitted by genital contact.

genotype The particular assortment or combination of genes of an individual.

German measles See *rubella*.

germ cell A spermatozoon or an ovum.

gerontology The scientific study of aging, including its sociological, clinical, and biological aspects.

gestation See *pregnancy*.

gigantism Abnormal overgrowth; excessive size and stature.

gland A group of cells that separates elements from the blood and produces from them a specific substance for the body to use.

glans The sensitive erectile body at the end of the clitoris or penis.

glaucoma A condition of the eye marked by increased pressure within the eyeball.

glomerulonephritis Inflammation of the capillary loops in the kidney glomeruli.

glomerulus (pl. **glomeruli**) The numerous tiny capillary coils or tufts in the kidney, each projecting into the expanded end, or capsule, of a uriniferous tubule. From it blood wastes are filtered into the tubule.

glycogen A complex sugar, formed from carbohydrate (such as starches), found in many body tissues (such as those of the embryo and in muscle), and stored in the liver, where, as the body requires, it is converted to a simpler sugar, glucose.

glycolysis The breakdown of the sugar glucose to lactic acid, a fatigue toxin.

glucose A simple sugar. It is in this form that carbohydrate is carried in the blood to be metabolized in the tissues.

goiter An enlargement of the thyroid gland, primarily due to iodine deficiency.

Golgi complex A structure within a cell, part of the endoplasmic reticulum, the surface of which is always smooth and which has sacs; its purpose seems to be to store and release protein enzymes manufactured at the ribosomes.

gonad A gland that produces gametes; the ovary or testis.

gonadotropic hormone Any hormone that influences a gonad.

gonadotropin A hormone that stimulates or has an affinity for the gonads.

gout An inborn error of metabolism of uric acid (a chemical waste product) in the blood, marked by the formation of chalky deposits in the joints and by recurrent attacks of acute arthritis.

Graafian follicle A tiny sac or pouch in the ovary that contains the maturing ovum, releasing it at ovulation.

group therapy (group psychotherapy) Treatment for emotional problems given to a group of patients by a professional therapist. It is based not only on the effect of the group upon the individual but also on the individual's interaction with the group. It has been used in the treatment of a variety of conditions, among them alcoholism and other drug dependencies, and in the treatment of persons who wish to change or better understand their homosexual behavior.

group practice A systemic relationship among several professional people, such as physicians and dentists, formally organized to provide health services.

H

half life The time it takes the radioactivity originally associated with an isotope to lessen by half as a result of radioactive decay.

hallucinogen An agent or drug that produces hallucinations or the perception of sights and sounds that are not actually present.

haploid Having one set of unpaired chromosomes, as is normal in the gametes of the human being.

health insurance The pooling of funds by a group from which amounts are withdrawn to pay, or to assist in paying, unpredictable health care expenses of the members of the group.

heart attack A lay term for damage to the heart muscle that results from the blockage of a coronary artery by either a thrombus or an embolus.

helminth A worm or wormlike parasite.

hemoglobin The pigment that is the primary constituent of red blood cells and that carries oxygen and carbon dioxide.

hemophilia A hereditary disease in which the blood cannot clot.

hepatitis A viral inflammation of the liver caused by two distinct types of infection, called *hepatitis A* (or *infectious hepatitis*) and *hepatitis B* (or *serum hepatitis*).

heredity The transmission of physical and emotional traits and characteristics from parents to offspring.

hermaphrodite An individual who possesses tissues of both male and female sex organs.

hermaphroditism A condition in which tissues of both male and female sex organs exist in one individual. In the human it is characterized by the presence of both ovarian and testicular tissue and reproductive organs that are not typical of one gender.

heroin A white, crystalline powder derived from morphine; it is a powerful narcotic.

herpes genitalis (herpes progenitalis) A common viral disorder causing a disease often marked by small fluid-filled sacs upon patchy areas of red skin. It is commonly transmitted by sexual intercourse.

herpes simplex A viral disease marked by blisters on the skin and mucous membranes. Also called *cold sore*.

herpes zoster (shingles) A viral disease, usually of adults, caused by the same virus responsible for chickenpox. It is marked by inflammation of nerves and painful, blisterlike lesions on the skin or on mucous membranes in which the nerves end.

heterosexual behavior Sexual interest or activity that is directed toward individuals of the opposite sex.

histamine A chemical released by body tissues

in allergic reactions; it causes capillaries to dilate.

Hodgkin's disease A progressive, formerly fatal enlargement of the spleen, lymph nodes, and general lymphoid tissue.

homosexual behavior Sexual interest or activity that is directed toward individuals of the same sex.

hormone A chemical substance secreted by an endocrine (ductless) gland into the circulatory system and having a specific effect on a certain target organ.

host An animal or plant that harbors or nourishes another organism.

hydrocarbon An organic compound that contains only hydrogen and carbon.

hydrocortisone A steroid produced by the adrenal glands or prepared in the laboratory to be used in treatment of certain acute infections and allergic states. It acts like cortisone but is much more active.

hymen The membrane that partly or entirely covers the external opening of the vagina in some females who have never had sexual intercourse.

hyperkinetic Pertaining to abnormally increased mobility or activity.

hyperplasia An abnormal increase in the number of cells of a given tissue; often associated with malignant tumors.

hypersensitivity See *allergy*.

hypertension Persistent abnormally high blood pressure.

hyperthyroidism Excessive activity of the thyroid gland, characterized by severe nervousness, weight loss, and sometimes protruding eyeballs.

hypertrophy An increase in the size of a tissue or organ without relation to general body growth, and resulting from an increase in the size, not the number, of cells.

hypochondriasis Undue and severe anxiety about one's health.

hypothalamus A portion of the brain that regulates many basic body functions, such as water balance, temperature, and sleep. It also produces certain hormones that stimulate the anterior lobe of the pituitary to produce and release hormones. In addition, it may produce chemicals to regulate the amount of hormones it produces.

I

immunity The ability of the body to resist the development of a disease or infection. See also *active immunity, passive immunity*.

implantation The process by which the blastocyst penetrates the surface layer of the uterus and becomes embedded in the endometrium. This occurs six or seven days after fertilization of the ovum.

impotence Inability of the male to have satisfactory sexual intercourse; usually, the inability to achieve or maintain an erection.

incest Sexual intercourse between close relatives, such as mother and son, father and daughter, or sister and brother.

indemnity benefits Insurance benefits in the form of cash payments rather than services. The indemnity insurance policy usually defines specifically what services are and are not included and the maximum amount that will be paid for the various services covered.

infarct An area of dead tissue that results from lack of oxygenated blood caused by a circulatory obstruction such as a clot.

infection The invasion of the body by a disease-causing organism and the reaction of the tissues to the presence of the organism and its toxins.

infectious hepatitis One of the two best-known types of viral hepatitis; the infectious agent is often called IH or A virus.

infectious mononucleosis A usually benign viral disease marked by irregular fever, sore throat, painful swelling of lymph nodes, enlarged spleen, and an increase of lymphocytes in the blood.

inferior vena cava The large venous blood vessel that drains blood from the pelvic and abdominal organs and the lower extremities and empties into the right atrium of the heart. See also *superior vena cava*.

inflammation A condition that occurs in tissues as a result of injury, characterized by redness, pain, heat, and swelling.

influenza An acute viral respiratory disease characterized by headache, fever, depression, muscular pain (in adults), and sore throat.

instinct A natural tendency that urges a human being or animal, without the exercise of reason, to perform actions that are usually useful or beneficial.

insulin A hormone produced by the islet cells of Langerhans in the pancreas and secreted into the blood, where it regulates sugar metabolism.

interferon A protein formed by animal cells during their interaction with viruses. It has the ability to confer on fresh animal cells of the same animal species resistance to infection by other viruses.

intrauterine Within the uterus.

intromission Insertion of the penis into the vagina.

ischemia Lack of sufficient blood to a body part, due to obstruction of a blood vessel.

islet cells of Langerhans The specific cells in the pancreas that produce the hormone insulin.

isometric contraction A contraction in which a muscle cannot shorten. Tension develops, but it is dissipated as heat. Neither movement nor work is performed.

isotonic contraction A contraction in which a muscle shortens against a load, leading to work and movement.

isotope A form of a chemical element that has the same number of nuclear protons as another form of that element, but has a different number of nuclear neutrons.

J

jaundice A symptom of many diseases, such as viral hepatitis, that lead to an excess of bile in the blood; it is characterized by a yellowing of the skin and the whites of the eyes.

joint An articulation; a body location where two bones are connected to each other in a way that allows them to move.

K

karyotype A chart showing the typical characteristics (such as number, size, and form) and systematic arrangement of the chromosomes of a cell of an individual or species.

Klinefelter's syndrome A genetic disorder in which the mature sex cells of the individual have two X-chromosomes and one Y-chromosome (XXY). The individual may appear normal, but he is usually tall, has underdeveloped sexual structures, is usually sterile, and is often mentally retarded.

L

lactation The secretion of milk by the breast.

lactic acid The toxic end product of anaerobic metabolism of glucose or glycogen.

lead poisoning (plumbism) A poisoning due to prolonged ingestion or absorption of lead or lead-containing materials. Colic, permanent brain damage, extensive nerve damage, and severe anemia may result.

leprosy An infectious disease of variable communicability, believed to be caused by a bacillus. There are two forms of the disease, one more communicable than the other. The body parts most frequently affected are skin and nerves.

lesion An injury, damage, or other change in an organ or tissue that may result in loss or impairment of function.

lethal Deadly; fatal.

leukemia A cancer of the blood-forming organs that may be either chronic or acute and is marked by a great increase in the number of white blood cells and by enlargement of the lymphatic tissue and bone marrow.

leukocyte See *white blood cell*.

libido Sexual desire; the motivational force of sexuality.

ligament A fibrous connective tissue that holds bone joints together or supports organs.

lobe A more or less rounded, well-defined part of an organ or gland.

lockjaw See *tetanus*.

lobule A small lobe or a part of a lobe.

lumen The channel or cavity within a tubular organ.

luteinizing hormone (LH) A substance secreted and released by the anterior lobe of the pituitary gland that causes the mature Graafian follicle to rupture, releasing the ovum. In the male, this hormone is involved in the production of testosterone.

luteinizing-hormone–releasing hormone/follicle-stimulating-hormone–releasing hormone (LH-RH/FSH-RH) A substance that originates in the hypothalamus of the brain and that stimulates the anterior lobe of the pituitary gland to produce and release both luteinizing hormone and follicle-stimulating hormone.

lymph A clear, yellowish liquid collected from the tissue spaces once it has entered the lymph vessels. It transports back to the blood protein molecules that seep into the extracellular spaces. It also contains white cells loaded with wastes that are filtered out by the lymph nodes.

lymphatic system A system of vessels (separate from but accessory to the blood circulatory system) and masses of other tissue (filtering lymph nodes) used to transport lymph and certain waste products.

lymph node One of a number of masses of lymphoid tissue situated along the course of lymphatic vessels. They filter cellular debris and other wastes from lymph. They are involved in immunity. In them, lymphocytes are manufactured and plasma cells make antibodies.

lymphocyte A type of white blood cell on which the body's immune response depends. Manufactured largely in the bone marrow, lymphocytes enter the blood stream to be differentiated into B lymphocytes and T lymphocytes. B lymphocytes play the major role in the antibody immune response. T lymphocytes (called "killer cells") are more active in the cell-mediated immune response, directly attacking and destroying many organisms that invade the body. In this activity, they are joined by another type of white blood cell, the macrophage.

lymphoma A new growth, usually cancerous, of lymphatic tissues.

lysosomes Tiny organelles found inside a cell that contain digestive enzymes capable of breaking down complex nutrients into simpler substances that the cell can use.

M

macrophage A type of cell that assists T lymphocytes in the cell-mediated immune response, functioning as a phagocyte, engulfing and ingesting foreign particles or cells (such as bacteria) that harm the body.

major medical insurance An insurance policy that covers unusually high health care expenses, as for a long illness. Such insurance is usually offered by commercial insurance companies.

malaria An infectious disease that is transmitted by the bite of a mosquito and is therefore most common in tropical areas. It is characterized by recurring fever alternating with chills.

malignant Cancerous; dangerous to health or life.

malocclusion Improper alignment of the upper and lower rows of teeth.

Mantoux test A test for tuberculosis that involves an injection of tuberculin (a growth product of the tubercle bacillus) into the skin. If a local allergic reaction occurs, the test is positive—meaning that the person has active tuberculosis or the infection has occurred and the disease is self-healed and thus not active. If there is no allergic reaction, the test is negative.

measles See *rubella, rubeola.*

Medicaid A program that provides federal grants of money to the states to operate medical assistance programs for people who were already receiving some assistance from the federal government.

Medicare A program of health insurance for people aged sixty-five or older.

medulla The middle or innermost part of an organ, gland, or structure; for example, the medulla of the adrenal gland.

meiosis A type of cell division that occurs only in the maturation process of sex cells; each daughter nucleus receives one-half the number of chromosomes normally found in a somatic (body) cell. See also *mitosis.*

membrane A thin layer of tissue that divides a space or an organ or that covers a surface.

menarche The onset of menstruation.

meninges The three membranes that enclose the brain and spinal cord.

menopause The cessation of menstruation in the female, usually occurring between the ages of forty-five and fifty.

messenger RNA A type of ribonucleic acid that transfers information from a portion of the nuclear DNA to a ribosome of a cell, where proteins are formed.

metabolism All the chemical and physical processes by which living substance is produced and maintained; the process by which energy is made available to the cell.

metastasis The transfer of disease (usually cancer) from one organ or site to another.

methadone A narcotic drug used as a substitute for heroin.

microbe A microscopic organism, especially a bacterium.

microorganism A microscopic organism, especially a bacterium or one-celled protozoan.

migraine Severe periodic headaches, often accompanied by nausea, vomiting, and various sensory or motor disturbances.

migration In this text, apparently spontaneous movement of cells.

mineral A nonorganic substance found naturally in the earth. Some principal minerals in the human body are: calcium, phosphorus, chlorine, potassium, sodium, sulfur, iodine, iron, and magnesium. Among those also present in the body are: copper, manganese, cobalt, zinc, fluorine, molybdenum, selenium, and chromium.

miscarriage A lay term for the premature and spontaneous expulsion from the uterus of the products of conception; a spontaneous abortion.

mitochondrion (pl. **mitochondria**) Any of the organelles in the cytoplasm of a cell that convert the chemical energy of cellular nutrients into a high-energy compound called adenosine triphosphate (ATP). They also contain their own DNA.

mite A tiny, sometimes microscopic animal, related to spiders, that is often parasitic to man, other animals, insects, or plants.

mitosis A type of cell division in which each daughter nucleus receives the exact number and complement of chromosomes that the parent somatic (body) cell has. See also *meiosis.*

mold Any of a group of very small fungi that live on living, decaying, or dead matter and can cause moldiness on food.

molecule The smallest particle of a compound or element that has the characteristics of that compound or element.

Mongolism See *Down's syndrome.*

moniliasis An infection caused by a fungus. It may occur in the genital tract, the skin, or the mouth (where it is called *thrush*). Also called *candidiasis.*

monosomy The absence of one chromosome from the normal number of chromosomes of a diploid cell.

morbidity The condition of being diseased.

mosaicism The presence within the same individual of cells with different chromosomal makeup.

mucosa Mucous membrane; thin body tissue that has a moist surface.

mucous Pertaining to mucus.

mucus The slimy, protective material of the mucous membranes that contains their secretions and various other materials, such as dead cells.

multiple sclerosis A chronic degenerative disease of the central nervous system.

mumps A contagious viral disease, often marked by inflammation and swelling of the parotid and other salivary glands, fever, and pain beneath the ear. In males, it may be complicated by swelling of the testes; in the female, the ovary may be involved.

mutation A change in form or other characteristic; often refers to a spontaneous change in the genetic makeup of an organism.

myocardial infarction Death of a part of the heart muscle as a result of an obstruction of the blood supply to that area.

myocardium The heart muscle.

myofibril One of the structures, containing nuclei and mitochondria, that make up striated muscle. Each consists of two kinds of filaments, thick and thin, that overlap, giving striated muscle its characteristic striped appearance.

myopia A visual disorder marked by the ability to see near objects more clearly than far ones and caused by a lengthening of the diameter of the eye from front to back, which causes images to fall in front of the retina. Also called *nearsightedness.*

N

narcolepsy A disorder marked by an uncontrollable desire for sleep or by sudden attacks of sleep. Often associated with obesity.

narcotic A drug that, when properly used, relieves pain, produces sleep, and diminishes feeling. Overdose may result in stupor, coma, convulsions, or death.

nausea A feeling of sickness in the stomach area with a tendency to vomit.

nearsightedness See *myopia.*

neighborhood health center A community health center established to provide comprehensive health care in poverty areas.

neonatal Pertaining to a newborn infant.

nephron One of the very small filtering units of the kidney that produce urine. It is composed of a glomerulus (a capillary tuft) and a kidney tubule.

nerve deafness Impairment of hearing due to an injury or damage to the auditory nerve.

neurasthenia A group of symptoms, of a neurotic nature, marked by chronic fatigue, aches and pains, and sometimes exhaustion.

neuron A complete nerve cell, including all its projections and terminations; regarded as the basic structural unit of the nervous system.

neurosis (pl. **neuroses**) An emotional disorder that variously interferes with an individual's ability to deal effectively with reality. It is marked by anxiety and impairment of functioning in some areas of the individual's life. It is usually the result of an attempt to resolve unconscious emotional conflicts. Unlike the psychotic, the neurotic has not lost contact with reality.

neutron An electrically neutral particle of matter existing along with protons in the nuclei of atoms.

nocturnal emission Involuntary ejaculation of semen during sleep; "wet dream."

nonarticular rheumatism Inflammation of any of the connective tissue structures of the body, excluding the joints.

nondisjunction Failure of paired chromosomes to separate during cell division (usually meiosis) so that one daughter nucleus receives both members of the pair, and the other daughter nucleus lacks that particular chromosome.

nucleic acid Any of the class of proteins found in the nucleus and cytoplasm of a cell and consisting of ribonucleic acids and deoxyribonucleic acids.

nucleus A spherical body found within a cell and consisting of several characteristic organelles, such as a nuclear membrane, nucleoli, granules of chromatin, and diffuse protoplasm. Also within the nucleus are the chromosomes.

nurse A professionally trained individual who cares for the sick, wounded, or invalid. There are specialists in the nursing field, such as public health nurses and psychiatric nurses; less trained than these are licensed practical nurses, licensed vocational nurses, and nurses' aides. Also, to suckle an infant.

nursing home An institution organized to provide health care services for people who must be in-patients but do not need regular hospital care.

nutrient A substance that yields energy, is used as a building material by the body, and is obtained from foods.

O

Oedipus complex A conscious or unconscious emotional and psychological attachment of a son to his mother. The term may also refer to a similar attachment of a daughter to her father. See also *Electra complex.*

oöcyte A developing egg that has not finished its maturation process.

oögenesis The process of origin and maturation of the ovum.

oögonium The primordial cell from which an ovum derives; its divisions produce oöcytes.

opiate A drug derived from opium; it also may mean any drug that induces sleep.

oral contraceptive A tablet that is swallowed for the purpose of preventing pregnancy; the birth control "pill."

organelle A particular type of organized living material, usually with a specific function, that is present in most cells; among these are the nucleus, ribosomes, mitochondria, endoplasmic reticulum, and Golgi complex.

organ A differentiated part of the body that performs a special function.

organic (1) Having organs. (2) Of living organisms. (3) In chemistry, pertaining to compounds containing carbon. (4) Pertaining to physical, rather than emotional, sources of symptoms. (5) Pertaining to foods grown and produced without artificial substances, such as pesticides or additives.

organ of Corti A spiral-shaped organ located within the cochlea of the ear; it contains the ciliated cells, the nerves which carry sound vibrations to the auditory nerve and thus to the brain.

osmosis The flow of a pure liquid through a membrane from the greater to the lesser concentration of a solution. It is usually by this method that nutrients are absorbed by cells and wastes are excreted.

osteoarthritis A chronic joint disease marked by the deterioration of cartilage and bone.

outpatient An individual who comes to a hospital, clinic, doctor's office, or other facility for diagnosis or treatment but does not occupy a bed there; an ambulatory patient.

ovary The female gonad; the reproductive gland of the female in which the ova (eggs) develop.

oviduct The tube that extends from the ovary to the uterus and through which the ovum (egg) travels. Also called *Fallopian tube, uterine tube.*

ovulation The discharge of a mature ovum from the Graafian follicle of the ovary.

ovum (pl. **ova**) The mature female reproductive cell, or egg, which after fertilization by a spermatozoon develops into a new individual of the same species.

oxidation The union of a compound or substance with oxygen. Also, the chemical process in which the positive charges of an atom increase or negative charges are lost.

oxide Any compound of oxygen with an element or a radical (a group of two or more atoms that act as a single atom).

oxygen A gaseous element existing in air. It is the essential agent in the respiration of animals and plants.

oxygenation The loose, readily reversible combination of oxygen with blood hemoglobin.

oxygen debt The amount of oxygen that is required in the recovery period after exercise to reverse the anaerobic reactions that occurred during the exercise. It is the difference between the amount of oxygen required to do a certain task, and the amount taken in during the actual performance of the task.

oxyhemoglobin Hemoglobin loosely combined with oxygen.

oxytocin A chemical hormone stored and released from the posterior lobe of the pituitary gland but manufactured in the brain's hypothalamus. Its principal action is to stimulate the uterus to contract, but it also stimulates the production of milk.

P

pacemaker An area of the heart tissue specialized to trigger rhythmic contractions of the heart muscle. Also, a device to do this.

Papanicolaou test ("Pap smear") A painless diagnostic test for cancer of the uterine cervix. The test can also be applied to other easily accessible areas to detect cancer cells.

pandemic A widespread, even worldwide epidemic.

paralysis Loss or impairment of movement or feeling due to a lesion of the muscular or nerve mechanism.

paranoia A chronic, slowly progressing, serious emotional disturbance marked by the development of suspicions (or sometimes ambitions) into systematized delusions of persecution (or grandeur), which are built up in an apparently logical form.

parasite An animal or plant that lives within or upon another living organism (the host), at whose expense the parasite obtains some advantage without the host receiving compensation.

parasympathetic nervous system One of the two divisions of the autonomic nervous system; it is composed of ganglia located on either side of the spinal cord and innervates various muscles, glands, and organs. When a person is relaxed, the parasympathetic division dominates. After the sympathetic nervous system has altered various body functions, the parasympathetic nervous system returns these functions to their normal state. Sometimes the sympathetic and parasympathetic systems work together; for example, during the male sexual act, erection is parasympathetic in origin and ejaculation is sympathetic. See also *autonomic nervous system, sympathetic nervous system.*

parathyroid gland One of four small glands, situated beside the thyroid gland in the neck, that control the metabolism of calcium and phosphorus.

passive immunity Immunity that is acquired by the administration of preformed antibody; it is borrowed immunity and does not last long.

penis The male organ of sexual intercourse and the external organ of urination.

perinatal period The period beginning with the birth of a fetus at twenty weeks or more of pregnancy and ending seven to twenty-eight days later.

perineum The area between the genital organs and the rectum. It is sometimes defined as the whole area at the pelvic outlet, including the anus and the internal genitals.

peripheral nervous system The portion of the nervous system not included in the brain and spinal cord. It consists of the twelve pairs of cranial nerves and the autonomic nervous system.

peristalsis The wormlike or wavelike contractions by which tubular organs, such as the Fallopian tubes and the alimentary canal, propel their contents.

pH The symbol for the degree of acidity or alkalinity in a solution; a pH of 7 is neutral (neither acid nor alkaline); pH values from 0 to 7 indicate acidity; pH values from 7 to 14 indicate alkalinity.

phagocyte A cell produced by the body that can engulf and digest disease-causing organisms.

phenotype The visible expression of the hereditary or genetic makeup of an individual.

phenylketonuria (PKU) A genetic disorder of the metabolism of phenylalanine, an amino acid essential for growth in infants, caused by the absence of the enzyme necessary to metabolize this amino acid. The disorder may be associated with mental retardation.

phosphagens Adenosine triphosphate and creatinine, the two chemical compounds in the muscle cells that are the basic sources of energy for muscle contraction.

physical fitness A very general term referring to the individual's ability to adjust dynamically to various environmental stresses. *Specific fitness* refers to the ability to do a specific task, like running or weight lifting. *General fitness* implies the ability to meet adequately with all the tasks of life, including its emergencies, without enough residual energy at the end of the day to enjoy individual ways of relaxation. The basic elements of physical fitness are strength, endurance, and flexibility.

physician's assistant A person who, having received some training and working under a physician's supervision, relieves the physician of certain routine duties.

pica A hunger for nonfood substances; it may occur during pregnancy, emotional disturbance, or malnutrition.

pineal gland (pineal body) A single, pea-sized organ near the center of the brain; it sends messages to the nervous system that influence the body's biological rhythms. Melatonin, one of its chemicals, affects the sexual cycle in animals.

pituitary gland A small gland of enormous importance, located at the base of the brain; it has a profound effect on the function of certain other glands, especially the thyroid, adrenals, and sex glands. It is dependent for its function on the nearby hypothalamus of the brain.

placenta The organ in the uterus that connects the fetus to the mother by means of the umbilical cord; through it, the fetus is nourished and wastes are removed. Also called *afterbirth*.

plaque Fatty deposits on the lining of arteries, characteristic of atherosclerosis. Also, a deposit of hardened debris on the surface of a tooth, which may serve as a medium for the growth of bacteria and play a role in tooth decay.

plasma cell A cell present in lymphoid tissue and derived from lymphocytes (a type of white blood cell); it is involved in the production of antibodies.

plasma membrane The porous organelle that surrounds a cell and allows only certain kinds and amounts of materials to enter and leave the cell.

platelet A colorless disk present in blood and involved in the coagulation of blood and the formation of blood clots.

poliomyelitis An acute viral disease that can occur in varying degrees of severity. In the mild form, there is fever, headache, aching muscles, and diarrhea; unless the infective agent is identified, this form is not usually recognized as polio. The second form is called nonparalytic; it is characterized by temporary paralysis of the limbs. The final form is called paralytic; it can produce permanent deformity caused by muscular atrophy and is sometimes fatal.

polychlorinated biphenyls (PCBs) Chemical compounds used for a variety of industrial purposes. Have been a pollutant in the United States, but use is now limited to avoid further pollution.

polycystic kidney A usually hereditary condition marked by enlargement of the kidneys, which develop many cysts.

polyunsaturated fats Fats that are usually vegetable rather than animal. See also *saturated fats*.

postnatal Immediately following birth.

postpartum After delivery or birth.

posture The position of the body as a whole; the way in which the segments of the body rest on one another.

pregnancy The period during which a female has a developing embryo or fetus in her uterus.

premature ejaculation The expulsion of semen prior to or immediately after insertion of the penis into the vagina.

prenatal Before birth.

prepayment plan A health insurance plan in which premiums are paid in advance into a fund used to pay for health services when they are needed. The term includes nonprofit plans, insurance contracts, self-insured plans, and health and welfare plans.

prepuce In the uncircumcised male, the fold of skin that covers the head of the penis (glans); in the female, the fold formed by the labia minora that covers the glans of the clitoris. Also called *foreskin*.

primary team A group of health personnel who replace the single-physician concept. The team may include a physician internist, pediatrician, nurse practitioner, and family health worker.

primordial germ (sex) cell One of the reproductive cells having a diploid number of chromosomes (forty-six, in humans) and from which the gametes (secondary sex cells) arise by means of meiosis.

progesterone The hormone secreted by the corpus luteum; its basic function is to ready the uterus for the reception and development of a fertilized ovum.

progestin The name for certain brands of synthetic progesterone.

prolactin A hormone manufactured and released by the anterior lobe of the pituitary gland; it stimulates milk production.

promiscuity In this text, engagement in sexual intercourse indiscriminately or casually with many people; sexual activity without rules.

prophylaxis Prevention of disease.

protein One of a group of compounds made up mostly of amino acids that are the main component of protoplasm.

protoplasm A semiliquid, translucent material that is the essential matter of all plant and animal cells.

protozoon (pl. **protozoa**) Any of a group of one-celled animals, such as an amoeba.

psychoactive drug Any drug that produces temporary changes in the physiological functions of a person's nervous system, affecting thoughts, feelings, mood, or behavior. These "mind-bending" drugs include sedatives and tranquilizers ("downers") and stimulants ("uppers"). Also called *psychotropic drug*.

psychedelic drug Any "mind-expanding" drug, usually a hallucinogen, that induces a state of altered perception, thought, and feeling that may otherwise be experienced only in dreams or during times of religious exaltation.

psychomotor epilepsy A type of epilepsy in which, during a seizure, the individual performs complex and purposeful acts but cannot remember them afterward.

psychosis (pl. **psychoses**) Severe emotional disorder, especially a deep, far-reaching, and long-term behavior disturbance manifested, in part, by withdrawal from reality.

psychosomatic Pertaining to physical symptoms of an emotional origin.

psychosurgery Treatment of severe chronic mental disorders by surgical interruption or removal of certain pathways or areas of the brain.

psychotherapy Treatment of emotional disorders by psychological methods such as suggestion, persuasion, reassurance, re-education, group therapy, hypnosis, and psychoanalysis.

psychotropic drug Any drug that exerts an effect on the mind or is capable of changing emotional activity.

puberty The period of time during which secondary sex characteristics appear; the stage of physical development when sexual reproduction first becomes possible.

pubes The hair growing in the pubic area. Also, the plural of *pubis*, the pubic bone.

pubescence The period of individual arrival at puberty during which the secondary sex characteristics begin to appear and sexual functioning begins to mature.

pulmonary artery The artery that extends from the right ventricle of the heart to the lungs and carries the blood to the lungs to receive oxygen.

pus The thick, usually yellowish or greenish liquid product of an infection.

Q

quinine A drug used mainly to treat malaria, but also a common and often fatal adulterant of heroin.

R

race Any of the major divisions of mankind, based on color of skin, texture of hair, stature, and other bodily properties.

radiation Any form of energy that is sent out in rays from its source.

radioactive Giving off, or capable of giving off, energy in the form of rays. These rays result from the spontaneous disintegration of the nucleus of certain atoms, for example plutonium.

red blood cell A very small, nonnucleated disk both faces of which are concave, and which contains hemoglobin and carries oxygen to and carbon dioxide away from the tissues. Also called *erythrocyte*.

reflex arc The arrangement of sensory input pathway, nerve center, and motor output pathway that causes reflex actions, for example the immediate removal of a finger from a hot object before the brain can consider the action.

refractory period A term used by Masters and Johnson to describe the temporary state of male disinterest in further sexual stimulation immediately following orgasm.

rehabilitation The restoration of a handicapped or disabled person to the fullest possible mental, physical, social, and economic usefulness.

remission A decrease of the signs and symptoms of a disease.

REMs (rapid eye movements) Eye movements that occur at fairly regular intervals during sleep and that usually indicate that the individual is dreaming.

renal Pertaining to the kidney.

resistance The ability of an individual to ward off the harmful effects of agents such as toxins (poisons) and, especially, disease-causing microorganisms.

respiratory center A group of nerve cells in the medulla of the brain that controls the contractions of the muscles of respiration and, thus, controls the rate and depth of breathing.

reverse tolerance The apparent ability to obtain the same effect with decreasing doses of a drug (such as marihuana) as was obtained with the initial dose.

Rh blood disease See *erythroblastosis fetalis*.

rheumatic heart disease The most important result of untreated rheumatic fever, marked by inflammatory changes resulting in scarring and deformation of the heart valves.

rheumatism A disorder marked by inflammation of the connective tissues of the body, especially the joints and muscles. See also *nonarticular rheumatism*.

rheumatoid arthritis A chronic joint disorder, usually affecting many joints, and marked also by involvement of connective tissue throughout the body.

ribosomal RNA The ribonucleic acid that is found in or that makes up the ribosome; it composes 70 to 80 percent of the total RNA.

ribosome A cellular organelle at which proteins are constructed or synthesized. It is not believed to be stationary and is thought to actively participate in protein formation.

RNA (ribonucleic acid) A substance that is a template of portions of the DNA and functions in the cytoplasm of a cell. There are three types of RNA: messenger RNA (mRNA); ribosomal RNA (rRNA); and transfer RNA (tRNA).

rod One of the light-sensitive cells of the retina of the eye that contain a chemical substance called rhodopsin and that react to low-intensity light. See also *cone*.

rubella (German measles) A highly contagious viral infection of young people that is usually mild in nature. Signs and symptoms include rash, fever, and swollen nodes in the back of the neck. It lasts about three days. When a pregnant woman is exposed in the first trimester, the danger is to the unborn child.

rubeola (regular measles) A potentially dangerous viral infection that, despite an effective vaccine, is still common in children. It is marked by a sore throat, nasal discharge, and rash.

S

"safe period" The part of a woman's menstrual cycle when it is believed that she is infertile.

sarcoma Cancer arising in connective tissue such as bone, cartilage, or muscle.

saturated fats Fats that contain in their chemical formula a maximum number of hydrogen atoms. They are usually animal fats. See also *polyunsaturated fats*.

scabies A contagious skin disease caused by a mite; the most prominent symptom is itching. Also called *"the itch."*

schizophrenia A type of psychosis in which the individual sometimes becomes apathetic and withdrawn, and sometimes has delusions and hallucinations. The variety of these behavior patterns is so great that many experts in the field are reluctant to use this single term to describe them.

scopolamine A central nervous system depressant, used primarily as a sedative, as well as to dilate the pupil of the eye.

scrotum The external pouch or sac that contains the male testes and related organs.

sebaceous gland One of the skin glands that secrete sebum, an oily, lubricating substance.

secondary sex characteristics The physical features, other than the genitalia, that distinguish female and male.

sedative A drug that causes a quieting effect on the central nervous system, yet does not produce sleep nor relief from pain.

semen The thick, whitish secretion produced by the male that is ejaculated at orgasm and, in fertile males, contains spermatozoa.

seminal vesicles The paired pouches attached to the urinary bladder that join the vas deferens to form the ejaculatory duct.

seminiferous tubules Passages in the testis in which sperm develop and through which they leave the testis.

serum hepatitis See *hepatitis*.

sex chromosome One of the pair of chromosomes that determine an organism's genetic sex. See also *autosome*.

sex drive Desire for sexual expression.

sexual intercourse See *coitus*.

sickle cell disease (sickle cell anemia) A chronic genetic disorder occurring mostly in blacks and in some whites. It is marked by acute attacks of abdominal pain, severe anemia, pain and ulcerations of the lower extremities. It is caused by a defective chemical arrangement of the hemoglobin in the red blood cells. Insufficient oxygen causes the red blood cells to be sickle-shaped.

sign Any objective, observable evidence of a disease. Compare *symptom*.

sinus A cavity or hollow space.

smallpox An acute, highly contagious viral disease marked by fever, headache, abdominal pain, and disfiguring pockmarks. It is transmitted by direct contact with an infected person.

smooth muscle An involuntary muscle consisting of nonstriated, spindle-shaped muscle fibers. It appears in such structures as the intestines and the blood vessels. See also *striated muscle*.

soft palate The rear, fleshy part of the palate.

somatic Of the body; physical.

somatotherapy Treatment aimed at curing body ills.

specialties

MEDICAL:

Allergy deals with abnormal body reactions resulting from undue sensitivity to a wide variety of substances, including various foods, dusts, and pollens. A recently defined area of study is of particular interest to allergists; it is *pharmacogenetics*—the study of inherited sensitivities to drugs.

Cardiovascular diseases is concerned with the heart and blood vessels.

Dermatology is the skin specialty. Few diseases are without some skin manifestations. Like other specialists, therefore, the dermatologist must have a wide knowledge of general medicine.

Gastroenterology is concerned with the stomach and intestines.

Internal medicine involves the diagnosis and nonsurgical treatment of diseases of the internal organs.

Pediatric allergy deals with the sensitivities of children to various substances.

Pediatric cardiology is concerned with childhood diseases of the heart and blood vessels.

Pediatrics deals with the development and care of the normal child and with the diagnosis

specialties (continued)
and treatment of the diseases of childhood. The pediatrician treats children from infancy to the age of fourteen to sixteen.
Pulmonary diseases deals with lung conditions.

SURGICAL:

Colon and rectal surgery involves the lower intestine.
General surgery involves all kinds of surgical procedures. However, the general surgeon may, when he considers it necessary, consult with a specialist within this specialty, such as a neurological or thoracic surgeon.
Neurological surgery is that of the nervous system.
Obstetrics and gynecology: *obstetrics* is that branch of surgery dealing with the management of pregnancy, labor, and the period of confinement after labor; *gynecology* deals with disorders of the female reproductive system.
Ophthalmology concerns the eye and its diseases. (*Oculist* is the old term for ophthalmologist; it is now being discarded.) An ophthalmologist will usually prescribe glasses or contact lenses, but is capable of performing much more complex procedures.
Orthopedic surgery is that of the bones and joints.
Otolaryngology treats of the ear and throat.
Plastic surgery is concerned with the restoration or reconstruction of a body structure damaged by disease or injury or for cosmetic reasons.
Thoracic surgery is limited to the chest.
Urology is concerned with the urinary tract of both sexes, and with the male genital organs.

OTHER:

Anesthesiology is the complex study of the use of a wide variety of anesthetics. It is the anesthesiologist who decides which anesthetic is best for the individual patient. The anesthesiologist's competence also includes methods of resuscitation and maintenance of a clear airway.
Aviation medicine is the specialty of the space age. It deals with all the physical and emotional problems associated not only with ordinary flight but also with travel in outer space.
Child psychiatry deals with the emotional problems of children.
Diagnostic radiology uses X-rays and other rays to diagnose disease.
Forensic pathology deals with the application of medical knowledge to legal questions. The forensic pathologist is usually both a physician and a lawyer.
Neurology is concerned with diseases of the nervous system.
Occupational medicine deals with health problems associated with work in industry.
Pathology deals with the structural or functional changes in the body (organs, tissues, and cells) that cause or are caused by disease.
Physical medicine and rehabilitation employs physical means in the diagnosis and treatment of various disorders. Thus, water, heat, cold, electricity, light, manipulation, massage, exercise, or mechanical devices may be used to restore a sick or injured patient to the highest attainable self-sufficiency.
Preventive medicine is concerned with methods of preventing illness.
Psychiatry is concerned with emotional problems.
Public health is a subspecialty of preventive medicine concerned primarily with preventing disease and promoting health by means of the mobilization of community resources.
Radiology involves the diagnosis and treatment of disease by means of the specialized use of X-rays, radium, and radioactive isotopes. A *roentgenologist* is a specialist who diagnoses and treats solely by means of X-rays.
Therapeutic radiology uses X-rays and other rays to treat disease.

DENTAL:

Endodontics is concerned with the prevention, diagnosis, and treatment of diseases that affect the tooth pulp and the tissues surrounding the tooth root.
Oral pathology is the diagnosis and treatment of tumors and other lesions of the mouth.
Oral surgery involves operative procedures on the teeth, mouth, and adjacent structures.
Orthodontics aims basically to correct poorly positioned teeth so that they make proper contact during chewing.
Periodontics deals with diseases of the tissues that surround and support the teeth.
Prosthodontics is concerned with the art and science of making dental appliances and substitutes, such as artificial dentures, bridges, and crowns.

sperm, spermatozoon (pl. **sperm, sperms, spermatozoa**) A mature male germ or sex cell that is capable of fertilizing an ovum.
spermacide A contraceptive substance designed to kill sperm.
spermatogenesis The production and development of spermatozoa.
spermatogonium A primordial male germ cell that originates in a seminal tubule; it divides into two primary spermatocytes.
sphincter A ringlike band of muscle fibers that surrounds a natural body opening and can open or close it by expanding or contracting.
spinal cord The part of the nervous system contained in the vertebral canal.
spleen An organ situated in the upper abdomen immediately below the diaphragm on the left side. It destroys old red blood cells, thus setting free hemoglobin, and it also produces lymphoid cells.
sterile Not fertile; incapable of producing young.
steroid Any of a group of compounds that resemble cholesterol in chemical structure and include sex hormones and other substances.
stillbirth The birth of a dead child.
stimulant A drug or agent that temporarily increases the activity of some organ or vital process.
stimulus satiation One method of aversion therapy used in attempting to help smokers quit the habit. The number of cigarettes smoked is increased drastically for several days until eventually even one cigarette becomes overwhelmingly distasteful.
stress A stimulus, or succession of stimuli, of enough magnitude to possibly disrupt the integrated, steady, coordinated functional processes of the body. Not all stress need be considered harmful.
striated muscle A voluntary skeletal muscle consisting of muscle fibers that under a microscope appear striped. When it contracts, it produces movement of bones. See also *smooth muscle.*
stroke A sudden brain injury that is usually caused by a rupture of a blood vessel or by an embolus.
strychnine A central nervous system stimulant.
subfertility The state of being relatively sterile or less than normally fertile.
superior vena cava The large venous blood vessel that drains blood from the head, upper extremities, and chest and empties into the right atrium of the heart. See also *inferior vena cava.*
sweating phenomenon In this text, the appearance of small drops of a lubricating liquid on the vaginal walls, occurring in the excitement phase of female sexual response.
symbiosis The close association of two dissimilar organisms to the benefit or harm of both. In some cases the organisms are so dependent on each other that they cannot live apart.
sympathetic nervous system The part of the autonomic nervous system composed of nerve fibers and ganglia and concerned with emotions. When a person is under stress, the sympathetic division takes over from the parasympathetic division, which predominates when the person is relaxed. See also *autonomic nervous system, parasympathetic nervous system.*
symptom Any functional evidence of a disease; it cannot be observed but rather is felt or experienced by the individual. Compare *sign.*
synapse The region of contact between projections of two adjacent neurons, forming the area where a nervous impulse is transmitted from one neuron to another.
syndrome A set or group of symptoms that occur together.
synovial fluid Clear fluid, resembling egg white, found in various joints, bursa, and the sheaths of tendons.
synovial membrane The lining of a synovial cavity; it consists of connective tissue cells.
systole The period of contraction of the heart. Compare *diastole.*

T

tachycardia Excessively rapid heart rate.
temperature The degree of intensity of body heat, usually as measured by a scale thermometer.

tendon A strong, fibrous cord at the end of a muscle that attaches the muscle to a bone.
teratogen An agent (as a chemical or disease) causing malformation of an embryo or fetus.
testis (pl. **testes**) The male gonad, which produces spermatozoa; it is an egg-shaped gland contained in the scrotum. Also called *testicle.*
testosterone The hormone produced by the testis that induces and maintains the male secondary sex characteristics.
tetanus An acute bacterial infection caused by a toxin produced by a microbe. It is marked by headache, fever, and spasms of the jaw muscles, followed by painful spasms of the back muscles, eventual stiffening of the entire body, and, in about 35 percent of cases, death. Also called *lockjaw.*
tetrahydrocannabinol ("THC") The principal active ingredient of marihuana.
thoracic Pertaining to the chest.
thorax The portion of the body between the neck and the respiratory diaphragm, enclosed by the ribs; the chest.
thrombosis The formation of a thrombus.
thrombus A plug or a clot in a blood vessel or in the heart.
thrush A fungus infection marked by whitish spots in the mouth, followed by small sores that can spread to the groin, buttocks, and other body parts. See also *moniliasis.*
thymus gland A small ductless gland located in the chest behind the breast bone. While in the thymus gland, lymphocytes mature into T lymphocytes.
thyroid gland A large ductless gland that straddles the trachea and larynx; it governs the rate of body metabolism.
tissue A group of cells organized and specialized to perform a particular function.
tolerance The adaptation of the body to a specific drug that necessitates increased doses of the drug in order to produce the same effect.
tonsil One of two spongy lymph tissues situated in the back of the mouth on either side of the throat and believed to supply the mouth and pharynx with bacteria-destroying phagocytes.
toxic Pertaining to, or of the nature of, a poison.
toxic psychosis An acute emotional or organic brain disorder caused by the ingestion of toxic agents such as alcohol, lead, opium, carbon tetrachloride, or, very rarely, marihuana.
toxin A poison; frequently used to refer to a poison produced by a disease-causing bacterium.
trachea The windpipe; a membranous, cartilaginous tube descending from the larynx to the bronchi.
trade name Name given to a drug by its manufacturer so that it may be more readily identified by consumers.
tranquilizer A drug or agent used as a depressant in controlling and relieving various emotional disturbances.
transfer RNA A type of ribonucleic acid that, instructed by DNA, combines with a specific amino acid and transfers it to the ribosome in the process of protein synthesis.
translocation The shifting of a fragment or segment of one chromosome into another part of a similar chromosome, or sometimes into a dissimilar chromosome.
trauma An injury or wound.
trichomoniasis An infection caused by *Trichomonas vaginalis,* a type of parasitic protozoon. It usually occurs in the female genital tract and the male urinary tract.
trisomy The presence of an extra (third) chromosome of one type in a diploid cell.
trisomy 21 syndrome See *Down's syndrome.*
tubal ligation The application of a thread or wire to close the Fallopian tube as a means of birth control.
tubal pregnancy A pregnancy in which the fertilized ovum is implanted and develops in the Fallopian tube instead of in the uterus.
tuberculosis A communicable disease caused by a bacillus and marked by the formation of tubercles (nodules) in the affected tissue.
tumescence Swelling, usually with blood.
Turner's syndrome A genetic abnormality that results from nondisjunction, in which the individual has only an X-chromosome (OX); it is characterized by retarded physical growth and sexual development.
typhoid fever An acute, communicable bacterial infection marked by a wide variety of signs and symptoms, including fever, headache, cough, rose-colored spots on the skin, and diarrhea or constipation. It may be transmitted via water, milk, or other foods contaminated by infected feces or urine of a carrier or by direct contact with a sick individual.
typhus fever An acute rickettsial infection marked by fever, a rash, and headache. The two major forms of typhus fever, epidemic louse-borne and endemic flea-borne, differ in mode of transmission and severity of symptoms. The disease is transmitted from rats to humans via the feces of feeding fleas or lice.

U

ulcer Loss of substance on a skin or mucous surface that gradually causes the death of the tissue.
uterine tube See *oviduct.*

V

vaccination Generally, the inoculation or ingestion of weakened or killed organisms or the inoculation of inactivated toxins to induce antibody production. More specifically, the inoculation of vaccinia virus to protect against smallpox.
vaccinia virus A laboratory-prepared virus related to both the smallpox and cowpox viruses. It is the material now used for vaccination against smallpox.
vacuum aspiration A method of removing tissue or other material from the wall of the uterus by means of suction. The method now used most frequently for abortion.
vagina The canal-like organ in the female that extends from the neck (lowest part) of the uterus to the vulva (external genital region) and that receives the penis in sexual intercourse.
vasectomy A method of birth control involving surgical removal of all or (usually) part of the vas deferens; the excretory duct of the testes.
vasocongestion Congestion of the blood vessels.
vasopressin A hormone stored in and released from the posterior lobe of the pituitary gland but manufactured in the nearby hypothalamus. It contracts arterioles and capillaries and limits water excretion by the kidneys.
vein A vessel through which blood passes from different organs and body parts back to the heart.
ventricle One of the lower pair of chambers, with thick, muscular walls, that compose the bulk of the heart.
villus (pl. **villi**) Any small vascular fingerlike projection of tissue, for example those in the lining of the small intestine.
viral hepatitis See *hepatitis.*
virulence The degree to which a microorganism is able to produce disease.
virus A very small (usually ultramicroscopic) infective agent that is characterized by a lack of its own metabolism; it can multiply only within living cells.
vitamin Any of a group of organic compounds present in foods and necessary for normal growth and metabolism.
vulva The external genital organs of the woman.

W

wart A nonmalignant viral tumor of the outermost layer of the skin.
"wet dream" See *nocturnal emission.*
white blood cell A small, colorless cell found in the blood, lymph, and tissues. It is concerned with destroying disease-causing organisms. Also called *leukocyte.*

X

X-chromosome The sex chromosome carried by one-half of the male gametes and all of the female gametes. The male carries one X-chromosome; the female, two.

Y

Y-chromosome The sex chromosome carried by one-half of the male gametes and none of the female gametes. The male carries one Y-chromosome; the female, none.
yeast A type of fungus that germinates and multiplies in the presence of sugar or starch.
yellow fever An acute infectious viral disease transmitted by a mosquito.

Z

zygote The single-celled fertilized ovum that results from the union of the male and female gametes.

Jonathan Cape, Ltd., for an excerpt from George Seferis, "Mythistorema," from George Seferis, *Collected Poems, 1924–1955,* tr., ed., and intro. by Edmund Keeley and Philip Sherrard, published by Jonathan Cape, Ltd., in the British Commonwealth and Canada.

M. Edward Davis, for Table 19-1, "Stages of Labor," from M. Edward Davis and Reva Rubin, *De Lee's Obstetrics for Nurses,* 18th ed. (1966), published by W. B. Saunders Company.

Doubleday & Company, Inc., for a poem by Issa from *An Introduction to Haiku,* by Harold G. Henderson. Copyright © 1958 by Harold G. Henderson. Reprinted by permission of Doubleday & Company, Inc.

Norma Millay Ellis for an excerpt from "Sonnet CXXXVII" by Edna St. Vincent Millay, from *Collected Poems* (Harper & Row). Copyright 1939, 1967 by Edna St. Vincent Millay and Norma Millay Ellis.

M. Evans & Co., Inc., for Table 23-2, "Standards at Various Ages for Cooper's Twelve-Minute Field Test for Men," from Kenneth H. Cooper, *The New Aerobics* (1970), and for Table 23-3, "Standards for Cooper's Optional Twelve-Minute Field Test for Women," from Mildred Cooper and Kenneth H. Cooper, *Aerobics for Women* (1972). Reprinted by permission of M. Evans & Co., Inc.

W. H. Freeman and Company, for excerpts from Bruno Bettelheim, "Joey: A 'Mechanical Boy,'" *Scientific American,* Vol. 200, No. 3 (March 1959), pp. 117–27. Copyright © 1959 by Scientific American, Inc. All rights reserved.

David Belais Friedman, for Table 12-1, "Parent and Child Development," from David Belais Friedman, "Parent Development," *California Medicine,* Vol. 86, No. 1 (January 1957), pp. 25–28.

Harcourt Brace Jovanovich, Inc., for Table 10-1, "Some Human Endocrine Glands and Hormones and Some of Their Effects," adapted from *Life: An Introduction to Biology,* 2nd ed., by George Gaylord Simpson and William S. Beck, copyright © 1957, 1965, by Harcourt Brace Jovanovich, Inc., and reproduced with their permission.

Gerald A. Heidbreder, for Table 7-2, "Natural History of Acquired Syphilis," and for Table 7-3, "Natural History of Acquired Gonorrhea," courtesy of Gerald A. Heidbreder, retired Deputy Director, Community Health Services, Department of Health Services of the County of Los Angeles.

Holt, Rinehart and Winston, Inc., for data used in Table 22-1, "A Dozen Leading Nutrients," and Table 22-2, "Caloric Values for Representative Foods, Classified by Food Groups," adapted and reprinted from Ethel Austin Martin, *Nutrition in Action,* 2nd ed. Copyright © 1963, 1965 by Holt, Rinehart and Winston, Inc. Adapted and reprinted by permission of Holt, Rinehart and Winston, Inc.

Hospital Tribune, for "Health Planning, 1972," by Michael M. Stewart, M.D., from *Hospital Tribune,* Vol. 7, No. 1 (January 1, 1973), p. 22.

Indiana University Press, for Table 20-1, "Estimate of Births in Three Periods of Human History," and for Table 20-2, "Estimated World Population: A.D. 1000–A.D. 2000," from Annabelle Desmond, "How Many People Have Ever Lived on Earth?" in Stuart Mudd, ed., *The Population Crisis and the Use of World Resources* (The Hague, 1964).

Alfred A. Knopf, Inc., for an excerpt from "On Children," reprinted from *The Prophet,* by Kahlil Gibran, with permission of the publisher, Alfred A. Knopf, Inc. Copyright 1923 by Kahlil Gibran; renewal copyright 1951 by Administrators C.T.A. of Kahlil Gibran Estate, and Mary G. Gibran.

John Lear, for an excerpt from "Spinning the Thread of Life" by John Lear, in *Saturday Review* (April 5, 1969), pp. 63–64. Reprinted by permission of John Lear.

J. B. Lippincott Company, for Table 22-3, "Caloric Values for Common Snacks," and for Table 22-5, "A Typical Female College Student's Activities for One Day," adapted from Helen S. Mitchell *et al., Cooper's Nutrition in Health and Disease,* 15th ed. (1968); for a poem by an Oklahoma high school boy, quoted in Evelyn Duvall, *Family Development,* 4th ed., copyright 1971; and for Table 14-1, "Comparative Strengths of LSD and Other Hallucinogens (Approximate)," from Sidney Cohen, "Pot, Acid and Speed," *Medical Science,* Vol. 19, No. 2 (February 1968), p. 31. Reprinted by permission of the publisher, J. B. Lippincott Company.

Little, Brown and Company, for quotes used in Table 12-1, "Parent and Child Development": From "Tarkington, Thou Should'st Be Living in This Hour," from Ogden Nash, *Verses from 1929 On,* copyright 1947 by Ogden Nash (originally appeared in *The New Yorker*); from "Pediatric Reflection," copyright 1931 by Ogden Nash; from Ogden Nash, "The Kitten," copyright 1940 by Curtis Brown Publishing Co.; from "A Child's Guide to Parents," copyright 1936 by Ogden Nash; from "The Parent," copyright 1933 by Ogden Nash. All from Ogden Nash, *Family Reunion.* For an excerpt from "Allergy Met a Bear," from Ogden Nash, *I'm a Stranger Here Myself,* copyright 1938 by Ogden Nash. Acknowledgment also for excerpts from William H. Masters and Virginia E. Johnson, *Human Sexual Response* (1966). All by permission of Little, Brown and Company.

County of Los Angeles Health Department, for Table 7-2, "Natural History of Acquired Syphilis," and for Table 7-3, "Natural History of Acquired Gonorrhea," courtesy of the Records and Statistics Division, County of Los Angeles Health Department, May 1969.

The Macmillan Company for Table 23-1, "Energy Expenditures for Various Everyday Activities," adapted from C. M. Taylor, Grace MacLeod, and M. D. S. Rose, *Foundations of Nutrition,* 5th ed. Reprinted with permission of The Macmillan Company. © by The Macmillan Company, 1956. For an excerpt from W. B. Yeats, "A Prayer for My Daughter," reprinted with permission of The Macmillan Company from W. B. Yeats, *Collected Poems.* Copyright 1924 by The Macmillan Company, renewed in 1952 by Bertha Georgie Yeats.

Josiah Macy, Jr., Foundation, for excerpts from Erik H. Erikson, "Growth and Crises of the Healthy Personality," in Clyde Kluckhohn, Henry A. Murray, and David Schneider, eds., *Personality in Nature, Society and Culture* (1953). Reprinted by permission of the Josiah Macy, Jr., Foundation.

Metropolitan Life Insurance Company, for Table 22-6, "Desirable Weights in Pounds for People Twenty-Five or Over," based on data of the Build and Blood Pressure Study, Society of Actuaries, 1959.

National Dairy Council, for data used in Table 22-1, "A Dozen Leading Nutrients," adapted from Ruth M. Leverton, *A Girl and Her Figure* (National Dairy Council, 1955). Courtesy, National Dairy Council.

The National Foundation–March of Dimes, for Table 18-2, "The More Common Birth Defects," adapted from a booklet (PR-45-5) published by The National Foundation–March of Dimes.

New American Library, Inc., for a poem by Marie Ford, "The Junkies," from *36 Children* by Herbert Kohl. Copyright © 1967 by Herbert Kohl. Reprinted by arrangement with the New American Library, Inc., New York, New York.

The New York Times Company, for quotes from *The New York Times.* © 1966 by The New York Times Company. Reprinted by permission.

Postgraduate Medicine, for Table 13-1, "Some Common Deceptions in the Illicit Drug Market," from Edward A. Wolfson and Donald B. Louria, "Prevention of Drug Abuse," *Postgraduate Medicine,* Vol. 51, No. 1 (January 1972), p. 164.

Princeton University Press, for an excerpt from George Seferis, "Mythistorema," from George Seferis, *Collected Poems, 1924–1955,* tr., ed., and intro. by Edmund Keeley and Philip Sherrard. Copyright © 1967 by Princeton University Press. Reprinted by permission of Princeton University Press.

W. B. Saunders Company, for Table 19-1,

"Stages of Labor," from M. Edward Davis and Reva Rubin, *De Lee's Obstetrics for Nurses,* 18th ed. (1966).

G. D. Searle & Co., for Table 21-1, "A Summary of Birth Control Methods," adapted from *Your Future Family* (G. D. Searle & Co., 1971), pp. 12–17.

Smith, Kline, & French Laboratories, for data used in Table 22-3, "Caloric Values for Common Snacks."

Michael M. Stewart, M.D., for "Health Planning, 1972" by Michael M. Stewart, from *Hospital Tribune,* Vol. 7, No. 1 (January 1, 1973), p. 22.

A. P. Watt & Son, for an excerpt from "A Prayer for My Daughter" by W. B. Yeats, from W. B. Yeats, *Collected Poems.* Reprinted by permission of Mr. M. B. Yeats, Miss Anne Yeats, and The Macmillan Company of Canada.

The Western Journal of Medicine, for Table 12-1, "Parent and Child Development," from David Belais Friedman, "Parent Development," *California Medicine,* Vol. 86, No. 1 (January 1957), pp. 25–28.

ILLUSTRATIONS

Key to abbreviations

NIH: National Institute of Health
UPI: United Press International
USDA: United States Department of Agriculture
UN: United Nations
WHO: World Health Organization

b: bottom
c. center
l: left
r: right
t: top

PART 1: p. 1, Bausch and Lomb Optical Company

Chapter 1: p. 2, Gerry Cranham/Rapho Guillumette; 5, Tony Rollo/*Newsweek;* 10, courtesy Edouard Kellenberger; 11, courtesy Helmut A. Gordon, M.D., from *Triangle,* the Sandoz Journal of Medical Science, Vol. 7, No. 3 (1965), p. 115; 13, New York Daily News; 15, Radio Times Hulton Picture Library; 16, Mansell Collection; 20*l,* American Museum of Natural History; 20*r,* W. Luthy/De Wys Inc.

Chapter 2: p. 22, WHO; 23, USDA; 28*tl,* Wayne Miller/Magnum; 28*tr,* WHO; 28*bl,* Bettmann Archive; 28*br,* Yale–New Haven Hospital; 29*t,* Roger-Viollet; 29*b,* Ciccione/Rapho Guillumette; 30, Mansell Collection; 32, UPI; 36, Mansell Collection.

PART 2: p. 39, Alinari/Madeline Grimoldi, Rome.

Chapter 3: p. 40, Library of Congress; 44, Stephenson Blake; 46, Bettmann Archive; 47, Harbrace; 49, Wide World; 54, Mansell Collection; 55, UPI; 57, Wide World; 60, Everett Johnson/De Wys Inc.; 63, UN; 69*t,* Wide World; 69*b,* Corning Glass Works; 73, UPI.

Chapter 4: p. 76, Bill Saidez/Stock, Boston; 78*t,* Wide World; 78*b,* WHO; 79, USDA; 83, UPI; 85, Wide World; 95, courtesy Eastman Kodak Company, from *Medical Radiography and Photography,* published by Radiography Markets Division; 97, Pacific Gas and Electric News Bureau; 103, courtesy David M. Lipscomb.

PART 3: p. 109, USDA.

Chapter 5: p. 110, The National Gallery of Art, Washington, D.C., Rosenwald Collection; 112, WHO; 114, British Museum; 115, Mansell Collection; 116, woodcut by Mich. Wohlgemuth, 1493; 119, Mansell Collection; 120, Bodleian Library, Oxford; 121, Mansell Collection; 123*t,* New York Academy of Medicine; 123*b,* County of Los Angeles Health Dept.; 129*t, b,* Mansell Collection.

Chapter 6: p. 134, Dr. Lee Simon, Institute for Cancer Research, Philadelphia; 135, New York Academy of Medicine; 136*t,* E. R. Squibb & Sons; 136*c,* The Upjohn Co.; 136*b,* Lewis M. Druscan, M.D., and George B. Chapman, M.D.; 137*t,* WHO; 137*bl,* U.S. Dept. HEW; 137*br,* U.S. Public Health Service; 140, *Harper's Weekly;* 141, Bettmann Archive; 142*c, b,* courtesy Dr. Aaron Pollicak, Sloan-Kettering Institute for Cancer Research; 144*l, r,* courtesy R. M. Albrecht; 147, courtesy Ny Carlsberg Glyptothek, Copenhagen; 155, 156, courtesy Dr. R. W. Horne; 157*t,* courtesy Dr. Lee Simon; 157*bl, br,* courtesy Dr. R. W. Horne; 161*t,* King Features Syndicate; 161*b,* Division of Virology, National Institute for Medical Research, London; 166*t,* NIH; 166*b,* courtesy Dr. June D. Almeida, The Wellcome Research Laboratories.

Chapter 7: p. 169, Bibliotheque Nationale, Paris; 171, Jacob A. Riis Collection, Museum of the City of New York; 172, The Upjohn Co.; 177, Bibliotheque Nationale, Paris; 178*t,* E. R. Squibb & Sons; 178*b,* Society of American Bacteriologists; 185, Ronald Glaser, JAMA Medical News; 188, Peter B. Armstrong, David W. Deamer, and John J. Mais, University of California at Davis.

PART 4: p. 191, "Comfort in the Gout" by Thomas Rowlandson, National Gallery of Art, Washington, D.C., Addie Burr Clark Collection.

Chapter 8: p. 192, Wide World; 194, Jean-Paul Revel, California Institute of Technology; 197, Culver; 198, Ewing Galloway; 199, University of Bristol; 203, American Cancer Society; 205*t, b,* NIH; 209*t, c, b,* Sloan-Kettering Institute for Cancer Research; 210, Dr. Albert J. Dalton, National Cancer Institute.

Chapter 9: p. 215, Thames & Hudson, Ltd.; 218, adapted from James E. Crouch, *Functional Human Anatomy* (Philadelphia, 1965), with permission of Lea & Febiger; 219, courtesy Eugene L. Gottfried, M.D.; 220, Keith R. Porter, M.D., and Clifton Van Zandt Hawn, M.D.; 221, adapted from James E. Crouch, *Functional Human Anatomy* (Philadelphia, 1965), with permission of Lea & Febiger; 222, Bettmann Archive; 224*tl, tr,* courtesy, Carl A. Smith, M.D.; 224*b,* from H. S. Mayerson, "The Lymphatic System," copyright © 1963 by Scientific American, Inc., all rights reserved; 229*l, c, r,* American Heart Assoc.; 230, New York University Medical Center; 231*t, b,* C. Walton Lillehei, M.D.; 240, Ron Sherman, Medical World News; 244, adapted from Theodore W. Torrey, *Morphogenesis of the Vertebrates,* 2nd ed. (New York, 1967), with permission of John Wiley & Sons, Inc.; 245, courtesy W. S. Hammond, M.D.; 246, Henry E. Huntington Library.

Chapter 10: p. 248, Clay-Adams, Inc.; 249*l, c, r,* Smithsonian Institute National Museum of Natural History; 252, *Harper's Weekly;* 253*b,* courtesy Austin Johnson, M.D.; 258, UPI; 263*tr,* UPI; 265, José M. R. Delgado, M.D., from "Evolution of Physical Control of the Brain," James Arthur Lecture on the Evolution of the Human Brain, The American Museum of Natural History, New York, 1965; 266, R. Sternback/Photo Researchers, Inc.; 268, from Ernest R. Hilgard and Richard D. Atkinson, *Introduction to Psychology,* 4th ed., copyright, 1953, 1957, 1962, 1967, by Harcourt Brace Jovanovich, Inc., and reproduced with their permission; 269, Wide World; 275, courtesy Eckhard H. Hess, University of Chicago; 276*t,* National Society for the Prevention of Blindness; 277*bl,* Historical Pictures Service, Chicago; 277*br,* St. Louis Art Museum.

PART 5: p. 281, UN.

Chapter 11: p. 282, Fred Plaut; 284*l,* Historical Pictures Service, Chicago; 284*r,* Culver; 287, Bruno Bettelheim, Ph.D.; 288, W. Eugene Smith; 289, Eve Arnold/Magnum; 290, photo by Lennart Nilsson, from *A Child Is Born;* 291, Mark Haven; 292, Barbara Morgan; 297, Bill Bridges/Globe Photos; 302, U.S. Army Photo; 312–13, drawing by Olfin, © October 29, 1973, The New Yorker Magazine, Inc.; 318, W. Eugene Smith.

Chapter 12: p. 321, WHO; 322, Seán Kernan; 326, Charles Harbutt/Magnum; 334*t,* Ken Heyman; 334*bl, br,* Regional Primate Research Center, University of Wisconsin; 335*t, br,* Regional Primate Research Center, University of Wisconsin; 335*bl,* WHO; 336, Leon Levinstein; 340, Suzanne Szasz; 346, Wide World.

Chapter 13: p. 353, Michael Weisbrot/Black Star; 356, Arthur Tress; 362, Arents Collection, The New York Public Library, Astor, Lenox, and Tilden Foundations; 369, Archie Lieberman/Black Star; 377, Metropolitan Museum of Art, Egyptian Expedition; 378, Newberry Library, Chicago; 379, Museum of the City of New York, gift of Dr. Arthur Hunter; 384, Wide World; 385, Bettmann Archive; 391*t,* from Julius Comroe, "The Lung," Copyright © 1966, by Scientific American, Inc., all rights reserved; 391*b,* courtesy Eastman Kodak Company, from

Medical Radiography and Photography, published by Radiography Markets Division; 392*t, c, b,* courtesy Oscar Auerbach, M.D., and L. J. Walker; 400, Wide World.

Chapter 14: p. 402, Arthur Tress; 404, Suzanne Szasz; 405*t, b,* N.C. Dept. of Mental Health; 411, Sansoni; 415, Harbrace; 422, Culver; 434, St. Paul *Dispatch.*

PART 6: p. 437, British Information Service/Tate Gallery.

Chapter 15: 438, Tympanum, Rottweil, Kapellenkirsche; Landesbildestelle Würteinberg, Stuttgart; 439, Jean Prevost; 442, © *Punch,* London; 451, courtesy, National Gallery of Art, Washington, D.C., Rosenwald Collection; 459, Ken Heyman; 461, Charles Harbutt/Magnum; 463, Bettmann Archive.

Chapter 16: p. 465, courtesy Landrum B. Shettles, M.D.; 469, adapted from Robert Latou Dickinson, *Atlas of Human Sex Anatomy,* 2nd ed., copyright 1949, with permission of Williams & Wilkins Co., Baltimore, Md. 21202; 471*b,* courtesy Dr. L. J. D. Zaneveld, Dept. of Obstetrics and Gynecology, University of Chicago, and Dr. K. Gould, Yerkes Primate Center, Emory University, Atlanta, from *J. Reprod. Med.,* Vol. 6, No. 4 (1971), p. 147.

Chapter 17: p. 487, sculpture by Gustav Vigeland, photo by David Finn; 491, Burk Uzzle/Magnum; 492*l,* Giraudon, Paris; 493*r,* Marc Riboud/Magnum; 496–97, sculpture by Gustav Vigeland, photos by David Finn.

Chapter 18: p. 519, WHO; 522, courtesy Albert E. Vatter, M.D.; 523*tl,* courtesy Dorothy Warburton, Ph.D., and W. Roy Breg, M.D.; 523*tr,* The Upjohn Company; 523*b,* courtesy Jon Beckwith, M.D., and Lorne MacHattie, M.D.; 524*t,* © 1973 by CIBA Pharmaceutical Company, Division of CIBA-Geigy Corporation, reproduced with permission from the *Clinical Symposia* illustrated by John A. Craig, M.D., all rights reserved; 524*b,* courtesy Hidejiro Yokoo, M.D., Veterans Administration Research Hospital, Chicago; 529*l,* courtesy Dorothy Warburton, Ph.D., and W. Roy Breg, M.D.; 531*l,* courtesy O. L. Miller, Jr., and Barbara R. Beatty, Biology Division, Oak Ridge National Laboratory; 531*r,* O. L. Miller, Jr. and Aimee H. Bakken, Biology Division, Oak Ridge National Laboratory; 532*t, b,* courtesy Albert E. Vatter, M.D.; 534, from Masayasu Nomura, "Ribosomes," copyright © 1969 by Scientific American, Inc., all rights reserved; 538, courtesy Eva McGilvray, M.D.; 539*l, t, b,* Bruce Roberts/Rapho Guillumette; 543, courtesy O. J. Miller, M.D.; 547, courtesy National Foundation–March of Dimes; 556, courtesy David H. Baker, M.D.

Chapter 19: p. 570, Elliott Erwitt/Magnum; 573, *Medical Tribune;* 574, from B. M. Patten, *Human Embryology,* 3rd ed., copyright © 1968 by McGraw-Hill, Inc., used with permission of McGraw-Hill Book Company; 575*l, c, r,* Carnegie Institute of Washington; 575*tr,* photo by Lennart Nilsson, from *A Child Is Born;* 575*br,* Donald Yeager/Camera MD Studios; 576, photo by Lennart Nilsson, from *A Child Is Born;* 583, photographs courtesy Museum of Science and Industry, Chicago; 588, Ken Heyman.

Chapter 20: p. 598, Ben Ross; 599, Paolo Koch/Rapho Guillumette; 601, UN; 606, Radio Times Hulton Picture Library.

Chapter 21: p. 615, Michaud/Rapho Guillumette; 616, from Norman E. Himes, *History of Contraception,* copyright © 1963 by Gamut Press, used with permission of Gamut Press; 631, courtesy Nuri Sagiroglu, M.D., *J. Reprod. Med.,* Vol. 7, No. 5 (1971); 633, Daniel Budnik/Woodfin Camp Assoc.

PART 7: p. 647, WHO.

Chapter 22: p. 648, Bettmann Archive; 649, Carl Strüwe/Monkmeyer; 654, Granger Collection; 656, Bettmann Archive; 667, The Byron Collection, Museum of the City of New York; 668, Raimondo Borea; 670, *Harper's Weekly;* 679, American Dental Association; 686, National Library of Medicine; 689*l,* photo by Anthony M. Kuzma, from *Medical Tribune;* 689*tr, br,* Dr. Johnson L. Thistle and Alan F. Hofmann of the Mayo Clinic, from the *New England Journal of Medicine;* 690, adapted from James E. Crouch, *Functional Human Anatomy* (Philadelphia, 1965), with permission of Lea & Febiger; 691*t, b,* courtesy Roche Laboratories and William Douglas McAdams, Inc.

Chapter 23: p. 693, Ashmolean Museum, Oxford; 694, Radio Times Hulton Picture Library; 695, courtesy University of Nebraska at Lincoln; 698*l,* Wide World; 698*r,* Bob Sánchez/Harbrace; 701*l,* from Harold B. Falls, Earl L. Wallis, and Gene A. Logan, *Foundations of Conditioning,* copyright © 1970 by Academic Press, Inc.; 701*r,* General Biological Supply House; 705, Novosti Press Agency; 706, Harbrace photos; 707, Byron Collection, Museum of the City of New York; 711, Bob Sánchez; 714, Historical Pictures Service, Chicago; 715, from Marion Broer, *Efficiency of Human Movement,* copyright © 1973 by permission of W. B. Saunders Co.; 719, from A. E. Brown and H. A. Jeffcott, Jr., *Absolutely Mad Inventions,* copyright © 1932 by A. E. Brown and H. A. Jeffcott, Jr. Published by Dover Publications Inc., 1970.

Chapter 24: p. 722, Mansell Collection; 723, Historical Pictures, Chicago; 724, Library of Congress; 727, Lynn McLaren/Rapho Guillumette; 732, Michael Alexander; 738, Bruce Roberts/Rapho Guillumette; 746*tl,* Denver Public Library, Western History Dept.; 746*tr,* Seattle Historical Society; 746*b,* Ben Ross/Photo Trends; 747*tl,* Culver; 747*tr,* Jules Zalon/DPI; 747*bl,* Denver Public Library, Western History Dept.; 747*br,* Franklynn Peterson/Black Star; 754, Granger Collection.

PART 8: p. 759, Roger Malloch/Magnum.

Chapter 25: p. 760, WHO; 764, Wide World; 765, Wide World; 766, courtesy Michael E. DeBakey, M.D.; 767, *Medical Tribune;* 770, courtesy Arthur Kornberg, M.D.; 779, Henri Cartier-Bresson/Magnum; 780, Harvey Stein; 783, WHO; 784*l,* Ralph Bredland/NIH; 784*r,* Raymond F. Chen, M.D., Ph.D./NIH; 788, Wide World; 790, Mary Ann Erickson, *Medical World News.*

index

Page numbers in *italics* refer to illustrations; body chart references are to the color insert; *n* refers to footnotes.

A 4 B 5 C 6 D 7 E 8 F 9 G 0 H 1 I 2 J 3